Practical Early Orthodontic Treatment

Practical Early Orthodontic Treatment

A Case-Based Review

Thomas E. Southard, DDS, MS
Department of Orthodontics
University of Iowa College of Dentistry
Iowa City, Iowa, USA

Steven D. Marshall, DDS, MS
Department of Orthodontics
University of Iowa College of Dentistry
Iowa City, Iowa, USA

Laura L. Bonner, DDS, MS
Department of Orthodontics
University of Iowa College of Dentistry
Iowa City, Iowa, USA

Kyungsup Shin, PhD, DMD, MS
Department of Orthodontics
University of Iowa College of Dentistry
Iowa City, Iowa, USA

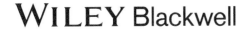

Registered Office
John Wiley & Sons, Inc., 111 River Street, Hoboken, NJ 07030, USA

Editorial Office
111 River Street, Hoboken, NJ 07030, USA

For details of our global editorial offices, customer services, and more information about Wiley products visit us at www.wiley.com.

Wiley also publishes its books in a variety of electronic formats and by print-on-demand. Some content that appears in standard print versions of this book may not be available in other formats.

Limit of Liability/Disclaimer of Warranty
The contents of this work are intended to further general scientific research, understanding, and discussion only and are not intended and should not be relied upon as recommending or promoting scientific method, diagnosis, or treatment by physicians for any particular patient. In view of ongoing research, equipment modifications, changes in governmental regulations, and the constant flow of information relating to the use of medicines, equipment, and devices, the reader is urged to review and evaluate the information provided in the package insert or instructions for each medicine, equipment, or device for, among other things, any changes in the instructions or indication of usage and for added warnings and precautions. While the publisher and authors have used their best efforts in preparing this work, they make no representations or warranties with respect to the accuracy or completeness of the contents of this work and specifically disclaim all warranties, including without limitation any implied warranties of merchantability or fitness for a particular purpose. No warranty may be created or extended by sales representatives, written sales materials or promotional statements for this work. The fact that an organization, website, or product is referred to in this work as a citation and/or potential source of further information does not mean that the publisher and authors endorse the information or services the organization, website, or product may provide or recommendations it may make. This work is sold with the understanding that the publisher is not engaged in rendering professional services. The advice and strategies contained herein may not be suitable for your situation. You should consult with a specialist where appropriate. Further, readers should be aware that websites listed in this work may have changed or disappeared between when this work was written and when it is read. Neither the publisher nor authors shall be liable for any loss of profit or any other commercial damages, including but not limited to special, incidental, consequential, or other damages.

Library of Congress Cataloging-in-Publication Data

Names: Southard, Thomas E. author. | Marshall, Steven D., author. | Bonner,
  Laura L., author. | Shin, Kyungsup, 1973– author.
Title: Practical early orthodontic treatment : a case-based review /
  Dr. Thomas E. Southard, Dr. Steven D. Marshall, Dr. Laura Bonner,
  Dr. Kyungsup Shin.
Description: Hoboken, NJ : Wiley-Blackwell, 2023. | Includes
  bibliographical references and index.
Identifiers: LCCN 2021062806 (print) | LCCN 2021062807 (ebook) |
  ISBN 9781119793595 (cloth) | ISBN 9781119793601 (Adobe PDF) |
  ISBN 9781119793618 (epub)
Subjects: MESH: Malocclusion–therapy | Child | Dentofacial
  Deformities–therapy | Malocclusion–diagnosis | Dentofacial
  Deformities–diagnosis | Early Medical Intervention |
  Orthodontics–methods | Problems and Exercises | Case Reports
Classification: LCC RK523 (print) | LCC RK523 (ebook) | NLM WU 18.2 |
  DDC 617.6/43–dc23/eng/20220131
LC record available at https://lccn.loc.gov/2021062806
LC ebook record available at https://lccn.loc.gov/2021062807

Cover Design: Wiley
Cover Image: Courtesy of Thomas E. Southard

Set in 9.5/12.5pt STIXTwoText by Straive, Pondicherry, India

SKY10086207_092724

Brief Contents

Contents

Preface

Welcome to the world of early orthodontic treatment, an exciting and professionally satisfying area of our specialty. Every orthodontist should be proficient in this area: in assessing childhood malocclusions and dentofacial deformities, making appropriate decisions when dealing with these conditions, and providing superlative care based upon these decisions.

Many orthodontic residency programs provide first-rate early treatment education. Unfortunately, others do not. When Steve, Laura, Kyungsup, and I began practicing after graduation, we quickly realized that most patient consultations were for children, that the early treatment education we had received during our residencies was lacking, and that we were often ill-prepared to answer simple consultation questions, such as:

- "Should I begin treatment on this child *now*, or should I recall the child in six to twelve months?"
- "If I choose to treat now, what are my treatment goals? What treatment should I provide to achieve those goals? What treatment should wait, and when should I provide treatment?"
- "If I choose *not* to treat this child now, what harm could result?"

We wrote this book so that you will be better prepared than we were. It will provide you with a solid foundation in the early management of malocclusions. This is the book we wish we had studied as residents.

Dr. Shin and I spoke at the American Association of Orthodontists' annual meeting on the topic "Practical Early Treatment." At the conclusion of our talk, an audience member asked, "Why *early* treatment? Can't I just treat patients later, comprehensively, after all their permanent teeth erupt?" The short answer is that you can wait until all permanent teeth erupt, but the patient may be harmed by waiting. For example, if the ectopic eruption of maxillary permanent canines is not corrected early, then resorption of adjacent teeth roots may occur. Further, you may increase the complexity of the case by waiting until all

permanent teeth erupt. If you do not begin early orthopedics in certain patients, you may miss an opportunity to modify a patient's growth to their advantage. However, there are times when you can (and should) wait to begin treatment until all permanent teeth erupt. One purpose of this textbook is to provide you with the knowledge needed to determine when you should initiate early orthodontic treatment and when you can wait.

This book is divided into six chapters: Foundations, Crowding, Eruption Problems/Missing Succedaneous Teeth/First Permanent Molar Extractions, Anteroposterior Problems, Vertical Problems, and Transverse Problems, as well as an Appendix. In the Foundations chapter, we provide an overview of general early treatment principles along with important craniofacial growth and development concepts. In the Crowding chapter, we provide overall treatment principles along with specific diagnostic and treatment recommendations in the Introduction. The cases that follow in the Crowding chapter encompass a wide range of crowded patients illustrating the application of these principles and recommendations. Some consultation patients are presented with minimal records, and you are asked to assess the patient and provide recommendations during one visit. Other patients are presented with full records and you are asked to use these records to treat the patient from initial assessment through completion of early (and comprehensive) treatment. The organization of this chapter is repeated for subsequent chapters.

The Appendix presents a cephalometric analysis primer, the Iowa AP Classification Primer, useful tables, and abbreviations.

We wish to note that every case we present was painstakingly chosen from a cumulative practice experience of over seventy years with the intent of illustrating principles by applying those principles to a broad range of problems. In summary, you will become intimately involved in the diagnosis and treatment planning of more than 50 patients early in their development.

Like our previous book (*Orthodontics in the Vertical Dimension: A Case-Based Review. Wiley Blackwell, 2015*), the format of this book is based on a question-answer style of teaching – as experienced during an orthodontic residency. This question-answer format keeps you intellectually involved, encourages critical thinking, offers you the opportunity to reflect on our questions and your answers, and gauges the progress of your understanding. Using this format, we will coach you to address a spectrum of challenging clinical problems and formulate appropriate treatment decisions. To grasp the principles upon which we focus, we recommend that you study each case at one sitting, from beginning to end. Carefully think through the answer to each question we present (ideally, by writing down your answer), and make the best decision you can. You should do this *before* you refer to the answer we provide. Answer each question as thoughtfully as you would if you were with a patient.

After you have finished studying one case, go back and review the questions you were not comfortable with. Try answering them again. Then, *close your eyes. Visualize a child coming to you with a condition similar to the one you just studied. Visualize how you would recommend treating that child.* Finally, return to those same questions a week or so later. Your orthodontic diagnostic, treatment planning, and in-treatment decision-making abilities will strengthen in direct proportion to your efforts to work through each problem presented.

The practice of orthodontics and dentofacial orthopedics is a cognitive discipline which requires exceptional intelligence, the ability to apply the best science combined with practical principles of growth and development, anatomy, physiology, diagnosis, and biomechanics, and an uncompromising desire to care for the patient. Every patient is different, and every patient's individual response to treatment will vary. However, the principles established in this text are applicable for every child and will serve you over a lifetime of clinical practice.

These principles are emphasized and applied repeatedly throughout this book – just as during a residency. The principles will instill in you patterns of analysis and habits of rational decision making. You will learn to apply these principles over a diverse patient population until they become an inherent part of your thought processes in daily practice.

"Repetitio mater studiorum est."
(Repetition is the mother of all learning.)

The answers we provide for the cases presented are based upon our many years of teaching, literature review, and clinical experience at the University of Iowa and in private practice. This does not mean, however, that our answers are necessarily, or always, correct. Everything taught in our specialty must be constantly challenged and questioned. If our ideas cannot withstand the rigor of scrutiny and the test of time, then we must modify our position. If you disagree with concepts in this text, please discuss them with your colleagues, attending faculty, or us. Constructive dialogue makes us better orthodontists, results in better care for our patients, and strengthens our specialty.

Included in this text are important references for many clinical and scientific concepts, but this book was not written as a systematic review reference source. The treatment principles contained herein will be valid for your lifetime, but the specific scientific and clinical study references may evolve over the years.

We wish to acknowledge the diagnostic skill, treatment outcomes, and patient care provided by Dr. Karin A. Southard who kindly allowed us to include many of her cases. Karin is a clinician's clinician and an educator's educator. We thank her for her teaching and her many contributions to excellent patient care. We wish to thank Dr. Michael L. Swartz for his permission to use Orthodontic Clipart in developing many of the illustrations in this text, and Ms. Chris White for her thorough review and many insightful suggestions.

Our goal is your goal – we want you to become the best orthodontist you can be. As teachers, Steve, Laura, Kyungsup, and I always strive to help you become a better orthodontist than we are. We experience no greater professional joy than when our students rise above us.

From conception to completion, we invested seven years in composing this textbook. If you learn one thing, our years of preparation and writing will have been worthwhile.

This book is dedicated to you, the doctor who strives daily to become proficient in the art and science of early orthodontic treatment, and who endeavors to provide uncompromising care to his or her patients. Doctor, we salute you.

About the Companion Website

Don't forget to visit the companion website for this book:

www.wiley.com/go/southard/practical

It contains:

- a 200-slide PowerPoint presentation covering the principles
- video clips of lectures using a question-and-answer format

1

Foundations

General Principles

The problems you will face in treating early malocclusions vary widely and are ever-changing. However, the principles presented in this section are enduring and will serve as your foundation for dealing with those problems.

Q: What is early orthodontic treatment?

A: Early orthodontic treatment (early limited treatment, early interceptive treatment, or Phase I treatment) is the treatment provided during the *primary or mixed dentition* stages of dental development. Comprehensive orthodontic treatment (Phase II treatment) is provided in the adult dentition.

Q: What is the goal of early orthodontic treatment?

A: The goal is to correct developing problems to get the patient *back on track (back to normal) for their stage of development*. This includes treatment to prevent complications, reduce future comprehensive treatment complexity, and reduce/eliminate unknowns.

Q: Can you provide examples of early treatment to prevent complications or reduce future treatment complexity?

A: Early treatment can prevent root resorption or tooth impaction in some cases of ectopic tooth eruption. Early treatment can eliminate the need for permanent tooth extractions or orthognathic surgery in some cases of skeletal discrepancies.

Q: Can you provide examples of unknowns which can be reduced/eliminated with early treatment? Why are reducing/eliminating unknowns important?

A: Examples of unknowns include:
- Magnitude and direction of future jaw growth
- Undetected CR-CO shifts
- Patient cooperation with headgears, functional appliances, elastics, hygiene, etc.
- Ectopic tooth eruption

Reducing/eliminating unknowns enables the orthodontist to more effectively plan final treatment and achieve desired outcomes. Let's consider one quick example. Assume that a child presents to you in the late mixed dentition with a bilateral Class II molar relationship of 4 mm. Further assume that, after careful analysis, you settle upon two treatment options – either Class II orthopedics or extraction of maxillary first premolars (masking the underlying skeletal discrepancy). It would be prudent to reduce unknowns first by *attempting* Class II orthopedics and monitor the response you get, before you decide on a final treatment plan (finish with orthopedics or treat irreversibly with extractions).

Key principle: After you have defined the patient problems you hope to address, always force yourself to answer the following questions: *What unknowns are present in treating this patient, and what unknowns should I eliminate before I define my final treatment plan or do something irreversible*?

Always explain unknowns to patients and parents. Informing them early of uncertainties in your plan will foster a smooth transition if you later need to modify your treatment plan due to unanticipated growth or treatment response. Always reduce/eliminate unknowns before committing to irreversible treatment. To do otherwise is to gamble on your patient's outcome.

Practical Early Orthodontic Treatment: A Case-Based Review, First Edition. Thomas E. Southard, Steven D. Marshall, Laura L. Bonner, and Kyungsup Shin.
© 2023 John Wiley & Sons, Inc. Published 2023 by John Wiley & Sons, Inc.
Companion website: www.wiley.com/go/southard/practical

Finally, many unknowns exist for each patient. We will highlight only the most pertinent and important.

Q: Another principle we will emphasize is this: Proper diagnosis should identify the patient's *primary problems* in each dimension (anteroposterior, vertical, transverse) plus other major problems (e.g. crowding, ectopic tooth eruption, thin periodontal biotype). Why is this important?

A: These are the problems which will impact your treatment goals and treatment outcome the most. Some will require early treatment. Others are best managed later in development. You must identify primary problems in your diagnosis and develop a treatment plan to address them. During the time you manage each early treatment patient, make it a point to stay focused on the major problems you are facing. If you focus on major problems, then you can gradually reduce these problems and next focus on lesser problems. If you fail to focus on major problems, then the major problems could remain or worsen and detract from the desired outcome.

During your initial patient evaluation, and *as you examine the patient at each appointment*, always ask yourself: "What are this patient's primary anteroposterior, vertical, and transverse problems (plus other major problems), and what is my plan to address these problems?" Then, regularly reassess these major problems as you get the child back on track.

Q: Is early treatment beneficial?

A: It can be. A recent study was conducted with 300 children (mean age nine years) who received treatment via numerous treatment modalities, including 2x4 fixed appliances, cervical or high-pull headgears (CPHGs, HPHGs), reverse pull headgears (RPHGs), functional appliances, lip bumpers, lower lingual holding arches (LLHAs), and serial extractions. Significant reductions in the American Board of Orthodontics Discrepancy Index were observed [1].

Of course, this does not mean that early treatment is always beneficial. Benefit is maximized when diagnosis is accurate and appropriate treatment is applied. In this book, we will illustrate conditions where early treatment should be considered.

Q: Can early treatment add to *total* treatment time?

A: Yes. You must weigh the benefits of early treatment against the cost – including the possible increase in total treatment time. Remember, the cost can be influenced by unknowns that may be revealed after you begin treatment (e.g. aberrant growth or poor compliance). Reducing unknowns is key to weighing benefit vs. cost.

Q: An orthodontist in your study club complains, "I used to perform a lot of early treatment. I do a lot less now because those cases seemed to drag on and on. I ended up doing most of the treatment in the permanent dentition anyway, and the children complained that they were in braces forever!" How would you respond?

A: We think this orthodontist makes a good point. *Early orthodontic treatment should address very specific problems, with a clearly defined endpoint.* With the exception of orthopedics for anteroposterior (and open bite) skeletal discrepancies, early treatment should generally begin and end within six to nine months, not drag on for years and years.

Let's consider a few short examples. Assume a healthy eight-year-old boy presents in the early mixed dentition with a Class I molar relationship and displaying one maxillary central incisor tipped lingually and in traumatic edge-to-edge occlusion with a mandibular incisor (incisal edge wear noted). A reasonable early treatment of short duration (3–4 months) would be to move the maxillary incisor labially out of traumatic edge-to-edge occlusion, and then place the patient in a clear maxillary retainer. Correcting the incisor trauma will get the patient *back on track* for his stage of development, and eliminating the incisor trauma has a *clearly defined endpoint*.

Now assume another healthy eight-year-old boy presents in the early mixed dentition and displays a bilateral 5 mm Class II molar relationship secondary to mandibular skeletal hypoplasia. Here, it may be best *not* to begin early treatment for the Class II problem (Class II orthopedics) *unless the boy demonstrates good statural growth velocity*. Why is this prudent? If growth velocity is slow, then a defined endpoint is less clear and years could be added to his total treatment time. All prospective clinical trials report no advantage in attempting Class II correction in the early mixed dentition (except for possible incisal trauma reduction) [2]. Therefore, unless you can reduce this unknown and establish that your patient has good growth velocity, it may be best to wait to begin treatment.

Our point is that there are many times when you should begin early treatment. There are also many times when you should not begin early treatment. One of the purposes of this text is to provide you with a foundation in making the decision to begin or recall.

Q: What questions should you ask yourself at every early treatment consultation?

A: *Do I need to do anything now? What harm will come if I simply monitor the patient at this time and recall in six to twelve months?* If the answer to your question is *no harm*, then your best treatment may be to monitor only and re-evaluate later.

Q: Can you list specific conditions that might warrant early orthodontic treatment?

A: We already mentioned incisor trauma due to edge-to-edge relationships or anterior crossbite relationships. Other conditions include dental crowding, eruption problems, excess overjet, skeletal Class II malocclusions in the late mixed dentition (or early mixed dentition if the patient exhibits good statural growth velocity), skeletal Class III malocclusions in the early or late mixed dentition (depending upon severity), deep bites with palatal incisor impingement/pain/tissue trauma upon closing, dental anterior open bites, skeletal anterior open bites (depending upon severity), and posterior crossbites with lateral shifts.

Let's invite our first patient in for a consultation and make a decision whether to provide early treatment or recall. Theo (Figure 1.1) is an eight-year-old boy who presents to us with his parents' chief complaint, "Theo has a cross bite that we want corrected." Past medical history (PMH) and Past dental history (PDH) are within the range of normal (WRN). Temporomandibular joint (TMJs) are WRN, and CR = CO.

Q: What do you notice about the position of the permanent maxillary canines in the lateral cephalometric radiograph (Figure 1.2)?

A: There appears to be a slight difference in their anteroposterior and vertical position.

Q: What could this be due to?

A: Lack of perfect superimposition of bilateral paired structures on a cephalometric radiograph can be due to:
- The effect of radiographic enlargement on bilateral structures
- Inaccurate patient positioning due to misalignment of the cephalostat or improper patient positioning in the cephalostat
- Marked asymmetry between right and left paired structures
- Marked size differences between right and left paired structures

Q: What is your assessment of this issue for Theo?

A: First, exact superimposition of right and left paired structures is confounded to a small degree by radiographic enlargement. Enlargement has the greatest impact on bilateral structures farthest from the sagittal midline (e.g. mandibular condyles and gonial angles) [3]. For maxillary canines, which lie closer to the sagittal midline, enlargement of the right vs. left canine in a standard cephalometric radiograph is ~0.15 mm. So, we conclude that the amount of anteroposterior difference in maxillary canines seen in Theo's cephalometric radiograph (~3 mm) has little contribution from enlargement.

Patient positioning can have dramatic effect on the superimposition of bilateral structures. Rotation of the cephalostat (or rotation of the patient by improper positioning in the cephalostat) by ~10° results in ~5 mm of anteroposterior image separation of the right and left maxillary canines and a larger (~8 mm) separation of the maxillary second molars (due to their greater distance from the mid-sagittal plane).

Looking at Theo's cephalometric radiograph, the ear-rods appear well aligned and the maxillary second molars show minimal (~2 mm) anteroposterior asymmetry. This suggests the anteroposterior image separation of Theo's maxillary canines does not have a significant contribution from patient rotation and may be due to spatial position asymmetry or size asymmetry of the maxillary canines.

Theo's panoramic radiograph suggests a vertical height difference in the right and left maxillary canines, supporting the similar finding on the cephalometric radiograph. Finally, bilateral tooth size asymmetry is not apparent.

Taking the cephalometric and panoramic information together, it may indicate a true difference exists in the anteroposterior and vertical positions of the right and left maxillary permanent canines.

Q: Why is this important?

A: In orthodontic diagnosis, asymmetry in spatial position of bilateral paired structures is a common finding. However, for developing maxillary canines, asymmetry in spatial position may be a clue to impending palatal or facial ectopic eruption and should be investigated further. This evaluation can include manual palpation of the maxillary alveolus from the facial in the area of the developing maxillary canine crowns to detect a difference in right and left prominence in the labial cortical plate, by periapical radiographic assessment using Clark's rule [4] or by 3-D radiography. None of these additional evaluations were performed on Theo.

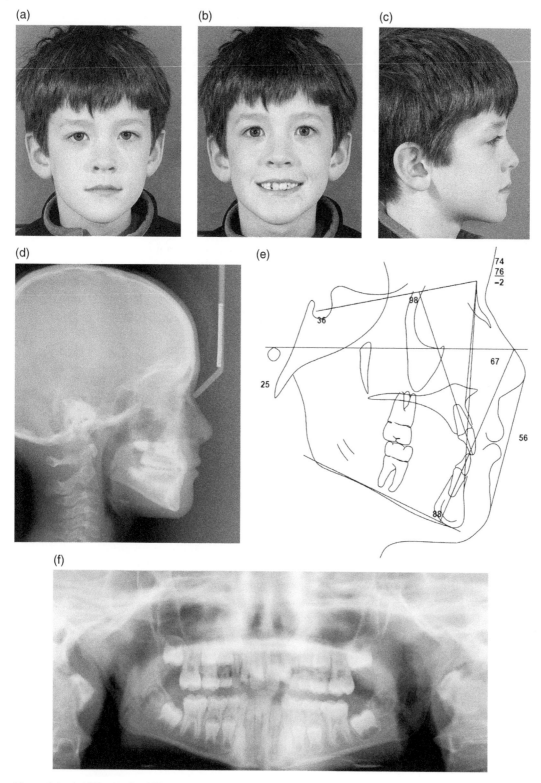

Figure 1.1 Initial records of Theo: (a–c) facial photographs, (d–e) lateral cephalometric radiograph and tracing, (f) pantomograph, (g–k) intraoral photographs.

(g) (h) (i)

(j) (k)

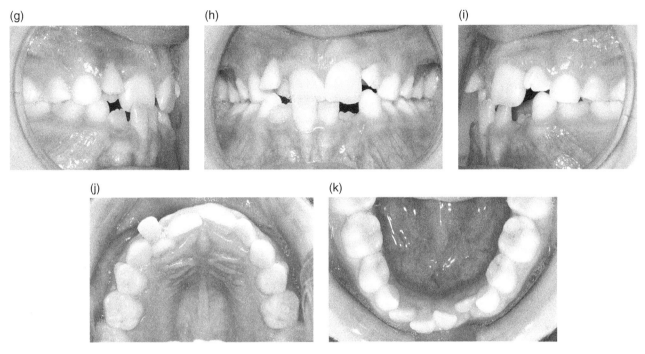

Figure 1.1 (Continued)

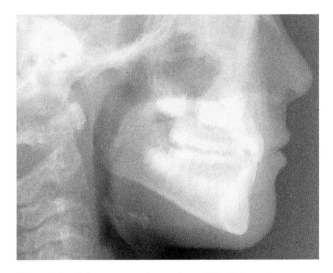

Figure 1.2 Enlargement of a portion of Theo's lateral cephalometric radiograph.

Q: What is meant by the term *apical base*? Are the terms *apical base discrepancy* and *skeletal discrepancy* interchangeable?

A: The term *apical base* refers to the junction of the alveolar and basal bones of the maxilla and mandible in the region of the apices of the teeth [5]. We will use the terms apical base discrepancy and skeletal discrepancy interchangeably.

Q: List your diagnostic findings and problems for Theo and make your diagnosis.

A:

Table 1.1 Diagnostic findings and problems list for Theo *(apical base/skeletal discrepancies italicized).*

Full face and profile	**Frontal view**
	Slight chin deviation to right
	Vertical facial proportions WRN (soft tissue Glabella-Subnasale approximately equal to Subnasale – soft-tissue Menton)
	Lip competence
	UDML WRN
	Mildly inadequate gingival display in posed smile (central incisor gingival margins apical to vermillion border of maxillary lip)

(Continued)

Table 1.1 (Continued)

	Profile view
	Straight to mildly concave profile
	Obtuse nasolabial angle (NLA) with upturned nose
	Chin projection WRN
	Chin-throat length WRN
	Acute lip-chin-throat angle
Ceph analysis	**Skeletal**
	Maxillary anteroposterior skeletal position is *retrusive/deficient* (A-Point lies behind Nasion-perpendicular line, ANB = −2°)
	Mandible also appears to be skeletally *retrusive/deficient*
	Skeletal LAFH WRN (LAFH/TAFH × 100% = 56%; normal = 55%, sd = 2%)
	Mandibular plane angle WRN (FMA = 25°; SNMP = 36°)
	Effective bony Pogonion (Pogonion lies on extended Nasion-B Point line)
	Dental
	Upright maxillary incisors (U1 to SN = 98°)
	Mandibular incisor inclination WRN (FMIA = 67°)
Radiographs	Early mixed dentition stage of development
	Slight overlap of maxillary left permanent canine crown over maxillary left permanent lateral incisor root (possible ectopic eruption)
Intraoral photos and models	Angle Class III subdivision left
	Iowa Classification: I I III (1–2 mm) III (1–2 mm)
	OB 20%
	Maxillary permanent right central and right lateral incisors in lingual crossbite
	5 mm maxillary permanent incisor crowding (moderate crowding, Figure 1.1j)
	6 mm mandibular permanent incisor crowding (moderate crowding, Figure 1.1k)
	LDML to right of UDML by 2 mm
	Maxillary and mandibular arches are symmetric (Figures 1.1j – 1.1k)
	Thin labial periodontal biotype of mandibular right central incisor (Figure 1.1h)
	Traumatized maxillary central incisors edges (Figure 1.1h)
	Retained maxillary right primary lateral incisor
Other	None
Diagnosis	Angle Class III subdivision left with anterior crossbite and moderate anterior crowding

Q: We judged Theo's mandibular skeletal anteroposterior position to be deficient, in spite of the fact that his ANB angle is −2° (an ANB value usually associated with mandibular anteroposterior excess). Why did we judge his mandibular skeletal anteroposterior position to be deficient?

A: If Theo's maxilla was in a normal anteroposterior position, then A-Point would lie on the Nasion-perpendicular line, and we could use ANB angle to judge his mandibular anteroposterior position. However, as discussed in the Appendix, because his maxillary position is *deficient* (A-Point lies behind Nasion-perpendicular line), we cannot use his ANB angle to judge his mandibular anteroposterior position.

Instead, we use the angle formed between the Nasion-perpendicular line itself and the Nasion B-Point line to judge his mandibular skeletal anteroposterior position.

If we measure this angle (Figure 1.3), we find that it equals 5°, indicating that his mandible is skeletally deficient. In other words, Theo has a skeletally deficient maxilla *and* mandible.

Q: But Theo has a straight, even a mildly concave, profile. He does not have a convex profile, which generally indicates a deficient mandible. Furthermore, he has a left side Class III dental relationship – not a Class II dental relationship indicative of a deficient mandible. How do you explain this?

A: The explanation is found in his deficient maxilla. Although Theo's mandible is deficient relative to Nasion-perpendicular line, his mandible is excessive *relative* to his deficient maxilla (ANB angle = −2°). It is not unusual for patients with normal mandibles to appear mandibular excessive when they have a

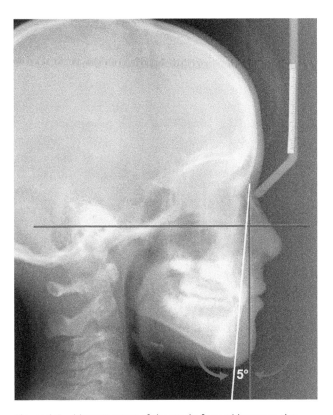

Figure 1.3 Measurement of the angle formed between the Nasion-perpendicular line (red vertical line) and the Nasion B-Point line (yellow line). This angle was found to be 5° indicating that the mandibular skeletal anteroposterior position is deficient. Therefore, both Theo's maxilla and mandible are deficient anteroposteriorly.

deficient maxilla. We must remain cognizant of this inconsistency as we treatment plan Theo and as we monitor his future growth.

Q: Theo is eight years old with an upturned nasal tip, adequate chin projection, and adequate chin-throat length. What changes do you anticipate in his nasal tip, chin projection, and chin-throat length as he grows and develops?

A: We anticipate that Theo's nasal tip angle will *decrease* with age [6] and both his chin projection and chin-throat length will *increase* with age [7].

Q: We noted that Theo exhibits a thin labial periodontal biotype covering his mandibular right central incisor. What does this mean? What is our concern with having a thin labial biotype during orthodontic treatment? How would you deal with this finding?

A: A thin labial biotype is characterized by a narrower zone of attached keratinized tissue than normal and a thinner facial-lingual gingival dimension than normal. A thick biotype is characterized by a wider zone of

attached keratinized tissue and a thicker facial-lingual gingival dimension [8–12]. If mandibular incisor roots are covered by periodontium exhibiting a thin biotype, then gingival recession may occur If the Incisor roots are moved labially or rotated (stressing the tissue). On the other hand, less than 1 mm of attached gingiva may be compatible with gingival health [13–17].

Based upon these points, and because Theo has *some* keratinized attached gingival tissue labial to his mandibular central incisor, we recommend monitoring Theo's mandibular anterior gingival tissues for now. However, his parents should be informed that the need for a future gingival graft exists if recession occurs at this site.

Q: Look at the photographs (Figures 1.1h – 1.1i). What do you note regarding the angulation of the maxillary left permanent lateral incisor? Why could this be important?

A: The maxillary left permanent lateral incisor appears to have its crown inclined to the labial and the root inclined to the lingual. Given the partial overlap of the maxillary left permanent canine crown and maxillary left permanent lateral incisor root (Figure 1.1f), this suggests the crown of the developing maxillary left permanent canine could be positioned to the labial of the lateral incisor root. Orthodontic movement of the lateral incisor root to the labial may cause root resorption.

Q: We stated that Theo's Angle Classification was Class III subdivision left and that his Iowa Classification was: I I III (1–2 mm) III (1–2 mm). What do we mean by Iowa Classification?

A: For years, we were frustrated using the Angle Classification system because it fails to quantify – that is to provide the orthodontist with a sense of discrepancy *magnitude*. In other words, when a patient is said to be Angle Class II does that mean that the patient is slightly Class II or severely Class II? The orthodontist is left without any sense of whether the patient needs Class II elastic wear or orthognathic surgery. Furthermore, we feel that canine anteroposterior relationships are just as important as molar relationships. The Angle Classification system lacks this detail.

We decided to modify the Angle system by quantifying the anteroposterior discrepancy at the patient's right molar, right canine, left canine, and left molar. (Please see the Appendix). For Theo that results in an Iowa Classification of: I I III (1–2 mm) III (1–2 mm).

Q: What are Theo's *primary*, or major, problems in each dimension, plus other problems that you need to remain focused on?

A:

Table 1.2 Primary problems list for Theo *(apical base/skeletal discrepancies italicized)*.

AP	Angle Class III subdivision left
	Iowa Classification: I I III (1–2 mm) III (1–2 mm)
	Maxillary and mandibular skeletal anteroposterior deficiency
Vertical	-
Transverse	-
Other	Anterior crossbite
	Possible ectopic eruption of maxillary left permanent canine
	Moderate anterior crowding in both arches

Q: Discuss Theo in the context of three principles applied to every early treatment patient.

1) The goal of early treatment is to correct developing problems – get the patient *back to normal for their stage of development* (including preventing complications such as resorption of adjacent tooth roots, reducing later treatment complexity, or reducing/eliminating unknowns). Theo's anterior crossbite, left Class III relationship, maxillary left permanent canine possible ectopic eruption, and moderate anterior crowding would need to be corrected to get him back to normal.

2) Early treatment should be applied to correct *very specific problems with a clearly defined endpoint*, usually within six to nine months (except for anteroposterior skeletal and skeletal open-bite orthopedics). Correction of Theo's anterior crossbite has a clearly defined endpoint and could be accomplished with fixed orthodontics in a few months. His moderate anterior crowding has a clearly defined endpoint, but improvement/correction could take longer than six to nine months (using space maintenance/fixed appliances) depending upon how long it takes his permanent canines and premolars to erupt. Correction of his possible ectopically erupting maxillary left permanent canine could take longer than nine months. Finally, correction of Theo's left Class III relationship could take years of orthopedic treatment, depending upon his future growth and compliance.

3) Always ask: Is it necessary that I treat the patient now? *What harm will come if I choose to do nothing?* It is important to treat Theo's anterior crossbite now to prevent additional incisor trauma/wear.

Without early treatment anterior crowding will remain, and unerupted permanent canines could become impacted or erupt blocked out. The risk of maxillary left permanent canine impaction is of special concern to us (note overlap of the maxillary left permanent canine crown across the maxillary left lateral incisor root, Figure 1.1f). Further, the maxillary left permanent canine crown could resorb the maxillary left permanent lateral incisor root.

Without Class III orthopedic treatment, maxillary deficient forward growth (relative to mandibular forward growth) could worsen Theo's left Class III relationship. Worsening of Theo's left Class III relationship could also result from mandibular permanent first molar mesial drift if an LLHA is not placed before exfoliation of his mandibular primary canines and molars.

Q: We noted that Theo's chin is deviated slightly to the right, CR = CO, his LDML is to the right of his UDML and face, and he is Class III on the left by 1–2 mm. What do these findings suggest?

A: These findings suggest that his mandible may be growing asymmetrically, with slight excess left mandibular forward growth.

Q: What unknowns do you face with Theo's care?

A: His future jaw growth (magnitude and direction), treatment compliance, and a potential undetected CR-CO shift are significant unknowns.

Q: What early treatment option(s) would you consider for Theo?

A: Early treatment options could include:

- *Recall (monitor only) and re-evaluate in one year – is not a recommended option.* Why? Risks include additional incisor trauma, increasing ectopic eruption of Theo's maxillary left permanent canine (increasing the risk of canine impaction and/or lateral incisor root resorption [16]), and continued Class III skeletal growth.

- *Anterior crossbite correction – is recommended* and could be performed in a number of ways. After extracting his maxillary right primary lateral incisor, you could: (i) ask Theo to close gently on a tongue blade covered with gauze (or on a soft suction tip) throughout the day in order to advance his right maxillary incisors; (ii) ask Theo to wear a removable maxillary biteplate with finger springs to advance his maxillary incisors; or (iii) place fixed orthodontic appliances to advance his maxillary right incisors. Also, some anterior crossbites will self-correct from tongue pressure alone if the patient's bite is first opened with bilateral band cement bonded on the permanent first molar occlusal surfaces.

Note: advancing the maxillary right lateral incisor crown forward will tend to drive its root reciprocally into the erupting canine crown – potentially resorbing the lateral incisor root. This must be explained to the parents. If you advance the lateral incisor crown, do so gently and slowly.

- *Extracting his maxillary primary canines and maxillary primary first molars – is a viable option when his maxillary first premolar roots are at least half developed.* Why? Eruption of the maxillary first premolars would be accelerated, which would make room for the maxillary permanent canines to erupt, thereby lessening the chance that his maxillary left permanent canine will be impacted [18, 19]. Generally, *a primary tooth should not be removed until its permanent successor has at least half of its root length formed* [20, 21]. Earlier primary tooth extraction can cause delayed eruption and emergence of its successor, probably as a result of scar tissue forming a mechanical barrier [22].
- *Space maintenance – is recommended, but not yet.* Placement of an LLHA could (i) prevent/minimize worsening of Theo's left Class III relationship due to permanent first molar mesial drift as his mandibular primary teeth exfoliate; and (ii) reduce mandibular anterior crowding as primary teeth exfoliate (leeway space). However, since the roots of his mandibular permanent canines and premolars are less than half formed (Figure 1.1f), their eruption is not imminent and placement of an LLHA would be premature [23].
- *Extraction of mandibular primary canines –* to permit spontaneous mandibular incisor alignment. We do not recommend this option since mandibular incisor crowding is not a concern for Theo or his parents. If you decided to extract mandibular primary canines, then we would strongly recommend placement of an LLHA to maintain arch perimeter and reduce mesial molar drift (worsening of the left Class III relationship).
- *Orthopedic treatment (e.g. reverse pull face mask therapy) –* is a possible option to improve/correct Theo's left Class III molar relationship by advancing his maxilla/maxillary teeth. Note: orthopedic treatment *will not normalize* Theo's growth. If Theo's maxilla is advanced orthopedically, then its position will need to be overcorrected in anticipation of future deficient maxillary growth, or he will need to be placed in a high-pull chin cup (or temporary anchorage device (TAD)-supported Class III elastics) to maintain the

correction – until he is finished growing. If excess left asymmetric mandible forward growth is identified, then asymmetric orthopedics (TAD supported Class III elastics) may be required on his left.
- *Extraction of his retained maxillary right primary lateral incisor –* is recommended if it does not exfoliate spontaneously.

Q: Based upon the above discussion, do you recommend recalling Theo in nine to twelve months (no treatment, monitoring only), or, do you recommend early treatment? If you recommend early treatment, what treatment would you perform?

A: We extracted Theo's maxillary right primary lateral incisor. Our early treatment objective was to correct his maxillary right central incisor crossbite by advancing it with fixed appliances and compressed open coil springs placed between his central incisors and primary canines (Figure 1.4). Band cement was bonded to the occlusal surfaces of his maxillary first permanent molars as a bite plate to open his bite and allow his maxillary right central incisor to advance, unimpeded.

We did not bracket the maxillary lateral incisors because they were not in traumatic occlusion and because we were concerned about possibly driving their roots reciprocally into the erupting permanent canine crowns (potential root resorption). Surprisingly, the maxillary right permanent lateral incisor *spontaneously* shifted forward out of lingual crossbite following extraction of the maxillary right primary lateral incisor

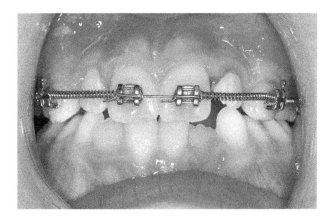

Figure 1.4 Maxillary fixed appliances were placed to advance Theo's maxillary right central incisor out of crossbite. We did not advance his maxillary right permanent lateral incisor for fear that moving its crown forward would drive its root reciprocally into the erupting permanent canine crown (potentially causing lateral incisor root resorption). Surprisingly, the maxillary right lateral incisor *spontaneously* shifted forward out of lingual crossbite following extraction of the maxillary right primary lateral incisor. We speculate that this movement resulted from either tongue pressure or transeptal fiber pull.

and advancement of the maxillary right permanent central incisor (Figure 1.4).

We decided to delay placement of an LLHA until Theo's mandibular permanent canines and premolars were closer to eruption. Also, we decided to postpone Class III orthopedic treatment. Why? Although Theo's anteroposterior relationship would be monitored, orthopedic treatment was deemed aggressive at this time considering his mild unilateral Class III magnitude (1–2 mm).

Finally, we decided not to extract Theo's maxillary primary canines and maxillary primary first molars. Why? The maxillary left permanent canine crown overlap of the maxillary left lateral incisor root was minimal (Figure 1.1f), and his first premolar roots were less than half developed.

Q: Look at Theo's early treatment deband photographs (Figure 1.5). Was our early treatment successful? Did we achieve our goals?

A: Yes and no. We achieved our goal to correct Theo's anterior crossbite. However, he is still Class III on his left side, he still has mandibular anterior crowding, and his maxillary left permanent canine is still erupting ectopically. These are problems that we must continue to monitor and eventually address to get him back on track.

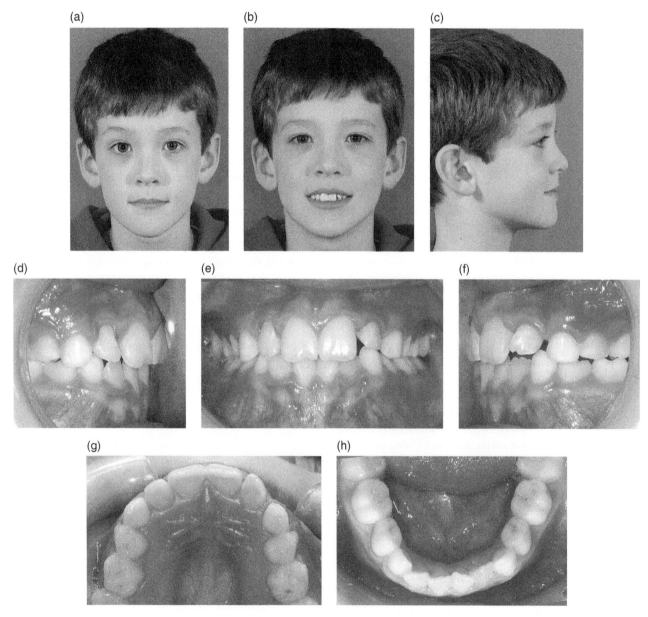

(a)   (b)   (c)

(d)   (e)   (f)

(g)   (h)

Figure 1.5 (a–h) Early treatment deband photographs of Theo. Previous incisal wear, especially of the maxillary right central incisor, is clearly evident.

Q: How do you recommend proceeding?

A: We made Theo an appointment to return in one year. At that time, we planned to make another panoramic radiograph. If Theo's maxillary left permanent canine crown was seen to overlap his maxillary permanent lateral incisor root more than on the initial panoramic radiograph, then we would extract his maxillary primary canines and primary first molars (assuming the premolar roots were at least half developed). These extractions would accelerate eruption of the first premolars and thus create an eruption path for the permanent canines.

We planned to place an LLHA when Theo approached exfoliation of his mandibular primary canines and primary molars. Finally, we planned to monitor his left Class III relationship, instituting orthopedic treatment (RPHG, high-pull chin cup, or TAD-supported Class III elastics), if his left Class III relationship worsened.

Q: Despite repeated attempts to schedule Theo to return to our clinic, he failed to do so until he was fifteen years old (Figure 1.6). List changes that have occurred since we last saw him (Figure 1.5).

A: Changes include:
- Most permanent teeth have erupted, but the maxillary right primary canine and mandibular left primary canine are retained.
- Theo had significant Class III dental compensation changes. His maxillary incisors proclined (U1 to SN angle increased from 98° to 108°, compare (Figures 1.1e and 1.6e) while his mandibular incisors uprighted (FMIA increased from 67° to 77°).
- Worsening of his *right* occlusal relationship to Class III (1 mm), and slight improvement on his left side from Class III (1–2 mm) to nearly Class I. Why? One possible explanation is that Theo grew Class III skeletally but had more available space in his upper left quadrant from lateral incisor to molar (Figure 1.5g) than in his upper right quadrant, which allowed him to obtain dental Class I on the left during permanent tooth eruption and mesial drift.
- Maxillary left permanent canine, the canine that initially concerned us, erupted normally. However, the maxillary *right* permanent canine became palatally impacted (Figure 1.6f). Note the slight palatal soft-tissue bulge covering the impacted maxillary right permanent canine (Figure 1.6j).
- Both mandibular canines erupted into 90° rotated positions (Figure 1.6k). The mandibular left canine erupted lingually.
- A moderate amount of mandibular anterior crowding exists (~6 mm of total mandibular permanent canine crowding)
- The mandibular anterior labial periodontal biotype appears to have thickened (Figure 1.6h)
- We noted that Theo's maxillary lateral incisors were small mesiodistally. His parents were informed that he would possibly need composite veneers to give them a more ideal mesiodistal width.

Q: Could we have prevented palatal impaction of the maxillary right permanent canine?

A: Possibly. If further investigation of the noted asymmetry of the maxillary permanent canines had been done, our findings may have prompted us to be more aggressive toward improving the potential for its normal eruption. Theo's lack of appointment compliance also limited our ability to monitor and evaluate its development.

This raises an important point. Early treatment always involves a *monitor and evaluate* component, be it when you decide no early treatment is needed and place your patient on recall, or when you have completed a focused early treatment and continue to monitor the patient. You must always stress to the parents of early treatment patients that *periodic observation is important to minimize developing problems*. We may have been able to lessen Theo's developing maxillary canine problem if periodic observation had been maintained.

Q: We noted that Theo's mandibular anterior labial periodontium appears to have thickened. What does the literature say about maxillary and mandibular anterior labial keratinized gingival widths in children six to twelve years of age?

A: In well-aligned teeth, *increases in width* of the facial keratinized and attached gingiva can take place [13].

Q: Was Theo's early treatment warranted?

A: Yes. Correction of Theo's anterior incisor crossbite was effective and necessary.

Q: What else should have been done during the years that Theo failed to return to clinic?

A: An LLHA should have been placed before exfoliation of Theo's primary canines and primary molars in order to:
- Prevent mesial drift of mandibular molars. If mandibular molar mesial drift had been prevented, then Theo could now be in a bilateral Class I molar relationship instead of Class III on his right.
- Provide leeway space for improved mandibular anterior teeth alignment (especially mandibular canine alignment)

In addition, periodic panoramic radiographs should have been made in order to evaluate the eruption path

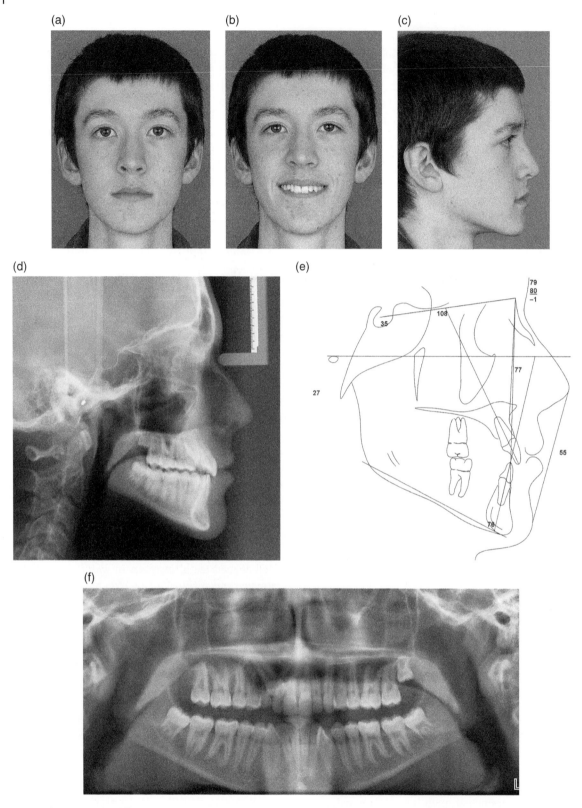

Figure 1.6 Records of Theo when he returned to our clinic at age fifteen years: (a–c) facial photographs, (d–e) lateral cephalograph and tracing (note that his dental arches were slightly separated when the cephalometric radiograph was made), (f) pantomograph, (g–k) intraoral photographs.

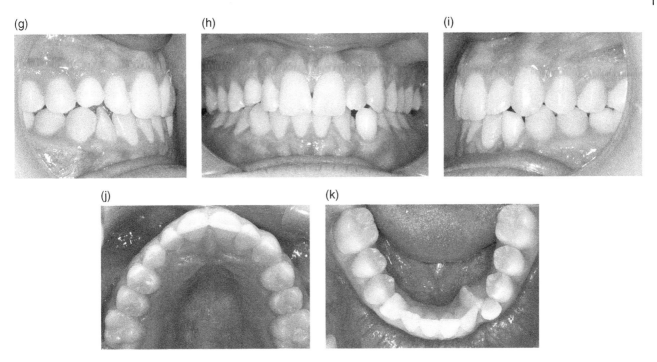

(g) (h) (i)

(j) (k)

Figure 1.6   (Continued)

of the permanent maxillary canines. We would have likely seen the earlier ectopic path of the maxillary left permanent canine improving with growth. The eventual ectopic path of the maxillary right permanent canine would have been seen earlier in Theo's development, allowing steps to be taken to improve the path of eruption prior to the full development of his adolescent dentition.

Also, Theo's growth should have been monitored, annually. We were lucky that Theo did not grow more Class III than he did. *Periodic observation is important to minimize the difficulty of developing problems.*

Q: Except for two retained primary teeth, Theo is now in the permanent dentition and ready for comprehensive orthodontic treatment. Although comprehensive treatment is not the focus of this book, do you have any recommendations on how to proceed?

A: Theo's mandibular incisors are upright, their labial periodontium has thickened, and he exhibits approximately 6 mm of mandibular anterior crowding. For these reasons, we decided to attempt comprehensive *nonextraction* treatment by aligning the mandibular anterior teeth. As they are aligned, the incisors will procline and tend to move into anterior crossbite. To avoid this, overjet would need to be created by proclining the maxillary incisors (spaces would be opened for composite veneers on the distal of the small maxillary lateral incisors). A reasonable alternative treatment

would be to extract a mandibular incisor to gain space for alignment. This treatment would result in less maxillary incisor proclination but more upright mandibular incisors.

Treatment began. To address the impacted maxillary right permanent canine, a transpalatal arch was placed, and a distal elastic traction force applied to the impacted maxillary right canine after it was surgically exposed. This force pulled the maxillary right canine crown *away* from the maxillary right lateral incisor root before the canine was moved laterally into arch alignment. We did this in order to avoid resorption of the lateral incisor root by the canine crown. The two retained primary canines were extracted. Maxillary fixed orthodontic appliances were placed. Using elastics, the maxillary right permanent canine was moved laterally into alignment within the arch (Figure 1.7a).

Anterior overjet was next created by making spaces between the maxillary lateral incisors and maxillary canines using open coil springs. This overjet would allow alignment (proclination) of mandibular anterior teeth without creating an anterior crossbite. A few months later, we noticed that Theo had grown more Class III (2 mm). He was placed on a high-pull chin cup (Figure 1.7b, 250 grams per side) to reduce and redirect mandibular forward growth while hoping maxillary forward growth would continue. He wore it from eight pm each night until morning.

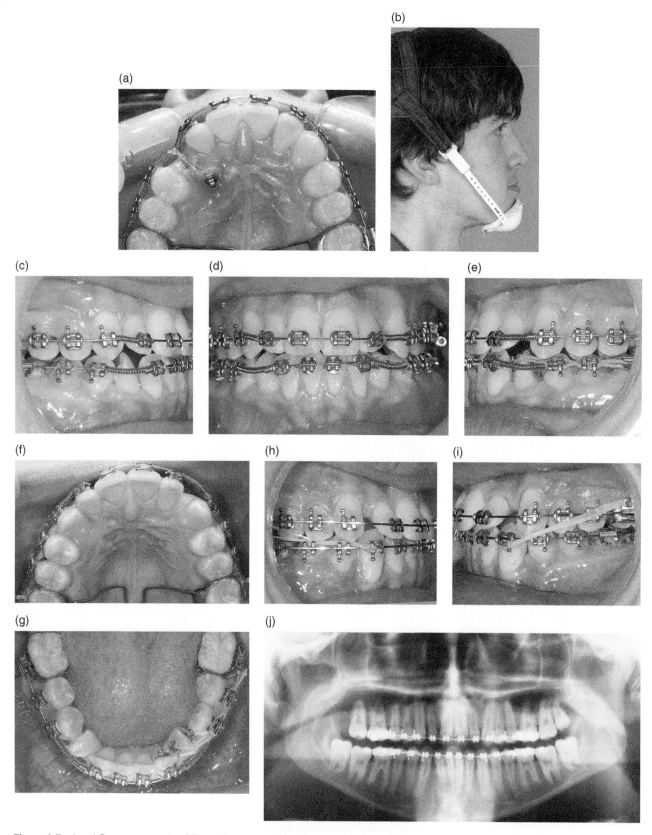

Figure 1.7 (a–u) Progress records of Theo. The panoramic radiograph in J was made one month prior to deband, and we did not make a panoramic image after deband because of radiation hygiene. (k–u) Deband records of Theo. The cephalometric superimposition (p) illustrates the bony and dental changes which occurred during comprehensive treatment.

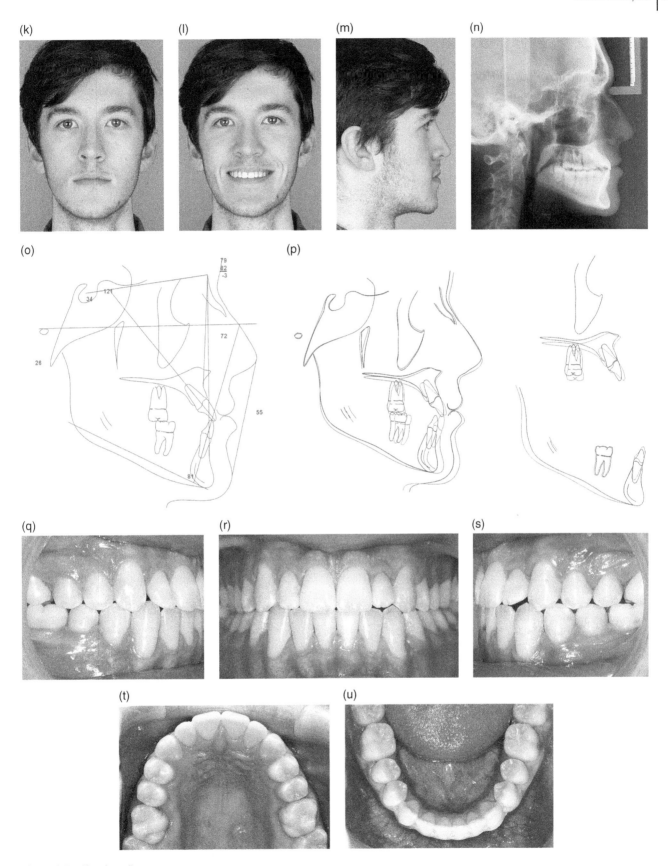

Figure 1.7 (Continued)

Theo was very compliant with chin cup wear. Mandibular-fixed orthodontic appliances were placed, and both arches were leveled and aligned (Figure 1.7c–g). Note in Figure 1.7g that space is being created for the mandibular right canine using a compressed open coil spring inserted between the lateral incisor and first premolar, and the mandibular left canine is being rotated with a couple (equal but opposite elastic forces on the buccal and lingual canine surfaces). Because of his excellent chin cup wear, Theo's Class III molar and canine relationships did not worsen, and we felt comfortable using Class III elastics to correct his 2 mm Class III relationship (Figures 1.7h–1.7i).

We began closing maxillary anterior spaces until anterior overjet was eliminated. The black triangle between his maxillary central incisors (Figure 1.7d) was eliminated by enameloplasty of the mesio-incisal corners of the central incisors followed by space closure. Because Theo's maxillary lateral incisors were small, we anticipated him needing maxillary lateral incisor composite veneers at the end of treatment to fill in residual spaces and give his maxillary lateral incisors the correct mesiodistal widths. However, we found that when a Class I canine relationship was achieved, we were able to close all maxillary spaces. This probably occurred because his mandibular incisors were upright (mandibular incisal edges were further back requiring less overjet than if they were proclined).

Theo's height was monitored throughout comprehensive treatment. By age seventeen he had stopped growing. Comprehensive orthodontic treatment, including finishing, was completed by age eighteen (deband records are shown in Figures 1.7k–1.7u). He was placed in maxillary and mandibular Hawley retainers.

We were pleased with Theo's final facial esthetics, smile, function, and occlusion. As expected, Theo had significant facial growth during comprehensive treatment (cephalometric superimpositions, Figure 1.7p). His maxilla underwent anterior rotation as a result of growth and treatment moving downward posteriorly and showing very little forward growth overall. His mandible grew downward and forward with mild anterior rotation.

We were not pleased with the uprightness of his mandibular incisors nor with the proclination of his maxillary incisors (Figures 1.7n and 1.7o), which reflect dental compensations for his differential maxillo-mandibular growth (mandible grew forward significantly, maxilla grew forward considerably less). We were not pleased with the second-order angulation of his maxillary left second premolar and his mandibular right lateral incisor (Figure 1.7j). His maxillary left

lateral incisor also displays too much mesial and lingual root angulation, contributing to the appearance of a shorter clinical crown. This was the clinical position of this tooth at the start of early treatment, and we neglected to focus on this problem during comprehensive treatment.

Finishing imperfections notwithstanding, Theo and his parents were ready to have his braces removed. We recommended that Theo have his maxillary left lateral incisor lengthened slightly with a composite veneer, but Theo declined.

In summary, Theo's *early* treatment consisted of anterior crossbite correction, which was completed by nine years of age and which prevented further incisor damage. However, we failed to place an LLHA at that time, we wish we had instituted Class III orthopedic treatment sooner than we did, but Theo disappeared for six years.

Q: Theo was included as an example in this section in order to underscore important concepts about early treatment diagnosis, treatment planning, and treatment delivery. Can you suggest other important concepts that his case illustrates?

A: These concepts are as follows:
- *Early treatment is only one piece of total orthodontic care.* Early treatment can be critically important. However, even if you get your patient back on track with early treatment, total treatment is incomplete until you have achieved excellent adult occlusion, function, tissue health, and facial esthetics. In addition, even after you successfully complete comprehensive treatment in the adult dentition, you must monitor the patient in retention. We did the right thing by treating Theo's anterior crossbite early, but we were committed to caring for him until his comprehensive treatment was complete as an adult – and beyond.
- Orthodontic treatment, including early orthodontic treatment, relies heavily on patient compliance. Theo failed to return to our clinic for years, during which time important early treatment opportunities (growth modification, space maintenance, and management of ectopically erupting teeth) were missed. *Periodic observation is important to minimize the difficulty of developing problems.*
- Cephalometric findings should corroborate clinical observations. When inconsistencies are noted between cephalometric findings and clinical observations, pay special attention. According to his cephalometric analysis, Theo presented with an anteroposterior mandibular deficiency (relative to Nasion-perpendicular line). Clinically, he appeared

to be developing a Class III malocclusion presumably due to greater mandibular anteroposterior skeletal growth than maxillary anteroposterior skeletal growth. Our cephalometric indicators may have suggested mild mandibular skeletal hypoplasia, but our initial clinical impression was correct.

- Due to his initial slight chin deviation to the right, lower dental midline to the right, Class III on the left by 1–2 mm, and CR = CO, we would have expected Theo to continue mandibular left asymmetric excess growth. Such an asymmetric growth pattern was not evident long term. Close monitoring during treatment allows for change of treatment plan in response to unanticipated growth or treatment response.

Q: Which early treatment cases are best *avoided*?

A: Be wary of *severe* skeletal Class II, severe skeletal Class III, or severe skeletal open-bite discrepancies. For example, a recent study reported that early, two-phase treatment for severe Class II high-angle patients offered no skeletal or dental advantage over later 1-phase treatment [24]. Exceptions to this guideline include severe skeletal discrepancy patients where there is a clear psychosocial (cosmetic) benefit to be gained from early treatment, when early treatment will dramatically simplify future (surgical) treatment, or when risk of dental injuries due to excess overjet is a concern [25, 26].

Q: Why is the above guideline important?

A: Skeletal jaw discrepancies in the anteroposterior, vertical, or transverse dimensions are treated in one of three ways: *orthopedics, masking, or surgery*. Dentofacial orthopedics uses forces to modify jaw growth and correct skeletal discrepancies. Masking (camouflage) corrects the occlusion dentally without correcting the underlying skeletal discrepancy. An example of masking would be skeletal Class II treatment via extraction of maxillary first premolars to create space for retracting maxillary canines from Class II into a Class I relationship. Masking and orthognathic surgery are generally considered only in the permanent dentition after growth is complete or nearly complete.

Orthopedics is the early treatment of choice for skeletal discrepancies. Whenever considering orthopedic treatment, you must reflect on the *magnitude* of the skeletal discrepancy and the *time* remaining to correct it.

Magnitude:
- For *mild* skeletal discrepancies: orthopedic correction may be possible with reasonable growth amount, direction, and patient cooperation.
- For *moderate* anteroposterior and skeletal open-bite discrepancies: orthopedic correction is less likely,

but improvement with orthopedics may be enough to permit successful masking. In other words, a final *dental* correction with reasonable facial esthetics may be achieved if early orthopedic skeletal improvement is first obtained. When successful, this generally minimizes the need to consider surgical correction as part of comprehensive treatment of the adolescent dentition.

- For *severe* anteroposterior and skeletal open-bite discrepancies: orthopedic correction is unlikely. If attempting orthopedics in these severe skeletal discrepancy patients, you must ensure that irreversible dental compensations are not placed, which would make later surgical correction difficult. We have made this mistake ourselves by placing a Class II patient with severe mandibular deficiency on a headgear only to find that dental correction was made by distal movement of the maxillary dentition. When the patient later requested a mandibular advancement osteotomy to improve her chin projection, the surgical advancement was limited because the maxillary teeth had been retracted.

With severe skeletal discrepancies, a decision must be made whether to attempt early orthopedics to the point where masking is possible (with good facial esthetics) or to postpone (surgical) treatment until after growth is complete. If we attempt early orthopedics in severe skeletal discrepancy cases it is with the parent's understanding that we will closely monitor to see what response we get (reduce unknowns) and that future orthognathic surgery is likely.

Time:
- Time of remaining growth can be your friend and your enemy.
- Time is your friend because the potential for orthopedic growth modification is maximized if you have years of growth remaining.
- Time is your enemy because most patients are not infinitely compliant. They may cooperate for months, or even years, but they will eventually stop. Beyond that point, additional orthopedic growth modification usually ends.
- Time is your enemy because *orthopedic treatment does not normalize the underlying jaw growth pattern*. In other words, assume you begin orthopedic treatment, the skeletal correction is made, and you stop orthopedic treatment. If the patient is still growing, then the previous growth pattern will return, and the patient may grow out of your correction.

Q: Jack (Figure 1.8) is ten years old and presents to you with the parents' CC: "Jack needs orthodontic treatment." PMH includes hydrocephaly, Goldenhar

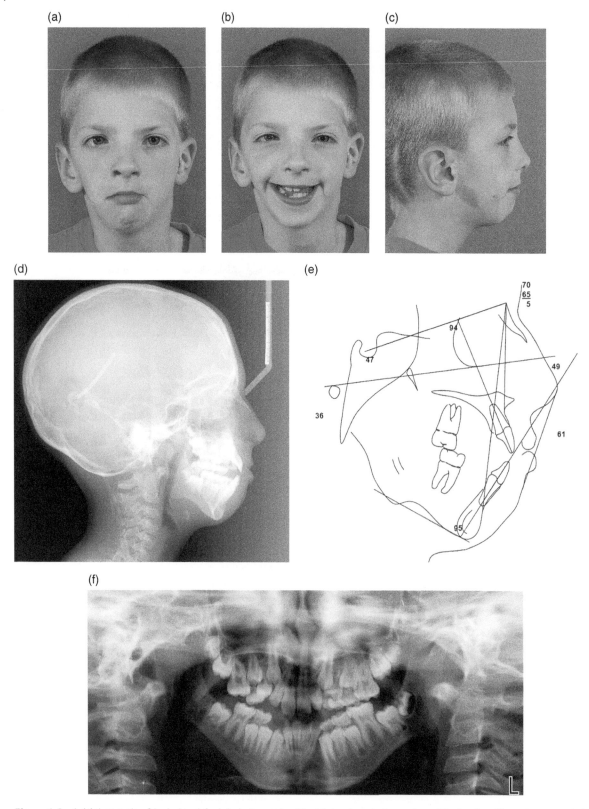

Figure 1.8   Initial records of Jack: (a–c) facial photographs, (d–e) lateral cephalograph and its tracing, (f) pantomograph, (g–k) intraoral photographs.

(g)   (h)   (i)

(j)   (k)

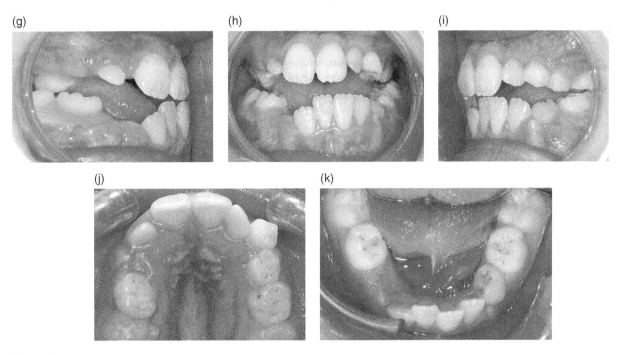

Figure 1.8 (Continued)

syndrome (oculo-auriculo-vertebral syndrome), hypoplastic left pinna, antimongoloid slant of palpebral tissues, right-to-left nares imbalance, fusion of atlas-axis, antibiotic prophylactic coverage required for dental procedures, and hemophilia. PDH and TMJ evaluations are WRN. CR-CO left lateral shift of 2 mm. Dentally, he is in the transition between early and late mixed dentitions. List your diagnostic findings and problem list for Jack.

A:

Table 1.3 Diagnostic findings and problem list for Jack.

Full face and profile	**Frontal view**
	Face is symmetric
	Long soft-tissue LAFH (soft-tissue Glabella-Subnasale < Subnasale – soft-tissue Menton)
	Mentalis strain to achieve lip competence
	UDML 3 mm to right of facial midline
	Large buccal corridors
	Inadequate gingival display in posed smile (central incisor gingival margins apical to vermillion border of maxillary lip)
	Profile view
	Convex profile
	Obtuse NLA
	Retrusive chin
	Mildly procumbent mandibular lip
Ceph analysis	**Skeletal**
	Maxillary anteroposterior *retrusion* (as indicated by A-Point being positioned behind Nasion-perpendicular line. However, Jack's syndrome may prevent us from using this measure to judge maxillary position. In fact, his maxillary anteroposterior position looks reasonably normal in the natural head position (Figure 1.8e).
	Mandibular anteroposterior *deficiency/retrusion*
	Long skeletal LAFH (LAFH/TAFH100% = 61%)
	Steep MPA (FMA = 36°, SNMP = 47°)
	Pronounced antegonial notching
	Vertical maxillary excess (VME)
	Ineffective bony Pogonion (Pogonion lies behind extended Nasion B-Point line)

(Continued)

Table 1.3 (Continued)

	Dental
	Maxillary incisor angulation appears WRN relative to natural head position (Figure 1.8e), but U1 to SN angle = 94° indicating upright maxillary incisors
	Proclined mandibular incisors (FMIA = 49°)
Radiographs	Hydrocephaly shunt (Figure 1.8d)
	Right condylar hypoplasia or absence (difficult to see due to superimposition of other bony structures (Figure 1.8f)
	Left condyle is flattened
	Ectopic eruption of maxillary right permanent first molar
	Transition between early and late mixed dentition stages of development
Intraoral photos and models	Angle Class III subdivision right
	Iowa Classification: III (4 mm) X I I (X indicates that right canine is missing)
	Anterior open bite extending posteriorly to the permanent first molars
	Bilateral posterior lingual crossbite
	UDML 3 mm right of LDML
	Mandibular transverse dental compensations (Figure 1.8h, mandibular permanent first molar lingual crown torque)
	Severe maxillary and mandibular anterior dental crowding
Other	-
Diagnosis	Angle Class III subdivision right skeletal open bite with VME, mandibular skeletal anteroposterior hypoplasia, bilateral posterior lingual crossbite due to maxillary transverse skeletal deficiency, and severe crowding

Q: What are Jack's *primary* problems you must stay focused on?

A:

Table 1.4 Primary problems list for Jack *apical base/skeletal discrepancies italicized.*

AP	Angle Class III subdivision right with *mandibular skeletal retrusion*
Vertical	*Skeletal open bite (VME, skeletal long LAFH)*
Transverse	*Maxillary transverse skeletal deficiency* with bilateral lingual crossbite
Other	Severe maxillary and mandibular anterior crowding

Q: Jack has skeletal problems in all three facial dimensions. Let's start with the vertical and anteroposterior dimensions. Should you begin early (orthopedic) treatment to address these? If yes, what treatment would you recommend?

A: The skeletal and dental problems confronting Jack are severe. In the vertical dimension, an attempt to orthopedically close his skeletal anterior open bite (and to maintain closure of the open bite) would require exceptionally long treatment with an uncertain outcome. Even if you placed TADs in both arches as anchors to intrude his posterior teeth, or simply to prevent eruption of his posterior teeth (relative intrusion), the TADs would need to remain in place until Jack completed growth. The effects of such a treatment on his developing airway are unknown.

Compared to his vertical skeletal discrepancy, Jack's anteroposterior skeletal discrepancy is more moderate. As Jack is entering the late mixed dentition stage of development, an attempt could be made to improve his anteroposterior skeletal relationship using orthopedics. However, high-pull headgear wear is prohibited because the headgear straps could occlude Jack's hydrocephaly shunt (tubing is palpable). Further, we do not recommend Class II functional appliance wear because it would further procline his mandibular incisors and promote a deleterious backward mandibular rotation [27].

For the above reasons, we decided not to attempt orthopedics in the vertical or anteroposterior dimensions but instead chose to wait until Jack had completed growth. Surgery would be the treatment option of choice at that time.

Q: What about Jack's transverse dimension? Should you begin early orthopedic treatment to address his posterior crossbite?

A: Yes, limited early transverse treatment could simplify future comprehensive treatment. If Jack's maxillary transverse deficiency can be corrected now with orthopedics, then the need for a future *multiple-piece* maxillary osteotomy (MPMO) to widen his maxilla, or the need for a future surgically assisted rapid maxillary expansion (SARME) procedure, could be eliminated. In other words, if Jack's maxilla can be widened now with RME, then a maxillary *one-piece* impaction osteotomy could someday correct his skeletal open bite – dramatically reducing the complexity of the maxillary surgery.

For these reasons, the maxillary right primary second molar and maxillary left primary first molar were extracted. After the ectopically erupting maxillary right permanent first molar and both maxillary first premolars erupted, a Hyrax expansion appliance was delivered and RME begun (Figure 1.9). An expanded LLHA (with labial molar crown torque) was also inserted to upright the mandibular first permanent molars (Figure 1.9e) and allow maximum expansion of the maxilla by removing the mandibular transverse compensations.

Finally, in an attempt to maintain the vertical dimension as much as possible, Jack was asked to chew gum (exercise) every day. Previous studies have shown that daily chewing exercises resulted in a significant decrease in the mandibular plane angle or assisted in orthodontic treatment to close anterior open bites [28, 29]. Jack developed recurrent coagulopathy problems, and his mother decided to discontinue orthodontic treatment until he was an adult.

Q: Caden (Figure 1.10) is nine years and seven months old. He was referred to you by his pediatric dentist for orthodontic treatment. Caden tells you, "I do not want braces." His mother says Caden had a small jaw when he was born and that, "Caden is not the best at cooperating." PMH, PDH, and TMJ evaluations are WRN and CR = CO. Caden cries during your examination and when your staff makes records. What are Caden's *primary* problems in each dimension (plus other problems)?

A:

Table 1.5 Primary problems list for Caden *apical base/skeletal discrepancies italicized.*

AP	Angle Class II division 2 Iowa Classification: II (7 mm) X X II (6 mm) *Mandibular skeletal deficiency*
Vertical	90% OB
Transverse	-
Other	Potentially impacted maxillary permanent canines Poor hygiene Localized juvenile spongiotic gingival hyperplasia (maxillary left anterior)

Q: We have one specific question. Would you begin early (orthopedic) treatment to address Caden's Class II

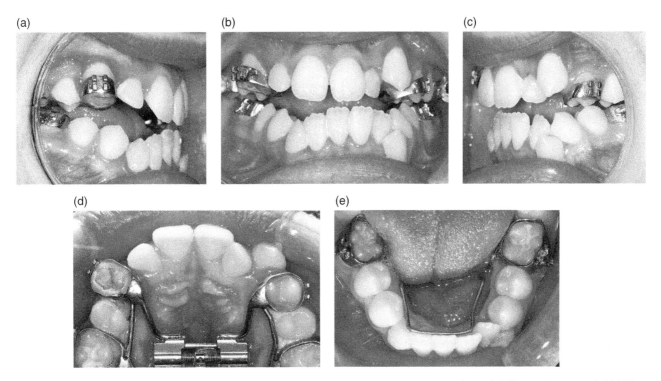

Figure 1.9 (a–e) Progress records of Jack illustrating RME to correct his maxillary transverse skeletal deficiency. An expanded LLHA was also placed to upright his mandibular permanent first molars.

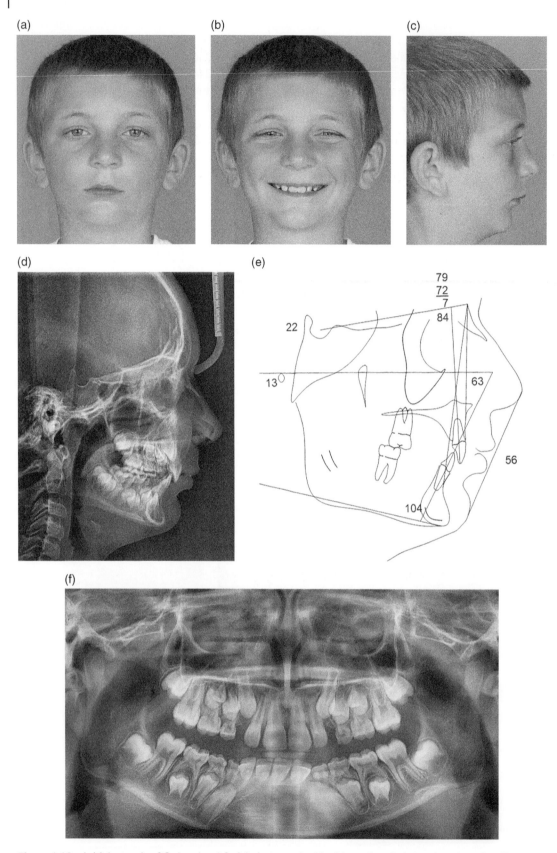

Figure 1.10 Initial records of Caden: (a–c) facial photographs, (d–e) lateral cephalograph and tracing, (f) pantomograph, (g–k) intraoral photographs, (l–p) intraoral scans.

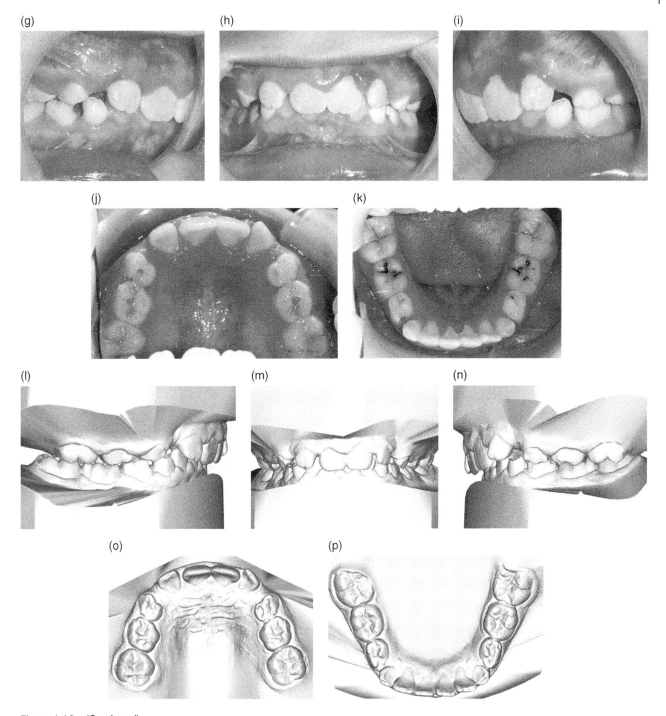

Figure 1.10   (Continued)

skeletal discrepancy? If yes, what treatment would you recommend?

A: Because Caden has a *severe* mandibular skeletal deficiency, a negative attitude toward orthodontic treatment, a history of mediocre cooperation, and evidence of poor oral hygiene, we *do not* recommend attempting orthopedic treatment. We recommend waiting until he reaches maturity when, if he is interested in treatment, a mandibular advancement osteotomy could be considered.

Q: Do you recommend avoiding other types of cases?

A: We are reluctant to treat patients with *severe* disabilities unless they are able to perform all functions needed to secure a successful outcome. Otherwise, treatment is frustrating for patient and doctor. Also, we recommend that you confirm treatment is something the *child* wants. You are providing care for the child, not the parent. A desire for treatment must come from the child.

Q: Can you suggest general principles to follow regarding patient *compliance* during early treatment?

A: General principles include the following:
- "Each patient is blessed with one cup of compliance." (Dr. Mike Callan). When it is gone, it is gone. *Design your treatment to be as efficacious as possible over the shortest time possible.* For some treatments (e.g. Class III orthopedics), the patient may need to exhibit super-human compliance over many years until they are finished growing.
- *Always have a fallback plan* (contingency plan) if your primary treatment plan fails due to lack of cooperation. For example, in Class III treatment, you may be forced to offer permanent tooth extractions or orthognathic surgery if the patient's response to orthopedic treatment is less than desired.

Q: Let's briefly discuss the need for early treatment in terms of esthetics and self-esteem. Dylan, a seven-year-old boy, presents for a consultation (Figure 1.11) with his mother's CC, "Dylan is teased at school because his front tooth sticks out. He is very self-conscious about it. I went to another orthodontist who refused to do anything about it. He said it was too early. *I want his front tooth corrected.*" You examine Dylan. PMH, PDH, TMJ's, and periodontal tissues are normal. CR = CO. What do you observe?

A: Overall, Dylan appears to be developing normally. His face is symmetric with a normal LAFH and mildly convex profile. He is in the early mixed dentition and exhibits a mesiodens (Figure 1.11d). He has a Class I canine and molar relationship, normal OB of the maxillary right central incisor, and 50% OB of the maxillary left central incisor. He has a normal transverse relationship (but large buccal corridors, Figure 1.11b), mild mandibular anterior crowding, and premature loss of mandibular right primary first molar with the space being maintained by a band and loop appliance (Figure 1.11i). His maxillary left central incisor is severely rotated/proclined, and he has a large diastema between his maxillary central incisors. There is an absence of either hard or soft-tissue damage resulting from this malalignment.

Q: What is the cause of the misaligned incisor?

A: The etiology is unknown. However, the presence of a mesiodens may have contributed to the ectopic eruption of the maxillary left permanent central incisor.

Q: Do issues of poor self-esteem, such as Dylan's, warrant early orthodontic intervention?

A: Generally, no. [30] For instance, in Class II patients, *early* treatment had no effect on self-esteem [26]. However, orthodontic treatment can improve self-concept and decrease negative social experiences [31, 32]. So, *the question of whether to provide early treatment in the hope of improving self-concept (everything you know about yourself) or self-esteem (how you rate what you know about yourself) must be dealt with on a case-by-case basis.* If a child is being teased about their dental condition, then this could be justification for early treatment.

Q: His mother's chief complaint offers us an important "take-home pearl". What is it?

A: Be cautious about letting parents dictate orthodontic treatment. You should treat only if you consider the treatment to be of benefit, reasonable, and what you would want for your own child.

Q: You decide to provide early treatment to address the malpositioned maxillary left central incisor. What treatment would you recommend?

A: The supernumerary tooth between the maxillary central incisors (Figure 1.11d) was surgically removed, fixed orthodontic appliances were bonded to the maxillary central incisors and maxillary primary second molars, the diastema was closed, and the maxillary left central incisor was aligned (Figure 1.12). A circumferential supracrestal fiberotomy (CSF, Figure 1.12e) was then performed.

Q: Why did we request a CSF for Dylan?

A: Severing the gingival fibers around the sulcus of a tooth (to the alveolar crest) may reduce posttreatment relapse. CSFs have been shown to be more effective in *alleviating pure rotational relapse* than in reducing labiolingual relapse [33] *and more successful in reducing relapse in the maxillary anterior segment* than reducing relapse in the mandibular anterior segment. With his severe maxillary left central incisor rotation, Dylan was the perfect candidate for a CSF.

Q: In addition to requesting a CSF, how else would you recommend retaining his maxillary central incisor's corrected alignment?

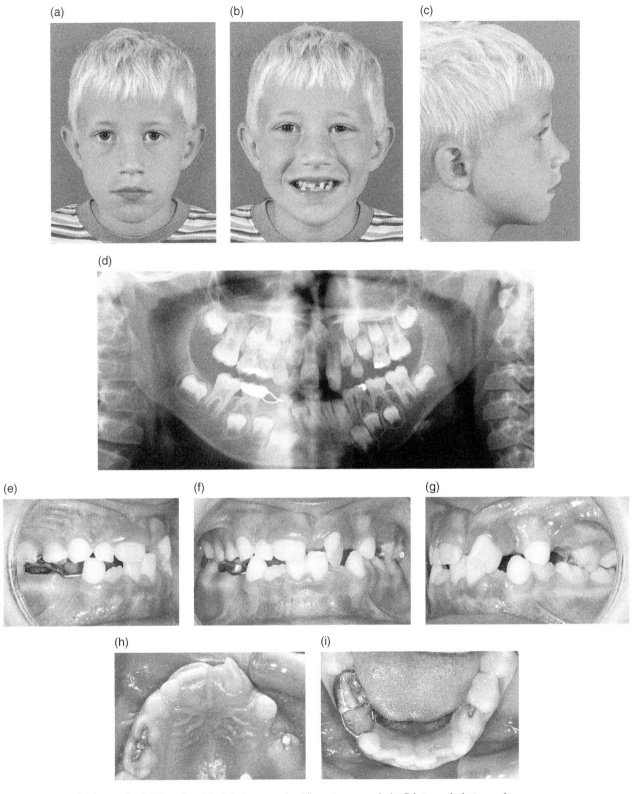

Figure 1.11 Initial records of Dylan: (a–c) facial photographs, (d) pantomograph, (e–i) intraoral photographs.

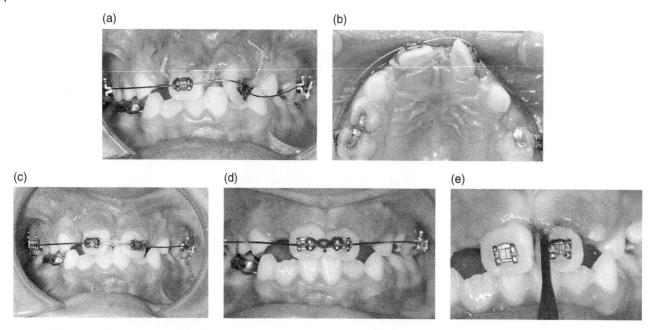

Figure 1.12 (a–d) Progress records of Dylan, (e) circumferential supracrestal fiberotomy (CSF).

A: We placed a fixed lingual retainer/wire bonded between Dylan's maxillary central incisors.

Notes: (i) OB must be shallow (not deep) in order to bond a fixed maxillary lingual retainer so that the mandibular incisors do not occlude against it; and (ii) it is a good idea to bond the fixed maxillary lingual retainer at least one month before the debanding appointment in order to monitor that it will remain attached. A clear, vacuum-formed retainer covering his palate and maxillary incisors was also given to Dylan to be worn at night until additional permanent teeth erupt.

Q: Figure 1.13 shows Dylan at deband. What changes do you observe?

A: The severe rotation of his maxillary left central incisor has been corrected resulting in significant improvement of Dylan's smile esthetics. He will be monitored for additional early treatment (e.g. placement of an LLHA to help alleviate mandibular anterior crowding) and later comprehensive treatment.

Q: Was Dylan's early treatment warranted?

A: Early treatment to improve a child's self-concept or self-esteem must be made on a case-by-case basis. On the one hand, you could argue that no tissue damage was occurring from the malaligned maxillary left central incisor and that correction of the malaligned tooth could have been postponed until comprehensive treatment in the adult dentition. On the other hand, Dylan and his mother were delighted with the correction and

stated that the teasing at school had stopped. We feel like his treatment was warranted.

Q: What are your "take-home pearls" from this section?

A: "Take-home pearls" include the following:

- The goal of early treatment is to correct developing problems – get the patient *back to normal for their stage of development* (including preventing complications, reducing later treatment complexity, and reducing/eliminating unknowns).
- Early treatment should be applied to correct *very specific problems with a clearly defined end point*, usually within six to nine months. Early treatment should generally not drag out for years and years into comprehensive treatment. There are exceptions to this guideline, including orthopedic treatment of some developing skeletal problems, such as skeletal Class III malocclusions.
- When deciding whether to begin early treatment, always ask, "Is it necessary that I treat the child now? *What harm can come if I choose to do nothing now – if I recall the patient in 6–12 months?*" One of the hardest things for orthodontists to do is to wait.
- Focus on the patient's primary problems in each dimension (plus other major problems).
- Before beginning treatment, always ask, "What unknowns am I facing?" Whenever possible, reduce your unknowns first – before establishing a final treatment plan but especially before doing anything irreversible (e.g. extracting permanent teeth).

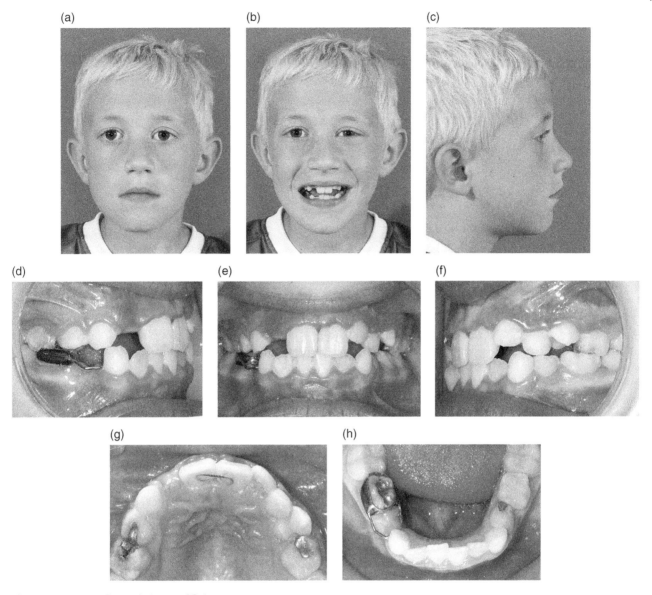

Figure 1.13   (a–h) Deband photos of Dylan.

- Always have a *fallback plan* (contingency plan) if your primary treatment plan fails due to lack of patient compliance or unfavorable growth.
- Early treatment involves frequent monitoring of patients. Adjustments to plans are made as you deem appropriate.
- When considering orthopedic treatment, reflect on the *magnitude* of the skeletal discrepancy and the *time* (potential growth) remaining to address it.
- As a rule, avoid early orthopedic treatment of *severe* skeletal Class II, severe skeletal Class III, or severe skeletal open-bite discrepancies. In such severe cases, some limited early treatment may be recommended to improve the patient's appearance (psychosocial benefit) or if *early treatment will dramatically simplify*

future treatment. We will often recommend early correction of severe maxillary transverse skeletal deficiencies in order to avoid later (surgical) maxillary expansion.
- Masking (camouflage) and orthognathic surgery are generally not considered as early treatment options. Orthopedics is the skeletal discrepancy early treatment of choice.
- Be wary of early treatment cases when the patient is *severely* disabled unless the patient has expressed a strong desire for treatment and is able to perform all necessary functions to insure a successful outcome.
- Decisions to provide early treatment to improve a child's self-concept or self-esteem are made on a case-by-case basis.

- Early treatment can offer significant benefits. However, it can also result in prolonged treatment times, worse final clinical assessments, and increased incidences of patient/parent "burn-out." [34] Be selective when applying early treatment. This text will provide a foundation for helping you to decide when to do so.

Growth and Development of the Craniofacial Complex

Background

An in-depth understanding of craniofacial growth and development is essential to the practice of our specialty. Patients are often evaluated for early orthodontic intervention at a time when their facial skeleton and associated soft tissues are experiencing significant growth. Thus, foundational knowledge of post-natal craniofacial growth, heritable and environmental influences on jaw growth and tooth development, and potential response of the growing jaws and teeth to intervention is crucial to provide effective early treatment to patients, and to assess early treatment outcomes. This section provides a brief review of important craniofacial growth and development concepts, with an emphasis on the facial skeleton, the airway, and the dentition. The development of other key soft tissues that support neural activity, respiration, mastication, and deglutition undoubtedly have an important influence on the growth and development of the facial skeleton. For more additional information on the growth and development of craniofacial soft tissues, the reader is referred to more comprehensive treatises on this subject [35–37].

Normal Skeletal Growth and Development, Abnormal Growth, and Growth Velocity

Q: Do we have a complete understanding of the underlying mechanisms responsible for craniofacial growth and development?

A: Despite advances in our knowledge of craniofacial growth and development, a complete understanding of the underlying mechanisms has not yet been elucidated. The prevailing theory posits genetic control, whereby molecular signaling processes that dictate the temporal and spatial expression of key developmental genes, and environmental factors that modulate these control mechanisms operate in concert to influence craniofacial development [38]. The functional matrix hypothesis of Moss, a mechanistic description of the process of craniofacial growth and development, is the main conceptual framework understood by orthodon-

tists [39, 40]. Future research on the genetic control theory will elucidate the mechanism of the functional matrix hypothesis. Comprehensive treatment of these concepts can be found elsewhere [39–44].

Q: What is meant by craniofacial growth and development?

A: The term growth describes a change in size or quantity. In the context of craniofacial development, this occurs by cell proliferation leading to tissue enlargement. The term *development* describes changes in form and function based on changes in the specialization of cells, tissues, and organs [45].

Q: What drives the growth and development of the craniofacial skeleton?

A: Growth and development of the craniofacial skeleton is under genetic control and modified by environmental factors. This growth control system mediates the specialization and enlargement of craniofacial skeletal tissue in concert with the specialization and enlargement of the tissues supporting neural activity, respiration, mastication, and deglutition. Craniofacial development is controlled by complex gene-regulatory networks. For example, HOX and DLX genes are responsible for patterning of the vertebrate head in rostro-caudal and dorso-ventral axes, respectively [46]. Other key genes expressing transcription control factors and growth factors are responsible for mediating the growth, development, and maintenance of skeletal and soft tissues throughout embryogenesis and postnatal development [40, 42, 47].

Q: In general terms, how does the facial skeleton grow?

A: The growing facial skeleton is a composite of *cranial base growth, individual facial bone growth, and eruption and drift of the teeth*. Each of these components has its own unique pattern of change, in space and time, driven by growth and development of associated key soft tissues and sensory organs. The unique shape and size characteristics of the facial skeleton are not generated independently. Change in size and shape of each growing facial bone is the result of complex genetic, spatial, temporal, and functional interrelationships among the essential functional components of the craniofacial region [41–43]. A composite of the growth and development changes for the cranial base and facial bones in the sagittal view is depicted in Figure 1.14.

Q: What are the underlying osteogenic mechanisms responsible for facial bone size and shape changes?

A: Underlying osteogenic mechanisms include:

(a) 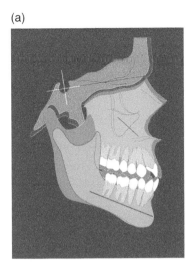 (b)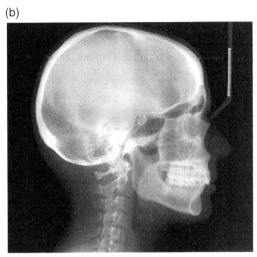

Figure 1.14   (a) Changes in size, shape, and position of the major skeletal components contributing to the growth of the face as viewed in the sagittal. Approximate outline of the cranial base (gray), the maxilla (green) and the mandible (blue) as seen on a lateral cephalogram. Darker shades of color indicate the approximate location and direction of changes in size and shape due to drift and displacement of the cranial base, maxilla, mandible, and teeth during growth (*Source*: From Duterloo and Planche [48]. Figure 3-23. Reproduced with permission from Quintessence Publishing Company Inc, Chicago); (b) the location of the cranial base (gray), maxilla (green), and mandible (blue) on a lateral cephalogram.

- Bone formation by both intramembranous and endochondral ossification.
- Intramembranous ossification is the mechanism for modeling and remodeling of the majority of the facial skeleton. Bone modeling drives spatial displacement of the cortical surfaces of intramembranous bone during which bone deposition and resorption of the periosteal and endosteal cortical surfaces occurs.
- Endochondral ossification replaces a cartilage template with bone. This is the mechanism for formation of the bony cranial base from the primary cartilage precursor. It is also the mechanism for growth of the condyle from adaptive secondary cartilage of the condyle.
- Bone modeling at the facial bone *surfaces* causing individual facial bone enlargement and change in shape. This is defined as facial bone *surface drift*.
- Bone modeling at the facial bone *sutures* coordinated with spatial displacement of investing functional tissues. This displacement is termed *primary displacement* of the facial bones and is often referred to as "sutural growth" of the craniofacial skeleton.
- Interstitial growth of cartilage in the synchondroses of the cranial base and nasal septal cartilage associated with spatial displacement of the adjoining bones of the face. Facial bone displacement by the enlargement and/or translation of adjoining facial bones is termed *secondary displacement*.

- Chondrogenesis and endochondral ossification of secondary cartilage of the mandibular condyle associated with primary displacement of the mandible.

With the possible exception of secondary displacement mediated by growth at synchondroses and the nasal septal cartilage, bone displacement and drift does not cause bones to "push" against each other. Facial bone displacement and drift is, by and large, mediated by biochemical and biomechanical signals during growth and development of the enveloping soft tissues [41, 42, 49].

The following questions provide a brief overview of the growth and development of the cranial base, the nasomaxillary complex, the mandible, and the airway. For more comprehensive reviews of these processes, we refer the reader to some excellent references [35, 47].

Q: How does the cranial base grow? How does cranial base growth contribute to facial growth? Provide a detailed review.

A: The cranial base provides the foundation for postnatal facial development. In the midline, the cranial base undergoes lengthening by primary displacement to accommodate the growing brain. Frontal and temporal lobe brain expansion corresponds with the endochondral bone replacement of cartilage in the main growth centers of the cranial base, the spheno-ethmoidal and spheno-occipital synchondroses. Frontal and temporal lobe expansion also drives anterior and middle cranial fossae anteroposterior, vertical, and lateral enlargement via sutural growth and drift (see Figure 1.15). Details of cranial base spatial and temporal growth are found elsewhere [50].

The resulting forward movement of the anterior cranial base has a forward displacement (secondary) effect on the nasomaxillary complex. The forward growth of the anterior cranial base reaches adult dimension sooner than the posterior cranial base, reaching 90% of adult size by ~five years of age. The portion measured from *sella turcica* to foramen cecum ceases anteroposterior growth by ~seven years of age. Nasion continues forward growth through puberty influenced by expansion of the frontal sinus and, as some have suggested, growth of the nasal septal cartilage [51].

The pterygoid processes move downward by drift and displacement. As frontal lobe expansion and sphenoethmoidal synchondrosis growth cease (approximately age seven), temporal lobe expansion continues, displacing the frontal lobe anteriorly with a continued secondary displacement effect on the anterior cranial base and the nasomaxillary complex. Temporal lobe expansion laterally and vertically also influences the position of the glenoid fossae, which are displaced posteriorly and inferiorly until approximately age fifteen to sixteen

years [52, 53], and to a greater degree during adolescence compared to childhood [54]. Numerous studies across different ethnic populations have shown that a more obtuse cranial base angle (angle formed by Nasion-Sella and Sella-Basion) and/or a long anterior (relative to posterior) cranial base length is associated with a skeletal Class II relationship. A more acute cranial base angle and/or a short anterior cranial base length is associated with a skeletal Class III relationship [55]. A composite of these growth movements in the sagittal view is depicted in Figure 1.16.

Q: How does the nasomaxillary complex grow?
A: Growth expansion of the nasal septal cartilage, the investing soft tissues, and the airway displace the nasomaxillary complex downward and forward with primary displacement at the circummaxillary sutures adjoining the frontal, zygomatic, ethmoid, nasal, lacrimal, and palatine bones (see Figure 1.17).

Airway and soft-tissue expansion directs bilateral displacements with growth at the intermaxillary sutures. In relative terms, the greatest amount of growth displacement of the nasomaxillary complex is displacement in vertical height, followed by displacement in anteroposterior depth, followed by displacement in transverse width [47]. Downward and forward growth of the anterior cranial base contributes early to nasomaxillary

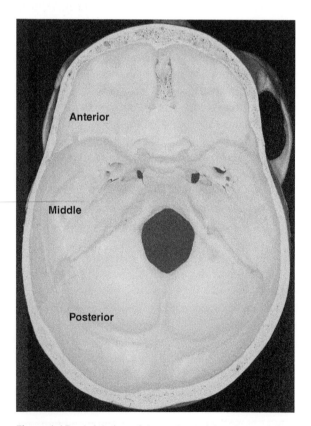

Figure 1.15 Axial view of the endocranial surfaces of the cranial base. Shaded areas refer to the anterior, middle and posterior cranial fossae.

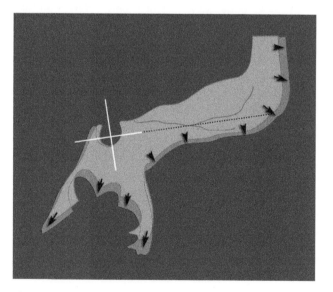

Figure 1.16 Changes in size, shape, and position of the cranial base during growth – as viewed in the sagittal. The intersection of the white lines indicates Sella point. Darker gray and dark arrows indicate approximate magnitude and direction of changes due to growth-driven drift and displacement. (*Source*: From Duterloo and Planche [48]. Figure 3-25. Reproduced with permission from Quintessence Publishing Company Inc., Chicago.)

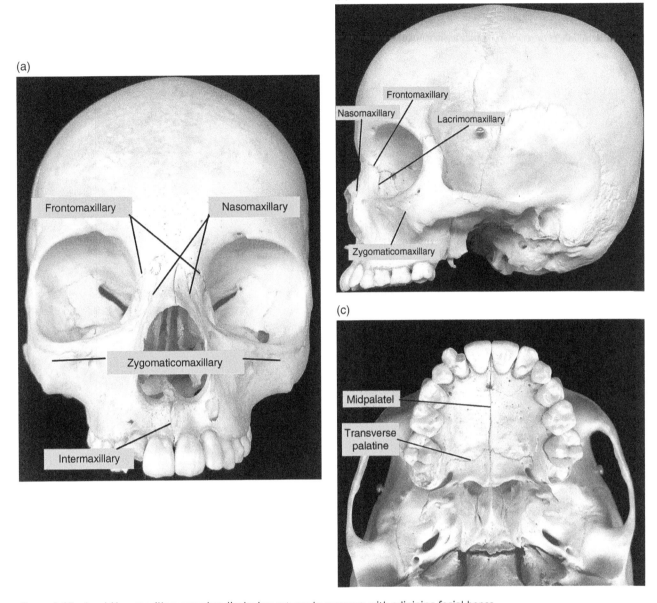

Figure 1.17 (a–c) Nasomaxillary complex displaying sutures in common with adjoining facial bones.

displacement, diminishing at ~ age seven, as continued displacement is directed by enlargement of the airway, investing soft tissue and the nasal septal cartilage [42, 51]. This is accompanied by backward downward drift at the posterior maxilla (tuberosity) with new bone available for eruption of permanent molar teeth and downward directed drift of the hard palate. Nasomaxillary surface drift occurs in response to changing soft tissue and facial bone spatial relationships. Palatal inferior drift and vertical drift of the maxillary permanent teeth contribute approximately 66% of the vertical height change in the maxilla [56, 57]. Vertical drift of maxillary teeth is controlled by forces of

eruption (exact mechanism unknown) and forces opposing eruption (e.g. functional/parafunctional loading with mandibular teeth). A composite of these growth movements in the sagittal view is depicted in Figure 1.18.

The contribution of nasal septal cartilage interstitial growth to downward forward translation of the nasomaxillary complex remains controversial. Many believe the growth expansion of the nasal septal cartilage drives nasomaxillary downward and forward displacement [58–60]. Others believe the expansion of the nasal septal cartilage is adaptive to the functional demands directing the expansion of the airway

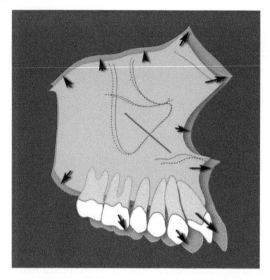

Figure 1.18 Changes in size, shape, and position of the maxilla and maxillary teeth during growth – as viewed in the sagittal. Darker color and dark arrows indicate approximate magnitude and direction of changes due to growth-driven drift and displacement. (*Source*: From Duterloo and Planche [48]. Figure 3-29. Reproduced with permission from Quintessence Publishing Company Inc., Chicago.)

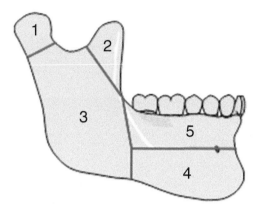

Figure 1.19 The mandible consists of five regions: (1) condyle, (2) coronoid process, (3) ramus, (4) corpus, and (5) alveolar process.

according to the functional matrix hypothesis [61, 62]. Some authors have suggested the role of the nasal septum as a growth center is attenuated at the time the junction of the ethmoid and sphenoid bones transition from a cranial base growth center (synchondrosis) to a cranial base growth site (suture) [63].

Q: How does the mandible grow?

A: The mandible is carried downward and forward by growth expansion of the enveloping soft tissues. In response, the mandible grows upward and backward largely by a combination of bone surface drift (intramembranous ossification) and primary displacement at the condyle (endochondral replacement of secondary cartilage).

Q: The mandible consists of five developmentally important regions. What are they, and what role does each play?

A: The mandible consists of the condyle, coronoid process, ramus, corpus, and alveolar process (Figure 1.19). The role of each is as follows: [42]

- Condyle: along with the ramus, it is a major site of compensatory mandibular growth during downward and forward facial soft-tissue expansion. It provides articulation with the temporal bone to mediate function between the maxillary and mandibular teeth. It performs these roles by virtue of the condylar cartilage, a specialized secondary cartilage allowing endochondral bone growth to occur in the presence of masticatory compressive forces on the condylar head. The arrangement of secondary cartilage allows condylar growth to be adaptive, facilitating change in growth direction as pressure and tension on the condylar head change, and to maintain the relationship of the condyle and glenoid fossa as the mandible is carried downward and forward.

- Coronoid process: provides attachment of the temporalis muscle, which supports the process of mastication. The coronoid process undergoes extensive drift upward, backward and laterally during the downward and forward translation of the mandible.

- Ramus: as a major site of adaptive growth and growth compensations, it is of equal importance to the condyle during downward and forward translation of the mandible. In order to maintain the appropriate spatial and functional relationship of the mandibular dentition with the maxillary dentition during growth, the ramus undergoes complex changes in width, depth, height, and uprighting (gonial angle becoming more acute). Although it is common to encounter the term "condylar growth," signifying the condyle as the most important mandibular growth center, the importance of ramus growth is co-equal in establishing balance or imbalance in mandibular position. Also, the ramus provides attachment for the masseter and medial pterygoid muscles.

- Corpus: supports the alveolar process and teeth during development and mastication; provides attachment for many muscles, include the mentalis muscle.

- Alveolar process: provides a bony housing for the eruption, drift, and function of teeth.

Q: Describe the anatomy of the pharynx at birth, and the changes that occur during growth and development to adolescence.

A: In the newborn, the pharynx, uvula, and epiglottis are in proximity to allow the independent functions of suckling and breathing. During the period from approximately eighteen months of age until adolescence, vertical growth causes the relative descent of the larynx, increasing the cumulative vertical length of the nasopharynx, oropharynx, and laryngopharynx twofold from ~7–8 mm to ~15–16 mm, ultimately stretching vertically between the sphenoid bone superiorly and the level of the fifth cervical vertebrae inferiorly (Figure 1.20) [64, 65] This change in length is thought to be an anatomical prerequisite for human speech [66]. As this vertical growth ensues, the pharynx develops three specialized functions: deglutition, during which the pharyngeal constrictors and tongue are employed to transport food from the oral cavity into the esophagus; phonation, during which the pharynx changes length and shape to alter the sounds passing from the larynx; and respiration, during which the pharynx must become more rigid to avoid collapse to allow adequate passage of air.

Q: Describe the anatomy of the adolescent pharynx.

A: The pharynx is divided into three anatomic regions (Figure 1.21): (i) The nasopharynx is bounded by the soft palate inferiorly, the pharyngeal tonsils superiorly, the superior pharyngeal constrictor posteriorly and the nasal choanae anteriorly. (ii) The oropharynx is bounded by the soft palate superiorly and the epiglottis inferiorly. The palatoglossal arches and the posterior third of the tongue form the anterior boundary. The posterior wall of the oropharynx is formed by the superior, middle, and inferior constrictor muscles. The lateral pharyngeal walls are formed by the hyoglossus, styloglossus, stylohyoid, stylopharyngeus, palatoglossus, palatopharyngeus, and the lateral aspects of the superior, middle, and inferior pharyngeal constrictor muscles.

In the midsagittal view, the oropharynx is subdivided into the retropalatal region, bounded by the hard palate superiorly and the caudal margin of the soft palate inferiorly, and the retroglossal, bounded by the caudal margin of the soft palate superiorly and the tip of the epiglottis inferiorly. In infants and young children, the retropalatal region is larger in relative size, because the soft palate and the epiglottis are in proximity (Figure 1.20). (iii) The laryngopharynx is bounded by the epiglottis and by the pharyngoepiglottic fold superiorly and the upper esophageal sphincter inferiorly.

Q: From an orthodontic point of view, characterize "normal" and "abnormal" craniofacial growth and development.

A: Craniofacial growth and development that is considered "normal" results in a range of intermaxillary skeletal and dental relationships that do not create impediments to the major elements of craniofacial function: brain function, nerve function, respiration,

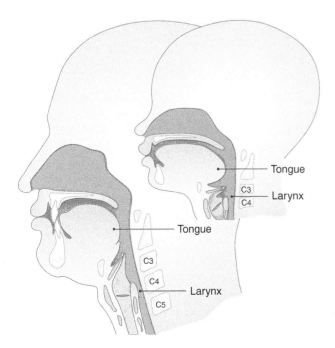

Figure 1.20 The development of the pharynx from childhood to adolescence.

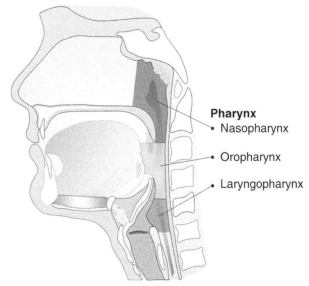

Figure 1.21 The anatomical divisions of the mature pharynx.

mastication, or deglutition (i.e. development with an absence of superimposed pathogenesis) [67]. In orthodontic terms, "normal" is a spectrum of variation that includes normal occlusion and ideal occlusion. Ideal occlusion describes ideal tooth alignment and maximum intercuspation of the dentition in the presence of balanced maxillo-mandibular interrelationships in three planes of space. Normal occlusion describes a range of tooth alignment relationships that have Class I molar relationship in common. Normal occlusion occurs in a wide range of diverse anteroposterior, transverse, and vertical skeletal relationships [68, 69]. Normal craniofacial pattern describes a range of intermaxillary and interocclusal relationships associated with normal craniofacial function.

However, "abnormal" is also a term used in orthodontics to describe a range of malocclusion stemming from mild to moderate discrepancies of intermaxillary skeletal and dental relationships not impacting craniofacial function that are routinely treated by orthodontists. The extremes of "abnormal" skeletal discrepancies are severe dentofacial deformities and syndromic craniofacial dysmorphism that are treated by craniofacial orthodontists as part of a craniofacial clinical team. In this book, when we use the term "abnormal" we are referring to mild to moderate growth and development-related intermaxillary and interocclusal discrepancies for which the goal is to employ routine orthodontic treatment to improve these discrepancies WRN. Information on the diagnosis and management of craniofacial anomalies can be found elsewhere [70].

Q: How does "normal" development of the facial skeleton occur?

A: "Normal" relationships of the facial skeleton arise from a sequential coordination of the major elements of the craniofacial growth process:

- Cranial base growth.
- Downward and forward translation of the maxilla with adaptive growth at the circummaxillary and intermaxillary sutures and vertical drift of the palate/nasal floor.
- Posteriorly and superiorly directed adaptive growth of the mandibular corpus, ramus and condyle.
- Maxillary and mandibular growth rotation (clockwise or counterclockwise).
- Vertical dentoalveolar development.

These processes are directed by complex interrelationships between factors under genetic control and environmental (epigenetic) factors influencing this control.

Q: Is "normal" skeletal development a prerequisite for "normal" interocclusal dental relationships?

A: No. A Class I molar relationship is considered "normal" as is 1–2 mm of incisor overjet, and 10–20% of incisor overbite. However, "normal" interocclusal dental relationships develop in individuals with a wide range of "normal" skeletal relationships. For example, it is estimated that 50–55% of the United States population has Class I malocclusion [71], yet Class I molar relationship is associated with a variety of anteroposterior, vertical, or transverse skeletal relationships (in addition to dental problems, such as crowding) [69, 72].

Among all human populations, there are individuals who vary significantly from others in both vertical, anteroposterior, and transverse skeletal relationships, yet have similar interocclusal relationships [73].

Q: The preceding answer raises the following question: what is the growth mechanism providing "normal" interocclusal dental relationships despite significant variation in skeletal relationships?

A: Simply put, it is the *compensatory growth potential* of each major element of the facial growth process. In other words, compensatory growth of one element can overcome unbalanced growth of another element, allowing for attainment and maintenance of normal interocclusal relationships [42]. For example, decreased cranial base flexure can be associated with skeletal mandibular hypoplasia which, in turn, is often associated with an abnormal interocclusal relationship. However, decreased cranial base flexure combined with compensating increased ramus depth growth can produce a normal interocclusal relationship.

Q: In addition, what is the *dental* mechanism which provides normal interocclusal dental relationships despite significant variation in skeletal relationships?

A: The path for tooth eruption is dictated, labiolingually/buccolingually, by a balance of soft-tissue pressures between the tongue and cheeks/lips. This path provides a dental compensatory mechanism to permit the teeth to erupt together in spite of the presence of skeletal relationship variation. For instance, in the case of a hypoplastic mandible (Figures 1.22a and 1.22b), the mandibular incisors will erupt between the tongue and lips with a *proclined* inclination in order to contact with the maxillary incisors. In the case of a hyperplastic mandible (Figures 1.22c and 1.22d), the mandibular incisors will erupt between the tongue and lips with a *retroclined* inclination in order to contact the maxillary incisors.

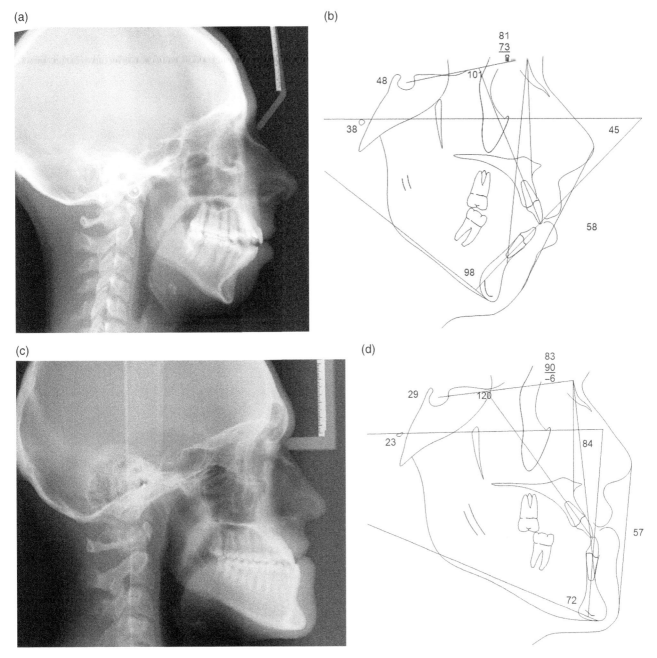

Figure 1.22 (a, b) Patient exhibiting a normal maxilla and hypoplastic/deficient mandible. Note compensatory proclination of mandibular incisors. (c, d) Patient exhibiting a normal maxilla and a hyperplastic/excessive mandible. Note compensatory retroclination of mandibular incisors and compensatory proclination of maxillary incisors.

Q: Our knowledge of the transverse morphologic changes which occur during growth and development is far greater than our understanding of the biology underlying those changes. Can you describe the pattern of transverse *bone* changes which occur during maxillary and mandibular growth and development?

A: A pattern of bony width changes in the alveolar bone supporting the teeth occurs as a *gradient* in the vertical dimension [73]. As illustrated in Figure 1.23, the greatest width change occurs more superiorly (Jugale point), and the least width change occurs inferiorly (mid-alveolar point of the mandible). Divorced from this pattern are the transverse mandibular basal bone changes, measured as bi-gonion and bi-antegonion.

Q: Can you describe the transverse *dental* (permanent molar) movements which occur during growth and development.

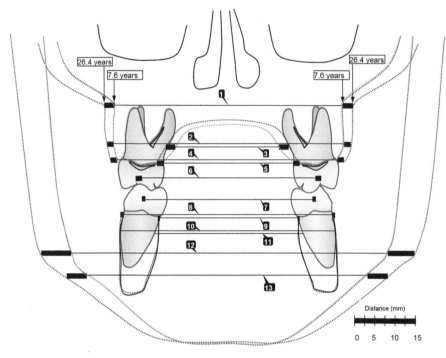

Figure 1.23 Mean transverse basilar, cross arch alveolar, and inter molar changes from age 7.5 years to 26.4 years: (1) maxillary basilar width; (2) maxillary cross arch width mid-alveolar buccal; (3) maxillary cross arch width mid-alveolar palatal; (4) maxillary cross arch width alveolar crest buccal; (5) maxillary cross arch width alveolar crest palatal; (6) maxillary intermolar width; (7) mandibular intermolar width; (8) mandibular cross arch width alveolar crest buccal; (9) mandibular cross arch width alveolar crest lingual; (10) mandibular cross arch width mid-alveolar buccal; (11) mandibular cross arch width mid-alveolar lingual; (12) mandibular basilar width (bi-gonion); and (13) mandibular basilar width (bi-antegonion). Horizontal bars indicate average change in width measured in millimeters from 7.5 years to 26.4 years.

A: Maxillary molars erupt with buccal crown torque and upright with age as the maxilla widens (Figure 1.24). Mandibular molars erupt with lingual crown torque and upright with age. These molar crown torque changes are accompanied by concurrent increases in maxillary and mandibular intermolar widths. On average, the basal bone of the maxilla increases in width by 5.4 mm; maxillary intermolar width increases by 3.0 mm; mandibular intermolar width increases by 2.0 mm; and mandibular cross arch crest-level alveolar width increases by 1.6 mm [73, 74].

Q: What does the above finding mean in terms of dental treatment goals?

A: The finding provides support for the American Board of Orthodontics' requirement that ideal finishing treatment include *upright* posterior teeth.

Q: What are *transverse* posterior dental compensations?

A: Transverse posterior dental compensations are excessive buccal or lingual torques resulting from transverse apical base discrepancies between the jaws. Figure 1.25a illustrates excessive maxillary first molar buccal crown torque, and excessive mandibular lingual crown torque,

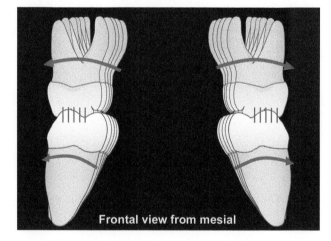

Figure 1.24 Average transverse molar movements from ages seven to twenty six years.

resulting from either inadequate maxillary transverse growth or excessive mandibular transverse growth. Figure 1.25b illustrates excessive maxillary first molar lingual crown torque, and excessive mandibular buccal crown torque, resulting from either excessive maxillary transverse growth or inadequate mandibular transverse growth.

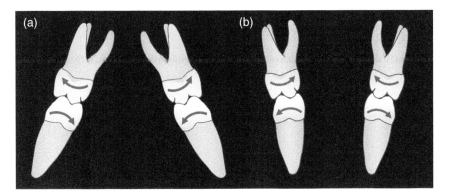

Figure 1.25   (a–b) Transverse posterior dental compensations.

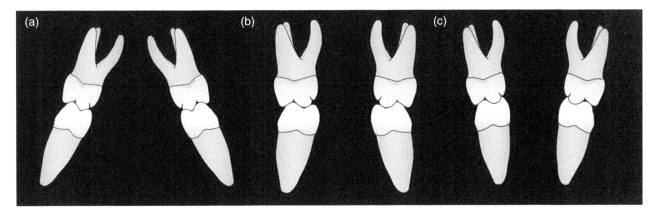

Figure 1.26   Variation in transverse skeletal widths in the absence of crossbites: (a) small maxillary skeletal width compared to a large mandibular skeletal width (maxillary buccal crown torque and mandibular lingual crown torque compensations), (b) comparable maxillary and mandibular skeletal widths (relatively upright molars), and (c) large maxillary skeletal width compared to a small mandibular skeletal width (maxillary lingual crown torque and mandibular buccal crown torque compensations).

Q: How do transverse dental compensations develop?

A: Transverse dental compensations develop in the same way, and for the same reasons, that anteroposterior dental compensations develop. Teeth tend to erupt throughout life until sufficient occlusal, or soft tissue, load prevents further eruption. They erupt along their long axes, but their buccal-lingual direction is influenced by the soft tissue envelop (tongue-cheeks-lips) in order to bring them into occlusion with teeth from the opposing jaw. In the presence of a hypoplastic maxilla, the tongue will tend to tip the maxillary incisors forward, and the mandibular lip will tend to tip the mandibular incisors lingually (anteroposterior compensations). In that way, the incisors will be brought into occlusion. In a similar fashion, in the presence of a hypoplastic maxilla, the tongue will tend to tip the maxillary molars buccally, and the cheeks will tend to tip the mandibular molars lingually (transverse compensations). In that way, the molars will erupt into occlusion.

Q: Is there any research to support the above concepts?

A: Yes. A recent study [67] found there is a large variation in transverse skeletal widths (and transverse dental compensations) in the absence of crossbites ranging from:
- small maxillary skeletal widths compared to large mandibular skeletal widths (Figure 1.26a), to
- comparable maxillary and mandibular skeletal widths (Figure 1.26b), to
- large maxillary skeletal widths compared to a small mandibular skeletal width (Figure 1.26c).

Q: How can differential maxillary and mandibular anteroposterior jaw growth affect transverse relationships?

A: Let's begin with the jaws in a Class II relationship (mandibular anteroposterior deficiency or maxillary anteroposterior excess, Figure 1.27a). Further, assume that excess posterior overjet exists.

If the mandible begins to outgrow the maxilla (Figure 1.27b), then a wider part of the mandibular arch

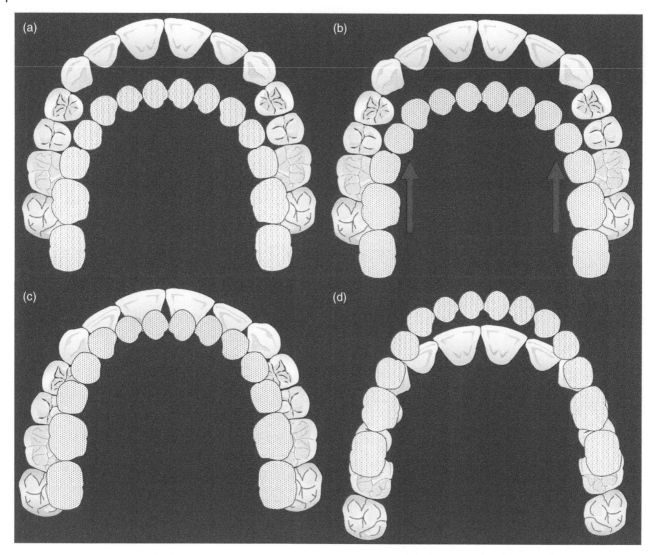

Figure 1.27 Effect of differential anteroposterior jaw growth on the transverse jaw relationship: (a) if excess posterior overjet initially exists in a patient with a deficient mandible, then if the mandible outgrows the maxilla (b); (c) a more ideal posterior overjet can result; or (d) inadequate posterior overjet can result if the mandible continues growing forward.

is growing into a narrower part of the maxillary arch. A more ideal transverse relationship can result (Figure 1.27c). If the mandible continues to outgrow the maxilla, then insufficient posterior overjet could even result as the molars become Class III (Figure 1.27d).

Q: What is the mechanism for *abnormal* craniofacial growth and development?

A: By and large, there is not one *single* causative mechanism for abnormal development of the craniofacial complex. Developmental problems of the craniofacial skeleton are multifactorial, and *abnormal* skeletal relationships arise from aberrations in genetic and/or environmental influences. Aberrations produce altered growth intensity and/or altered temporal coordination of one or more major growth elements. Aberrations, sufficient in magnitude and/or duration to disrupt the interrelationships of these elements, result in adaptive growth movements of the maxilla and mandible that may lead to abnormal changes in the spatial relationship of the jaws [42, 43]. Aberrations are normally intrinsic, but may also be induced. For example, certain early surgical interventions to improve abnormal dentoskeletal relationships in cleft palate patients can actually impede maxillary skeletal growth [75].

Q: What are the temporal relationships among the growing components of the facial skeleton during maturation of facial size and shape?

A: Maturation of facial size and shape occurs, by and large, along a superior-inferior (cephalo-caudal) temporal gradient [42]. Measuring the change in the craniofacial skeleton with growth and development, cranial structures mature first, followed by cranial base structures, then facial bones, and finally the mandible completes its maturation after the maxilla. Aberrations in the temporal sequence result in significant craniofacial deformities. Some have characterized the gradient with distinct tiers (cranial, cranial base, facial), while others have argued for a continuous gradient with maturation of anatomic structures between tiers showing overlap [53]. Adding to the complexity of facial growth, maturation of the mediolateral structures of the cranial base do not mature in the same "tier," or at the same time, as those along the superior–inferior gradient. Midline cranial base structures, presumably influenced by maturation of the spheno-occipital synchondrosis, appear to mature well in advance of structures in the lateral cranial floor. Lateral cranial floor structures mature in a similar timeframe to the mandible, suggesting a possible functional integration of the masticatory apparatus and the development of lateral cranial floor [53]. Additionally, there are authors who believe in the growth of the craniofacial skeleton being integrated, whereby growth in time and dimension of the earlier maturing portions (cranium, cranial base) dictate some shape constraints to the later maturing portions (face) [76]. An example being a retruded mandible with obtuse gonial angle, decreased corpus height, vertically oriented symphysis, and pronounced sigmoid notch is associated with the cranial base variations seen in dolichocephalic subjects [42, 76]. Others believe there is little integration between maturation of the cranium-cranial base and the face [77].

Q: Given the complex orchestration of temporal and spatial development of the craniofacial skeleton, variations in the pattern of the facial skeleton are the norm. Extreme variations in *vertical* growth and displacement of the facial skeleton are often referred to as "skeletal open-bite pattern" and "skeletal deep-bite pattern." How would you describe the growth and displacement of the major units of the facial skeleton in these two extreme craniofacial patterns?

A: Skeletal open bites may result from:
- Decreased cranial base flexure leading to superior spatial positioning of the temporomandibular fossae. However, this influence is not well understood and requires more study before it can be used reliably in diagnosis.

- Excessive sutural lowering (vertical growth/descent) of the maxilla.
- Diminished vertical growth of the mandibular condyles (posterior-superior condylar growth).
- Backward mandibular (apparent) rotation.
- Excessive vertical drift of the posterior dentoalveolar complex (excessive posterior tooth eruption).

Skeletal deep bites may result from:
- Increased cranial base flexure leading to inferior spatial positioning of the temporomandibular fossae. However, this influence is not well understood and requires more study before it can be used reliably in diagnosis.
- Deficient sutural lowering (vertical growth/displacement) of the maxilla.
- Excessive vertical growth of the mandibular condyles.
- Forward mandibular (true/internal) rotation.
- Deficient vertical drift of the posterior dentoalveolar complex.

Q: With respect to craniofacial development in the vertical dimension, discrepant skeletal relationships are characterized using various cephalometric measures. Can you list, and describe, four of these measures?

A: Cephalometric measures describing vertical development include:
- Ratio of posterior face height (linear measurement from Sella to Gonion) to anterior face height (linear measurement from Nasion to Menton) or PFH/AFH, viewed in the sagittal plane. A reduced PFH/AFH ratio is associated with greater divergence between the mandibular plane and cranial base, indicating a "skeletal open-bite" facial pattern. Conversely, a large PFH/AFH ratio tends to indicate a "skeletal deep-bite" facial pattern [78].
- Ratio of lower anterior face height to total anterior face height (linear measurement from Menton to ANS superimposed on the linear measurement of Menton to Nasion) or LAFH/TAFH. A reduced LAFH/TAFH ratio indicates a skeletal deep-bite facial pattern, and a large ratio is associated with greater facial divergence and a skeletal open-bite pattern.
- Angular measurement between the Sella-Nasion line and mandibular plane, or SN-MP angle. An elevated SN-MP angle indicates greater facial divergence and skeletal open-bite facial pattern. A reduced SN-MP angle indicates a skeletal deep bite facial pattern.
- The junction of the posterior surface of the ramus and the inferior mandibular border forms the gonial

angle. An average gonial angle measurement is ~130°. A more obtuse gonial angle (>130°) is associated with vertical skeletal hyperdivergence.

Q: According to Schudy [79], how does vertical condylar growth relate to the sum of vertical maxillary descent, plus maxillary/mandibular molar eruption during normal, hyperdivergent, and hypodivergent facial development?

A: Schudy suggests:
- When vertical condylar growth *matches* the sum of maxillary descent and posterior dentoalveolar development – *normal vertical development results.*
- With diminished vertical condylar growth relative to the sum of maxillary descent and posterior dentoalveolar development – facial hyperdivergence, decreased PFH/AFH, increased LAFH/TAFH, increased SN-MP, and a skeletal open-bite pattern result.
- With excessive vertical condylar growth relative to the sum of maxillary descent and posterior dentoalveolar development – facial hypodivergence, increased PFH/AFH, decreased LAFH/TAFH, decreased SN-MP, and a skeletal deep-bite pattern result.
- It is noteworthy that extreme patterns of vertical skeletal growth develop early and, by and large, remain relatively stable throughout craniofacial growth.

Q: In terms of craniofacial growth, how do discrepancies in anteroposterior skeletal relationships occur?

A: Discrepancies in anteroposterior skeletal relationships of the maxilla and mandible occur primarily as the result of three mechanisms acting individually or together. By and large, postnatal downward and forward displacement of the mandible is influenced by the growth of the cranial base, the growth of investing soft tissues, and the growth of the oronasal capsule that is coordinated with nasomaxillary displacements [47, 80].

Displacement of the mandible during postnatal growth is closely associated with the growth of the posterior cranial base and middle cranial fossa via the posterior and inferior displacements of the glenoid fossae [42, 47]. Individuals with more obtuse cranial base angles and/or larger anterior and posterior cranial base lengths display mandibular hypoplasia. Individuals with more acute cranial base angles and/or smaller anterior and posterior cranial base lengths display mandibular hyperplasia.

As noted by Shudy, the relative vertical displacement of the nasomaxillary complex compared to the vertical displacement of the mandibular ramus and condyle also plays a role [79]. Vertical displacement of the nasomaxillary complex in excess of concurrent vertical displacement of the mandibular ramus can result in backward (clockwise) mandibular rotation resulting in reduced chin projection in profile and greater discrepancy in anteroposterior maxillo-mandibular relationship. Supporting this, a study of French-Canadian children followed longitudinally found that individuals showing increases in anteroposterior maxillo-mandibular skeletal discrepancies with growth also displayed increases in vertical skeletal discrepancies [81].

Additionally, lack of displacement of the mandible, secondary to deficient condylar growth response or deficient corpus growth response to the growth of investing soft tissues results in increased maxillo-mandibular anteroposterior discrepancy.

Q: In terms of craniofacial growth how do discrepancies in transverse skeletal relationships occur?

A: Transverse skeletal discrepancies mainly occur as a result of maxillary transverse skeletal deficiency, but the underlying mechanism is not clear. The degree of maxillary transverse enlargement has been shown to relate to craniofacial pattern when studied longitudinally in untreated subjects [82]. Hyperdivergent individuals were shown to have less maxillary transverse skeletal growth and smaller maxillary intermolar widths compared to hypodivergent individuals.

Muscle weakness and mouth breathing have a statistical association with maxillary transverse deficiency, but the underlying mechanism for this association remains unknown [83–85].

Q: Do we know the *exact* mechanisms by which aberrations in craniofacial growth processes create skeletal abnormalities?

A: No. The exact mechanisms by which aberrations in craniofacial growth processes create skeletal abnormalities remains unknown. Environmental factors are thought to influence the interrelationship of these processes, but this influence is not well understood.

As one example, structural and/or environmental conditions that restrict nasal breathing have long been associated with facial hyperdivergence (skeletal open bite). Enlarged adenoids being a conspicuous etiologic agent for restricted breathing, the term "adenoid facies" was widely used to describe the clinical picture of affected individuals. Extreme facial hyperdivergence, narrow maxillary arch, and lip incompetence are prominent clinical features. The theory of environmental influence proposed for the development of this skeletal pattern has been largely mechanistic: restricted nasal breathing demands mouth breathing, mouth breathing alters the tongue position, mandibular posture, and head posture. Altered postures lead to muscle imbalance, and muscle imbalance influences craniofacial growth, leading to decreased vertical condylar growth, increased sutural growth of the upper face and increased posterior dentoalveolar development with negative (elongating) effects on vertical facial growth [86–90]. Although much study has been applied to this theory, a direct cause-and-effect relationship remains equivocal [91].

More recently, a new theory has been proposed that suggests restricted nasal breathing may be related to abnormal nocturnal secretion of growth hormone (GH) [92]. Children with obstructive sleep apnea (OSA) share similar craniofacial characteristics to those earlier characterized with "adenoid facies" and also show abnormal nocturnal GH secretion. GH is known to have a positive mediating effect on mandibular ramus height during growth [93]. Further, recent information suggests that faulty GH receptors are a genetic marker for reduced ramus height during growth in certain populations [94–96]. Taken together, this information suggests that the mechanism by which restricted nasal breathing affects craniofacial form is due to a more complex sequence of genetic, epigenetic, or environmental events than envisioned previously. Our point is that, even using one example, the *exact* mechanisms by which aberrations in craniofacial growth processes create skeletal abnormalities remain unknown.

Q: Is there a direct relationship between craniofacial abnormalities and breathing problems in children?

A: There is not a direct cause and effect relationship between craniofacial form and breathing problems in children. There is an association between abnormalities in craniofacial form that results in a narrowing of the pharyngeal segment of the airway and pediatric obstructive sleep apnea. However, current research suggests that the primary reason for OSA in children is hypertrophy of soft tissue (adenotonsillar hypertrophy) and/or reduced muscular tone of the pharyngeal airway. In children, a narrow pharyngeal airway predisposes those with adenotonsillar hypertrophy and/or reduced pharyngeal muscle tone to OSA. A summary of risk factors contributing to pediatric airway collapse is shown in Figure 1.28 [97].

Q: What is the orthodontist's role in managing pediatric OSA?

A: Because there is limited scientific information on the treatment of OSA in pediatric patients, the orthodontist's primary role in managing pediatric OSA is screening and appropriate referral. The orthodontist may participate in care as approved by the physician directing the patient's treatment of OSA. Clearly defined treatment goals, focusing on the orthodontic and orthopedic changes, should be articulated to the physician, parents, and patient. Improvement of the OSA should not be conveyed as a certainty. There is currently no evidence-based information that orthodontic treatment provides resolution to OSA or improves obstructed breathing long-term. Outcomes related to improved breathing or OSA resolution by orthodontic

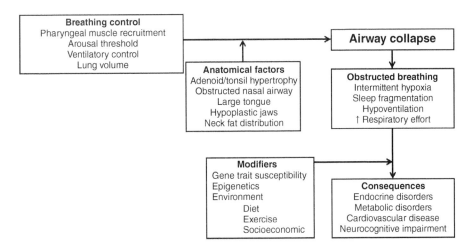

Figure 1.28 Diagram of the pathophysiology of pediatric obstructive sleep apnea and its potential consequences. (*Source*: Adapted from Katz [97]).

treatment cannot be guaranteed. Therefore, success in OSA resolution should not be implied in communication of anticipated outcomes [98].

Q: What is the effect of rapid maxillary expansion (RME) on the airway in children?

A: A recent systematic review analyzed eight clinical studies measuring either dimensional or volume changes in the nasal cavity, nasopharynx, or the oropharynx using 2-D or 3-D radiography, or changes in nasal resistance using acoustic rhinometry to rapid maxillary expansion using a variety of fixed rapid maxillary expanders. The authors found seven of the eight studies to be of poor methodological quality (low or critically low) and concluded that although increases in nasal cavity width and nasal cavity volume were reported, no conclusions can be drawn regarding measurable improvement in nasal breathing. Data for dimensional changes in the nasopharynx or oropharynx in response to RME provided controversial results. The authors concluded there is potential improvement in nasal cavity dimensions in response to RME, but evidence is not sufficient to use RME to improve nasal breathing in the absence of orthodontic indications [99].

Q: Can RME resolve obstructed breathing in children? What is the evidence?

A: At this time there is not sufficient evidence that RME can resolve obstructed breathing in children. RME has been shown to improve nasal cavity dimensions and decrease nasal resistance. Some reports show short-term improvement in the apnea-hypopnea index (AHI) for those diagnosed with OSA by polysomnography, others do not [66]. A recent meta-analysis of these studies suggests that publication bias, small sample sizes, and inconsistent methodologies limit the generalizability of their findings. Randomized controlled trials with large sample sizes are needed [100]. Some reports combining RME and adenotonsillectomy suggest favorable improvement of OSA in some patients [101].

Q: Is there a relationship between masticatory function and vertical facial dimensions?

A: Yes, variation in vertical facial dimensions is closely associated with masticatory performance. Studies have documented that an increase in the relative height of the anterior lower facial skeleton is predictably associated with a decrease in bite force magnitude, smaller cross-sectional area of the masticatory adductors (i.e. masseter, medial pterygoid and tempo-

ralis), and reduced masticatory muscle activity. The precise influence of masticatory performance on facial form is not well understood, and there is debate regarding the causal nature of this relationship [102]. In a manner similar to habitual mouth breathing, reduced muscle function may alter the posture of the mandible and thus affect the pattern of mandibular rotation during development resulting in a long-face phenotype [103].

Q: What is meant by *growth rotation* of the jaws?

A: Viewed in the sagittal plane, the maxilla and mandible undergo patterns of rotation during facial growth and development. Björk [104, 105] identified three components of mandibular rotation and remodeling (matrix, intramatrix and total rotation, Figure 1.29 illustrates an example) that has been more recently redefined [71].

- Apparent rotation ("matrix" rotation) is a measure of angular changes of the mandibular inferior

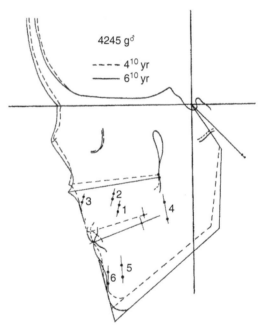

Figure 1.29 Overall superimposition of cephalometric tracings depicting two years of growth in a young male. Black dots indicate location of implant markers. Numbers 1, 2, and 3 indicate maxillary implant markers. Numbers 4, 5, and 6 indicate mandibular implant markers. Black lines bisecting dot pairs indicate the direction of implant marker displacement during growth. Note the equivalence in magnitude and direction of maxilla implant displacement indicating nominal true rotation. In contrast, the pattern of changes in magnitude and direction of the mandibular implants indicates true mandibular anterior rotation. The pattern of inferior mandibular border change suggests nominal apparent mandibular rotation due to angular remodeling. (*Source*: Reproduced from Björk [104], with permission from Taylor & Francis Ltd.)

border relative to the anterior cranial base (usually measured as changes in SN-MP in degrees). It is the absolute change in mandibular plane angle during growth.

- Angular remodeling ("intramatrix" rotation) is a measure of change (in degrees) of the mandibular plane relative to the mandibular reference line representing the mandibular corpus (determined by mandibular structures stable during growth). It reflects remodeling along the mandibular lower border during growth.

- True rotation ("total" rotation, "internal" rotation) is a measure of change (in degrees) of the mandibular reference line (mandibular corpus) relative to cranial base reference line. True rotation (in degrees) is the sum of the change (in degrees) of apparent rotation and the change in angular remodeling (in degrees) during growth. (e.g. true rotation (deg) = Δ apparent rotation (deg) + Δ angular remodeling (deg)). Apparent rotation is often less than true rotation due to the angular remodeling that changes the shape of the mandibular inferior border and minimizes SN-MP change during growth.

Q: How does growth rotation of the jaws influence the vertical dimension of the face?

A: Björk was the first to discover true growth rotation, defined as rotation of the maxillary or mandibular corpus relative to the cranial base, measured from stable references (implanted bone markers) in the sagittal view [105–107]. His studies demonstrated a relationship between true mandibular growth rotation and condylar growth:

- Greater true forward mandibular growth rotation is associated with vertical condylar growth of larger magnitude directed more anteriorly.

- Greater backward mandibular growth rotation is associated with vertical condylar growth of smaller magnitude directed more posteriorly.

- True forward mandibular rotation during growth is also associated with decreases in the gonial angle [108–111], decreases in mandibular plane angle [112], and increases in posterior face height [106]. True forward rotation results in adaptive modeling of the mandible, including increased posterior ramus deposition, increased posterior lower border resorption, and increased anterior lower border deposition [113, 114].

- Extremes of true forward or backward mandibular rotation are associated with skeletal deep bite and skeletal open bite respectively [78].

Q: What is the occurrence of forward or backward growth rotation of the jaws?

A: Measurement of selected populations longitudinally have suggested that *true mandibular growth rotation is, by and large, forward for most* individuals [115–117]. High-angle (increased SN-MP angle) subjects show less forward true rotation (degrees per year) and less condylar growth magnitude (mm per year) compared with low-angle (decreased SN-MP angle) subjects. In addition, these studies support the findings of Björk [104–107], namely that apparent forward rotation (decreasing SN-MP) during growth occurs even for hyperdivergent subjects. The take-home message is that the vast majority of individuals with hyperdivergent skeletal patterns experience net forward jaw rotation during growth.

Q: Is rotation of the jaws uniform during craniofacial growth?

A: No. In a manner similar to the velocity of condylar growth, individuals show variation in amount, duration, and direction of growth rotation [110, 112, 115]. This means that some hyperdivergent individuals that experience a net forward rotation may experience backward rotation during some period of growth.

Q: Are there diagnostic indices that foretell an individual's maxillary or mandibular future growth rotation?

A: No. Björk identified seven specific structural features that might develop as a result of remodeling during a particular type of growth rotation. His suggestions for predicting condylar rotation have, however, not been widely used by the specialty because (i) some of the indicators cannot be easily seen on the average cephalogram, (ii) the use of the indicators is very time-consuming for the clinician, and (iii) there has been no scientific validation of the suggested indicators because of difficulties encountered in study design [118–120]. It has been suggested the Y-axis angle, the acute cephalometric angle formed at the intersection of the Frankfort Horizontal line and the Sella-Gnathion line can be used as a guide to a patient's downward and forward mandibular translation during growth [121]. Numerous studies suggest the Y-axis covaries with vertical skeletal pattern, particularly SN-MP. However, the change in Y-axis with growth does not consistently differ between subjects with widely differing vertical skeletal pattern [122–125]. This suggests it can be used as a guide for the anticipated vector of downward and forward mandibular translation, but, by and large, may not predict mandibular rotation.

Q: Does growth rotation affect dentoalveolar development?

A: Yes. Greater mandibular forward tipping of incisors and molars, forward shift of the dental arch in relation to jaw base, and relatively greater mandibular molar than incisor eruption have been related to greater true forward rotation [106, 126].

Q: Does dentoalveolar development and tooth eruption *cause,* or only adapt to, skeletal problems in the vertical dimension?

A: Dentoalveolar development and tooth eruption *adapt* to skeletal problems in the vertical dimension. Issacson [127] was the first to report on dentoalveolar development in three groups of subjects—those with short anterior face height (hypodivergent), those with average anterior face height, and those with excessive anterior face height (hyperdivergent). Maxillary posterior alveolar development was found to decrease with decreasing SN-MP angle, with a difference of 5.1 mm of dentoalveolar development between hypodivergent and hyperdivergent individuals. This finding has subsequently been confirmed by others [128, 129]. Björk [106] suggested dentoalveolar development was coupled to vertical facial growth, a suggestion later verified in a longitudinal female sample. In this study, eruption of mandibular teeth followed vertical growth displacement of the mandible. Also, mandibular molar eruption showed greater plasticity than vertical mandibular growth, indicating that molar eruption *adapts* to vertical mandibular growth displacement [130].

Q: What causes abnormalities in *vertical* dentoalveolar development?

A: Vertical dentoalveolar development abnormalities manifest as supra-eruption or infra-eruption of teeth. Since vertical dentoalveolar development/tooth eruption are controlled by forces of eruption (exact mechanism unknown) and forces opposing eruption (e.g. functional/parafunctional occlusal loading), any disturbance of these forces may create abnormalities. Such disturbances may include:

- Diminished masticatory performance/diminished loading: this has been shown to be associated with increased posterior alveolar development, increased posterior tooth eruption, severe hyperdivergence, skeletal open bite, and may influence tooth eruption and jaw growth [102].
- Altered spatial relationship of the jaws: can result in teeth left unopposed and absence of forces opposing eruption. For example, in a large Class II discrepancy patient (mandibular hypoplasia, large ANB angle), the mandibular incisors are unopposed by the maxillary incisors. The mandibular incisors can supra-erupt creating an exaggerated curve of Spee.
- Tongue interposition, digit sucking, and lip biting habits: can increase the duration/magnitude of forces opposing tooth eruption and result in anterior or posterior open bites.
- Ankylosis or tooth loss: results in elimination of forces opposing eruption and supra-eruption of teeth in the opposing arch.

Q: Is facial growth coordinated with statural growth?

A: Yes. By and large, the temporal sequence of maturation is synchronized throughout the body. General body (somatic) growth, measured by change in stature with time (growth velocity), is an indicator of velocity changes in craniofacial dimensions during growth [131, 132]. This is in contrast to the neurocranium which is more closely coordinated with neural growth.

Q: Do facial and statural growth proceed with constant velocity during development?

A: No. A typical plot of statural growth velocity (Figure 1.30) shows that change is not uniform. One-half of adult stature is attained within the first two years of life during a rapid deceleration of growth velocity. After two years, a much slower deceleration of growth velocity occurs until the onset of puberty. The inflection point where deceleration of growth velocity changes to acceleration is the beginning of pubertal growth acceleration, often termed the "pubertal growth spurt." This pubertal growth acceleration increases growth velocity to a maximum, termed the peak height velocity (PHV), followed by a rapid deceleration in growth velocity [131, 133].

Q: What is the duration of pubertal growth acceleration?

A: Approximately two to two and a half years between onset and PHV [131].

Q: Does pubertal growth acceleration occur at the same age for males and females?

A: No. On average, females reach PHV at age of 11.5–12 years and males reach PHV at age of 14 years. Pubertal growth acceleration is slightly longer in males compared to females [131, 133, 134].

Q: Is peak *facial* growth velocity coordinated with PHV?

A: Yes. On average, females reach peak facial growth velocity at 10.9–12.3 years and males reach peak facial growth velocity at 14.1–14.3 years, supporting the close association between change in stature and the growth of the face [87, 135–137].

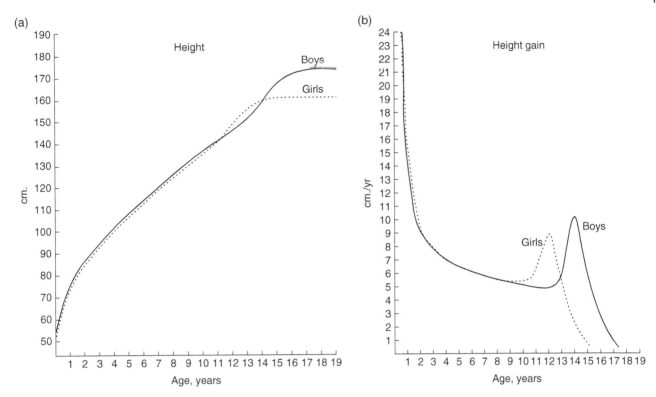

Figure 1.30 (a) Plot of change in stature with age. (b) Plot of change in growth velocity with age. (*Source*: Reproduced from Tanner et al. [133], with permission from BMJ Publishing Group Ltd.)

Q: How much growth occurs during pubertal growth acceleration?

A: On average, males add 20 cm in stature and females add 16 cm in stature. On average, the chin moves downward and forward, away from the cranial base (measured Sella to Gnathion), 1.8–2.0 cm in males and 1.1–1.2 cm in females [138].

Q: Are males and females similar in the downward and forward facial growth pattern during pubertal growth acceleration?

A: Possibly not. A recent longitudinal study of 111 untreated French-Canadian females demonstrated that during the period of pubertal growth acceleration, beginning at approximately 11.5 years of age, measures of vertical skeletal change showed acceleration, but measures of horizontal skeletal change did not. Moreover, in this sample, measures of horizontal skeletal change decelerated during adolescence. For this sample, female pubertal growth acceleration did not provide anteroposterior improvement in chin projection [139].

Q: Is the pattern and rate of forward and downward growth during the pubertal growth acceleration the same as found prior to puberty?

A: No. Studies have shown that horizontal and vertical translation of the chin varies between prepubertal and pubertal growth periods [81, 140–144]. Growth-driven *anterior* movement of the chin has a greater velocity during childhood compared to the period of adolescence. In contrast, growth-driven *inferior* movement of the chin has less velocity during childhood compared to the period of adolescence. These findings suggest a tendency for face height to increase more than facial depth during adolescence compared to childhood [144–146].

Q: Is there a measurable indicator of pubertal growth acceleration and PHV?

A: There is no one best indicator of pubertal growth acceleration and PHV. Maturation of hand-wrist and cervical spine bones have been studied as potential predictors of PHV, but give unreliable estimates of PHV timing and peak facial growth velocity [135, 147–152]. Skeletal development of hand and wrist bones has been shown to be useful in estimating whether the pubertal growth acceleration has already occurred [135], but the method of assessing a patient's skeletal development by hand/wrist radiography against a radiographic atlas of normal hand-wrist skeletal development has low sensitivity in predicting whether the pubertal growth acceleration is impending or ongoing [131, 147]. That being said, measurement of growth acceleration itself, measured as *change in stature with time, may be considered the least invasive and most reliable predictor of pubertal growth acceleration and PHV* [135, 153].

Q: Can other periods of growth acceleration occur before puberty?

A: Yes. Statural growth acceleration has been reported to occur in the age range 6.5–8.5 years for some individuals (termed the mid-growth spurt) [154, 155]. Reports on the magnitude of change in statural growth velocity vary in characterization from "less deceleration" to mild acceleration, and of considerably lower magnitude, compared to pubertal growth acceleration [154–157]. Mid-growth spurts in facial growth velocity have also been shown in some individuals [135, 141, 158].

Q: Does the timing of puberty have an effect on final statural height?

A: Possibly. A study of longitudinal records in various populations suggests early pubertal onset exerts a negative effect on overall height and a late pubertal onset exerts a positive effect on final height [159, 160].

Q: What is the relationship of menarche to PHV in girls?

A: The onset of menarche is highly correlated with PHV in girls, occurring nine and twelve months after PHV. With estimates of pubertal deceleration being ~ two years, the *onset of menarche foretells approximately twelve to fifteen months of pubertal growth remaining* [161, 162].

Q: Do all patients undergo an adolescent growth spurt?

A: No. For example, Figure 1.31 illustrates the statural height of a daughter of one of our colleagues, made over a thirteen-year period. She exhibited continual, linear, growth and not an adolescent growth spurt.

Q: Why is the presence (or absence) of an adolescent growth spurt important for timing orthopedic treatment?

A: Because most patients are compliant for only limited amount of time – so, it is important to utilize that compliance during the time of most growth (i.e. the growth spurt).

Development of the Primary Dentition, Transitional Dentition, and Occlusion. Developmental Anomalies, Crowding, and Habits

Q: What is meant by tooth eruption? What is meant by tooth emergence?

A: Tooth eruption is a continuous process, commencing with the developing tooth translocating from its formative position in the jaw to a functional position in the oral cavity.

   Tooth emergence is a point in time during tooth eruption when the enamel of the tooth crown pierces the gingiva and enters the oral cavity [163].

Q: What is the age range for emergence of all twenty primary teeth?

A: The age range for emergence of all twenty primary teeth begins, on average, with the emergence of the mandibular primary central incisors at six months and ends, on average, with the maxillary primary second molars at approximately thirty months [164]. The emergence estimates are shown in Table 1.6.

Q: What is the timing and sequence for the emergence and exfoliation of the primary teeth?

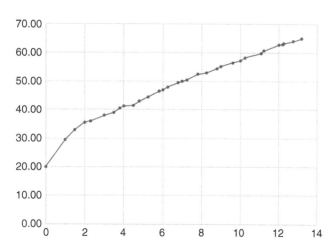

Figure 1.31 A growth chart recording statural height measurements of a girl made from birth to age thirteen years. Note a continual, linear, pattern of growth and an absence of an adolescent growth spurt.

A:

Table 1.6   The timing of eruption and exfoliation of the primary Dentition[a].

	Eruption		Exfoliation	
	Maxillary	Mandibular	Maxillary	Mandibular
Central incisors	8–12 mo	6–10 mo	6–7 yr	6–7 yr
Lateral incisors	9–13 mo	10–16 mos	7–8 yr	7–8 yr
Canines	16–22 mo	17–23 mo	10–12 yr	9–12 yr
First molars	13–19 mo	14–18 mo	9–11 yr	9–11 yr
Second molars	25–33 mo	23–31 mo	10–12 yr	10–12 yr

[a] ADA 2012 Retrieved and adapted from https://www.mouthhealthy.org/en/az-topics/e/eruption-charts

Q: Is emergence of the first primary tooth predictive of the emergence of the first permanent tooth?

A: No. Two studies on Swedish children showed only a weak correlation ($r = 0.2$–0.4) between the timing of the emergence of primary teeth and the subsequent emergence of permanent teeth [165, 166].

Q: Is the timing of primary and permanent tooth eruption subject to secular trends?

A: Yes. Studies have suggested secular trends across different ethnic and/or racial populations and within the same population over time [167–171]. For example, tooth emergence is advanced in African-American children compared to Chinese and Japanese children, and advanced in American Indian children compared to American Caucasian and African-American children. Studies on children in Finland, Germany, Japan, and China suggest tooth emergence is advanced in current populations compared to older population samples within the same countries. When comparing the median age of tooth emergence for each permanent tooth (except third molars) across samples from nine countries, the age of gingival emergence differed between a minimum of 0.5 years (maxillary second molars) and a maximum of 1.5 years (maxillary premolars) [171].

Q: What is primate space? What is primary tooth spacing? What is the importance of both?

A: Primate space is a diastema between primary lateral incisor and primary canine in the maxillary arch, and between primary canines and primary first molars in the mandibular arch. Studied across many populations, primate space is more prevalent in the maxillary arch compared to the mandibular arch. Mandibular primate space may contribute to early mesial shift of the mandibular permanent first molar during the transitional dentition [172, 173].

Primary tooth spacing (i.e. intra-arch spacing between primary teeth) includes primate spaces and spacing between the primary incisors. Primary tooth spacing is thought to compensate for the discrepancy between the sizes of deciduous and permanent teeth. Primary teeth that do not display interdental spacing may be predisposed to crowding in the transition from primary to permanent teeth [172]. Studied across many populations, primary tooth spacing is more prevalent in males, more prevalent in the maxillary arch, and has range of prevalence between 68 and 98% depending on the population studied [174, 175].

Q: Is spacing in the primary dentition a useful indicator of the degree of permanent tooth crowding during development?

A: No. There is not a predictable relationship between primary tooth size, primary spacing, and permanent tooth crowding during development. Measurements of tooth-size arch length discrepancy (TSALD) can be performed with much greater accuracy in the mixed dentition [176].

Q: Is primary tooth mesiodistal dimension a useful predictor of permanent tooth mesiodistal dimension?

A: No. The correlation between size of primary teeth and size of permanent successors is approximately $r = 0.5$, meaning primary tooth size would be expected to predict permanent tooth successor in 25 of 100 individuals [177–179].

Q: What are the vertical *occlusal* characteristics of the full primary dentition?

A: The full primary dentition has a flat to mild mandibular curve of Spee and maxillary compensating curve ranging in depth from 0 to 1 mm [180, 181].

Q: What are the features of a normal primary dentition?

A: The features of a normal primary dentition include [45]:
- Spacing of the maxillary and mandibular anterior teeth.
- Upright vertical inclination of the maxillary and mandibular anterior teeth.
- Presence of primate spaces.
- Minimal overbite and overjet.
- Straight terminal plane occlusal relationship of the primary second molars.
- Class I canine relationship.

Q: How are the stages of permanent tooth eruption defined?

A: There are three major stages of permanent tooth eruption. The *pre-eruptive stage*, during which small positional changes are seen in the developing tooth crown, the *active eruption stage*, commencing when crown formation is complete within the jaw and concluding after the tooth is in function and the root formation is complete; and the *passive eruption stage*, occurring mainly during postadolescent maturation of the jaws, characterized by apical migration of the dentogingival attachment toward and beyond the cementoenamel junction.

The *active eruption stage*, during which the developing tooth is translocated into the oral cavity, is further subdivided into four distinct stages: The *intraosseous stage*, including the developing tooth below the alveolar crest and subsequent elimination of the alveolar crest to create an eruption pathway, the *supra-osseous stage*, with the simultaneous lengthening of the tooth root and the translocation of the developing tooth through the gingival margin; the *supra-gingival stage,* with the clinical crown emerging through gingival tissue prior to antagonist tooth contact; and the *functional stage*, commencing with antagonist tooth contact and finishing with completion of root formation [182, 183].

Q: What is the rate of tooth eruption in the intraosseous and supra-osseous stages?

A: The rate of tooth eruption differs when comparing the intraosseous stage and the supra-osseous stage. Estimates for the rate of intraosseous tooth eruption range from 0.03 to 0.3 mm/month. Estimates for the rate of supra-osseous tooth eruption range from 0.75 to 2.25 mm/month [184].

Q: At what point does a permanent tooth emerge into the oral cavity?

A: Permanent tooth emergence is closely associated with maturation of the permanent tooth root [153, 154]. In a study of 874 individuals, Grøn found 77–100% of maxillary incisors, and mandibular teeth (incisor to second molar) displayed tooth emergence when root length had reached between ½ and ¾ final root length. Some mandibular canines (16%) and mandibular second molars (24%) tended to emerge later, when their roots were between ¾ and 100% of final root length [154]. A small percentage of mandibular incisors (3.5%) and first molars (6%) tended to emerge earlier, when their roots were between ¼ and ½ root length.

Q: Is tooth movement during eruption a continuous process?

A: No. There are periods of measurable movement and periods of little or no detectable movement. Nearly, all tooth eruption occurs between 8 pm and midnight, and often some intrusion occurs during the early morning [185, 186].

Q: How does permanent tooth root maturation help determine delayed tooth emergence?

A: If a tooth has developed more than ¾ root length and has not yet emerged, you should consider the tooth having delayed emergence [163, 187]. For canines and premolars, permanent tooth root maturation is closely associated with root resorption of the primary predecessor. Loss of the primary predecessor is associated with eruption of the permanent successor that has at least ½ final root length. Therefore, loss of a primary predecessor prior to the permanent successor reaching ½ final root length is considered *premature exfoliation*, and retention of a primary predecessor after the permanent successor root is complete is considered *delayed exfoliation* [188]. The latter can predispose permanent teeth to delayed emergence.

Q: What can be used to assess root length development of permanent teeth?

A: Panoramic or periapical radiographs can be compared to diagrams depicting stages of tooth development as shown in Figure 1.32.

Q: What is the spatial relationship of the developing permanent teeth to their primary precursors?

A: The permanent incisors and canines develop *lingually* to the deciduous teeth and erupt toward the labial. Premolars develop between the roots of the deciduous molars and normally erupt in a vertical path [182].

Q: What is the sequence of emergence of the permanent teeth?

A: Studies of large populations find the most frequently occurring (modal) sequence of permanent tooth

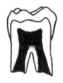 R 1/2: Root length is ≥ crown height.
The walls of the root canal approximate a triangle.
The apex of the root canal ends in a funnel shape.

 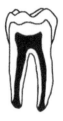 R 3/4: The walls of the root canal are parallel.
The apical end of the root canal is open with the
walls diverging at the apex.

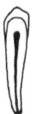 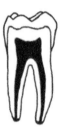 RC: Root length is complete.
The walls of the root canal are parallel at the apex.

Figure 1.32 Description of root development stages: one-half root formation (R 1/2), three-fourths root formation (R 3/4), and complete root formation (R C). *Source*: Adapted from AlQahtani et al. [189] and Demirjian A, et al. [190].

emergence in the maxilla is first molar, central incisor, lateral incisor, first premolar, canine, second premolar, and second molar (displayed as 6-1-2-4-[3-5]-7 using Palmer's tooth numbering system [191], with canine [3] and second premolar [5] often emerging simultaneously or in reverse order). The modal sequence in the mandible is first molar, central incisor, lateral incisor, canine, first premolar, second premolar, and second molar (displayed in Palmer tooth numbers as 6-1-2-3-4-[5-7], with second premolar [5] and second molar [7] often emerging simultaneously or in reverse order).

Other maxillary and mandibular eruption sequences include maintaining the initial emergence order first molar, central incisor, lateral incisor (6-1-2), but having other order combinations of canine, first premolar, second premolar, and second molar. These make up approximately 35% of the emergence order variation seen [192, 193]. Some populations studied have shown only 25% of children share one common eruption sequence [194, 195]. One study, following more than 3200 untreated Flemish children longitudinally, found only 19% shared one common eruption sequence [196]. Approximately, 45% of these children displayed emergence of mandibular second molars prior to mandibular second premolars.

At the University of Iowa, we have the benefit of a longitudinal growth study of subjects with normal occlusion. Figures 1.33–1.36 illustrate a time-lapse view of permanent tooth eruption from age five to thirteen for one individual in the study.

Q: Looking at Figure 1.35, what is/was the modal sequence of eruption for the maxillary and mandibular teeth?

A: The sequence of maxillary tooth eruption is central incisor, first molar, lateral incisor, canine, first premolar, second molar, second premolar (1-6-2-3-4-7-5). The right and left sides differ slightly in the timing of central incisor and first molar emergence. The sequence of mandibular tooth eruption is central incisor, first molar, lateral incisor, canine, first premolar, second molar, second premolar (1-6-2-3-4-7-5). Again, the right and left sides differ slightly in the timing of central incisor and first molar emergence.

Q: Looking at the position of the maxillary permanent lateral incisor roots between ages eight and twelve years, what do you note?

A: At age eight years, the roots appear to be positioned toward the midline (mesial) due to the influence of the permanent canine crowns developing in proximity to the lateral incisor roots. By age twelve years, the lateral incisor roots have uprighted toward the lateral (distal) as the permanent canines erupt and emerge through gingival tissue.

Q: Compare the mandibular primary first and second molars in Figure 1.33a and 1.34b. What do you note?

A: In Figure 1.33a, both mandibular primary first and second molars lie on the occlusal plane. In Figure 1.34b, the mandibular primary first molars are below the occlusal plane (infraocclusion).

Q: How is infraocclusion classified?

A: Infraocclusion is mild if the tooth occlusal surface is less than 2 mm below that of the adjacent teeth, moderate if the tooth occlusal surface is *at* the contact point of the adjacent tooth (teeth), and severe if the tooth occlusal surface is *below* the contact point of the adjacent tooth (teeth) [197]. The infraocclusion noted in Figure 1.34b would be classified as mild.

Q: What percentage of six-year-old children have all four permanent first molars erupted?

A: All molars erupted (20–30%), no permanent first molar eruption (20–30%) [198].

Q: Are there gender differences in the timing of permanent tooth eruption?

A: Yes. With the exception of third molars, permanent tooth eruption on average occurs five months earlier in females compared to males [199]. Interestingly, the gender variation in permanent tooth eruption timing is small compared to the gender variation in skeletal development [200].

Q: Is the timing of first permanent molar emergence affected by body mass index (BMI)?

A: Yes. Overweight (BMI-for-age value between 85th and –95th percentile) or obese (BMI > 95th percentile) individuals show earlier emergence of permanent first molars by six to twelve months compared to individuals with lower BMI [198, 201]. The emergence of later developing permanent teeth is similarly accelerated [202].

Q: Is the timing of first permanent molar emergence affected by the congenital absence of other permanent teeth?

A: No. Although there is an association between hypodontia and delayed development of mandibular premolars and permanent second molars, the timing of mandibular first permanent molar emergence is not affected by congenital absence of other permanent teeth [203].

Q: What is the timing of the sequence of emergence of the permanent teeth? At what age, on average, do permanent teeth emerge through gingival tissue?

A: A graph depicting the age variation in the sequence of eruption of the permanent teeth is shown in Figure 1.37. The left and right tails of the curve for each tooth show the earliest and latest ages when emergence is expected [182]. The peak of the curve for each tooth shows the average age of tooth emergence. Shown in this way, it is easy to visualize why variation in timing and sequence is not considered abnormal [193].

Q: What is meant by "straight terminal plane," "distal step," and "mesial step" of the primary second molars?

A: Straight (flush) terminal plane (Figure 1.38a), distal step (Figure 1.38b), and mesial step (Figure 1.38c) are interocclusal classifications defined by the relationship of lines drawn tangent to the distal surfaces of the maxillary and mandibular primary second molars and intersect perpendicular to the occlusal plane. In a straight (flush) terminal plane relationship, these lines coincide. In a distal step relationship, the mandibular line intersects the occlusal plane distal (posterior) to the maxillary line. In a mesial step relationship, the mandibular line intersects the occlusal plane mesial (anterior) to the maxillary line [172, 204].

Q: What is an approximate distribution of interocclusal relationships (straight terminal plane, distal step, mesial step) of the primary second molars in the primary dentition?

A: Based on a number of studies, 76–84% straight terminal plane, 10–14% distal step, 6–14% mesial step [172, 204, 205].

Q: What changes occur in these primary second molar interocclusal relationships between the primary and mixed dentition stages? What changes occur between the mixed dentition and permanent dentition stages?

A: In a study of 170 untreated children followed for five years, 79% of straight terminal planes transitioned to Class I permanent molar relationships, while 21% transitioned to Class II permanent molar relationships (Figure 1.39). Distal steps transitioned equally into 50% Class I and 50% Class II permanent molar relationships. Mesial steps transitioned to 87% Class I permanent molar and 13% Class III permanent molar relationships [206].

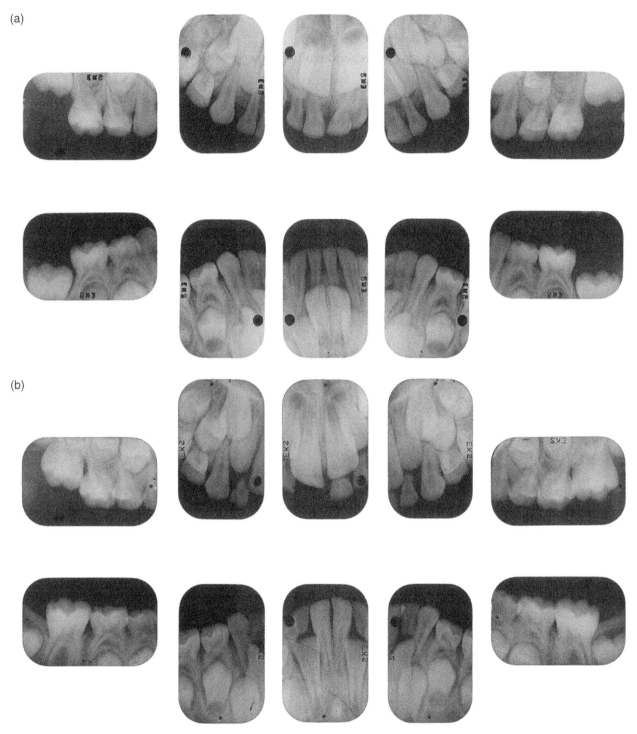

Figure 1.33 Longitudinal complete mouth series radiographs for subject F8 from the Iowa Facial Growth Study of developing normal occlusions. (a) Age five years, zero months. Complete primary dentition. Permanent central incisors just beginning root formation. Primary tooth roots not yet resorbing. (b) Age six years, six months. Emergence of mandibular permanent first molars and central incisors and maxillary right permanent central incisor. Primary lateral incisors all show resorbing roots. Mandibular permanent first molars have reached the occlusal plane. Maxillary permanent first molars are just emerging.

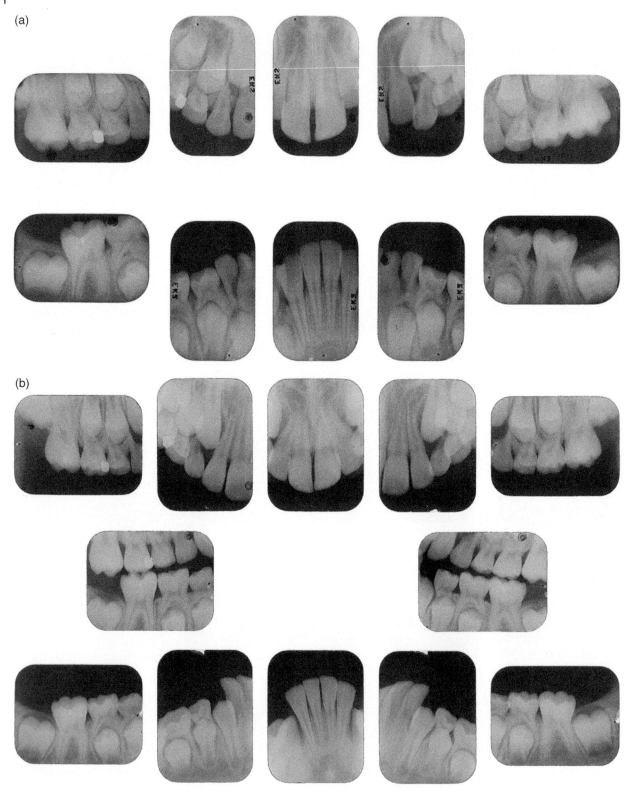

Figure 1.34 Longitudinal complete mouth series radiographs for a subject F8 from the Iowa Facial Growth Study of developing normal occlusions (continued). (a) Age seven years, six months. Maxillary permanent central incisors have erupted with a 2 mm diastema. Maxillary permanent first molars have reached the occlusal plane. Maxillary permanent lateral incisors are approaching the occlusal plane. Primary first molars show signs of apical root resorption. Mandibular primary canines show root resorption from mandibular permanent lateral incisor eruption. (b) Age eight years, six months. Maxillary permanent lateral incisor roots appear mesially inclined in response to maxillary permanent canine eruption. Maxillary primary canines and first molars show significant apical root resorption. Mandibular permanent canines are emerging. Mandibular second molars are beginning root formation and rising toward the alveolar crest.

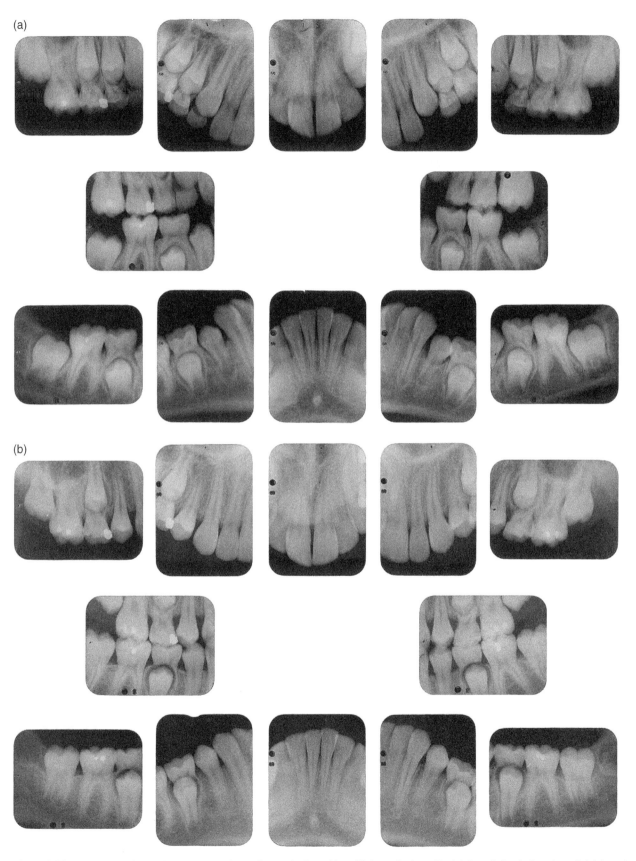

Figure 1.35 Longitudinal complete mouth series radiographs for subject F8 from the Iowa Facial Growth Study (continued). (a) Age nine years, six months. Maxillary permanent canines appear to be advancing toward emergence ahead of maxillary first premolars (alternate eruption sequence). Mandibular first premolars are emerging. Apical root resorption of primary second molars is evident. The permanent second molars are resorbing the alveolar crest. (b) Age eleven years, zero months. Maxillary permanent canines have emerged ahead of maxillary first premolars. The maxillary central diastema is reduced. Root resorption of primary second molars continues. Mandibular permanent second molars have emerged ahead of mandibular second premolars and are nearing the occlusal plane.

(a)

(b)

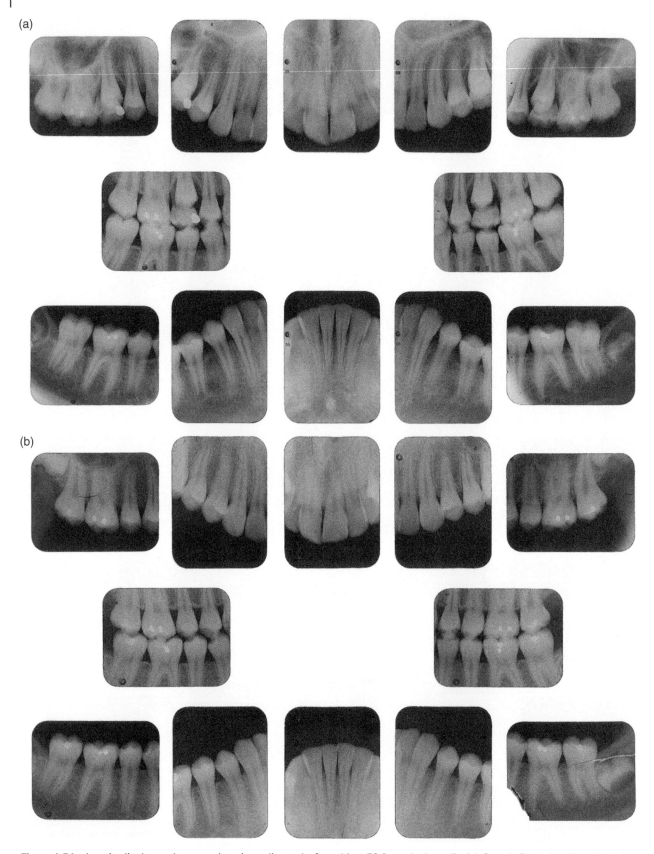

Figure 1.36 Longitudinal complete mouth series radiographs for subject F8 from the Iowa Facial Growth Study (continued). (a) Age twelve years, zero months. Maxillary permanent second molars have emerged ahead of maxillary second premolars and have reached the occlusal plane along with mandibular second premolars. Maxillary primary second molar exfoliation is imminent. (b) Age thirteen years, zero months. All permanent teeth, except third molars, have reached the occlusal plane.

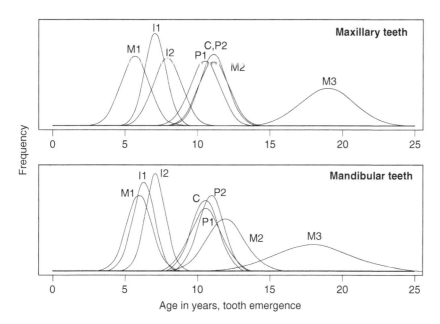

Figure 1.37   Density curves displaying the variation in age of emergence of permanent teeth. Tooth emergence is defined as the point in time when the tooth crown emerges through gingival tissue. (*Source*: Adapted from Liversidge [182]).

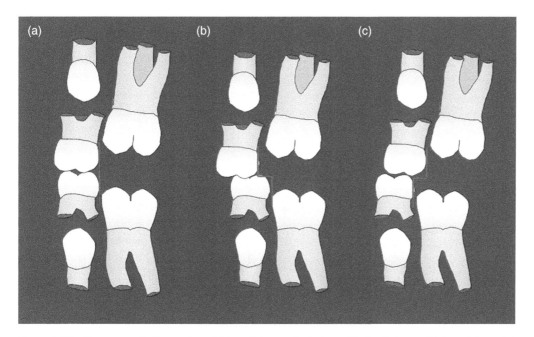

Figure 1.38   Diagrammatic illustration of (a) straight terminal plane, (b) distal step, and (c) mesial step interocclusal relationships.

Transitions from straight terminal plane or distal step relationships to Class I permanent first molar relationships in the early mixed dentition are thought to occur by simultaneous closure of the mandibular primate space and mesial movement of the mandibular permanent first molars termed *early mesial shift* [173].

In a study of 80 untreated individuals followed longitudinally from the early mixed dentition to the permanent dentition, 94% of early mixed dentition Class I molar relationships were stable in transition to the permanent dentition, with 6% becoming Class III molar; 60% of early mixed dentition Class II molar relationships were stable in transition to the permanent dentition, with 40% becoming Class I molar [207].

Transitions from Class II molar relationships in the early mixed dentition to Class I molar relationships in the permanent dentition are thought to occur by late mesial movement of the mandibular permanent first molar into mandibular leeway space. This is termed *late mesial shift* [173]. The study by Barros et al. [207] suggests that in the absence of early mesial shift, permanent first molars maintained in *mild* Class II relationships during their emergence to a functional relationship can transition to Class I molar relationships by late mesial shift (Figure 1.39).

Q: What is the Angle Classification of malocclusion? What is the Iowa Classification of malocclusion?

A: Edward H. Angle [208] defined malocclusion as any deviation from normal intra-arch tooth alignment and normal inter-arch occlusal relationships. He classified malocclusion into distinct groups, I, II, and III, based on the mesiodistal occlusal relationship between the maxillary first permanent molar and the mandibular first permanent molar.

Angle Class I molar relationship (normal occlusion) is defined by the mesiobuccal cusp tip of the maxillary first permanent molar in mesiodistal alignment with the buccal groove of the mandibular first permanent molar, measured with the teeth in occlusion.

Angle Class II molar relationship (distal occlusion) occurs when the buccal groove of the mandibular first permanent molar is distal to the mesiobuccal cusp tip of the maxillary first permanent molar by greater than one-half cusp width, measured with the teeth in occlusion.

Angle Class III molar relationship (mesial occlusion) occurs when the buccal groove of the mandibular first permanent molar is mesial to the mesiobuccal cusp tip of the maxillary first permanent molar by greater than one-half cusp width, measured with the teeth in occlusion.

Angle Class II has two divisions: Division 1 (protruded maxillary incisors) and Division 2 (retruded maxillary incisors). Angle Class II and Class III molar relationships that occur unilaterally are identified as subdivisions of the Angle Classification (e.g. Class II division 1 subdivision right for a unilateral Class II molar relationship on the patient's right, Class III subdivision left for a unilateral Class III molar relationship on the patient's left).

The Angle Classification system suffers from several weaknesses.

- It constrains the diagnosis of inter-arch occlusal relationships into discreet categories, but the range of inter-arch occlusal relationships is a continuum.
- It does not describe the magnitude of the anteroposterior discrepancy in inter-arch occlusal relationships.
- It does not classify inter-arch canine occlusal relationships.
- It cannot classify malocclusions that are Class II on one side and Class III on the other.

The Iowa Classification system is a modification of the Angle Classification system [209]. It measures, in millimeters, the mesiodistal discrepancy of the Angle first molar relationships and the mesiodistal discrepancy of the inter-arch canine occlusal relationships bilaterally with the teeth in occlusion. Noting the four measurements from right side to left side, the Angle molar relationship and canine relationship are

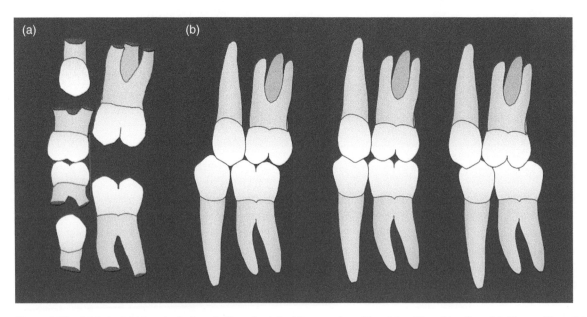

Figure 1.39 (a) A straight terminal plane in the mixed dentition can transition into either (b) a Class I (left), or a Class II (center, right) relationship in the permanent dentition.

displayed in sequence. For example, II(5) II(5) II(2) I describes the patient having an Angle Class II molar relationship on the right by 5 mm, a Class II canine relationship on the right by 5 mm, a Class II canine relationship on the left by 2 mm, and an Angle Class I molar relationship on the left. This approach permits ready communication and visualization of the patient's anteroposterior interocclusal relationships.

Q: What is the distribution of Angle Class I, Class II, and Class III molar relationships in the mixed dentition across different geographic locations?

A: In a systematic review of 53 studies involving >77,000 individuals worldwide, the global distribution of Angle molar relationship in the mixed dentition was shown to be significantly different by region (see Table 1.7) [210].

Table 1.7 Distribution (%) of mixed dentition molar interocclusal relationships by region[a].

Angle molar classification	Americas	Africa	Asia	Europe
Class I	70	90	72.8	64
Class II	27	7.5	21.4	32
Class III	3	2.5	5.8	4

[a] Adapted from Alhammadi et al. [210].

Q: What factors, other than the presence of a mesial step, distal step, or straight primary second molar terminal plane, determine the final permanent first molar anteroposterior relationship?

A: Maxillary anterior and vertical growth magnitude, mandibular anterior and vertical growth magnitude, molar eruption magnitude, mesiodistal widths of the permanent premolars and canines, and magnitude of tooth drift.

Q: What happens to the mandibular primary intercanine width during permanent incisor eruption? Why is this important?

A: As the permanent lateral incisors erupt, the *primary canines can move laterally and the intercanine width increase* (Figure 1.40) [211]. This is important because the primary canine lateral movement creates space for the erupting incisors.

Q: What happens to mandibular and maxillary *arch length* as permanent canines, first premolars, and second premolars erupt?

A: There is a *reduction in arch length* [211].

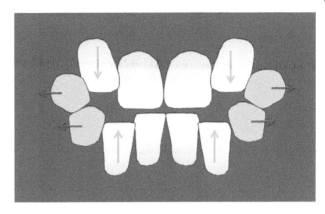

Figure 1.40 Intercanine width increase during permanent lateral incisor eruption.

Q: *Why* does this happen?

A: As the permanent canines, first premolars, and second premolars erupt, they drift mesially, reducing arch length (Figure 1.41, red solid arrows). In a reciprocal manner, the anterior teeth can drift distally (red dashed arrows). Both movements are likely caused by transeptal fiber contraction pulling the *mesiodistal narrower* permanent teeth together.

Q: How does this mesial drift affect orthodontic treatment?

A: It is important for orthodontists to anticipate this potential loss of arch length and understand that *arch length is not gained but is lost during posterior occlusion transition from primary to permanent dentition*. A decision must be made either: to *allow* the posterior teeth to drift forward unimpeded, thereby reducing arch length; to *reduce* the amount of forward drift of posterior teeth by placing an LLHA or Nance button (space maintenance); to *regain space* that has already been lost (say, by premature exfoliation of mandibular primary canines); or to *extract teeth* (serial extraction) in cases of severe crowding.

Q: What is the *most reliable* indicator of severe mandibular anterior crowding?

A: *Premature loss of primary canines – not* lack of interdental spacing. In crowded dental arches, the permanent lateral incisors often erupt and resorb the mesial portion of the root of deciduous canines, causing their premature loss [212].

Q: A mandibular primary canine, primary first molar, or primary second molar is exfoliated or extracted. What is the effect on the arch? What treatment should be considered?

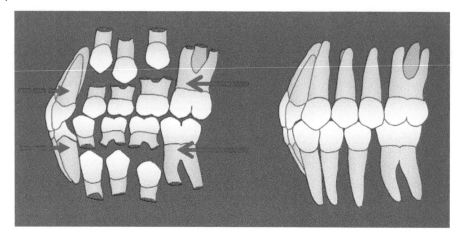

Figure 1.41 Mesial drift of permanent posterior teeth (red solid arrows) during eruption. Anterior teeth can drift distally (red dashed arrows).

A:

- Mandibular primary canine loss: Kau [213] reported that incisor angulation changes were similar for both primary canine extraction and nonextraction groups, but arch perimeter decreased more in the extraction group (attributed to mesial molar movement). Sjögren [214] agreed (decrease in mandibular incisor irregularity, decrease in mandibular arch length) with over 2 mm less arch perimeter found in extraction patients one year after primary canine loss. Sayin [215] challenged these findings, reporting a slight retrusion of lower incisors but no significant effect on arch length. However, he recorded one measurement immediately post-extraction, some measurements four months later, and other measurements eighteen months later. Yoshihara et al. [216] reported distal tipping of the incisors. Conclusion: Studies are somewhat conflicting. However, *if the possibility of mandibular arch perimeter loss, midline deviation due to incisal drift, or mandibular incisor retrusion will be detrimental to the patient, then place an LLHA if mandibular primary canines are lost.*
- Mandibular primary first molar loss (Figure 1.42): Tunison et al. [217] reported a 1.5 mm (per side) perimeter reduction (not statistically significant). Lin and Cha [218] reported a 0.68 mm total arch perimeter reduction (not statistically significant) following *unilateral* primary first molar extractions. They also reported a 1.2 mm space reduction (attributed to distal tipping of the primary canine) following extraction of *both* the primary first and second molars. Cuoghi et al. [219] reported that space reduction was primarily due to distal movement of the canine following primary first molar loss. Kumari and Retnakumari [220] reported < 0.5 mm

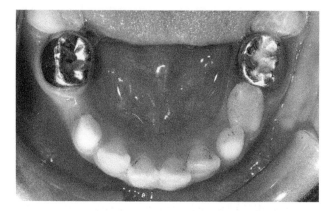

Figure 1.42 Loss of mandibular right primary first molar.

arch perimeter reduction (not statistically significant.), due to distal movement of the primary canines, after unilateral primary first molar extractions. Finally, in a systematic review, Macena et al. [221] claimed no significant arch perimeter changes or arch length changes following primary first molar extractions. Conclusion: Based upon the above, we would conclude that *a small, perhaps insignificant, perimeter reduction may occur following mandibular primary first molar loss. However, if the patient cannot afford arch perimeter reduction, then an LLHA should be placed when mandibular primary first molars are lost. Spurs, wrapping around the primary canine distal, should be soldered to the LLHA to prevent drifting of the primary canine, prn.*

- Mandibular primary second molar loss: first permanent molars move mesially [221]. Conclusion: *If loss of arch perimeter or risk of premolar impaction is a concern, place an LLHA.*

Q: Following tooth loss, the remaining teeth tend to drift into the edentulous space. Why?

A: Teeth drift toward the edentulous space probably as a result of transseptal fiber pull [222].

Q: A *maxillary* primary canine, primary first molar, or primary second molar is exfoliated or extracted. What is the effect on the arch? What treatment should be considered?

A:

- Maxillary primary canine loss: Sjögren [214] reported a significant reduction in maxillary arch length (~1 mm) and arch perimeter (~2 mm). Conclusion: *arch perimeter is reduced with maxillary primary canine extractions. If the patient cannot afford arch perimeter reduction, then a Nance holding arch should be placed when maxillary primary canines are lost.*

- Maxillary primary first molar loss: Tunison et al. [217] reported a 1 mm (per side) perimeter reduction (not clinically significant). Northway [223] and Lin et al [224] reported reductions in the extraction space (mesial movement of the second primary molar or distal movement of the primary canines) but no significant change in the first permanent molar position. Macena et al [220], Lin et al [224], and Park et al [225], reported no significant change in arch measurements. Conclusion: *space maintenance is probably unnecessary following maxillary primary first molar loss.*

- Maxillary primary second molar loss – following an initial reduction in space, Macena et al. [221] reported that a large portion of it was later recovered from growth. However, their follow-up was only 10 months, postextraction. Owen [226] reported that maxillary second primary molar spaces show the greatest closure, followed by mandibular primary second molar spaces: the longer the time available for space closure, the greater the closure,

particularly for primary second molar extractions before eruption of the first permanent molar. Conclusion: *If the patient cannot afford to have maxillary first permanent molar mesial drift, or cannot afford maxillary arch perimeter loss, then place a Nance holding arch when the maxillary primary second molar is lost (Figure 1.43).*

Q: Based upon the foregoing studies, what is the take-home message regarding the need for space maintenance following loss of maxillary or mandibular primary canines or primary molars?

A: Our recommendation: *If the patient cannot afford any permanent first molar mesial drift, or arch perimeter reduction, then place a space maintainer following primary canine or primary molar loss.*

Q: What if, following loss of a primary canine or primary molar (Figure 1.44), drifting/space closure has already occurred. Should a space maintainer be placed then?

A: The same principle applies as earlier: *If the patient cannot afford additional tooth drift or additional reduction*

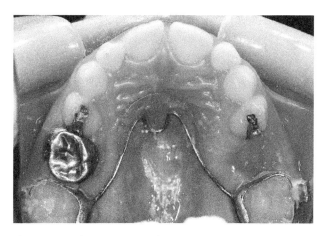

Figure 1.43 Premature loss of maxillary left primary second molar and subsequent placement of a Nance holding arch.

(a) (b)

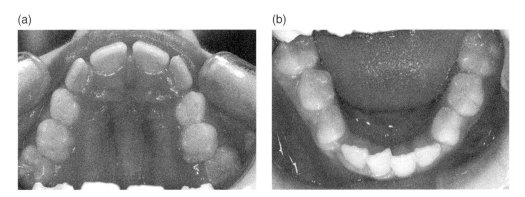

Figure 1.44 (a) Significant drift/space closure following loss of primary maxillary and mandibular (b) canines.

of arch perimeter, then consider placing a space maintainer. However, in arches where excessive drifting/space closure has already occurred, you must decide whether to maintain what space is left, to regain space that has been lost, or to consider serial extraction (in cases of severe crowding).

Q: How does one diagnose delayed tooth eruption?

A: According to Suri et al. [163], the diagnosis of delayed tooth eruption is determined by following a diagnostic sequence in which the clinician assesses: (i) the chronology of tooth eruption compared to chronologic norms; (ii) the presence or absence of factors adversely affecting or impeding tooth development; and (iii) the patient's dental age, using 2/3 root formation as the biologic norm for emergence of a tooth.

Delayed chronologic tooth eruption is defined as delay by more than two standard deviations from the average eruption time for a given tooth. *Delayed biologic eruption* occurs when a tooth has formed $\geq 2/3$ of final root length, but the tooth has failed to emerge. *Factors adversely affecting or impeding tooth development* include numerous genetic syndromic disorders [227], genetic tooth eruption disorders [227], and non-syndromic hypodontia [203, 228, 229].

Q: What is ankylosis?

A: Ankylosis is a failure of the tooth eruption process due to fusion of cementum and/or dentin of the tooth root structure to the adjacent alveolar bone, resulting in loss of the periodontal ligament space in the area of fusion. This definition is based on histological findings of ankylosed teeth after their removal from the oral cavity. The mechanism creating the aberration of the periodontal ligament is not fully understood. Trauma is thought to be causative for any tooth that has emerged and thus available to receive direct trauma. However, ankylosis also occurs during the intraosseous and/or supra-osseous stage of the tooth eruption process prior to tooth emergence by an unknown mechanism [230].

Clinically, ankylosis is suspected in a developing tooth if it fails to emerge or fails to complete normal vertical movement in the supra-gingival stage of tooth eruption. Tooth trauma may or may not be part of the clinical history. Partially or fully emerged teeth can be further evaluated by a percussion test to compare sound (sharp, solid tone) to percussion tests of adjacent teeth (softer tone) [231]. A check for immobility can also reveal tooth ankylosis. However, the gold standard for determining tooth ankylosis is radiographic evidence that the suspect tooth has not erupted compared to erupting adjacent teeth (difference in alveolar bone heights).

Q: What are the signs of primary molar ankylosis during the development of the transitional dentition?

A: Infraocclusion of the primary molar is the principal diagnostic indication of primary molar ankylosis. With respect to primary molars that have emerged through gingival tissue, infraocclusion can occur during eruption to the occlusal plane or after full eruption during continuing vertical alveolar development. Brearley classified infraocclusion by the magnitude of the vertical discrepancy between the affected primary molar and the adjacent teeth as: Slight (approximately 1 mm of discrepancy), Moderate (2–5 mm of discrepancy), and Severe (primary molar occlusal surface at or below the level of the interproximal gingivae of the adjacent teeth) [232].

However, because primary molar crowns are often shorter that permanent molar crowns, one must be careful in diagnosing ankylosis based upon a clinical difference in crown height relationship. Instead, the gold standard for determining primary molar ankylosis is radiographic evidence that the suspect tooth has not erupted compared to erupting adjacent teeth (difference in alveolar bone heights).

Q: What is the prevalence of primary molar ankylosis?

A: Frequency of occurrence has been reported between 24% and 38%. Males and females, right and left sides, primary first and second molars are affected equally. The incidence of moderate and severe infraocclusion increases from age eight to thirteen years. Mandibular primary molars are more commonly affected than maxillary primary molars, with some studies reporting fivefold greater mandibular frequency [232–237].

Q: What are treatment alternatives for primary molar ankylosis when permanent premolar successors are present?

A: *Monitoring is favored over extraction.* When a primary molar displays infraocclusion due to ankylosis and a premolar successor is present, the primary molar will likely exfoliate on time or within a six-month delay. Approximately 80% of primary molars displaying infraocclusion due to ankylosis undergo spontaneous exfoliation. Extraction should be pursued in cases of severe primary molar infraocclusion associated with adjacent tooth tipping and arch length loss, or when the premolar displays an unfavorable eruption path that will not promote complete root resorption of the precursor primary molar [237, 238].

Q: Does primary molar ankylosis affect future vertical alveolar growth of the bone surrounding the infraoccluded tooth?

A: No. Although a reduction in vertical growth of alveolar bone surrounding an infraoccluded tooth has been demonstrated (0.4 mm reduction over an eighteen-month period) [239], a majority of studies have shown no long-term effect on vertical growth of the alveolar bone surrounding an ankylosed primary molar, after extraction or spontaneously exfoliation [237].

Q: Is ankylosis of primary molars associated with other dental anomalies?

A: Yes. Associations have been observed between primary molar ankylosis and occurrence of tooth agenesis, microdontia of maxillary lateral incisors, palatally displaced canines, and distal angulation of developing mandibular second premolars suggesting a common genetic mechanism [240].

Q: What is primary failure of eruption? How is primary failure of eruption distinguished from ankylosis?

A: Beginning in the inter-osseous stage of tooth development, active tooth eruption requires bone resorption and gingival resorption above the dental follicle and root elongation at the apex of the dental follicle [241]. By an unknown mechanism, primary failure of eruption (PFE) is thought to result from a disruption of these processes mediated by mutations in the gene coding for parathyroid hormone receptor 1 (*PTH1R* gene) [227].

The clinical features of PFE include the following:
- Teeth emerge partially (supracrestally) and then cease to erupt further.
- Teeth may also show arrested eruption during the interosseous stage of development.
- Permanent first molars are most often affected.
- Posterior teeth are predominately affected.
- Primary teeth can also be affected.
- Can present unilaterally or bilaterally.
- Teeth ankylose after application of orthodontic force.
- A wide range of clinical variability thought to be the result of variation in the timing and intensity of the dysregulation.

Ankylosis is an eruption failure due to mechanical impedance to eruption by fusion of cementum and/or dentin of the tooth root structure to the adjacent alveolar bone, resulting in loss of the periodontal ligament space in the area of fusion. On the other hand, *PFE* is thought to be due to a defective eruption mechanism. Ankylosis can occur as a *result* of PFE when orthodontic force is applied to a tooth with a defective eruption mechanism, creating a fusion between cementum or dentin and alveolar bone [227, 242].

Q: What is the definition of hypodontia? Which teeth are most commonly missing in hypodontia?

A: Hypodontia is defined as the absence of one to five primary or permanent teeth excluding third molars [243]. It is a rare condition in the primary dentition with a prevalence <1.5% and no gender differences. Prevalence in the permanent dentition is 3.5–7%, with females more affected by a ratio of 3:2 [243].

Permanent teeth most commonly missing in approximate order of prevalence (excluding third molars) are mandibular second premolars (3–4%), maxillary lateral incisors (1–2.5%), maxillary second premolars (1–2%), and mandibular central incisors (<1%). [244, 245]

Q: What is the cause of hypodontia?

A: Hypodontia is a developmental anomaly that occurs as the result of failures at one of three early stages of tooth development: (i) the initiation of tooth formation, (ii) a decrease in the odontogenic potential of the cells in the dental lamina, or (iii) arrested development due to lack of formation of successional dental lamina, the extension of the dental lamina of the predecessor tooth forming during the early cap stage of tooth development [243]. Tooth agenesis occurs as an isolated event in otherwise "normal" individuals, but also has been associated with more than 150 syndromic conditions, particularly those involving defects in other ectodermal organs (e.g. ectodermal dysplasia and Rieger syndrome). Morphogenesis and cell differentiation of tooth forming cells is under strict genetic control with genes *WNT10A, MSX1*, and *PAX9* playing major roles in orchestrating the process of tooth formation. Nearly 50% of instances of tooth agenesis have been attributed to *WNT10A* mutations [246, 247].

Q: Is hypodontia associated with other dental or craniofacial anomalies?

A: Yes. Studies of tooth agenesis covariance with other dental anomalies have shown a strong association between the presence of tooth agenesis and the prevalence of maxillary lateral incisor microdontia, infra-eruption of deciduous molars, disto-angulation of erupting mandibular second premolars, and delayed tooth eruption [203, 213, 228, 229, 243, 248, 249].

In addition, congenital absence of mandibular second premolars has been associated with shorter mandibular corpus length, smaller mandibular cross-sectional dimension including the region of the first premolar and first molar, a more pronounced lingual alveolar plate and more distinct submandibular fossa beneath the mylohyoid line [250, 251].

Q: If second premolars are congenitally absent, can retained primary second molars teeth be preserved?

A: Yes. Longitudinal studies following retained primary second molars in subjects with hypodontia suggest that the preservation of primary second molars is a viable treatment alternative. Followed, on average, 11–12 years, 58–86% of retained primary second molars with congenitally absent permanent successors remained healthy and stable [252, 253].

Q: What is hyperdontia?

A: Hyperdontia is the presence of supernumerary teeth. It is not as common as hypodontia, occurring with <1% prevalence in the primary dentition and between 0.5 and 5.3% prevalence in the permanent dentition across various populations [254]. The most common supernumerary tooth is the mesiodens occurring in 0.15–1.9% of populations studied [255].

Similar to hypodontia, hyperdontia can occur in otherwise normal individuals as an isolated developmental anomaly or as part of a syndrome where different affected tissues share common mutations in their gene regulatory networks. Although the underlying mechanism remains unclear, it appears the genes *RUNX2* and *SOX2* play an important role [243].

Q: What is the prevalence of peg-shaped permanent maxillary lateral incisors?

A: Prevalence varies by gender and geographic populations. A survey of epidemiologic studies from sixteen countries found an overall prevalence of 1.8%, ranging from 1.3% (Caucasian) to 3.1% (Mongoloid). Incidence of unilateral and bilateral absence was similar. Left side unilateral absence was twice as common as right side unilateral absence. Across all populations, females are 1.35 times more likely to be affected compared to males [256].

Q: What is the prevalence of palatally displaced permanent maxillary canines?

A: Palatal displacement with impaction, of one or both permanent maxillary canines (termed palatally displaced canines, abbreviated PDCs) occurs in 2% of the general population. This is in contrast to the rate of occurrence of PDCs in subjects with other dental anomalies, where the incidence associated with, (i) small maxillary permanent lateral incisors is 25%, (ii) peg-shaped maxillary permanent lateral incisors is

12–17%, and (iii) missing maxillary permanent lateral incisors is 5–14%, suggesting a nonrandom association between PDCs and anomalous maxillary lateral incisors and the possible influence of genetic mechanisms.

Unilateral displacement is twice as common as bilateral displacement. Occurrence is more common in females for both unilateral (1.65:1) and bilateral (4:1) displacements compared to males. Anomalous maxillary lateral incisors are also more common in females (2.5:1). In addition, 85% of PDCs occur with adequate maxillary perimeter arch length, suggesting that maxillary dental arch crowding alone is not a major contributing factor to PDCs [257].

Q: What is the cause of palatally displaced permanent maxillary canines?

A: Mechanical obstruction of an erupting tooth due to the presence of hard-tissue impediments (e.g. supernumerary teeth) or soft-tissue lesions (e.g. dentigerous cysts) can cause a change in the path of eruption of any permanent tooth, including maxillary permanent canines. In the absence of mechanical obstruction, the underlying mechanism causing palatally displaced permanent maxillary canines remains unknown. Two working hypotheses to explain the mechanism are being pursued: (i) a direct genetic origin for the anomaly [258, 259] and (ii) a guidance mechanism theory, which postulates that local (neighboring) dental anomalies (diminutive or missing maxillary permanent lateral incisors) create a local environment causing palatal displacement of the maxillary permanent canine [260].

Ultimately, the complex mechanism may involve both postulates. The genetics of PDCs are not simple. The etiology is likely complex with more than one pathogenic model involving variable contributions from genetic factors, environmental factors, and individual responses to the interplay of these factors [261].

Q: What is the prevalence of ectopic (mesial) eruption of maxillary permanent first molars?

A: Studies of various populations of children have reported prevalence between 1 and 6% [261–268]. Children with cleft lip and palate (CLP) have a fivefold greater prevalence rate compared to normal children [42]. Siblings of children with CLP have a greater incidence (~20%) compared to the general population, suggesting a genetic influence [269].

Historically, this local eruption anomaly is characterized as reversible (self-correcting) or irreversible (requiring treatment). On average, 70% of ectopically erupting maxillary first permanent molars are self-correcting and 30% require treatment [267, 268].

Q: How is tooth crowding defined?

A Crowding of teeth in the dental arch is commonly referred to as tooth-size / arch length discrepancy (TSALD) where "arch length," a measurement of arch perimeter estimating the position of each tooth in ideal arch alignment, is compared to the sum of mesiodistal tooth sizes along that perimeter.

Q: What is the relative importance of tooth-size and arch perimeter in occurrence of tooth crowding?

A: A number of studies in various populations have shown tooth crowding has a stronger association to smaller dental arch dimensions rather than to larger mesiodistal tooth sizes [270–273].

Q: What is the etiology of tooth crowding?

A: Tooth crowding has a complex etiology. Tooth position is the result of an equilibrium of many forces acting on the tooth [274, 275]. These forces include eruptive forces, occlusal forces, soft-tissue forces, and forces from neighbor teeth [276]. Because forces acting on teeth change during growth, development, and aging, tooth position equilibrium is periodically altered. During these perturbations of tooth equilibrium, adaptive changes in tooth position occur and a new equilibrium is established. These adaptive changes often allow for maintenance of occlusal interdigitation between arches during changing skeletal relationships, the tenet of the dentoalveolar compensatory mechanism [276]. However, adaptive tooth position changes to perturbed equilibrium often result in tooth malposition and ultimately anterior tooth crowding [277].

Q: What are the major factors that contribute to the disruption of tooth position equilibrium?

A: Three major factors are thought to contribute to the disruption of tooth position equilibrium and contribute to anterior tooth crowding [278]: (i) loss of posterior arch space during the mixed dentition, (ii) the anterior component of occlusal force [278, 279], and (iii) vertical drift of mandibular anterior teeth associated with clockwise mandibular displacement during growth [280, 281]. The loss of posterior arch space must be considered in the transitional dentition. As discussed earlier, early loss of deciduous molars, or altered eruption sequence of the canine, premolar, and second molar teeth can contribute to loss of posterior arch length [277]. Vertical drift of mandibular anterior

teeth in response to vertical mandibular displacement must be considered well into the third decade of life. The anterior component of occlusal force promotes forces directed mesially along the dental arch throughout life [277].

Q: How is crowding assessed in the transitional dentition?

A: The most common method to assess crowding in the transitional dentition is the Mixed Dentition Analysis developed by Robert Moyers [282]. The method uses direct measurement on study casts and large-sample regression estimates of permanent premolar and canine size based on permanent incisor size. The method has been validated in a variety of samples [283]. The method in each dental arch involves the following steps:

1) Direct perimeter measurement of the dental arch in four segments and summation to arrive at *arch perimeter available* (see Figure 1.45).
2) Direct measurement and summation of the mesiodistal (M-D) width of each of four incisors.
3) Estimation of the sum of permanent premolar and canine M-D widths from the sum of the M-D width of the four incisors. The Tanaka-Johnston approach for this estimation uses $11\,\text{mm} + (\sum [\text{M-D incisor widths}]/2)$ and $10.5\,\text{mm} + (\sum [\text{M-D incisor widths}]/2)$ for maxillary and mandibular estimations respectively [284].
4) Summation of 2) and 3) above to arrive at *arch perimeter required*.
5) Subtraction of 4) from 1) above to arrive at arch perimeter deficit or excess.

Q: How do habits affect the development of malocclusion?

A: Oral habits, including thumb and finger sucking, nail and lip biting, and lateral or anterior tongue posture that presses the tongue against teeth or interposes the tongue between the maxillary and mandibular teeth have an effect on tooth position equilibrium. The effect is not based on force magnitude. Maximum effect is seen when light forces are present for extended times. Lack of vertical eruption of teeth and open-bite malocclusion is a primary response to oral habits (dental, or functional, open bite). Thumb and finger sucking has been associated with lingually directed movement of the posterior maxillary teeth. Posterior crossbite is seen in 7–15% of children in the primary dentition with thumb and finger sucking habits in various studies [285]. Cessation of the habit early allows self-correction of the negative effects in the majority of cases [286].

(a)

(b)

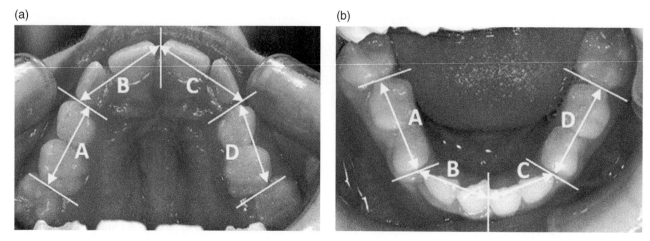

Figure 1.45 Perimeter measurement of the dental arch in four segments. (a) Maxillary arch. (b) Mandibular arch. A and D measurements: from the distal contact point of the second primary molar with the adjacent permanent molar to the mesial contact point of the most mesial primary tooth in the buccal segment (primary first molar or primary canine). B and C measurements: from the distal contact point of the permanent lateral incisor to the dental midline. Sum A+B+C+D = arch perimeter available. In this example, arch length perimeter available is greatly reduced by the early loss of all four primary canines.

"Mouth breathing" is often referred to as an oral habit. The relationship between mode of breathing and malocclusion remains controversial. Individuals with interferences in nasal breathing adopt an open mouth posture to allow simultaneous nasal and oral breathing. A cause-and-effect relationship between mouth breathing and malocclusion has been proposed largely based on the altered mandibular posture creating altered muscular balance that induces adaptive skeletal and dental changes during growth. [87, 287–294] Others do not support a direct cause-and-effect relationship, emphasizing that exposure to mouth breathing during development is associated with a considerable variation in inter-arch relationships ranging from normal relationships to severe discrepancies [91, 294–297].

References

1 Vasilakou, N., Araujo, E., Kim, K., and Oliver, D.R. (2016). Quantitative assessment of the effectiveness of phase 1 orthodontic treatment using the American Board of Orthodontics Discrepancy Index. *Am. J. Orthod. Dentofac. Orthop.* 150 (6): 997–1004.

2 Southard, T.E., Marshall, S.D., Allareddy, V. et al. (2013). An evidence-based comparison of headgear and functional appliance therapy for the correction of Class II malocclusions. *Semin. Orthod.* 19 (3): 174–195.

3 Newman, K.J. and Meredith, H.V. (1956). Individual growth in skeletal biogonial diameter during the childhood period from 5 to 11 years of age. *Am. J. Anat.* 99 (1): 157–187.

4 Clark, C.A. (1910). A method of ascertaining the relative position of unerupted teeth by means of film radiographs. *Proc. R. Soc. Med.* 3 (Odontol Sect): 87–90.

5 Sergl, H.G., Kerr, W.J., and McColl, J.H. (1996). A method of measuring the apical base. *Eur. J. Orthod.* 18 (5): 479–483.

6 Sforza, C., Grandi, G., De Menezes, M. et al. (2011). Age- and sex-related changes in the normal human external nose. *Forensic Sci. Int.* 204 (1-3): 205.e1–205.e9.

7 Bergman, R.T., Waschak, J., Borzabadi-Farahani, A., and Murphy, N.C. (2014). Longitudinal study of cephalometric soft tissue profile traits between the ages of 6 and 18 years. *Angle Orthod.* 84 (1): 48–55.

8 Muller, H.P. and Eger, T. (1997). Gingival phenotypes in young male adults. *J. Clin. Periodontol.* 24 (1): 65–71.

9 Muller, H.P., Heinecke, A., Schaller, N., and Eger, T. (2000). Masticatory mucosa in subjects with different periodontal phenotypes. *J. Clin. Periodontol.* 27 (9): 621–626.

10 Olsson, M. and Lindhe, J. (1991). Periodontal characteristics in individuals with varying form of the upper central incisors. *J. Clin. Periodontol.* 18 (1): 78–82.

11 Muller, H.P. and Eger, T. (2002). Masticatory mucosa and periodontal phenotype: a review. *Int. J. Periodontics Restorative Dent.* 22 (2): 172–183.

12 Zweers, J., Thomas, R.Z., Slot, D.E. et al. (2014). Characteristics of periodontal biotype, its dimensions, associations, and prevalence: a systematic review. *J. Clin. Periodontol.* 41 (10): 958–971.

13 Andlin-Sobocki, A. (1993). Changes of facial gingival dimensions in children. A 2-year longitudinal study. *J. Clin. Periodontol.* 20 (3): 212–218.

14 Wennström, J., Lindhe, J., and Nyman, S. (1982). The role of keratinized gingiva in plaque-associated gingivitis in dogs. *J. Clin. Periodontol.* 9 (1): 75–85.

15 Dorfman, H.S., Kennedy, J.E., and Bird, W.C. (1982). Longitudinal evaluation of free autogenous gingival grafts. A four-year report. *J. Periodontol.* 53 (6): 349–352.

16 Miyasato, M., Crigger, M., and Egelberg, J. (1977). Gingival condition in areas of minimal and appreciable width of keratinized gingiva. *J. Clin. Periodontol.* 4 (3): 200–209.

17 Kim, D.M., Bassir, S.H., and Nguyen, T.T. (2020). Effect of gingival phenotype on the maintenance of periodontal health: an American academy of periodontology best evidence review. *J. Periodontol.* 91 (3): 311–338.

18 Lindauer, S.J., Rubenstein, L.K., Hang, W.M. et al. (1992). Canine impaction identified early with panoramic radiographs. *J. Am. Dent. Assoc.* 123 (3): 91–97.

19 Bonetti, G.A., Zanarini, M., Parenti, S.I. et al. (2011). Preventive treatment of ectopically erupting maxillary permanent canines by extraction of deciduous canines and first molars: a randomized clinical trial. *Am. J. Orthod. Dentofac. Orthop.* 139 (3): 316–323.

20 Leonardi, M., Armi, P., Franchi, L., and Baccetti, T. (2004). Two interceptive approaches to palatally displaced canines: a prospective longitudinal study. *Angle Orthod.* 74 (5): 581–586.

21 Baccetti, T., Mucedero, M., Leonardi, M., and Cozza, P. (2009). Interceptive treatment of palatal impaction of maxillary canines with rapid maxillary expansion: a randomized clinical trial. *Am. J. Orthod. Dentofac. Orthop.* 136 (5): 657–661.

22 Fanning, E.A. (1962). Effect of extraction of deciduous molars on the formation and eruption of their successors. *Angle Orthod.* 32 (1): 44–53.

23 Grøn, A.M. (1962). Prediction of tooth emergence. *J. Dent. Res.* 41 (3): 573–585.

24 Cha, J.Y., Kennedy, D.B., Turley, P.K. et al. (2019). Outcomes of early versus late treatment of severe Class II high-angle patients. *Am. J. Orthod. Dentofac. Orthop.* 156 (3): 375–382.

25 Nguyen, Q.V., Bezemer, P.D., Habets, L., and Prahl-Andersen, B. (1999). A systematic review of the relationship between overjet size and traumatic dental injuries. *Eur. J. Orthod.* 21 (5): 503–515.

26 Batista, K.B., Thiruvenkatachari, B., Harrison, J.E., and O'Brien, K.D. (2018). Orthodontic treatment for prominent upper front teeth (Class II malocclusion) in children and adolescents. *Cochrane Database Syst. Rev.* 3 (3): CD003452.

27 Rogers, K., Campbell, P.M., Tadlock, L. et al. (2018). Treatment changes of hypo- and hyperdivergent Class II Herbst patients. *Angle Orthod.* 88 (1): 3–9.

28 Ingervall, B. and Bitsanis, E. (1987). A pilot study of the effect of masticatory muscle training on facial growth in long-face children. *Eur. J. Orthod.* 9 (1): 15–23.

29 English, J.D. and Olfert, K.D.G. (2005). Masticatory muscle exercise as an adjunctive treatment for open bite malocclusions. *Semin. Orthod.* 11 (3): 164–169.

30 Tulloch, J.F.C. (1995). Early versus late treatment of Class II malocclusion: preliminary results from the UNC clinical trial. In: *Orthodontic Treatment: Outcome and Effectiveness*, Craniofacial Growth Series (ed. J.A. McNamara Jr. and C.-A. Trotman), 113–138. Ann Arbor: Center for Human Growth and Development, University of Michigan.

31 O'Brien, K., Wright, J., Conboy, F. et al. (2003). Effectiveness of early orthodontic treatment with the Twin-block appliance: a multicenter randomized, controlled trial. Part 2: psychosocial effects. *Am. J. Orthod. Dentofac. Orthop.* 124 (5): 488–495.

32 O'Brien, K., Macfarlane, T., Wright, J. et al. (2009). Early treatment for Class II malocclusion and perceived improvements in facial profile. *Am. J. Orthod. Dentofac. Orthop.* 135 (5): 580–585.

33 Edwards, J.G. (1988). A long-term prospective evaluation of the circumferential supracrestal fiberotomy in alleviating orthodontic relapse. *Am. J. Orthod. Dentofac. Orthop.* 93 (5): 380–387.

34 Hsieh, T.J., Pinskaya, Y., and Roberts, W.E. (2005). Assessment of orthodontic treatment outcomes: early treatment versus late treatment. *Angle Orthod.* 75 (2): 162–170.

35 Sperber, G.H. (2001). *Craniofacial Development*. London: BC Decker.

36 Carlson, B.M. (2014). *Human Embryology and Developmental Biology*, 5e. Philadelphia: Elsevier.

37 Nanci, A. (2017). *Ten Cate's Oral Histology-e-book: Development, Structure, and Function*, 9e. Amsterdam: Elsevier Health Sciences.

38 Carlson, D.S. (2015). Evolving concepts of heredity and genetics in orthodontics. *Am. J. Orthod. Dentofac. Orthop.* 148 (6): 922–938.

39 Moss, M.L. (1997). The functional matrix hypothesis revisited. 3. The genomic thesis. *Am. J. Orthod. Dentofac. Orthop.* 112 (3): 338–342.

40 Carlson, D.S. (2005). Theories of craniofacial growth in the postgenomic era. *Semin. Orthod.* 11 (4): 172–183.

41 Dixon, A.D., Hoyte, D.A., and Ronning, O. (1997). *Fundamentals of Craniofacial Growth*, 1e. Boca Raton: CRC Press.

42 Enlow, D.H. and Hans, M.G. (2008). *Essentials of Facial Growth*, 2e. Ann Arbor: Needham Press.

43 Hartsfield, J.K. Jr., Morford, L.A., and Otero, L.M. (2014). Genetic factors affecting facial growth. In: *Orthodontics – Basic Aspects and Clinical Considerations* (ed. F. Bourzgui), 125–152. InTech: Rijeka.

44 Hallgrímsson, B., Jamniczky, H., Young, N.M. et al. (2009). Deciphering the palimpsest: studying the relationship between morphological integration and phenotypic covariation. *Evol. Biol.* 36 (4): 355–376.

45 Moyers, R.E. (1988). *Handbook of Orthodontics*, 4e. Chicago: Year Book Medical.

46 Minoux, M. and Rijli, F.M. (2010). Molecular mechanisms of cranial neural crest cell migration and patterning in craniofacial development. *Development* 137 (16): 2605–2621.

47 Carlson, D.S. and Buschang, P.H. (2017). Craniofacial growth and development: developing a perspective. In: *Orthodontics, Current Principles and Techniques*, 6e (ed. T.M. Graber, R.L. Vanarsdall, K.W.L. Vig and G.J. Huang), 1–30. St. Louis: Elsevier.

48 Duterloo, H.S. and Planche, P.G. (2001). *Handbook of Cephalometric Superimposition*. Quintessence: Hanover Park.

49 Hallou, A. and Brunet, T. (2020). On growth and force: mechanical forces in development. *Development* 147 (4): dev187302. https://doi.org/10.1242/dev.187302.

50 Venugopalan, S.R. and Van Otterloo, E. (2021). The skull's girder: a brief review of the cranial base. *J. Dev. Biol.* 9 (1): 3.

51 Al Dayeh, A.A., Rafferty, K.L., Egbert, M., and Herring, S.W. (2013). Real-time monitoring of the growth of the nasal septal cartilage and the nasofrontal suture. *Am. J. Orthod. Dentofac. Orthop.* 143 (6): 773–783.

52 Björk, A. (1955). Cranial base development. *Am. J. Orthod.* 41 (3): 198–225.

53 Bastir, M., Rosas, A., and O'Higgins, P. (2006). Craniofacial levels and the morphologic maturation of the human skull. *J. Anat.* 20 (5): 637–654.

54 Buschang, P.H. and Santos-Pinto, A. (1998). Condylar growth and glenoid fossa displacement during childhood and adolescence. *Am. J. Orthod. Dentofac. Orthop.* 113 (4): 437–442.

55 Almeida, K.C.M., Raveli, T.B., Vieira, C.I.V. et al. (2017). Influence of the cranial base flexion on Class I, II and III malocclusions: a systematic review. *Dental Press J. Orthod.* 22 (5): 56–66.

56 Björk, A. and Skieller, V. (1977). Growth of the maxilla in three dimensions as revealed radiographically by the implant method. *Br. J. Orthod.* 4 (2): 53–64.

57 Baumrind, S., Ben-Bassat, Y., Bravo, L.A. et al. (1996). Partitioning the components of maxillary tooth displacement by the comparison of data from three cephalometric superimpositions. *Angle Orthod.* 66 (2): 111–124.

58 Verwoerd, C.D., Urbanus, N.A., and Mastenbroek, G.J. (1980). The influence of partial resections of the nasal septal cartilage on the growth of the upper jaw and the nose: an experimental study in rabbits. *Clin. Otolaryngol. Allied Sci.* 5 (5): 291–302.

59 Wealthall, R.J. and Herring, S.W. (2006). Endochondral ossification of the mouse nasal septum. *Anat. Rec. A Discov. Mol. Cell Evol. Biol.* 288 (11): 1163–1172.

60 Hartman, C., Holton, N., Miller, S. et al. (2016). Nasal septal deviation and facial skeletal asymmetries. *Anat. Rec. (Hoboken)* 299 (3): 295–306.

61 Moss, M.L. and Salentijn, L. (1969). The primary role of functional matrices in facial growth. *Am. J. Orthod.* 55 (6): 566–577.

62 Melsen, B. (1977). Histological analysis of the postnatal development of the nasal septum. *Angle Orthod.* 47 (2): 83–96.

63 Goergen, M.J., Holton, N.E., and Grünheid, T. (2017). Morphological interaction between the nasal septum and nasofacial skeleton during human ontogeny. *J. Anat.* 230 (5): 689–700.

64 Arens, R. and Marcus, C.L. (2004). Pathophysiology of upper airway obstruction: a developmental perspective. *Sleep* 27 (5): 997–1019.

65 Vorperian, H.K., Wang, S., Chung, M.K. et al. (2009). Anatomic development of the oral and pharyngeal portions of the vocal tract: an imaging study. *J. Acoust. Soc. Am.* 125 (3): 1666–1678.

66 Lieberman, D.E., McCarthy, R.C., Hiiemae, K.M., and Palmer, J.B. (2001). Ontogeny of postnatal hyoid and larynx descent in humans. *Arch. Oral Biol.* 46 (2): 117–128.

67 Vig, K.W. and Fields, H.W. (2000). Facial growth and management of orthodontic problems. *Pediatr. Clin. N. Am.* 47 (5): 1085–1123.

68 Miner, R.M., Al Qabandi, S., Rigali, P.H., and Will, L.A. (2012). Cone-beam computed tomography transverse analysis. Part I: normative data. *Am. J. Orthod. Dentofac. Orthop.* 142 (3): 300–307.

69 Kim, J.Y., Lee, S.J., Kim, T.W. et al. (2005). Classification of skeletal variation in normal occlusion. *Angle Orthod.* 75 (3): 311–319.

70 Markiewicz, M.R., Allareddy, V., and Miloro, M. (2020). Orthodontics for the oral and maxillofacial surgery patient. *Oral Maxillofac. Surg. Clin. North Am.* 32 (1): xiii–xiv.

71 Proffit, W.R., Fields, H.W., and Sarver, D.M. (2007). *Contemporary Orthodontics*, 4e. Mosby Elsevier Health Sciences: St. Louis.

72 Ikoma, M. and Arai, K. (2018). Craniofacial morphology in women with Class I occlusion and severe maxillary anterior crowding. *Am. J. Orthod. Dentofac. Orthop.* 153 (1): 36–45.

73 Hesby, R.M., Marshall, S.D., Dawson, D.V. et al. (2006). Transverse skeletal and dentoalveolar changes during growth. *Am. J. Orthod. Dentofac. Orthop.* 130 (6): 721–731.

74 Marshall, S.D., Dawson, D.V., Southard, K.A. et al. (2003). Transverse molar movements during growth. *Am. J. Orthod. Dentofac. Orthop.* 124 (6): 615–624.

75 Trotman, C.A., Long, R.E. Jr., Rosenstein, S.W. et al. (1996). Comparison of facial form in primary alveolar bone-grafted and non-grafted unilateral cleft lip and palate patients: intercenter retrospective study. *Cleft Palate Craniofac. J.* 33 (2): 91–95.

76 Alarcón, J.A., Bastir, M., García-Espona, I. et al. (2014). Morphological integration of mandible and cranium: orthodontic implications. *Arch. Oral Biol.* 59 (1): 22–29.

77 Wellens, H.L., Kuijpers-Jagtman, A.M., and Halazonetis, D.J. (2013). Geometric morphometric analysis of craniofacial variation, ontogeny and modularity in a cross-sectional sample of modern humans. *J. Anat.* 222 (4): 397–409.

78 Nielsen, I.L. (1991). Vertical malocclusions: etiology, development, diagnosis and some aspects of treatment. *Angle Orthod.* 61 (4): 247–260.

79 Schudy, F.F. (1964). Vertical growth versus anteroposterior growth as related to function and treatment. *Angle Orthod.* 34 (2): 75–93.

80 Moss, M.L., Bromberg, B.E., Song, I.C., and Eisenman, G. (1968). The passive role of nasal septal cartilage in mid-facial growth. *Plast. Reconstr. Surg.* 41 (6): 536–542.

81 Buschang, P.H. and Martins, J. (1998). Childhood and adolescent changes of skeletal relationships. *Angle Orthod.* 68 (3): 199–206. discussion 207-8.

82 Wagner, D.M. and Chung, C.H. (2005). Transverse growth of maxilla and mandible in untreated girls with low, average and high MP-SN angles: a longitudinal study. *Am. J. Orthod. Dentofac. Orthop.* 128 (6): 716–723. quiz 801.

83 Kiliaridis, S. (1995). Masticatory muscle influence on craniofacial growth. *Acta Odontol. Scand.* 53 (3): 196–202.

84 Weijs, W.A. and Hillen, B. (1986). Correlations between the cross-sectional area of the jaw muscles and craniofacial size and shape. *Am. J. Phys. Anthropol.* 70 (4): 423–431.

85 Gungor, A.Y. and Turkkahraman, H. (2009). Effects of airway problems on maxillary growth: a review. *Eur. J. Dent.* 3 (3): 250–254.

86 Solow, B. and Kreiborg, S. (1977). Soft-tissue stretching: a possible control factor in craniofacial morphogenesis. *Scand. J. Dent. Res.* 85 (6): 505–507.

87 Linder-Aronson, S. (1970). Adenoids: their effect on mode of breathing and nasal airflow and their relationship to characteristics of the facial skeleton and the dentition. A biometric, rhino-manometric and cephalometro-radiographic study on children with and without adenoids. *Acta Otolaryngol. Suppl.* 265: 1–132.

88 Linder-Aronson, S. (1979). Respiratory function in relation to facial morphology and the dentition. *Br. J. Orthod.* 6 (2): 59–71.

89 Solow, B., Siersbaek-Nielsen, S., and Greve, E. (1984). Airway adequacy, head posture, and craniofacial morphology. *Am. J. Orthod.* 86 (3): 214–223.

90 Behlfelt, K., Linder-Aronson, S., McWilliam, J. et al. (1990). Cranio-facial morphology in children with and without enlarged tonsils. *Eur. J. Orthod.* 12 (3): 233–243.

91 Vig, K.W. (1998). Nasal obstruction and facial growth: the strength of evidence for clinical assumptions. *Am. J. Orthod. Dentofac. Orthop.* 113 (6): 603–611.

92 Peltomäki, T. (2007). The effect of mode of breathing on craniofacial growth – revisited. *Eur. J. Orthod.* 29 (5): 426–429.

93 Vogl, C., Atchley, W.R., Cowley, D.E. et al. (1993). The epigenetic influence of growth hormone on skeletal development. *Growth Dev. Aging* 57 (3): 163–182.

94 Yamaguchi, T., Maki, K., and Shibasaki, Y. (2001). Growth hormone receptor gene variant and mandibular height in the normal Japanese population. *Am. J. Orthod. Dentofac. Orthop.* 119 (6): 650–653.

95 Zhou, J., Lu, Y., Gao, X.H. et al. (2005). The growth hormone receptor gene is associated with mandibular height in a Chinese population. *J. Dent. Res.* 84 (11): 1052–1056.

96 Tomoyasu, Y., Yamaguchi, T., Tajima, A. et al. (2009). Further evidence for an association between mandibular height and the growth hormone receptor gene in a Japanese population. *Am. J. Orthod. Dentofac. Orthop.* 136 (4): 536–541.

97 Katz, E.S. (2012). Pathophysiology of pediatric obstructive sleep apnea: putting it all together. In: *Sleep Disordered Breathing in Children: A Comprehensive Clinical Guide to Evaluation and Treatment (Respiratory Medicine)* (ed. L. Kheirandish-Gozal and D. Gozal), 151–158. New York: Springer.

98 Behrents, R.G., Shelgikar, A.V., Conley, R.S. et al. (2019). Obstructive sleep apnea and orthodontics: an American Association of Orthodontists White Paper. *Am. J. Orthod. Dentofac. Orthop.* 156 (1): 13–28.

99 Bucci, R., Montanaro, D., Rongo, R. et al. (2019). Effects of maxillary expansion on the upper airways: evidence from systematic reviews and meta-analyses. *J. Oral Rehabil.* 46 (4): 377–387.

100 Sánchez-Súcar, A.M., Sánchez-Súcar, F.B., Almerich-Silla, M. et al. (2019). Effect of rapid maxillary expansion on sleep apnea-hypopnea syndrome in growing patients. A meta-analysis. *J. Clin. Exp. Dent.* 1 (8): e759–e767.

101 Guilleminault, C., Monteyrol, P.J., Huynh, N.T. et al. (2011). Adenotonsillectomy and rapid maxillary distraction in pre-pubertal children, a pilot study. *Sleep Breath.* 15 (2): 173–177.

102 van Spronsen, P.H. (2010). Long-face craniofacial morphology: cause or effect of weak masticatory musculature? *Semin. Orthod.* 16 (2): 99–117.

103 Buschang, P.H., Heider, J., and Carrillo, R. (2013). The morphological characteristics, growth and etiology of the hyperdivergent phenotype. *Semin. Orthod.* 1: 19.

104 Björk, A. (1955). Facial growth in man, studied with the aid of metallic implants. *Acta Odontol. Scand.* 13 (1): 9–34.

105 Björk, A. (1963). Variations in the growth pattern of the human mandible: longitudinal radiographic study by the implant method. *J. Dent. Res.* 42 (1) Pt.2: 400–411.

106 Björk, A. and Skieller, V. (1972). Facial development and tooth eruption. An implant study at the age of puberty. *Am. J. Orthod.* 62 (4): 339–383.

107 Björk, A. and Skieller, V. (1983). Normal and abnormal growth of the mandible. A synthesis of longitudinal cephalometric implant studies over a period of 25 years. *Eur. J. Orthod.* 5 (1): 1–46.

108 Odegaard, J. (1970). Growth of the mandible studied with the aid of metal implant. *Am. J. Orthod.* 57 (2): 145–157.

109 Odegaard, J. (1970). Mandibular rotation studies with the aid of metal implants. *Am. J. Orthod.* 58 (5): 448–454.

110 Lavergne, J. and Gasson, N. (1977). Operational definitions of mandibular morphogenetic and positional rotations. *Scand. J. Dent. Res.* 85 (3): 185–192.

111 Sinclair, P.M. and Little, R.M. (1985). Dentofacial maturation of untreated normals. *Am. J. Orthod.* 88 (2): 146–156.

112 Lavergne, J. and Gasson, N. (1977). Direction and intensity of mandibular rotation in the sagittal adjustment during growth of the jaws. *Scand. J. Dent. Res.* 85 (3): 193–196.

113 Buschang, P.H. and Gandini Júnior, L.G. (2002). Mandibular skeletal growth and modelling between 10 and 15 years of age. *Eur. J. Orthod.* 24 (1): 69–79.

114 Mojdehi, M., Buschang, P.H., English, J.D., and Wolford, L.M. (2001). Postsurgical growth changes in the mandible of adolescents with vertical maxillary excess growth pattern. *Am. J. Orthod. Dentofac. Orthop.* 119 (2): 106–116.

115 Karlsen, A.T. (1995). Craniofacial growth differences between low and high MP-SN angle males: a longitudinal study. *Angle Orthod.* 65 (5): 341–350.

116 Chung, C.H. and Wong, W.W. (2002). Craniofacial growth in untreated skeletal Class II subjects: a longitudinal study. *Am. J. Orthod. Dentofac. Orthop.* 122 (6): 619–626.

117 Kim, J. and Nielsen, I.L. (2002). A longitudinal study of condylar growth and mandibular rotation in untreated subjects with Class II malocclusion. *Angle Orthod.* 72 (2): 105–111.

118 Björk, A. (1969). Prediction of mandibular growth rotation. *Am. J. Orthod.* 55 (6): 585–899.

119 Baumrind, S., Korn, E.L., and West, E.E. (1984). Prediction of mandibular rotation: an empirical test of clinician performance. *Am. J. Orthod.* 86 (5): 371–385.

120 Leslie, L.R., Southard, T.E., Southard, K.A. et al. (1998). Prediction of mandibular growth rotation: assessment of the Skieller, Björk, and Linde-Hansen method. *Am. J. Orthod. Dentofac. Orthop.* 114 (6): 659–667.

121 Buschang, P.H., Roldan, S.I., and Tadlock, L.P. (2017). Guidelines for assessing the growth and development of orthodontic patients. *Semin. Orthod.* 23 (4): 321–335.

122 Ngan, P.W., Byczek, E., and Scheick, J. (1997 Dec). Longitudinal evaluation of growth changes in Class II division 1 subjects. *Semin. Orthod.* 3 (4): 222–231.

123 Lee, R.S., Daniel, F.J., Swartz, M. et al. (1987). Assessment of a method for the prediction of mandibular rotation. *Am. J. Orthod. Dentofac. Orthop.* 91 (5): 395–402.

124 Chung, C.H. and Mongiovi, V.D. (2003). Craniofacial growth in untreated skeletal Class I subjects with low, average, and high MP-SN angles: a longitudinal study. *Am. J. Orthod. Dentofac. Orthop.* 124 (6): 670–678.

125 Ochoa, B.K. and Nanda, R.S. (2004 Feb). Comparison of maxillary and mandibular growth. *Am. J. Orthod. Dentofac. Orthop.* 125 (2): 148–159.

126 Nanda, S.K. (1990). Growth patterns in subjects with long and short faces. *Am. J. Orthod. Dentofac. Orthop.* 9 (3): 247–258.

127 Isaacson, J.R., Isaacson, R.J., Speidel, T.M., and Worms, F.W. (1971). Extreme variation in vertical facial growth and associated variation in skeletal and dental relations. *Angle Orthod.* 41 (3): 219–229.

128 Kuitert, R., Beckmann, S., van Loenen, M. et al. (2006). Dentoalveolar compensation in subjects with vertical skeletal dysplasia. *Am. J. Orthod. Dentofac. Orthop.* 129 (5): 649–657.

129 Janson, G.R., Metaxas, A., and Woodside, D.G. (1994). Variation in maxillary and mandibular molar and incisor vertical dimension in 12-year-old subjects with excess, normal, and short lower anterior face height. *Am. J. Orthod. Dentofac. Orthop.* 106 (4): 409–418.

130 Liu, S.S. and Buschang, P.H. (2011). How does tooth eruption relate to vertical mandibular growth displacement? *Am. J. Orthod. Dentofac. Orthop.* 139 (6): 745.

131 Ranly, D.M. (1988). *A Synopsis of Craniofacial Growth*, 2e. Appleton and Lange: Norwalk.

132 Buschang, P.H. (2009). Craniofacial growth and development. In: *Mosby's Orthodontic Review* (ed. J.D. English, T. Peltomaki and K. Litschel), 1–12. St. Louis: Elsevier Mosby.

133 Tanner, J.M., Whitehouse, R.H., and Takaishi, M. (1966). Standards from birth to maturity for height, weight, height velocity, and weight velocity: British children, 1965. *Arch. Dis. Child.* 41 (219): 454–471.

134 Malina, R.M., Bouchard, C., and Beunen, G. (1988). Human growth: selected aspects of current research on well-nourished children. *Ann. Rev. Anthropol.* 17: 187–219.

135 Mellion, Z.J., Behrents, R.G., and Johnston, L.E. Jr. (2013). The pattern of facial skeletal growth and its relationship to various common indexes of maturation. *Am. J. Orthod. Dentofac. Orthop.* 143 (6): 845–854.

136 Bambha, J.K. and Van Natta, P. (1963). Longitudinal study of facial growth in relation to skeletal maturation during adolescence. *Am. J. Orthod.* 49 (7): 481–493.

137 Hunter, C.J. (1966). The correlation of facial growth with body height and skeletal maturation at adolescence. *Angle Orthod.* 36 (1): 44–54.

138 Mitani, H. (1973). Contributions of the posterior cranial base and mandibular condyles to facial depth and height during puberty. *Angle Orthod.* 43 (3): 337–343.

139 Buschang, P.H., Jacob, H.B., and Demirjian, A. (2013). Female adolescent craniofacial growth spurts: real or fiction? *Eur. J. Orthod.* 3 (6): 819–825.

140 Bishara, S.E. and Jakobsen, J.R. (1985). Longitudinal changes in three normal facial types. *Am. J. Orthod.* 88 (6): 466–502.

141 Nanda, R.S. (1955). The rates of growth of several facial components measured from serial cephalometric roentgenograms. *Am. J. Orthod.* 41 (9): 658–673.

142 Buschang, P.H., Tanguay, R., Demirjian, A. et al. (1989). Modeling longitudinal mandibular growth: percentiles for gnathion from 6 to 15 years of age in girls. *Am. J. Orthod. Dentofac. Orthop.* 95 (1): 60–66.

143 van der Beek, M.C., Hoeksma, J.B., and Prahl-Andersen, B. (1996). Vertical facial growth and statural growth in girls: a longitudinal comparison. *Eur. J. Orthod.* 18 (6): 549–555.

144 Chvatal, B.A., Behrents, R.G., Ceen, R.F., and Buschang, P.H. (2005). Development and testing of multilevel models for longitudinal craniofacial growth prediction. *Am. J. Orthod. Dentofac. Orthop.* 128 (1): 45–56.

145 Bishara, S.E., Peterson, L.C., and Bishara, E.C. (1984). Changes in facial dimensions and relationships between the ages of 5 and 25 years. *Am. J. Orthod.* 85 (3): 238–252.

146 van der Beek, M.C., Hoeksma, J.B., and Prahl-Andersen, B. (1991). Vertical facial growth: a longitudinal study from 7 to 14 years of age. *Eur. J. Orthod.* 13 (3): 202–208.

147 Houston, W.J. (1980). Relationships between skeletal maturity estimated from hand-wrist radiographs and the timing of the adolescent growth spurt. *Eur. J. Orthod.* 2 (2): 81–93.

148 Hägg, U. and Taranger, J. (1982). Maturation indicators and the pubertal growth spurt. *Am. J. Orthod.* 82 (4): 299–309.

149 Flores-Mir, C., Nebbe, B., and Major, P.W. (2004). Use of skeletal maturation based on hand-wrist radiographic analysis as a predictor of facial growth: a systematic review. *Angle Orthod.* 74 (1): 118–124.

150 Hunter, W.S., Baumrind, S., Popovich, F., and Jorgensen, G. (2007). Forecasting the timing of peak mandibular growth in males by using skeletal age. *Am. J. Orthop. Dentofacial. Orthod.* 131 (3): 327–333.

151 Gabriel, D.B., Southard, K.A., Qian, F. et al. (2009). Cervical vertebrae maturation method: poor reproducibility. *Am. J. Orthod. Dentofac. Orthop.* 136 (4): 478.e1–478.e7. discussion 478-80.

152 Nestman, T.S., Marshall, S.D., Qian, F. et al. (2011). Cervical vertebrae maturation method morphologic criteria: poor reproducibility. *Am. J. Orthod. Dentofac. Orthop.* 140 (2): 182–188.

153 Baume, R.M., Buschang, P.H., and Weinstein, S. (1983). Stature, head height, and growth of the vertical face. *Am. J. Orthod.* 83 (6): 477–484.

154 Tanner, J.M. and Cameron, N. (1980). Investigation of the mid-growth spurt in height, weight and limb circumferences in single-year velocity data from the London, 1966-67 growth survey. *Ann. Hum. Biol.* 7 (6): 565–577.

155 Gasser, T., Müller, H.G., Köhler, W. et al. (1985). An analysis of the mid-growth and adolescent spurts of height based on acceleration. *Ann. Hum. Biol.* 12 (2): 129–148.

156 Molinari, L., Largo, R.H., and Prader, A. (1980). Analysis of the growth spurt at age seven (mid-growth spurt). *Helv. Paediatr. Acta.* 35 (4): 325–334.

157 Sheehy, A., Gasser, T., Molinari, L., and Largo, R.H. (1999). An analysis of variance of the pubertal and midgrowth spurts for length and width. *Ann. Hum. Biol.* 26 (4): 309–331.

158 Buschang, P.H., Tanguay, R., Demirjian, A. et al. (1988). Mathematical models of longitudinal mandibular growth for children with normal and untreated Class II, division 1 malocclusion. *Eur. J. Orthod.* 10 (3): 227–234.

159 Onland-Moret, N.C., Peeters, P.H.M., van Gils, C.H. et al. (2005). Age at menarche in relation to adult height: the EPIC study. *Am. J. Epidemiol.* 162 (7): 623–632.

160 Limony, Y., Koziel, S., and Friger, M. (2015). Age of onset of a normally timed pubertal growth spurt affects the final height of children. *Pediatr. Res.* 78 (3): 351–355.

161 Demirjian, A., Buschang, P.H., Tanguay, R., and Patterson, D.K. (1985). Interrelationships among measures of somatic, skeletal, dental, and sexual maturity. *Am. J. Orthod.* 88 (5): 433–438.

162 Magarey, A.M., Boulton, T.J., Chatterton, B.E. et al. (1999). Bone growth from 11 to 17 years: relationship to growth, gender and changes with pubertal status including timing of menarche. *Acta Paediatr.* 88 (2): 139–146.

163 Suri, L., Gagari, E., and Vastardis, H. (2004). Delayed tooth eruption: pathogenesis, diagnosis, and treatment: a literature review. *Am. J. Orthod. Dentofac. Orthop.* 126 (4): 432–445.

164 Lunt, R.C. and Law, D.B. (1974). A review of the chronology of calcification of deciduous teeth. *J. Am. Dent. Assoc.* 89 (3): 599–606.

165 Lysell, L., Magnusson, B., and Thilander, B. (1969). Relations between the times of eruption of primary and permanent teeth. A longitudinal study. *Acta Odontol. Scand.* 27 (3): 271–281.

166 Hamano, Y. and Hägg, U. (1988). Inter-relationships among ages of emergence of teeth A prospective longitudinal study of Swedish children from birth to 18 years. *Eur. J. Orthod.* 10 (3): 273–280.

167 Jayaraman, J., Wong, H.M., King, N., and Roberts, G. (2013). Secular trends in the maturation of permanent teeth in 5 to 6 years old children. *Am. J. Hum. Biol.* 25 (3): 329–334.

168 Eskeli, R., Lösönen, M., Ikävalko, T. et al. (2016). Secular trends affect timing of emergence of permanent teeth. *Angle Orthod.* 86 (1): 53–58.

169 Jayaraman, J. and Roberts, G.J. (2018). Comparison of dental maturation in Hong Kong Chinese and United Kingdom Caucasian populations. *Forensic Sci. Int.* 292: 61–70.

170 Warren, J.J., Fontana, M., Blanchette, D.R. et al. (2016). Timing of primary tooth emergence among U.S. racial and ethnic groups. *J. Public Health Dent.* 76 (4): 259–262.

171 Almonaitiene, R., Balciuniene, I., and Tutkuviene, J. (2012). Standards for permanent teeth emergence time and sequence in Lithuanian children. *Stomatologija* 14 (3): 93–100.

172 Baume, L.J. (1950). Physiological tooth migration and its significance for the development of occlusion. I. The biogenetic course of the deciduous dentition. *J. Dent. Res.* 29 (2): 123–132.

173 Baume, L.J. (1950). Physiological tooth migration and its significance for the development of the occlusion: the biogenesis of the accessional dentition. *J. Dent. Res.* 29 (3): 331–337.

174 Janiszewska-Olszowska, J., Stepien, P., and Syrynska, M. (2009). Spacing in deciduous dentition of Polish children in relation to tooth size and dental arch dimensions. *Arch. Oral Biol.* 54 (5): 397–402.

175 Sun, K.T., Li, Y.F., Hsu, J.T. et al. (2018). Prevalence of primate and interdental spaces for the primary dentition in 3-to 6-year-old children in Taiwan. *J. Formos. Med. Assoc.* 117 (7): 598–604.

176 Bishara, S.E., Khadivi, P., and Jakobsen, J.R. (1995). Changes in tooth size – arch length relationships from the deciduous to the permanent dentition: a longitudinal study. *Am. J. Orthod. Dentofac. Orthop.* 108 (6): 607–613.

177 Hixon, E.H. and Oldfather, R.E. (1958). Estimation of the sizes of unerupted cuspid and bicuspid teeth. *Angle Orthod.* 28 (4): 236–240.

178 Moorrees, C.F. and Chadha, J.M. (1962). Crown diameters of corresponding tooth groups in deciduous and permanent dentitions. *J. Dent. Res.* 41: 466–470.

179 Moorrees, C.F. and Reed, R.B. (1964). Correlations among crown diameters of human teeth. *Arch. Oral Biol.* 9 (6): 685–697.

180 Marshall, S.D., Caspersen, M., Hardinger, R.R. et al. (2008). Development of the curve of Spee. *Am. J. Orthod. Dentofac. Orthop.* 134 (3): 344–352.

181 Imai, H., Yakushiji, M., and Shintani, S. (2010). Longitudinal observation of the changes of the consecutive curve of the incisal edge, tip and cusp tip from deciduous to permanent dentition. *Ped. Dent. J.* 20 (2): 131–151.

182 Liversidge, H.M. (2015). Tooth eruption and timing. In: *A Companion to Dental Anthropology*, 1e (ed. J.D. Irish and G.R. Scott), 159–171. West Sussex, UK: John Wiley & Sons.

183 Richman, J.M. (2019). Shedding new light on the mysteries of tooth eruption. *Proc. Natl. Acad. Sci.* 116 (2): 353–355.

184 Marks, S. and Schroeder, H.E. (1996). Tooth eruption: theories and facts. *Anat. Rec.* 245 (2): 374–393.

185 Lee, C.F. and Proffit, W.R. (1995). The daily rhythm of human premolar eruption. *Am. J. Orthod. Dentofac. Orthop.* 107 (1): 38–47.

186 Risinger, R.K. and Proffit, W.R. (1996). Continuous overnight observation of human premolar eruption. *Arch. Oral Biol.* 41 (8-9): 779–789.

187 Becker, A. (1998). *The Orthodontic Treatment of Impacted Teeth*. London: Martin Dunitz.

188 Haralabakis, N.B., Yiagtzis, S.C., and Toutountzakis, N.M. (1994). Premature or delayed exfoliation of deciduous teeth and root resorption and formation. *Angle Orthod.* 64 (2): 151–157.

189 AlQahtani, S.J., Hector, M.P., and Liversidge, H.M. (2010). Brief communication: the London atlas of human tooth development and eruption. *Am. J. Phys. Anthropol.* 142 (3): 481–490.

190 Demirjian, A., Goldstein, H., and Tanner, J.M. (1973). A new system of dental age assessment. *Hum. Biol.* 45 (2): 211–227.

191 Palmer, C. (1891). Palmer's dental notation. *Dent. Cosmos.* 33: 194–198.

192 Lo, R.T. and Moyers, R.E. (1953). Studies on the etiology and prevention of malocclusion I. The sequence of eruption of the permanent dentition. *Am. J. Orthod.* 39 (6): 460–467.

193 Smith, B.H. and Garn, S.M. (1987). Polymorphisms in eruption sequence of permanent teeth in American children. *Am. J. Phys. Anthropol.* 74 (3): 289–303.

194 Knott, V.B. and Meredith, H.V. (1966). Statistics on the eruption of the permanent dentition from serial data for North American white children. *Angle* 36 (1): 68–79.

195 Savara, B.S. and Steen, J.C. (1978). Timing and sequence of eruption of permanent teeth in a longitudinal sample of children from Oregon. *J. Am. Dent. Assoc.* 97 (2): 209–214.

196 Leroy, R., Cecere, S., Lesaffre, E., and Declerck, D. (2008). Variability in permanent tooth emergence sequences in Flemish children. *Eur. J. Oral Sci.* 116 (1): 11–17.

197 Kennedy, D.B. (2009). Treatment strategies for ankylosed primary molars. *Eur. Arch. Paediatra Dent.* 10 (4): 201–210.

198 Pahel, B.T., Vann, W.F. Jr., Divaris, K., and Rozier, R.G. (2017). A contemporary examination of first and second permanent molar emergence. *J. Dent. Res.* 96 (10): 1115–1121.

199 Garn, S.M., Lewis, A.B., Koski, K., and Polacheck, D.L. (1958). The sex difference in tooth calcification. *J. Dent. Res.* 37 (3): 561–567.

200 Garn, S.M. and Rohmann, C.G. (1966). Interaction of nutrition and genetics in the timing of growth. *Pediat. Clin. North Am.* 13 (2): 353–359.

201 Hilgers, K.K., Akridge, M., Scheetz, J.P., and Kinane, D.E. (2006). Childhood obesity and dental development. *Pediatr. Dent.* 28 (1): 18–22.

202 Nicholas, C.L., Kadavy, K., Holton, N.E. et al. (2018). Childhood body mass index is associated with early dental development and eruption in a longitudinal sample from the Iowa Facial Growth Study. *Am. J. Orthod. Dentofac. Orthop.* 154 (1): 72.

203 Dhamo, B., Vucic, S., Kuijpers, M.A. et al. (2016). The association between hypodontia and dental development. *Clin. Oral Investig.* 20 (6): 1347–1354.

204 Almeida, E.R., Narvai, P.C., Frazão, P., and Guedes-Pinto, A.C. (2008). Revised criteria for the assessment and interpretation of occlusal deviations in the deciduous dentition: a public health perspective. *Cad. Saude Publica* 24 (4): 897–904.

205 Vegesna, M., Chandrasekhar, R., and Chandrappa, V. (2014). Occlusal characteristics and spacing in primary dentition: a gender comparative cross-sectional study. *Int. Sch. Res. Notices* 2014: 512680.

206 da Silva, L.P. and Gleiser, R. (2008). Occlusal development between primary and permanent dentitions: a 5-year longitudinal study. *J. Dent. Child (Chic.)* 75 (3): 287–294.

207 Barros, S.E., Chiqueto, K., Jansen, G., and Ferreira, E. (2015). Factors influencing molar relationship behavior in the mixed dentition. *Am. J. Orthod. Dentofac. Orthop.* 148 (5): 782–792.

208 Angle, E.H. (1907). *Treatment of Malocclusion of the Teeth*, 3e. Philadelphia: S.S. White Dental Manufacturing.

209 Southard, T.E., Marshall, S.D., and Bonner, L.L. (2015). *Orthodontics in the Vertical Dimension. A Case-Based Review*. Hoboken, NJ: John Wiley & Sons.

210 Alhammadi, M.S., Halboub, E., Fayed, M.S. et al. (2018). Global distribution of malocclusion traits: a systematic review. *Dent. Press J. Orthod.* 23 (6): 40e1–40e10.

211 Moorrees, C.F. and Reed, R.B. (1965). Changes in dental arch dimensions expressed on the basis of tooth eruption as a measure of biologic age. *J. Dent. Res.* 44 (1): 129–141.

212 Martins-Júnior, P.A. and Marques, L.S. (2012). Clinical implications of early loss of a lower deciduous canine. *Int. J. Orthod. Milwaukee* 23 (3): 23–27.

213 Kau, C.H., Durning, P., Richmond, S. et al. (2004). Extractions as a form of interception in the developing dentition: a randomized controlled trial. *J. Orthod.* 31 (2): 107–114.

214 Sjögren, A., Arnrup, K., Lennartsson, B., and Huggare, J. (2012). Mandibular incisor alignment and dental arch changes 1 year after extraction of deciduous canines. *Eur. J. Orthod.* 34 (5): 587–594.

215 Sayin, M.O. and Türkkahraman, H. (2006). Effects of lower primary canine extraction on the mandibular dentition. *Angle Orthod.* 76 (1): 31–35.

216 Yoshihara, T., Matsumoto, Y., Suzuki, J. et al. (2000). Effect of serial extraction alone on crowding: spontaneous changes in dentition after serial extraction. *Am. J. Orthod. Dentofac. Orthop.* 118 (6): 611–616.

217 Tunison, W., Flores-Mir, C., ElBadrawy, H. et al. (2008). Dental arch space changes following premature loss of primary first molars: a systematic review. *Pediatr. Dent.* 30 (4): 297–302.

218 Lin, Y.T. and Chang, L.C. (1998). Space changes after premature loss of the mandibular primary first molar: a longitudinal study. *J. Clin. Pediatr. Dent.* 22 (4): 311–316.

219 Cuoghi, O.A., Bertoz, F.A., de Mendonca, M.R., and Santos, E.C. (1998). Loss of space and dental arch length after the loss of the lower first primary molar: a longitudinal study. *J. Clin. Pediatr.* 22 (2): 117–120.

220 Padma Kumari, B. and Retnakumari, N. (2006). Loss of space and changes in the dental arch after premature loss of the lower primary molar: a longitudinal study. *J. Indian Soc. Pedod. Prev. Dent.* 24 (2): 90–96.

221 Macena, M.C., Tornisiello Katz, C.R., Heimer, M.V. et al. (2011). Space changes after premature loss of deciduous molars among Brazilian children. *Am. J. Orthod. Dentofac. Orthop.* 140 (6): 771–778.

222 Moss, J.P. and Picton, D.C. (1982). Short-term changes in the mesiodistal position of teeth following removal of approximal contacts in the monkey Macaca fascicularis. *Arch. Oral Biol.* 27 (3): 273–278.

223 Northway, W.M. (2000). The not-so-harmless maxillary primary first molar extraction. *J. Am. Dent. Assoc.* 131 (12): 1711–1720.

224 Lin, Y.T., Lin, W.H., and Lin, Y.T. (2011). Twelve-month space changes after premature loss of a primary maxillary first molar. *Int. J. Pediatr. Dent.* 21 (3): 161–166.

225 Park, K., Jung, D.W., and Kim, J. (2009). Three-dimensional space changes after premature loss of a maxillary primary first molar. *Int. J. Ped. Dent.* 19 (6): 383–389.

226 Owen, D.G. (1971). The incidence and nature of space closing following premature extraction of deciduous teeth: a literature survey. *Am. J. Orthod.* 59 (1): 37–49.

227 Frazier-Bowers, S.A., Puranik, C.P., and Mahaney, M.C. (2010). The etiology of disruption disorders – further evidence of a genetic paradigm. *Semin. Orthod.* 16 (3): 180–185.

228 Badrov, J., Lauc, T., Nakas, E., and Galic, I. (2017). Dental age and tooth development in orthodontic patients with agenesis of permanent teeth. *Biomed. Res. Int.* 2017: 8683970. https://doi.org/10.1155/2017/8683970. Epub 2017 Feb 26. PMID: 28331854; PMCID: PMC5346386.

229 Park, M.K., Shin, M.K., Kim, S.O. et al. (2017). Prevalence of delayed tooth development and its relation to tooth agenesis in Korean children. *Arch. Oral Biol.* 73: 243–247.

230 Ducommun, F., Bornstein, M.M., Bosshardt, D. et al. (2018). Diagnosis of tooth ankylosis using panoramic views, cone beam computed tomography, and histological data: a retrospective observational case series study. *Eur. J. Orthod.* 40 (3): 231–238.

231 de Souza, R.F., Travess, H., Newton, T., and Marchesan, M.A. (2015). Interventions for treating traumatised ankylosed permanent front teeth. *Cochrane Database Syst. Rev.* 2015 (12): CD007820.

232 Brearley, L.J. and McKibben, D.H. Jr. (1973). Ankylosis of primary molar teeth. I. Prevalence and characteristics. *ASDC J. Dent. Child.* 40 (1): 54–63.

233 Messer, L.B. and Cline, J.T. (1980). Ankylosed primary molars: results and treatment recommendations from an eight-year longitudinal study. *Pediatr. Dent.* 2 (1): 37–47.

234 Kurol, J. and Thilander, B. (1984). Infraocclusion of primary molars and the effect on occlusal development: a longitudinal study. *Eur. J. Orthod.* 6 (4): 277–293.

235 Kurol, J. and Koch, G. (1985). The effect of extraction of infraoccluded deciduous molars: a longitudinal study. *Am. J. Orthod.* 87 (1): 46–55.

236 Kurol, J. and Olson, L. (1991). Ankylosis of primary molars--a future periodontal threat to the first permanent molars? *Eur. J. Orthod.* 13 (5): 404–409.

237 Tieu, L.D., Walker, S.L., Major, M.P., and Flores-Mir, C. (2013). Management of ankylosed primary molars with premolar successors. *J. Am. Dent. Assoc.* 144 (6): 602–611.

238 Arhakis, A. and Boutiou, E. (2016). Etiology, diagnosis, consequences and treatment of infraoccluded primary molars. *Open Dent. J.* 30 (10): 714–719.

239 Dias, C., Closs, L.Q., Fontanella, V., and de Araujo, F.B. (2012). Vertical alveolar growth in subjects with infraoccluded mandibular deciduous molars. *Am. J. Orthod. Dentofac. Orthop.* 141 (1): 81–86.

240 Shalish, M., Peck, S., Wasserstein, A., and Peck, L. (2010). Increased occurrence of dental anomalies associated with infraocclusion of deciduous molars. *Angle Orthod.* 80 (3): 440–445.

241 Cahill, D.R. and Marks, S.C. Jr. (1980). Tooth eruption: evidence for the central role of the dental follicle. *J. Oral Path.* 9 (4): 189–200.

242 Grippaudo, C., Cafiero, C., D'Apolito, I. et al. (2018). Primary failure of eruption: clinical and genetic findings in the mixed dentition. *Angle Orthod.* 88 (3): 275–282.

243 Juuri, E. and Balic, A. (2017). The biology underlying abnormalities of tooth number in humans. *J. Dent. Res.* 96 (11): 1248–1256.

244 Kreiborg, S. and Jensen, B.L. (2018). Tooth formation and eruption – lessons learnt from cleidocranial dysplasia. *Eur. J. Oral Sci.* 126 (Suppl 1): 72–80.

245 Brook, A.H., Jernvall, J., Smith, R.N. et al. (2014 Jun). The dentition: the outcomes of morphogenesis leading

to variations of tooth number, size and shape. *Aust. Dent. J.* 59 (Suppl 1): 131–142.

246 Boeira Junior, B.R. and Echeverrigaray, S. (2012). Polymorphism in the MSX1 gene in a family with upper lateral incisor agenesis. *Arch. Oral Biol.* 57 (10): 1423–1428.

247 Balic, A. and Thesleff, I. (2015). Tissue interactions regulating tooth development and renewal. *Curr. Top. Dev. Biol.* 115: 157–186.

248 Garib, D.G., Peck, S., and Gomes, S.C. (2009). Increased occurrence of dental anomalies associated with second-premolar agenesis. *Angle Orthod.* 79 (3): 436–441.

249 Garib, D.G., Alencar, B.M., Lauris, J.R., and Baccetti, T. (2010). Agenesis of maxillary lateral incisors and associated dental anomalies. *Am. J. Orthod. Dentofac. Orthop.* 137 (6): 732.e1–732.e6.

250 Kreczi, A., Proff, P., Reicheneder, C., and Faltermeier, A. (2011). Effects of hypodontia on craniofacial structures and mandibular growth pattern. *Head Face Med.* 7: 23–28.

251 Bertl, M.H., Bertl, K., Wagner, M. et al. (2016). Second premolar agenesis is associated with mandibular form: a geometric morphometric analysis of mandibular cross-sections. *Int. J. Oral Sci.* 8 (4): 254–260.

252 Sletten, D.W., Smith, B.M., Southard, K.A. et al. (2003). Retained deciduous mandibular molars in adults: a radiographic study of long-term changes. *Am. J. Orthod. Dentofac. Orthop.* 124 (6): 625–630.

253 Hvaring, C.L. and Birkeland, K. (2019). The long-term fate of persisting deciduous molars and canines in 42 patients with severe hypodontia: a 12-year follow-up. *Eur. J. Orthod.* 42 (6): cjz090.

254 Wang, X.P. and Fan, J. (2011). Molecular genetics of supernumerary tooth formation. *Genesis* 49 (4): 261–277.

255 Van Buggenhout, G. and Bailleul-Forestier, I. (2008). Mesiodens. *Eur. J. Med. Genet.* 51 (2): 178–181.

256 Hua, F., He, H., Ngan, P., and Bouzid, W. (2013). Prevalence of peg-shaped maxillary permanent lateral incisors: a meta-analysis. *Am. J. Orthod. Dentofac. Orthop.* 144 (1): 97–109.

257 Rutledge, M.S. and Hartsfield, J.K. Jr. (2010). Genetic factors in the etiology of palatally displaced canines. *Semin. Orthod.* 16 (3): 165–171.

258 Peck, S. (2016). Misleading article on palatally displaced canines. *Am. J. Orthod. Dentofac. Orthop.* 149 (2): 149–150.

259 Chung, D.D., Weisberg, M., and Pagala, M. (2011). Incidence and effects of genetic factors on canine impaction in an isolated Jewish population. *Am. J. Orthod. Dentofac. Orthop.* 139 (4): e331–e335.

260 Becker, A. and Chaushu, S. (2015). Etiology of maxillary canine impaction: a review. *Am. J. Orthod. Dentofac. Orthop.* 148 (4): 557–567.

261 Cheyne, V.D. and Wessels, K.E. (1947). Impaction of permanent first molar with resorption and space loss in region of deciduous second molar. *J. Am. Dent. Assoc.* 35 (11): 774–787.

262 Young, D.H. (1957). Ectopic eruption of the first permanent molar. *J. Dent. Child.* 24: 153–162.

263 O'Meara, W.F. (1962). Ectopic eruption pattern in selected permanent teeth. *J. Dent. Res.* 41: 607–616.

264 Pulver, F. (1968). The etiology and prevalence of ectopic eruption of the maxillary first permanent molar. *ASDC J. Dent. Child.* 35 (2): 138–146.

265 Bjerklin, K. and Kurol, J. (1981). Prevalence of ectopic eruption of the maxillary first permanent molar. *Swed. Dent. J.* 5 (1): 29–34.

266 Kimmel, N.A., Gellin, M.E., Bohannan, H., and Kaplan, A.L. (1982). Ectopic eruption of maxillary first permanent molars in different areas of the United States. *ASDC J. Dent. Child.* 49 (4): 294–299.

267 Chintakanon, K. and Boonpinon, P. (1998). Ectopic eruption of the first permanent molars: prevalence and etiologic factors. *Angle Orthod.* 68 (2): 153–160.

268 Barberia-Leache, E., Suarez-Clúa, M.C., and Saavedra-Ontiveros, D. (2005). Ectopic eruption of the maxillary first permanent molar: Characteristics and occurrence in growing children. *Angle Orthod.* 75 (4): 610–615.

269 Bjerklin, K. (1994). Ectopic eruption of the maxillary first permanent molar. An epidemiological, familial, etiological and longitudinal clinical study. *Swed. Den. J. Suppl.* 100: 1–66.

270 Howe, R.P., McNamara, J.A. Jr., and O'Connor, K.A. (1983). An examination of dental crowding and its relationship to tooth size and arch dimension. *Am. J. Orthod.* 83 (5): 363–373.

271 Sayin, M.O. and Türkkahraman, H. (2004). Factors contributing to mandibular anterior crowding in the early mixed dentition. *Angle Orthod.* 74 (6): 754–758.

272 Agenter, M.K., Harris, E.F., and Blair, R.N. (2009). Influence of tooth crown size on malocclusion. *Am. J. Orthod. Dentofac. Orthop.* 136 (6): 795–804.

273 Arif, A., Rasheed, T., and Ali, A. (2014). Dental crowding and its relationship to tooth size and arch dimensions. *J. Nat. Sci. Res.* 4 (10): 133–136.

274 Weinstein, S., Haack, D.C., Morris, L.Y. et al. (1963). On an equilibrium theory of tooth position. *Angle Orthod.* 33 (1): 1–26.

275 Proffit, W.R. (1978). Equilibrium theory revisited: Factors influencing position of the teeth. *Angle Orthod.* 48 (3): 175–186.

276 Solow, B. (1980). The dentoalveolar compensatory mechanism: background and clinical implications. *Br. J. Orthod.* 7 (3): 145–161.

277 Buschang, P.H. (2014). Class I malocclusions – the development and etiology of mandibular malalignments. *Semin. Orthod.* 20 (1): 3–15.

278 Southard, T.E., Behrents, R.G., and Tolley, E.A. (1989). The anterior component of occlusal force. Part 1. Measurement and distribution. *Am. J. Orthod. Dentofac. Orthop.* 96 (6): 493–500.

279 Southard, T.E., Behrents, R.G., and Tolley, E.A. (1990). The anterior component of occlusal force. Part 2. Relationship with dental malalignment. *Am. J. Orthod. Dentofac. Orthop.* 97 (1): 41–44.

280 Driscoll-Gilliland, J., Buschang, P.H., and Behrents, R.G. (2001). An evaluation of growth and stability in untreated and treated subjects. *Am. J. Orthod. Dentofac. Orthop.* 120 (6): 588–597.

281 Goldberg, A.I., Behrents, R.G., Oliver, D.R., and Buschang, P.H. (2013). Facial divergence and mandibular crowding in treated subjects. *Angle Orthod.* 83 (3): 381–388.

282 Moyers, R.E. (1973). *Handbook of Orthodontics for the Student and General Practitioner*, 3e. Chicago: Year Book Medical Publishers.

283 Luu, N.S., Mandich, M.A., Tieu, L.D. et al. (2011). The validity and reliability of mixed-dentition analysis methods: a systematic review. *J. Am. Dent. Assoc.* 142 (10): 1143–1153.

284 Tanaka, M.M. and Johnston, L.E. (1974). The prediction of the size of unerupted canines and premolars in a contemporary orthodontic population. *J. Am. Dent. Assoc.* 88 (4): 798–801.

285 Larsson, E. (1983). Prevalence of crossbite among children with prolonged dummy- and finger-sucking habit. *Swed. Dent. J.* 7: 115–119.

286 Larsson, E. (1987). The effect of finger-sucking on the occlusion: a review. *Eur. J. Orthod.* 9 (1): 279–282.

287 Ricketts, R.M. (1968). Respiratory obstruction syndrome. *Am. J. Orthod.* 54 (7): 495–507.

288 Paul, J.L. and Nanda, R.S. (1973). Effects of mouth breathing on dental occlusion. *Angle Orthod.* 43 (2): 201–206.

289 Schendel, S.A., Eisenfeld, J., Bell, W.H. et al. (1976). The long face syndrome: vertical maxillary excess. *Am. J. Orthod.* 70 (4): 398–408.

290 Rubin, R.M. (1980). Mode of respiration and facial growth. *Am. J. Orthod.* 78 (5): 504–510.

291 McNamara, J.A. Jr. (1981). Influence of respiratory pattern on craniofacial growth. *Angle Orthod.* 51 (4): 269–300.

292 Cheng, M.C., Enlow, D.H., Papsidero, M. et al. (1988). Developmental effects of impaired breathing in the face of the growing child. *Angle Orthod.* 58 (4): 309–320.

293 Bresolin, D., Shapiro, P.A., Shapiro, G.G. et al. (1983). Mouth breathing in allergic children: its relationship to dentofacial development. *Am. J. Orthod.* 83 (4): 334–340.

294 Vig, P.S. (1985). Respiration, nasal airway, and orthodontics: a review of current clinical concepts and research. In: *New Vistas in Orthodontics* (ed. L.E. Johnston Jr.), 76–102. Philadelphia: Lea & Febiger.

295 Güray, E. and Karaman, A.I. (2002). Effects of adenoidectomy on dentofacial structures: a 6-year longitudinal study. *World J. Orthod.* 3 (1): 73–81.

296 Preston, B. (2005). The upper airway and cranial morphology. In: *Orthodontics: Current Principles and Techniques* (ed. L. Graber, R. Vanarsdall and K.W.L. Vig), 117–143. St. Louis: Mosby.

297 Souki, B.Q., Pimenta, G.B., Souki, M.Q. et al. (2009). Prevalence of malocclusion among mouth breathing children: do expectations meet reality? *Int. J. Pediatr. Otorhinolaryngol.* 73 (5): 767–773.

2

Crowding

Introduction

Recent graduates tell us, "Decisions related to crowding are the most frequent early treatment decisions I have to make." This section provides a review of the diagnosis and treatment of early crowding. By studying this chapter carefully, you will establish a framework for making decisions to either monitor (recall), employ space maintenance, institute space regaining, or begin serial extraction for children with crowding.

Q: In order to estimate how much space is needed for tooth eruption or alignment, it is helpful to memorize the average widths of permanent teeth – at least the anterior teeth and premolars. What are the *average* mesiodistal widths (in millimeters) of each *permanent* maxillary and mandibular tooth? [1]

A:

Maxillary Central Incisor	8.5	Mandibular Central Incisor	5.0
Maxillary Lateral Incisor	6.5	Mandibular Lateral Incisor	5.5
Maxillary Canine	7.5	Mandibular Canine	7.0
Maxillary First Premolar	7.0	Mandibular First Premolar	7.0
Maxillary Second Premolar	7.0	Mandibular Second Premolar	7.0
Maxillary First Molar	10.0	Mandibular First Molar	11.0
Maxillary Second Molar	9.0	Mandibular Second Molar	10.5

Q: What are the *average* mesiodistal widths (in millimeters) of each *primary* maxillary and mandibular tooth? [1]

A:

Maxillary Central Incisor	6.5	Mandibular Central Incisor	4.2
Maxillary Lateral Incisor	5.1	Mandibular Lateral Incisor	4.1
Maxillary Canine	7.0	Mandibular Canine	5.0
Maxillary First Molar	7.3	Mandibular First Molar	7.7
Maxillary Second Molar	8.2	Mandibular Second Molar	9.9

Q: How do you estimate maxillary and mandibular anterior crowding?

A: One simple technique is to add together all the space needed to align the teeth at each contact – from distal of left canine to distal of right canine. In other words, *estimate how much tooth enamel would need to be removed* in order to provide room to align the teeth.

Let us illustrate this technique using the mandibular arch drawing shown in Figure 2.1a, which includes an unerupted mandibular right lateral incisor.

Contact	Estimated crowding (space needed)
Left Canine – Left First Premolar (Figure 2.1b)	0.2 mm (slight canine rotation)
Left Lateral Incisor – Left Canine (Figure 2.1c)	2.0 mm
Left Central Incisor – Left Lateral Incisor (Figure 2.1d)	1.0 mm
Right Central Incisor – Left Central Incisor (Figure 2.1e)	1.0 mm
Since the right lateral incisor is unerupted, we compare its anticipated mesiodistal width (5.5 mm) with the 5 mm space, which is currently present (Figure 2.1f)	0.5 mm
Right First Premolar – Right Permanent Canine (Figure 2.1g)	1.0 mm (right canine rotated)
Total	*5.7 mm*

Practical Early Orthodontic Treatment: A Case-Based Review, First Edition. Thomas E. Southard, Steven D. Marshall, Laura L. Bonner, and Kyungsup Shin.
© 2023 John Wiley & Sons, Inc. Published 2023 by John Wiley & Sons, Inc.
Companion website: www.wiley.com/go/southard/practical

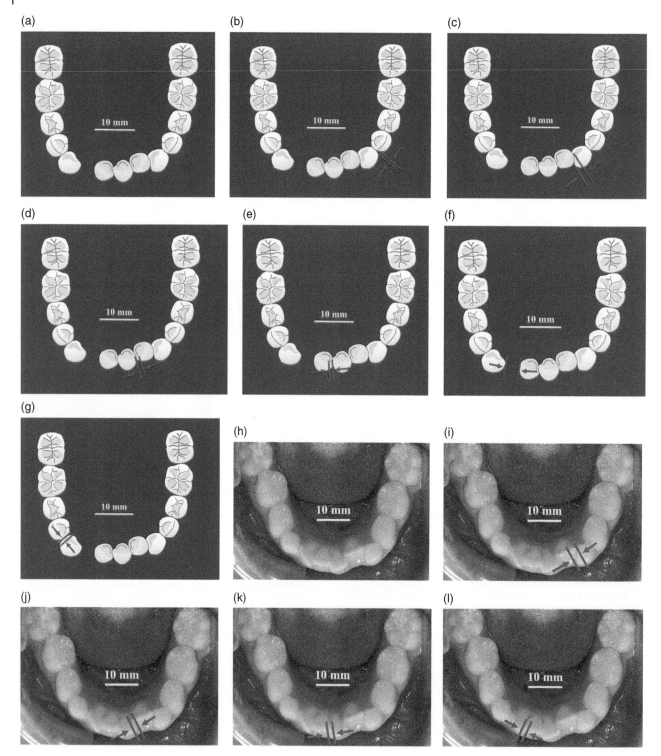

Figure 2.1 (a-q) Estimating anterior crowding.

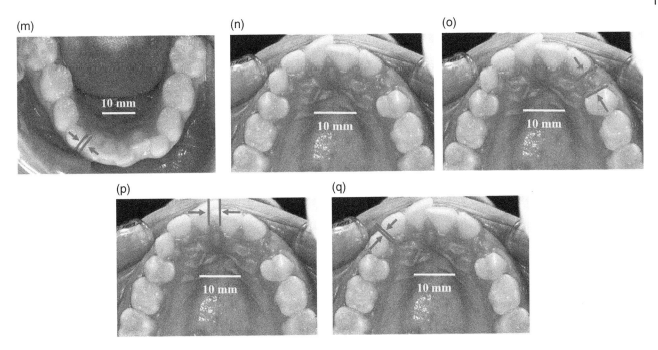

(m) (n) (o) (p) (q)

Figure 2.1 (Continued)

We calculated 5.7 mm of anterior crowding in this drawing. Next, repeat this technique using the arch starting with Figure 2.1h.

Contact	Estimated crowding (space needed)
Left Primary Canine – Left Primary First Molar (Figure 2.1h)	0.0 mm (teeth are aligned)
Left Lateral Incisor – Left Primary Canine (Figure 2.1i)	2.0 mm
Left Central Incisor – Left Lateral Incisor (Figure 2.1j)	1.0 mm
Right Central Incisor – Left Central Incisor (Figure 2.1k)	1.0 mm
Right Lateral Incisor – Right Central Incisor (Figure 2.1l)	1.0 mm
Right Lateral Incisor – Right Primary Canine (Figure 2.1m)	1.0 mm
Right Canine – Right Primary First Molar (Figure 2.1h)	0.0 mm (teeth are aligned)
Total	*6.0 mm*

We calculated 6 mm of mandibular anterior crowding. Finally, repeat this technique using the arch shown starting in Figure 2.1n.

Contact	Estimated crowding (space needed)
Since the left canine is unerupted, we compare its anticipated mesiodistal width (7.5 mm) with the 6.5 mm space, which is currently present (Figure 2.1o)	1.0 mm
Left Lateral Incisor – Left Central Incisor (Figure 2.1n)	0.0 mm (teeth are aligned)
Left Central Incisor – Right Central Incisor (Figure 2.1p)	3.5 mm
Right Central Incisor – Right Lateral Incisor (Figure 2.1n)	0.0 mm (teeth are aligned)
Right Lateral Incisor – Right Primary Canine (Figure 2.1q)	0.1 mm
Right Primary Canine – Right Premolar (Figure 2.1n)	0.0 mm (teeth are aligned)
Total	*4.6 mm*

We calculate 4.6 mm of maxillary anterior crowding in Figure 2.1n. With practice, this technique is accurate and quick.

Q: What would be a reasonable *millimetric* range of mild, moderate, and severe anterior tooth crowding?

A: *Mild (1–3 mm), moderate (4–8 mm), severe (≥9 mm)*

Q: What is a reliable indicator of *severe* mandibular anterior crowding?

A: A reliable indicator of severe developing mandibular anterior crowding is *premature loss of primary canines – not* lack of interdental spacing. Why? In crowded mandibular arches, the permanent lateral incisors often erupt and resorb the mesial portion of the root of deciduous canines, causing their premature loss [2].

Q: Can you suggest general principles (guidelines) to follow when managing crowding in the primary, early mixed, and late mixed dentitions?

A: *Principle: for most patients, first attempt non-extraction treatment.*

- *Consider monitoring (recalling) patients with crowding in the primary/early mixed dentition.* This is assuming that the permanent canine and premolar roots are immature (less than ½ developed) – that is, that the canines and premolars are not close to eruption. This is also assuming that you judge the potential harm from monitoring to be minimal (e.g. the probability of root resorption from ectopically erupting teeth to be minimal).
- *Consider space maintenance* for patients with mild-to-moderate crowding in the late mixed dentition. Space maintenance (LLHA or Nance holding arch) can provide room (leeway space or "E-space") for permanent teeth to erupt and align in many patients without extraction of permanent teeth.
- *Generally, defer extraction decisions until permanent canines and premolars erupt* whenever possible *(reduce unknowns before committing to irreversible treatment – including extractions).* Once the permanent canines and premolars erupt, a more accurate assessment of crowding (and a clearer decision to extract) can be made.
- *Generally, defer extraction decisions until anteroposterior growth is addressed (reduce unknowns before committing to irreversible treatment).* Get future growth under control before extracting permanent teeth! Once you extract permanent teeth, those teeth cannot be put back even if the patient grows out of your correction.
- Exceptions to the above, when extraction of primary or permanent teeth should be considered, include cases of space regaining, ectopic eruption, incisor dehiscence, eruption into nonkeratinized gingiva, and severe crowding.
- We generally recommend serial extraction in early mixed dentition patients with *severe anterior crowding and only if the patient is normal otherwise (anteroposteriorly, vertically, and transversely).*

Q: Can you briefly state four options for dealing with anterior dental crowding in children?

A: Options include:

- Monitoring (recall)
- Space maintenance
- Space regaining
- Eliminating tooth mass to create space by extraction of teeth or interproximal reduction (IPR) of enamel

Q: What is *space maintenance*?

A: Space maintenance is the prevention of arch perimeter loss (arch length loss) subsequent to primary tooth exfoliation. One important role of primary teeth is to hold space for permanent successors. When a primary tooth is lost, the adjacent erupted teeth are pulled together by transseptal fibers. They drift into the lost primary tooth space. This drifting may diminish arch perimeter, create undesirable occlusal changes, and impact erupting permanent teeth. Space maintenance seeks to prevent drifting.

Q: Figure 2.2 illustrates mandibular anterior crowding in a patient entering the late mixed dentition stage of development. Can you estimate the mandibular anterior crowding?

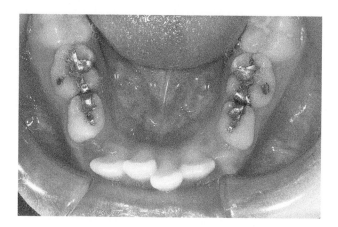

Figure 2.2 Mandibular anterior crowding in a mixed dentition patient.

A: Let us repeat the analysis we just performed:

Contact	Estimated crowding (space needed)
Since the left permanent canine is unerupted, we compare its anticipated mesiodistal width (7mm) with the 3.5mm space currently present	3.5mm
Left Lateral Incisor – Left Central Incisor	0.2mm

Contact	Estimated crowding (space needed)
Left Central Incisor – Right Central Incisor	1.5 mm
Right Central Incisor – Right Lateral Incisor	0.0 mm
Right Canine – since it is unerupted, we compare its anticipated mesiodistal width (7 mm) with the 3.5 mm space present	3.5 mm
Total estimated anterior crowding	8.7 mm

Q: How would you manage the mandibular anterior crowding shown in Figure 2.2?

A: We attempted non-extraction treatment by employing space maintenance. We fabricated and cemented an LLHA. As the primary molars exfoliated, premolars replaced them, and crowding decreased (Figure 2.3a). Note the residual ~3 mm of crowding (rotated mandibular canines).

A mandibular model from another patient with mild anterior crowding is illustrated in Figure 2.3b. How would you manage this crowding? Again, employing space maintenance with an LLHA resulted in spontaneous incisor alignment (Figure 2.3c).

Q: Spontaneous improved alignment of crowded mandibular incisors in mixed dentition patients is achieved by placing LLHAs. *Where* does the space come from that permits this spontaneous alignment?

A: The sum of the mesiodistal widths of mandibular primary canines plus mandibular primary first molars plus mandibular primary second molars is greater than the sum of the mesiodistal widths of their permanent successors. By maintaining the distance from the permanent first molars to the incisors with an

(a)

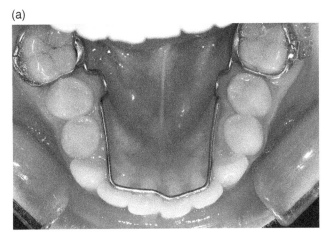

(b)

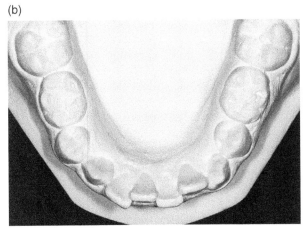

(c)

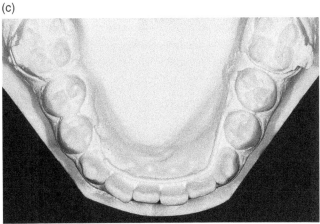

Figure 2.3 Effect of mandibular space maintenance using LLHAs (lower lingual holding arches). (a) Patient from Figure 2.2 after LLHA placement and eruption of permanent teeth, (b) initial model of another patient in the late mixed dentition, and (c) after placement of an LLHA, exfoliation of mandibular primary second molars, eruption of second premolars, and spontaneous incisor alignment.

LLHA, residual space remains when the primary teeth exfoliate and their successors replace them. This is where the space comes from. This space is called *leeway space*.

Q: Using the average mesiodistal widths of primary and permanent teeth we listed earlier [1], can you estimate the potential leeway space available in mandibular and maxillary arches?

A: Start by calculating the average *mandibular* leeway space per side:
- Sum of mandibular primary canine, primary first molar, and primary second molar mesiodistal widths = 5.0 mm + 7.7 mm + 9.9 mm = 22.6 mm.
- Sum of mandibular permanent canine, first premolar, and second premolar mesiodistal widths = 7.0 mm + 7.0 mm + 7.0 mm = 21.0 mm.
- Average mandibular leeway space = 22.6 mm – 21.0 mm = *1.6 mm per side of arch*.

Now, calculate the average *maxillary* leeway space per side:
- Sum of maxillary primary canine, primary first molar, and primary second molar mesiodistal widths = 7.0 mm + 7.3 mm + 8.2 mm = 22.5 mm.
- Sum of maxillary permanent canine, first premolar, and second premolar mesiodistal widths = 7.5 mm + 7.0 mm + 7.0 mm = 21.5 mm.
- Average maxillary leeway space = 22.5 mm – 21.5 mm = *1.0 mm per side of arch*.

In other words, the average *mandibular leeway space is 1.6 mm per side* (3.2 mm for the mandibular arch), and the average *maxillary leeway space is 1.0 mm per side* (2 mm for the maxillary arch). This value is less than the value reported by Moyers [3, 4] (2.5 mm per side or 5 mm for the mandibular arch), but we will use our value (calculated from Wheeler's data) because it provides a more conservative estimate of future available space. Of course, *the leeway space found in any individual patient will depend upon the actual size of their primary and permanent teeth.*

Q: We have explained the concept of leeway space. What is "E-space"?

A: "E-space" is the difference in mesiodistal widths between primary second molars and their permanent successors (second premolars).

Q: Can you calculate mandibular "E-space"?

A: Mandibular "E-space" equals the difference in mesiodistal widths between mandibular primary second molars and mandibular second premolars, or: 9.9 mm – 7.0 mm = *2.9 mm per side*.

Q: Can you calculate maxillary "E-space"?

A: Maxillary "E-space" equals the difference in mesiodistal widths between maxillary primary second molars and maxillary second premolars, or: 8.2 mm – 7.0 mm = *1.2 mm per side*.

Q: Why is the concept of "E-space" important?

A: Children will often present with erupted permanent canines and erupted first premolars but unerupted second premolars (see Figure 2.3b). In these cases, leeway space is no longer valid, but "E space" can provide an estimate of future space available (for spontaneous incisor alignment if space maintenance is employed).

Q: Does a "D-space" also exist?

A: Yes, it is smaller than "E-space," but for the mandible, it would equal 7.7 mm – 7.0 mm = 0.7 mm per side (the difference in mesiodistal widths between mandibular primary first molars and mandibular first premolars).

Q: *How* does spontaneous alignment of crowded mandibular anterior teeth occur after LLHA placement in the mixed dentition?

A: First, examine what happens *without* an LLHA (Figure 2.4a, top left and bottom left). When the mandibular primary canines and primary molars exfoliate (Figure 2.4a, top center and bottom center), leeway space is created because the sum of the primary teeth mesiodistal widths exceeds the sum of their permanent successor mesiodistal widths. Probably, as a result of transseptal fiber contraction, mandibular molars drift mesially (yellow arrows), canines and incisors drift distally (red arrows), posterior spaces close, and incisors align minimally and upright [5, 6].

This mesial molar drift can benefit an "end-on" molar relationship, moving mandibular molars into a Class I relationship. However, mesial molar drift uses up leeway space that could be used to align crowded anterior teeth, and mandibular incisors are left crowded (Figure 2.4a, top right and bottom right).

Next, examine what happens *with* an LLHA. Once again, when mandibular primary canines and primary molars exfoliate (Figure 2.4b, top center and bottom center), leeway space is created. However, in this case mandibular molars attempt to drift mesially, but the molars are inhibited from doing so by the lower lingual arch pressing against the incisor lingual surfaces. Instead, transseptal fiber contraction closes the leeway space by retracting canines and retracting/aligning incisors (Figure 2.4b, top right and bottom right).

(a)

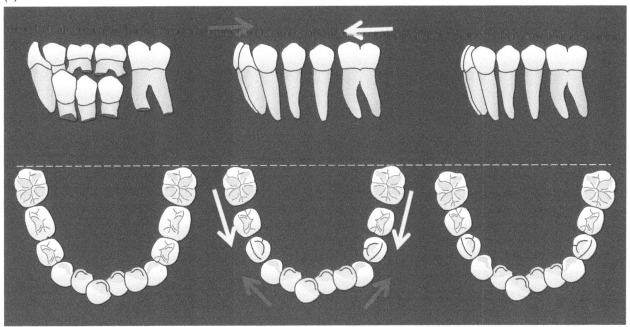

(b)

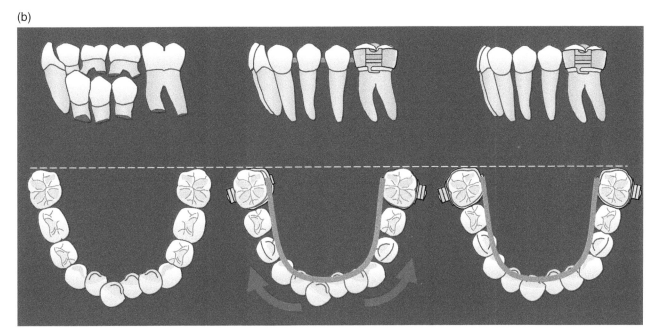

Figure 2.4 Transition between mixed and permanent dentitions. (a) Crowded mandibular arch *without* an LLHA. Note mesial molar drift with minimal improvement of mandibular anterior crowding. (b) Crowded mandibular arch *with* an LLHA in place. Note improved alignment of mandibular anterior teeth.

On the one hand, with an LLHA in place, an end-on Class II molar relationship will *not* improve by mesial permanent molar mesial drift. Instead, the end-on Class II relationship must be corrected by some other means (headgear, Class II functional appliance, Class II elastics, etc.). On the other hand, in patients with Class III molar relationships, an LLHA can prevent mesial molar drift and worsening of the Class III molar relationship.

One final note: mandibular first permanent molars do move *slightly* to the mesial with an LLHA in place. As they do this, they push the mandibular incisors slightly forward with the lingual arch bar (proclining the incisors) [5, 7]. But, *the primary effect of the LLHA is spontaneous improvement of incisor alignment.*

Q: How did spontaneous alignment of crowded mandibular anterior teeth with LLHA occur for the patient shown in Figures 2.2 and 2.3a?

A: Our original estimate of mandibular anterior crowding for the patient in Figure 2.2 was 8.7 mm. If we assume 2.9 mm of "E-space" per side with an LLHA (5.8 mm total), and 0.7 mm "D-space" per side (1.4 mm total), then upon complete emergence of mandibular premolars and canines, the remaining anticipated crowding was 1.5 mm, which is close to the actual ~3 mm found.

Remember, leeway space, "E-space", and "D-space" are based on average values. Every patient is different.

Q: When was use of the LLHA first reported?

A: Dewey [6] and Mershon [8] first reported use of the LLHA in 1916–1917.

Q: What percentage of mixed-dentition patients may be treated to satisfactory mandibular anterior alignment, without extraction of permanent teeth, using an LLHA?

A: It is estimated that *76% of patients can be treated non-extraction in the mandible with use of an LLHA* [9, 10]. If 2 mm or less of crowding is permitted, this percentage increases to 84% [11]. These success percentages are the reason why we recommend first attempting non-extraction treatment in mixed dentition patients.

Q: What is the effect of an LLHA on the developing *vertical* dimension? In other words, what is the effect of an LLHA on mandibular permanent first molar eruption? When can this effect be beneficial?

A: One study reported that LLHAs are effective in *reducing mandibular first permanent molar eruption by 1–2 mm over a 1–2 year period*, compared with controls [11]. In growing patients, reduction of mandibular first permanent molar eruption can reduce downward and backward mandibular plane rotation, reduce LAFH, increase chin projection, and improve Class II relationships.

Q: What do you observe in Figure 2.5? Assuming the patient is skeletally normal, has a Class I molar relationship, and has normal mandibular incisor angulation, what early treatment would you recommend?

A: The patient is in the early mixed dentition stage of dental development with moderate mandibular incisor crowding (~6 mm anterior crowding, blocked out mandibular left lateral incisor). Placement of an LLHA

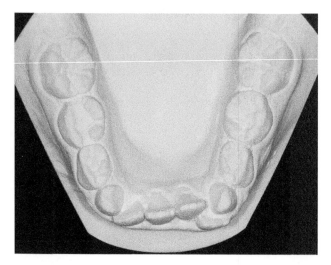

Figure 2.5 Mandibular arch model.

before exfoliation of the primary teeth would permit some spontaneous alignment (~3.2 mm of leeway space) during the transition from mixed to permanent dentition.

Q: We placed an LLHA. Figure 2.6 shows the same patient following permanent tooth eruption. What do you observe now?

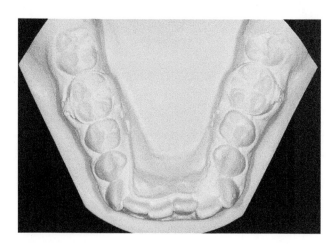

Figure 2.6 The same mandibular arch of Figure 2.5 after placement of an LLHA and eruption of permanent teeth.

A: There has been significant improvement in mandibular anterior teeth alignment.

Q: Should an LLHA be removed once all permanent teeth erupt?

A: Not necessarily. Consider leaving the LLHA until *after* placement of fixed orthodontic appliances. Why? Alignment is maintained.

(a)

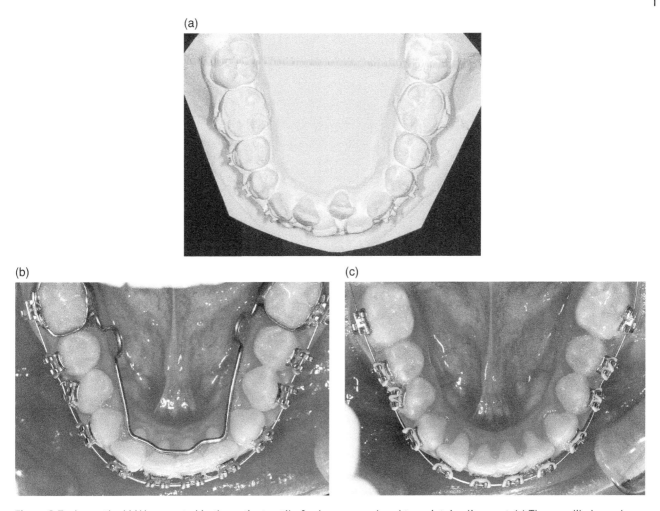

(b)   (c)

Figure 2.7 Leave the LLHA cemented in the patient until *after* braces are placed to maintain alignment. (a) The mandibular arch shown in Figure 2.6 on the day braces were placed six months after the LLHA was removed. Note the increased incisor crowding compared with Figure 2.6 (b, c) A different patient showing our recommended removal of the LLHA *after* braces are bonded. Alignment was maintained.

We ignored this recommendation for the patient in Figures 2.5 and 2.6. Instead, we removed the LLHA, and significant crowding occurred by the time brackets were placed (Figure 2.7a).

However, following this recommendation for another patient (Figure 2.7b), you see that the LLHA was left in place until the mandibular arch was bonded with fixed appliances. At that time, the LLHA was removed (Figure 2.7c) and the permanent first molars were bonded. Anterior alignment was maintained.

Q: You screen a nine-year-old patient (Figure 2.8). His mandibular left primary second molar recently exfoliated, his right primary first molar is ready to exfoliate, and his right primary second molar is very mobile. Your lab may take weeks to fabricate an LLHA. What can you do to prevent mesial molar drift until placement of an LLHA?

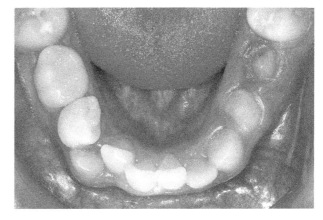

Figure 2.8 Mandibular left primary second molar recently exfoliated. We are concerned that the left permanent first molar will drift mesially by the time our lab can fabricate an LLHA.

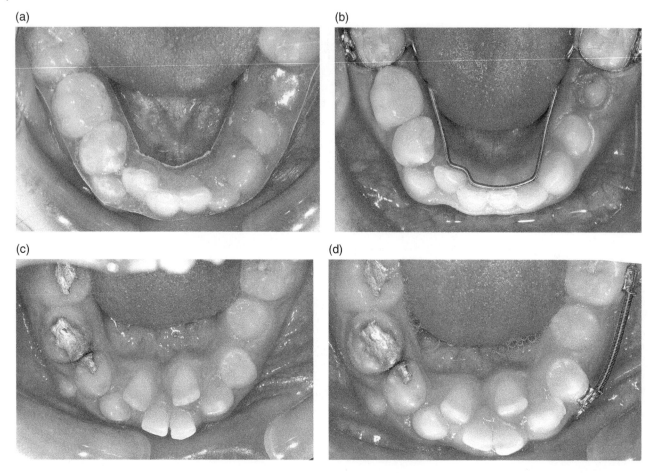

(a) (b) (c) (d)

Figure 2.9 Recent loss of a mandibular left primary second molar. (a) To prevent first permanent molar mesial drift, fabricate a vacuum-formed temporary retainer until (b) placement of an LLHA. (c, d) Alternatively, you can insert a segmental archwire with closed coil spring.

A: Make an alginate impression or intraoral scan and fabricate a vacuum-formed temporary retainer (Figure 2.9a) to hold the leeway space until you can deliver an LLHA (Figure 2.9b). Or, you can insert a segmental wire with a closed coil spring between brackets bonded on the left first premolar and left first permanent molar (Figures 2.9c and 2.9d). However, this latter approach does not prevent mesial drift of the right permanent molar when the right primary molars exfoliate.

Q: Discuss other uses of an LLHA.

A: In addition to maintaining arch perimeter and achieving spontaneous incisor alignment via leeway space, an LLHA can:

- Expand or constrict first molar arch width (Figure 2.10a). We wish to emphasize that this effect is *bilateral*. An LLHA cannot expand or constrict unilaterally (cross bite elastic wear is more suitable for *unilateral* arch expansion or constriction).
- Apply buccal or lingual first molar crown torque (Figure 2.10b) bilaterally, or unilaterally.

- Help eliminate an anterior tongue interposition habit (causing a dental open bite) by soldering spurs (reminders) to the anterior wire (Figure 2.10c).
- Prevent mesial molar drift in Class III patients in order to prevent worsening of the Class III relationship. If an LLHA is placed in a Class III mixed dentition patient to prevent mesial molar drift, then later the erupted premolars and anterior teeth can be retracted *distally* through the leeway space using TADs, J-hook headgear, or Class III elastics as anchorage.

Q: What is mixed dentition space analysis?

A: Mixed dentition space analysis (e.g. Moyers space analysis [3, 12]) evaluates the likely degree of dental crowding following permanent tooth eruption, using prediction of mesiodistal permanent premolar and canine tooth widths based on mesiodistal mandibular incisor widths.

Q: Should you perform a mixed dentition space analysis before placing an LLHA?

(a)

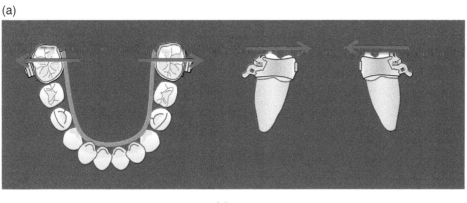

(b)

(c)

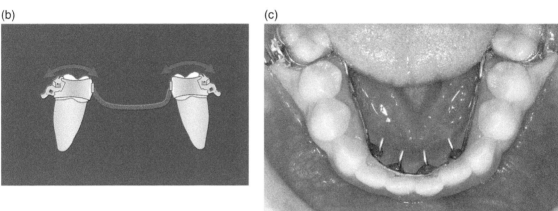

Figure 2.10   LLHA uses: (a) first molar *bilateral* expansion or constriction, (b) placement of first molar buccal or lingual crown torque, and (c) as an aid during interpositional tongue habit cessation using soldered spurs.

A: Although Moyer's and many other space analyses exist (radiographic, non-radiographic, and combinations of radiographic and chart analyses), we recommend caution in using them. Why? First, methods based on interpretation of radiographs suffer from errors due to lack of standardization in taking radiographs. Even with good radiographic technique, it can be difficult to judge the size of unerupted premolars and canines [13]. Second, prediction methods are based on the use of average tooth-sizes. Secular trends in tooth-size may result in different average tooth-size values for the same tooth across different populations. This could result in estimation errors for your patient. In particular, Moyer's analysis is based on data derived from a Caucasian population [3]. Normal biologic variation of tooth sizes exists between individuals of different racial backgrounds and between individuals of the same racial background, resulting in small but significant differences in tooth-size values in prediction tables [14, 15].

Our approach is to *use these methods as an additional guide to estimate permanent tooth crowding but not to use them to make irreversible decisions to relieve* *permanent tooth crowding*. When there is less than severe mixed dentition crowding, we recommend space maintenance (LLHA or a Nance holding arch). Exact dental arch space analysis can be performed *after* permanent teeth erupt.

Q: Does placement of an LLHA increase the likelihood of mandibular second molar impaction?

A: Yes. First permanent molar mesial drift is minimal with an LLHA in place. As a result, second molar impaction is 10–20 times more likely (8%) in LLHA patients compared with the general population [16, 17]. Note in Figures 2.11a and 2.11b how the patient's mandibular right second molar became impacted under the LLHA band (compared with normal eruption of the patient's left second molar).

How would you deal with the impacted mandibular right second molar shown in Figure 2.11b? A simple solution (Figure 2.11c, left) is to remove the LLHA and *bond* the mandibular first molar when the remaining arch is bonded (Figure 2.11c, right). Or, the LLHA can be removed and a clear, vacuum-formed, retainer worn by the patient until you bond the arch.

(a)

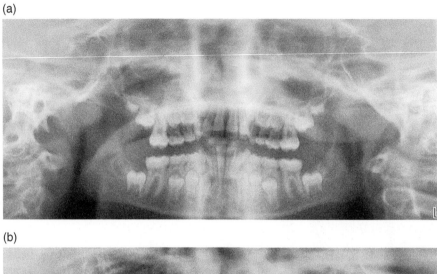

(b)

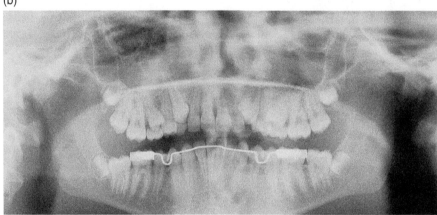

(c)

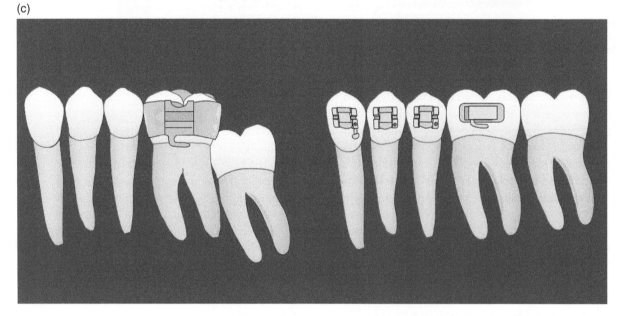

Figure 2.11 Mandibular right permanent second molar impaction under an LLHA band: (a) radiograph showing dentition before placement of an LLHA; (b) mandibular left second molar has erupted into occlusion, but the mandibular right second molar has become impacted under the LLHA band; (c) simple correction can be achieved by removing the LLHA and bonding the first permanent molar.

Q: Following premature loss of mandibular primary canines, you place an LLHA. How can the LLHA be modified in order to prevent *lateral incisor distal drift* (potentially blocking permanent canine eruption)?

A: Lateral incisor distal drift can be prevented by soldering spurs (clasps) to the LLHA to wrap around the distal of the lateral incisors (Figure 2.12). Note that the right permanent canine is beginning to erupt and will be blocked out by the soldered spur. The left soldered spur will similarly block the left permanent canine. How would you deal with this? You can either: remove the LLHA, grind away the spurs, and re-cement the LLHA, or, you could remake the LLHA without spurs.

Q: If one mandibular primary canine is lost prematurely, is it necessary to extract the contralateral primary canine in order to maintain arch symmetry?

A: No. *If the posterior segments are symmetric, do not extract the contralateral primary canine.* Instead, simply place an LLHA to prevent loss of arch perimeter. Solder a spur on the side with the lost primary canine to prevent incisor distal drift.

Q: The following is a brainteaser. Assume that a child's mother is unhappy with the child's mandibular incisor crowding and asks you to align the incisors (Figure 2.13, top left, early mixed dentition). You could extract the mandibular primary canines which would create space for the mandibular incisors to drift distally and align. But if you extract the mandibular primary canines, then the mandibular posterior teeth could drift forward (reducing arch perimeter) – which you may not want. Assuming that you *want* to maximize use of the child's leeway space for incisor alignment but without mesial molar drift, can you suggest a solution?

A: Yes. If you extract a child's mandibular primary canines to achieve improved incisor alignment (Figure 2.13,

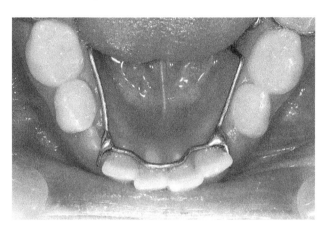

Figure 2.12   LLHA with spurs to prevent distal incisor drift.

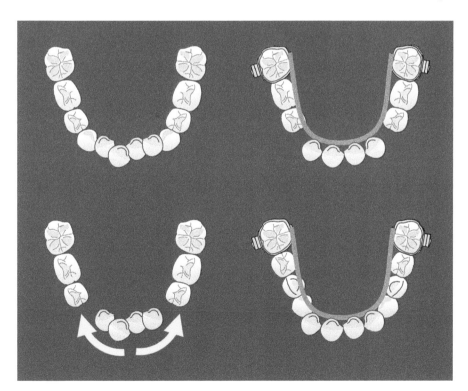

Figure 2.13   Extraction of mandibular primary canines results in spontaneous incisor alignment (top left to bottom left) but may also result in arch perimeter loss as the posterior teeth drift mesially. *If you chose to extract primary canines in order to achieve mandibular incisor alignment, then we recommend simultaneously placing an LLHA so that arch perimeter is maintained* (top right to bottom right).

bottom left), then you should *simultaneously place an LLHA* [18] (Figure 2.13, top right and bottom right) to prevent (reduce) mandibular first permanent molar mesial drift and to prevent arch perimeter loss. Once the incisors have drifted into improved alignment, consider fabricating another LLHA with spurs (clasps) distal to the lateral incisors to prevent further incisor drift.

Note: Some orthodontists would argue that the same final incisor alignment may be achieved by simply placing an LLHA, waiting for eruption of permanent teeth, and avoiding canine extractions. *Be careful not to allow parents to dictate treatment.*

Q: A nine-year-old girl presents with "end-on" first permanent molar occlusion and an LLHA cemented to her mandibular *primary* second molars (Figures 2.14a and 2.14b). Her mandibular primary left second molar will exfoliate soon. Why was her LLHA made with bands

(a)

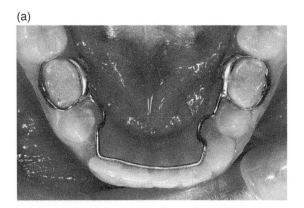

(b)

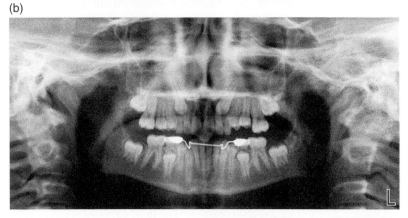

(c)

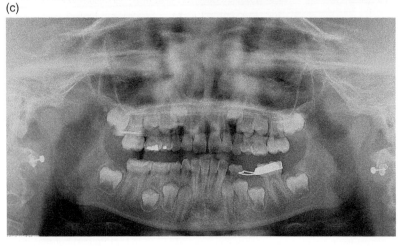

Figure 2.14 Space maintainers we do *not* recommend include (a, b) LLHAs cemented to mandibular primary second molars, or (c) band and loop appliances cemented to permanent first molars with arms extending to the primary first molars.

cemented to the primary second molars instead of with bands cemented to the *permanent* first molars? Another nine-year-old girl (Figure 2.14c) presents with a band and loop appliance whose arms extend to the primary first molar. Why do we generally not recommend either of these space maintainer designs?

A: The LLHA (Figures 2.14a and 2.14b) was probably placed to prevent mesial drift of mandibular primary second molars and permanent first molars following premature loss of mandibular primary canines and/or primary first molars. The doctor probably banded the primary second molars either because the first permanent molars had not yet erupted or to avoid cement washout/decalcification of banded first permanent molars.

We generally do not recommend banding primary second molars for an LLHA. Why? Look at what you are now facing in this patient. The left primary second molar is close to exfoliation. If you do not remove the LLHA soon, the left primary second molar will become mobile. The child could bite on the loose appliance, possibly breaking it, and swallowing/aspirating it. For this reason, *we recommend attaching LLHAs to permanent first molars and not to primary second molars*. If you are concerned with potential cement washout, then recall the patient frequently to check for cement integrity.

In a similar fashion, the mandibular left primary first molar (Figure 2.14c) will soon exfoliate. When it does, the mandibular left permanent first molar will drift mesially, and arch perimeter will be lost – defeating the purpose of having a space maintainer. In this patient, we ordered removal of the band and loop appliance and placement of an LLHA cemented to the permanent first molars.

Q: How should you proceed with the patient shown in Figure 2.14?

A: Let us examine the facts first:
- Mandibular incisors are aligned.
- Mandibular left permanent canine is erupted.
- Inadequate space exists for the mandibular right permanent canine to erupt (by about 2–3 mm).
- Mandibular left first premolar is rotated and needs about 1 mm of space to be aligned properly.
- Both mandibular first premolars are partially erupted with over 2/3's root length developed.
- "E space" of about 2.9 mm per side is present (5.8 mm total).
- "End-on" first permanent molar occlusion.

Based upon these facts, we recommended removing the LLHA and not replacing it, since the second

premolars should erupt very quickly. The permanent first molars will drift mesially – hopefully placing the patient in Class I molar occlusion. The first premolars will drift distally – providing space for mandibular left first premolar alignment and mandibular right permanent canine eruption.

Q: What other problem can you detect in this patient's panoramic radiograph (Figure 2.14b)?

A: The erupting maxillary permanent canine crowns overlap the maxillary permanent lateral incisor roots – significantly. You should address this problem now to reduce the chances of the maxillary permanent canines not erupting or resorbing the lateral incisor roots. Early treatment would include making space for the maxillary permanent canines, providing a path for their eruption, and possibly surgical exposure.

Q: What concept does this observation reinforce?

A: No matter what specific orthodontic condition you are evaluating, always step back and look for other problems the patient presents with. *If you are not seeing other problems, you are not looking.*

Q: LLHAs prevent (significantly reduce) mesial molar drift so that mandibular leeway space or "E space" can be used to spontaneously diminish mandibular anterior crowding. What is the analogous space maintenance appliance for the maxilla?

A: The Nance holding arch is the analogous space maintenance appliance for the maxillary arch. It consists of a trans-palatal arch (TPA) soldered to maxillary first molar bands and combined with an acrylic button covering the anterior palate rugae (Figure 2.15a). A Nance holding arch can prevent mesial drift of the maxillary first molars when the maxillary primary canines or primary molars exfoliate. The average leeway space provided by an LLHA is ~1.6 mm per side, and the average leeway space provided by a Nance holding arch is ~1 mm per side.

We prefer using a Nance holding arch for maxillary space maintenance, as opposed to using a band and loop appliance attached to primary teeth. Why? Look at the radiograph in Figure 2.15b. The maxillary primary first molar will exfoliate soon. When it does, the maxillary first permanent molar will drift mesially, arch perimeter will be lost, impaction of the second premolar may occur, and the patient could swallow/aspirate the band and loop appliance. In this patient, we ordered removal of the band and loop appliance and placement of a Nance holding arch with bands cemented to the maxillary first permanent molars.

(a)

(b)

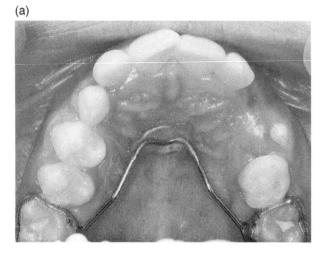
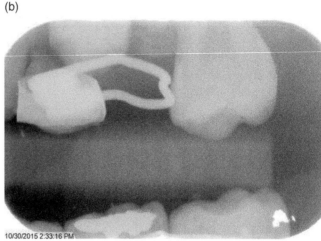

Figure 2.15 Maxillary space maintainers: (a) Nance holding arch appliance, (b) band and loop appliance. As shown, the problem with this band and loop appliance is that the primary first molar will exfoliate soon, and the maxillary first permanent molar will drift mesially – possibly impacting the second premolar and decreasing arch perimeter. We recommended extraction of the primary first molar (removal of the band and loop appliance) and placement of a Nance holding arch.

Q: Space maintenance is intended to prevent (reduce) undesirable tooth drift and arch perimeter loss following primary tooth exfoliation/loss. What is *space regaining*?

A: Space regaining is orthodontic tooth movement designed to *reverse space loss* resulting from tooth drift following premature primary tooth loss, tooth drift into extensive carious lesions of adjacent teeth; or ectopic tooth eruption. Techniques to regain space include the use of removable appliances, fixed appliances, or headgear.

Q: An eight-year-old boy presents to you for a consultation. His parents state that their dentist is concerned because a permanent molar has not erupted. You make a panoramic image (Figure 2.16). What do you observe?

A: The boy is in the early mixed dentition stage of dental development. His maxillary right permanent first molar is erupting ectopically (mesially) and is impacted under his maxillary right primary second molar. Arch perimeter has been lost.

Q: Would you recommend early treatment for this condition or would you monitor (recall) him in one year? What harm could occur from only monitoring him?

A: We recommend treatment of this condition *now*. Potential harm includes continued arch perimeter loss as the maxillary right permanent first molar drifts mesially (resorbing the primary second molar) and impaction of the maxillary right second premolar beneath the first permanent molar.

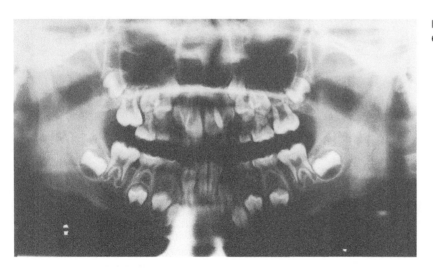

Figure 2.16 Panoramic image of an eight-year-old boy.

Q: What early treatment would you recommend?

A: Space regaining – moving the maxillary right permanent first molar distally. In doing so, arch perimeter (space) would be regained.

Q: Can you suggest three space-regaining options for the patient shown in Figure 2.16? Which option do you recommend?

A: Options include:

- *Insertion of an elastomeric separator* between the maxillary right primary second molar and maxillary right permanent first molar to free the trapped permanent molar and push it distally. This option is not recommended here because of poor access. The mesial of the maxillary right permanent first molar is buried very apically and fitting a separator between the two teeth would be problematic. In a similar fashion, if access were available, a brass wire could be inserted around the contact and twisted to push the permanent first molar distally. Local anesthetic would most likely be required if this were attempted.
- *Extraction of the maxillary right primary second molar* to free the maxillary right permanent first molar and allow it to erupt. After the maxillary right permanent first molar erupts sufficiently to allow application of force, a fixed or removable appliance could be used to distalize the maxillary right permanent first molar and regain lost space. *Extraction of a primary second molar may be the only choice in a case where the impacted permanent first molar is completely subgingival.*
- If the maxillary right primary second molar is non-mobile, and if you have partial access to the crown of the maxillary right permanent first molar, then *bond orthodontic brackets and place a segmental archwire* to de-impact and distalize the permanent first molar (Figures 2.17a and 2.17b). You may need to trap a compressed open coil spring between the permanent first molar and the primary second molar brackets to help distalize the permanent first molar. This was the option we chose.
- A *Halterman appliance* (Figures 2.17c–2.17e) consists of metal hooks soldered to molar bands. The hooks usually extend to the tuberosity or retromolar pad areas. A button is bonded to the tooth that needs movement. Elastomeric power chain applies tension between the hook and the button to move the tooth (see red arrows in Figure 2.17d).
- If the maxillary primary second molar has exfoliated, and if the permanent first molar has erupted and drifted mesially, then a simple removable spring appliance can be used (Figures 2.17f and 2.17g) to move the maxillary permanent molar distally and regain space. This same appliance can then be worn as a retainer. A headgear could also be used to move the maxillary molar distally – without reciprocal mesial movement of the primary teeth.

Q: When faced with a partially erupted maxillary first permanent molar impacted under a primary second molar, how does patient compliance affect your decision to use a *removable* appliance versus *fixed* appliances to achieve space regaining by distalizing the molar?

A: If you have a compliant patient, then either a removable (spring) appliance or fixed appliances may be considered. If you have a noncompliant patient, then fixed appliances should be chosen.

Q: Once you move the impacted maxillary right molar (Figure 2.16) distally and regain space (Figure 2.18), how should you retain the permanent molar in its corrected position? Specifically, how will *mobility* of the maxillary right *primary* second molar affect your retention decision?

A: Retention options include the following:

- If the maxillary right primary second molar is *non-mobile*, then leave it in place as a space maintainer. The maxillary right second premolar should erupt normally.
- If the maxillary right primary second molar is *mobile*, then place a Nance holding arch or other retainer to maintain the regained space and prevent mesial drift of the maxillary right permanent molar.

Q: Space regaining can be applied anywhere in the dental arch. Can you suggest two techniques for regaining space following premature exfoliation of *mandibular* primary second molars (subsequent to mesial drift of the mandibular permanent first molar and distal drift of the primary first molar)?

A: A fixed appliance option (Figure 2.19a) to regain lost primary second molar space consists of banding the permanent first molar and bonding a bracket (terminal tube) to the primary first molar (or primary first molar *and* primary canine). A compressed open coil spring is inserted along a segmental archwire between the two teeth (leave some extra wire length at the ends but anneal and turn down the wire ends so they will not slip out of the brackets). Space is regained (Figure 2.19b) as the compressed spring pushes the permanent molar distally and the primary first molar mesially. An LLHA with soldered spur (clasp) wrapping around the primary first molar (Figure 2.19c) is then inserted to hold the regained space.

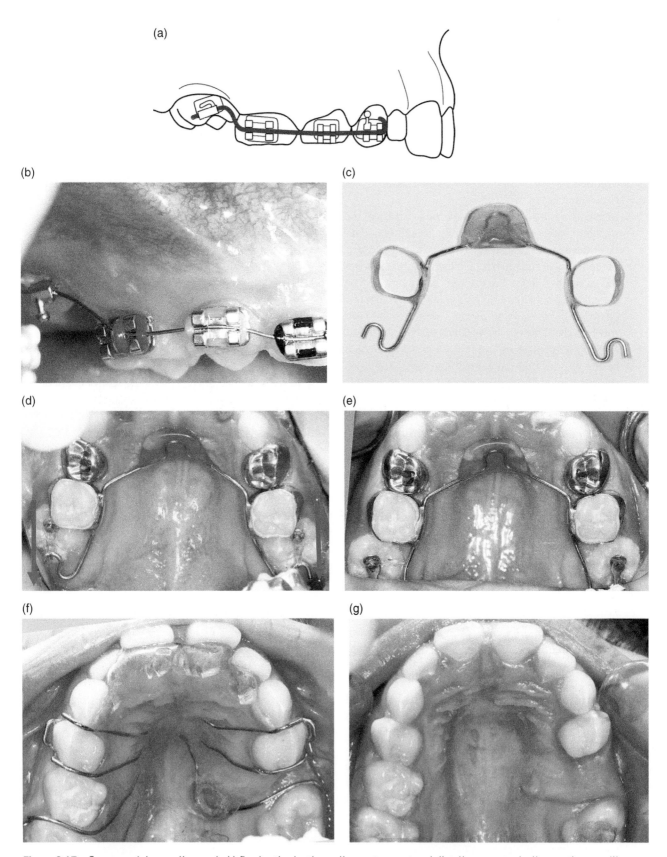

Figure 2.17 *Space regaining appliances:* (a, b) fixed orthodontic appliances to erupt and distalize an ectopically erupting maxillary right permanent first molar. This technique is viable when the maxillary right primary second molar is nonmobile and can be used as anchorage; (c–e) a Halterman appliance to distalize two ectopically erupting maxillary first permanent molars. In this design, we incorporated a palatal acrylic button to increase anchorage and reduce reciprocal mesial movement of primary teeth; (f, g) if the primary second molar has exfoliated, and if the permanent first molar has drifted mesially, then a simple removable spring appliance can be used to move the maxillary permanent molar distally. Subsequently, the spring appliance can be adjusted and worn as a passive retainer.

Figure 2.18 Same patient as in Figure 2.16 after ectopically erupted maxillary right permanent first molar was moved distally (lost space regained).

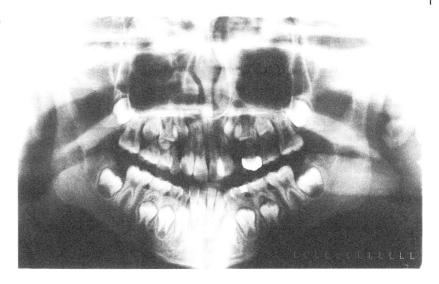

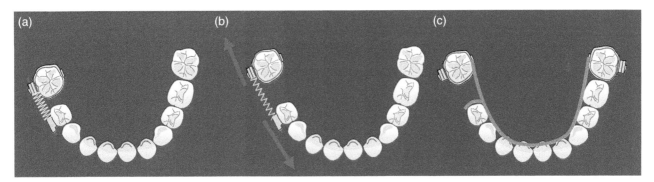

Figure 2.19 Mandibular space regaining following premature loss of the mandibular right primary second molar (space was lost by mesial drift of the right permanent first molar and distal drift of the right primary first molar). (a, b) An open coil spring is compressed between fixed appliances to regain the lost space. (c) An LLHA with a spur (clasp) distal to the primary first molar is placed to maintain the regained space.

A removable option is a split plate space regaining appliance (Figure 2.20) incorporating an expansion screw. The screw is opened 0.25–0.50 mm (one–two turns) per week. Opening the screw pushes the mandibular right permanent first molar distally and the mandibular right primary first molar mesially which regains the lost space. The passive appliance can then be worn as a retainer.

Q: Thus far, we have introduced monitoring (recall), space maintenance, and space regaining as options for managing early crowding. Occasionally, sensible early treatment includes extraction of teeth to create enough space to eliminate crowding. What is *serial extraction*? Can you describe the ideal serial extraction patient?

A: Serial extraction is the guidance of the developing dentition by sequential extraction of primary and permanent teeth. Serial extraction is usually performed to eliminate severe crowding. The ideal serial extraction patient is in the early mixed dentition stage of development and exhibits a:

- *Severe amount of anterior crowding* (≥9 mm per arch). The more severe the crowding, the less residual space closure will be required after incisors are aligned.
- *Normal anteroposterior relationship* (Class I). If the patient presents with a Class II or Class III molar relationship, we recommend that you do not extract permanent teeth until a Class I molar relationship has been achieved – unless you are sure that future growth will maintain balance between maxillary and mandibular skeletal relationships, and that extraction of permanent teeth will help correct the Class II or Class III dental relationship.

Some authors report successful serial extraction in Class II patients (maxillary arch treatment) and Class III patients (mandibular arch treatment) [19]. However, we recommend that it is always best to

(a)

(b)

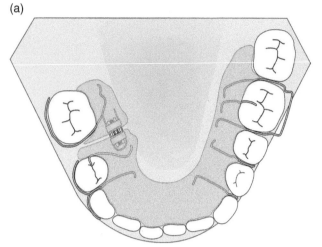

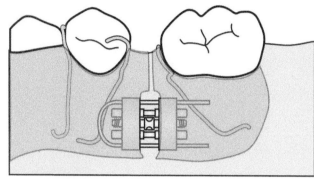

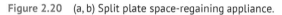

Figure 2.20 (a, b) Split plate space-regaining appliance.

reduce unknowns before doing anything irreversible, including extracting permanent teeth. Therefore, *we strongly recommend that Class II or III anteroposterior growth be addressed before serial extraction is instituted. Ideally, a Class I molar relationship should be present with minimal uncertainty regarding future jaw growth.*

- *Normal vertical relationship* (minimal OB). The vertical incisor overbite will deepen (increase) following premolar extractions as incisors are retracted and uprighted. For this reason, the patient should have *normal vertical skeletal relationships or have a slightly long soft tissue and skeletal LAFH, steep mandibular plane angle, and minimal OB or possibly a mild open bite but never a deep bite.*

- *Normal transverse relationship* (well-coordinated maxillary and mandibular arch widths without cross bites; minimal transverse compensations such as maxillary molar buccal crown torque or mandibular molar lingual crown torque). Why is this important? If the patient's transverse relationship is normal, then you have one less problem to deal with post-extractions.

- *Normal incisor angulation or proclined incisors (protrusive lips), but not upright incisors.* Why? Incisors tend to upright as they are retracted during premolar extraction space closure.

Q: Now is a good time to discuss space requirements to reduce *incisor proclination*. Not only is space needed to eliminate dental crowding (the discrepancy between teeth sizes and arch perimeter/length), but space may also be needed to retract/upright proclined incisors. For example, the patient (cephalometric tracing) in Figure 2.21a presents with proclined mandibular incisors (FMIA = 58°) and proclined maxillary incisors (U1 to SN = 116°). A treatment goal for this patient was to retract/upright her mandibular incisors to an ideal inclination of FMIA = 68°. How can you estimate the space needed to accomplish this incisor retraction/uprighting?

A: Let us assume a one-to-one correspondence between the actual size of the patient and the size of the cephalometric tracing (no magnification difference). Further, assume that her mandibular incisors are already aligned. Draw a line (dotted red line, Figure 2.21b) from the mandibular incisor apex to FH so that an angle of 68° is formed (FMIA = 68°), and measure the distance from the current mandibular incisal edge tip (along the solid red line) to its future anticipated position along the dotted red line. Here, we find that distance equals 5 mm. To retract the mandibular anterior teeth by 5 mm (Figure 2.21c, left top and left bottom) requires 5 mm of space on *both* the right and left sides for a total of 10 mm of space needed. This space requirement (to reduce incisor proclination) is in addition to any space needed to alleviate dental crowding.

10 mm of mandibular space is much greater than can be gained from leeway space. For this reason, a decision was made in this patient to extract her right and left mandibular first premolars (and maxillary first premolars). First premolar extractions provided 14 mm of space (two premolars × 7 mm per premolar) in each arch to retract incisors (Figure 2.21c, right top and right bottom). Following maxillary and mandibular first premolar extractions, and space closure with fixed orthodontic appliances (Figure 2.21d), her mandibular incisors uprighted to an FMIA of 69° (maxillary incisors uprighted slightly to U1 to SN = 115°).

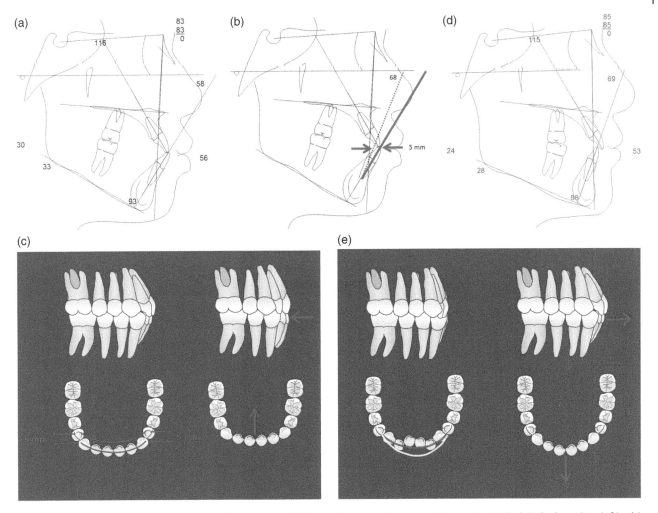

Figure 2.21 (a–d). Estimating space needed to retract/upright proclined mandibular anterior teeth. (e) Upright incisors (top left) with a thick labial periodontal biotype are often *proclined* to a more normal angulation to gain space and reduce crowding. The arch perimeter is thereby increased (bottom left) from a shorter (red) anterior arch perimeter to a longer (yellow) anterior arch perimeter by incisor proclination (right top and right bottom).

Dr. Charles Tweed provided a simple technique to calculate the space needed to upright mandibular incisors, as follows: *0.8 mm lower incisor retraction space is needed for every 1° increase in FMIA desired* [20]. For our example that works out to 8 mm of retraction space needed for the patient shown in Figure 2.21a ($68° - 58° = 10° \times 0.8 \, \text{mm}/° = 8 \, \text{mm}$). This estimate assumes minimal changes in arch form during premolar extraction space closure. When arch form changes are anticipated, a mathematical formula is available to calculate arch space used for mandibular incisor retraction [21].

Now, if a patient presents with *upright* incisors, then space to reduce dental crowding may be gained by proclining anterior teeth (Figure 2.21e) to a more normal incisor angulation. Incisor proclination *increases* arch perimeter and reduces crowding. Proclining incisors stresses the labial gingiva covering the incisor roots, and ideally the patient should have a thick labial periodontal biotype to support this movement.

Q: What is the extraction sequence followed during serial extraction?

A: There is no single serial extraction sequence. However, in one common sequence, the primary canines are first extracted (Figure 2.22a) when the permanent canines have attained at least one-half of their final root length. This will create space for spontaneous alignment of permanent incisors. Permanent incisors drift distally into the extraction space, and posterior teeth may drift mesially into the extraction space. The bite may deepen as the incisors upright (Figure 2.22b).

When the first premolar roots have attained at least one-half of their final root length, extraction of the first

(a) (b) (c)

(d) (e) (f)

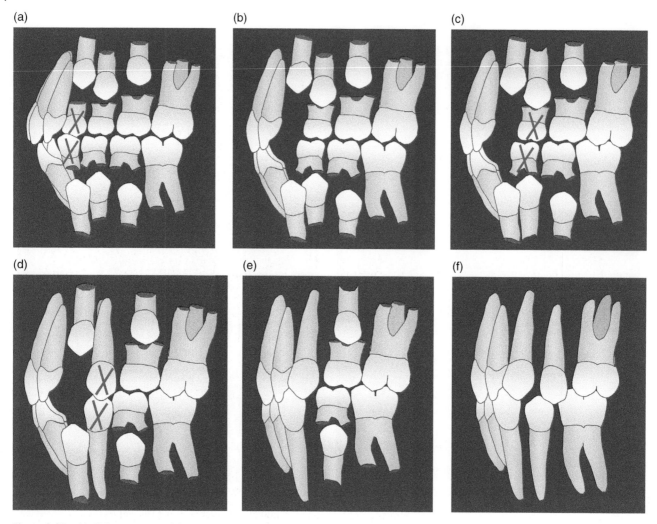

Figure 2.22 (a–f) A common serial extraction sequence used to treat an otherwise normal Class I patient with severe anterior crowding.

primary molars accelerates their eruption (Figure 2.22c). As the permanent canines erupt, extraction of permanent teeth (usually the first premolars, Figure 2.22d) facilitates canine eruption and canine distal drift (Figure 2.22e). Depending upon the magnitude of crowding, space closure will be required after the second premolars erupt (Figure 2.22f). In cases where the permanent canines erupt before the first premolars, the first premolars may be enucleated concurrently with primary first molar extractions.

Q: What is the principal problem with serial extraction?

A: *Poor patient selection*, such as performing serial extraction on marginally crowded patients. Extraction of teeth for any purpose is never taken lightly. Mild mandibular anterior crowding of 3 mm or less can usually be treated with space maintenance and preservation of leeway space. Interproximal tooth reduction (IPR) is

another way to create space without tooth extractions. Extraction of permanent teeth in cases of mild anterior crowding may result in excess residual space, over-retraction of anterior teeth during closure of these residual spaces, excessive uprighting of incisors, and bite deepening.

Figures 2.23a and 2.23b illustrate the trade-offs between serial extraction, crowding, incisor proclination, and the need for post-extraction orthodontic space closure. In Figure 2.23a (left), serial extraction is performed on a mandibular arch with severe initial anterior *crowding* and severe incisor *proclination*. The post-extraction result is improved incisor inclination and the need for minimal residual space closure after eruption of permanent teeth (Figure 2.23a, right). In this case, serial extraction was an excellent choice. In Figure 2.23b (left), serial extraction is performed on a mandibular arch with minimal crowding and normal incisor

Figure 2.23 Serial extraction in a Class I patient who initially presents with severe anterior crowding and proclined incisors (a) results in minimal space closure and improved incisor angulation after all permanent teeth erupt; (b) serial extraction in a Class I patient who initially presents with mild anterior crowding and normal incisor inclination results in the need for large residual space closure and upright incisors.

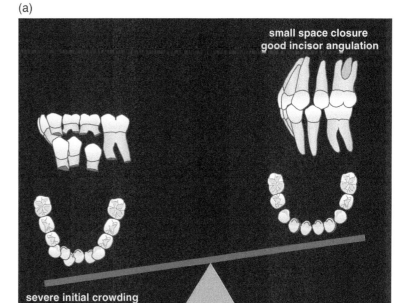

(a)

small space closure
good incisor angulation

severe initial crowding
severe proclination

(b)

mild initial crowding
normal angulation

large space closure
upright incisors

inclination. The post-extraction result is very upright incisors and large residual spaces that must be closed (Figure 2.23b, right). In this case, serial extraction was a poor choice.

Even in patients where mandibular primary canines have been prematurely lost due to excessive crowding, prediction of severe crowding is difficult before all permanent canines and premolars have erupted. So, the ultimate question is, how early should you decide to extract permanent teeth?

As a general rule, except in cases of ectopic eruption, incisor dehiscence, incisor eruption into nonkeratinized *gingiva, or where you are sure the patient presents with severe crowding, it is prudent to place an LLHA until the permanent teeth have erupted to accurately assess the need for permanent teeth extractions.*

Q: What is the difference in outcome between patients treated with serial extraction and patients treated with later conventional premolar extractions?

A: Excluding cases of ectopic eruption, *no difference in treatment outcome is found* [22, 23]. Also, serial extraction might reduce active treatment time, but significant observation time precedes active treatment [23].

Q: Are mandibular arches treated with serial extraction more stable (less likely to crowd post-treatment)?

A: No. Incisor stability of serial extraction cases equals incisor stability of later premolar extraction cases, but *mixed dentition mandibular arches (having favorable leeway space) treated with LLHAs are more stable* [24, 25].

Q: Is there a difference in external apical root resorption in patients treated with serial extraction versus patients treated with later extractions?

A: No. Serial extraction followed by orthodontic tooth movement does *not* reduce apical root resorption compared with treatment with later extractions [26].

Q: Emma (Figure 2.24) is 8 years and 11 months old. She presents to you with her parent's CC, "Emma needs braces." Her PMH, TMJ, and periodontal evaluations are WRN. CR = CO. List diagnostic findings and problems. What is your diagnosis?

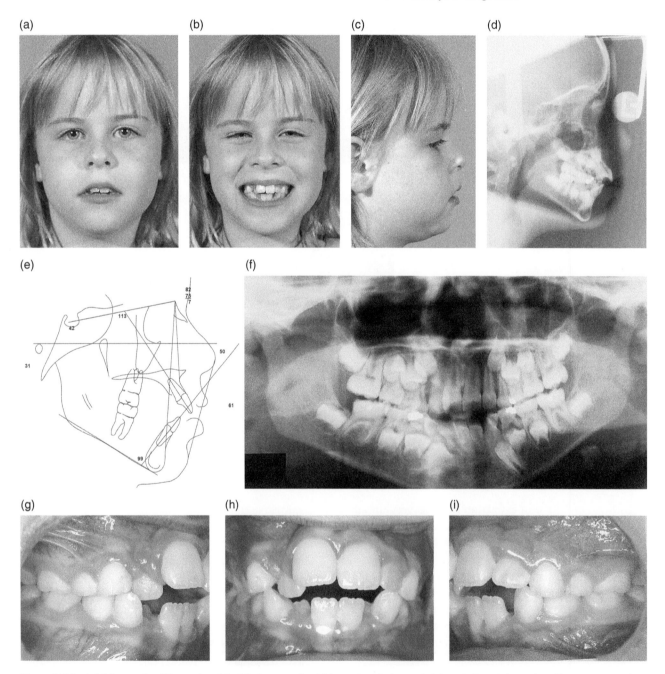

Figure 2.24 Initial records of Emma (a–c) facial photographs, (d) lateral cephalograph, (e) cephalometric tracing, (f) pantomograph, (g–i) intraoral photographs, and (j–p) model photographs.

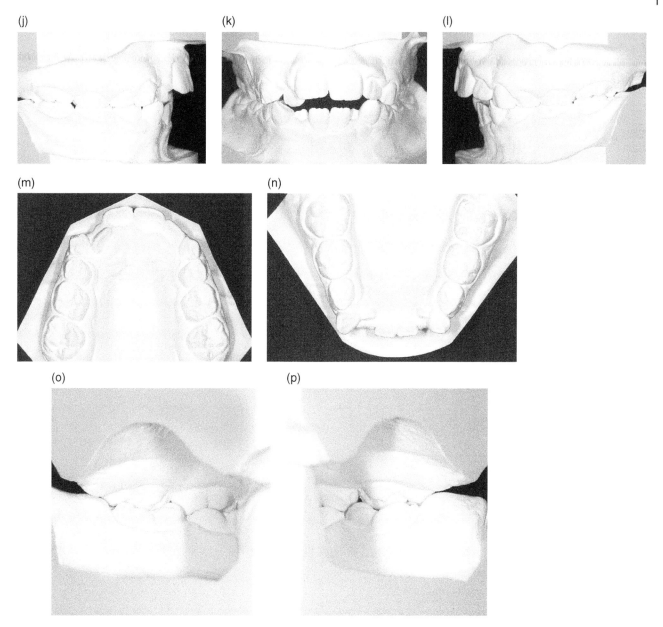

Figure 2.24   (Continued)

A:

Table 2.1   Diagnostic findings and problem list for Emma.

Full face and profile	**Frontal view**
	Face is symmetric
	Long LAFH (soft tissue Glabella-Subnasale < Subnasale-soft tissue Menton)
	ILG: 6–7 mm
	Acceptable incisal display at rest
	Accentuated Cupid's bow (maxillary lip length at philtrum is ~6 mm shorter than maxillary lip length at commissures; ideal philtrum length-commissure height difference is only 2–3 mm)
	Inadequate incisal display in posed smile (maxillary central incisor gingival margins are apical to the maxillary lip; maxillary incisors are stepped *up* relative to posterior teeth)
	UDML WRN

(*Continued*)

Table 2.1 (Continued)

	Profile view
	Convex profile and retrusive chin
	Upturned nose
	Obtuse NLA
	Obtuse lip-chin-throat angle
Ceph analysis	**Skeletal**
	Maxilla slightly protrusive (A-Point slightly ahead of Nasion-perpendicular line)
	Mandible severely retrusive (ANB = 7°)
	Long skeletal LAFH (LAFH/TAFH × 100% = 61%; over two standard deviations greater than the average 55%, sd = 2°)
	Vertical maxillary excess (VME)
	Steep MPA (FMA = 31°; SNMP = 42°)
	Short posterior face height
	Lips protrusive to the E-plane
	Dental
	Very proclined maxillary incisors (U1 to SN = 113°)
	Very proclined mandibular incisors (FMIA = 50°)
Radiographs	Early mixed dentition
	Premature resorption of mandibular primary canine roots
Intraoral photos and models	Angle Class II division 1
	Iowa Classification: II (2 mm) II (2 mm) II (1 mm) II (1–2 mm)
	Class I molar relationships when viewed from the lingual (Figures 2.24o and 2.24p)
	OJ 4 mm
	Cross bite maxillary right lateral incisor
	Anterior open bite extending to primary canines
	Maxillary incisors stepped up relative to posterior teeth
	Mandibular incisors stepped down relative to mandibular posterior teeth
	Mild COS
	Mild maxillary incisor crowding (~3 mm)
	Severe mandibular crowding (~9 mm)
	Maxillary first molars are rotated mesially
	Prominent mandibular central incisor roots and thin attached tissue (Figure 2.24h)
Other	Anterior tongue interposition habit
Diagnosis	Angle Class II division 1 malocclusion
	Skeletal open bite

Q: What is a reliable indicator of severe mandibular anterior crowding?

A: *Premature loss of primary canines* [2]. Lack of interdental spacing is *not* a reliable indicator of severe mandibular anterior crowding. Emma exhibits premature resorption of mandibular primary canine roots.

Q: Is Emma a candidate for serial extraction?

A: To answer this question, we will consider Emma in the light of each criterion that makes an ideal serial extraction candidate. The ideal serial extraction patient is in the early mixed dentition stage of development and exhibits a:

- *Normal anteroposterior relationship* (Class I). At first, you would conclude that Emma does *not* meet this criterion because she is Class II by 1–2 mm, bilaterally. However, you would be wrong. While it is true that Emma appears slightly Class II from the buccal (Figures 2.24j and 2.24l), in fact Emma is really Class I.

  How do we conclude this? When Emma is viewed from the lingual (Figure 2.24o and p), her permanent molars are Class I. In other words, her maxillary first permanent molars are *rotated mesially* (Figure 2.24m) which results in them appearing Class II when viewed from the buccal. If we simply rotate her maxillary first permanent molars around their lingual roots (rotating buccal surfaces toward the distal), then she will be Class I when viewed from both the buccal and from the lingual.

Always check for molar rotations. Ask how the molar rotations affect your molar anteroposterior classification. Always view molars from the lingual. Emma meets the criteria of having Class I molars (although she is Class II skeletally).

- *Normal vertical relationship* (minimal OB). Emma presents with a long skeletal LAFH, ILG, steep MPA, and mild anterior open bite. These features are not ideal but should not preclude serial extraction since the open bite will tend to close as incisors are rotated/uprighted following premolar extractions. Emma meets this criterion.
- *Normal transverse relationship* (coordinated arch widths without cross bites; minimal transverse compensations). Emma has a reasonable transverse relationship and meets this criterion.
- *Severe amount of anterior crowding* (≥9 mm per arch). Emma meets this criterion in her mandibular arch.
- *Normal incisor angulation or proclined incisors (protrusive lips), but not upright incisors.* Emma meets this criterion.

In conclusion, Emma is a candidate for serial extraction. The one feature that we find disconcerting is her severely retruded mandible (skeletal Class II relationship). We would feel more comfortable with her as a serial extraction candidate if her mandible was normal.

Q: Should you place an LLHA in Emma?

A: No. Emma has severe mandibular anterior crowding (9 mm) coupled with severe mandibular incisor proclination. Even with space maintenance, treating her non-extraction would increase incisor proclination and thereby worsen her open bite.

Q: What treatment do you recommend for Emma?

A: Emma's parents stated that she was not growing noticeably at this time. We asked them to measure her height each month. Emma was asked to keep her tongue away from her incisors in the hope that the incisors would erupt. We decided to treat her with serial extraction. She was referred for primary canine extractions. Nine months later, Emma's parents stated that she was growing. We asked Emma to wear a HPHG which she wore until her molars were slightly Class III. Headgear wear served us two purposes. First, moving her maxillary molars distally to slightly Class III would give us extra anchorage when we eventually began to retract her anterior teeth posteriorly. Second, restricting her maxillary growth, while permitting her mandible to continue growing forward, would improve her profile.

Her primary first molars were extracted when the roots of her first permanent premolars were ½ formed. Her permanent first premolars were extracted when they erupted. Emma was placed in fixed appliances, her arches leveled and aligned, and treatment finished. Her deband photographs are shown in Figure 2.25a–k. Note that her profile has improved, incisors have uprighted, anterior open bite has closed, lips are no longer protusive, lip competence attained, and arch alignment achieved. Serial extraction treatment for Emma was appropriate and successful.

(a) 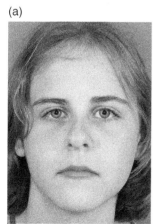 (b) 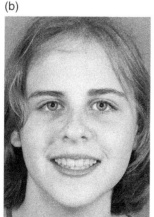 (c) 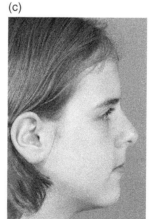 (d)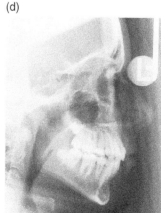

Figure 2.25 (a–k) Emma's deband records.

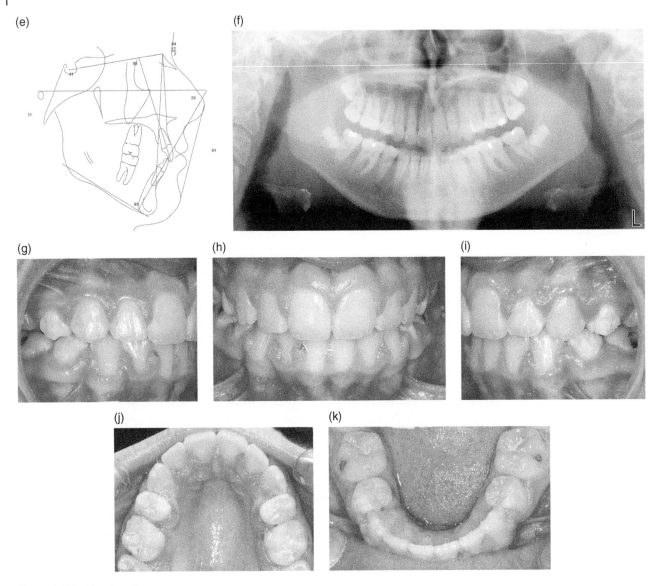

(e) (f)

(g) (h) (i)

(j) (k)

Figure 2.25 (Continued)

Q: Amelia is seven years and six months old (Figure 2.26). She presents to you with her parent's chief complaint, "We were referred for orthodontic treatment by our family dentist." Her PMH, PDH, periodontal evaluation, and TMJ evaluation are WRN. CR = CO. Compile your diagnostic findings and problem list for Amelia. Also, state your diagnosis.

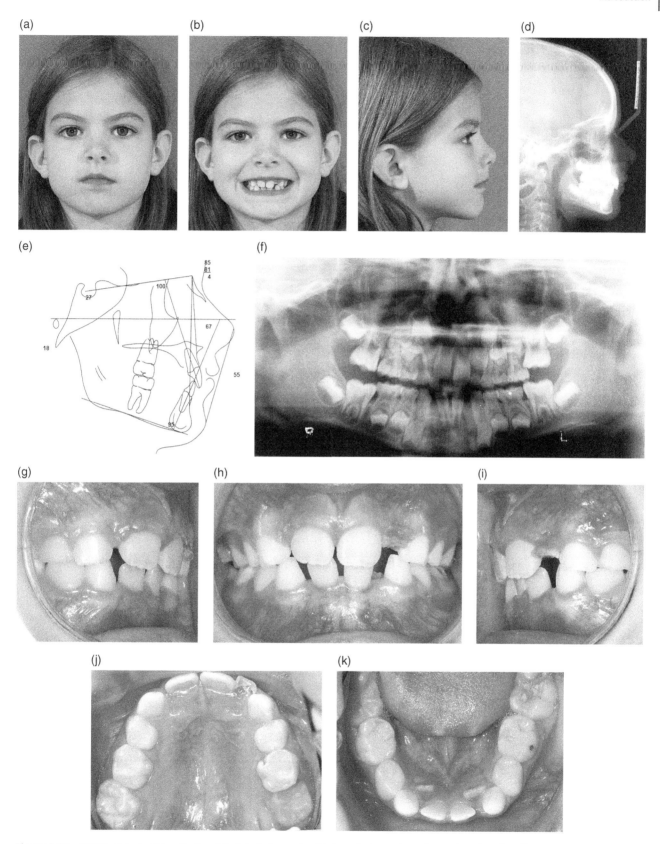

Figure 2.26 Initial records of Amelia (a–c) facial photographs, (d, e), cephalometric radiograph and tracing, (f) pantomograph, and (g–k) intraoral photographs.

A:

Table 2.2 Diagnostic findings and problem list for Amelia.

Full face and profile	*Frontal view* Face is symmetric (philtrum tilted to the right) Soft tissue LAFH WRN (soft tissue Glabella – Subnasale approximately equal to Subnasale – soft tissue Menton) Lip competence UDML ~1 mm right Gingival display in posed smile WRN Mild right-to-left occlusal cant *Profile view* Relatively straight profile Chin projection WRN Upturned nose Obtuse NLA Lip-chin-throat angle WRN
Ceph analysis	*Skeletal* Maxillary anteroposterior position mildly protrusive (A-Point lies ahead of Nasion-perpendicular line) Mandibular anteroposterior position WRN (ANB angle = 4° but maxillary anteroposterior position mildly protrusive) Skeletal LAFH WRN (ANS-Menton/Nasion-Menton × 100% = 55%) Flat MPA (FMA = 18°; SNMP = 27°) Effective bony pogonion (Pogonion lies ahead of extended Nasion-B Point line) *Dental* Maxillary incisors slightly upright (U1 to SN = 100°) Mandibular incisors WRN (FMIA = 67°)
Radiographs	Early mixed dentition Maxillary left permanent first molar is ectopically erupting (resorbing maxillary left primary second molar)
Intraoral photos and models	Angle Class II Iowa Classification: II (1 mm) II (1 mm) II (1 mm) II (1 mm) OJ ~ 1 mm OB 20–30% Maxillary permanent lateral incisors potentially impacted Mandibular permanent lateral incisors erupting and blocked to the lingual 5.0 mm of maxillary anterior spacing is currently present but maxillary permanent lateral incisors are unerupted, so the current anterior crowding is ~8 mm. 6.0 mm of maxillary arch crowding is anticipated following eruption of all permanent teeth (if proper space maintenance is employed). 3.0 mm of mandibular incisor spacing is currently present but mandibular permanent lateral incisors are erupting and blocked to the lingual, so the current anterior crowding is ~8 mm. 4.8 mm of mandibular arch crowding is anticipated following eruption of all permanent teeth (if proper space maintenance is employed). Midlines are not coincident (LDML to left of UDML by ~1–2 mm) Maxillary and mandibular dental arches are symmetric Anterior biotype WRN
Other	None
Diagnosis	Mild Class II malocclusion with moderate anterior crowding and ectopically erupting maxillary left permanent first molar

Q: Provide a detailed dental arch space analysis for Amelia's maxillary and mandibular arches. In other words, how were the anticipated 6.0 mm maxillary arch crowding and 4.8 mm mandibular arch crowding calculated (*if proper space maintenance is employed*)?

A:

Average mesiodistal widths of permanent teeth (mm) [3]:

Maxillary Central Incisor	8.5	Mandibular Central Incisor	5.0
Maxillary Lateral Incisor	6.5	Mandibular Lateral Incisor	5.5
Maxillary Canine	7.5	Mandibular Canine	7.0
Maxillary First Premolar	7.0	Mandibular First Premolar	7.0
Maxillary Second Premolar	7.0	Mandibular Second Premolar	7.0
Maxillary First Molar	10.0	Mandibular First Molar	11.0
Maxillary Second Molar	9.0	Mandibular Second Molar	10.5

Average mesiodistal widths of *primary* teeth (mm) [3]:

Maxillary Central Incisor	6.5	Mandibular Central Incisor	4.2
Maxillary Lateral Incisor	5.1	Mandibular Lateral Incisor	4.1
Maxillary Canine	7.0	Mandibular Canine	5.0
Maxillary First Molar	7.3	Mandibular First Molar	7.7
Maxillary Second Molar	8.2	Mandibular Second Molar	9.9

MAXILLARY ARCH
+5.0 mm of incisor spacing currently present, including nearly exfoliated maxillary left primary lateral incisor (Figure 2.26j).
−6.5 mm of space needed for potentially impacted maxillary right permanent lateral incisor.
−6.5 mm of space needed for potentially impacted maxillary left permanent lateral incisor.
+2 mm of anticipated leeway space (1 mm/side).
Balance = +5.0 mm − 6.5 mm − 6.5 mm + 2 mm = −6.0 mm.

MANDIBULAR ARCH
+3.0 mm of incisor spacing currently present (Figure 2.26k).
−5.5 mm of space needed for mandibular left permanent lateral incisor.
−5.5 mm of space needed for mandibular right permanent lateral incisor.

+3.2 mm of anticipated leeway space (1.6 mm/side).
Balance = +3.0 mm − 5.5 mm − 5.5 mm + 3.2 mm = −4.8 mm.

That is, *6.0 mm of maxillary arch crowding and 4.8 mm of mandibular arch crowding is anticipated following eruption of all permanent teeth (if proper space maintenance is employed).*

Q: What are Amelia's *primary* problems in each dimension (that we must stay focused on), plus other problems?

A:

Table 2.3   Primary problems list for Amelia.

AP	Class II (1 mm)
Vertical	–
Transverse	–
Other	Maxillary permanent lateral incisors potentially impacted
	Mandibular permanent lateral incisors erupting to the lingual
	Moderate (8 mm) maxillary and mandibular anterior crowding
	Ectopic eruption of maxillary left first permanent molar

Q: Discuss Amelia in the context of three principles applied to every early treatment patient.

A:

- The goal of early treatment is to correct developing problems – get the patient *back to normal for their stage of development* (including preventing complications such as resorption of adjacent tooth roots, reducing later treatment complexity, or reducing/eliminating unknowns). Correcting the ectopic eruption of her maxillary left first permanent molar, correcting her mild Class II relationship, and alleviating her anterior crowding would get her back to normal.

- Early treatment should address *very specific problems with a clearly defined end point*, usually within six to nine months (except for some orthopedic problems). Distal movement (de-impacting) of her ectopically erupting maxillary left first permanent molar is a clearly defined objective which could be managed in a few months using fixed orthodontic appliances. Correcting her mild Class II relationship with orthopedics could be readily corrected with cooperation once Ameila exhibits good (statural) growth velocity. Providing room for her erupting incisors is a clearly defined solution which, with extraction of primary canines, could be managed in a short time. However, to prevent risk of arch perimeter loss, an LLHA and Nance holding arch should be placed concurrently with primary canine extractions. Finally, even with space maintenance, we estimate 6.0 mm of maxillary arch crowding and 4.8 mm of mandibular arch crowding once all permanent teeth erupt.

- Always ask: Is it necessary that I treat the patient now? *What harm will come if I chose to do nothing now?* It is necessary to institute early treatment now. If we do not correct her ectopically erupting maxillary left permanent first molar, then the first molar will continue to resorb the maxillary left primary second molar, erupt to the mesial, reduce arch perimeter, and impact the maxillary left second premolar.

  On the other hand, it is *not* necessary to deal with Amelia's mild Class II relationship yet (her parents measure her height regularly and state that she is not growing appreciably). Nor is it necessary to address Amelia's anterior crowding immediately (permanent canines and premolars are years from erupting). If we chose to recall in one year, then her maxillary lateral incisors will remain potentially impacted or erupt blocked out from her maxillary dental arch. Her mandibular lateral incisors will remain blocked out in a lingual position.

Q: In terms of anterior crowding, is Amelia currently a good candidate for space maintenance?

A: Yes and no. On the one hand, if you choose to extract her four primary canines in order to alleviate permanent incisor crowding/facilitate permanent incisor eruption, then placement of an LLHA and Nance holding arch would be prudent to prevent possible permanent first molar mesial drift and arch perimeter loss. On the other hand, if you do not extract primary canines, then space maintenance to reduce anterior crowding (via leeway space) would be unnecessary at this time since permanent canine and premolar eruption is years away.

Q: In terms of anterior crowding, is Amelia a good candidate for space regaining?

A: Possibly. If we regain lost primary lateral incisor space *now* for permanent lateral incisors, then we need about 8 mm of additional anterior space in each arch (we cannot include leeway space now because primary canines and molars are still present).

8 mm of anterior space per arch could be regained via ~4 mm of central incisor proclination (i.e. ~4 mm regained on both right and left sides). 4 mm of incisor proclination seems reasonable because the labial gingival biotype of both arches is WRN (Figure 2.26h), maxillary incisors are upright (Figure 2.26e), and mandibular incisors exhibit normal angulation. However, periapical radiographs should be made of the central incisor roots to ensure a reasonable amount of root development and caution must be exercised during space regaining to ensure that bonded central incisor roots do not drive unerupted lateral incisor roots into permanent canine crowns.

Q: Can you list factors that suggest Amelia is an ideal candidate for serial extraction? Can you list factors that suggest she is not?

A: Factors suggesting that Amelia is a candidate for serial extraction include the fact that she:

- Is in the early mixed dentition stage of development.
- Is vertically normal (OB is 20–30%).
- Exhibits a normal posterior transverse relationship.

The factor that disqualifies Amelia as an ideal candidate for serial extraction is her moderate crowding magnitude (8 mm, not severe). Further, if we include leeway space (space maintenance), only 6.0 mm of maxillary crowding and 4.8 mm of mandibular crowding is anticipated following eruption of all permanent teeth. Another factor which disqualifies her is that she is slightly Class II.

The ideal serial extraction patient is in the early mixed dentition stage of development and normal in every way, except for the presence of *severe anterior crowding (≥9 mm anterior crowding in each arch)*. We conclude that Amelia is not an ideal candidate for serial extraction.

Q: Should you start (early) treatment now or recall Amelia? If you start treatment, what treatment would you recommend?

A: We decided to institute early treatment now. We began by bonding her maxillary left posterior teeth with fixed orthodontic appliances and trapping a compressed open coil spring between her maxillary left permanent first molar and primary second molar (Figure 2.27a). The permanent first molar was de-impacted from under the primary second molar, thus correcting its ectopic eruption. We checked the

(a)   (b)

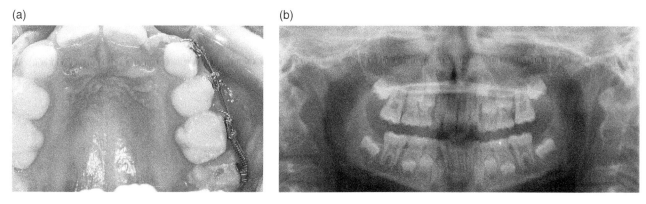

Figure 2.27 Progress records of Amelia (a) de-impacting her maxillary left permanent first molar using fixed appliances, (b) panoramic radiograph made later. The maxillary left permanent first molar is in a good position and the nonmobile maxillary left primary second molar is acting as a space maintainer.

mobility of the maxillary left primary second molar and found it to be nonmobile. We removed the fixed orthodontic appliances and retained the maxillary left primary second molar as a space maintainer (Figure 2.27b).

Later, as Amelia was beginning to enter the late mixed dentition stage of development, she was placed on a high-pull headgear to correct her mild Class II relationship. We planned to extract Amelia's maxillary primary canines in order to permit her maxillary permanent lateral incisors to erupt, and we planned to monitor Amelia and evaluate for mandibular space maintenance or lateral incisor space regaining.

However, Amelia never followed up for treatment in spite of repeated requests to do so.

Q: De-impacting Amelia's ectopically erupting maxillary left first molar was an example of what form of treatment?

A: *Space regaining.* Arch perimeter (space) was lost during the molar's ectopic eruption into the maxillary left primary second molar. This lost space was regained during correction of the ectopic eruption.

Q: Amelia returned to our clinic five years later and records were made (Figure 2.28a–k). What changes do you note?

(a)   (b)   (c)

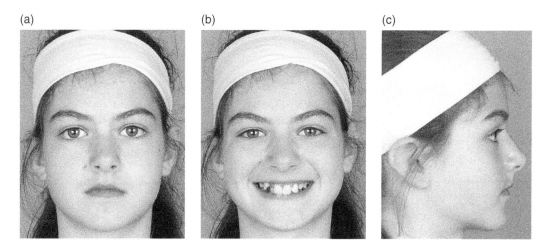

Figure 2.28 (a–k) Progress records of Amelia at 12 years of age.

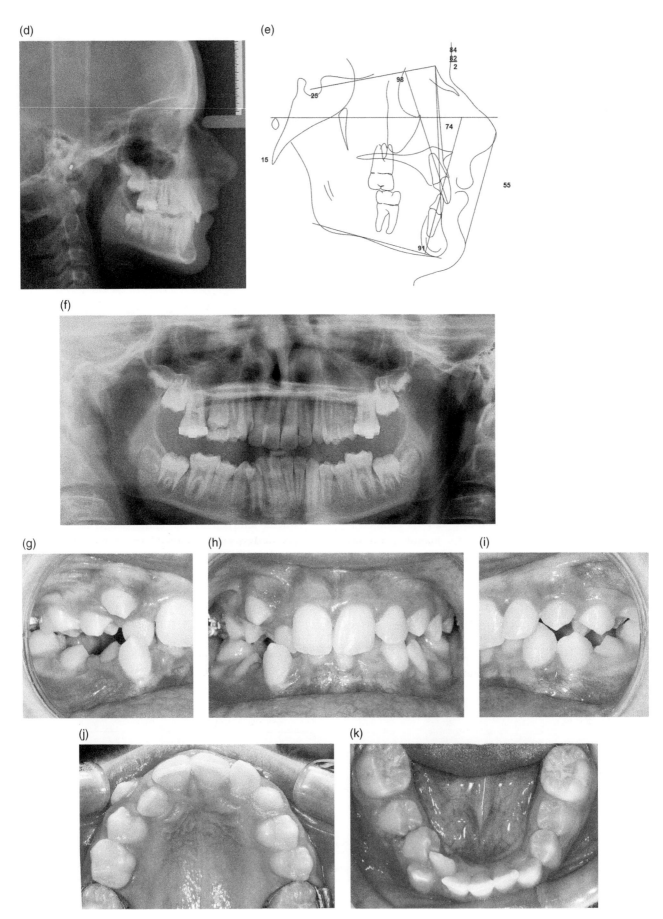

Figure 2.28   (Continued)

A: Changes include:

- Excess gingiva displayed in posed smile (maxillary incisors appear stepped down relative to maxillary posterior occlusal plane).
- Relatively straight profile.
- ANB angle has decreased from 4° to 2°.
- Mandibular incisors are now upright (FMIA = 74°).
- Maxillary incisors have uprighted (maxillary incisor long axis to SN line = 98°).
- Permanent dentition is now present (maxillary right primary second molar is close to exfoliation) and she is Class I at her molars.
- OB has increased to 70–80%.
- Maxillary permanent lateral incisors have erupted.
- Maxillary right permanent lateral incisor is in lingual cross bite.
- Both right permanent canines are blocked out of the arches.
- Thin labial periodontal biotype of right permanent canines and mandibular left permanent central incisor is noted (Figure 2.28g and h).
- ~6.5 mm of maxillary anterior crowding is present.
- ~5.5 mm of mandibular anterior crowding present.

Q: Since we are now in the permanent dentition, further treatment is no longer *early* treatment. However, what treatment options can you suggest at this point?

A: Treatment options include:

- *Recall* (no treatment, monitor) – re-evaluate in one year. We do not recommend this option. It is time to begin comprehensive fixed appliance orthodontic treatment.
- *Non-extraction treatment* – leveling and aligning both arches with fixed appliances to create room for the blocked out right permanent canines. This option is appealing because Amelia's incisors are upright, and because she has an obtuse NLA. That is, aligning her maxillary arch will procline her maxillary incisors and increase her maxillary lip support. Further, she still has maxillary right "E-space."

  Our concern with non-extraction treatment is that her anterior periodontal tissues will be stressed as spaces for the right canines are opened, and areas of gingival recession could result. A periodontal consult (gingival grafting) would be recommended if this option was pursued.
- *Extraction of first or second premolars* – will provide space to alleviate the moderate (5.5–6.5 mm) anterior crowding without stressing periodontal tissues. However, Amelia's incisors are already upright.

Space closure following four premolar extractions would probably upright her incisors even more – potentially dishing in her profile.
- *Mandibular single incisor extraction* – could be a viable alternative if an anterior Bolton analysis reveals a significant mandibular anterior tooth-size excess. If a significant (3–5 mm) mandibular anterior Bolton excess is *not* present, then excess anterior OJ will remain following comprehensive treatment. Maxillary periodontal tissue stress will still occur if the maxillary arch is treated non-extraction.
- *Maxillary arch alignment first* – then re-evaluation for extractions. This option offers the advantage of reducing treatment unknowns before an extraction decision is made. Using this approach, you can monitor the maxillary right permanent canine labial gingiva *and* observe how much anterior OJ is created following maxillary arch alignment.

Q: What important principle can you take home from these comprehensive treatment options?

A: *Exhaustively consider all options (non-extraction, extraction of anterior teeth, extraction of posterior teeth) before making your final comprehensive treatment decision.*

Q: What treatment do you now recommend?

A: A decision was made to reduce unknowns before making a non-extraction/extraction decision. Amelia's maxillary right primary second molar was removed, and her maxillary right second premolar erupted. Her maxillary permanent teeth (except for her maxillary right lateral incisor) were bonded with fixed orthodontic appliances, and a compressed open coil spring was trapped between her maxillary right canine and maxillary right central incisor to create room for her maxillary right lateral incisor. This was done slowly while the maxillary right canine labial gingiva was monitored.

When enough space had been created for her maxillary right lateral incisor, Amelia was placed on a posterior biteplate (orthodontic cement bonded to the occlusal surfaces of her maxillary first molars) to open her anterior bite and permit clearance for her maxillary right lateral incisor to be advanced out of cross bite. The lateral incisor was then bonded, and the cross bite was corrected.

Q: Progress records were made and are shown in Figures 2.29a–2.29e. What changes do you observe?

(a) (b) (c)

(d) (e)

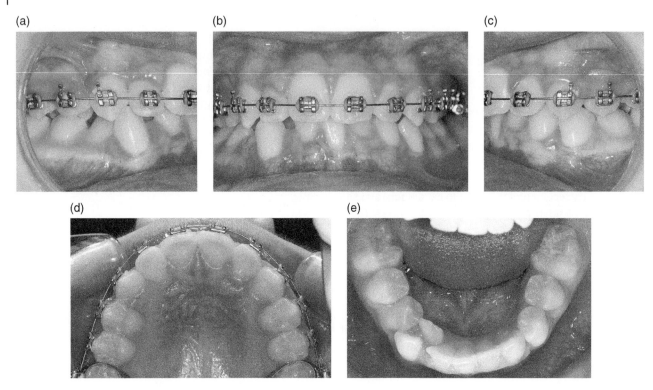

Figure 2.29 (a–e) Progress records of Amelia.

A: Changes include:

- Anterior cross bite has been corrected.
- Maxillary right permanent canine labial gingiva appears intact.
- Anterior OJ is minimal, ~1 mm.
- Maxillary arch is aligned and maxillary spaces are closed.
- Thin labial gingiva is noted labial to the mandibular right canine and mandibular left central incisor.
- Mandibular right permanent canine is still blocked out of the arch.

Q: Was it smart to align her maxillary arch first (reduce unknowns)? What treatment do you recommend now, and why?

A: As is so often the case, it was wise to reduce unknowns first (align her maxillary arch). We now recommended extraction of Amelia's mandibular right central incisor to provide 5 mm of mandibular anterior space. This extraction would be followed by placement of fixed mandibular orthodontic appliances, leveling and aligning of the mandibular arch, and shifting the mandibular right lateral incisor and right canine toward the left. Why did we choose this treatment plan?

With minimal anterior OJ (Figure 2.29a), extraction of a mandibular central incisor would:

- Provide 5 mm of space to permit aligning mandibular anterior teeth.
- Avoid stressing mandibular anterior labial periodontium which would occur with non-extraction mandibular arch alignment.
- Avoid proclining mandibular anterior teeth into anterior cross bite which could occur with non-extraction alignment.
- Avoid the need for maxillary anterior space creation (plus veneers to fill the spaces created), or significant mandibular interproximal enamel reduction, to create overjet with non-extraction alignment.
- Avoid dishing in Amelia's profile with four premolar extraction treatment.

Q: Deband records are shown in Figure 2.30. What do you observe?

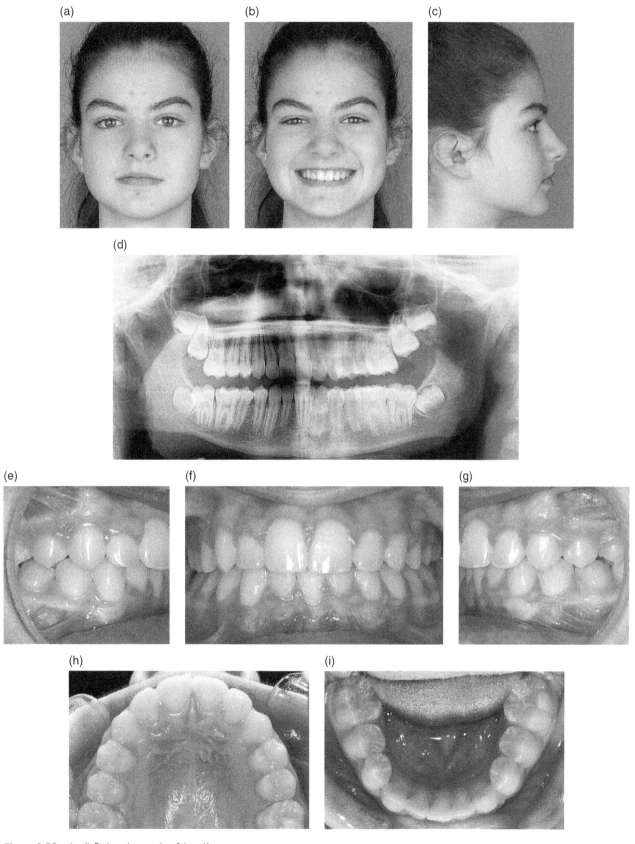

Figure 2.30 (a–i) Deband records of Amelia.

A: Amelia ended with a beautiful smile and well interdigitated Class I occlusion. Additional observations include:

- A mild right-to-left occlusal cant still exists.
- Her profile is straight.
- The panoramic image is magnified on the left compared with the right; maxillary second molars are unerupted; mandibular second molars are tipped distally; mandibular right second premolar's root is tipped distally; and third molars are developing.
- Her right maxillary central incisor gingival margin is slightly apical compared with her left.
- Her right maxillary lateral incisor gingival margin is slightly incisal compared with her left.
- 20% OB.
- <1 mm OJ.
- Mandibular left central incisor labial periodontal biotype is still thin and will be monitored.
- Her maxillary midline overlays the *center* of her mandibular central incisor (to be expected in a mandibular incisor extraction case).
- Mandibular right lateral incisor is slightly rotated (Figure 2.30i).

Q: Should we have extracted another incisor, instead of the mandibular right central incisor?

A: You could certainly argue that extraction of the mandibular right *lateral* incisor would have been a better choice. Why? The crowding (blocked out mandibular right canine) was closer to the right lateral incisor than to the right central incisor. This would have made post-extraction alignment and space closure easier. Of course, extraction of the mandibular right lateral incisor would have meant that slightly more extraction space would have been created, leading to slightly more anterior OJ at the end of treatment.

You could also argue that extracting the mandibular *left* central incisor would have been a better choice. Why? The labial periodontium covering the mandibular left central incisor was (and is) of a thinner biotype than the other incisors. Of course, extraction of the mandibular left central incisor would have made space closure (shifting the mandibular right central incisor and right lateral incisor to the left) more difficult.

Q: What retention protocol would you recommend for Amelia?

A: She will wear Hawley retainers every night, for life. Only with lifelong retention can alignment of teeth be guaranteed. The maxillary Hawley retainer includes an anterior biteplate to disclude her posterior teeth slightly when she wears it, which should help prevent her OB from deepening. A mandibular fixed canine-to-canine retainer could also have been used instead of a removable mandibular retainer.

Q: Can you suggest "take-home pearls" regarding Amelia's treatment?

A: "Take-home pearls" include the following:

- It was prudent to correct Amelia's ectopically erupting maxillary left permanent first molar with *early treatment*. Why? If we had not moved her maxillary left permanent first molar distally, then her maxillary left second premolar could have become impacted by the ectopic mesial eruption of the permanent first molar.
- Amelia exemplifies the following *principle: always ask if there are unknowns which can be eliminated before performing irreversible treatment*. It was smart to level and align Amelia's maxillary arch first with fixed orthodontic appliances (to gage resulting anterior OJ) before a decision was made regarding permanent tooth extractions. Because only minimal anterior OJ resulted after maxillary arch alignment, extraction of a mandibular incisor seemed reasonable in order to correct ~5.5 mm of mandibular anterior crowding present. If a large anterior OJ had resulted following maxillary arch alignment, then extracting a mandibular incisor would have been less desirable.
- Amelia exemplifies the following *principle: exhaustively consider all non-extraction and extraction options before making your final comprehensive treatment decision*. There are always trade-offs to consider in various extraction (or non-extraction) options. Force yourself to consider the cost/benefit of treating the patient non-extraction, non-extraction with IPR, with extraction of various anterior teeth, and with extraction of various combinations of posterior teeth. Combined with the patient's desires, consideration of all options will usually reveal the best course of treatment.
- In cases of early crowding always consider monitoring (recall only), space maintenance, space regaining, and permanent tooth extraction. All options should be considered.

Q: Let us finish with two questions. Can you list factors which influence your management of early crowding? What are the general principles, or guidelines, to follow when managing early crowding?

A: Factors influencing your management of early crowding include:
- *Crowding magnitude*
- Developmental stage
- Presence of leeway space or E-space
- Labial periodontal biotype
- Incisor proclination or uprightness
- Presence of deepbite or openbite
- Degree of lip protrusion and presence of lip incompetence
- LAFH
- Anteroposterior and transverse relationships
- Profile straightness or convexity

- *Principle for managing early crowding – for the majority of patients, first attempt non-extraction treatment.*
- *Consider monitoring (recalling) patients with crowding in the primary/early mixed dentitions* – assuming that the permanent canine/premolar roots are immature (less than ½ developed so they are not close to eruption) and assuming that you judge the potential harm from monitoring to be minimal (e.g. the probability of root resorption from ectopically erupting teeth to be minimal).
- *Consider space maintenance* for patients with mild-to-moderate crowding in the late mixed dentition. Space maintenance (LLHA or Nance holding arch) can provide room (leeway space or "E-space") for permanent teeth to erupt and align in many patients without extraction of permanent teeth.
- *Generally, defer extraction decisions until permanent canines and premolars erupt whenever possible (reduce unknowns before committing to irreversible treatment, including extractions).* Once the permanent canines and premolars erupt, a more accurate assessment of crowding (and a clearer decision to extract) can be made.
- *Generally, defer extraction decisions until anteroposterior growth is addressed (reduce unknowns before committing to irreversible treatment).* Get future growth under control before extracting permanent teeth! Once you extract permanent teeth, those teeth cannot be put back even if the patient grows out of your correction.
- Exceptions to the above – when extraction of primary or permanent teeth should be considered include cases of ectopic eruption, incisor dehiscence, eruption into nonkeratinized gingiva, and severe crowding.
- We generally recommend serial extraction in early mixed dentition patients with *severe anterior crowding and only if the patient is normal otherwise (anteroposteriorly, vertically, and transversely).*

Case Jasmine

Q: Jasmine is eight years old (Figure 2.31) and presents to you for a consultation. Her parents' chief complaint is, "We were referred because of Jasmine's crowding." Her PMH, PDH, periodontal evaluation, and TMJ evaluation are WRN and CR = CO. Do you need any additional records in order to decide whether to perform early treatment, or recall Jasmine?

A: No. You can decide to treat or recall using these records.

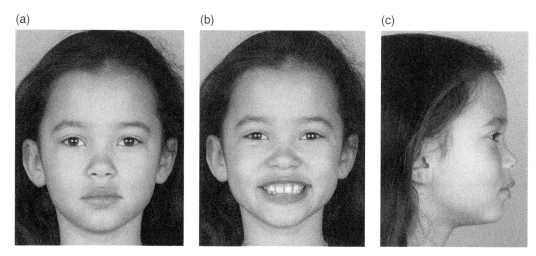

(a) (b) (c)

Figure 2.31 Initial records of Jasmine: (a–c) facial photographs, (d) pantomograph, and (e–i) intraoral photographs.

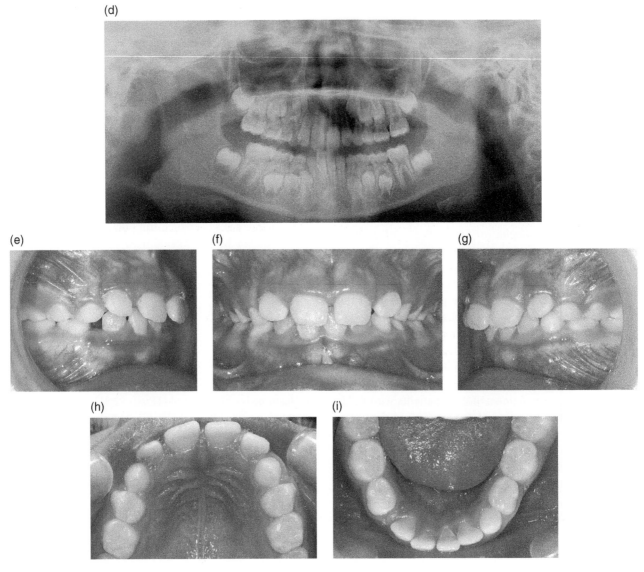

Figure 2.31 (Continued)

Q: Compile your diagnostic findings and problem list for Jasmine. Also, state your diagnosis.

A:

Table 2.4 Diagnostic findings and problem list for Jasmine.

Full face and profile	*Frontal view*
	Face is symmetric
	Soft tissue LAFH WRN (soft tissue Glabella – Subnasale approximately equal to Subnasale – soft tissue Menton)
	Lip competence
	UDML WRN
	Gingival display in posed smile is excessive (maxillary central incisor gingival margins are 5–6 mm below the maxillary lip)
	Profile view
	Relatively straight profile

Table 2.4   (Continued)

	Chin projection WRN
	Tipped-up nose
	NLA ~90° but only because maxillary lip is protrusive
	Lip-chin-throat angle WRN
Radiographs	Early mixed dentition
Intraoral photos and models	Angle Class I
	Iowa Classification: I I I I
	OJ ~ 4 mm
	OB 100 % (mandibular incisor palatal impingement but without pain or tissue damage), (Figure 2.31f and h)
	3 mm of maxillary anterior space is currently present
	5 mm of maxillary arch space is anticipated following eruption of all permanent teeth (if appropriate space maintenance is employed)
	3 mm of mandibular anterior space is present, but the 5 mm wide mandibular right primary canine is missing, so 2 mm of anterior crowding is actually present
	1.2 mm of mandibular arch space is anticipated following eruption of all permanent teeth (if appropriate space maintenance is employed
	LDML has shifted to Jasmine's right by ~2 mm and is to the right of her UDML
	Unerupted mandibular right permanent canine
	Maxillary arch asymmetry – maxillary left posterior appears slightly ahead of right (H), but the left-to-right occlusion does not reflect an asymmetry (right and left molars are Class I)
	Mandibular arch appears symmetric (Figure 2.31i)
	Maxillary central incisors are stepped down relative to her maxillary posterior teeth (Figure 2.31f)
	Maxillary midline diastema
	Poor hygiene
Other	None
Diagnosis	Class I malocclusion with mandibular anterior crowding

Q: Provide a detailed dental arch space analysis for Jasmine's maxillary and mandibular arches. In other words, how were the 5 mm of maxillary arch spacing and 1.2 mm of mandibular arch spacing calculated (if proper space maintenance is employed)?

A:

Average mesiodistal widths of permanent teeth (mm) [1]:

Maxillary Central Incisor	8.5	Mandibular Central Incisor	5.0
Maxillary Lateral Incisor	6.5	Mandibular Lateral Incisor	5.5
Maxillary Canine	7.5	Mandibular Canine	7.0
Maxillary First Premolar	7.0	Mandibular First Premolar	7.0
Maxillary Second Premolar	7.0	Mandibular Second Premolar	7.0
Maxillary First Molar	10.0	Mandibular First Molar	11.0
Maxillary Second Molar	9.0	Mandibular Second Molar	10.5

Average mesiodistal widths of *primary* teeth (mm) [1]:

Maxillary Central Incisor	6.5	Mandibular Central Incisor	4.2
Maxillary Lateral Incisor	5.1	Mandibular Lateral Incisor	4.1
Maxillary Canine	7.0	Mandibular Canine	5.0
Maxillary First Molar	7.3	Mandibular First Molar	7.7
Maxillary Second Molar	8.2	Mandibular Second Molar	9.9

MAXILLARY ARCH

+3 mm of anterior space is currently present (Figure 2.31h).

+2 mm of anticipated leeway space (1 mm/side).

Balance = +3 mm + 2 mm = +5.0 mm.

MANDIBULAR ARCH

+3 mm of anterior space present (Figure 2.31i).

−5 mm of space is needed for missing mandibular right primary canine.

+3.2 mm of anticipated leeway space (1.6 mm/side) if mandibular right primary canine was still present. Balance = +3 mm − 5 mm + 3.2 mm = +1.2 mm.

That is, *5.0 mm of maxillary arch space and 1.2 mm of mandibular arch space is anticipated following eruption of all permanent teeth (if appropriate space maintenance is employed).*

Q: What are Jasmine's *primary* problems in each dimension, plus other problems?

A:

Table 2.5 Primary problems list for Jasmine *(apical base/skeletal discrepancies italicized).*

AP	–
Vertical	OB 100% (palatal impingement, but without pain or tissue damage)
Transverse	–
Other	Mild (2 mm) mandibular anterior crowding currently present

Q: Discuss Jasmine in the context of three principles applied to every early treatment patient.

- The goal of early treatment is to correct developing problems – get the patient *back to normal for their stage of development* (including preventing complications such as resorption of adjacent tooth roots, reducing later treatment complexity, or reducing/eliminating unknowns). Regaining lost space for her mandibular right permanent canine to erupt, shifting her mandibular midline to the left to be coincident with her maxillary midline, and reducing her deep overbite would bring Jasmine back to normal for her stage of development.

- Early treatment should address *very specific problems with a clearly defined end point*, usually within six to nine months (except for some orthopedic problems). We can reduce her deep bite by placing fixed orthodontic appliances (braces) and leveling her arches with increasingly larger arch wires to intrude her maxillary and mandibular incisors. Her mandibular midline can be shifted to the left (space regaining) by using the same mandibular fixed appliances and trapping an open coil spring between her mandibular right primary first molar and mandibular right permanent lateral incisor. An LLHA (with a soldered spur to prevent lateral incisor drift) can then maintain this midline correction and allow her mandibular right permanent canine to erupt. This focused early treatment could be completed in six to nine months.

- Always ask: Is it necessary that I treat the patient now? *What harm will come if I choose to do nothing now?* It is *not* necessary to treat Jasmine now. If we do not treat her early, then her mandibular right permanent canine may remain unerupted, erupt ectopically, or (if the mandibular right primary first molar exfoliates) erupt over the mandibular right first premolar (possibly impacting it). The probability of her mandibular right permanent canine causing lateral incisor root resorption is low. Finally, since her mandibular incisor palatal impingement is causing neither pain nor tissue damage, we can treat her deep bite later. We anticipate no harm by waiting.

Q: Would you begin early treatment or recall Jasmine? If you start treatment, what treatment options would you consider?

A: Your options include the following:
- *Recall* (no treatment, monitor only) – re-evaluate in six to nine months. No harm is anticipated by monitoring Jamison. Eruption of her permanent teeth should continue normally, except for her mandibular right permanent canine, which may remain unerupted, erupt over the mandibular right first premolar, or erupt ectopically.

- *Space maintenance* – placement of an LLHA (and possibly Nance holding arch) would gain us leeway space on her maxillary left, maxillary right, mandibular left, and "E space" plus "D space" on her mandibular right when her remaining primary teeth exfoliate. However, her permanent canine and premolar roots appear to be less than ½ developed so their eruption is not imminent.

- *Space regaining* – opening space for Jasmine's mandibular right permanent canine using fixed orthodontic appliances (trapping an open coil spring between her mandibular right primary first molar and mandibular right permanent lateral incisor). Overjet may first need to be increased by placing fixed maxillary appliances, leveling her arches, and opening her bite. Later, after space is created for the mandibular right permanent canine, the space could be held using an LLHA with spurs soldered to prevent distal drifting of the permanent right lateral incisor.

- *Extraction of her mandibular right primary first molar* – would provide room for eruption of the mandibular right permanent canine (which is erupting ahead of her mandibular right first premolar), but could result in arch perimeter loss as the right permanent first molar drifts mesially. If an LLHA is placed at the time of primary first molar extraction, then arch perimeter loss could be prevented. Later, fixed appliances could be used to shift the mandibular midline to the left and regain space for her mandibular right first premolar. Because Jasmine's mandibular right premolar root is <½ developed, extraction of her mandibular right primary first molar will likely *delay* its eruption.

- *Serial extraction* – is not a reasonable option. As calculated above, Jasmine could eventually have anterior spacing in both arches if space maintainers are placed. Serial extraction should be considered in cases of severe anterior crowding.

- *Placement of fixed appliances (braces) to level the arches, open the deep bite, and eliminate mandibular incisor palatal impingement* – would be a recommended option if her mandibular incisor palatal impingement was causing tissue damage or pain. In such a case, a quicker and less expensive solution would be to fabricate a maxillary clear retainer that covered the palate and anterior teeth only (no coverage of posterior teeth). If she wore the retainer full time, then pain and further tissue damage would be eliminated, and posterior teeth would continue to erupt – opening the anterior bite.

Q: If you decide to place an LLHA, then should you solder a clasp (spur) which wraps around the distal of the mandibular right lateral incisor to prevent further distal drift?

A: In our opinion, no. Why? Look closely at the mandibular right permanent canine in Figure 2.31d. It has erupted so far occlusally that its crown should block further distal drift of the mandibular right lateral incisor.

Q: What is your recommended treatment for Jasmine at this consultation? How would you proceed?

A: We decided to monitor and *recall Jasmine in six to nine months*. At that time, if her mandibular left primary canine is mobile, then we will fabricate and cement an LLHA. We anticipate no additional early treatment for Jasmine.

Q: Would it be smarter to place an LLHA *now*?

A: It would be reasonable to place an LLHA now. Why? If Jasmine fails to show up for her recall appointment, then we will lose arch perimeter as the premolars and permanent canines erupt and posterior teeth drift mesially (and incisors upright).

On the other hand, we do not feel that an LLHA is necessary now because the remaining permanent teeth are not ready to erupt and because we worry about band cement "washout"/enamel decalcification if we place an LLHA too early. This is an example of the options and trade-offs you face with early crowding management.

Q: In contrast to Jasmine, look at another patient in Figures 2.32a and 2.32b. Would you place an LLHA in this patient (with a clasp wrapping around the distal of the mandibular *left* lateral incisor)?

A: In our opinion, yes. Why? The mandibular left permanent canine has erupted less than Jasmine's right permanent canine, and the mandibular left lateral incisor is likely to continue drifting to the distal without a spur holding it.

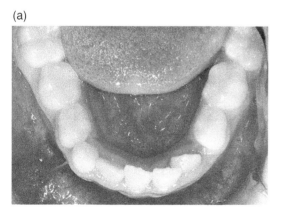
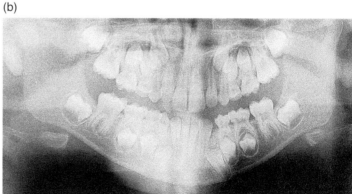

Figure 2.32   (a, b) A different patient with a clinical situation similar to Jasmine's.

Case Bella

Q: Bella is six years old (Figure 2.33). You are asked to provide a consultation for her pediatric dentist. Her parents state, "Our dentist referred us because Bella lost a lower front tooth." Her PMH, PDH, periodontal, mucogingival, and TMJ evaluations are WRN. CR = CO. *Compile your diagnostic findings and problem list*. State your *diagnosis*.

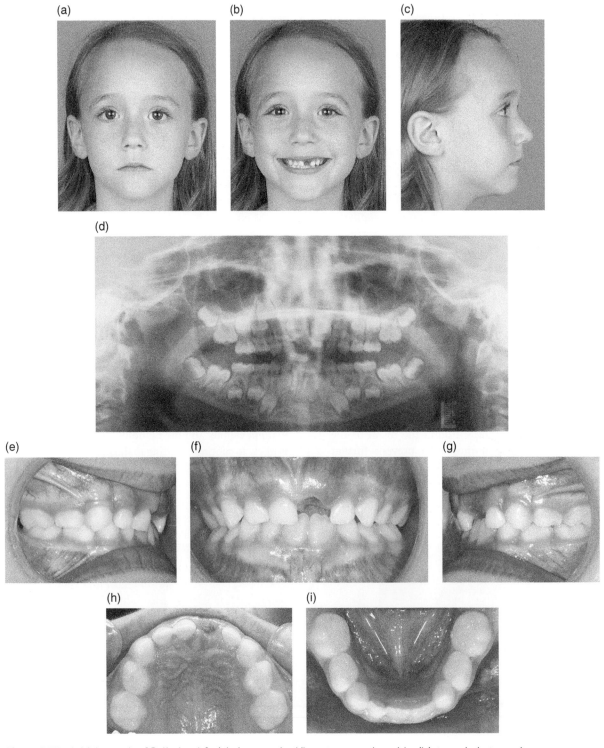

Figure 2.33 Initial records of Bella (a–c) facial photographs, (d) pantomograph, and (e–i) intraoral photographs.

A:

Table 2.6 Diagnostic findings and problem list for Bella.

Full face and profile	*Frontal view*
	Face is symmetric
	Soft tissue LAFH WRN (soft tissue Glabella – Subnasale ≈ Subnasale – soft tissue Menton)
	Lip competence
	UDML WRN
	Profile view
	Relatively straight profile
	Upturned nose
	NLA WRN
	Chin position WRN
	Lip-chin-throat angle WRN
	Chin-throat length WRN
Radiographs	Early mixed dentition (permanent first molars are unerupted, but permanent mandibular central incisors are erupted)
	Missing mandibular left primary lateral incisor
	Missing maxillary left primary central incisor
	Ectopically erupting mandibular left permanent lateral incisor
Intraoral photos and models	Angle Class I
	Iowa Classification: I I I I
	LDML 2 mm left of UDML
	Symmetric dental arches
	5.8 mm maxillary permanent incisor crowding currently present (calculated based upon 7.5 mm of space present, widths of primary incisors, and anticipated widths of permanent incisors)
	3.8 mm of maxillary arch crowding is anticipated following eruption of all permanent teeth (if proper space maintenance is employed)
	7.9 mm mandibular permanent incisor crowding currently present (based upon width of right primary lateral incisor, and anticipated widths of two permanent lateral incisors)
	4.7 mm of mandibular arch crowding is anticipated following eruption of all permanent teeth (if proper space maintenance is employed)
	Recently exfoliated maxillary left primary central incisor
	Missing mandibular left primary lateral incisor
	OJ 0 mm
	OB 30%
	Thick labial maxillary and mandibular periodontal biotype
Other	—
Diagnosis	Class I malocclusion with moderate anterior crowding
	Ectopically erupting mandibular left permanent lateral incisor

Q: Why is Bella's mandibular midline to the left of her maxillary midline?

A: Following loss of her mandibular left primary lateral incisor, her mandibular permanent central incisors erupted/drifted to the left (Figure 2.33i), closing the missing primary lateral incisor space and shifting the midlines to the left. Anterior teeth drift distally, and posterior teeth drift mesially, probably as a result of transseptal fiber pull [27].

Q: Do you need any additional records to decide whether to recall Bella or to perform early treatment?

A: No additional records are needed to make this decision. However, we would recommend making a periapical radiograph (or limited field of view CT scan) of the ectopically erupting mandibular left permanent lateral incisor in order to better visualize it. This was not done.

Q: Look at the panoramic radiograph (Figure 2.33d). Are any of Bella's permanent first molars ectopically erupting (impacted) under their primary second molars? Do you anticipate that her permanent first molars will erupt normally?

A: None of her permanent first molars appear to be ectopically erupting. At this time, we anticipate that her permanent first molars will erupt normally. However, we can never be certain that any tooth will erupt normally until eruption is complete.

Q: Would you recommend monitoring her permanent first molar eruption, or would you recommend early treatment to enhance their eruption (e.g. surgical exposure with forced orthodontic eruption)?

A: We would recommend monitoring eruption of her permanent first molars.

Q: Provide a detailed space analysis for Bella's maxillary and mandibular arches. In other words, how were the anticipated 3.8 mm of maxillary arch crowding and 4.7 mm of mandibular arch crowding calculated (following eruption of all permanent teeth if proper space maintenance is employed).

A: Below are space estimates:

Average mesiodistal widths of permanent teeth (mm) [1]:

Maxillary Central Incisor	8.5	Mandibular Central Incisor	5.0
Maxillary Lateral Incisor	6.5	Mandibular Lateral Incisor	5.5
Maxillary Canine	7.5	Mandibular Canine	7.0
Maxillary First Premolar	7.0	Mandibular First Premolar	7.0
Maxillary Second Premolar	7.0	Mandibular Second Premolar	7.0
Maxillary First Molar	10.0	Mandibular First Molar	11.0
Maxillary Second Molar	9.0	Mandibular Second Molar	10.5

Average mesiodistal widths of *primary* teeth (mm) [1]:

Maxillary Central Incisor	6.5	Mandibular Central Incisor	4.2
Maxillary Lateral Incisor	5.1	Mandibular Lateral Incisor	4.1
Maxillary Canine	7.0	Mandibular Canine	5.0
Maxillary First Molar	7.3	Mandibular First Molar	7.7
Maxillary Second Molar	8.2	Mandibular Second Molar	9.9

MAXILLARY ARCH

+7.5 mm of anterior space is currently present (Figure 2.33h).
−8.5 mm anticipated width of left permanent central incisor required.
+6.5 mm width of right primary central incisor.
−8.5 mm width of right permanent central incisor required.
+5.1 mm width of right primary lateral incisor.
−6.5 mm width of right permanent lateral incisor required.
+5.1 mm width of left primary lateral incisor.
−6.5 mm width of left permanent lateral incisor required.
+2 mm anticipated leeway space (1 mm/side).
Balance = +7.5 mm − 8.5 mm + 6.5 mm − 8.5 mm + 5.1 mm − 6.5 mm + 5.1 mm − 6.5 mm + 2 mm = −3.8 mm.

MANDIBULAR ARCH

−1 mm of incisor crowding is currently present, but the left primary lateral incisor is missing (Figure 2.33i).
−5.5 mm anticipated width left permanent lateral incisor.
+4.1 mm width right primary lateral incisor.
−5.5 mm anticipated width right permanent lateral incisor.
+3.2 mm of anticipated leeway space (1.6 mm/side).
Balance = −1 mm − 5.5 mm + 4.1 mm − 5.5 mm + 3.2 mm = −4.7 mm.

That is, *3.8 mm of maxillary arch crowding and 4.7 mm of mandibular arch crowding is anticipated following eruption of all permanent teeth (if proper space maintenance is employed).*

Q: What are Bella's primary problems in each dimension, plus other problems, that you should focus on at every appointment?

A:

Table 2.7 Primary problems list for Bella *(apical base/skeletal discrepancies italicized).*

AP	—
Vertical	—
Transverse	—
Other	Moderate maxillary (5.8 mm) and mandibular (7.9 mm) anterior crowding
	Ectopically erupting mandibular left permanent lateral incisor

Q: Discuss Bella in the context of three principles applied to every early treatment patient.

- The goal of early treatment is to correct developing problems – get the patient *back to normal for their stage of development* (including preventing complications such as resorption of adjacent tooth roots, reducing later treatment complexity, and reducing/eliminating unknowns). Ensuring that all of Bella's permanent teeth erupt would get her back to normal for her stage of development.

- Early treatment should address *very specific problems with a clearly defined end point*, usually begun and ended within six to nine months (not protracted over many years, except for select orthopedic problems). Bella's anterior crowding and ectopically erupting mandibular left permanent lateral incisor are specific problems with clearly defined end points. However, if space maintenance is employed for leeway space, then correction will take longer than nine months because permanent canines and premolars are years away from erupting.

- Always ask: Is it necessary that I treat the patient now? *What harm will come if I chose to do nothing now?* It is not necessary to treat Bella now, and you could choose to monitor her permanent tooth eruption. The risk of monitoring is that her mandibular left permanent lateral incisor could continue to erupt ectopically, become impacted, or possibly resorb the left central incisor root.

Q: Let us review our guidelines for dealing with early mandibular anterior crowding. Are the following six statements true or false?

1) For most patients, first attempt non-extraction treatment.

2) Generally, monitor (recall) patients with crowding in the primary/early mixed dentitions.

3) Generally, consider space maintenance for patients with mild-to-moderate crowding in the late mixed dentition. By employing an LLHA and taking advantage of mandibular leeway space (3.2 mm total in the arch), spontaneous crowding reduction can occur during the transition to permanent dentition.

4) Reduce unknowns. Generally, postpone extraction decisions until premolars and permanent canines erupt. Then, you can better judge their size and the magnitude of crowding.

5) Reduce unknowns. Postpone extraction decisions until anteroposterior growth is addressed/under control.

6) Consider serial extraction, or other extraction of primary and permanent teeth, in cases of:
   a) ectopic eruption
   b) incisor dehiscence
   c) eruption in nonkeratinized gingiva
   d) severe crowding (obvious extraction case)

A: All six statements are true.

Q: Bella's mandibular left permanent lateral incisor is erupting ectopically, and there is inadequate space for her mandibular right permanent lateral incisor to erupt into alignment. Should we treat Bella with serial extraction? Does she exhibit features of an ideal serial extraction patient?

A: No, we should not treat Bella with serial extraction. Let us discuss Bella in the context of each feature which would define an ideal serial extraction patient (*normal in every way, except severe anterior crowding*):

- *Class I first molars.* Bella is Class I in her primary second molars and primary canines.

- *Vertically normal to slightly long soft tissue and skeletal LAFH, with minimal OB or possibly a mild open bite, but <u>not</u> a deep bite.* Bella is normal vertically (soft tissue), but her OB is mildly deep (30%).

- *Normal incisor angulation or proclined incisors, but <u>not</u> upright incisors.* We do not have a cephalometric radiographic to accurately measure Bella's incisor angulation. Further, only her mandibular permanent central incisors are erupted.

- *Normal posterior transverse relationship (good posterior interdigitation; absence of posterior cross bites; and absence of significant transverse compensations).* Bella has a normal transverse relationship.

- *Severe (≥9 mm) anterior crowding* – Bella does not meet this criterion. We anticipate 3.8 mm of maxillary arch crowding and 4.7 mm of mandibular arch crowding following eruption of all permanent teeth (if proper space maintenance is employed).

Based upon the above features, Bella is *not* an ideal candidate for serial extraction.

Q: What treatment options would you consider for Bella? Exhaustively discuss the benefits and costs of each.

A: Treatment options include the following:

- *Recall* (monitor) – in nine to twelve months to evaluate tooth eruption. Since the mandibular left permanent lateral incisor does not appear to be causing problems (dehiscence or root resorption), monitoring Bella would seem reasonable. But if we choose this option, then we must explain the risks to her parents (mandibular left permanent lateral incisor continuing to erupt ectopically, becoming impacted, or possibly resorbing the left central incisor root). Further, we should consider additional imaging to better judge the mandibular left permanent lateral incisor situation.

- *Space maintenance* – placement of an LLHA and Nance holding arch as soon as the first permanent molars erupt. Because Bella's permanent canine and premolar roots are minimally developed (their eruption is years away), and because her primary canine and primary molar roots are not resorbing (exfoliation not imminent), there is no pressing need to place space maintainers yet. Space maintainers should be placed when she approaches the late mixed dentition stage of development.

  We wish to emphasize that the 3.2 mm of anticipated mandibular leeway space could go a long way toward resolving her anterior crowding, so the importance of Bella returning for annual recall visits must be emphasized. In our clinical opinion, *it is better to place space maintainers too early (and risk band cement washout) than to place them too late (and lose arch perimeter from mesial molar drift)*.

- *Extraction of mandibular left primary canine* – would aid in eruption of the mandibular left permanent lateral incisor. This is a reasonable extraction option since the mandibular left permanent lateral incisor is erupting ectopically (Figure 2.33d). Recall our guideline: *early extraction of primary and permanent teeth should be considered in patients with ectopic incisor eruption, dehiscence of tissue covering incisors, incisors erupting into nonkeratinized gingiva, and severe crowding*.

  If extraction of the mandibular left primary canine is the option chosen, then we would wait until both mandibular permanent first molars erupted to proceed. Why? Following extraction of the left primary canine, we would band the permanent first molars and place an LLHA with a soldered spur wrapping around the distal of the left central incisor – to prevent mesial drift of the left molars (loss of arch perimeter) and to prevent further distal drift of the mandibular left lateral incisor.

- *Extraction of both right and left mandibular primary canines plus extraction of the mandibular right primary lateral incisor* – would aid in eruption and alignment of mandibular permanent lateral incisors. Once again, if this were the option chosen, then we would wait until the permanent first molars erupted before proceeding. And please remember, there is a little girl attached to this option who would require bilateral mandibular anesthesia to proceed.

- *Space regaining* – opening space for the ectopically erupting mandibular left permanent lateral incisor is not recommended at this time. Why? Bella lacks anterior overjet. In other words, in order to create space for the mandibular left permanent lateral incisor, we will need to *procline* the mandibular central incisors. But, in order to procline the mandibular central incisors, we must have anterior overjet. Without overjet, you will procline/advance her mandibular incisors into cross bite.

  Space regaining *may* be an option once her maxillary permanent incisors erupt, but space regaining is not recommended now. Why? Because in order to create overjet, maxillary primary incisors must be proclined, and their roots will be driven reciprocally into the permanent incisor crowns.

  If space is eventually regained for the mandibular left permanent lateral incisor, then you will need to place an LLHA (with a soldered spur distal to the mandibular left central incisor) to order to maintain the opened space.

- *Extraction of maxillary primary canines* and remaining primary incisors – could be a viable option if the permanent incisors fail to erupt or if Bella's maxillary permanent canine crowns begin to overlap her maxillary permanent lateral incisor roots on a panoramic image (ectopic eruption). We do not recommend this option now.

- *Serial extraction* – would not be appropriate for Bella. We anticipate only 3.8 mm of maxillary arch crowding and 4.7 mm of mandibular arch crowding following eruption of all her permanent teeth (if proper space maintenance is employed). Serial extraction patients should present with severe crowding (≥9 mm).

Q: After considering the above options, do you recommend recalling (monitoring) Bella or do you recommend early treatment at this consultation? If you recommend early treatment, what treatment do you recommend?

A: We recommended extraction of the mandibular left primary canine and placement of an LLHA with soldered spur wrapping around the distal of the mandibular left central incisor.

Q: One year later, Bella presented for a follow-up appointment (Figure 2.34). What changes do you note from this radiograph?

Figure 2.34 Panoramic image of Bella one year later.

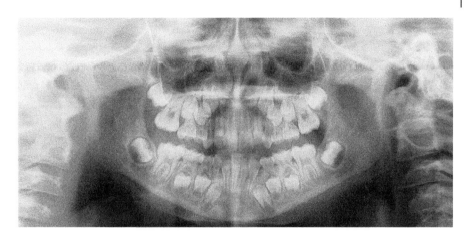

A: Changes include:
- Exfoliation of all primary incisors, eruption of all permanent incisors, and eruption of all permanent first molars.
- Continuation of permanent canine and premolar root development.

Our request for an LLHA (with spur distal to the mandibular left central incisor) was ignored. Note that the mandibular left lateral incisor has continued to drift to the distal and is now contacting the mandibular left primary first molar.

Q: A decision was now made by the pediatric dentist to extract the mandibular *right* primary canine. What can you gain by this extraction? What can you lose?

A: You can gain mandibular midline improvement if her mandibular incisors drift/shift to the right as a result of this extraction. You can lose arch perimeter if an LLHA is not placed with the extraction and if the posterior teeth drift mesially.

Q: Bella moved away, and no additional records were made. Can you suggest "take-home pearls" for Bella's treatment?

A: "Take-home pearls" include:
- Additional imaging of Bella's ectopically erupting mandibular left permanent lateral incisor may have been helpful to better visualize the situation we were initially dealing with. Practice radiation hygiene, but always request the imaging you need to properly care for your patients.
- Since all four maxillary incisors erupted normally, and since the maxillary permanent canines appear to be reasonably positioned (Figure 2.34), the decision *not* to extract the maxillary primary canines and remaining primary incisors appears to have been

correct. It is important that Bella's tooth eruption continues to be monitored regularly.
- The decision to monitor permanent first molar eruption was correct.
- Whenever you are concerned with arch perimeter loss in the mixed dentition following loss of primary teeth, consider including a space maintainer in your treatment plan.
- We generally do not recommend extracting primary canines in order to achieve incisor alignment or midline improvement. However, if a primary canine is extracted for those purposes, then we recommend placing an LLHA to prevent arch perimeter loss.

Case Evan

Q: Evan is a 10-year-old boy with a clinical situation similar to Jasmine's in the previous case (Class I, deep bite, missing mandibular right primary molar). He presents to you for a consultation. His parents' chief complaint is "crowding." What do you tell his parents at this consultation? Should you monitor (recall) him? Do you wish to perform early treatment? If you wish to perform early treatment, what treatment do you recommend? (Figure 2.35)

A: We recommended *immediate* placement of an LLHA and Nance holding arch (Figure 2.36). Why? Compared with Jasmine, Evan's premolar and permanent canine root development is more advanced. In fact, Evan's maxillary left first premolar has already erupted. By placing an LLHA and Nance holding arch now, we will utilize leeway space/"E-space"/"D-space" to reduce anterior crowding. Progress photographs (Figure 2.37) show Evan after all permanent teeth have erupted (early treatment complete). Note spontaneous improvement in maxillary anterior teeth alignment and spontaneous eruption of mandibular right permanent canine.

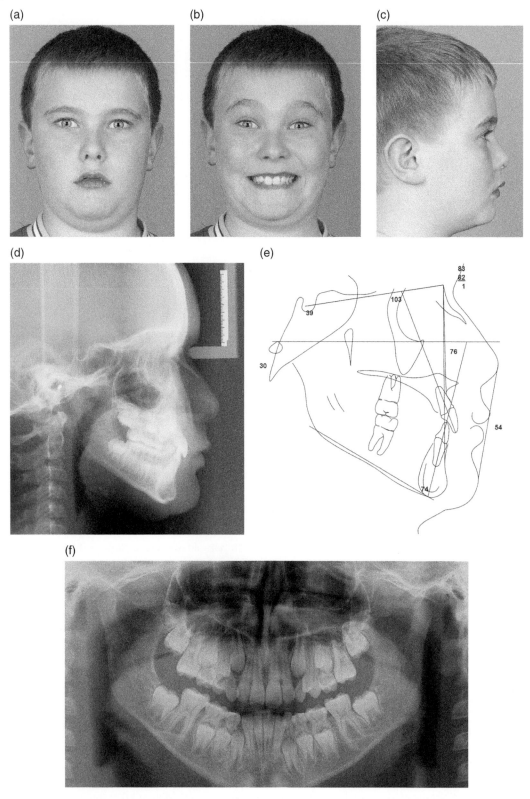

Figure 2.35 Initial records of Evan: (a–c) facial photographs, (d, e) lateral cephalometric radiograph and tracing, (f) pantomograph, and (g–k) intraoral photographs.

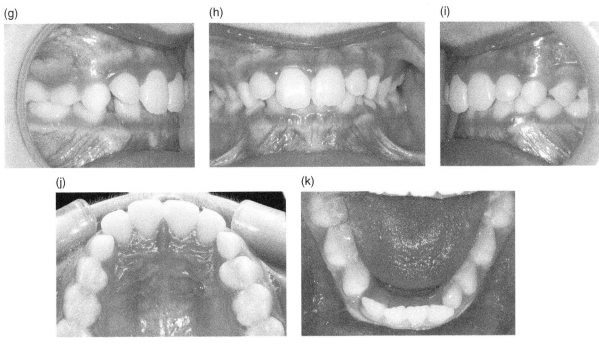

Figure 2.35 (Continued)

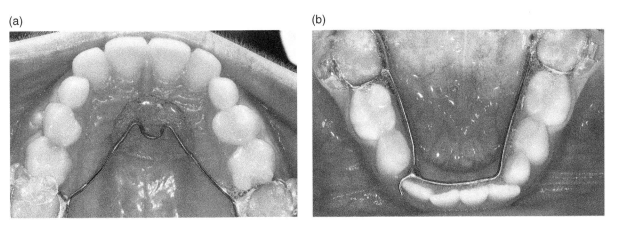

Figure 2.36 (a) Cementation of a Nance holding arch and (b) an LLHA in Evan.

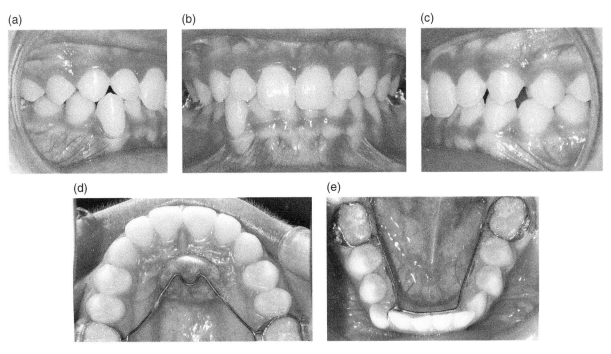

Figure 2.37 (a–e) Progress photographs of Evan following eruption of all permanent teeth.

Q: Was Evan's early treatment warranted?

A: Evan's early treatment was necessary and successful.

Q: Can you suggest a "take-home pearl" regarding Evan's early treatment?

A: Evan's treatment underscores the importance of space maintenance. By utilizing leeway space/"E-space"/ "D-space," all of Evan's permanent teeth erupted and his mandibular right canine now requires only a few millimeters of space to be aligned.

Q: How would you recommend proceeding with comprehensive treatment? Would you recommend non-extraction treatment, extraction of anterior teeth, or extraction of posterior teeth?

A: Because Evan's mandibular labial periodontium has a thick biotype and his mandibular incisors are upright (Figure 2.35e, FMIA = 76°), we anticipate Evan can now undergo non-extraction comprehensive treatment by removing the space maintainers, placing fixed orthodontic appliances, leveling his arches with wires to open his bite (which will increase his anterior overjet), and aligning his arches. His upright mandibular incisors will procline to a more normal angulation as his mandibular right canine is aligned with the arch.

Case Amber

Q: Amber is nine years and six months old (Figure 2.38). She is referred to you for orthodontic treatment. PMH includes asthma, PDH is WRN, TMJs are WRN, periodontal/mucogingival tissues are healthy, and CR = CO. *Compile your diagnostic findings and problem list.* State your *diagnosis.*

(a)　　　　　　　(b)　　　　　　　(c)

(d)　　　　　　　(e)

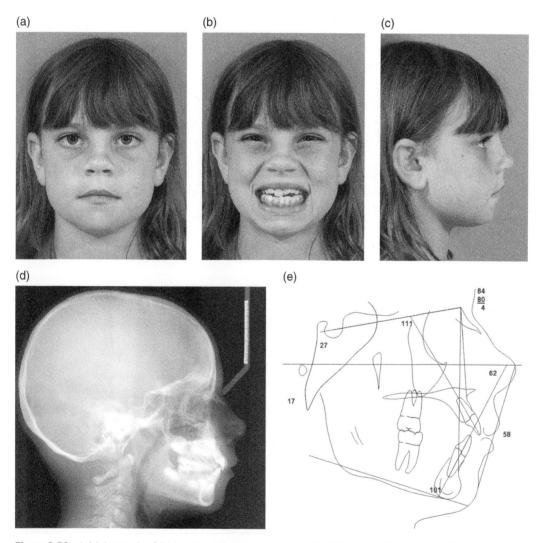

Figure 2.38 Initial records of Amber: (a–c) facial photographs, (d, e) lateral cephalometric radiograph and tracing, (f) pantomograph, and (g–k) intraoral photographs.

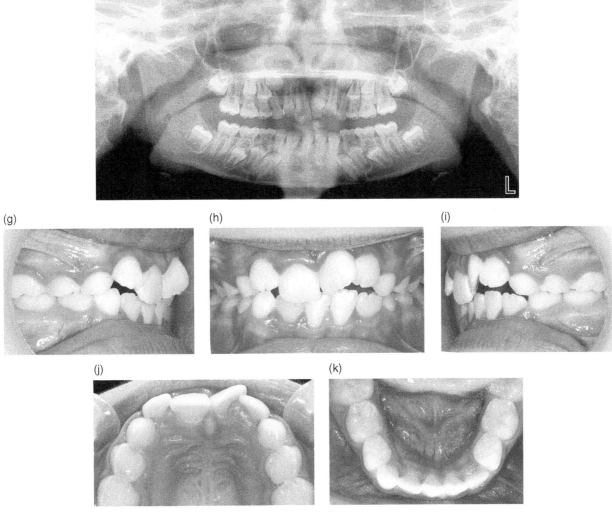

(f)

(g) (h) (i)

(j) (k)

Figure 2.38 (Continued)

A:

Table 2.8 Diagnostic findings and problem list for Amber.

Full face and profile	*Frontal view*
	Face is symmetric
	Long soft tissue LAFH (soft tissue Glabella – Subnasale < Subnasale – soft tissue Menton)
	Lip competence
	UDML to left of face by 1–2 mm
	Incisal display during posed smile WRN for maxillary right central incisor (Figure 2.38b, maxillary right central incisor gingival margin congruent with the maxillary lip)
	Wide buccal corridors
	Profile view
	Convex profile
	Upturned nose
	Obtuse NLA
	Retrusive chin position
	Obtuse lip-chin-throat angle
	Short chin-throat length

(Continued)

Table 2.8 (Continued)

Ceph analysis	*Skeletal* Maxillary anteroposterior position WRN (A-Point lies approximately on Nasion-perpendicular line) Deficient mandibular anteroposterior position (ANB = 4° with normal maxilla) Mildly long skeletal LAFH (LAFH/TAFH× 100% = 58%; normal = 55% with a 2% sd) Flat MPA (FMA = 17°, SN-MP = 27°) Effective bony Pogonion (Pogonion lies anterior to extended Nasion – B-Point line) *Dental* Proclined maxillary incisors (maxillary left central incisor is traced with U1 to SN = 111°; maxillary right central incisor angle is more acute to SN) Mildly proclined mandibular incisors (FMIA = 62°)
Radiographs	Early mixed dentition Potentially impacted mandibular left permanent canine Mild overlap of maxillary left permanent canine crown over root of maxillary left permanent lateral incisor
Intraoral photos and models	Angle Class I Iowa Classification: I I X I OJ 0 mm at right central incisor, 2–3 mm at maxillary lateral incisors Open bite at maxillary lateral incisors OB 30% at right central incisor 5 mm maxillary anterior crowding currently present 3 mm of maxillary arch crowding is anticipated following eruption of all permanent teeth (if appropriate space maintenance is employed) 5.5 mm mandibular anterior crowding currently present (1 mm incisor crowding, 0.5 mm spacing distal to left lateral incisor, and missing 5 mm mandibular left primary canine) 2.3 mm of mandibular arch crowding is anticipated following eruption of all permanent teeth (if appropriate space maintenance is employed) Premature loss of mandibular left primary canine LDML 2 mm left of UDML Dental arches symmetric in posterior Adequate periodontal biotype thickness labial to maxillary and mandibular incisors
Other	
Diagnosis	Class I malocclusion with moderate maxillary and mandibular anterior crowding, proclined incisors, and potentially impacted mandibular left permanent canine

Q: Do you require additional records to assess Amber's need for early treatment?

A: Since the mandibular incisor roots cannot be adequately evaluated from the panoramic image (Figure 2.38f), periapical radiographs of these teeth could be helpful. Periapical radiographs were not made.

Q: If her maxillary arch is symmetric in the posterior, then why is her maxillary midline to the left of her face? Why is her mandibular midline to the left of her maxillary midline?

A: As far as her UDML is concerned, we can only speculate that Amber's maxillary right permanent central incisor erupted ahead of the left. Being larger than the maxillary primary central incisors, the right permanent central incisor took up some of the left permanent central incisor's space – leaving the UDML to the left of the face and forcing the maxillary left permanent central incisor to erupt into a rotated position. As far as her LDML is concerned, following loss of her mandibular left primary canine, her mandibular incisors drifted to her left as a result of transseptal fiber pull [27].

Q: Provide a detailed space analysis for Amber's maxillary and mandibular arches. In other words, how were the 3 mm of anticipated future maxillary arch crowding and 2.3 mm of future mandibular arch crowding calculated (if space maintenance is employed)?

A: Below are space analysis estimates:
Average mesiodistal widths of permanent teeth (mm) [1]:

Maxillary Central Incisor	8.5	Mandibular Central Incisor	5.0
Maxillary Lateral Incisor	6.5	Mandibular Lateral Incisor	5.5
Maxillary Canine	7.5	Mandibular Canine	7.0
Maxillary First Premolar	7.0	Mandibular First Premolar	7.0
Maxillary Second Premolar	7.0	Mandibular Second Premolar	7.0
Maxillary First Molar	10.0	Mandibular First Molar	11.0
Maxillary Second Molar	9.0	Mandibular Second Molar	10.5

Average mesiodistal widths of *primary* teeth (mm) [1]:

Maxillary Central Incisor	6.5	Mandibular Central Incisor	4.2
Maxillary Lateral Incisor	5.1	Mandibular Lateral Incisor	4.1
Maxillary Canine	7.0	Mandibular Canine	5.0
Maxillary First Molar	7.3	Mandibular First Molar	7.7
Maxillary Second Molar	8.2	Mandibular Second Molar	9.9

MAXILLARY ARCH
−5 mm of anterior crowding is currently present (Figure 2.38j).
+2 mm of anticipated leeway space (1 mm/side).
Balance = −5 mm + 2 mm = −3 mm.

MANDIBULAR ARCH (cannot use *left* leeway space due to absence of primary canine)
+0.5 mm of spacing is present distal to the mandibular left lateral incisor (Figure 2.38k).
−1 mm of incisor crowding currently present.
+1.6 mm of anticipated leeway space on the right.
−7.0 mm width of left permanent canine required.
+7.7 mm width of left primary first molar.
−7.0 mm width of left first premolar required.
+9.9 mm width of left primary second molar.
−7.0 mm width of left second premolar required.
Balance = +0.5 mm − 1 mm + 1.6 mm − 7 mm + 7.7 mm − 7 mm + 9.9 mm − 7.0 mm = −2.3 mm.

That is, *3 mm of maxillary arch crowding and 2.3 mm of mandibular arch crowding is anticipated following eruption of all permanent teeth (if proper space maintenance is employed).*

Q: What is a reliable indicator of *severe* mandibular anterior crowding in the early mixed dentition?
A: Premature loss of primary canines. However, we calculate that Amber has only moderate crowding in both arches (and mild residual crowding if proper space maintenance is employed).

Q: Always focus on the patient's *primary* problems in each dimension, plus other primary problems, at every appointment. What are Amber's primary problems?
A: Amber's primary problems are:

Table 2.9 Primary problems list for Amber *(apical base/skeletal discrepancies italicized).*

AP	*Mandibular anteroposterior skeletal deficiency* (but Class I dentally)
Vertical	*Mildly long LAFH*
Transverse	—
Other	Moderate maxillary (5 mm) and moderate mandibular (5.5 mm) anterior crowding Proclined incisors

Q: Let us consider Amber's mandibular skeletal deficiency. She exhibits a convex profile and retrusive chin. Would you attempt Class II orthopedics to improve her chin projection?
A: It depends. First, Amber is Class I dentally and discussions with her parents reveal that they are happy with her profile. Therefore, we would not recommend Class II orthopedics for Amber. (Please be sensitive when discussing esthetics with patients and parents.)

If Amber was Class II dentally, then we would employ Class II orthopedics at some time. However, she is in the early mixed dentition, and research has demonstrated no advantage to beginning Class II treatment in the early mixed dentition (except for a possible reduction in incisor trauma) [28–37]. We generally follow this guideline, but since dental age may not coincide with skeletal age, we will consider Class II orthopedics *in the early mixed dentition if the patient has good statural growth velocity (growing continuously or is in their adolescent growth spurt).*

In Amber's case, her parents said that she is not growing. Therefore, we would not recommend Class II orthopedic treatment at this time if Amber was Class II dentally.

Q: Next, let us consider her vertical dimension. Amber exhibits a long soft tissue LAFH, a long skeletal LAFH, and open bites at both maxillary lateral incisors. Are you worried that Amber could be developing a skeletal open bite?

A: No. Although it is true that Amber's soft tissue and skeletal LAFHs are longer than normal, she lacks other features of a skeletal open bite. Amber exhibits lip competence (not lip incompetence), a flat MPA (not a steep MPA), her posterior face height appears normal (not short), and she has 30% OB at her right central incisor. We feel that her lateral incisor open bites are temporary due to their stage of eruption and/or due to crowding, and we recommend monitoring only in the vertical dimension.

Q: Amber demonstrates maxillary and mandibular dental proclination plus moderate maxillary and mandibular anterior crowding. Based upon these features, the need for permanent tooth extractions should be considered. Can you describe the features of an *ideal* serial extraction patient? Does Amber exhibit these ideal features, and is she a good candidate for serial extraction?

A: The ideal serial extraction patient is in the early mixed dentition stage of development and is *normal in every way, except severe anterior crowding (≥9 mm per arch)*. The patient should present with:

- *Class I first molars*: Amber presents with this feature.
- *Vertically normal to slightly long soft tissue and skeletal LAFH, with minimal OB or possibly a mild open bite, but not a deep bite*: Amber presents with these features.
- *Normal incisor angulation or proclined incisors, but not upright incisors*: Amber presents with this feature.
- *Normal posterior transverse relationship (normal inter-molar arch widths with good posterior interdigitation; absence of posterior cross bites; and absence of significant transverse compensations)*: Amber presents with this feature.
- *Severe (≥9 mm) anterior crowding*: Amber lacks this feature. She currently exhibits only moderate anterior crowding (5 mm maxillary anterior crowding and 5.5 mm mandibular anterior crowding). Furthermore, only 3 mm of maxillary arch crowding and 2.3 mm of mandibular arch crowding is anticipated if appropriate space maintenance is employed.

Based upon the above features, Amber is *not* an ideal candidate for serial extraction.

Q: We generally recommend monitoring patients with mild-to-moderate crowding in the primary/early mixed dentitions and space maintenance for patients with mild-to-moderate crowding in the late mixed dentition. Once all permanent teeth erupt, we recommend re-evaluating crowding severity and the need for extractions.

What if, instead, serial extraction is performed in patients with only mild-to-moderate crowding? What is the drawback of performing serial extraction on a mixed dentition patient *without severe crowding*?

A: The drawback is that the less anterior crowding the patient initially has, the less premolar extraction space will be used to align the anterior teeth, and the more residual extraction space will remain. This residual extraction space can be used to retract/upright proclined incisors. However, if incisors are not initially proclined, then closing this residual extraction space can upright incisors too much.

Q: Discuss Amber in the context of three principles applied to every early treatment patient.

1) The goal of early treatment is to correct developing problems – get the patient back to normal for their stage of development (including preventing complications such as resorption of adjacent tooth roots, reducing later treatment complexity, or reducing/eliminating unknowns). Amber's mandibular skeletal deficiency, excessive vertical growth, moderate maxillary and mandibular crowding, incisor proclination, and mandibular midline shift to the left are not normal for her stage of development and would need to be corrected to get her back on track.

2) Early treatment should address *very specific problems with a clearly defined end point*, usually beginning and ending within six to nine months (not protracted over many years), except for some orthopedic problems. Since Amber is Class I dentally without profile concerns, her growth will be monitored only. If anteroposterior or vertical orthopedic treatment is later desired, then it would probably take longer than nine months.

   Her crowding is a specific problem which has a clearly defined end point. Placement of a Nance holding arch and LLHA could utilize leeway space/"E space"/"D space" to reduce crowding during the transition to the permanent dentition. However, placement of an LLHA will prevent uprighting of her mildly proclined mandibular incisors and could slightly *increase their proclination* [5, 7]. This space maintenance could take longer than nine months depending upon permanent canine and premolar eruption.

3) Always ask: Is it necessary that I treat the patient now? *What harm will come if I choose to do nothing now?* It is *not* necessary to do anything now, because Amber's remaining permanent teeth are not expected to erupt within six months, and because she is not growing. If we chose to recall, then her permanent teeth will continue to erupt (except for the mandibular left permanent canine which will remain potentially impacted), erupt ectopically, or resorb the mandibular left lateral incisor root.

However, if we wait *longer* than six months, then Amber's first permanent molars may drift mesially into the leeway space/"E space" as the remaining primary teeth exfoliate – and that space will not be available for incisor alignment.

Q: What unknowns do you face with Amber's future treatment?

A: Magnitude and direction of future jaw growth are significant unknowns, along with the presence of an undetected CR–CO shift, patient compliance, and actual sizes of permanent canines and premolars.

Q: Should you start early treatment or recall? If you start treatment, what treatment would you suggest?

A: Your options include the following:

- *Recall* in six months (no early treatment, monitor only) – evaluate tooth eruption at that time. The risk of this approach is that the mandibular left permanent canine will either remain potentially impacted, erupt ectopically, or resorb the mandibular left permanent lateral incisor root.

- *Space maintenance* – place an LLHA and Nance holding arch before exfoliation of additional primary teeth. From our space analysis, it appears that Amber can probably be treated non-extraction with this option, if we are willing to leave her incisors mildly proclined.

  If we choose space maintenance, then it will not be necessary to solder an LLHA spur distal to the mandibular left lateral incisor to prevent drifting because the space distal to the mandibular left lateral incisor is nearly closed. Also, because the mandibular posterior quadrants appear symmetric (Figure 2.38k), the mandibular left midline deviation could be dealt with after the permanent canines and premolars erupt, at which time a final determination of tooth size, crowding, and need for permanent tooth extractions can be made. Finally, if her mandibular left canine does not erupt, then fixed appliances can be placed after premolar eruption, space opened for the mandibular left canine, and the mandibular midline shifted to the right. If space maintainers are placed now, then we would recommend periodically examining the appliances for cement washout (or asking the family dentist to do the same).

- *Space regaining* – open space for the missing mandibular left primary canine. In order to regain mandibular space, fixed appliances must first be placed on the maxillary teeth, and the maxillary anterior teeth aligned to create OJ. Next, fixed appliances are placed on the mandibular teeth, and mandibular anterior teeth aligned. Then, space is regained (space opened) where the mandibular left primary canine was lost by trapping a compressed open coil spring between the left lateral incisor and left primary first molar. Finally, the fixed appliances are removed, an LLHA placed (with spur soldered to prevent the left lateral incisor from drifting distally again), and a maxillary retainer worn to maintain alignment until all permanent teeth erupt. A potential risk with this approach is possible lateral incisor root resorption (by the unerupted maxillary and mandibular permanent canine crowns) as the lateral incisors are moved orthodontically.

- *Extraction of the mandibular right primary canine* – would provide spontaneous mandibular incisor alignment and shifting of the mandibular midline to the right. However, there is also the potential of mandibular arch perimeter loss (and less space for the permanent canines) if the right permanent molar drifts forward [38, 39]. Placing an LLHA would prevent/reduce this mesial molar drifting and loss of arch perimeter. However, because the mandibular incisors will spontaneously align if an LLHA is placed and the right primary canine exfoliates normally, we are not enthusiastic about putting Amber through a primary canine extraction with this approach.

- *Extraction of mandibular permanent left lateral incisor or IPR of her mandibular anterior teeth* – would provide room for eruption of her potentially impacted mandibular left permanent canine. However, based upon our space analysis, only 2.3 mm of mandibular arch crowding will remain if an LLHA is placed. Further, lateral incisor extraction (or anterior IPR) treatment could create a significant anterior Bolton discrepancy – leaving a large anterior OJ and lack of permanent canine coordination at the end of comprehensive treatment.

- *Extraction of maxillary primary canines or extraction of both maxillary primary canines and maxillary primary first molars* – to decrease the likelihood of her maxillary left permanent canine becoming impacted (mild overlap of canine crown and lateral incisor root seen on panoramic image) would not be recommended at this time. Why? The roots of the maxillary permanent canines and first premolars are <½ developed, and extraction of their primary predecessors could delay their eruption.

- *Alignment of maxillary incisors with fixed appliances to improve smile esthetics* – is not recommended because this is not a concern for Amber and her parents. Further, orthodontic movement could result in maxillary lateral incisor root resorption as their roots are forced into her unerupted maxillary permanent canine crowns.

- *Serial extraction* – is not recommended. Although Amber presents with some features which make her a serial extraction candidate (Class I first molars; slightly long soft tissue and skeletal LAFH, minimal OB or possibly a mild open bite; proclined incisors; normal posterior transverse relationship), she lacks the most important feature, *severe anterior crowding*. If you employ space maintenance now, then you can make a final decision regarding permanent tooth extractions later, after all of Amber's permanent teeth erupt.

Q: After considering the above options, how do you recommend proceeding?

A: A decision was made to recall Amber in six months to monitor eruption of permanent teeth. Unfortunately, Amber did not return for two and one-half years at which time records were made (Figure 2.39). What changes do you note?

Changes include:
- Facial features are largely unaltered.
- UDML appears to have shifted to the left following loss of maxillary left primary canine.
- Midlines coincident and to the left of facial midline.
- Late mixed dentition stage of development.

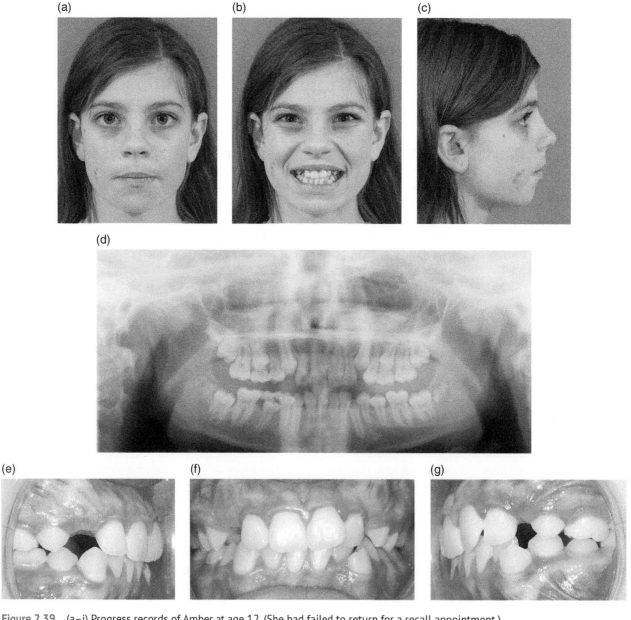

(a) (b) (c)

(d)

(e) (f) (g)

Figure 2.39 (a–i) Progress records of Amber at age 12. (She had failed to return for a recall appointment.)

(h)

(i)

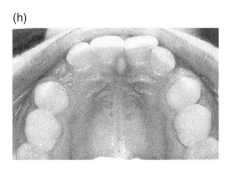
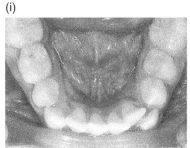

Figure 2.39   (Continued)

- Primary canines have exfoliated.
- Maxillary left permanent canine is possibly impacted.
- Mandibular left permanent canine is blocked out to the facial, but did not resorb the mandibular left lateral incisor root.
- Maxillary first premolars are Class II (distocclusion) of their ideal position relative to the mandibular first premolars. On her right side, the maxillary first premolar is Class II by 1–2 mm relative to the mandibular first premolar. On her left side, the maxillary first premolar is Class II by 3–4 mm.
- Moderate maxillary and mandibular anterior crowding is still present.
- Maxillary primary second molars and mandibular right primary second molar are still present.
- Maxillary left lateral incisor is in cross bite with mandibular left canine.

Q: Now that Amber has entered the late mixed dentition stage of development, would you consider addressing her Class II relationship (mandibular skeletal deficiency)? If you would, what suggestions could you make?

A: Of the three approaches to correcting a skeletal jaw discrepancy (orthopedics, masking, and surgery), an attempt to correct Amber's mandibular skeletal deficiency with orthopedics is reasonable. Orthopedics could be performed by either restricting maxillary growth (while permitting the mandible to continue growing forward) or by accelerating mandibular growth. Orthopedic options include headgear or Class II functional appliance treatment.
  - Headgears: in growing individuals, high-pull headgears restrict maxillary forward growth, distalize maxillary molars, and possibly reduce maxillary corpus descent and maxillary molar eruption. Cervical-pull headgears restrict maxillary forward growth, distalize maxillary first molars, create anterior palatal plane downward rotation, and erupt maxillary first molars by less than 1 mm [40–43].

  - Class II functional appliances: with mildly proclined mandibular incisors, Amber would not be an ideal candidate for a Class II functional appliance (e.g. Twin Block, Bionator, or Herbst appliance) since these appliances would cause additional mandibular incisor proclination. Class II functional appliances posture the mandible forward, distracting the condylar head out of the glenoid fossa. As the mandible is held forward, the stretched musculature and other soft tissues attempt to retract the mandible, producing the following effects in growing individuals to varying degrees: restriction of maxillary forward growth, retraction of maxillary posterior teeth, uprighting of maxillary incisors, mesial movement of mandibular posterior teeth, proclination of mandibular incisors, acceleration of condylar growth, and anterior displacement of the glenoid fossae. Functional appliances *do* accelerate mandibular growth in growing individuals. However, functional appliances do *not* enhance mandibular horizontal growth beyond that found in control subjects [44–49].

Q: Can you offer suggestions for dealing with Amber's anterior crowding at this point?

A: If orthopedics (headgear or Herbst appliance treatment) were applied, then maxillary molars would be distalized and maxillary space created (including maxillary "E-space") for her maxillary canines. Placing an LLHA before exfoliation of the mandibular right primary second molar would be prudent (providing right "E-space"). A final decision regarding permanent tooth extraction, or non-extraction, could be made after all permanent teeth erupt.

Q: How would you proceed?

A: Following discussions with Amber and her parents, a decision was made to *attempt* non-extraction orthopedic treatment and re-evaluate for possible premolar extractions after all permanent teeth erupted. Amber was placed on an HPHG to *overcorrect* her molars/premolars from Class II to Class III by 1–2 mm. Overcorrection is a common goal employed in orthodontic treatment since some treatment rebound will be anticipated.

Maxillary dental retraction with HPHG would provide room for her maxillary permanent canines to erupt, and the headgear force against her maxillary molars would restrict forward maxillary corpus growth while her mandible continued to grow forward. Amber would be held in this overcorrected relationship (with reduced headgear force and time) until all permanent teeth erupted.

An LLHA would be placed before exfoliation of the mandibular right primary second molar. After the mandibular right second premolar and remaining permanent teeth erupted, early treatment would be complete, and comprehensive treatment would begin. Fixed appliances would be placed, Amber's arches leveled and aligned, space created for her mandibular left permanent canine, and a final decision made (based upon incisor proclination/lip protrusion/patient desires) to either continue non-extraction or with extractions. One final note: if Amber creates, and maintains, an overcorrected Class III relationship with headgear, then Class III elastics could be used later to upright her mandibular incisors by tipping her occlusal plane CCW.

Q: Progress records made at the time her arches were leveled and aligned are shown in Figure 2.40a–h. What changes do you note?

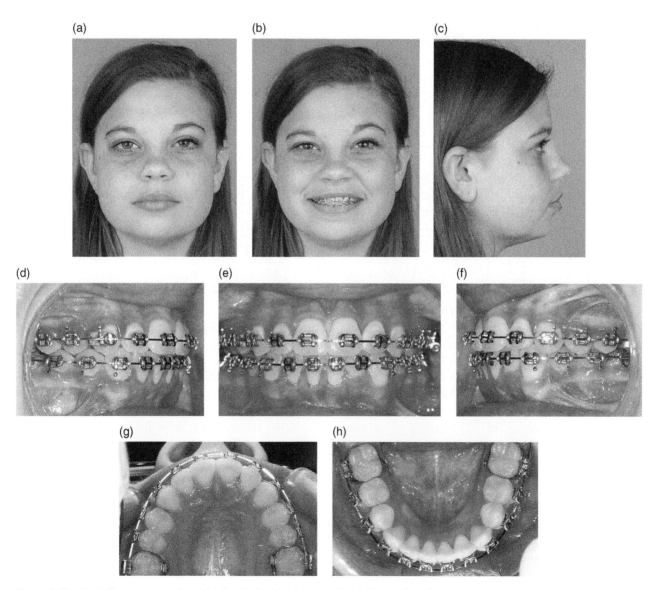

(a) (b) (c)

(d) (e) (f)

(g) (h)

Figure 2.40 (a–h) Progress records made after Amber's arches were leveled and aligned.

A: Changes include:
- An increase in Amber's facial fullness.
- Marginally inadequate incisal display in a posed smile.
- Downward descent of her nasal tip accompanied by a decrease in NLA.
- Increase in lip fullness.
- Deepening of labiomental sulcus.
- Increased chin projection.
- UDML WRN.
- LDML ~1 mm to right of UDML.
- Permanent dentition present.
- Class II (1 mm) right canines (Figure 2.40d).
- Class I left.
- Arches are leveled and aligned.

Q: A discussion was held with Amber and her mother to either continue non-extraction treatment or to extract four premolars. What are your thoughts?

A: Evidence-based orthodontic practice dictates that clinical decisions be founded on: (i) the best scientific evidence available; (ii) the orthodontist's experience and clinical judgment; and (iii) the patient's desires. Premolar extractions, in conjunction with incisor retraction, will reduce Amber's lip protrusion and increase her NLA [50–53].

In our opinion, Amber's maxillary lip currently exhibits attractive profile esthetics while her mandibular lip appears full and mildly protrusive. Premolar extractions may be beneficial in reducing her lower lip protrusion, but premolar extractions could open her NLA and create a less esthetic maxillary lip.

Amber and her mother were adamant – they loved her current esthetics and did not want premolars extracted. For these reasons, a decision was made to finish Amber's treatment non-extraction.

Q: Deband records are shown in Figure 2.41. What changes do you observe, apart from those noted above?

A: Changes noted include:
- Amber's treatment resulted in a dramatic improvement in her facial esthetics.
- Improved chin projection.
- ANB angle has reduced from 4° to 2°.
- Class I occlusion.

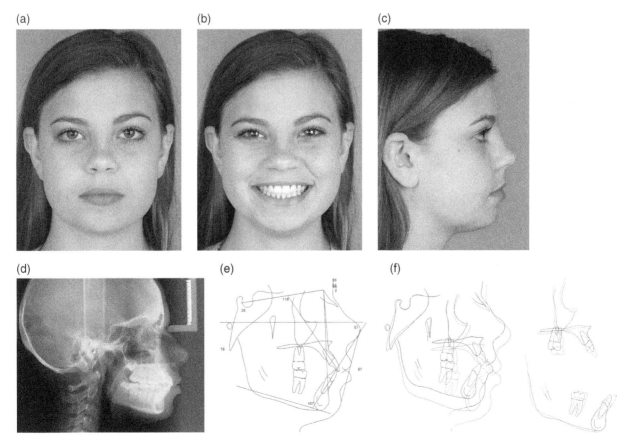

(a) (b) (c)

(d) (e) (f)

Figure 2.41 (a–l) Deband records of Amber.

(g)

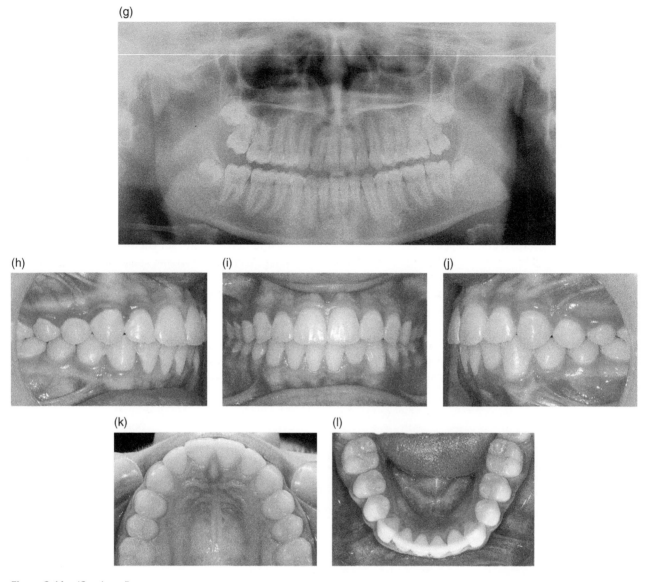

(h)　(i)　(j)

(k)　(l)

Figure 2.41 (Continued)

- Maxillary midline to left of mandibular midline by approximately 1 mm.
- Maxillary and mandibular incisors proclined during treatment.
- Maxillary and mandibular first molars erupted and drifted to the mesial.

Q: Do you have any suggestions regarding retention of her proclined mandibular incisors?

A: Yes. Orthodontic retention is as important as orthodontic diagnosis and treatment. Due to the proclination of her incisors, we decided to place a *fixed mandibular 3–3 retainer* (Figure 2.42). In addition, we asked her to wear a mandibular removable retainer at night and a maxillary Hawley retainer at night.

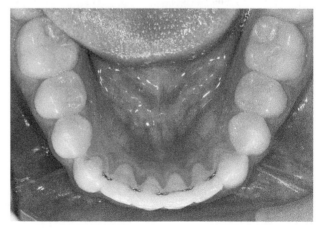

Figure 2.42 Mandibular fixed retainer in Amber.

Q: Can you suggest any "take-home pearls" for Amber?

A: "Take-home pearls" include the following:

- Amber was nine years old when she presented as Class I dentally (Class II skeletally) with moderate (~5 mm) crowding in both arches. Early and comprehensive treatment resulted in an esthetic, healthy, and functionally successful outcome. It employed HPHG (Class II orthopedic treatment) and non-extraction fixed appliance therapy.

- The biggest mistake in Amber's treatment was her not returning to our clinic for a recall appointment following her initial consultation. If she had returned six to nine months following her initial examination, then we could have placed her on space maintenance appliances (LLHA, Nance holding arch) and reduced her crowding via leeway space to an estimated 2–3 mm. Non-extraction treatment could then have resulted in less incisor proclination than she ended with.

- Emphasize the need for patients to return at designated recall times. Despite our best efforts, Amber did not return for over two years. By that time, leeway space was probably lost with mesial permanent first molar drift.

- It is better to place LLHAs and Nance holding arches too early rather than too late. The problem of placing one too early is band cement washout, but patients can always be recalled to check for this, and bands can always be re-cemented. The problem of placing space maintainers too late is loss of arch perimeter from permanent first molar mesial drift.

- *Reduce unknowns* whenever possible before committing to irreversible treatment (such as extraction of permanent teeth). We reduced unknowns with headgear wear and fixed appliances (to correct her Class II relationship and level/align arches) before we made a final non-extraction/extraction decision.

- As an orthodontist, you must decide whether extraction treatment or non-extraction treatment will create the best overall facial, occlusal, functional, healthy, and stable outcome. This decision is your professional opinion. But the patient's opinion (once you have informed them of the best scientific evidence and your opinion) has equal weight in the final decision. This is the foundation of an evidence-based orthodontic practice.

Case Kate

Q: Kate is 10 years old (Figure 2.43) and presents to you with her parents' chief complaint, "We were sent here by our family dentist. Kate has delayed dental development and may need braces." Her PMH and TMJ evaluation are WRN. PDH includes familial Class III development. CR = CO. *Compile your diagnostic findings and problem list. State your diagnosis.*

(a)

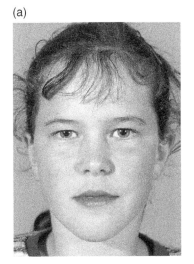

(b)

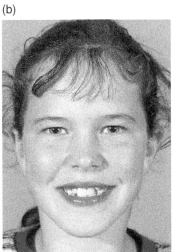

(c)

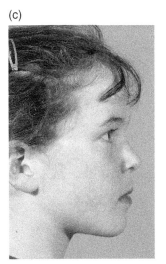

Figure 2.43 Initial records of Kate: (a–c) facial photographs, (d, e) lateral cephalometric radiograph and tracing, (f) pantomograph, (g–i) intraoral photographs, and (j–n) models.

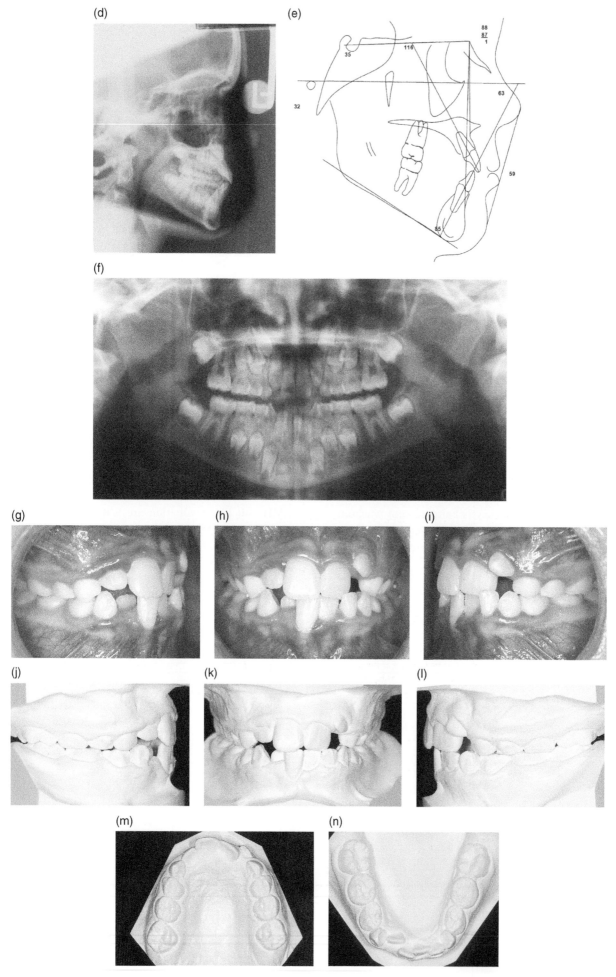

Figure 2.43 (Continued)

A:

Table 2.10 Diagnostic findings and problem list for Kate.

Full face and profile	*Frontal view*
	Face is symmetric
	Long soft tissue LAFH (soft tissue Glabella – Subnasale < Subnasale – soft tissue Menton)
	Lip competence
	UDML left of philtrum by 1 mm
	Incisal display during smile WRN (maxillary central incisor gingival margins slightly below the maxillary lip)
	Profile view
	Straight profile
	Upturned nose
	Obtuse NLA
	Chin position WRN
	Lip-chin-throat angle WRN
	Chin-throat length WRN
Ceph analysis	*Skeletal*
	Maxillary anteroposterior position WRN (A-Point lies on Nasion-perpendicular line)
	Mandibular anteroposterior position WRN (ANB angle = 1° with maxilla WRN)
	Long skeletal LAFH (LAFH/TAFH × 100% = 59%)
	Steep MPA (FMA = 32°, SN-MP = 35°)
	Effective bony Pogonion (Pogonion lies along or ahead of line extended from Nasion through B-Point)
	Dental
	Proclined maxillary incisors (U1 to SN = 116°)
	Slightly proclined mandibular incisors (FMIA = 63°)
Radiographs	Early mixed dentition
Intraoral photos and models	Angle Class I
	Iowa Classification: I I I I
	OJ: 0 mm
	OB: 10%
	3 mm current maxillary anterior crowding
	1 mm of maxillary crowding is anticipated following eruption of all permanent teeth (if appropriate space maintenance is employed)
	7.4 mm mandibular anterior crowding is currently present (including rotated primary canines and unerupted left permanent lateral incisor)
	4.2 mm of mandibular arch crowding is anticipated following eruption of all permanent teeth (if appropriate space maintenance is employed)
	Dental arches are symmetric
	Maxillary first molars are rotated mesially
	Maxillary and mandibular dental midlines are coincident
	Maxillary left permanent lateral incisor is erupting labially
	Mandibular right permanent lateral incisor is erupting lingually
	Mandibular left permanent lateral incisor is unerupted
	Mandibular left primary lateral incisor is retained and is in cross bite with the maxillary left central incisor
	Absence of keratinized gingival tissue labial to the mandibular right central incisor root
Other	—
Diagnosis	Class I malocclusion with proclined maxillary incisors, moderate mandibular anterior crowding, and absence of keratinized gingival tissue labial to mandibular right central incisor

Q: Do you wish to make any additional records?

A: Yes, a periapical radiograph of the mandibular left primary lateral incisor (Figure 2.44) could be helpful in clarifying the position of the permanent lateral incisor.

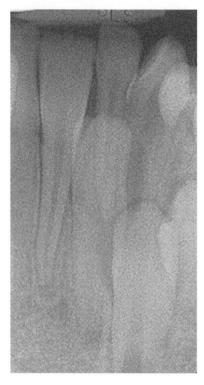

Figure 2.44 Periapical radiograph of Kate's erupting mandibular left permanent lateral incisor.

Q: How can we conclude that Kate has a steep MPA when SN-MP = 35°?

A: While it is true that SN-MP = 35° (exceeding an average SN-MP angle of 32° by only 3°), Sella is high (Figure 2.43e) which significantly reduces SN-MP. In Kate's case, FMA reflects the steepness of MPA more closely. Since her FMA (32°) is *7° greater than average*, we conclude that Kate has a steep MPA.

Q: Provide a detailed space analysis for Kate's maxillary and mandibular arches. In other words, how were the 1 mm of anticipated future maxillary arch crowding and 4.2 mm of future mandibular arch crowding calculated (if space maintenance is employed)?

A:

Below are space estimates:
Average mesiodistal widths of permanent teeth (mm) [1]:

Maxillary Central Incisor	8.5	Mandibular Central Incisor	5.0
Maxillary Lateral Incisor	6.5	Mandibular Lateral Incisor	5.5
Maxillary Canine	7.5	Mandibular Canine	7.0
Maxillary First Premolar	7.0	Mandibular First Premolar	7.0
Maxillary Second Premolar	7.0	Mandibular Second Premolar	7.0
Maxillary First Molar	10.0	Mandibular First Molar	11.0
Maxillary Second Molar	9.0	Mandibular Second Molar	10.5

Average mesiodistal widths of *primary* teeth (mm) [1]:

Maxillary Central Incisor	6.5	Mandibular Central Incisor	4.2
Maxillary Lateral Incisor	5.1	Mandibular Lateral Incisor	4.1
Maxillary Canine	7.0	Mandibular Canine	5.0
Maxillary First Molar	7.3	Mandibular First Molar	7.7
Maxillary Second Molar	8.2	Mandibular Second Molar	9.9

MAXILLARY ARCH
−3 mm of anterior crowding is currently present (Figure 2.43m).
+2 mm of anticipated leeway space (1 mm/side).
Balance = −3 mm + 2 mm = −1 mm.

MANDIBULAR ARCH
−6 mm of anterior crowding including rotated primary canines (Figure 2.43n).
+4.1 mm width of mandibular left primary lateral incisor.
−5.5 mm anticipated width of mandibular left permanent lateral incisor.
+3.2 mm of anticipated leeway space (1.6 mm/side).
Balance = −6 mm + 4.1 mm − 5.5 mm + 3.2 mm = −4.2 mm.

That is, *1 mm of maxillary arch crowding and 4.2 mm of mandibular arch crowding is anticipated following eruption of all permanent teeth (if proper space maintenance is employed).*

Q: It was noted that Kate's maxillary first molars are Class I but *mesially rotated* (Figure 2.43m). What is the effect of this mesial rotation on the *true* first molar anteroposterior relationship?

A: As Kate's maxillary first molar mesial rotation is eventually eliminated, the crowns will rotate distally and the mesiobuccal cusps will move into a more distal position. This rotation could leave Kate with a Class III molar relationship.

Q: It was noted (Figure 2.43h) that Kate presents with an *absence of keratinized gingival tissue* labial to her mandibular right permanent central incisor. Further, this incisor has a very prominent root. How would you classify the gingival tissue covering this root?

A: This tissue would be classified as having a *thin biotype* [54–59].

Q: What is the difference between thin and thick biotype? Which biotype is better for orthodontic tooth movement? Why?

A: Thin labial biotype has shorter attached tissue height, thinner attached tissue width, and thinner alveolar bone thickness. Thick biotype has longer attached tissue height, thicker attached tissue width, and thicker alveolar bone thickness.

It is better to have thick biotype covering a root when the tooth undergoes orthodontic tooth movement. Why? A thick periodontal biotype will lessen the chance of developing periodontal recession, or dehiscence, over that root during the stress of tooth movement.

Q: What are Kate's *primary* problems?
A:

Table 2.11 Primary problems list for Kate.

AP	–
Vertical	Long soft tissue and skeletal LAFH
Transverse	—
Other	Moderate (7.4 mm) current mandibular anterior crowding
	Proclined maxillary incisors
	Anterior cross bite of mandibular left primary lateral incisor and maxillary left permanent central incisor

Q: Discuss Kate in the context of three principles applied to every early treatment patient.

- The goal of early treatment is to correct developing problems – get the patient *back to normal for their stage of development* (including preventing complications such as resorption of adjacent tooth roots, reducing later treatment complexity, or reducing/eliminating unknowns). Alleviating Kate's mandibular anterior crowding, permitting her mandibular left permanent lateral incisor to erupt, uprighting her proclined maxillary incisors, and correcting her left anterior cross bite would bring Kate back to normal.
- Early treatment should address *very specific problems with a clearly defined end point*, usually begun

and ended within six to nine months (not protracted over many years with the exception of some orthopedic problems). Extraction of Kate's retained mandibular left primary lateral incisor (combined with LLHA) should eliminate her anterior cross bite, permit left lateral incisor eruption, and improve anterior tooth alignment as her remaining primary teeth exfoliate. However, since the premolar roots are < ½ developed (Figure 2.43f), we do not expect the primary molars to exfoliate within the next nine months.

- Always ask: Is it necessary that I treat the patient now? *What harm will come if I choose to do nothing now?* It is not necessary to treat Kate now, and we could choose to monitor her permanent tooth eruption. However, if we choose to monitor, then Kate's:
  - Mandibular molars could drift mesially into a Class III relationship when her primary canines and primary molars exfoliate.
  - Mandibular anterior crowding could be worse than if we instituted space maintenance (leeway space being partially used up by mandibular first permanent molar mesial drift).
  - Mandibular left permanent lateral incisor could remain unerupted or erupt ectopically.
  - Mandibular left primary lateral incisor could create wear of her maxillary left permanent central incisor crown.
  - Prominent mandibular right central incisor root could develop recession.

Q: As a brief review, what guidelines do you recommend for dealing with mandibular anterior crowding in the mixed dentition?

A: For most patients, attempt non-extraction treatment. Utilizing mandibular leeway space (1.6 mm per side or 3.2 mm total in the arch) or "E-space" with an LLHA can result in spontaneous improvement of mandibular incisor alignment after primary canine and primary molar exfoliation. Following second premolar eruption, and after anteroposterior molar correction has been addressed, a clearer decision regarding extraction of permanent teeth can be made. In summary, we generally:

- *Monitor (recall) patients with crowding in the early mixed dentition.*
- *Employ space maintenance in patients with mild-to-moderate crowding in the late mixed dentition* to utilize leeway space/"E-space."
- Defer extraction decisions until after premolars and permanent canines erupt in order to *reduce unknowns* (e.g. actual size of permanent teeth).

- Defer extraction decisions until anteroposterior growth is addressed in order to *reduce unknowns* (get Class II or Class III jaw growth, and molar relationships, under control before committing to irreversible treatment).

Exceptions (where extraction of primary and permanent teeth should be considered) include cases of ectopic tooth eruption, incisor dehiscence or eruption in nonkeratinized gingiva, and severe crowding (obvious extraction case).

Q: Kate demonstrates mild (3 mm) maxillary anterior crowding and moderate (7.4 mm) mandibular anterior crowding with maxillary incisor proclination. We should discuss the possibility of treating her with permanent tooth extractions. That decision could be postponed until all premolars erupt, but what do you think about serial extraction now? Can you list all features of the *ideal* serial extraction patient? Does Kate exhibit these features?

A: The ideal serial extraction patient is in the early mixed dentition stage of development and is *normal in every way, except severe anterior crowding (≥9 mm per arch)*. Specifically, the patient should present with:

- *Class I first permanent molars.* Kate is Class I (but remember, her maxillary molars are rotated mesially).
- *Vertically normal to slightly long soft tissue and skeletal LAFH, with minimal OB or possibly a mild open bite, but not a deep bite.* Kate exhibits these features. She has a long soft tissue and skeletal LAFH with minimal OB (10%).
- *Normal incisor angulation or proclined incisors, but not upright incisors.* Kate exhibits this feature. Her maxillary incisors are proclined, and her mandibular incisors are slightly proclined (FMIA = 63°).
- *Normal posterior transverse relationship (normal inter-molar arch widths with good posterior interdigitation; absence of posterior cross bites; and absence of significant transverse compensations).* Kate has a normal transverse relationship.
- *Severe (≥9 mm) anterior crowding:* Kate does not exhibit this feature. We anticipate 1 mm of maxillary arch crowding and 4.2 mm of mandibular arch crowding following eruption of all permanent teeth if proper space maintenance is employed.

Based upon the above features, Kate is *not* an ideal candidate for serial extraction.

Q: Should you recall or start early treatment? If you start, what treatment options would you consider?

A: Options include:

- *Recall* (no early treatment, monitor only) in one year to evaluate tooth eruption. As previously stated,

this is a possible option with the following risks: mandibular permanent molars drifting mesially into a Class III relationship as her primary canines and primary molars exfoliate; anterior crowding could be worse than if we employed space maintenance; mandibular left permanent lateral incisor could remain unerupted or erupt ectopically; mandibular left primary lateral incisor could create wear of her maxillary left permanent central incisor crown; and recession could develop over her prominent mandibular right permanent central incisor root.

- *Space maintenance* – placement of an LLHA, and possibly a Nance holding arch, before exfoliation of any mandibular primary teeth is reasonable since Kate's anterior crowding is moderate. However, an LLHA will prevent uprighting of mandibular anterior teeth and actually procline them *slightly* [5, 7].
- *Space maintenance with extraction of mandibular anterior primary teeth* – placing an LLHA *plus* extracting the mandibular left primary lateral incisor and mandibular primary canines would permit eruption of the mandibular permanent left lateral incisor, improved alignment of mandibular permanent incisors, and elimination of the maxillary left central incisor cross bite.
- *Space maintenance accompanied by mandibular anterior IPR after all permanent teeth erupt* – would reduce mandibular anterior crowding without extraction of permanent teeth. Care must be taken to ensure that an anterior Bolton discrepancy is not created.
- *Space regaining* – opening space for the maxillary left permanent lateral incisor and mandibular left permanent lateral incisor would procline Kate's incisors further and stress the thin labial tissue covering her mandibular right central incisor. Gingival recession could result.
- *Extraction of maxillary primary canines and possibly maxillary primary first molars* – is not recommended because: (i) the maxillary permanent canine crowns do not overlap the maxillary permanent lateral incisor roots on a panoramic image (Figure 2.43f), and (ii) the maxillary permanent canine roots are <½ formed (eruption not imminent).
- *Extraction of Kate's permanent mandibular right central incisor with poor labial biotype to provide 5 mm of anterior space* – may be a reasonable option to reduce anterior crowding in the future but not at this time. Instead, it would be prudent to employ space maintenance first (reduce unknowns).

Later, if her mandibular anterior crowding warrants extraction (after all permanent teeth erupt), then we could consider extracting a mandibular incisor.

This would make sense if an anterior Bolton discrepancy exists – *if her maxillary lateral incisors are small.* If an anterior Bolton discrepancy does not exist (maxillary and mandibular anterior teeth have normal proportions), then extracting a mandibular incisor could result in large anterior overjet and lack of canine coordination.

- *Serial extraction* – although Kate presents with some features which make her a serial extraction candidate (Class I, minimal OB, proclined incisors, and normal transverse relationship), she lacks severe anterior crowding. We do not recommend serial extraction.

Q: Do you wish to proceed with early treatment or monitor? If you wish to proceed, then what treatment would you recommend?

A: Kate's treatment did not proceed according to our recommendation. With her moderate mandibular anterior crowding (7.4 mm), steep MPA, and thin mandibular central incisor labial periodontal biotype, the attending orthodontist chose to treat Kate with serial extractions. Our initial evaluation suggested did not fit the criteria of severe mandibular crowding.

Kate's maxillary primary canines, mandibular primary canines, and mandibular left primary lateral incisor were extracted. Her maxillary and mandibular primary first molars were extracted when the roots of her first premolars were >½ developed. Eruption checks of the first premolars continued.

One year later, as a result of concern that Kate's first permanent molars were shifting into a Class III relationship, an LLHA was placed (Figure 2.45a). One year

(a)

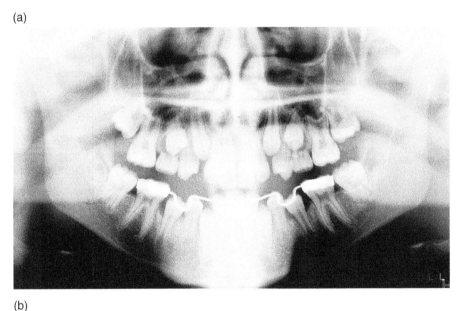

(b)

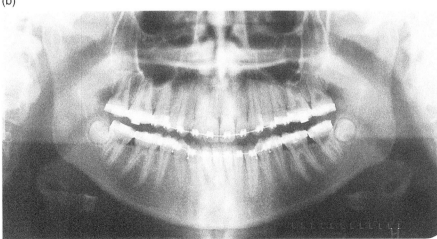

Figure 2.45 (a, b) Progress panoramic radiographs of Kate.

after that, Kate's first permanent molars appeared to be in an ideal Class I relationship and all second premolars had erupted (early treatment was complete). A decision was made to treat Kate non-extraction. Fixed appliances were placed (Figure 2.45b), arches leveled/aligned, spaces closed, and arches finished.

Q: Deband records are shown in Figure 2.46. (A panoramic film taken prior to deband is shown in Figure 2.45b.) What treatment changes do you note?

A: Changes include the following:
- An excellent outcome in terms of facial esthetics, occlusion, function, and tissue health.

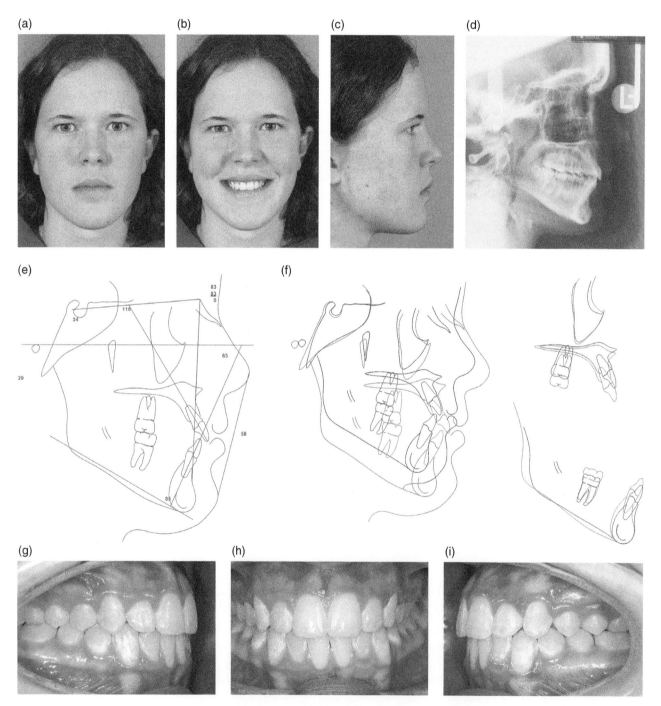

Figure 2.46 Deband records of Kate: (a–c) facial photographs, (d, e) lateral cephalometric radiograph and tracing, (f) cephalometric superimposition of initial to deband time points, (g–k) intraoral photographs, and (l–p) models.

(j)   (k)

(l)   (m)   (n)

(o)   (p)

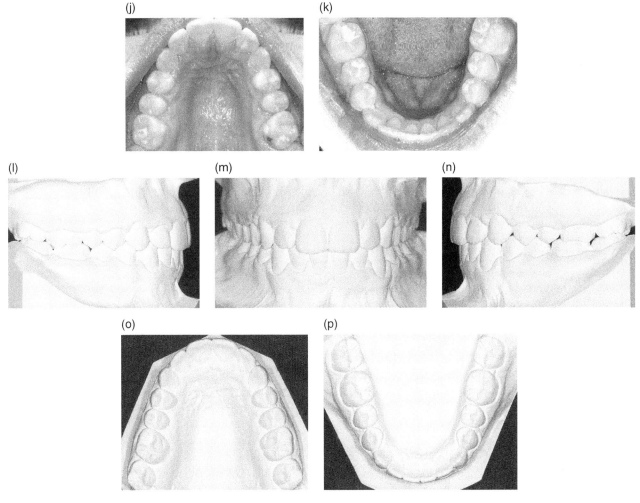

Figure 2.46 (Continued)

- Class I canine and molar relationships, adequate OB, and a reasonable transverse relationship is noted.
- Buccal corridors are prominent and her posterior overjet appears minimal – or "tight."
- Significant mandibular growth (Figure 2.46f) resulted in pronounced soft tissue chin projection.
- Mandibular incisors uprighted to an FMIA of 65° probably as a result of leeway space closure and slight CCW rotation of her mandibular plane.
- Maxillary and mandibular midlines are not coincident by about 0.5 mm with the mandibular midline to the left of the maxillary midline.
- A root dilaceration of the mandibular right permanent lateral incisor is noted (Figure 2.45b).
- A thin labial band of attached keratinized tissue developed over her mandibular right permanent central incisor (Figure 2.46h).

Q: Kate initially lacked keratinized attached tissue labial to the root of her mandibular permanent right central incisor (Figure 2.43h). However, at deband, she was found to have a thin labial band of keratinized attached tissue over the root of that tooth. How can that be? Is it unusual to find an increase in width of labial keratinized attached gingiva during childhood?

A: No, it is not unusual. In a two-year longitudinal study of children 6–12 years of age with well-aligned maxillary and mandibular teeth, increases in widths of facial keratinized and attached gingiva took place. The authors recommended a conservative, monitoring approach prior to a corrective, surgical intervention in children of this age who present with a minimal zone *or absence* of attached gingiva [60].

Q: Can you suggest "take-home pearls" regarding Kate's treatment?

A: "Take-home pearls" include:

- Kate presented at 10 years of age with mild (3 mm) maxillary anterior crowding, moderate (7.4 mm) mandibular anterior crowding, a long LAFH, a steep MPA, minimal OB, and thin (non-keratinized) tissue labial to her mandibular permanent right central incisor.

    The attending orthodontist chose to begin with serial extractions for a number of reasons: extraction of four first premolars would provide space to retract/upright incisors; uprighting incisors would have deepened Kate's overbite as her incisor crowns retracted/rotated around their root apicies; and retracting her incisors would have reduced stress on the labial periodontal tissue covering her mandibular permanent right central incisor.

    We recommended eventual space maintenance because only 4.2 mm of mandibular crowding was anticipated if an LLHA was used. Furthermore, Kate presented with an obtuse NLA which may have become more obtuse (unesthetic) if her maxillary incisors/maxillary lip were retracted. In other words, like many patients, Kate presented with features which made her a four premolar extraction candidate and features which made her a non-extraction candidate.

- We feel fortunate that a final decision to extract permanent teeth was postponed until after the second premolars had erupted (unknowns reduced). At that time, Kate was deemed a less-than-ideal premolar extraction candidate and was treated non-extraction.
- We feel that an LLHA should have been placed *immediately* when her maxillary and mandibular primary canines and mandibular left primary lateral incisor were extracted. Why? This would have prevented her mandibular molars from drifting mesially toward a Class III relationship, and it would have allowed using the leeway space for incisor alignment. The reason you generally do not place an LLHA in serial extraction cases is because you *want* molars to drift mesially – closing some of the extraction space.
- We were fortunate that a band of attached keratinized tissue developed labial to Kate's mandibular right central incisor. If instead, recession had occurred, then referral to a periodontist for a gingival graft would have been indicated.
- Never lose sight of the big picture. Kate's parents stated that their family has a Class III history. *You need to monitor Kate's growth until she has finished growing.* If Kate begins to grow Class III, then consider placing her on a high-pull chin cup or TAD-supported Class III elastics to halt/reduce mandibular forward growth.

Case Dillon

Q: Dillon is seven years and six months old (Figure 2.47) and presents with his parent's chief complaint, "Dillon has a missing front tooth." His PMH, PDH, and TMJ evaluations are WRN. He is without periodontal problems and CR = CO. Do you need additional records to decide whether to recall Dillon or to perform early treatment?

A: No additional records are needed. However, a lateral cephalometric radiograph and complete mouth survey of dental images were made (Figure 2.48).

(a) (b) (c)

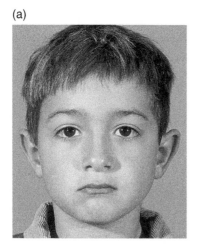 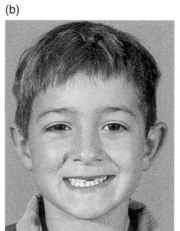 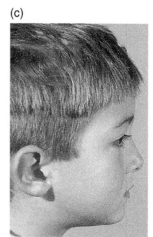

Figure 2.47 Initial records of Dillon: (a–c) facial photographs, (d) pantomograph, and (e–i) intraoral photographs.

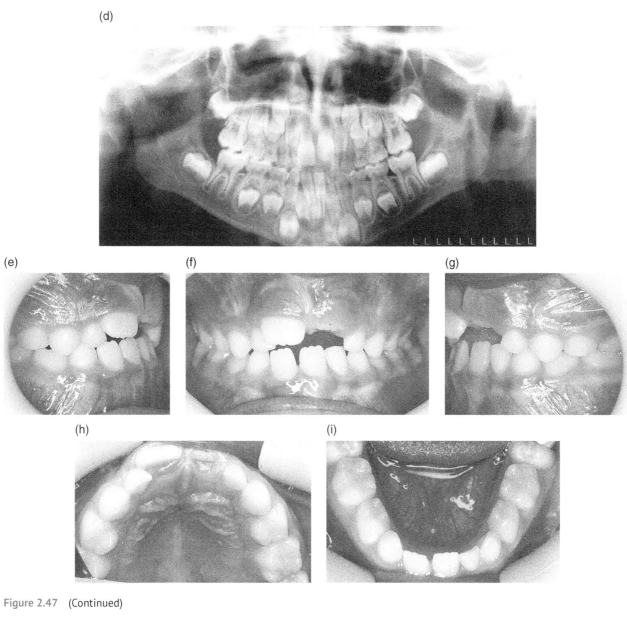

Figure 2.47 (Continued)

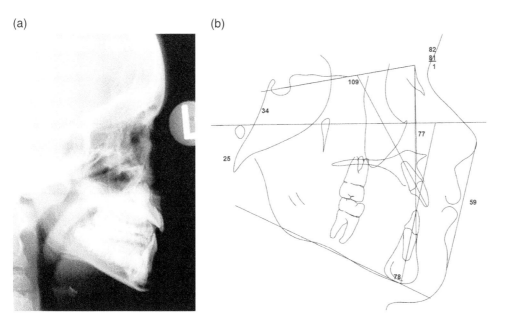

Figure 2.48 Additional records of Dillon. Lateral cephalometric radiograph (a), lateral cephalometric tracing (b), and complete mouth survey (c).

(c)

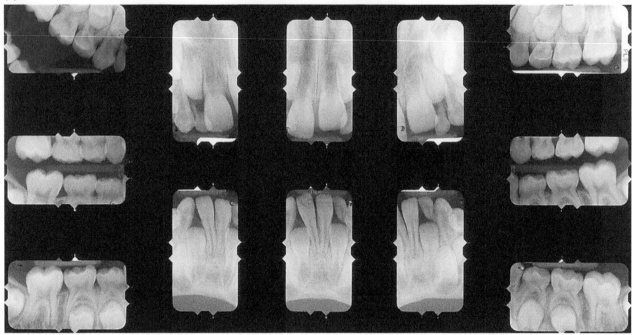

Figure 2.48 (Continued)

Q: Compile your diagnostic findings and problem list for Dillon. Also, state your diagnosis.

A:

Table 2.12 Diagnostic findings and problem list for Dillon.

Full face and profile	*Frontal view*
	Face is symmetric
	Short soft tissue LAFH (Glabella-Subnasal > Subnasal-soft tissue Menton)
	Lip competence
	UDML WRN
	Inadequate incisal display when smiling (border of maxillary lip rests below maxillary central incisor gingival margins)
	Profile view
	Mildly convex profile
	Obtuse NLA
	Chin projection WRN
	Lip-chin-throat angle WRN
Ceph analysis	*Skeletal*
	Maxillary anteroposterior position WRN (A-Point lies on Nasion-perpenidcular line)
	Mandibular anteroposterior position WRN (ANB = 1° with normal maxilla)
	Long skeletal LAFH (ANS-Menton/Nasion-Menton×100% = 59%, normal = 55%, sd = 2%)
	MPA WRN (FMA = 25°, SNMP = 34°)
	Dental
	Proclined maxillary incisors (U1 to SN = 109°)
	Upright mandibular incisors (FMIA = 77°)

Table 2.12 (Continued)

Radiographs	Early mixed dentition
	Unerupted permanent lateral incisors (potentially impacted mandibular right lateral)
	Unerupted maxillary permanent left central incisor
Intraoral photos and models	Angle Class I
	Iowa Classification: I I I I
	OJ ~1–2 mm
	Anterior open bite
	Mandibular dental midline shifted to right
	5.3 mm maxillary anterior crowding is currently present
	3.3 mm of maxillary arch crowding is anticipated following eruption of all permanent teeth (if appropriate space maintenance is employed)
	6.4 mm mandibular crowding is currently present
	3.2 mm of mandibular arch crowding is anticipated following eruption of all permanent teeth (if appropriate space maintenance is employed)
	Maxillary and mandibular dental arches are symmetric
	Thick periodontal biotype is present in the anterior of both arches (Figure 2.47f)
Other	—
Diagnosis	Class I malocclusion with potentially impacted mandibular right lateral incisor

Q: Dillon's parents are concerned with his anterior open bite and the fact that his maxillary left permanent central incisor has not erupted. What should you tell them?

A: Tell them that the anterior open bite appears to be temporary as a result of the transition from primary to permanent dentition. Below are the average ages (in years) for permanent anterior tooth eruption (Table 2.13).

Table 2.13 Timing of permanent tooth eruption.

Permanent tooth			Age (years)
Maxillary first molars	Mandibular first molars	Mandibular central incisors	6–7
Maxillary central incisors	Mandibular lateral incisors		7–8
Maxillary lateral incisors			8–9
Mandibular canines			9–10
Maxillary canines			11–12

As shown, the average eruption age for a maxillary permanent central incisor is between seven and eight years, so Dillon is on track. However, there is always the possibility that the central incisor may not be erupting, so it should be monitored.

Q: There are inconsistencies between Dillon's facial and cephalometric features. Can you identify them? How might they impact Dillon's treatment?

A: In the frontal view, Dillon's soft tissue LAFH appears shorter than his midface height. But cephalometrically, he demonstrates a long skeletal LAFH. Because his MPA is WRN, we feel that Dillon is normal and that his long skeletal LAFH is partially due to a tipped-up ANS.

In profile, Dillon appears mildly convex. But skeletally (cephalometrically) both jaws appear normal. We feel that Dillon is normal anteroposteriorly (as reflected by his bilateral Class I dental relationship). His borderline effective Pogonion (Pogonion lies *on* a line extending from Nasion through B-Point) could be contributing to the mildly convex profile.

These vertical and anteroposterior inconsistencies should be monitored. But for now, Dillon should be treated as normal.

Q: Provide a detailed space analysis for Dillon's maxillary and mandibular arches. In other words, how were the 3.3 mm of anticipated maxillary arch crowding and 3.2 mm of anticipated mandibular arch crowding calculated (if appropriate space maintenance is employed)?

A: Below are space estimates:

Average mesiodistal widths of permanent teeth (mm) [1]:

Maxillary Central Incisor	8.5	Mandibular Central Incisor	5.0
Maxillary Lateral Incisor	6.5	Mandibular Lateral Incisor	5.5
Maxillary Canine	7.5	Mandibular Canine	7.0
Maxillary First Premolar	7.0	Mandibular First Premolar	7.0
Maxillary Second Premolar	7.0	Mandibular Second Premolar	7.0
Maxillary First Molar	10.0	Mandibular First Molar	11.0
Maxillary Second Molar	9.0	Mandibular Second Molar	10.5

Average mesiodistal widths of *primary* teeth (mm) [1]:

Maxillary Central Incisor	6.5	Mandibular Central Incisor	4.2
Maxillary Lateral Incisor	5.1	Mandibular Lateral Incisor	4.1
Maxillary Canine	7.0	Mandibular Canine	5.0
Maxillary First Molar	7.3	Mandibular First Molar	7.7
Maxillary Second Molar	8.2	Mandibular Second Molar	9.9

MAXILLARY ARCH (Figure 2.47h)

+5.1 mm width of maxillary right primary lateral incisor.

−6.5 mm anticipated space needed for erupting maxillary right permanent lateral incisor.

−2 mm crowding of maxillary right primary lateral incisor and permanent central incisor.

+8 mm of space for maxillary left permanent central incisor.

−8.5 mm anticipated space needed for erupting maxillary left permanent central incisor.

+5.1 mm width of maxillary left primary lateral incisor.

−6.5 mm anticipated space needed for erupting maxillary left permanent lateral incisor.

+2 mm of anticipated leeway space (1 mm/side).

Balance = +5.1 mm − 6.5 mm − 2 mm + 8 mm − 8.5 mm + 5.1 mm − 6.5 mm + 2 mm = −3.3 mm.

MANDIBULAR ARCH

+0.5 mm of anterior space is present (Figure 2.47i).

+4.1 mm width of mandibular left primary lateral incisor.

−5.5 mm anticipated space needed for erupting mandibular left permanent lateral incisor.

−5.5 mm anticipated space needed for erupting mandibular right permanent lateral incisor.

+3.2 mm of anticipated leeway space (1.6 mm/side).

Balance = +0.5 mm + 4.1 mm − 5.5 mm − 5.5 mm + 3.2 mm = −3.2 mm.

That is, *3.3 mm of maxillary arch crowding and 3.2 mm of mandibular arch crowding is anticipated following eruption of all permanent teeth (if proper space maintenance is employed).*

Q: Always focus on the patient's *primary* problems in each dimension, plus other primary problems, at every appointment. What are Dillon's *primary* problems?

A:

Table 2.14 Primary problems list for Dillon.

AP	—
Vertical	—
Transverse	—
Other	Potentially impacted mandibular right permanent lateral incisor
	Moderate maxillary (5.3 mm) and mandibular (6.4 mm) anterior crowding
	Upright mandibular incisors

Q: Discuss Dillon in the context of three principles applied to every early treatment patient.

1) The goal of early treatment is to correct developing problems – get the patient *back to normal for their stage of development* (including preventing complications such as resorption of adjacent tooth roots, reducing later treatment complexity, or reducing/eliminating unknowns). Providing room for Dillon's anterior teeth to erupt, and alleviating his moderate crowding, would get him back on track for this stage of development.

2) Early treatment should be used to treat *very specific problems with a clearly defined end point*, usually within six to nine months (except for some orthopedic problems). Treatment to regain (open) space for the potentially impacted mandibular right permanent lateral incisor could be completed in six to nine months (anterior OJ will need to be increased before mandibular space can be opened). A benefit of such

space regaining would be proclination of his upright mandibular incisors to a more normal angulation. If instead of space regaining, an LLHA is placed in the hope that enough leeway space exists to allow all mandibular permanent teeth to erupt, then it will take longer than six to nine months.

3) Always ask: Is it necessary that I treat the patient now? *What harm will come if I choose to monitor only?* It is *not* necessary to treat Dillon now. We could monitor his permanent tooth eruption (placing an LLHA/Nance holding arch to maintain leeway space as the permanent canine and premolar roots develop). If we choose to do nothing, then we run the risk of the blocked out/potentially impacted incisors remaining blocked out, becoming impacted, erupting ectopically, or impeding permanent canine eruption.

Q: Dillon exhibits moderate anterior crowding, and permanent tooth extractions to alleviate this crowding should be considered. Describe the features of the *ideal* serial extraction patient. Does Dillon exhibit these features? Is Dillon a candidate for serial extraction?

A: The ideal serial extraction patient is in the *early mixed dentition stage of development and is <u>normal in every way, except severe anterior crowding (≥9 mm per arch)</u>.* The patient should present with:

- *Class I first molars.* Dillon presents with Class I molars.
- *Vertically normal to slightly long soft tissue and skeletal LAFH, with minimal OB or possibly a mild open bite, but <u>not</u> a deep bite.* Although Dillon exhibits a mildly short soft tissue LAFH, his skeletal LAFH is long, and he has an anterior open bite. Therefore, Dillon exhibits this feature.
- *Normal incisor angulation or proclined incisors, but <u>not</u> upright incisors.* Dillon presents with proclined maxillary incisors but upright mandibular incisors. However, if his permanent mandibular lateral incisors were erupted into the arch, then the central incisors would need to be proclined to make space for them – leaving the incisors at a normal angulation. Therefore, Dillon exhibits this feature.
- *Normal posterior transverse relationship (normal inter-molar arch widths with good posterior interdigitation; absence of posterior cross bites; and absence of significant transverse compensations).* Dillon exhibits this feature.
- *Severe (≥9 mm) anterior crowding.* Dillon does *not* exhibit this feature. He currently has 5.3 mm of maxillary and 6.4 mm of mandibular anterior crowding. We anticipate 3.3 mm of maxillary arch crowding

and 3.2 mm of mandibular arch crowding following eruption of all permanent teeth (if proper space maintenance is employed).

Based upon the above points, Dillon is *not* a good candidate for serial extraction.

Q: Should you start treatment now or recall? If you start treatment, what treatment options would you consider?

A: Your treatment options include the following:

- *Recall* (no treatment, monitor only) – evaluate tooth eruption in six to twelve months. The risks of monitoring include the blocked out/potentially impacted incisors remaining blocked out, becoming impacted, erupting ectopically, or impeding permanent canine eruption.

- *Space maintenance* – placing an LLHA/Nance holding arch and monitoring tooth eruption. Only 3.3 mm of maxillary arch crowding and 3.2 mm of mandibular arch crowding is anticipated following eruption of all permanent teeth if space maintenance is employed. So, we should be able to treat Dillon non-extraction with space maintenance only.

- *Space regaining* – open space lost as a result of mandibular right primary lateral incisor exfoliation. Also, open spaces for other permanent lateral incisors to erupt. We recommend waiting a few months to see if the maxillary left permanent central incisor erupts before proceeding with this option.

  1) *If the maxillary left central incisor erupts*, then bond both arches with fixed orthodontic appliances and open space for the mandibular right permanent lateral incisor. Open additional space for all other permanent lateral incisors. After regaining space, maintain the opened spaces with the fixed appliances until the permanent lateral incisors erupt. Then, place an LLHA and Nance holding arch, or wear temporary (vacuum-formed) retainers, until all permanent canines and premolars erupt.

  2) *If the maxillary left central incisor does not erupt*, then extract the maxillary *primary* lateral incisors to make additional room for the maxillary central incisor and maxillary permanent lateral incisors. If the maxillary left central incisor still does not erupt, then the gingiva covering it could be preventing its eruption, or it could be ankylosed. If thick gingiva (which could be removed with a laser) is not the cause, and if you conclude that it is ankylosed, then a decision should be made either to luxate the maxillary left central incisor and attempt erupting it orthodontically, or to extract it. Place fixed appliances and open spaces in both arches for the permanent lateral incisors. Proceed as in (1) above.

- *Extraction of all remaining primary canines and primary lateral incisors* – would provide room for eruption of all permanent lateral incisors but could also result in arch perimeter loss as primary and permanent molars drift mesially. An LLHA and Nance holding arch could prevent/reduce this mesial molar drift.

  We are not enthusiastic about this option. Extraction of these primary teeth is an added surgical procedure for Dillon, and we would strongly recommend verifying that the permanent lateral incisor root lengths are at least ½ developed before considering it.

- *Serial extraction* – as discussed earlier, Dillon is *not* a good candidate for serial extraction.

Q: Which of the above treatment options would you choose and why?

A: The uprightness of Dillon's mandibular incisors, coupled with the fact that he had a thick anterior labial periodontal biotype (Figure 2.47f), led to us attempting space regaining. Fortunately, Dillon's maxillary left central incisor erupted spontaneously. Fixed orthodontic appliances were placed, and space was created with compressed open coil springs for all permanent lateral incisors by proclining the permanent *central* incisors.

Q: Observe (Figure 2.47c) that Dillon's maxillary permanent incisor roots are incompletely developed. Does orthodontic tooth movement of immature roots shorten the roots?

A: Deflection of Hertwig's epithelial sheath during orthodontic movement may create *dilacerations* of incompletely developed roots [61]. However, one study reported that incompletely developed maxillary incisor roots reached a significantly *greater* length following orthodontic treatment than fully developed roots following orthodontic treatment [62]. The authors concluded that a mechanism exists which protects younger roots against apical resorption during orthodontic treatment and advised initiating orthodontic correction of the incisors at a young age during the mixed dentition. The finding that immature teeth are at a much *lower* risk of apical root resorption was recently corroborated by Li et al. [63].

Q: Figure 2.49 illustrates Dillon's space regaining with fixed orthodontic appliances in the mandibular right lateral incisor area plus space opening for the other permanent lateral incisors. Once space has been regained, how do you recommend proceeding?

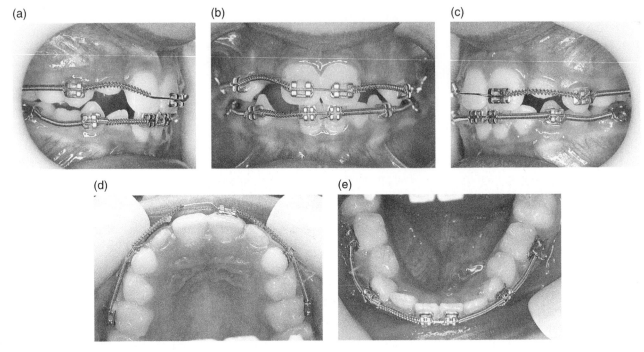

Figure 2.49 (a–e) Progress records of Dillon showing space regaining for the mandibular right lateral incisor plus additional space creation for the other lateral incisors. Space was created by proclining his maxillary and mandibular central incisors.

A: Proceed by maintaining the space you created. Fixed appliances were removed, and an LLHA plus Nance holding arch were placed to maintain the Class I molar relationship and utilize leeway space/"E-space"/"D-space." Panoramic images, subsequently made, are shown in Figure 2.50. Note the LLHA soldered "spur" wrapping around distal to the mandibular right permanent lateral incisor to prevent drifting of that tooth.

Q: No additional treatment was provided following eruption of all Dillon's permanent teeth. In his parents' words, "Thank you so much, doctor, for giving Dillon a wonderful smile with only early braces." Space maintainers were removed, and final records are shown in Figure 2.51a–h. (Since no additional treatment was provided, no additional radiographs were made.) What changes do you note?

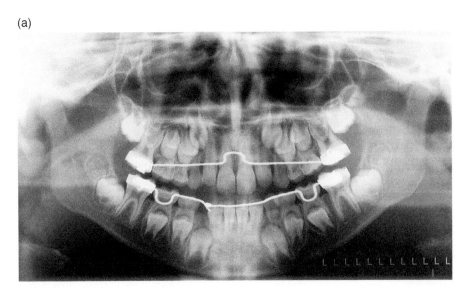

Figure 2.50 (a, b) Progress records of Dillon following space regaining.

(b)

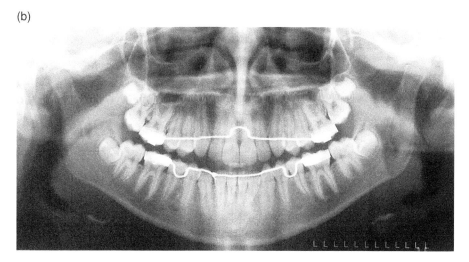

Figure 2.50   (Continued)

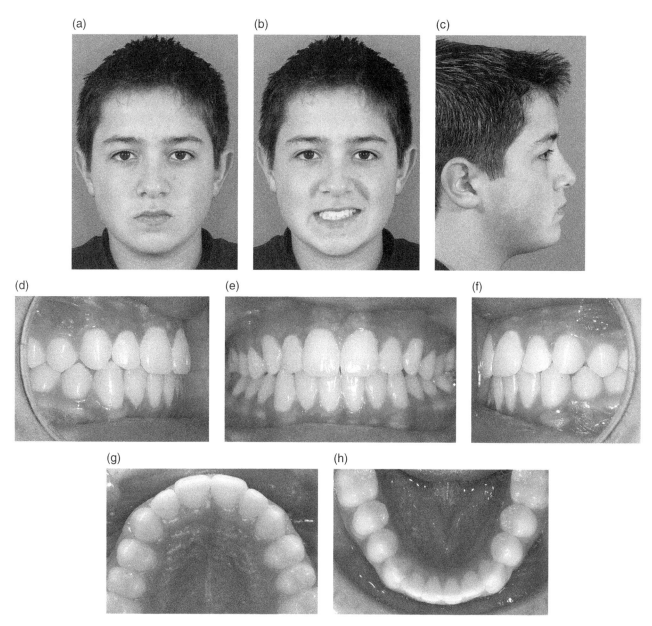

Figure 2.51   (a–h) Final records of Dillon after all permanent teeth erupted and the LLHA and Nance button were removed. The patient and his parents were happy with the result and elected not to have comprehensive treatment.

A: Changes include:
- An excellent esthetic, occlusal, functional, and healthy outcome was achieved through a combination of space regaining, space creation, and space maintenance early treatment. The outcome was achieved without comprehensive orthodontic treatment.

    Maxillary and mandibular midlines are now coincident and aligned with Dillon's facial midline.
- Criticisms of the result include:
a) Inadequate incisal display during posed smile (in part due to Dillon's minimal facial musculature activity).
b) Gingival margin of the maxillary left permanent central incisor is slightly more incisal than the gingival margin of the maxillary right permanent central incisor.
c) Distal of the maxillary right permanent canine is not coordinating with the mandibular right first premolar (Figure 2.51d).
d) Maxillary anterior teeth are stepped up relative to maxillary posterior teeth (Figure 2.51e).
e) Mandibular anterior teeth roots are not parallel (Figure 2.50b). A dilaceration of the mandibular left lateral incisor appears to be present.

Q: Were Dillon's initially incompletely formed maxillary incisor roots harmed with orthodontic tooth movement?

A: No (Figure 2.50b). The incompletely developed roots were *not* harmed. The roots appear normal.

Q: Can you suggest "take-home pearls" regarding Dillon's early treatment?

A: "Take-home pearls" include:
- Dillon presented at seven years and six months of age with a Class I molar and canine relationship, potentially impacted mandibular right permanent lateral incisor, moderate maxillary (5.3 mm) and mandibular (6.4 mm) anterior crowding, and upright mandibular incisors. He was an excellent example of early treatment reducing later treatment complexity. By regaining/creating space for his lateral incisors, the need for comprehensive orthodontic treatment was eliminated.
- A number of factors played a role in the successful use of space regaining/space creation for Dillon.
1) Only 3.3 mm of maxillary arch crowding and 3.2 mm of mandibular arch crowding was anticipated following eruption of all permanent teeth if space maintenance alone was employed. Therefore, the amount of final incisor proclination was probably minimal.
2) Mandibular central incisors were initially very upright (FMIA = 77°).
3) A thick periodontal tissue biotype was present labial to his incisors. This thick tissue could better resist the stress of incisor proclination.
- An equally successful result may have occurred if only space maintenance was employed until all permanent canines and premolars had erupted. At that time, any remaining mild crowding could have been resolved with fixed appliances during comprehensive treatment.

Case Madison

Q: Madison is eight years and two months old (Figure 2.52). She presents to you with her parents' chief complaint, "We are concerned that Madison's teeth are crowded." Her PMH, PDH, periodontal evaluation, and TMJ evaluation are WRN. CR = CO. Compile your diagnostic findings and problem list for Madison. Also, state your diagnosis.

(a) (b) (c)

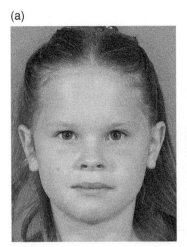 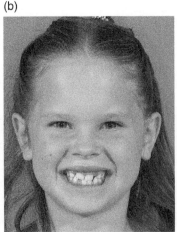 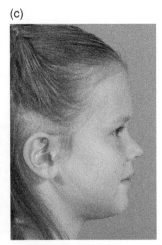

Figure 2.52 Initial records of Madison: (a–c) facial photographs, (d, e) lateral cephalometric radiograph and tracing, (f) pantomograph, (g–k) intraoral photographs, and (l) right-to-left occlusal cant.

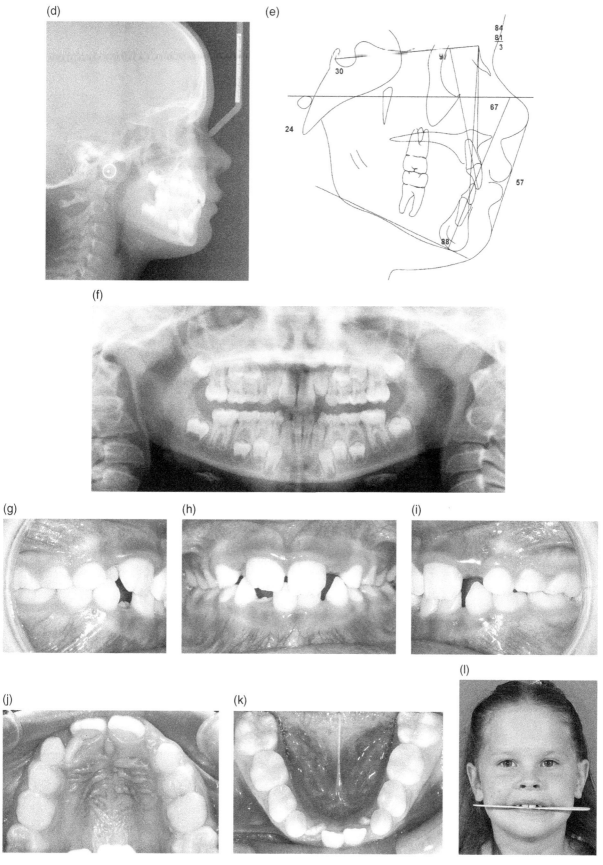

Figure 2.52 (Continued)

A:

Table 2.15 Diagnostic findings and problem list for Madison.

Full face and profile	*Frontal view*
	Face is symmetric
	Soft tissue LAFH WRN (soft tissue Glabella – Subnasale approximately equal to Subnasale – soft tissue Menton)
	Lip competence
	UDML 1 mm right of facial midline
	Gingival display in posed smile excessive (maxillary central incisor gingival margins below the maxillary lip)
	Left to right occlusal cant (Figure 2.52b)
	Profile view
	Straight profile
	Nose is tipped up slightly
	NLA WRN
	Chin projection WRN
	Lip-chin-throat angle WRN
Ceph analysis	*Skeletal*
	Maxillary anteroposterior position WRN (A-Point lies approximately on Nasion-perpendicular line)
	Mandibular anteroposterior position WRN (ANB angle = 3° with maxilla WRN)
	Skeletal LAFH WRN (ANS-Menton/Nasion-Menton × 100% = 57%)
	Mandibular plane angle WRN (FMA = 24°; SNMP = 30°)
	Effective bony Pogonion (Pogonion lies on a line extended from Nasion through B-point)
	Dental
	Upright maxillary incisors (U1 to SN = 97°)
	Mandibular incisor inclination WRN (FMIA = 67°)
Radiographs	Early mixed dentition
	Right and left mandibular borders are not coincident (Figure 2.52d)
Intraoral photos and models	Angle Class I
	Iowa Classification: I I I I
	OJ ~0 mm
	OB 30–50%
	4.5 mm of maxillary anterior crowding is currently present
	2.5 mm of maxillary arch crowding is anticipated following eruption of all permanent teeth (if proper space maintenance is employed)
	7.5 mm of mandibular anterior crowding is currently present
	4.3 mm of mandibular arch crowding is anticipated following eruption of all permanent teeth (if proper space maintenance is employed)
	Maxillary right lateral incisor is in cross bite (no trauma/tissue damage noted)
	Unerupted/potentially impacted maxillary and mandibular lateral incisors
	Ectopic eruption of maxillary and mandibular right lateral incisors
	Midlines are not coincident (LDML to left of UDML by ~ 2 mm)
	Maxillary and mandibular dental arches are symmetric
Other	None
Diagnosis	Class I malocclusion with moderate anterior crowding

Q: Madison has a left to right occlusal cant (Figure 2.52l), but her face appears symmetric. What other feature corroborates the fact that she has an occlusal cant? How would you deal with the cant?

A: The fact that her left and right mandibular borders do not superimpose on a lateral cephalometric radiograph (Figure 2.52d) corroborates the fact that she has an occlusal cant and indicates that Madison has more vertical ramus growth on her left side than right side. In addition, we could also look for asymmetry in the length of her condyles on a panoramic radiograph (Figure 2.52f). However, we do not see an overt condylar length difference, probably because the vertical asymmetry is mild. For now, we would recommend monitoring Madison's occlusal cant. If it worsens, then we may need to treat it with orthopedics or orthognathic surgery.

Q: How large must a right-to-left occlusal cant be in order to be noticeable by lay persons?

A: At least 3 mm [64].

Q: Provide a detailed space analysis for Madison's maxillary and mandibular arches. In other words, how were the anticipated 2.5 mm maxillary arch crowding and 4.3 mm mandibular arch crowding calculated *(if proper space maintenance is employed)*?

A:

Average mesiodistal widths of permanent teeth (mm) [1]:

Maxillary Central Incisor	8.5	Mandibular Central Incisor	5.0
Maxillary Lateral Incisor	6.5	Mandibular Lateral Incisor	5.5
Maxillary Canine	7.5	Mandibular Canine	7.0
Maxillary First Premolar	7.0	Mandibular First Premolar	7.0
Maxillary Second Premolar	7.0	Mandibular Second Premolar	7.0
Maxillary First Molar	10.0	Mandibular First Molar	11.0
Maxillary Second Molar	9.0	Mandibular Second Molar	10.5

Average mesiodistal widths of *primary* teeth (mm) [1]:

Maxillary Central Incisor	6.5	Mandibular Central Incisor	4.2
Maxillary Lateral Incisor	5.1	Mandibular Lateral Incisor	4.1
Maxillary Canine	7.0	Mandibular Canine	5.0
Maxillary First Molar	7.3	Mandibular First Molar	7.7
Maxillary Second Molar	8.2	Mandibular Second Molar	9.9

MAXILLARY ARCH

−3 mm of right lateral incisor crowding (Figure 2.52j).

+5 mm of space is present for maxillary left permanent lateral incisor.

−6.5 mm of space is needed for the potentially impacted maxillary left permanent lateral incisor.

+2 mm of anticipated leeway space (1 mm/side).

Balance = −3 mm + 5 mm − 6.5 mm + 2 mm = −2.5 mm.

MANDIBULAR ARCH

−3 mm of incisor crowding (Figure 2.52k, left central incisor to right lateral incisor).

+1 mm of space is present for mandibular left permanent lateral incisor.

−5.5 mm of space is needed for mandibular left permanent lateral incisor.

+3.2 mm of anticipated leeway space (1.6 mm/side).

Balance = −3 mm + 1 mm − 5.5 mm + 3.2 mm = −4.3 mm.

That is, *2.5 mm of maxillary crowding and 4.3 mm of mandibular crowding is anticipated following eruption of all permanent teeth (if proper space maintenance is employed).*

Q: What are Madison's *primary* problems in each dimension, plus other problems?

A:

Table 2.16 Primary problems list for Madison *(apical base/ skeletal discrepancies italicized).*

AP	Cross bite of the maxillary right lateral incisor
Vertical	OB 30–50%
Transverse	—
Other	Potentially impacted/unerupted maxillary and mandibular lateral incisors
	Moderate anterior crowding in both arches

Q: What unknowns do you face in treating Madison?

A: Future jaw growth magnitude and direction, an undetected CR–CO shift, cooperation, and the actual size of her unerupted permanent teeth (actual leeway space, final amount of crowding).

Q: Discuss Madison in the context of three principles applied to every early treatment patient.

A:

- The goal of early treatment is to correct developing problems – get the patient *back to normal for their stage of development* (including preventing complications, reducing later treatment complexity, and reducing/eliminating unknowns). Alleviating Madison's anterior crowding, permitting her permanent lateral incisors to erupt/aligning them, eliminating her anterior cross bite, and reducing her deep overbite would bring Madison back to normal for her stage of development.

- Early treatment should address *very specific problems with a clearly defined end point*, usually within six to nine months (not protracted over many years, except for some orthopedic problems). Extraction of Madison's primary canines, combined with placement of an LLHA and Nance holding arch to reduce/prevent mesial posterior tooth drift and arch perimeter loss, could provide space for eruption of her permanent lateral incisors. Limited fixed orthodontic appliances (maxillary 2 × 6 appliance – braces placed on first molars, canines, and incisors) could then be used to align her maxillary anterior teeth and correct her anterior cross bite. This focused early treatment could be completed in six to nine months. Residual crowding could be dealt with later, during comprehensive treatment, after all permanent teeth erupted.

- Always ask: Is it necessary that I treat the patient now? *What harm will come if I choose to do nothing now?* It is not necessary to treat Madison now. Why? If we do not treat her now, then her lateral incisors will simply remain unerupted or erupt malaligned. Furthermore, her maxillary right lateral incisor is not in traumatic occlusion, her permanent lateral incisors have erupted enough that we should not be concerned with resorption of adjacent roots, and her premolars and permanent canines are many months away from erupting.

Q: Can you list three factors that suggest Madison is a candidate for serial extraction? Can you list three factors that suggest Madison is not a candidate for serial extraction? Is Madison a candidate for serial extraction?

A: Factors that would qualify Madison as a candidate for serial extraction include the fact that she:

- Is in the early mixed dentition stage of development.
- Presents with a normal Class I molar relationship.
- Presents with a normal posterior transverse relationship.

Factors that would disqualify Madison as a candidate for serial extraction include the fact that she:

- Presents with only moderate, not severe (≥9 mm), maxillary and mandibular anterior crowding.
- Is normal vertically (soft tissue and skeletal LAFH WRN) but has 30–50% OB. That is, her bite will deepen even more if first premolars are extracted and incisors are retracted/uprighted around their apices.
- Has normal mandibular incisor inclination (FMIA = 67°) but *maxillary* incisors that are upright (U1 to SN = 97°). Furthermore, she has a high Sella – so, her maxillary incisors are more upright than U1 to SN indicates. Maxillary incisors will tend to upright even more with premolar extractions/incisor retraction.

Remember, the ideal serial extraction patient is in the *early mixed dentition stage of development and is normal in every way, except has severe anterior crowding (≥9 mm anterior crowding in each arch)*. Based upon the above factors, Madison is not an ideal candidate for serial extraction.

Q: Should you start early treatment now or recall Madison? If you start treatment, what treatment options would you consider?

A: Options include the following:

- *Recall* (no treatment, monitor only) – re-evaluate in one year. No harm is anticipated by monitoring Madison. Her lateral incisors will either remain unerupted or will erupt ectopically – but they should not cause root resorption since they are already erupting through the gingiva. The roots of her canines and premolars are <½ developed, so their eruption is not imminent.
- *Space maintenance only* – placement of an LLHA, and possibly a Nance holding arch, could reduce Madison's crowding in the maxilla to 2.5 mm and in the mandible to 4.3 mm after all permanent teeth erupt. However, because Madison's canine and premolar roots are <½ developed, their eruption is not imminent and there is no need to place space maintainers yet.
- *Space regaining* – opening spaces for Madison's permanent lateral incisors using fixed orthodontic appliances (2 × 6 appliances) in both arches. This reasonable treatment would procline and align her incisors (and correct her right lateral incisor cross bite). However, the necessity for doing this now is questionable because there is no traumatic damage to her maxillary right lateral incisor.
- *Extraction of all maxillary and mandibular primary canines* – would provide room for eruption of all permanent incisors but could result in arch perimeter loss if primary molars and permanent molars drift mesially. To reduce/prevent arch perimeter loss, an LLHA and Nance holding arch should be placed if this option is chosen. In Madison's case, placing these space maintainers could increase our chances of future non-extraction treatment.
- *Serial extraction* – because Madison has only moderate (not severe) anterior crowding, 30–50% OB, and upright maxillary incisors, she is not an ideal candidate for serial extraction.

Q: What is your recommended treatment? How would you proceed?

A: At her case presentation appointment, Madison's Class I relationship was confirmed. A decision was made to extract all four primary canines to make room for her permanent lateral incisors to erupt, but *neither an LLHA nor a Nance holding arch were placed to prevent mesial drift of molars (arch perimeter loss).* In retrospect, this was a mistake. A recall appointment was scheduled.

Q: One year later, records were made (Figure 2.53). What changes do you note?

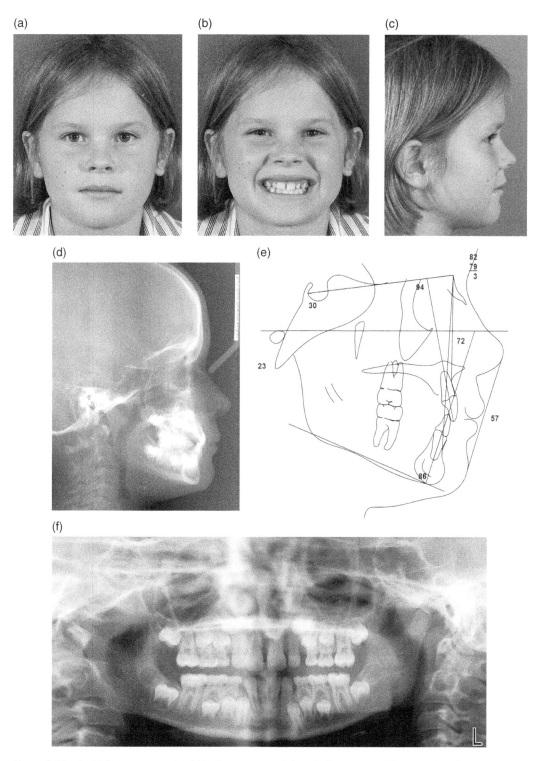

(a)

(b)

(c)

(d)

(e)

(f)

Figure 2.53   (a–k) Progress records of Madison one year later at nine years and two months of age.

(g)   (h)   (i)

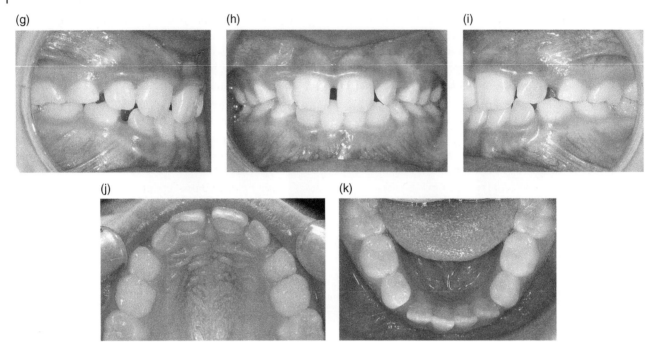

(j)   (k)

Figure 2.53 (Continued)

A: Changes include:
- All four permanent lateral incisors have erupted with improved alignment.
- Maxillary and mandibular incisors have uprighted (U1 to SN angle has decreased from 97° to 94°, while FMIA has increased from 67° to 72°).
- Permanent canine and premolar roots are lengthening.
- Minimal space exists for eruption of potentially impacted permanent canines.
- Maxillary right lateral incisor cross bite spontaneously corrected.
- Her maxillary permanent canine crowns are beginning to overlap the roots of her maxillary lateral incisors (Figure 2.53f).
- Keratinized gingiva labial to the mandibular right central incisor was deemed thin when Madison was clinically examined.

Q: Can you suggest a possible reason why the cross bite of her maxillary right lateral incisor corrected spontaneously?

A: We suspect that, following removal of primary canines, tongue pressure advanced the maxillary right lateral incisor out of cross bite.

Q: Since so much has changed, could you please perform a new space analysis for Madison?

A:

Average mesiodistal widths of permanent teeth (mm) [1]:

Maxillary Central Incisor	8.5	Mandibular Central Incisor	5.0
Maxillary Lateral Incisor	6.5	Mandibular Lateral Incisor	5.5
Maxillary Canine	7.5	Mandibular Canine	7.0
Maxillary First Premolar	7.0	Mandibular First Premolar	7.0
Maxillary Second Premolar	7.0	Mandibular Second Premolar	7.0
Maxillary First Molar	10.0	Mandibular First Molar	11.0
Maxillary Second Molar	9.0	Mandibular Second Molar	10.5

Average mesiodistal widths of *primary* teeth (mm) [1]:

Maxillary Central Incisor	6.5	Mandibular Central Incisor	4.2
Maxillary Lateral Incisor	5.1	Mandibular Lateral Incisor	4.1
Maxillary Canine	7.0	Mandibular Canine	5.0
Maxillary First Molar	7.3	Mandibular First Molar	7.7
Maxillary Second Molar	8.2	Mandibular Second Molar	9.9

MAXILLARY ARCH (Since primary canines are missing, we cannot use leeway space.
Instead, we must calculate crowding as follows)

+5 mm of anterior space is present (Figure 2.53j).

−7.5 mm anticipated width of right permanent canine.

−7.5 mm width of left permanent canine.

+7.3 mm width of right primary first molar.

−7 mm width of right first premolar required.

+7.3 mm width of left primary first molar.

−7 mm width of left first premolar required.

+8.2 mm width of right primary second molar.

−7 mm width of right second premolar required.

+8.2 mm width of left primary second molar.

−7 mm width of left second premolar required.

Balance = +5 mm − 7.5 mm − 7.5 mm + 7.3 mm − 7 mm + 7.3 mm − 7 mm + 8.2 mm − 7 mm

+8.2 mm − 7 mm = −7 mm.

7.0 mm additional maxillary arch space is required for eruption/alignment of all teeth if space maintenance is used.

MANDIBULAR ARCH

+2 mm of anterior space is present (K).

−1 mm of incisor crowding currently present.

−7 mm anticipated width of right permanent canine.

+7.7 mm width of right primary first molar.

−7 mm width of right first premolar required.

+9.9 mm width of right primary second molar.

−7 mm width of right second premolar required.

−7 mm anticipated width of left permanent canine.

+7.7 mm width of left primary first molar.

−7 mm width of left first premolar required.

+9.9 mm width of left primary second molar.

−7 mm width of left second premolar required.

Balance = +2 mm − 1 mm − 7 mm + 7.7 mm − 7 mm + 9.9 mm − 7 mm

−7 mm + 7.7 mm − 7 mm + 9.9 mm − 7 mm = −5.8 mm.

5.8 mm additional mandibular arch space is required for eruption/alignment of all teeth if space maintenance is used.

We conclude that space maintenance alone will be *inadequate* to address Madison's crowding.

Q: If space maintenance (LLHA and Nance holding arch) had been initially employed, then 2.5 mm of maxillary arch crowding and 4.3 mm of mandibular arch crowding was anticipated following eruption of all permanent teeth. But these values have increased to 7 and 5.8 mm, respectively, if space maintenance is now employed. How do you account for this change?

A: The increase in anticipated crowding is due to incisor uprighting/retraction and probably mesial molar drift.

Q: What treatment options can you suggest at this time?

A: Options include the following:

- *Recall* (no treatment, monitor) – re-evaluate in one year. We do not recommend this option. We anticipate Madison's premolars continuing to erupt normally. However, if we do nothing, then her canines will remain unerupted, could erupt ectopically, could resorb her lateral incisor roots, or could become impacted (maxillary permanent canine crowns overlap lateral incisor roots, Figure 2.53f).

- *Space maintenance* – is not recommended because moderate crowding (7 mm maxillary, 5.8 mm mandibular) is anticipated if we maintain space only, and the same potential canine problems will exist with space maintenance that would exist if we monitored only.

- *Space regaining* – opening spaces for Madison's permanent canines using fixed orthodontic appliances. Based upon our current space maintenance analysis, Madison will need to have 7 mm of additional maxillary space and 5.8 mm of additional mandibular space for eruption of her permanent canines (additional space beyond what space maintenance can provide). This means that her maxillary and mandibular incisors will also need to be advanced approximately 3.5 and 2.9 mm, respectively (opening right and left spaces between lateral incisors and canines). Since her maxillary and mandibular incisors are upright, this is reasonable. However, advancing her mandibular incisors 2.9 mm will place stress on her thin mandibular anterior labial periodontal tissue – possibly resulting in gingival recession. If we choose this option, then we would want to consult a periodontist for a possible gingival graft.

- *Serial extraction* – Madison is not an ideal candidate for serial extraction. She has only moderate crowding in both arches (if space maintenance is now employed), her maxillary and mandibular incisors are upright, and she has 30–40% OB.

- *Extraction of primary first molars* – would accelerate first premolar eruption since the roots of the first premolars are ≥½ developed. As the first premolars erupt, space will be created at their apices for canines to erupt somewhat further. By choosing this option, a decision to extract permanent teeth can be postponed until after the first premolars erupt.

Q: Considering these options, what additional early treatment do you recommend?

A: We extracted primary first molars and recalled Madison one year later.

Q: By extracting primary first molars, what treatment protocol have we initiated?

A: We have initiated serial extraction. When we extracted Madison's primary canines, we were not yet committed to successive extraction decisions and may have been able to treat her non-extraction if space maintainers had been placed. With extraction of primary first molars, we have taken the second step toward serial extraction.

Q: Would it be prudent to place space maintainers now?

A: An LLHA and Nance holding arch would reduce/prevent mesial molar drift and arch perimeter loss following first primary molar extractions. We could then assess crowding after the first premolars erupted *before* we committed to the third stage of serial extraction treatment – first premolar extractions. However, we placed neither an LLHA nor a Nance holding arch.

Q: Madison returned when she was 11 years and 1 month old, and we made records (Figure 2.54). What changes do you note?

A: Changes include:
- Maxillary first premolars have erupted.
- Mandibular left first premolar is erupting.
- Mandibular right first premolar is impacted under her mandibular right second primary molar.
- Maxillary permanent canines appear impacted, and mandibular left canine is blocked to the labial (Figure 2.54i).
- Mandibular right canine has erupted.
- All permanent canines and premolars have roots >½ developed.
- Clinically, gingiva labial to the mandibular right central incisor now appears normal.

Q: Can you discuss all early treatment options at this time?

A: The options have not changed significantly:
- *Recall* (no treatment, monitor) – re-evaluate in one year. We do not recommend this option. Madison's canines appear impacted and could resorb her lateral incisor roots or erupt ectopically.
- *Space maintenance* – placement of an LLHA and Nance holding arch could reduce Madison's crowding by utilizing "E-space," or the difference between mesiodistal widths of her primary second molars and her second premolars. However, please observe that Madison's unerupted permanent second premolars do *not* appear to be narrow, mesiodistally (Figure 2.54f). That is, space maintenance alone will be inadequate to address the remaining crowding.

- *Space regaining* – opening spaces for Madison's permanent canines using fixed orthodontic appliances. Let us list the pros and cons of this option:

    Pros – Madison's maxillary and mandibular incisors are upright. Opening space (proclining maxillary and mandibular incisors) would result in a more normal inclination for these teeth.

    Cons – Look at the panoramic image in Figure 2.54f. The *action* of proclining Madison's maxillary lateral incisor crowns could result in a *reaction* of driving their roots into the permanent canine crowns – resorbing the lateral incisor roots.

- *Serial extraction* – Let us list the pros and cons:

    Pros – Extraction of Madison's mandibular primary second molars would allow impacted/blocked out mandibular first premolars to erupt. Then, extraction of all four first premolars would create adequate space to allow permanent canines to erupt.

    Cons – Madison has upright maxillary and mandibular incisors. Incisors will tend to upright more as we close residual extraction spaces.

Q: Wait a minute! When we considered space regaining to create room for the maxillary canines, we missed a very important concept. Can you suggest what that concept is?

A: Yes. Consider Figure 2.54f and j. If we place braces and compressed springs to make room for the maxillary canines at the level of the erupted *teeth crowns*, an equal amount of space at the level of the erupted teeth *apices* is not likely to be created. It is at the erupted teeth apices where the permanent canines need space now.

Space at the erupted teeth apices can be created by extraction of permanent teeth or by RME to widen the midpalatal suture. However, widening the maxilla significantly will move Madison's maxillary posterior teeth into bilateral buccal cross bite.

Q: What treatment do you recommend?

A: In spite of the uprightness of Madison's incisors, we decided to proceed with serial extraction.
- To prevent mandibular first permanent molars from tipping (mesially) over second premolars, an LLHA was placed.
- To prevent maxillary first permanent molars from drifting mesially, we asked Madison to wear a high-pull headgear when sleeping.
- As soon as Madison demonstrated headgear compliance, her maxillary right and left first premolars, mandibular left first premolar, and both mandibular primary second molars were extracted. We extracted

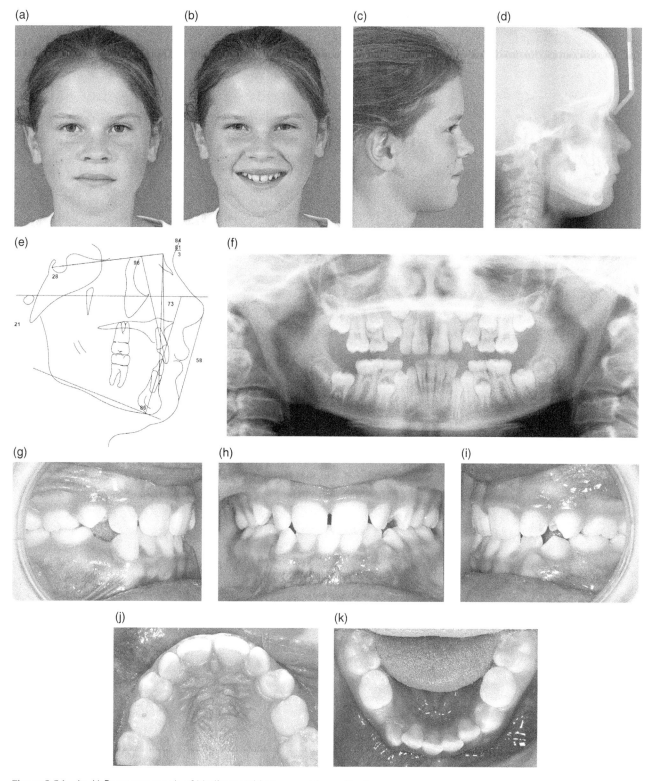

Figure 2.54   (a–k) Progress records of Madison at 11 years and 1 month of age.

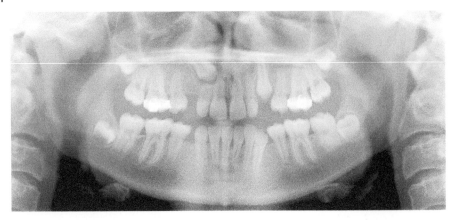

Figure 2.55 Progress panoramic image of Madison at 12 years and 3 months of age.

her mandibular right first premolar as soon as it erupted. We hoped that extraction of her first premolars would encourage normal eruption of her permanent canines by providing space and a pathway for them to erupt.

Q: We made a panoramic image one year and two months later (Figure 2.55). What do you observe?

A: Since only permanent teeth are now present, *early orthodontic treatment is complete.* However, we will follow Madison through completion of comprehensive treatment.

　The most significant finding is the ectopic eruption of Madison's maxillary right permanent canine. It is resorbing her maxillary right permanent lateral incisor root and very likely impacted. Following extraction of her maxillary first premolars, Madison's maxillary left permanent canine began erupting in a more *vertical* direction, but her maxillary right permanent canine began erupting in a more *horizontal* direction. (Compare Figures 2.54f and 2.55). Also, residual extraction space is observed in her mandibular right quadrant.

Q: What is the rate of maxillary permanent canine impaction during eruption?

A: About 1–2% [65–69].

Q: Are most maxillary impacted canines buccal or palatal?

A: Most are *palatal (85%)* – due to a positional anomaly. Only 15% are buccal – due to inadequate space [70].

Q: What percentage of maxillary incisor roots undergo resorption from ectopically erupting canines?

A: About 50% [71, 72].

Q: What are your options for dealing with root resorption of Madison's maxillary right lateral incisor?

A: Options include:
- *Monitor* – we do not recommend this option because the right canine could continue resorbing the right lateral incisor root and possibly the central incisor root.
- *Extract the maxillary right lateral incisor* – is a reasonable option but not our first choice. If we extract the lateral incisor, and if the canine erupts into the lateral incisor position, then the canine could be:
  1) Substituted for the lateral incisor (with an implant placed in the correct canine position), or
  2) Retracted into the correct canine position and the maxillary right lateral incisor restored with a bridge or implant.

  　If we extracted the right lateral incisor and the right canine did not erupt properly, then it may be necessary to surgically expose the canine to bring it into the arch or to extract the canine if it becomes ankylosed.
- *Surgically expose the maxillary right permanent canine and move it into the arch* – is a reasonable option, and our option of choice.

Q: Assume that we surgically expose the maxillary right canine and attempt to move it into the arch. Can you describe a common mistake made during such initial canine movement?

A: A common mistake consists of dragging the ectopically erupting maxillary canine crown *across the root* of an adjacent tooth – an error which can result in resorption of the adjacent tooth root [73].

　Instead, it is prudent to first move the ectopically erupting canine crown *away* from the adjacent tooth root. Figure 2.56a, b illustrates this point in another patient. Initially, we moved this patient's maxillary right canine crown distally, away from the incisor root (Figure 2.56a). Once the canine crown was distanced

(a)

(b)

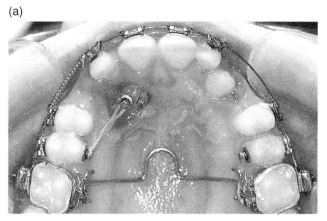

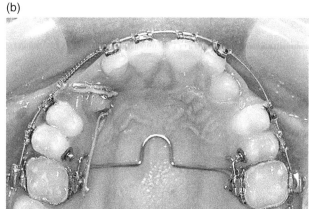

Figure 2.56 (a, b) To prevent lateral incisor root resorption following canine surgical exposure, (a) first move an ectopically-erupting maxillary canine crown away from the incisor root before (b) moving the canine crown buccally into the arch.

from the incisor roots, it was moved laterally (Figure 2.56b) into its proper arch position.

Q: If Madison's maxillary right canine is surgically exposed, and if its crown is moved away from the maxillary right lateral incisor root, then what will happen to the lateral incisor's resorbed root? Will resorption continue or stop? Can the lateral incisor be moved, and does it require root canal therapy to prevent additional resorption?

A: Resorption of the lateral incisor root *ends* after the canine crown is moved away from it. After the canine is moved away, the maxillary lateral incisor can be moved with minimal risk of increased resorption. Root canal therapy to decrease further resorption is unnecessary [74]. In one study of such clinical situations, no resorbed incisors were lost during a 2–10 year follow-up period [75].

Q: Considering the above discussion, what *comprehensive* treatment do you recommend?

A: Maxillary and mandibular fixed appliances were placed, except for Madison's maxillary right lateral incisor, and her maxillary right canine was surgically exposed. An elastic force was initially applied to move the palatal canine crown distally, toward a TPA that had been placed, and *away from her lateral incisor root*. Later, the canine was brought into its correction position (Figure 2.57a, b).

Q: Why was Madison's maxillary right lateral incisor not initially bonded?

A: If her maxillary right lateral incisor had been bonded, and engaged in the archwire, then its root could have been forced into the crown of the impacted canine, causing further root resorption. In situations like Madison's, *do not bond the maxillary lateral incisor*

(a)

(b)

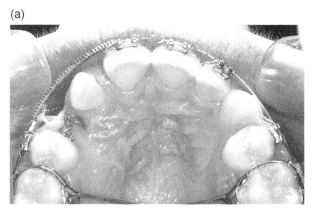

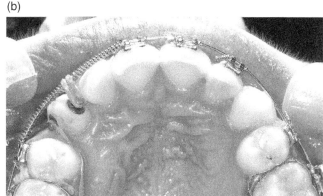

Figure 2.57 (a, b) Progress maxillary occlusal photographs illustrating forced eruption of Madison's maxillary right permanent canine. An elastic force (not shown) was first directed from the surgically exposed canine crown to the TPA in order to distance the canine crown away from the lateral incisor root. Next, (a) the canine crown was pulled to the buccal. Finally, elastic forces (b) were used to generate a couple to the crown to rotate it into correct position.

until the impacted canine crown is distanced from the lateral incisor root (Figure 2.57).

Q: Madison's arches were leveled, aligned, and all spaces closed. Her deband records are shown in Figure 2.58. What changes do you note?

A: Changes include:
- Her nose, lips, chin, maxilla, and mandible have all grown downward and forward (Figure 2.58f). Her mandible underwent significant growth, resulting in a reduction of ANB from 3° to 0°. Her maxillary molars, mandibular molars, and incisors have

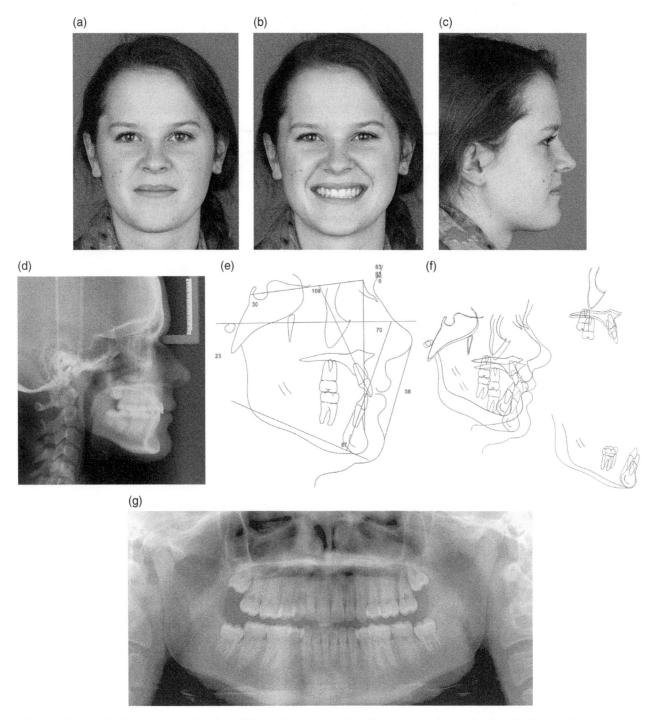

Figure 2.58 (a–l) Deband records of Madison, (f) Lateral cephalometric radiograph superimposition from initial records to deband.

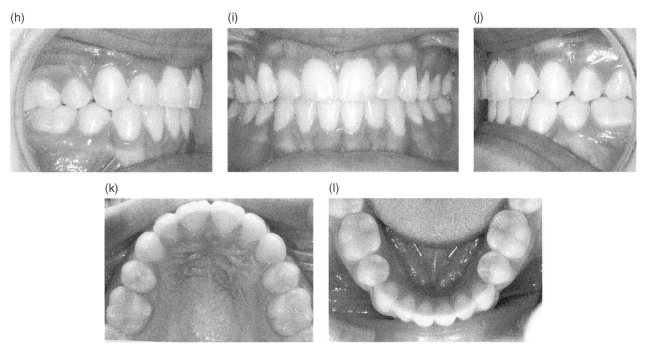

(h)　(i)　(j)

(k)　(l)

Figure 2.58　(Continued)

erupted. Maxillary and mandibular molars translated mesially, maxillary incisors proclined, and mandibular incisors uprighted.

- Her molars and right canines are Class I, but her left canines and left second premolars are Class II by 1 mm.
- OB has decreased to 10% (Figure 2.58i).
- Ectopically erupting maxillary right canine was brought into the arch.
- Significant root resorption of the maxillary right lateral incisor is noted (Figure 2.58g). However, the root resorption does not appear to have worsened since it was first observed (Figure 2.55).
- Mandibular right second premolar root is tipped distally (instead of being parallel with other roots).
- Crowding was eliminated.
- UDML appears coincident with the facial midline, but LDML is to the left of UDML by ~ 1 mm.
- Madison still presents with a mild right-to-left occlusal cant (Figure 2.58b). However, this cant has not worsened since she first presented at age eight years (Figure 2.52l).
- Development/eruption of her wisdom teeth will be monitored.

Q: Madison finished slightly Class II at her left canines and second premolars. How could this Class II relationship have been corrected?

A: Class II elastic wear on her left side could have readily corrected this problem by translating her mandibular left teeth to the mesial slightly and translating her maxillary left teeth to the distal slightly. Correcting the left Class II relationship could also have corrected her 1 mm midline discrepancy. However, in order to correct her left canine and premolar occlusion to precisely Class I, Madison would need to have had adequate overjet and her left first permanent molars would have been finished slightly Class III (Figure 2.58j).

Q: If Madison does not have overjet, how could adequate overjet be created?

A: Overjet could be created by:
- Performing IPR on her mandibular anterior teeth and then closing those spaces – which would retract the mandibular anterior teeth.
- Proclining maxillary incisors by opening spaces distal to the lateral incisors (these spaces would be closed later with composite veneers).

Note: you *could not* create OJ by opening Madison's bite. Why? She only has 10% OB. Any additional anterior bite opening would create an anterior open bite.

Q: Even with premolar extractions, Madison finished with *proclined* (not upright) maxillary incisors. How was this possible?

A: Note Madison's significant mandibular forward growth (Figure 2.58f). Proclination of her maxillary incisors is most likely explained as *dental compensation for this Class III growth pattern* (decrease in her ANB angle from 3° to 0°). The only other possible explanation is that maxillary lingual root torque (buccal crown torque) was generated by the preadjusted (straight-wire) appliance used during fixed appliance therapy.

Q: What retention protocol would you recommend for Madison?

A: She was placed in removable Hawley retainers and asked to wear them at night for life. Lifelong retention is the only guarantee that alignment of teeth can be maintained. The maxillary Hawley retainer has an anterior biteplate to disclude her posterior teeth slightly when she wears it. This feature could help prevent deepening of her OB. A mandibular lingual fixed canine-to-canine retainer could also have been used instead of a mandibular Hawley retainer.

Q: Was reduction of Madison's initial 30–50% OB to 10% OB a good idea?

A: Yes. For individuals with an initial deep bite, it is best to end with a shallow OB in anticipation of some relapse (OB deepening). Likewise, for individuals with an initial open bite, it is best to end with a deep bite (OB $\geq$ 20–30%).

Q: Can you suggest "take-home pearls" regarding Madison's treatment?

A: "Take-home pearls" include the following:
- Madison was eight years and two months old when she presented with her parents' chief complaint, "We are concerned that Madison's teeth are crowded." Clinical and radiographic evaluation revealed a Class I malocclusion, cross bite of the maxillary right lateral incisor, OB 30–50%, potentially impacted/unerupted maxillary and mandibular lateral incisors, and moderate anterior crowding in both arches. Her treatment evolved into serial extraction of four first premolars. She had an excellent esthetic, occlusal, and functional result.
- When we took into account the amount of initial incisor crowding, the anticipated leeway space, and the amount of space needed for permanent lateral incisors, we estimated that Madison would end up with 2.5 mm of maxillary arch crowding and 4.3 mm of mandibular arch crowding *if proper space maintenance was employed*. A decision was made to extract all four primary canines to aid in eruption of permanent lateral incisors. However, neither an LLHA nor a Nance holding arch was placed to prevent mesial drift of the permanent molars, incisor uprighting, and arch perimeter loss.

  Results of studies are mixed regarding the effect of primary canine extractions on permanent first molar mesial drift. However, based upon the fact that Madison's incisors uprighted (compare Figures 2.52e with 2.53e), we can assume that her posterior teeth probably drifted to the mesial in a reciprocal fashion. Both movements resulted in arch perimeter loss. Did mesial molar drift/incisor uprighting force us into extracting four premolars later? Yes, quite possibly.

  The point is that *we should have placed an LLHA and a Nance holding arch when Madison's primary canines were extracted in order to reduce/prevent mesial molar drift, incisor uprighting, and arch perimeter loss*.
- With initially upright maxillary incisors and normally inclined mandibular incisors, placement of an LLHA and Nance holding arch would have been a smart way to *reduce unknowns*. Then, a decision to treat either non-extraction or with extractions could have been made after all permanent teeth erupted and after a final crowding assessment had been made.
- In cases of early crowding, all options (monitoring, space maintenance, space regaining, and extractions) must be considered.
- If you chose an extraction option remember: the more initial crowding present, the less residual space you will need to close following extractions and anterior alignment; the less initial crowding present, the more residual space you will need to close following extractions and anterior alignment.
- Space regaining for Madison's maxillary permanent canines was not a viable option (Figure 2.53f). Why? Her maxillary permanent canines were too high – their crowns were at the level of the lateral incisor root apices. Without significant RME (in the range of 15 mm) or extraction of permanent teeth, there was simply no way to create 7.5 mm of anterior space for each maxillary canine crown *at the level of the lateral incisor root apices*.
- Always move ectopically erupting teeth crowns away from adjacent tooth roots *first* following surgical exposure. Then, and only then, begin moving the ectopically erupting teeth crowns into ideal positions. *Never drag ectopically erupting teeth crowns across adjacent tooth roots* – as this can cause root resorption.

- A word about treatment time. To date, Madison has been followed for 10 years, including periods of monitoring, extraction/eruption of teeth, surgical exposure of an ectopically erupting canine, and fixed orthodontic treatment. This lengthy treatment time underscores one important pearl – serial extraction may reduce *active* treatment time, but serial extraction can increase *total* treatment time as significant observation time often precedes active treatment time [23, 24].

Case Muriel

Q: Muriel, a seven-year-old girl (Figure 2.59), presents with her parents for a consultation. They state their chief complaint: "Our dentist says Muriel is missing a tooth." Her PMH, PDH, periodontal, and TMJ evaluations are WRN, and CR = CO. Do you need any additional records in order decide whether to recall Muriel or to perform early treatment?

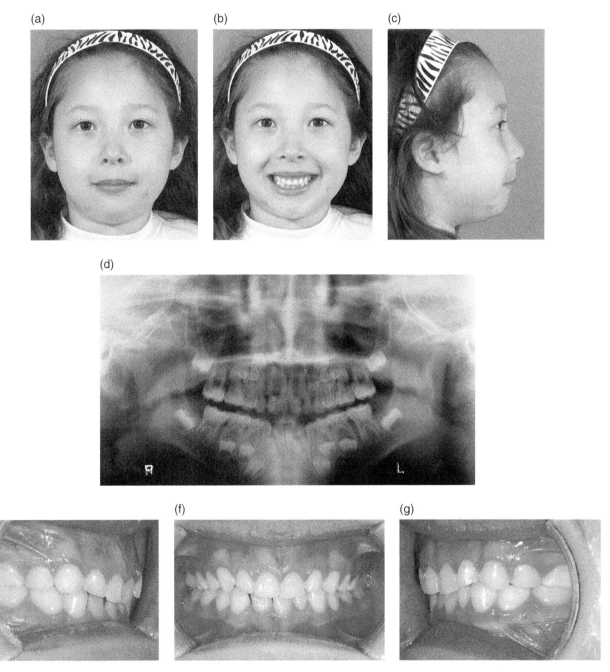

Figure 2.59 Initial records of Muriel: (a–c) facial photographs, (d) pantomograph, and (e–i) intraoral photographs.

(h)

(i)

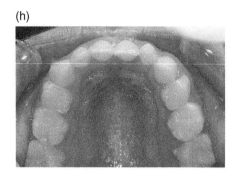
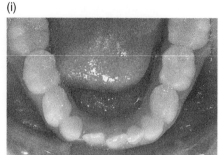

Figure 2.59 (Continued)

A: No additional records are not needed at this consultation.

Q: Compile your diagnostic findings and problem list. State your diagnosis.

A:

Table 2.17 Diagnostic findings and problem list for Muriel.

Full face and profile	*Frontal view*
	Facial symmetry
	Soft tissue LAFH WRN (soft tissue Glabella – Subnasale ≈ Subnasale – soft tissue Menton)
	UDML WRN
	Excess gingival display during posed smile (gingival margin should be congruent with maxillary lip)
	Lip competence
	Large buccal corridors in posed smile
	Profile view
	Convex profile
	Upturned nose
	Obtuse NLA
	Retrusive chin position
	Obtuse lip-chin-throat angle
	Chin-throat length appears WRN
Radiographs	Early mixed dentition (mandibular permanent central incisors have erupted)
	Unerupted maxillary permanent incisors
	Missing mandibular right primary lateral incisor
	Unerupted mandibular lateral incisors
Intraoral photos and models	Angle Class II subdivision right
	Iowa Classification: II (1 mm) II (1 mm) I I
	Mandibular dental midline 2 mm right of maxillary dental midline
	OB 30–40%
	Dental arches are symmetric (Figures 2.59h and 2.59i)

Table 2.17 (Continued)

	1 mm of maxillary primary incisor crowding is currently present, but an additional 6.8 mm of space will be needed for the permanent incisors to erupt aligned
	5.8 mm of maxillary arch crowding is anticipated following eruption of all permanent teeth (is space maintenance is employed)
	0 mm of mandibular anterior crowding is currently present, but 6.9 mm of additional space will be needed for permanent incisors to erupt aligned
	3.7 mm of mandibular arch crowding is anticipated following eruption of all permanent teeth (if space maintenance is employed)
	Missing mandibular right primary lateral incisor
	Maxillary central incisors are stepped down relative to maxillary posterior teeth (Figure 2.59f)
Other	—
Diagnosis	Class II subdivision right (1 mm) malocclusion with missing mandibular right primary lateral incisor, unerupted maxillary permanent incisors, and unerupted mandibular lateral incisors

Q: Is there a potential flaw in our diagnostic findings of Muriel's gingival display?

A: Yes. Although we have appropriately measured the relationship between the labial gingival margins of the maxillary primary incisors and the maxillary lip in her smile photo and note the excessive gingival display, values for incisal display are by and large from studies of adolescents and adults.

One study in children noted excessive gingival display was common [76]. This may relate to the finding of some authors that the amount of gingival display during smile shows moderate correlation to the vertical height of the incisor crowns (shorter crowns associated with increased incisal display) [77]. Although our analysis is correct, a more meaningful time to evaluate incisal display is after permanent maxillary incisors have fully erupted.

Q: Provide a detailed space analysis for Muriel's maxillary and mandibular arches. In other words, how were the 5.8 mm of anticipated maxillary arch crowding and 3.7 mm of anticipated mandibular arch crowding calculated (if appropriate space maintenance is employed)?

A:

Average mesiodistal widths of permanent teeth (mm) [1]:

Maxillary Central Incisor	8.5	Mandibular Central Incisor	5.0
Maxillary Lateral Incisor	6.5	Mandibular Lateral Incisor	5.5
Maxillary Canine	7.5	Mandibular Canine	7.0
Maxillary First Premolar	7.0	Mandibular First Premolar	7.0
Maxillary Second Premolar	7.0	Mandibular Second Premolar	7.0
Maxillary First Molar	10.0	Mandibular First Molar	11.0
Maxillary Second Molar	9.0	Mandibular Second Molar	10.5

Average mesiodistal widths of *primary* teeth (mm) [1]:

Maxillary Central Incisor	6.5	Mandibular Central Incisor	4.2
Maxillary Lateral Incisor	5.1	Mandibular Lateral Incisor	4.1
Maxillary Canine	7.0	Mandibular Canine	5.0
Maxillary First Molar	7.3	Mandibular First Molar	7.7
Maxillary Second Molar	8.2	Mandibular Second Molar	9.9

MAXILLARY ARCH

−1 mm of primary incisor crowding is currently present (Figure 2.59h).

+13 mm primary central incisor mesiodistal widths = +6.5 mm + 6.5 mm.

+10.2 mm primary lateral incisor mesiodistal widths = +5.1 mm + 5.1 mm.

−17 mm anticipated permanent central incisor space needed = −8.5 mm − 8.5 mm.

−13 mm anticipated permanent lateral incisor space needed = −6.5 mm − 6.5 mm.

+2 mm of anticipated leeway space (1 mm/side).

Balance = −1 mm + 13 mm + 10.2 mm − 17 mm − 13 mm + 2 mm = −5.8 mm.

MANDIBULAR ARCH

+1 mm space present between mandibular right primary canine and mandibular right permanent central incisor (Figure 2.59i).

−1 mm incisor crowding currently present.

+4.1 mm left primary lateral incisor mesiodistal width.

−11 mm anticipated permanent right and left lateral incisor mesiodistal widths = −5.5 mm − 5.5 mm

+3.2 mm of anticipated leeway space (1.6 mm/side).

Balance = +1 mm − 1 mm + 4.1 mm − 11 mm + 3.2 mm = −3.7 mm.

That is, *5.8 mm of maxillary arch crowding and 3.7 mm of mandibular arch crowding is anticipated once all permanent teeth erupt (if space maintenance to prevent loss of leeway space is instituted).*

Q: Always focus on the patient's *primary* problem in each dimension, plus other significant problems. Do this at every appointment. What are Muriel's primary problems?

A:

Table 2.18 Primary problems list for Muriel *(apical base/skeletal discrepancies italicized).*

AP	Slight (1 mm) Class II on right side
Vertical	OB 30–40%
Transverse	—
Other	Inadequate space for eruption/alignment of permanent incisors (7.8 mm needed for maxillary permanent incisors, 6.9 mm needed for mandibular permanent incisors)

Q: Muriel's dental arches appear symmetric (Figures 2.59h and 2.59i), but a dental or skeletal asymmetry *must* exist. Why?

A: Because she is Class II (1 mm) on the right side and Class I on the left side without a CR–CO shift. Whenever a patient has an anteroposterior relationship on the right side which differs from the left side, an underlying skeletal or dental arch asymmetry must exist to explain the difference. However, Muriel's right-to-left difference is so small that its origin is undefinable.

Q: Discuss Muriel in the context of three principles applied to every early treatment patient.

- The goal of early treatment is to correct developing problems – get the patient *back to normal for their stage of development* (including preventing complications such as resorption of adjacent tooth roots, reducing later treatment complexity, or reducing/eliminating unknowns). Treatment to ensure eruption of all permanent teeth, alleviate her crowding, plus correct her deep bite, midlines, and slight right Class II relationship would get her back on track.

- Early treatment should address *very specific problems with a clearly defined end point*, usually begun and ended within six to nine months (not protracted over many years, except for some orthopedic problems). Inadequate space for permanent incisor eruption/alignment could be quickly corrected by extracting primary canines and left primary lateral incisor, but we consider this option premature because the permanent lateral incisor roots are <½ developed. Further, if extraction of primary canines was performed, then space maintainers should be concurrently placed to prevent/reduce arch perimeter loss.

Ensuring eruption of permanent canines and premolars will take years because their roots are underdeveloped and eruption is not imminent. Her deep bite could be opened by intruding stepped down maxillary primary incisors using fixed appliances, but we do *not* recommend intruding primary incisor roots against permanent incisor crowns as resorption of the roots could accelerate (Figure 2.59d) and because overbite of permanent incisors cannot be predicted by overbite of primary incisors. It is best to assess OB after permanent incisors erupt.

Her midlines could be readily corrected by regaining space (opening space) for her mandibular right lateral incisor using fixed appliances. Finally, her slight right Class II relationship could be readily corrected with any number of Class II correctors.

- Always ask: Is it necessary that I treat the patient now? *What harm will come if I choose to do nothing now?* It is not necessary to treat Muriel now, and we could recall her in one year to monitor tooth eruption. If we choose to recall Muriel, then the permanent lateral incisors may remain unerupted or erupt ectopically. Her deep bite could worsen, or disappear, once the permanent maxillary incisors erupt. However, since she does not exhibit mandibular incisor palatal impingement/tissue damage/pain, there is no compelling reason to address the deep bite now. Lastly, no harm is anticipated from leaving the slight right Class II, or noncoincidence of midlines, untreated.

Q: Muriel is in the early mixed dentition. Can you state our guideline for dealing with crowding in the primary and early mixed dentitions?

A: *We generally recommend monitoring (recalling) patients with crowding in the primary/early mixed dentition.* This is assuming that the permanent canine and premolar roots are immature (less than ½ developed), and their eruption is not imminent. This is also assuming that you judge the potential harm from monitoring to be minimal (e.g. the probability of root resorption from ectopically erupting teeth to be minimal).

Q: Why is Muriel not an ideal serial extraction patient?

A: The ideal serial extraction patient presents in the early mixed dentition stage of development and is *normal in every way, except for the presence of severe anterior crowding (≥9 mm anterior crowding in both arches).* Let us review each of the ideal serial extraction patient features and see if Muriel exhibits these features.

- *Class I first molars:* Yes, she exhibits this feature. Although Muriel is Class II on her right side by a millimeter, she is essentially Class I.
- *Vertically normal (or slightly long soft tissue and skeletal LAFH, minimal OB or possibly a mild open bite – but not a deep bite):* Muriel has a deep bite and does not exhibit this feature. However, this could change once her maxillary permanent central incisors erupt.
- *Normal incisor angulation or proclined incisors, but not upright incisors:* It is unknown whether Muriel's permanent maxillary incisors will exhibit this feature. However, her primary maxillary incisors appear upright (Figure 2.59e and g).
- *Normal transverse relationship*: Muriel exhibits this feature.
- *Severe (≥9 mm) anterior crowding*: Muriel does not exhibit this feature. She currently exhibits moderate crowding for her permanent incisors to erupt aligned.

Based upon the above features, Muriel is not an ideal serial extraction candidate.

Q: What early treatment options would you consider for Muriel?

A: Options include the following:

- *Recall* (monitor, no early treatment now) – recall Muriel in one year and evaluate tooth eruption. This option would follow our general guideline for dealing with crowding in the early mixed dentition, and we anticipate no harm if we choose it.
- *Space maintenance* – placing an LLHA/Nance holding arch. There is no immediate need for space maintenance in either arch now because the roots of Muriel's permanent canines and premolars are

underdeveloped (their eruption is not imminent). However, failure to place space maintainers before the transition from early mixed to late mixed dentition could result in molars drifting mesially, loss of arch perimeter, and less space for crowding reduction.

- *Space regaining* (opening space for the mandibular right permanent lateral incisor). As you open space, mandibular arch perimeter will increase, and mandibular incisors will procline. Therefore, you would also need to create maxillary space/procline maxillary incisors to maintain overjet and avoid creating an anterior cross bite. We generally do not recommend proclining maxillary *primary* incisors at this developmental stage, except in some Class III cross bites. Consequently, we do not recommend space regaining as an option for Muriel.
- *Extraction of mandibular primary canines and mandibular left primary lateral incisor* – would result in accelerated eruption of mandibular permanent lateral incisors because the lateral incisor roots are ≥ ½ developed. However, arch perimeter could subsequently be lost as mandibular molars drift mesially. Placing an LLHA would greatly reduce/prevent this arch perimeter loss, but the LLHA will need to be in place for years before the mandibular permanent canines and premolars erupt (cement washout could be a problem).

  Remember – extraction of primary and permanent teeth should generally be considered in patients with ectopic eruption, dehiscence of crestal alveolar bone supporting permanent teeth, permanent incisors or canines erupting into nonkeratinized gingiva, and *severe* crowding.
- *Extraction of maxillary primary canines and primary lateral incisors* – could be a viable option if the permanent lateral incisor crowns fail to resorb the primary lateral incisor roots or if Muriel's maxillary permanent canine crowns begin to overlap her maxillary permanent lateral incisor roots on a panoramic image (ectopic eruption). However, we feel it is too early to extract the maxillary primary canines and primary incisors at this time. Why? Her maxillary permanent lateral incisor roots appear to be < ½ developed (Figure 2.59d), so extraction of the maxillary primary canines and primary lateral incisors could *slow* permanent lateral incisor eruption.

- *Serial extraction* – Muriel is not an ideal patient for serial extraction.

Q: After considering the above, what would you recommend at this consultation? Would you monitor or recommend early treatment? If you recommend early treatment, what is your plan?

A: A decision was made to recall Muriel in a year. The risk that the permanent lateral incisors would remain unerupted, or erupt ectopically, was not considered a serious risk. Furthermore, her deep bite, slight right Class II relationship, and UDML/LDML difference could be dealt with in the late mixed or adult dentition. Muriel moved away and did not return for a recall appointment.

Case Mudathir

Q: Mudathir is eight years and eight months old (Figures 2.60a–2.60i) and presents to you for a consultation. His pediatric dentist is concerned with his mandibular crowding. His PMH, PDH, periodontal, mucogingival, and TMJ evaluations are WRN. CR = CO. *Compile your diagnostic findings and problem list.* State your *diagnosis*.

(a)   (b)   (c)

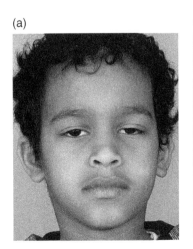 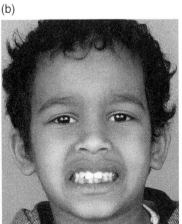 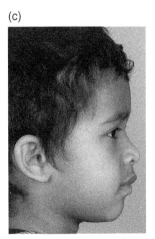

Figure 2.60 Initial records of Mudathir: (a–c) facial photographs, (d) pantomograph, and (e–i) intraoral photographs.

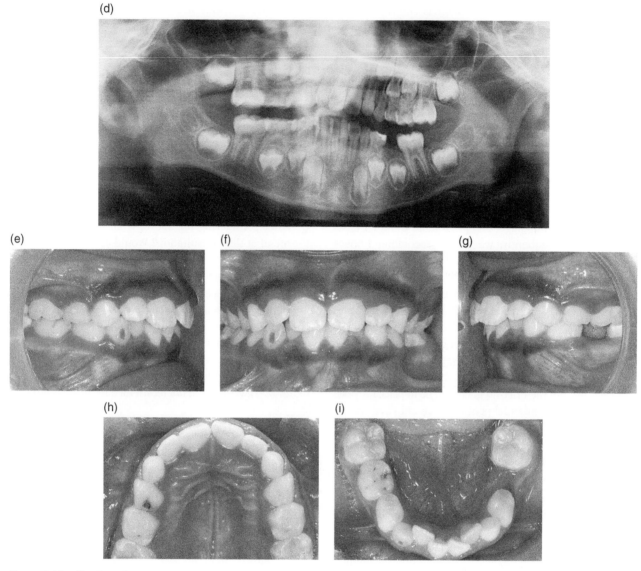

Figure 2.60 (Continued)

A:

Table 2.19 Diagnostic findings and problem list for Mudathir.

Full face and profile	*Frontal view*
	Face is symmetric
	Full lips
	Long soft tissue LAFH (soft tissue Glabella – Subnasale < Subnasale – soft tissue Menton)
	Lip competence
	UDML WRN
	Midlines are coincident
	Mudathir would not smile for us. B is a grimace and cannot be used to judge his posed smile incisal/gingival display nor his buccal corridors
	Profile view
	Convex profile

Table 2.19 (Continued)

	Upturned nose
	NLA WRN
	Lips protrusive relative to the E plane
	Retrusive chin position
	Obtuse lip-chin-throat angle
	Short chin-throat length
Radiographs	Early mixed dentition
	Right side of panoramic image is distorted
	Missing mandibular left primary second molar
	Mandibular left permanent first molar is tipped mesially
	Mandibular left second premolar potentially impacted by mesially tipped mandibular left first permanent molar
Intraoral photos and models	Angle Class III subdivision left
	Iowa Classification: I I I III (3 mm) (the maxillary left permanent molar is not visible in G, and the maxillary left primary second molar is used as a reference)
	OJ 2–3 mm
	OB 40%
	Small maxillary midline diastema
	Maxillary arch is symmetric
	Mandibular arch is asymmetric with left permanent first molar ahead of the right by 3 mm and slight distal drift of the primary left first molar
	1.0 mm of maxillary anterior crowding is currently present
	1.0 mm of maxillary arch spacing is anticipated following eruption of all permanent teeth (if proper space maintenance is employed)
	7.0 mm of mandibular anterior crowding is currently present
	8.7 mm of mandibular arch crowding is anticipated following eruption of all permanent teeth (if proper space maintenance is employed)
	Missing mandibular left primary second molar
	Thick labial anterior maxillary and mandibular periodontal biotype
Other	Visible tooth decay
Diagnosis	Class III subdivision left malocclusion with moderate mandibular arch crowding

Q: Do you need additional records to decide whether to recall or treat Mudathir early?

A: Yes. The distorted panoramic image should be remade to give a clearer view of Mudathir's maxillary right quadrant. An alternate option would be to make periapical radiographs of his maxillary right teeth. These records were not made.

Q: Mudathir exhibits a Class III (3 mm) left permanent first molar relationship. Is this Class III relationship a skeletal, or dental, problem?

A: It is a *dental* problem. Mudathir exhibits a convex profile (not a concave profile indicative of a Class III skeletal growth pattern), facial symmetry, bilateral Class I canine relationships, asymmetry of his mandibular first permanent molars (left first molar ahead of right), and mesial tipping of his left permanent first molar into the edentulous space (Figure 2.60d). It is the mesial tipping of the mandibular left permanent first molar that has resulted in the left Class III molar relationship.

Q: What is the most likely explanation for Mudathir's left Class III molar relationship?

A: Considering the present tooth decay, the most likely explanation is that he lost his mandibular left primary second molar from decay, and the mandibular left first permanent molar drifted mesially.

Q: Provide a detailed space analysis for Mudathir's maxillary and mandibular arches. In other words, how were the anticipated 1.0 mm of maxillary arch spacing and

8.7 mm of mandibular arch crowding calculated (following eruption of all permanent teeth, if proper space maintenance is employed)?

A:

Below are space estimates:

Average mesiodistal widths of permanent teeth (mm) [1]:

Maxillary Central Incisor	8.5	Mandibular Central Incisor	5.0
Maxillary Lateral Incisor	6.5	Mandibular Lateral Incisor	5.5
Maxillary Canine	7.5	Mandibular Canine	7.0
Maxillary First Premolar	7.0	Mandibular First Premolar	7.0
Maxillary Second Premolar	7.0	Mandibular Second Premolar	7.0
Maxillary First Molar	10.0	Mandibular First Molar	11.0
Maxillary Second Molar	9.0	Mandibular Second Molar	10.5

Average mesiodistal widths of *primary* teeth (mm) [1]:

Maxillary Central Incisor	6.5	Mandibular Central Incisor	4.2
Maxillary Lateral Incisor	5.1	Mandibular Lateral Incisor	4.1
Maxillary Canine	7.0	Mandibular Canine	5.0
Maxillary First Molar	7.3	Mandibular First Molar	7.7
Maxillary Second Molar	8.2	Mandibular Second Molar	9.9

MAXILLARY ARCH
−1.0 mm of anterior crowding is currently present (Figure 2.60h).
+2 mm of anticipated leeway space (1 mm/side).
Balance = −1.0 mm + 2 mm = +1.0 mm.

MANDIBULAR ARCH
−7.0 mm of incisor crowding is currently present (Figure 2.60i).
+1.6 mm anticipated leeway space on the right.
+5.0 mm width of mandibular left primary canine.
−7.0 mm anticipated width of mandibular left permanent canine.
+7.7 mm width of mandibular left primary first molar.
−7.0 mm anticipated width of mandibular left first premolar.
+5.0 mm space available for mandibular left second premolar.
−7.0 mm anticipated width of mandibular left second premolar.

Balance = −7.0 mm + 1.6 mm + 5.0 mm − 7.0 mm + 7.7 mm − 7.0 mm + 5.0 mm − 7.0 mm = −8.7 mm.

That is, *1.0 mm of maxillary arch space and 8.7 mm of mandibular arch crowding is anticipated following eruption of all permanent teeth (if proper space maintenance is employed).*

Q: What are Mudathir's primary problems in each dimension, plus other primary problems, that you must focus on at every appointment?

A:

Table 2.20   Primary problems list for Mudathir.

AP	Class III subdivision left malocclusion (permanent first molar relationship)
	Premature loss of mandibular left primary second molar with mesial drift of mandibular left permanent first molar
Vertical	40% OB
Transverse	—
Other	Moderate (7.0 mm) mandibular anterior crowding currently present
	Mesial tip of mandibular left first permanent molar
	Due to mandibular left permanent first molar mesial drift/tip and distal drift of mandibular left primary first molar, 8.7 mm of mandibular arch crowding is anticipated if proper space maintenance is employed
	Mandibular left second premolar potentially impacted by the permanent first molar tooth decay

Q: Discuss Mudathir in the context of three principles applied to every early treatment patient.

- The goal of early treatment is to correct developing problems – get the patient *back to normal for their stage of development* (including preventing complications such as resorption of adjacent tooth roots, reducing later treatment complexity, or reducing/eliminating unknowns). Correcting Mudathir's left unilateral Class III molar relationship, creating an eruption path for the potentially impacted mandibular left second premolar, correcting his deep overbite, moderate mandibular anterior crowding, and poor hygiene/decay – would get him back on track for his stage of development.
- Early treatment should address *very specific problems with a clearly defined end point*, usually begun and ended within six to nine months (not protracted over many years, except for some orthopedic

treatments). Since the unilateral left Class III molar relationship is a *dental* problem (not a skeletal growth problem), it could be corrected in less than nine months by uprighting/distalizing the mandibular left permanent first molar. If the mandibular left permanent first molar is uprighted/distalized 3 mm into a Class I relationship, then the mandibular left leeway space would be regained (except for the distal drift of the mandibular left primary first molar) – which would reduce the anticipated arch crowding. Also, a path for eruption of the mandibular left second premolar would be created. Mudathir's deep overbite could be reduced to normal (10–20%) using fixed orthodontic appliances to level the arches in six to nine months.

- Always ask: Is it necessary that I treat the patient now? *What harm will come if I choose to do nothing now?* If Mudathir's mandibular left permanent first molar is not uprighted/distalized, then it could continue tipping mesially, impacting his mandibular left second premolar and leaving his maxillary left permanent first molar unopposed and super-erupting.

  Since the roots of his permanent canines and premolars are underdeveloped, their eruption is not imminent and improving his mandibular arch crowding via space maintenance can be postponed without harm. However, an LLHA should be placed if the mandibular left permanent first molar is uprighted/distalized in order to hold that correction.

Q: Mudathir currently has 7.0 mm of mandibular anterior crowding. Is he a good candidate for serial extraction? Why or why not?

A: No, Mudathir is not a good candidate for serial extraction. Let us examine Mudathir in the context of each ideal serial extraction feature (*normal in every way, except severe anterior crowding*):

- *Class I first molars.* Mudathir does not exhibit this feature as he is Class III subdivision left.
- *Vertically normal to slightly long soft tissue and skeletal LAFH, with minimal OB or possibly a mild open bite, but* not *a deep bite.* Mudathir does not exhibit this feature. Although he has a long soft tissue LAFH, he also has a deep 40% OB.
- *Normal incisor angulation or proclined incisors, but* not *upright incisors.* We suspect that he exhibits this feature. We do not have a cephalometric radiographic to measure Mudathir's incisal angulation, but they do not appear upright in his clinical photographs.

- *Normal posterior transverse relationship (normal inter-molar arch widths with good posterior interdigitation; absence of posterior cross bites; and absence of significant transverse compensations).* Mudathir exhibits this feature.
- Severe (≥9 mm) anterior crowding: Mudathir does not exhibit this feature. He currently has 1 mm of maxillary anterior crowding and 7.0 mm of mandibular anterior crowding.

  However, we anticipate 8.7 mm of mandibular arch crowding after all his permanent teeth erupt if we rely solely on an LLHA (not space regaining). This would be reduced to 5.7 mm if we uprighted his mandibular left permanent first molar by 3 mm to Class I.

Based upon these features, Mudathir is *not* an ideal candidate for serial extraction.

Q: What treatment options would you consider for Mudathir?

A: Options include the following:

- *Recall* (monitor) in one year – is not recommended. Why? Mudathir's mandibular left permanent first molar will continue to tip/drift to the mesial, impacting his mandibular left second premolar and eventually leaving his maxillary left permanent first molar unopposed and super-erupting.
- *Space maintenance* – is not recommended. Placing an LLHA will prevent further mandibular left permanent first molar mesial drift and prevent worsening of the left Class III molar relationship, but the permanent first molar has already drifted to the point where it will impact the mandibular left second premolar (Figure 2.60d). Further, Mudathir's permanent canine and premolar roots are minimally developed, their eruption is not imminent, and there is no pressing need to place space maintainers for the purpose of maintaining leeway space in either arch.
- *Space regaining (mandibular left) followed by space maintenance* – is recommended and would involve uprighting/distalizing the mandibular left permanent first molar. A removable screw-type or spring-type space-regaining appliance could apply a distal force against the left permanent first molar (while permitting proper hygiene), but a reciprocal mesial force would be applied against the mandibular left primary first molar moving it to the mesial and worsening Mudathir's incisor crowding.

  Fixed orthodontic appliances could be placed on the mandibular arch and a compressed open coil spring trapped between the mandibular left permanent first molar and primary first molar. Again, the reciprocal force against the primary first molar would move it forward and worsen anterior crowding.

Or, a TAD could be placed in the left ascending ramus (a heroic TAD placement option to avoid teeth buds) which could provide anchorage for elastics to upright/retract the mandibular left permanent first molar without applying a reciprocal force against the primary first molar. Considering Mudathir's caries history, we are concerned that placement of fixed orthodontic appliances will worsen his hygiene.

- *Extraction of mandibular primary canines* – is not recommended. It would result in spontaneous distal drift of mandibular incisors, improving incisor alignment. However, this option requires a minor surgical procedure and offers no long-term space advantage. If you ever extract mandibular primary canines, say, in order to satisfy a parental demand for aligned incisors, please place an LLHA to prevent mesial molar drift/arch perimeter loss.
- *Extraction of maxillary primary canines (and possibly maxillary primary first molars)* – is not recommended. On the other hand, because the maxillary permanent canine crowns overlap the maxillary lateral incisor root apices *slightly* (Figure 2.60d), an argument can be made for extracting the maxillary primary canines and primary first molars in order to create space and decrease the chances the maxillary permanent canines will become impacted. On the other hand, the maxillary permanent canine and premolar roots are <½ developed, so their eruption is not imminent. We recommend monitoring the maxillary permanent canines for now.
- *Serial extraction* – Mudathir is not an ideal serial extraction patient.
- Hygiene and disease control – should be emphasized on every patient, but especially on Mudathir.

Q: Of the above options, what would you tell the parents at this consultation?

A: We recommended mandibular left space regaining using a removable screw-type space-regaining appliance. Following mandibular left permanent first molar uprighting/distalization, and correction of the left Class III molar relationship, an LLHA would be placed. Caries control and hygiene would be emphasized. After his permanent teeth erupt, records will be made followed by a decision of whether or not to

extract permanent teeth. Mudathir and his parents never returned for treatment despite repeated attempts to contact them.

Q: Can you suggest any "take-home pearls" for Mudathir?

A: "Take-home pearls" include the following:
- Mudathir presented at eight years and eight months of age with a Class III subdivision left malocclusion secondary to premature loss of the mandibular left primary second molar and mesial drift of the permanent first molar. He had a 40% OB, moderate mandibular anterior crowding, potentially impacted mandibular left second premolar, and tooth decay.
- Mudathir underscores the impact of oral disease. The loss of his mandibular left primary second molar, subsequent development of a left Class III molar relationship, and potential impaction of his mandibular left second premolar were probably due to poor oral hygiene. Emphasize proper oral hygiene with all patients. Reinforce the need for them to seek regular dental care during orthodontic treatment.
- The advantage of recommending a *removable* space-regaining appliance to upright/distalize his mandibular left permanent first molar was that he could take out the appliance to clean his teeth.
- Another option would be to place an LLHA with adjustment loops. You could distalize the mandibular left permanent first molar by opening the left adjustment loop. However, the reciprocal LLHA force would push against, and procline, incisors.
- Whoever extracted his mandibular left primary second molar should have immediately placed an LLHA to prevent mesial drift/tipping of the mandibular left permanent first molar. Please educate your family dentists about the need for this.

Case Lucas

Q: Lucas, a six-year-old boy (Figure 2.61), presents to you for a consultation with his parent's chief complaint, "Our dentist says Lucas needs orthodontics." His PMH, periodontal, and TMJ evaluations are WRN. He has a 1–2 mm left lateral shift from CR to CO. *Compile your diagnostic finding and problem list.* State your *diagnosis.*

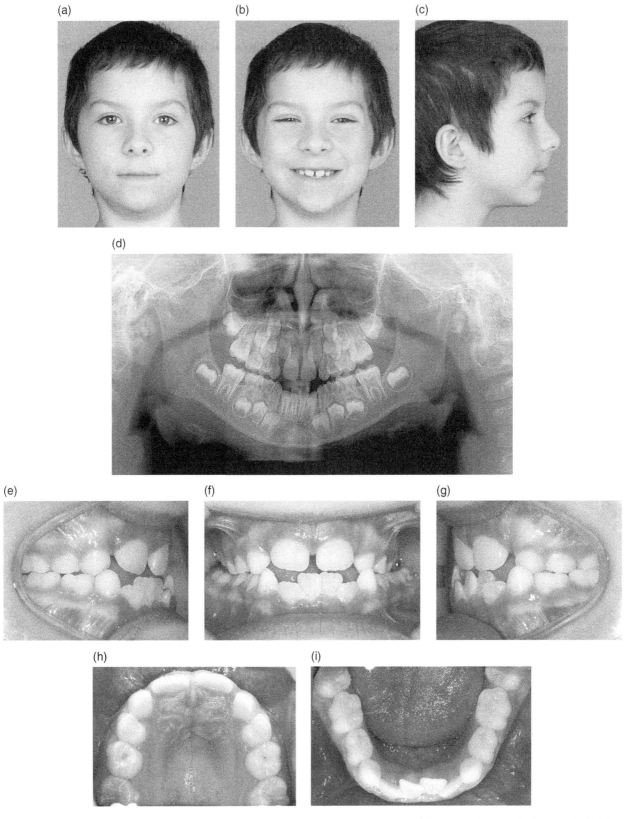

Figure 2.61 Initial records of Lucas: (a–c) facial photographs, (d) pantomograph, and (e–i) intraoral photographs (e–g made in CO).

A:

Table 2.21 Diagnostic findings and problem list for Lucas.

Full face and profile	*Frontal view*
	Chin deviated slightly to left of facial midline
	Mildly long soft tissue LAFH (soft tissue Glabella – Subnasale < Subnasale – soft tissue Menton)
	Lip competence
	UDML WRN
	Incisal display during posed smile less than ideal (central incisal gingival margins should be congruent with maxillary lip)
	Profile view
	Convex profile
	Upturned nose
	Obtuse NLA
	Retrusive chin position
	Lip-chin-throat angle mildly obtuse
	Chin-throat length WRN
Radiographs	Early mixed dentition
	Potentially impacted maxillary lateral incisors
Intraoral photos and models	Angle Class I
	Iowa Classification (in CO): I I I I
	Anterior open bite
	Stepped up maxillary central incisors
	Stepped down mandibular lateral incisors
	Maxillary midline diastema
	Maxillary right central incisor erupting into lingual cross bite
	Maxillary left central incisor erupting edge-to-edge
	Mandibular dental midline 2–3 mm left of maxillary dental midline
	Dental arches symmetric (Figures 2.61h and 2.61i)
	9.0 mm maxillary anterior crowding currently present (4 mm space present but 13 mm needed for potentially impacted permanent lateral incisors)
	7.0 mm maxillary arch crowding is anticipated following eruption of all permanent teeth (if proper space maintenance is employed)
	6.0 mm mandibular anterior crowding currently present
	2.8 mm mandibular arch crowding is anticipated following eruption of all permanent teeth (if proper space maintenance is employed)
	Bilateral posterior cross bite at the first permanent molars (Figure 2.61f)
	Unilateral left posterior cross bite of primary canines and primary second molars
	Thick periodontal biotype labial to maxillary and mandibular incisors (Figure 2.61f)
	Left lateral CR-CO shift 1–2 mm
Other	Poor hygiene
Diagnosis	Class I malocclusion with bilateral posterior cross bite, severe maxillary anterior crowding, moderate mandibular anterior crowding, and left lateral shift from CR–CO

Q: Do you wish to make any additional records?

A: No. We do not need to make additional records in order to decide whether to recall Lucas or begin early treatment.

Q: Provide a detailed space analysis for Lucas's maxillary and mandibular arches. In other words, how were the anticipated 7.0 mm of maxillary arch crowding and 2.8 mm of mandibular arch crowding calculated (following eruption of all permanent teeth if proper space maintenance is employed)?

A: Below are space estimates:

Average mesiodistal widths of permanent teeth (mm) [1]:

Maxillary Central Incisor	8.5	Mandibular Central Incisor	5.0
Maxillary Lateral Incisor	6.5	Mandibular Lateral Incisor	5.5
Maxillary Canine	7.5	Mandibular Canine	7.0
Maxillary First Premolar	7.0	Mandibular First Premolar	7.0
Maxillary Second Premolar	7.0	Mandibular Second Premolar	7.0
Maxillary First Molar	10.0	Mandibular First Molar	11.0
Maxillary Second Molar	9.0	Mandibular Second Molar	10.5

Average mesiodistal widths of *primary* teeth (mm) [1]:

Maxillary Central Incisor	6.5	Mandibular Central Incisor	4.2
Maxillary Lateral Incisor	5.1	Mandibular Lateral Incisor	4.1
Maxillary Canine	7.0	Mandibular Canine	5.0
Maxillary First Molar	7.3	Mandibular First Molar	7.7
Maxillary Second Molar	8.2	Mandibular Second Molar	9.9

MAXILLARY ARCH

+4.0 mm of anterior spacing is currently present (Figure 2.61h).

−6.5 mm of space needed for maxillary left permanent lateral incisor.

−6.5 mm of space needed for maxillary right permanent lateral incisor.

+2 mm of anticipated leeway space (1 mm/side).

Balance = +4.0 mm − 6.5 mm − 6.5 mm + 2 mm = −7.0 mm.

MANDIBULAR ARCH

−6.0 mm of anterior crowding is currently present (Figure 2.61i).

+3.2 mm of anticipated leeway space (1.6 mm/side).

Balance = −6.0 mm + 3.2 mm = −2.8 mm.

That is, *7.0 mm of maxillary arch crowding and 2.8 mm of mandibular arch crowding is anticipated following eruption of all permanent teeth (if proper space maintenance is employed).*

Q: What are Lucas's *primary* problems?

A:

Table 2.22   Primary problems list for Lucas.

AP	–
Vertical	Anterior open bite
Transverse	Bilateral posterior cross bite at first permanent molars
	Unilateral posterior cross bite of left primary canines and left primary second molars
Other	Severe (9.0 mm) maxillary anterior crowding
	Moderate (6.0 mm) mandibular anterior crowding
	Edge-to-edge relationship of left central incisors and developing lingual cross bite of right central incisors
	Poor hygiene
	Left lateral CR–CO shift 1–2 mm
	Potentially impacted maxillary lateral incisors

Q: Lucas exhibits a mildly long soft tissue LAFH and anterior open bite. Are you worried that Lucas could be growing into a skeletal open bite? Should you treat his open bite?

A: Lucas's soft tissue LAFH is slightly longer than ideal, but he exhibits lip competence – a key feature indicating he is vertically normal. His anterior open bite is due to stepped up maxillary permanent central incisors and stepped down mandibular permanent lateral incisors. These teeth are erupting normally consistent with his dental stage of development (maxillary permanent central incisors and mandibular permanent lateral incisors erupt between seven and eight years of age) [78]. For now, we recommend observation of his anterior open bite, not treatment.

Q: We noted that Lucas exhibits less than the ideal maxillary incisal display when smiling. What factors contribute to inadequate maxillary incisal display when smiling? Can you suggest the reason *why* he displays so little maxillary incisor when smiling?

A: Factors contributing to inadequate incisal display in a posed smile include:
- Inadequate vertical (downward) maxillary skeletal growth
- A long maxillary lip
- Stepped up maxillary incisors

(a)

(b)

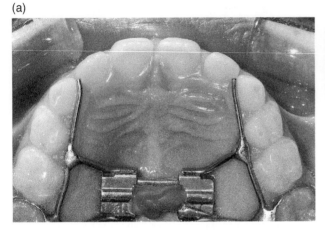 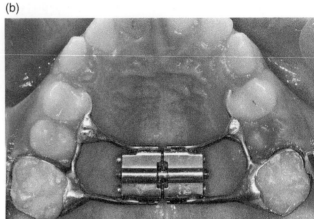

Figure 2.62 Modified RMEs to gain additional anchorage: (a) arms extending mesially to the maxillary primary canines and (b) arms extending mesially to, and bonded to, partially erupted maxillary first premolars.

- Maxillary incisal edge wear
- Excessive gingival overgrowth
- Hypoactivity of (smiling) facial muscles

Lucas demonstrates inadequate incisal display simply because his maxillary central incisors are not fully erupted.

Q: Lucas presents with a bilateral posterior cross bite at the permanent first molars and a left lateral CR-CO shift of 1–2 mm. His posterior cross bite is due to a constricted maxillary arch relative to the width of his mandibular arch. If we use orthopedics (maxillary expansion) to correct his posterior cross bite, *when* should we do this?

A: We should expand his maxilla *now*. Unlike Class II orthopedics, where the best evidence suggests waiting to treat until the late mixed dentition (or until we observe good statural growth velocity), expansion to correct a constricted maxilla can begin earlier. We recommend:
- Generally waiting until the *early* mixed dentition to begin RME so that the maxillary first permanent molars are available as RME appliance anchors and so you have better cooperation than from someone very young.
- Correcting Lucas's cross bite now so that you eliminate his shift and prevent development of a mandibular jaw asymmetry (as a result of the lateral shift).
- Correcting Lucas's cross bite now in order to maximize *skeletal* expansion (you will achieve less RME skeletal correction if you expand post-puberty).

Q: The typical RME appliance has bands fitted to the maxillary first molars and maxillary first premolars. But Lucas has only permanent first molars and primary molars in the maxillary posterior. How can you gain additional anchorage for his RME appliance if you decide to use one?

A: Ways to gain additional anchorage include:
- You can extend soldered heavy wire arms from the maxillary permanent first molars mesially (Figure 2.62a) to contact the lingual surfaces of all the primary teeth. These arms can be *bonded* to the lingual surfaces of the primary teeth.
- You can *band* the maxillary primary second molars (if immobile) in addition to the maxillary first permanent molars.
- Finally, in patients where the maxillary first premolars are partially erupted, you can bond the wire arms to their lingual surfaces (Figure 2.62b) instead of banding the first premolars.

Q: Discuss Lucas in the context of three principles applied to every early treatment patient.
- The goal of early treatment is to correct developing problems – get the patient *back to normal for their stage of development* (including preventing complications such as resorption of adjacent tooth roots, reducing later treatment complexity, or reducing/eliminating unknowns). Correcting his anterior open bite, lateral CR–CO shift, bilateral posterior cross bite, anterior cross bite, anterior crowding, potentially impacted maxillary lateral incisors, and permitting all his permanent teeth to erupt would get Lucas back on track for this stage of development.

- Early treatment should address *very specific problems with a clearly defined end point*, usually begun and ended within six to nine months (not protracted over many years, except for some orthopedic problems). Lucas's maxillary anterior crowding, potentially impacted maxillary lateral incisors, left lateral shift, and posterior cross bite are focused problems which could be readily corrected with RME.

  Limited fixed orthodontic appliances could correct his central incisor cross bite in a few months. Placement of an LLHA could reduce his 6.0 mm of mandibular anterior crowding to approximately 2.8 mm (depending upon the actual sizes of erupted mandibular permanent canines and premolars). However, this could take years since the permanent canines and premolars are not ready to erupt.

- Always ask: Is it necessary that I treat the patient now? *What harm will come if I chose to do nothing now?*

  If we choose to recall/monitor, then we run the risk of the:

  - Maxillary lateral incisors becoming impacted or erupting ectopically.
  - Maxillary permanent canines becoming impacted or resorbing the maxillary lateral incisor roots.
  - Maxillary central incisors becoming traumatized as they wear against the mandibular Incisors.
  - Mandibular molars drifting mesially as mandibular primary teeth exfoliate (long-term absence of LLHA), leaving less space for eliminating mandibular crowding.
  - Lucas developing a mandibular asymmetry due to the left lateral CR–CO shift.

Q: As a review, what guidelines do you recommend for early extraction of teeth?

A: We generally recommend early extraction of primary or permanent teeth in cases of permanent tooth ectopic eruption, dehiscence caused by crowding, eruption of permanent teeth into nonkeratinized gingiva, and severe crowding.

Q: Lucas currently exhibits severe (9.0 mm) maxillary anterior crowding and moderate (6.0 mm) mandibular anterior crowding. Do you consider Lucas to be a candidate for serial extraction?

A: No. The ideal serial extraction patient is in the early mixed dentition stage of development and is *normal in every way, except severe anterior crowding (≥9 mm per arch)*. Specifically, the patient should present with:

- *Class I first permanent molars.* Lucas does exhibit this feature.
- *Vertically normal to slightly long soft tissue and skeletal LAFH, with minimal OB or possibly a mild open bite, but not a deep bite.* Lucas exhibits this feature.
- *Normal incisor angulation or proclined incisors, but not upright incisors.* We do not have a cephalometric radiograph to quantify maxillary and mandibular incisor uprightness for Lucas. Clinically, Lucas's maxillary incisors appear upright. His mandibular incisor angulation is difficult to judge.
- *Normal posterior transverse relationship (normal inter-molar arch widths with good posterior interdigitation; absence of posterior cross bites; and absence of significant transverse compensations).* Lucas does not exhibit this feature. Furthermore, if his posterior cross bite is corrected with RME, then this expansion should reduce his maxillary crowding from severe to moderate.
- *Severe (≥9 mm) anterior crowding*: Lucas currently exhibits severe maxillary anterior crowding but only moderate mandibular anterior crowding. If we expand his maxilla with RME, then his maxillary arch crowding will reduce to moderate. Further, we anticipate only 2.8 mm of mandibular arch crowding following eruption of all permanent teeth if an LLHA is used.

Based upon the above features, Lucas is *not* an ideal candidate for serial extraction.

Q: Should you start early treatment or recall? If you begin treatment, what options would you consider?

A: Options include:

- *Recall* (no early treatment, monitor only) – we do not recommend this option. The risks of monitoring include: maxillary lateral incisors becoming impacted or erupting ectopically; maxillary permanent canines becoming impacted or resorbing the maxillary lateral incisor roots; maxillary central incisors becoming traumatized as they wear against the mandibular incisors; mandibular molars drifting mesially as mandibular primary teeth exfoliate leaving less space for eliminating mandibular arch crowding; and Lucas developing a mandibular asymmetry due to the left lateral CR–CO shift.

- *Space maintenance* – placement of an LLHA will be ideal at a future date. However, Lucas's mandibular permanent canine and premolar roots are immature, so there is no need to place an LLHA now. Future space maintenance in the maxillary arch may likewise be beneficial (1 mm maxillary leeway space per side) but would be inadequate to alleviate his severe maxillary arch crowding.

- *Mandibular space maintenance combined with extraction of mandibular primary canines* – would result in improved alignment of mandibular incisors while avoiding arch perimeter loss due to permanent first molar mesial drift. However, extraction of mandibular primary canines is an additional (unnecessary) surgical procedure with little long-term benefit.
- *RME (regaining space lost following exfoliation of the maxillary primary lateral incisors)* – is strongly recommended in order to correct the bilateral posterior cross bite, correct the left lateral CR–CO shift, and provide anterior space for eruption of the potentially impacted maxillary lateral incisors. However, depending upon the amount of expansion, RME may not provide enough space for eruption of the lateral incisors.
- *Extraction of maxillary primary canines* – would provide space for eruption of the maxillary permanent lateral incisors. However, long-term we will still face severe maxillary arch crowding.
- *Placement of fixed maxillary orthodontic appliances* – to advance maxillary incisors out from a developing cross bite. We would consider this option if RME and tongue pressure do not correct the developing cross bite spontaneously.
- *Serial extraction* – is not recommended. Although Lucas presents with severe maxillary anterior crowding, only moderate mandibular anterior crowding is present, and he is in bilateral posterior cross bite. Lucas is not an ideal serial extraction candidate.

Q: Of the above options, which do you recommend?
A: We spoke to Lucas's mother at the end of his consultation appointment and recommended:
- Extracting maxillary primary canines in order to permit eruption of maxillary permanent lateral incisors.
- RME to correct his bilateral posterior cross bite, correct his lateral shift, and create maxillary anterior space.
- Placement of limited fixed orthodontic appliances to correct his anterior cross bite – if the anterior cross bite is still present after RME.
- Later removal of the fixed appliances and RME appliance, placement of a Nance holding arch, placement of an LLHA, and monitoring of permanent teeth eruption. This would end early orthodontic treatment.

Q: Can you suggest "take-home pearls" for Lucas?
A: "Take-home pearls" include the following:
- Lucas's severe maxillary anterior crowding resulted from a constricted maxillary arch.
- Correcting his bilateral cross bite with RME will provide space for his permanent maxillary lateral incisors to erupt and will eliminate his left lateral shift.
- You must correct lateral shifts during growth to help prevent asymmetric mandibular growth.
- Should we request extracting his maxillary primary *first molars* in addition to his maxillary primary canines? We do not recommend this. Why? Looking at Figure 2.61h, we see that there will be adequate room for his maxillary permanent lateral incisors to erupt following extraction of his maxillary primary canines. Furthermore, the roots of his maxillary first premolars are underdeveloped (Figure 2.61d) – extracting the primary first molars this early could result in their delayed eruption.
- Based upon our space analysis, his moderate (6.0 mm) mandibular anterior crowding can be reduced to 2.8 mm with space maintenance. However, there is no urgent need to place an LLHA yet. Instead, we recommend placing an LLHA when the mandibular permanent canine and premolar roots are more developed and closer to erupting.
- However, *it is better to place an LLHA too early* (and deal with cement "washout" by periodically re-cementing the LLHA) *than to place one too late* (and deal with loss of arch perimeter through mandibular permanent molar mesial drift).
- You must address Lucas' poor hygiene! As is true of all orthodontic patients, you should consider poor oral hygiene to be a *primary* problem. You are a dentist first and an orthodontist second.

Case Jeff

Q: Jeff is nine years and six months old (Figure 2.63). He presents to you with his parents' chief complaint, "Jeff has crowded teeth." His PMH, PDH, and TMJ evaluation are WRN. He has mild gingivitis and CR = CO. *Compile your diagnostic findings and problem list*. Also, state your *diagnosis*.

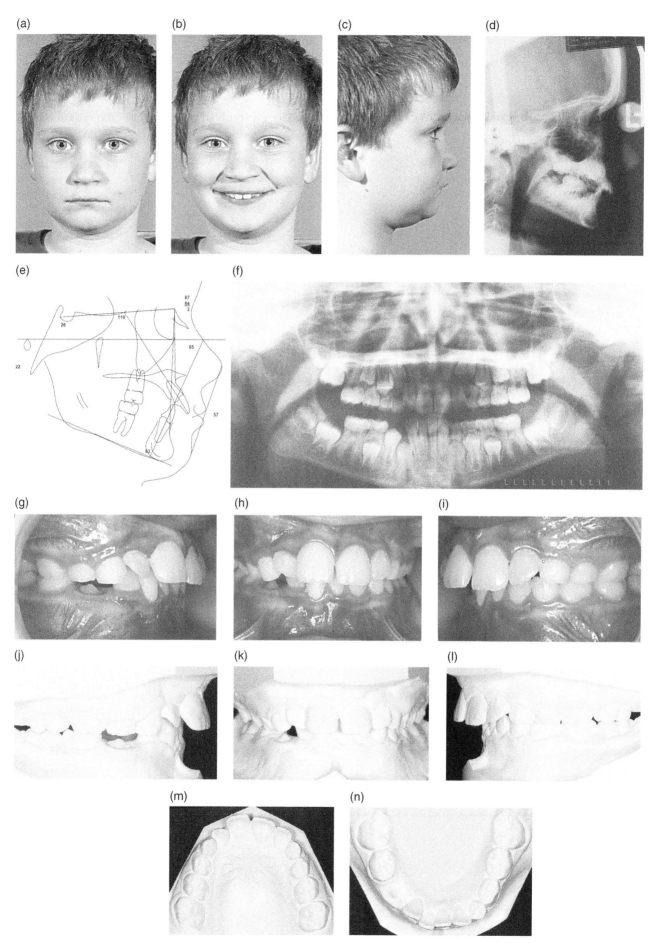

Figure 2.63   Initial records of Jeff: (a–c) facial photographs, (d, e) lateral cephalometric radiograph and tracing, (f) pantomograph, (g–i) intraoral photographs, and (j–n) models.

A:

Table 2.23 Diagnostic findings and problem list for Jeff.

Full face and profile	*Frontal view* Face is symmetric Short soft tissue LAFH (soft tissue Glabella – Subnasale < Subnasale – soft tissue Menton) Lip competence UDML WRN Inadequate gingival display in posed smile (central incisor gingival margins sit above the maxillary lip) *Profile view* Convex profile Retrusive chin Obtuse NLA Deep labiomental sulcus Obtuse lip-chin-throat angle
Ceph analysis	*Skeletal* Maxillary skeletal anteroposterior position WRN (A-Point lies on Nasion-perpendicular line) Mandibular skeletal anteroposterior WRN (ANB = 3° with maxilla WRN) Skeletal LAFH WRN (ANS-Menton/Nasion-Menton × 100% = 57%) Flat mandibular plane (FMA = 22°; SNMP = 26°) Effective bony Pogonion (Pogonion lies ahead of a line extended from Nasion to B-point) *Dental* Proclined maxillary incisors (U1 to SN = 119°) Mandibular incisors WRN (FMIA = 65°)
Radiographs	Late mixed dentition (premolars beginning to erupt) Loss of mandibular right primary canine and primary first molar Potentially impacted mandibular right permanent canine Maxillary permanent canine crowns overlap the roots of the lateral incisors
Intraoral photos and models	Angle Class II division 1 Iowa Classification: II (3–4 mm) II (3–4 mm) II (2–3 mm) II (2–3 mm) OJ 8 mm OB 100% (mandibular incisor palatal impingement, no pain or tissue damage) LDML deviation 1–2 mm to right of UDML secondary to loss of mandibular right primary canine and primary first molar (drifting of incisors to the right) 2 mm of maxillary anterior crowding is currently present 0 mm of maxillary arch crowding is anticipated following eruption of all permanent teeth (if appropriate space maintenance is employed) 5.5 mm of mandibular crowding is currently present (1.5 mm incisor crowding, 10 mm right space, 7 mm space needed for mandibular right canine, 7 mm needed for mandibular right first premolar) 1.0 mm of mandibular arch crowding is anticipated following eruption of all permanent teeth (if appropriate space maintenance is employed) Maxillary and mandibular dental arches symmetric in posterior
Other	Marginal gingivitis with plaque accumulation
Diagnosis	Class II division 1 malocclusion with 100% deep bite, maxillary dental protrusion, and moderate (5.5 mm) mandibular crowding

Q: Why is Jeff's anteroposterior relationship unusual?

A: Because he has a convex profile, is dentally Class II, but has a skeletally *normal* mandible and maxilla. We expected to find that his mandible was skeletally deficient, but it is normal.

Q: What impact will his Class II dental relationship, convex profile, but skeletally normal mandible have on your treatment goals?

A: In spite of his skeletally normal mandible, we will strive to correct his Class II dental relationship and improve his chin projection (profile) with Class II orthopedics. Cephalometric measurements are very important in diagnosing and treating patients. However, we are treating faces and occlusions, not cephalometric numbers.

Q: Do you require any additional records to decide whether to perform early treatment (or recall) Jeff?

A: No. An early treatment plan (or decision to recall) can be made using the above records.

Q: Provide a detailed space analysis for Jeff's maxillary and mandibular arches. In other words, how were the 0 mm of maxillary arch crowding and 1.0 mm of mandibular arch crowding calculated (if appropriate space maintenance is employed).

A: Below are space estimates:

Average mesiodistal widths of permanent teeth (mm) [1]:

Maxillary Central Incisor	8.5	Mandibular Central Incisor	5.0
Maxillary Lateral Incisor	6.5	Mandibular Lateral Incisor	5.5
Maxillary Canine	7.5	Mandibular Canine	7.0
Maxillary First Premolar	7.0	Mandibular First Premolar	7.0
Maxillary Second Premolar	7.0	Mandibular Second Premolar	7.0
Maxillary First Molar	10.0	Mandibular First Molar	11.0
Maxillary Second Molar	9.0	Mandibular Second Molar	10.5

Average mesiodistal widths of *primary* teeth (mm) [1]:

Maxillary Central Incisor	6.5	Mandibular Central Incisor	4.2
Maxillary Lateral Incisor	5.1	Mandibular Lateral Incisor	4.1
Maxillary Canine	7.0	Mandibular Canine	5.0
Maxillary First Molar	7.3	Mandibular First Molar	7.7
Maxillary Second Molar	8.2	Mandibular Second Molar	9.9

MAXILLARY ARCH

+1 mm of anterior space is present (Figure 2.63m).

−3 mm of incisor crowding.

+2 mm of anticipated leeway space (1 mm/side).

Balance = +1 mm − 3 mm + 2 mm = 0 mm.

MANDIBULAR ARCH (right leeway space cannot be used due to absence of right primary canine and primary first molar)

−1.5 mm of incisor crowding is currently present (Figure 2.63n).

+1.6 mm anticipated mandibular left leeway space.

+10 mm space between mandibular right primary second molar and right lateral incisor.

−7 mm space needed for the mandibular right permanent canine.

−7 mm space needed for the mandibular right first premolar.

+9.9 mm mesiodistal width of mandibular right primary second molar.

−7 mm space needed for mandibular right second premolar.

Balance = −1.5 mm + 1.6 mm + 10 mm − 7 mm − 7 mm + 9.9 mm − 7 mm = −1.0 mm.

That is, *0 mm of maxillary arch crowding and 1.0 mm of mandibular arch crowding is anticipated following eruption of all permanent teeth (if appropriate space maintenance is employed).*

Q: What are Jeff's primary problems in each dimension (plus other problems)?

A:

Table 2.24 Primary problems list for Jeff *(apical base/skeletal discrepancies italicized).*

AP	Angle Class II division 1
	Iowa Classification: II (3–4 mm) II (3–4 mm) II (2–3 mm) II (2–3 mm)
Vertical	100% OB (mandibular incisor palatal impingement)
Transverse	—
Other	Proclined maxillary incisors
	Potentially impacted mandibular right permanent canine
	Mild (2 mm) maxillary anterior crowding and moderate (5.5 mm) mandibular crowding is currently present

Q: What is a reliable indicator of *severe* mandibular anterior crowding? Does Jeff demonstrate this feature?

A: A reliable indicator of severe developing mandibular anterior crowding is *premature loss of primary canines – not* lack of interdental spacing. In crowded mandibular arches, the permanent lateral incisors often erupt and resorb the mesial portion of the primary canine root, causing their premature loss [2].

Jeff may have had premature loss of his mandibular right primary canine. Why? His mandibular incisors have drifted to the right (LDML to right) indicating that he lost the mandibular right primary canine some time ago. We asked Jeff's parents when he lost his mandibular right primary canine, but they could not remember when he did.

His current moderate (5.5 mm) mandibular crowding must be viewed together with the fact that he still has left mandibular leeway space and right mandibular "E space" – leaving him with an estimated 1.0 mm of mandibular arch crowding after all permanent teeth have erupted (if appropriate space maintenance is employed).

Q: Because Jeff demonstrates moderate (5.5 mm) mandibular crowding and maxillary incisor proclination, we should at least consider the possibility that he be treated with permanent teeth extractions. Can you describe the features of the *ideal* serial extraction patient? Does Jeff exhibit these features?

A: The ideal serial extraction patient is in the *early mixed dentition stage of development and is normal in every way, except severe anterior crowding (≥9 mm per arch)*. Specifically, the patient should present with:

- *Class I first molars:* Since Jeff is Class II by 2–4 mm, he does not exhibit this feature. We generally recommend that permanent tooth extraction decisions be deferred until the early treatment patient is first orthopedically corrected to Class I. Why? A final Class I relationship following extractions is easier to achieve if you begin with a Class I relationship. Extraction patterns to achieve Class I canines when beginning with Class II canines (e.g. extraction of maxillary first premolars only) should generally be considered as part of comprehensive, not early, orthodontic treatment.
- *Vertically normal to slightly long soft tissue and skeletal LAFH, with minimal OB or possibly a mild open bite, but not a deep bite.* Why? The patient's bite will deepen post-(premolar) extraction as incisors are retracted/uprighted around their apices during space closure. Unfortunately, Jeff does not exhibit this feature as he has palatal soft tissue lower incisor impingement – a 100% deep bite.
- *Normal incisor angulation or proclined incisors, but not upright incisors:* Why? Incisors tend to upright around their apices with retraction during extraction space closure. Jeff has proclined maxillary incisors and normally inclined mandibular incisors – so he does exhibit this feature.
- *Normal posterior transverse relationship* (normal inter-molar arch widths with good posterior interdigitation; absence of posterior cross bites; and absence of significant transverse compensations). If a cross bite is initially present, it should be corrected before serial extraction begins. Why? A final ideal transverse relationship will be much easier to achieve if you begin with an acceptable initial transverse relationship. Jeff has a normal transverse relationship.
- *Severe (≥9 mm)* anterior crowding. Jeff does not meet this criterion. We anticipate 0 mm of maxillary arch crowding and 1.0 mm of mandibular arch crowding after eruption of all Jeff's permanent teeth if appropriate space maintenance is employed.
- Lastly, Jeff is entering the late mixed dentition stage of development and is leaving the early mixed stage of development.

Based upon the above features, we conclude that Jeff is not an *ideal* candidate for serial extraction.

Q: If you are unsure whether anterior crowding warrants (permanent tooth) extractions, what should you do in the mixed dentition?

A: In the *early* mixed dentition, we generally recommend monitoring (recalling) the patient – assuming that the permanent canine and premolar roots are immature (less than ½ developed, eruption not imminent), and assuming that you judge the potential harm from monitoring to be minimal. Generally, avoid (serial) extractions in the early mixed dentition unless you are sure that anterior crowding is *severe*.

In the *late* mixed dentition, we generally recommend placement of space maintainers, deferring extraction decisions until permanent canines and premolars erupt, and deferring extraction decisions until anteroposterior growth is addressed (reducing unknowns). Once permanent canines and premolars erupt, make progress records to better ascertain the need for extractions.

Q: What is the biggest error orthodontists make with serial extraction patients?

A: *Poor patient selection*. Requesting serial extractions in a child with *mild* anterior crowding will result in large residual extraction spaces (once canines have been retracted and incisors aligned) – which must to be closed. Requesting serial extractions in a child with a Class II or Class III relationship can make correction to a Class I relationship very difficult. Requesting serial extractions in a deep bite patient with upright incisors can result in a worsening of the deep bite and further uprighting of the incisors during incisor retraction. The biggest error orthodontists make with serial extraction patients is *poor patient selection*.

Q: We noted that Jeff's maxillary permanent canine crowns overlap the roots of the lateral incisors (Figure 2.63f). Is this a concern?

A: Yes. As seen on a panoramic image, the more a maxillary permanent canine crown overlaps the lateral incisor root, the greater the chance that the canine will become impacted [79].

Q: Is *now* the appropriate time to address Jeff's Class II problem? Should we have addressed it earlier, or should we address it later?

A: Now is the appropriate time to address Jeff's Class II problem. Why? Jeff is entering the late mixed dentition stage of development. There is no advantage in treating Class II relationships in the *early* mixed dentition (except for a possible decrease in incisal trauma as a result of excess overjet) [27–33], and we subscribe to this guideline unless the patient shows good statural growth velocity (growing continuously or entering their adolescent growth spurt) in which case we will begin Class II treatment in the early mixed dentition. On the other hand, if we wait until all of Jeff's permanent teeth erupt to begin Class II treatment, then we may miss useful growth. Now is an ideal time to address Jeff's Class II problem.

Q: What are your options for treating Jeff's Class II relationship?

A: Even though Jeff is a *dental* Class II, we will treat him as a skeletal Class II because we are aiming for the same outcome – molar/canine correction to Class I plus improved chin projection. There are three general options for treating any anteroposterior, vertical, or transverse skeletal discrepancy: *orthopedics, masking, and surgery*. Class II masking (camouflage, achieving a functional and esthetic occlusion without addressing the underlying skeletal discrepancy) would include treatments such as Class II elastic wear or extraction of maxillary first premolars (in order to provide space to retract maxillary canines into a Class I relationship). Surgery would generally involve a mandibular advancement osteotomy. Usually, masking and surgery are reserved for comprehensive treatment in the adult dentition.

Orthopedics is a reasonable option and consists of either restricting Jeff's maxillary forward growth (while permitting the mandible to continue growing forward) and/or accelerating mandibular growth. Class II orthopedic options include headgear or functional appliance treatment.

- Headgears: high-pull headgears can correct Class II relationships in growing individuals by restricting maxillary forward growth, distalizing maxillary molars, and possibly reducing maxillary corpus descent and maxillary molar eruption. Cervical-pull headgears restrict maxillary forward growth, distalize maxillary first molars, create anterior palatal plane downward rotation, and erupt maxillary first molars by less than 1 mm [40–43].

- Functional appliances: Class II functional appliances can correct Class II relationships in growing individuals by restricting maxillary forward growth, retracting maxillary posterior teeth, advancing mandibular posterior teeth, accelerating condylar growth, and displacing the glenoid fossae anteriorly. Functional appliances do *not* enhance mandibular horizontal growth beyond that found in control subjects, and the *direction* of condylar growth with functional appliance wear may not correct the mandibular skeletal anteroposterior deficiency or improve chin projection [44–49, 80].

Q: When do you recommend early correction of deep bites? Do you recommend early correction of Jeff's deep bite?

A: We recommend early correction of deep bites when there is mandibular incisor palatal impingement with pain and/or tissue damage. Since Jeff exhibits neither, we do not feel that early correction of his deep bite is urgent. His deep bite can be corrected later, during comprehensive treatment in the adult dentition.

Q: Discuss Jeff in the context of three principles applied to every early treatment patient.

A:

1) The goal of early treatment is to correct developing problems – get the patient *back to normal for their stage of development* (including preventing complications such as resorption of adjacent tooth roots, reducing later treatment complexity, or reducing/eliminating unknowns). Jeff"s 2–4 mm Class II molar relationship, 100% OB with palatal impingement, potentially impacted mandibular right permanent canine, anterior crowding, mandibular midline deviation, and maxillary incisor protrusion need to be corrected to get him back on track.

2) Early treatment should address very specific problems with a clearly defined end point, usually within six to nine months and not protracted over many years (exceptions include some orthopedic treatments).

- Class II treatment would normally be addressed (orthopedically) in the late mixed dentition unless the patient exhibits good statural growth velocity in the early mixed. Since Jeff is entering his late mixed dentition stage of development, now is a good time to begin Class II orthopedics – which could take longer than six to nine months.

- Jeff's deep bite is a *dental* deep bite due to overeruption of his mandibular incisors (Figures 2.63d and 2.63j) and is not a skeletal deep bite (skeletal LAFH WRN). His deep bite can be corrected in six to nine months by intruding incisors/extruding posterior teeth with limited orthodontic appliances.
- Jeff's mild (2 mm) maxillary anterior crowding and moderate (5.5 mm) mandibular anterior crowding would improve in 9–12 months with permanent tooth eruption if a Nance holding arch and LLHA were placed now. Further, his potentially impacted mandibular right permanent canine could erupt spontaneously if an LLHA was placed.
- The mandibular midline deviation could be readily corrected via space regaining (mandibular incisors have drifted to the right following loss of the mandibular right primary canine and primary first molar). Using fixed orthodontic appliances, a compressed open coil spring could be inserted between the mandibular right primary second molar and mandibular right lateral incisor to do this.
- Early treatment to upright the proclined maxillary incisors will take longer than six to nine months and could involve retraction of maxillary teeth with a headgear or Herbst appliance.

3) Always ask: Is it necessary that I treat the patient now? What harm will come if I do nothing now?

- If you do not address Jeff's Class II relationship now, then you may miss out on significant mandibular growth, and the amount of Class II correction may be reduced.
- Since Jeff exhibits neither pain nor tissue damage as a result of his deep bite, we do not feel that *early* correction of his deep bite is necessary.
- If you do not place a Nance holding arch and LLHA now, then Jeff's permanent molars will drift mesially as he exfoliates his remaining primary teeth. This will reduce the amount of leeway space/"E space" available for crowding reduction.
- Since the mandibular posterior quadrant appears symmetric (Figure 2.63n), the anterior asymmetry (mandibular midline deviation) could be dealt with after the permanent second premolars erupt. Early treatment of the midline deviation is unnecessary.
- It is not necessary to deal with the maxillary incisor protrusion now. The protrusion could be dealt with during comprehensive treatment.

Q: What unknowns do you face with Jeff?
A: Unknowns include: future maxillary/mandibular growth magnitude and direction, an undetected CR–CO shift, and treatment compliance.

Q: What early treatment options would you consider?
A: Options include:
- *Recall* (monitor only) – get Jeff back in one year to evaluate permanent tooth eruption. We do not recommend this option. If Jeff exfoliates his remaining primary canines and primary molars, then his permanent molars will drift mesially – reducing leeway space/"E space" available for incisor alignment and eruption of his mandibular right canine. Also, depending upon how much jaw growth he has during the year, significant Class II orthopedic correction could be missed.
- *Space maintenance* – placing an LLHA (and possibly a Nance holding arch) before exfoliation of the remaining primary canines and primary molars. We consider this a viable option. Since 0 mm of maxillary arch crowding and 1.0 mm of mandibular arch crowding is anticipated following eruption of all permanent teeth (if space maintenance is employed), Jeff could possibly be treated non-extraction with space maintenance. Note: if Jeff wears a headgear or Herbst appliance to correct his Class II by distalizing his maxillary molars, then a Nance holding arch is unnecessary.
- *Space regaining* – placing fixed orthodontic appliances and regaining/opening space for the potentially impacted mandibular right permanent canine (space loss due to drift of mandibular incisors to the right after exfoliation of the mandibular right primary canine and primary first molar). We are not enthusiastic about space regaining as it will procline Jeff's mandibular incisors.
- *Extraction of mandibular left primary canine* – would improve alignment of the mandibular incisors and tend to shift the mandibular midline to the left as a result of transseptal fiber pull. However, extraction of the left primary canine may result in arch perimeter loss as the left molars drift forward. To prevent/reduce arch perimeter loss, place an LLHA if you extract the mandibular left primary canine.
- *Extraction of both maxillary primary canines and both maxillary primary first molars* – would be reasonable. First, as seen on Jeff's panoramic image, his maxillary permanent canine crowns overlap the roots of his maxillary permanent lateral incisors which increases the likelihood that the maxillary permanent canines may become impacted. Second, extracting the maxillary primary canines should increase the chances that the permanent canines will erupt normally (assuming there is adequate space for them). Third, extracting the maxillary primary first molars will accelerate eruption of the maxillary first

premolars since the roots of the maxillary first premolars are > ½ developed. The maxillary first premolar apices should then erupt away from the maxillary permanent canine crowns, leaving space and further encouraging the maxillary canines to erupt. If both maxillary primary canines and maxillary primary first molars are extracted, then a Nance holding arch should be placed to reduce the possibility that the maxillary first molars will drift mesially. However, if the patient is wearing a headgear or Herbst appliance, then a Nance holding arch would be unnecessary.

- *Serial extraction* – is not recommended. Why? Jeff has mild (not severe) maxillary crowding and moderate mandibular crowding, he is Class II (not Class I), and he has a 100% deep bite. It would be wiser to employ space maintenance and Class II orthopedics now – then, re-evaluate for permanent teeth extractions after all Jeff's permanent teeth erupt.
- *Class II orthopedics* – is recommended. We would typically use either a headgear (if the child will wear it) or a Herbst appliance.
- *Fixed orthodontic appliances to level arches, reduce the OB, and eliminate mandibular incisor palatal impingement* – would be recommended if mandibular incisor palatal impingement was causing pain or tissue damage, but it is not.

Q: Based upon the above options, would you provide early treatment or recall Jeff? If you treat, what treatment would you recommend?

A: Jeff was placed on a HPHG 12–14 hours per night, and an LLHA was delivered. Once first permanent molar overcorrection was achieved (molars corrected to Class III by ~1 mm), headgear wear was slowly tapered off and the molar correction monitored to ensure stability.

When all permanent canines and premolars erupted, early treatment ended. Discussions were held with Jeff and his parents regarding (premolar) extraction and non-extraction options. His parents asked if we could attempt non-extraction treatment and then re-evaluate after Jeff's arches were leveled and aligned.

Fixed orthodontic appliances were placed, and arches were leveled and aligned. At that time, Jeff and his parents stated emphatically that they did not want permanent teeth extracted. A connective tissue graft was required and placed over the root of the mandibular right permanent canine. All spaces were closed and treatment was finished.

Q: I am confused. If Jeff was Class II, then do not we *want* his mandibular molars to drift mesially? In other words, why would you place an LLHA in a Class II patient?

A: This is an excellent question. Yes, we would like Jeff's mandibular molars to drift mesially to aid in correcting his Class II molar relationship. However, if we allow mandibular molar mesial drift during the transition from mixed to permanent dentition, then we cannot use the leeway space/"E space" to help align anterior teeth. So, we placed an LLHA to help align mandibular anterior teeth, and we corrected Jeff's Class II relationship using a headgear (distalizing maxillary molars, restricting maxillary forward growth, allowing continued mandibular forward growth).

Q: Deband records are shown in Figure 2.64. What changes do you note?

A: Changes include:
- Inadequate incisal display during posed smile is still present (Figure 2.64b).
- Significant mandibular growth (Figure 2.64f), which contributed to Jeff''s improvement in profile/chin projection (compare Figures 2.63c and 2.64c).
- Mandibular incisors proclined (FMIA increasing from 65° to 57°), and maxillary incisors uprighted slightly (U1 to SN decreasing from 119° to 117°), leaving Jeff in bimaxillary protrusion.
- Class I molar and canine relationships achieved (Figures 2.64h and 2.64j) by restricting maxillary forward growth relative to mandibular forward growth (Figure 2.64f, A-Point grew forward less than B-Point).
- Coincidence of midlines achieved.
- 100% OB reduced to 10%.
- Blunting of premolar root tips (mild root resorption, Figure 2.64g).

Q: As seen in the initial to final lateral cephalometric superimposition (Figure 2.64f), the mandibular first molars erupted, and the maxillary corpus descended, significantly. How does molar eruption and maxillary corpus descent affect vertical and anteroposterior facial growth?

A: With *increased* molar eruption and increased maxillary descent (relative to mandibular growth), the mandible rotates down and back, increasing LAFH, decreasing B-point advancement, decreasing chin projection, and worsening a Class II relationship. Conversely, with *decreased* molar eruption and decreased maxillary descent (relative to mandibular growth), the mandible rotates up and forward, LAFH decreases, B-point advancement increases, chin projection increases, and a Class II relationship improves.

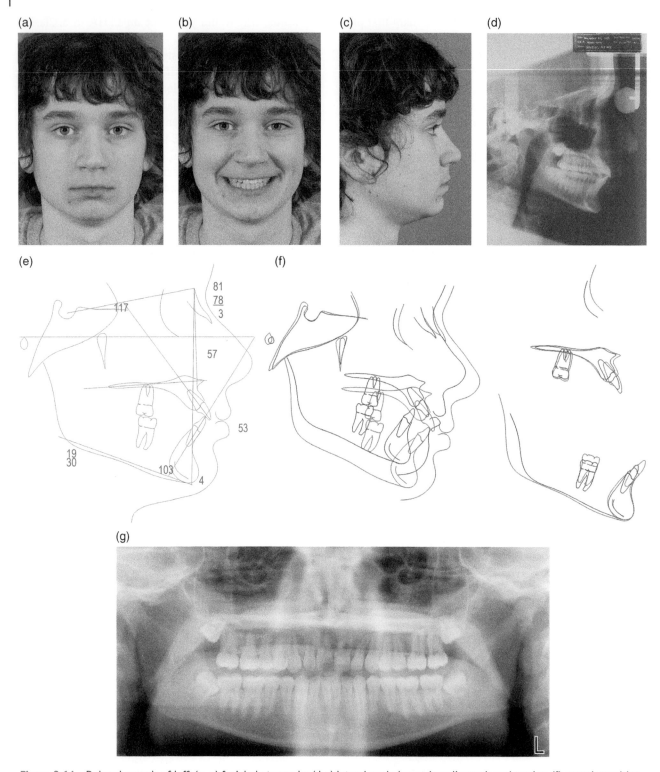

Figure 2.64 Deband records of Jeff: (a–c) facial photographs, (d, e) lateral cephalometric radiograph and tracing, (f) superimposition of initial to final cephalometric tracings, (g) pantomograph, and (h–l) intraoral photographs.

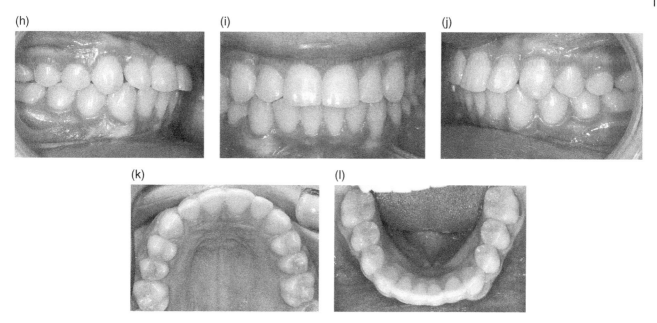

(h)　　　(i)　　　(j)

(k)　　　(l)

Figure 2.64　(Continued)

Q: Maxillary first molar eruption can be reduced with high-pull headgear wear, vertical-pull headgear wear, posterior biteplate wear (stretching the masseter/medial pterygoid muscles), or with TAD intrusion. Can you think of at least two ways to reduce *mandibular* molar eruption during growth?

A: Placement of an LLHA has been demonstrated to reduce mandibular molar eruption by 1–2 mm over a two-year period during adolescence [11]. Vertical-pull headgear or posterior biteplate wear can reduce mandibular molar eruption. TADs can be used to intrude mandibular molars.

Q: Jeff's maxillary permanent canine crowns initially overlapped his maxillary permanent lateral incisor roots on the panoramic image (Figure 2.63f), increasing the likelihood that the maxillary permanent canines would become impacted. And yet, the maxillary permanent canines erupted uneventfully. Why?

A: It is a matter of probabilities. Studies report that the more mesially positioned a maxillary canine crown is over the root of a lateral incisor (as viewed on a panoramic image), the more likely the canine will become impacted [70, 81]. Jeff's maxillary permanent canine crowns overlapped his lateral incisor roots by <½ their root thickness. Therefore, a greater chance existed for his maxillary permanent canines to erupt spontaneously than if the canine crowns had overlapped his lateral roots by >½ their root thickness. Of course, this is assuming that there was enough space for the permanent canines to erupt.

Q: Jeff's mandibular incisors *proclined* during treatment (Figure 2.64f). Can you suggest possible reasons why?

A: Possible reasons include the following:
- *Leveling the curve of Spee to open his deep bite* – As a curved line of fixed length is straightened, the ends of the line move outward. Similarly, as the curve of Spee is flattened/straightened, the mandibular incisors move forward (procline).
- *Effect of an LLHA* – Although placement of an LLHA in the mixed dentition greatly reduces permanent molar mesial drift as primary teeth exfoliate, mandibular first permanent molars still drift forward *slightly* – pushing the incisors forward (proclining them) through the LLHA wire [5, 7]. However, Jeff's mandibular molars did not move mesially (Figure 2.64f, bottom right).
- *Alignment of crowded anterior teeth* – Some mandibular anterior crowding was still anticipated even though an LLHA was employed. As crowded mandibular anterior teeth are aligned with an archwire, they procline.

Q: Jeff was treated non-extraction, but he finished with bimaxillary protrusion (proclination of both maxillary and mandibular incisors, Figure 2.64e). Should Jeff have been treated with extraction of four first premolars?

A: The answer to this question can be argued either way:
　Yes, a decision to extract four first premolars (following early Class II correction with headgear) would have provided space to retract/upright his proclined incisors

to more ideal inclinations, reduce mandibular lip protrusion (Figures 2.64a and 2.64c), and reduce labiomental sulcus depth.

No, non-extraction was the correct treatment. Why? The orthodontist must seriously weigh the patient's desires when considering treatment options. Jeff and his parents did not want permanent teeth extracted, and they were delighted with his facial esthetics. Further, non-extraction treatment provided a healthy and functional occlusion. Finally, Jeff had root resorption (root blunting) during treatment. We will never know the extent of root resorption Jeff would have had if he had been in treatment longer with premolar space closure.

Q: Can you suggest "take-home pearls" regarding Jeff's treatment?

A: "Take-home pearls" include the following:
- Jeff was nine years and six months old when he presented with a Class II relationship of 2–4 mm, a 100% deep bite (mandibular incisor palatal impingement), mild-to-moderate crowding, a potentially impacted mandibular canine, and maxillary incisor proclination. He was entering the late mixed dentition stage of development and underwent high-pull headgear and LLHA early treatment. Non-extraction comprehensive treatment resulted in a healthy, functional, and esthetic outcome. However, he ended with bimaxillary protrusion.
- All four treatment options for dealing with his early crowding were considered (monitoring, space maintenance, space regaining, and tooth extractions/serial extraction). Anterior crowding is like any other problem you face in practice or in life – exhaustively consider all options to solve it.
- Mandibular space maintenance was the early treatment option selected because calculations predicted

1.0 mm of mandibular arch crowding following eruption of all permanent teeth (if an LLHA was employed) and because his mandibular incisors had an ideal inclination (FMIA = 65°).
- After his arches were leveled and aligned in the adult dentition, Jeff and his parents insisted upon non-extraction treatment. His mandibular incisors proclined, probably as a result of curve of Spee leveling to open the deep bite and alignment of residual mandibular arch crowding. Space maintenance (leeway space/"E space") provided only enough room to alleviate most of his mandibular arch crowding and not enough room to permit uprighting of proclined incisors.
- In children presenting with maxillary permanent canine crowns overlapping maxillary lateral incisor roots (as seen on a panoramic image), you need to be concerned with possible future canine impaction. You can decrease the probability of maxillary permanent canine ectopic eruption/impaction by *creating space* for the canine and *creating a pathway* for it to erupt (e.g. extracting maxillary primary canines and maxillary primary first molars, RME, headgear wear, Herbst appliance wear, etc.). Surgical exposure may be required.

Case Kasandra

Q: Kasandra is 10 years old (Figure 2.65). She and her parents present to you with the chief complaint, "Missing bottom teeth." Her PMH, PDH, periodontal evaluation, and TMJ evaluation are WRN. CR = CO. Compile your diagnostic findings and problem list for Kasandra. Also, state your diagnosis.

(a)   (b)   (c)

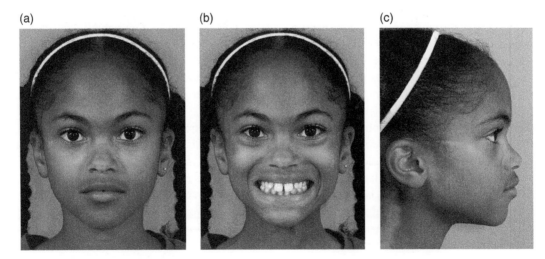

Figure 2.65 Initial records of Kasandra: (a–c) facial photographs, (d, e) lateral cephalometric radiograph and tracing, (f) pantomograph, and (g–k) intraoral photographs.

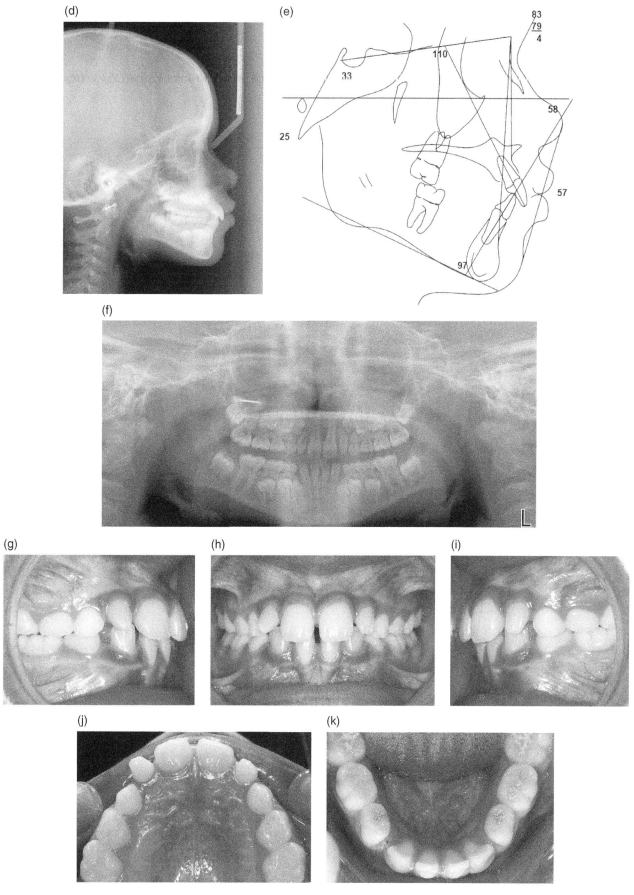

Figure 2.65 (Continued)

A:

Table 2.25 Diagnostic findings and problems list for Kasandra.

Full face and profile	*Frontal view* Face is symmetric Soft tissue LAFH WRN (soft tissue Glabella – Subnasale approximately equal to Subnasale – soft tissue Menton) Lip competence UDML WRN Gingival display in posed smile is less than average (maxillary central incisor gingival margins 2–3 mm above the maxillary lip) *Profile view* Mildly convex profile Acute NLA Protrusive lips relative to the E-plane Chin projection WRN Lip-chin-throat angle WRN
Ceph analysis	*Skeletal* Maxillary anteroposterior position WRN (A-Point lies on Nasion-perpendicular line) Mandibular anteroposterior position WRN (ANB angle = 4° with normal maxilla) Skeletal LAFH WRN (ANS-Menton/Nasion-Menton × 100% = 57%) Mandibular plane WRN (FMA = 25°; SN-MP = 33°) Effective bony Pogonion *Dental* Proclined maxillary incisors (U1 to SN = 110°) Proclined mandibular incisors (FMIA = 58°)
Radiographs	Early mixed dentition mandibular permanent canines are close to erupting) Maxillary permanent canines are pushing roots of maxillary lateral incisors to the mesial Mandibular permanent canines are potentially impacted Roots of first premolars and permanent canines are >½ developed
Intraoral photos and models	Angle Class III Iowa Classification: III (2 mm) X X III (2 mm) OJ ~ 3 mm OB 30–40% 6 mm of maxillary anterior space is currently present 8 mm of maxillary arch spacing is anticipated (if appropriate space maintenance is employed) 9 mm of mandibular anterior crowding is currently present (5 mm of spacing with two potentially impacted mandibular permanent canines requiring 14 mm) 1.8 mm of mandibular arch crowding is anticipated (if appropriate space maintenance is employed) Loss of mandibular primary canines with distal drift of mandibular permanent incisors Arches are symmetric Maxillary central incisors are stepped down relative to maxillary posterior teeth Maxillary and mandibular dental midlines are coincident Maxillary diastema Small permanent maxillary lateral incisors Good hygiene
Other	None
Diagnosis	Class III malocclusion with mandibular anterior crowding (potentially impacted/blocked out mandibular permanent canines)

Q: Is Kasandra a skeletal, or dental, Class III?

A: Kasandra is a *dental* Class III. Her profile is mildly convex (not concave as is typical of skeletal Class IIIs). Furthermore, when we look at her cephalometric tracing (Figure 2.65e), we see that her mandible is WRN (ANB angle = 4° with a normal maxilla).

Q: Why is this important?

A: Because as a dental Class III, Kasandra has normal jaw growth and should be easier to treat than if she was skeletally Class III.

Q: Can you speculate as to how Kasandra developed a dental Class III relationship?

A: Note the mandibular incisor distal drift that probably occurred as a result of premature primary canine loss (Figure 2.65k). We suspect that the transeptal fiber pull that caused this incisor distal drift also caused the molar mesial drift to Class III.

Q: How could this mandibular molar mesial drift have been prevented?

A: Placement of an LLHA at the time of mandibular primary canine loss prevents/reduces mesial molar drift. If an LLHA is placed, then soldered spurs should be wrapped around the distal of the lateral incisors to prevent their distal drift.

Q: Provide a detailed space analysis for Kasandra's maxillary and mandibular arches. In other words, how were the 8 mm of maxillary arch spacing and 1.8 mm of mandibular arch crowding calculated (if proper space maintenance is employed)?

A: Below are space estimates:

Average mesiodistal widths of permanent teeth (mm) [1]:

Maxillary Central Incisor	8.5	Mandibular Central Incisor	5.0
Maxillary Lateral Incisor	6.5	Mandibular Lateral Incisor	5.5
Maxillary Canine	7.5	Mandibular Canine	7.0
Maxillary First Premolar	7.0	Mandibular First Premolar	7.0
Maxillary Second Premolar	7.0	Mandibular Second Premolar	7.0
Maxillary First Molar	10.0	Mandibular First Molar	11.0
Maxillary Second Molar	9.0	Mandibular Second Molar	10.5

Average mesiodistal widths of *primary* teeth (mm) [1]:

Maxillary Central Incisor	6.5	Mandibular Central Incisor	4.2
Maxillary Lateral Incisor	5.1	Mandibular Lateral Incisor	4.1
Maxillary Canine	7.0	Mandibular Canine	5.0
Maxillary First Molar	7.3	Mandibular First Molar	7.7
Maxillary Second Molar	8.2	Mandibular Second Molar	9.9

MAXILLARY ARCH

+6.0 mm of anterior space is present (Figure 2.65j).
+2.0 mm of anticipated leeway space (1 mm/side).
Balance = +6.0 mm + 2.0 mm = +8.0 mm spacing.

MANDIBULAR ARCH (leeway space cannot be used because mandibular primary canines are missing)
+5.0 mm of anterior space is present (Figure 2.65k).
+9.9 mm width of mandibular left primary second molar.
−7.0 mm anticipated width of mandibular left second premolar.
+7.7 mm width of mandibular left primary first molar.
−7.0 mm anticipated width of mandibular left first premolar.
−7.0 mm space needed for mandibular left permanent canine.
−7.0 mm space needed for mandibular right permanent canine.
+7.7 mm width of mandibular right primary first molar.
−7.0 mm anticipated width of mandibular right first premolar.
+9.9 mm width of mandibular right primary second molar.
−7.0 mm anticipated width of mandibular right second premolar.
Balance = +5.0 mm + 9.9 mm − 7.0 mm + 7.7 mm − 7.0 mm − 7.0 mm − 7.0 mm + 7.7 mm − 7.0 mm + 9.9 mm − 7.0 mm = −1.8 mm crowding.

That is, *8 mm of maxillary arch spacing and 1.8 mm of mandibular arch crowding is anticipated following eruption of all permanent teeth (if appropriate space maintenance is employed).*

Q: Kasandra exemplifies the importance of estimating space. With 9 mm (severe) mandibular anterior crowding currently present (5 mm of space plus two potentially impacted mandibular permanent canines requiring 14 mm of space), how can space maintenance alone reduce that crowding to 1.8 mm? In other words, you only get 1.6 mm of leeway space per side, correct?

A: Since the mandibular primary canines are absent, we cannot use leeway space. Instead, we need to consider "E space" (and "D space"). If an LLHA is placed, the "E space" (mesiodistal widths of the mandibular primary second molars minus the widths of the second premolars) provides 9.9 mm minus 7 mm or nearly 3 mm of space per side. Add to that the additional millimeter of "D space" and future anticipated crowding is reduced from 9 to 1.8 mm. This is the beauty of space maintenance.

Q: What are Kasandra's *primary* problems in each dimension, plus other problems?

A:

Table 2.26 Primary problems list for Kasandra.

AP	Class III (2 mm)
Vertical	OB 30–40%
Transverse	—
Other	9 mm mandibular anterior crowding (potentially impacted mandibular permanent canines).

Q: Discuss Kasandra in the context of three principles applied to every early treatment patient.

  1) The goal of early treatment is to correct developing problems – get the patient *back to normal for their stage of development* (including preventing complications such as resorption of adjacent tooth roots, reducing later treatment complexity, or reducing/ eliminating unknowns). Correcting her Class III molar relationship, reducing her deep overbite, and correcting her anterior crowding (creating space for her potentially impacted mandibular permanent canines) would bring Kasandra back to normal for her stage of development.

  2) Early treatment should address *very specific problems with a clearly defined end point*, usually within six to nine months (not extended over many months, except for some orthopedic problems):
  • Her Class III (2 mm) dental relationship could be corrected in six to nine months using fixed appliances with Class III elastic wear. However, we would recommend waiting until comprehensive treatment in the permanent dentition to do this.
  • Her 30–40% OB could be corrected by leveling her curve of Spee (Figure 2.65d) with fixed appliances and archwires.

  • 4.5 mm per side of additional mandibular space could be regained by placing fixed appliances and trapping compressed open coil springs between her mandibular primary first molars and mandibular permanent lateral incisors. This space regaining, together with the 5 mm of space currently present (Figure 2.65k) provides the 14 mm of space required for the two potentially impacted canines to erupt. This could be completed in six to nine months.

  3) Always ask: Is it necessary that I treat the patient now? *What harm will come if I choose to do nothing now?* We feel that *it is necessary* to treat Kasandra now. If we do not, then her mandibular permanent first molars will drift further to the mesial when the primary molars exfoliate and her mandibular permanent canines may impact, erupt ectopically, or possibly resorb her mandibular lateral incisor roots. No harm will come from not treating her deep bite now as she exhibits neither pain nor tissue damage.

Q: Would you recall Kasandra or begin early treatment? If you start treatment, what treatment options would you consider?

A: Options include the following:
  • *Recall* (no treatment, monitor only) – re-evaluate in one year. We do *not* recommend this option. Kasandra's permanent canines and premolars are erupting. If an LLHA is not placed, then Kasandra's mandibular permanent first molars will drift to the mesial when her primary molars exfoliate – *worsening her Class III* relationship and reducing arch perimeter. Further, her potentially impacted mandibular permanent canines will remain unerupted, erupt ectopically, or possibly resorb the lateral incisor roots.
  • *Space maintenance* – placement of an LLHA would prevent worsening of Kasandra's Class III molar relationship as mandibular primary molars exfoliate. Further, space maintenance would provide us approximately 7.2 mm of mandibular "E space" and "D space." We do not recommend placement of a Nance holding arch since 6 mm of space is already present.
  • *Space regaining* – opening 4.5 mm of space bilaterally would provide the 14 mm total space needed for eruption of the mandibular permanent canines. OJ may first need to be created before these spaces are opened, and this OJ could be created by placing fixed appliances, leveling the maxillary arch (intruding stepped down maxillary incisors), and reducing Kasandra's deep bite.
    Compressed open coil springs could then be placed between Kasandra's mandibular primary first molars

(a) (b) (c)

(d) (e)

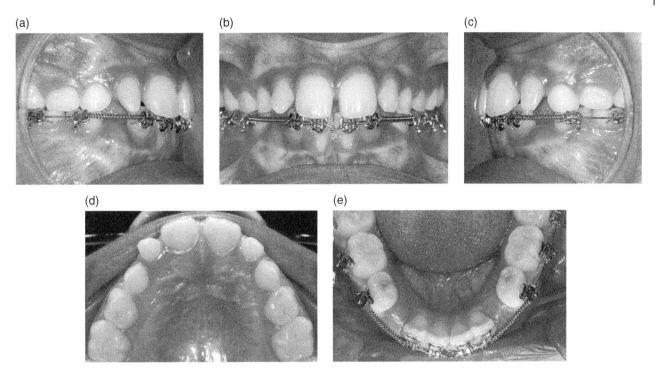

Figure 2.66 Progress records of Kasandra (a–e). Fixed orthodontic appliances were placed on the mandibular teeth and compressed open coil springs inserted to regain space needed for mandibular permanent canine eruption.

and her mandibular permanent lateral incisors. After space is created, the fixed appliances would be removed and an LLHA placed (with soldered spurs to prevent distal drifting of the lateral incisors). The LLHA would also prevent/reduce mandibular permanent first molar mesial drift and worsening of her Class III relationship.

- *Extraction of mandibular primary first molars* – would accelerate mandibular first premolar eruption since the roots of the first premolars are >½ developed. However, we see no advantage in this extraction pattern which could result in mesial molar drift and worsening of the Class III molar relationship – unless an LLHA is placed.

- *Extraction of maxillary primary canines and/or primary first molars* – is not necessary because the maxillary permanent canines appear to erupting normally (Figure 2.65d) and there appears to be adequate space for them (Figure 2.65j).

- *Serial extraction* – is *not* recommended. As was calculated above, Kasandra will eventually have excess maxillary space, and only mild (1.8 mm) mandibular crowding – if space maintenance is employed.

Q: Considering the above options, how would you proceed?

A: A decision was made to *regain* Kasandra's mandibular anterior space lost by exfoliation of primary canines (distal drift of incisors and probable mesial drift of molars). This was done using fixed appliances in the mandibular arch only (Figure 2.66).

Q: Now that you have regained the space needed for Kasandra's mandibular canines to erupt (Figure 2.66e), how would you proceed?

A: An LLHA with spurs soldered distal to her permanent mandibular lateral incisors was fabricated and delivered.

Q: Unfortunately, by the time the LLHA was delivered, some of the regained space was lost (Figure 2.67). How could this have been prevented? Is there enough space for the permanent canines to erupt?

A: Kasandra could have worn a clear (vacuum-formed) retainer to maintain the space until the LLHA was delivered. Or, the LLHA could have been made, and delivered, on the same day that the braces were removed.

There appears to be 8 mm of mandibular anterior space currently available. This is inadequate space for eruption of both canines. However, we will soon have an additional 3.6 mm of "E space" and "D space"

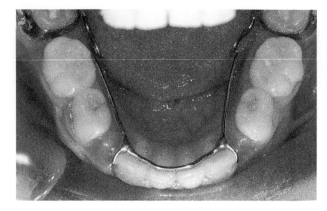

Figure 2.67 LLHA with spurs soldered to prevent distal incisor drift.

available on both sides of the arch after the primary molars exfoliate. This is more than enough room for both canines.

Q: Orthodontic crowding takes two forms. The first is the difference between arch perimeter and the sum of mesiodistal widths of the teeth (tooth size – arch length deficiency). The second is excessive proclination of teeth. In both forms, permanent teeth can be extracted in order to create space to align incisors and upright incisors.

Kasandra presented with incisor protrusion in both arches (bimaxillary protrusion). In addition, we regained lost space to make room for canines which increased mandibular incisor proclination even more. Should we have performed serial extraction in order to create space to upright incisors?

A: No, we should not have performed serial extraction in order to upright incisors. Why?

- Kasandra was not an ideal serial extraction patient. As calculated, Kasandra will eventually have excess maxillary space, and only mild (1.8 mm) mandibular crowding since an LLHA was placed and since significant "E space" and "D space" remains in the mandibular arch.
- Ethnicity plays a role in permanent teeth extraction decisions. Maxillary and mandibular incisors are naturally more protruded and proclined in black patients [82].
- She is a beautiful young lady with a very nice profile.

Instead of serial extraction, we recommend waiting until all permanent teeth erupt, evaluating the size of permanent canines and premolars, and discussing continued non-extraction or premolar extraction options with Kasandra and her parents.

Q: Can you suggest "take-home pearls" for Kasandra's early treatment?

A: "Take-home pearls" include the following:

- Kasandra was 10 years old when she presented with the chief complaint, "Missing bottom teeth." She was dentally Class III (2 mm) probably as a result of mandibular molar mesial drift following primary canine loss. Her mandibular permanent canines were potentially impacted.
- An LLHA should have been provided to Kasandra as soon as her mandibular primary canines were lost. This would have prevented/reduced drift and possibly left Kasandra in a Class I relationship.
- *LLHAs can be invaluable in skeletal Class III mixed dentition patients* – to prevent mesial molar drift and a worsening of the Class III molar relationship.
- Maintenance of Kasandra's LLHA is now critical. Why? The LLHA will prevent/diminish mesial drift of her mandibular permanent first molars, and worsening of her Class III relationship, following eventual loss of her primary molars. Furthermore, the LLHA will provide "D space" and "E space" for the mandibular canines.
- Once Kasandra's premolars and permanent canines erupt, she will be ready for comprehensive treatment. Because her incisors are proclined, premolar extractions to provide room to upright them will be considered. However, she has a beautiful profile, and because of her ethnicity we would be reluctant to treat her with premolar extractions.

During comprehensive treatment, Kasandra will be placed in fixed orthodontic appliances, her arches leveled, aligned, and most spaces closed. Because her maxillary lateral incisors are small, we anticipate that she will need cosmetic veneers to give them proper widths. Throughout her treatment, any potential for Class III growth will be monitored.

Case Clair

Q: Clair is nine years old (Figure 2.68) and presents to you with her parents' chief complaint, "Clair has crowded teeth." Her PMH, PDH, periodontal evaluation, and TMJ evaluation are WRN. CR = CO. *Compile your diagnostic findings and problem list. Also, state your diagnosis.*

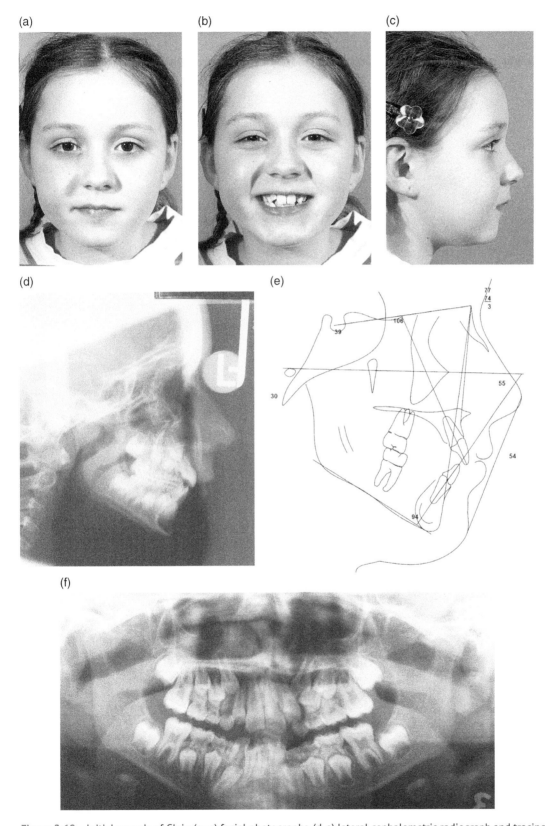

Figure 2.68 Initial records of Clair: (a–c) facial photographs, (d, e) lateral cephalometric radiograph and tracing, (f) pantomograph, (g–i) intraoral photographs, and (j–n) models.

(g) (h) (i)

(j) (k) (l)

(m) (n)

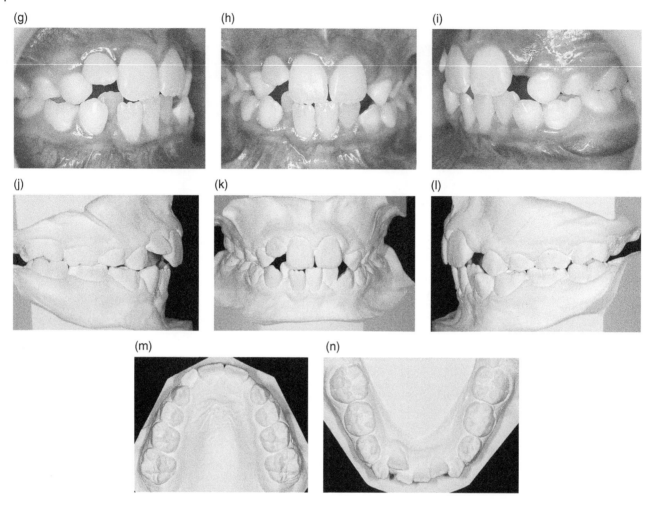

Figure 2.68 (Continued)

A:

Table 2.27 Diagnostic findings and problem list for Clair.

Full face and profile	*Frontal view* Face is symmetric Soft tissue LAFH WRN (soft tissue Glabella – Subnasale approximately equal to Subnasale – soft tissue Menton) Lip competence UDML left of facial midline by ~1 mm Gingival display in posed smile WRN (central incisor gingival margins approximately congruent with the maxillary lip) Moderate buccal corridors (Figure 2.68b) *Profile view* Mildly convex profile Retrusive chin Obtuse NLA Obtuse lip-chin-throat angle

Table 2.27 (Continued)

Ceph analysis	*Skeletal*
	Deficient maxillary anteroposterior position (A-Point lies behind Nasion-perpendicular line)
	Deficient mandibular anteroposterior position (ANB = 3° but with deficient maxilla)
	Skeletal LAFH WRN (ANS-Menton/Nasion-Menton × 100% = 54%)
	Steep mandibular plane angle (FMA = 30°; SNMP = 39°)
	Short posterior face height
	Effective bony Pogonion (Pogonion lies on a line extending from Nasion through B-Point)
	Dental
	Proclined maxillary incisors (U1 to SN = 106°)
	Proclined mandibular incisors (FMIA = 55°)
Radiographs	Early mixed dentition
	Ectopic eruption of mandibular right canine
Intraoral photos and models	Angle Class I
	Iowa Classification: I I I I
	OJ 2 mm
	Anterior open bite (Figure 2.68j)
	4.5 mm maxillary anterior crowding is currently present (potentially impacted maxillary left lateral incisor)
	2.5 mm maxillary arch crowding is anticipated following eruption of all permanent teeth (if appropriate space maintenance is employed)
	4 mm mandibular anterior crowding is currently present
	0.8 mm mandibular arch crowding is anticipated following eruption of all permanent teeth (if appropriate space maintenance is employed)
	Potentially impacted maxillary left lateral incisor
	Dental midlines are not coincident (LDML to right of UDML by 2 mm)
	Maxillary and mandibular dental arches are symmetric (Figure 2.68m and n)
	Thin periodontal biotype labial to mandibular incisors (Figure 2.68h)
Other	None
Diagnosis	Class I malocclusion with moderate anterior crowding

Q: We concluded that Clair has a deficient mandible even though she exhibits a normal ANB angle of ANB = 3°. How can this be?

A: As we discuss in the Appendix, the ANB angle can be used to judge mandibular anteroposterior position only when the maxilla is normal. When the maxillary anteroposterior position is not normal, you need to *relate the mandible to the Nasion perpendicular line*. Why? The angle formed between the Nasion perpendicular line and Nasion to B-Point line *would be the ANB* angle if the maxilla was normal (that is, if the N–A line was coincident with Nasion perpendicular line).

For Clair, the angle formed between the Nasion perpendicular line and Nasion to B-Point line is approximately 5–6° which indicates mandibular deficiency.

Couple this fact with the fact that Clair has a convex profile, and we conclude that she has a deficient mandible.

Q: Are there any additional records you would suggest taking?

A: Yes, occlusal and periapical radiographs (Figures 2.69a and 2.69b) of her mandibular right canine area reveal ectopic eruption of her mandibular right permanent canine. Of course, a CBCT would provide the same information.

Q: Can you determine the position of the ectopically erupting mandibular right permanent canine? Provide an explanation.

A: Using the periapical radiographs of A and B, we can apply Clark's rule [83], which compares the movement

(a)

(b)

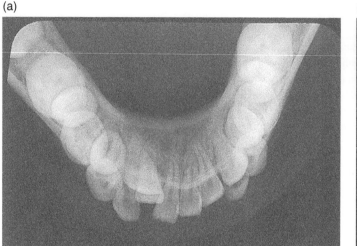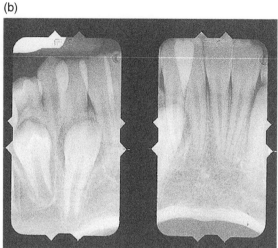

Figure 2.69 Additional radiographs of Clair: (a) mandibular occlusal radiograph and (b) periapical radiographs of her ectopically erupting mandibular right canine.

of the X-ray tube between two periapical films that expose the same group of teeth to the movement of tooth in question when viewing the two X-ray image frames. X-ray tube and tooth moving in the same direction means the tooth is lingually positioned. X-ray tube and tooth moving in opposite directions means the tooth is buccally positioned. This is abbreviated SLOB: Same Lingual Opposite Buccal. Clair's mandibular right canine is erupting to the buccal.

Q: Provide a detailed space analysis for Clair's maxillary and mandibular arches. In other words, how were the 2.5 mm maxillary arch crowding and 0.8 mm mandibular arch crowding calculated (if appropriate space maintenance is employed)?

A:

Below are space estimates:

Average mesiodistal widths of permanent teeth (mm) [1]:

Maxillary Central Incisor	8.5	Mandibular Central Incisor	5.0
Maxillary Lateral Incisor	6.5	Mandibular Lateral Incisor	5.5
Maxillary Canine	7.5	Mandibular Canine	7.0
Maxillary First Premolar	7.0	Mandibular First Premolar	7.0
Maxillary Second Premolar	7.0	Mandibular Second Premolar	7.0
Maxillary First Molar	10.0	Mandibular First Molar	11.0
Maxillary Second Molar	9.0	Mandibular Second Molar	10.5

Average mesiodistal widths of *primary* teeth (mm) [1]:

Maxillary Central Incisor	6.5	Mandibular Central Incisor	4.2
Maxillary Lateral Incisor	5.1	Mandibular Lateral Incisor	4.1
Maxillary Canine	7.0	Mandibular Canine	5.0
Maxillary First Molar	7.3	Mandibular First Molar	7.7
Maxillary Second Molar	8.2	Mandibular Second Molar	9.9

MAXILLARY ARCH

−1 mm of incisor crowding (right lateral incisor) (Figure 2.68m).

+3 mm of left anterior space is present.

−6.5 mm of space needed for maxillary left permanent lateral incisor.

+2 mm of anticipated leeway space (1 mm/side).

Balance = −1 mm + 3 mm − 6.5 mm + 2 mm = −2.5 mm.

MANDIBULAR ARCH

−4 mm of incisor crowding (N).

+3.2 mm of anticipated leeway space (1.6 mm/side).

Balance = −4 mm + 3.2 mm = −0.8 mm.

That is, *2.5 mm of maxillary arch crowding and 0.8 mm of mandibular arch crowding is anticipated following eruption of all permanent teeth (if appropriate space maintenance is employed).*

Q: What are Clair's *primary* problems?

A:

Table 2.28 Primary problems list for Clair.

AP	–
Vertical	Anterior open bite
	Steep MPA
Transverse	—
Other	Proclined maxillary and mandibular incisors
	Ectopically erupting mandibular right canine
	Moderate (4.5 mm) maxillary anterior crowding and moderate (4 mm) mandibular anterior crowding is currently present

Q: Discuss Clair in the context of three principles applied to every early treatment patient.

A:

- The goal of early treatment is to correct developing problems – get the patient *back to normal for their stage of development* (including preventing complications such as resorption of adjacent tooth roots, reducing later treatment complexity, or reducing/eliminating unknowns). Bringing Clair's ectopically erupting mandibular canine into a normal position, alleviating her anterior crowding, uprighting her incisors, and deepening her bite would bring Clair back to normal for her stage of development.

- Early treatment should address *very specific problems with a clearly defined end point*, usually within six to nine months. Extraction of primary canines, primary first molars, and possibly premolars could provide room for permanent tooth eruption plus incisor uprighting/bite deepening. Since the permanent canine roots, and most premolar roots, are >½ developed, their eruption will accelerate if their primary predecessors are extracted.

- Always ask if it is necessary to treat the patient now. *What harm will come if I choose to do nothing now?* It is *not* necessary to treat Clair immediately. However, if we choose to recall, then there is a risk that her permanent canines could remain unerupted, erupt ectopically, or become impacted. In addition, their crowns could resorb incisor roots, lateral incisors could erupt ectopically, or the maxillary left lateral incisor could remain potentially impacted. Lastly, if we chose to recall, then we will lose arch perimeter as primary teeth exfoliate and permanent molars drift mesially.

Q: Ignoring leeway space, Clair currently exhibits moderate (4.5 mm) maxillary anterior crowding and moderate (4 mm) mandibular anterior crowding. We should at least discuss the possibility of permanent tooth

extractions to alleviate this crowding. What features make Clair an *ideal* serial extraction patient? What features make Clair a poor serial extraction candidate?

A: The ideal serial extraction patient is in the *early mixed dentition stage of development and is* <u>normal in every way, except severe anterior crowding (≥9 mm anterior crowding in each arch)</u>. Ideally, the patient presents with:

- *Class I first permanent molars:* Clair presents with Class I molars and exhibits this feature. If Clair presented with a Class II or Class III molar relationship, then we would defer a decision to extract until after her anteroposterior relationship (growth) was addressed.

- *Vertically normal to slightly long soft tissue and skeletal LAFH, with minimal OB or possibly a mild open bite, but* <u>not</u> *a deep bite* (the bite will deepen post-premolar extraction as incisors are retracted/uprighted around their apices): Clair exhibits this feature. She has a normal soft tissue and skeletal LAFH (steep MPA), with a mild open bite (shallow OB).

- *Normal incisor angulation or proclined incisors, but* <u>not</u> *upright incisors* because incisors will tend to upright with extractions/incisor retraction: Clair presents with proclined maxillary and mandibular incisors and meets this criterion.

- *Normal transverse relationship* (normal inter-molar arch widths with good posterior interdigitation, absence of posterior cross bites, and absence of significant transverse compensations). Clair exhibits this feature. Although her posterior OJ appears minimal, she does not exhibit an overt posterior cross bite.

- *Severe (≥9 mm) anterior crowding*: Clair does not exhibit this feature as she currently has moderate anterior crowding in both arches. Also, she has leeway space.

Based upon the above features, Clair is *not* an ideal candidate for serial extraction.

Q: We recommend addressing Class II or III relationships (and growth) in children before extractions are considered. What principle does this underscore?

A: *Reduce unknowns before doing anything irreversible!* Future jaw growth magnitude and direction is a major unknown. If Class II or III relationships (and growth) are not addressed before extractions, then a major treatment error could result.

Q: What is the problem in performing serial extractions in a patient with mild-to-moderate (not severe) anterior crowding?

A: The problem is that, once canines are retracted through premolar extraction spaces and incisors aligned, excess residual space will remain to be closed compared to a patient with severe anterior crowding.

In patients with severe incisor *proclination*, this residual space can be used to retract/upright incisors. However, in patients with upright incisors, this retraction can over-retract incisors.

Q: What options would you consider for Clair?

A: Options include the following:

- *Recall* (monitor) – ask Clair to return in one year and evaluate permanent tooth eruption. The risk of recall includes the possibility that her permanent canines could remain unerupted or become impacted, their crowns could resorb incisor roots, they could erupt ectopically, lateral incisors could erupt ectopically, or the maxillary left permanent lateral incisor could remain potentially impacted.

  In addition, her primary canines and primary molars could be exfoliating during the next year. If we do not employ space maintenance, then we will lose arch perimeter as her permanent first molars drift mesially.

- *Space maintenance* – place an LLHA and Nance holding arch before exfoliation of primary canines and primary molars. Since only 2.5 mm of maxillary arch crowding and 0.8 mm of mandibular arch crowding is anticipated following eruption of all permanent teeth (if appropriate space maintenance is employed), Clair may possibly be treated non-extraction with space maintenance only. However, space maintenance will not upright her proclined incisors. As a matter of fact, an LLHA will increase proclination of Clair's mandibular incisors slightly.[5]

- *Space regaining* – opening space lost since Clair's maxillary left and mandibular right primary lateral incisors exfoliated (Figures 2.68m and 2.68n). However, opening these spaces will further increase Clair's incisor proclination.

- *Extraction of maxillary and mandibular primary canines* – would provide room for eruption/alignment of permanent incisors but may result in arch perimeter loss if permanent molars drift forward. To prevent/reduce arch perimeter loss, place an LLHA and Nance holding arch before/immediately after primary canine extraction.

- *Serial extraction* – Clair exhibits proclined incisors, mild open bite, and steep MPA but only moderate anterior crowding. So, the need for residual space closure would be expected if premolars were extracted. The benefit of residual space closure for Clair would be that incisors could be uprighted and her bite deepened.

If you initiate serial extraction by extracting primary canines/primary first molars, then you can re-evaluate the need for permanent tooth extractions once the first premolars erupt. Consider placing an LLHA and Nance holding arch to prevent arch perimeter loss until you are sure you wish to extract first premolars.

Q: As a review, can you state "rules of thumb" for space maintenance versus serial extraction?

A: Generally:

- Employ space maintenance during the late mixed dentition in cases of mild-to-moderate anterior crowding.

- Defer extraction decisions until after premolars and permanent canines erupt – *reduce unknowns*. Exceptions: cases of permanent tooth ectopic eruption, incisor dehiscences due to crowding, eruption in nonkeratinized gingiva, and severe crowding.

- Defer extraction decisions until after anteroposterior relationships are addressed – *reduce unknowns*. Address Class II/Class III relationships and jaw growth before extracting permanent teeth.

- Consider serial extraction in early mixed dentition patients who exhibit severe anterior crowding but are *normal in every other way*.

Q: Clair exhibits non-coincident midlines (Figure 2.68h). This is an anterior asymmetry resulting from her maxillary midline being shifted to her left (following loss of her maxillary left primary lateral incisor, M) and her mandibular midline being shifted to her right (following loss of her mandibular right primary lateral incisor, Figure 2.68n). However, the posterior quadrants of both arches are symmetric. Based upon these observations, will her midlines remain non-coincident following early and comprehensive treatment?

A: No. Because Clair has *symmetric posterior anchorage*, the anterior asymmetry should resolve once all permanent teeth erupt and are aligned. Because her arches are symmetric in the posterior, the maxillary and mandibular midlines should be coincident in the end (unless a tooth size discrepancy exists).

Q: What is your recommended treatment? How would you proceed?

A: Based upon her proclined incisors and moderate crowding, a decision was made to treat Clair with serial extractions. Since her permanent canines and first premolars (Figures 2.68f and 2.69b) had attained ½ of

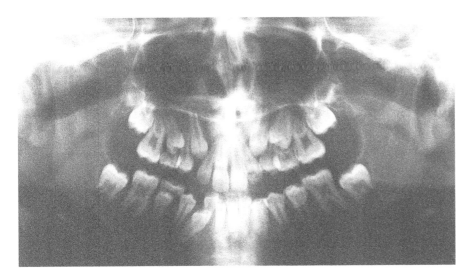

Figure 2.70 Progress radiograph of Clair one year later.

their final root length [84], the primary canines and primary first molars were extracted.

Q: Figure 2.70 is a panoramic radiograph of Clair one year later. What do you observe? What do you recommend now?

A: Her first premolars have erupted. The maxillary permanent canines are potentially impacted. These findings, together with her proclined incisors, mild open bite, and steep MPA led to a final decision to continue with serial extraction and extract first premolars. Clair was then monitored until all remaining permanent teeth erupted.

Q: Progress records were made at age 11 years 9 months (Figure 2.71). Comparing these records to her initial records, list the changes that have occurred following serial extraction.

A: Changes include:
- All remaining permanent teeth have erupted (early treatment is complete).
- Uprighting of incisors spontaneously occurred (U1 to SN angle has decreased from 106° to 102° and FMIA has increased from 55° to 64°).
- Deepening of bite spontaneously occurred from a mild open bite to an OB of ~ 40%.
- Adequate space is available in the maxilla for the erupting permanent canines.
- Excess mandibular residual space is now present (~ 4–5 mm of space bilaterally).
- The maxillary left lateral incisor is in cross bite.

(a)   (b)   (c)   (d)

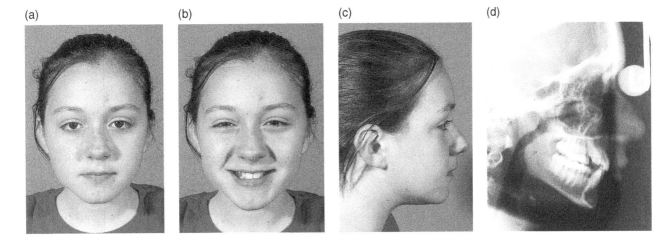

Figure 2.71 Progress records of Clair at 11 years and 9 months of age: (a–c) facial photographs, (d, e) lateral cephalometric radiograph and tracing, (f) pantomograph, (g) gull mouth series, (h–l) intraoral photographs, and (m–q) models.

(e)

(f)

(g)

(h)

(i)

(j)

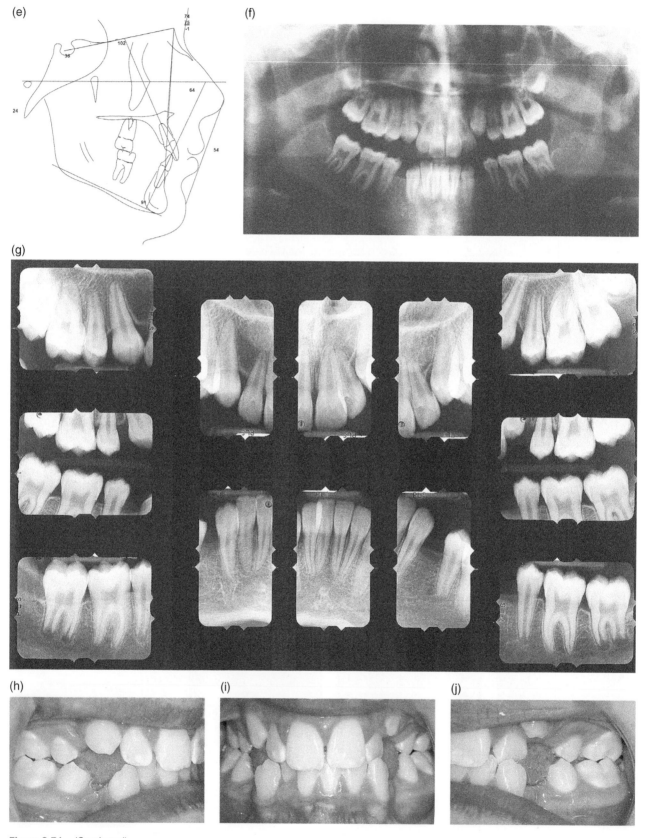

Figure 2.71 (Continued)

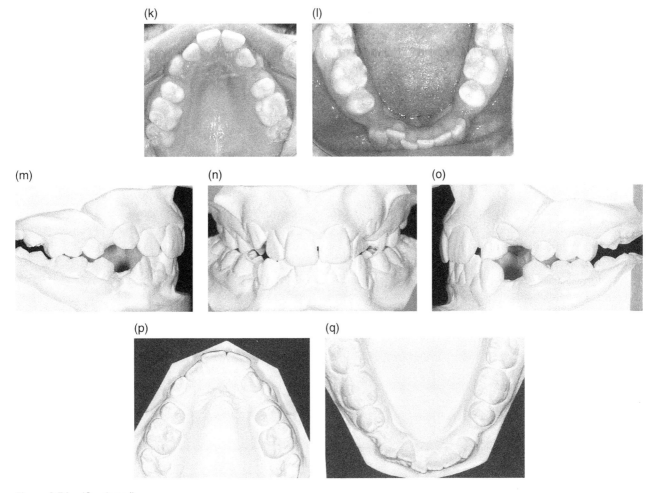

Figure 2.71 (Continued)

- Class I molar relationship is present on the right. The left molar is Class II by 1–2 mm.
- Her posterior OJ is minimal (Figure 2.71n, tight transverse relationship).

Q: What comprehensive treatment do you recommend at this time?

A: We placed fixed orthodontic appliances and leveled/aligned her arches. We retracted maxillary and mandibular permanent canines reciprocally into Class I relationships. Little maxillary space remained and minimal retraction of maxillary incisors was therefore necessary. Greater retraction/uprighting of her mandibular incisors was required. Following incisor retraction, the arches were finished.

Note: Clair's maxillary canines were tipped to the mesial before braces were placed (Figures 2.71m and 2.71o). This observation is important because it means that her maxillary canine roots were in a favorable position to move the crowns distally. In contrast, the mandibular canines were upright and their roots needed to be retracted further through bone during retraction. For this reason, her mandibular molars would be expected to move to the mesial during reciprocal space closure.

Q: Clair's deband images are in Figure 2.72. What changes do you observe?

A: Changes include the following:
- Clair has a beautiful and broad smile compared with her initial presentation (compare Figures 2.68b and 2.72b).
- Her profile is now relatively straight with excellent chin projection (Figure 2.72c).
- Bi-maxillary protrusion has been eliminated (Figure 2.72e).
- Maxillary and mandibular incisors were retracted (Figure 2.72f, right superimpositions).
- Maxillary incisor torque maintained during space closure.

- Class I molar and canine relationship achieved.
- Ectopically erupting mandibular right canine was brought into the arch.
- Arches aligned.
- Midline coincidence achieved.
- Anterior open bite eliminated – she now has 20% OB.
- Maxillary left lateral incisor cross bite was corrected although its root is tipped distally (Figures 2.72g and 2.72j).
- Minimal posterior OJ at permanent first molars ("tight" transverse).

Q: Was serial extraction the correct treatment?

A: Yes. Although we estimated Clair would have only 2.5 mm of maxillary arch crowding and 0.8 mm of mandibular arch crowding if we employed space maintenance, her resulting incisor proclination and anterior open bite may have been unacceptable if she was treated non-extraction. Serial extraction treatment allowed us to:

- Alleviate crowding
- Eliminate bimaxillary incisor protrusion
- Eliminate the open bite
- Provide and esthetic, functional, and healthy occlusion

Q: Should we have employed RME?

A: Possibly, considering the minimal posterior OJ at Clair's first permanent molars and the fact that her mandibular permanent molars appear lingually tipped (transverse compensations, Figure 2.72l). However, her final occlusion is very nice, and she exhibits minimal buccal corridors (Figure 2.72b) when smiling.

Q: Can you suggest any "take-home pearls" for Clair's treatment?

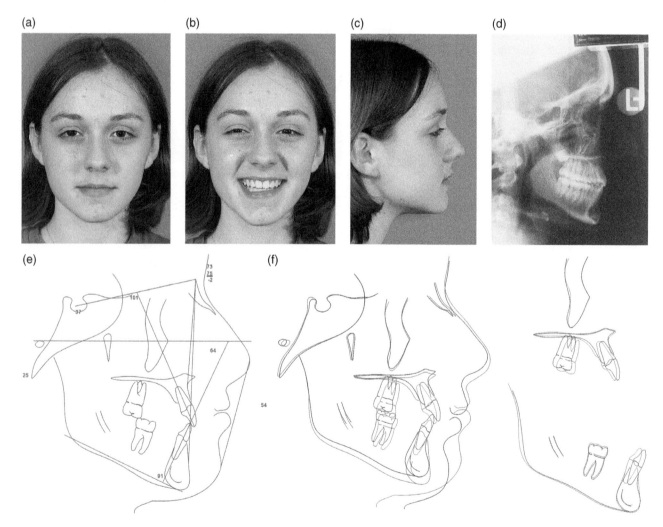

(a) (b) (c) (d)

(e) (f)

Figure 2.72 Deband records of Clair: (a–c) facial photographs, (d, e) lateral cephalometric radiograph and tracing, (f) cephalometric superimposition of initial to Deband time points, (g) pantomograph, (h–l) intraoral photographs, and (m–q) models.

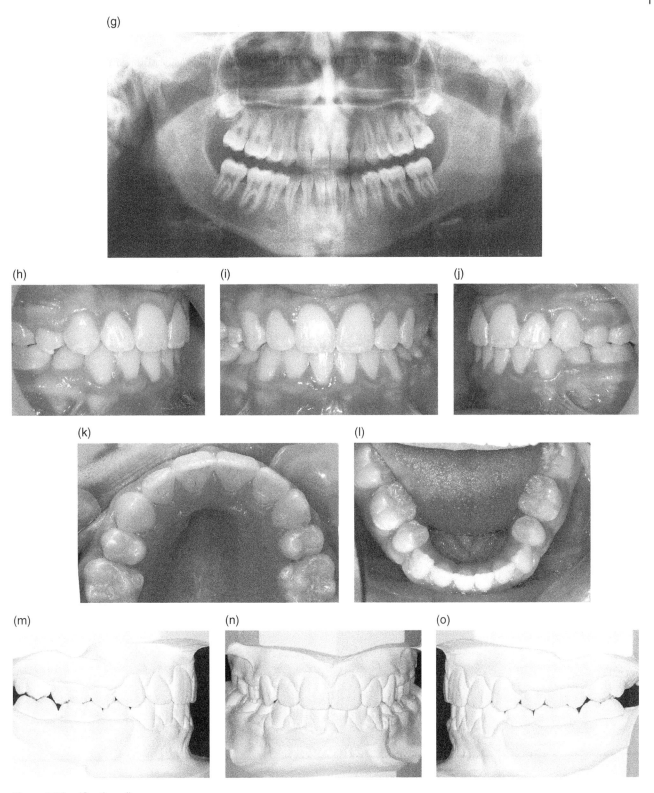

(g)

(h) (i) (j)

(k) (l)

(m) (n) (o)

Figure 2.72 (Continued)

(p) 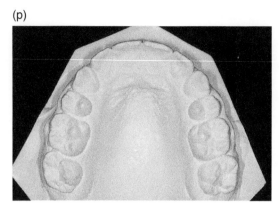 (q)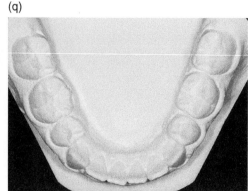

Figure 2.72 (Continued)

A: "Take-home pearls" include:

- Clair was nine years old when she presented with a complaint of crowded teeth. She was Class I with moderate anterior crowding in both arches, proclined incisors, an anterior open bite, and a steep MPA. She we successfully treated with serial extraction.
- In cases of early crowding, you must compare the cost/benefits of monitoring, space maintenance, space regaining, and serial extraction.
- Serial extraction was a reasonable option for Clair because of her *proclined incisors*, moderate crowding, open bite, and steep MPA.
- The *less* anterior crowding present, the more residual space will need to be closed following premolar extractions, canine retraction through the extraction spaces, and incisor alignment. The *more* anterior crowding present, the less space will need to be closed following premolar extractions, canine retraction, and incisor alignment. Excess space closure is used to upright proclined anterior incisors. Clair's mandibular incisors uprighted/retracted with serial extraction (Figure 2.72f).
- Should we have employed space maintenance and deferred a premolar extraction decision until *after* all of Clair's permanent teeth had erupted? We expect that if we had started with space maintenance and extraction of primary canines, then we would have ended up extracting premolars later due to Clair's incisor proclination, anterior open bite, and steep MPA. However, you could have started with space maintenance.

References

1 Wheeler, R.C. (1974). *Dental Anatomy, Physiology, and Occlusion*, 5the. PhiladelphiW.B. Saunders.
2 Martins-Júnior, P.A. and Marques, L.S. (2012). Clinical implications of early loss of a lower deciduous canine. *Int J Orthod Milwaukee.* 23 (3): 23–27.
3 Moyers, R.E. (1988). *Handbook of Orthodontics*, 4the, 109. Chicago: Year Book Medical Publishers, Inc.
4 Moyers, R.E., Van der Linden, F.P.G.M., and Riolo, M.L. (1976). *Standards of Human Occlusal Development.* Ann Arbor: Center for Human Growth and Development, University of Michigan.
5 Viglianisi, A. (2010). Effects of lingual arch used as space maintainer on mandibular arch dimension: a systematic review. *Am J Orthod Dentofacial Orthop* 138 (4): 382.e1–382.e4.
6 Dewey, M. (1916). The lingual arch in combination with the labial arch with extensions as used by Dr. Lloyd S. Lourie. *Int J Orthodontia.* 2 (10): 593–602.
7 Rebellato, J., Lindauer, S.J., Rubenstein, L.K. et al. (1997). Lower arch perimeter preservation using the lingual arch. *Am J Orthod Dentofacial Orthop.* 112 (4): 449–456.
8 Mershon, J.V. (1917). Band and lingual arch technique. *Int J Orthodontia.* 3 (4): 195–203.
9 Dugoni, S.A., Lee, J.S., Varela, J., and Dugoni, A.A. (1995). Early mixed dentition treatment: postretention evaluation of stability and relapse. *Angle Orthod.* 65 (5): 311–320.
10 Brennan, M.M. and Gianelly, A.A. (2000). The use of the lingual arch in the mixed dentition to resolve incisor crowding. *Am J Orthod Dentofacial Orthop* 117 (1): 81–85.

11 Villalobos, F.J., Sinha, P.K., and Nanda, R.S. (2000). Longitudinal assessment of vertical and sagittal control in the mandibular arch by the mandibular fixed lingual arch. *Am J Orthod Dentofacial Orthop.* 118 (4): 365–370.

12 Galvão, M., Dominguez, G.C., Tormin, S.T. et al. (2013). Applicability of Moyers analysis in mixed dentition: a systematic review. *Dental Press J Orthod.* 18 (6): 100–105.

13 Proffit, W.R. and Fields, H.W. (1986). *Contemporary Orthodontics*. St. Louis: CV Mosby.

14 Galvão, M., Dominguez, G.C., Tormin, S.T. et al. (2013). Applicability of Moyers analysis in mixed dentition: a systematic review. *Dental Press J Orthod.* 18 (6): 100–105.

15 Buwembo, W. and Luboga, S. (2004). Moyer's method of mixed dentition analysis: a meta-analysis. *Afr Health Sci.* 4 (1): 63–66.

16 Sonis, A. and Ackerman, M. (2011). E-space preservation. *Angle Orthod.* 81 (6): 1045–1049.

17 Rubin, R.L., Baccetti, T., and McNamara, J.A. Jr. (2012). Mandibular second molar eruption difficulties related to the maintenance of arch perimeter in the mixed dentition. *Am J Orthod Dentofacial Orthop.* 141 (2): 146–152.

18 Espinosa, D., da Vera, C.C., and Normando, D. (2020). The effect of extraction of lower primary canines in the morphology of dental arch: a systematic review and meta-analysis. *Int. J Paediatric Dentistry* https://doi.org/10.1111/ipd.12726.

19 Kjellgren, B. (2007). Serial extraction as a corrective procedure in dental orthopaedic therapy. *Eur J Orthod* 29 (Suppl 1): 37–50.

20 Tweed, C.H. (1954). The Frankfort mandibular incisor angle (FMIA) in orthodontic diagnosis, treatment planning and prognosis. *Angle Orthod.* 24 (3): 121–169.

21 Braun, S. and Hnat, W.P. (1997). Dynamic relationships of the mandibular anterior segment. *Am J Orthod Dentofacial Orthop* 111 (5): 518–524.

22 Ringenberg, Q.M. (1967). Influence of serial extraction on growth and development of the maxilla and mandible. *Am J Orthod.* 53 (1): 19–26.

23 O'Shaughnessy, K.W., Koroluk, L.D., Phillips, C., and Kennedy, D.B. (2011). Efficiency of serial extraction and late premolar extraction cases treated with fixed appliances. *Am J Orthod Dentofacial Orthop* 139 (4): 510–516.

24 Little, R.M. (2002). Stability and relapse: early treatment of arch length deficiency. *Am J Orthod Dentofacial Orthop.* 121 (6): 578–581.

25 Little, R.M., Riedel, R.A., and Engst, E.D. (1990). Serial extraction of first premolars – postretention evaluation of stability and relapse. *Angle Orthod.* 60 (4): 255–262.

26 Brin, I. and Bollen, A.M. (2011). External apical root resorption in patients treated by serial extractions followed by mechanotherapy. *Am J Orthod Dentofacial Orthop* 139 (2): e129–e134.

27 Moss, J.P. and Picton, D.C. (1982). Short-term changes in the mesiodistal position of teeth following removal of approximal contacts in the monkey Macaca fascicularis. *Arch Oral Biol.* 27 (3): 273–278.

28 Tulloch, J.F., Proffit, W.R., and Phillips, C. (2004). Outcomes in a 2-phase randomized clinical trial of early Class II treatment. *Am J Orthod Dentofacial Orthop.* 125 (6): 657–667.

29 Ghafari, J., Shofer, F.S., Jacobsson-Hunt, U. et al. (1998). Headgear versus function regulator in the early treatment of class II division 1 malocclusion: a randomized clinical trial. *Am J Orthod Dentofacial Orthop.* 113 (1): 51–61.

30 Keeling, S.D., Wheeler, T.T., King, G.J. et al. (1998). Anteroposterior skeletal and dental changes after early Class II treatment with bionators and headgear. *Am J Orthod Dentofacial Orthop.* 113 (1): 40–50.

31 Dolce, C., McGorray, S.P., Brazeau, L. et al. (2007). Timing of class II treatment: skeletal changes comparing 1-phase and 2-phase treatment. *Am J Orthod Dentofacial Orthop.* 132 (4): 481–489.

32 O'Brien, K. Is early treatment for Class II malocclusion effective? Results from a randomized controlled trial. *Am J Orthod Dentofacial Orthop.* 129 (4 Suppl): S64–S65.

33 O'Brien, K., Wright, J., Conboy, F. et al. (2009). Early treatment for Class II div 1 malocclusion with the Twin-block appliance: a multi-center, randomized, controlled trial. *Am J Orthod Dentofacial Orthop.* 135 (5): 573–579.

34 Thiruvenkatachari, B., Harrison, J., Worthington, H., and O'Brien, K. (2015). Early orthodontic treatment for Class II malocclusion reduces the chance of incisal traumresults of a Cochrane systematic review. *Am J Orthod Dentofacial Orthop* 148: 47–59.

35 Thiruvenkatachari, B., Harrison, J.E., Worthington, H.V., and O'Brien, K.D. (2013). Orthodontic treatment for prominent upper front teeth (Class II malocclusion) in children. *Cochrane Database Syst Rev* (11): CD003452. https://doi.org/10.1002/14651858.CD003452.pub3. Update in: Cochrane Database Syst. Rev. 2018;3: CD003452. doi: 10.1002/14651858.CD003452.pub4.

36 Batista, K.B., Thiruvenkatachari, B., Harrison, J.E., and O'Brien, K.D. (2018). Orthodontic treatment for prominent upper front teeth (Class II malocclusion) in children and adolescents. *Cochrane Database Syst Rev.* 3 (3): CD003452. https://doi.org/10.1002/14651858.CD003452.pub4.

37 Koroluk, L.D., Tulloch, J.F., and Phillips, C. (2003 Feb). Incisor trauma and early treatment for Class II Division 1 malocclusion. *Am J Orthod Dentofacial Orthop.* 123 (2): 117–125. discussion 125-6.

38 Kau, C.H., Durning, P., Richmond, S. et al. (2004 Jun). Extractions as a form of interception in the developing dentition: a randomized controlled trial. *J Orthod.* 31 (2): 107–114.

39 Sayın, M. and Türkkahraman, H. (2006 Jan). Effects of lower primary canine extraction on the mandibular dentition. *Angle Orthod.* 76 (1): 31–35.

40 Firouz, M., Zernik, J., and Nanda, R. (1992). Dental and orthopedic effects of high-pull headgear in treatment of Class II, division 1 malocclusion. *Am J Orthod Dentofacial Orthop.* 102 (3): 197–205.

41 Baumrind, S., Korn, E.L., Isaacson, R.J. et al. (1983). Quantitative analysis of the orthodontic and orthopedic effects of maxillary traction. *Am J Orthod.* 84 (5): 384–398.

42 Elder, J.R. and Tuenge, R.H. (1974). Cephalometric and histologic changes produced by extraoral high-pull traction to the maxilla in Macaca mulatta. *Am J Orthod.* 66 (6): 599–617.

43 Kirjavainen, M., Kirjavainen, T., Hurmerinta, K., and Haavikko, K. (2000). Orthopedic cervical headgear with an expanded inner bow in Class II correction. *Angle Orthod.* 70 (4): 317–325.

44 Pancherz, H. (1997). The effects, limitations, and long-term dentofacial adaptations to treatment with the Herbst appliance. *Semin Orthod.* 3 (4): 232–243.

45 Le Cornu, M., Cevidanes, L.H., Zhu, H. et al. (2013). Three-dimensional treatment outcomes in Class II patients treated with the Herbst appliance: a pilot study. *Am J Orthod Dentofacial Orthop.* 144 (6): 818–830.

46 Huang, G., English, J., Ferguson, D. et al. (2005). Ask Us – functional appliances and long-term effects on mandibular growth. *Am J Orthod Dentofacial Orthop* 128 (3): 271–272.

47 Pancherz, H., Ruf, S., and Kohlhas, P. (1998). "Effective condylar growth" and chin position changes in Herbst treatment: a cephalometric roentgenographic long-term study. *Am J Orthod Dentofacial Orthop.* 114 (4): 437–446.

48 Araujo, A.M., Buschang, P.H., and Melo, A.C. (2004). Adaptive condylar growth and mandibular remodeling changes with bionator therapy – an implant study. *Eur J Orthod.* 26 (5): 515–522.

49 Ruf, S., Baltromejus, S., and Pancherz, H. (2001). Effective condylar growth and chin position changes in activator treatment: a cephalometric roentgenographic study. *Angle Orthod.* 71 (1): 4–11.

50 Rudee, D.A. (1964). Proportional profile changes concurrent with orthodontic therapy. *Am J Orthodontics.* 50 (6): 421–434.

51 Lew, K.K. (1992). Changes in lip contour following treatment of maxillary protrusion with esthetic orthodontic appliances. *J Esthet Dent.* 4 (1): 16–23.

52 Drobocky, O.B. and Smith, R.J. (1989). Changes in facial profile during orthodontic treatment with extraction of four first premolars. *Am J Orthod Dentofacial Orthop.* 95 (3): 220–230.

53 Jacobs, J.D. (1978). Vertical lip changes from maxillary incisor retraction. *Am J Orthod.* 74 (4): 396–404.

54 Olsson, M. and Lindhe, J. (1991). Periodontal characteristics in individuals with varying form of the upper central incisors. *J Clin Periodontol.* 18 (1): 78–82.

55 Müller, H.P. and Eger, T. (1997). Gingival phenotypes in young male adults. *J Clin Periodontol.* 24 (1): 65–71.

56 Müller, H.P., Heinecke, A., Schaller, N., and Eger, T. (2000). Masticatory mucosa in subjects with different periodontal phenotypes. *J Clin Periodontol.* 27 (9): 621–626.

57 Müller, H.P. and Eger, T. (2002). Masticatory mucosa and periodontal phenotype: a review. *Int J Periodontics Restorative Dent.* 22 (2): 172–183.

58 Cook, D.R., Mealey, B.L., Verrett, R.G. et al. (2011). Relationship between clinical periodontal biotype and labial plate thickness: an in vivo study. *Int J Perio Restorative Dent.* 31 (4): 345–354.

59 Zweers, J., Thomas, R.Z., Slot, D.E. et al. (2014). Characteristics of periodontal biotype, its dimensions, associations and prevalence: a systematic review. *J Clin Periodontol.* 41 (10): 958–971.

60 Andlin-Sobocki, A. (1993). Changes of facial gingival dimensions in children. A 2-year longitudinal study. *J Clin Periodontol* 20 (3): 212–218.

61 Stenvik, A. and Mjör, A. (1970 Apr). Pulp and dentin reactions to experimental root intrusion. A histologic study of the initial changes. *Am J Orthod.* 57 (4): 370–385.

62 Mavragani, M., Bøe, O.E., Wisth, P.J., and Selvig, K.A. (2002). Changes in root length during orthodontic treatment: advantages for immature teeth. *Eur J Orthod.* 24 (1): 91–97.

63 Li, X., Xu, J., Yin, Y. et al. (2020). Association between root resorption and tooth development: a quantitative clinical study. *Am J Orthod Dentofacial Orthop.* 157 (5): 602–610.

64 Kokich, V.O. Jr., Kiyak, H.A., and Shapiro, P.A. (1999). Comparing the perception of dentists and lay people to altered dental esthetics. *J Esthet Dent.* 11 (6): 311–324.

65 Schindel, R.H. and Duffy, S.L. (2007). Maxillary transverse discrepancies and potentially impacted maxillary canines in mixed-dentition patients. *Angle Orthod.* 77 (3): 430–435.

66 Bishara, S.E. (1992). Impacted maxillary canines: a review. *Am J Orthod Dentofacial Orthop.* 101 (2): 159–171.

67 Shapira, Y. and Kuftinec, M.M. (1998 Oct). Early diagnosis and interception of potential maxillary canine impaction. *J Am Dent Assoc.* 129 (10): 1450–1454.

68 Ngan, P., Hornbrook, R., and Weaver, B. (2005). Early timely management of ectopically erupting maxillary canines. *Semin Orthod.* 11 (3): 152–163.

69 Bedoya, M.M. and Park, J.H. (2009 Dec). A review of the diagnosis and management of impacted maxillary canines. *J Am Dent Assoc.* 140 (12): 1485–1493.

70 Ericson, S. and Kurol, J. (1988 Nov). Early treatment of palatally erupting maxillary canines by extraction of primary canines. *Eur J Orthod.* 10 (4): 283–295.

71 Ericson, S. and Kurol, J. (2000). Incisor root resorptions due to ectopic maxillary canines imaged by computerized tomography: a comparative study in extracted teeth. *Angle Orthod.* 70 (4): 276–283.

72 Ericson, S. and Kurol, P.J. (2000). Resorption of incisors after ectopic eruption of maxillary canines: a CT study. *Angle Orthod.* 70 (6): 415–423.

73 Woloshyn, H., Årtun, J., Kennedy, D.B., and Joondeph, D.R. (1994). Pulpal and periodontal reactions to orthodontic alignment of palatally impacted canines. *Angle Orthod.* 64 (4): 257–264.

74 Becker, A. and Chaushu, S. (2005). Long-term follow-up of severely resorbed maxillary incisors after resolution of an etiologically associated impacted canine. *Am J Orthod Dentofacial Orthop.* 127 (6): 650–654. quiz 754.

75 Falahat, B., Ericson, S., Mark D'Amico, R., and Bjerklin, K. (2008 Sep). Root resorption due to ectopic maxillary canines. A long-term radiographic follow-up. *Angle Orthod.* 78 (5): 778–785.

76 Bernal-de Jaramillo, L.V., Zapata-Noreña, Ó., Tobón-González, C. et al. (2015). Smile characteristics in children with normal occlusion. *Rev Fac Odontol Univ Antioq.* 27 (1): 11–29.

77 Peck, S., Peck, L., and Kataja, M. (1992 Jun). Some vertical lineaments of lip position. *Am J Orthod Dentofacial Orthop.* 101 (6): 519–524.

78 ADA Division of Communications (2006). For the dental patient. Tooth eruption: the permanent teeth. *J Am Dent Assoc* 137 (1): 127.

79 Lindauer, S.J., Rubenstein, L.K., Hang, W.M. et al. (1992). Canine impaction identified early with panoramic radiographs. *J Am Dent Assoc.* 123 (3): 91–97.

80 Rogers, K., Campbell, P.M., Tadlock, L. et al. (2018). Treatment changes of hypo- and hyperdivergent Class II Herbst patients. *Angle Orthod.* 88 (1): 3–9.

81 Ericson, S. and Kurol, J. (1987 Jun). Radiographic examination of ectopically erupting maxillary canines. *Am J Orthod Dentofacial Orthop.* 91 (6): 483–492.

82 de Freitas, L.M., de Freitas, K.M., Pinzan, A. et al. (2010). A comparison of skeletal, dentoalveolar and soft tissue characteristics in white and black Brazilian subjects. *J Appl Oral Sci.* 18 (2): 135–142.

83 Clark, C.A. (1910). A method of ascertaining the relative position of unerupted teeth by means of film radiographs. *Proc R Soc Med* 3 (Odontol Sect): 87–90.

84 Moorrees, C.F.A., Fanning, E.A., and Gron, A.-M. (1963). The consideration of dental development in serial extraction. *Angle Orthod* 33 (1): 44–59.

3

Eruption Problems

Introduction

The development, eruption, and emergence of permanent teeth into the oral cavity is pivotal to facial growth and development. Problems that accompany ectopic permanent tooth eruption or permanent tooth absence must be dealt with thoughtfully and effectively. These problems are often diagnosed in the early and middle periods of the mixed dentition, but sometimes it is not practical to treat them early. This chapter addresses early diagnosis and treatment of tooth absence and eruption problems, as well as early diagnosis and later treatment of these problems. It provides you the foundation for addressing these problems.

Q: What is ectopic tooth eruption? Can you describe adverse sequelae that can result from ectopic tooth eruption?

A: Ectopic tooth eruption occurs when a tooth does not follow its normal eruption path (Figures 3.1a and 3.1b). Adverse sequelae of ectopic tooth eruption include loss of arch perimeter, tooth impaction, and root resorption.

Q: Discuss ectopic tooth eruption in the context of three principles applied to every early treatment patient.

A:

1) The goal of early treatment is to correct developing problems – to get the patient *back to normal for their stage of development*, thereby reducing unknowns, later treatment complexity, and preventing complications. Correcting ectopic tooth eruption is often essential to return the patient to a normal eruption pattern, prevent arch perimeter loss, prevent impaction of adjacent teeth, and prevent root resorption.

2) Early treatment should address *very specific problems with a clearly defined end point*, usually within six to nine months. Ectopic tooth eruption is a perfect example of a specific problem with a treatment of short duration and a clearly defined end point.

3) Always ask: Is it necessary that I treat the patient now? *What harm will come if I choose to do nothing now?* Without correction, ectopic eruption can result in arch perimeter loss, tooth impaction, and root resorption.

Q: Can you suggest general treatment principles to follow when correcting ectopically erupting permanent teeth?

A: Principles include:

- *Create space for the ectopic tooth to erupt – clear an eruption path*. This may include extracting teeth or creating space using headgear, RME, fixed orthodontic appliances, or a removable appliance.

- *Space regaining to move an ectopically erupting/erupted permanent tooth back to its correct position*, especially if arch perimeter has been lost. For example, if the patient in Figure 3.1a will be treated *non-extraction*, then you could attempt using either fixed appliances or a removable appliance to move the maxillary right permanent first molar distally (freeing it from under the primary second molar). Or, you could extract the maxillary right primary second molar, allow the maxillary right permanent first molar to erupt into a Class II molar relationship, then move the maxillary right permanent first molar distally using fixed appliances or a removable appliance. In some cases, surgical exposure may be required to place an orthodontic bracket on an ectopically erupting tooth so that space regaining forces can be applied.

- *Consider all possible anterior and posterior extraction patterns*. If the patient is clearly a case that will require extraction of permanent teeth, or in instances of severe root resorption of permanent teeth, exhaustively

Practical Early Orthodontic Treatment: A Case-Based Review, First Edition. Thomas E. Southard, Steven D. Marshall, Laura L. Bonner, and Kyungsup Shin.
Companion website: www.wiley.com/go/southard/practical

(a)   (b)

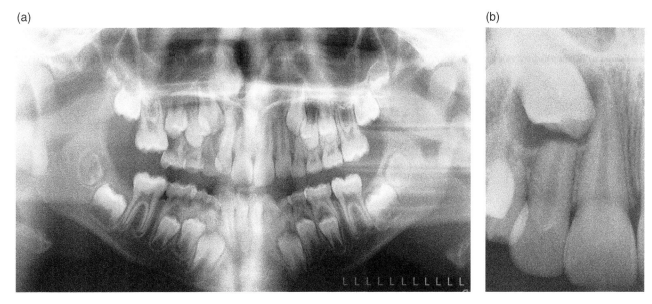

Figure 3.1 Examples of ectopic tooth eruption and associated adverse sequelae: (a) ectopic eruption of the maxillary right permanent first molar has resulted in its impaction under the primary second molar, arch perimeter loss, and maxillary right second premolar impaction; (b) maxillary right permanent canine ectopic eruption has resulted in severe root resorption of the maxillary right permanent lateral incisor root.

consider all possible extraction options. For example, if the patient in Figure 3.1a is an *extraction patient*, then you might extract the maxillary right primary second molar (allowing the maxillary right permanent first molar to erupt into a Class II molar relationship), then extract the impacted maxillary right second premolar, or first premolar, at a later date.

As another example, in Figure 3.1b you may consider extracting the maxillary right primary canine and primary first molar to provide room to move the maxillary right permanent canine distally following its surgical exposure. Or, you could consider extracting the maxillary right lateral incisor if it is deemed hopeless to permit the maxillary right permanent canine to erupt into the lateral incisor position. Then, you could leave the permanent canine in the lateral incisor position (canine substitution case) and retain the primary canine, or you could extract the primary canine and retract the permanent canine into its correct anteroposterior position (with prosthetic replacement of the missing lateral incisor). Our point is that there are many options you should exhaustively consider, in consultation with the restorative doctor, the parent, and perhaps an endodontist.

Q: What is the most common ectopic permanent tooth you will manage during the early and middle periods of the mixed dentition stage?

A: After third molars, the permanent maxillary canines are the most common tooth to display ectopic eruption during development [1–3]. Palatal displacement is more common than buccal displacement by approximately threefold [3, 4].

Q: How do you diagnose an ectopically erupting maxillary permanent canine in the mixed dentition?

A: Initial diagnosis of an early treatment patient may not provide a simple "yes or no" answer to the question of ectopic maxillary permanent canine eruption. Rather, diagnosis of ectopic eruption may be a developing scenario that is determined by establishing a baseline followed by careful periodic observation. This is for two reasons: (i) maxillary permanent canine development and eruption is occurring over the entire time period of the mixed dentition stage, and (ii) an ectopic path of eruption can occur at any stage during root development of the tooth [2].

Q: Can you name three important principles in making a diagnosis for maxillary permanent canine position in a patient considered for early treatment?

A: Principles include the following:
1) Because the timing of dentition development and chronologic age vary across individuals being considered for early treatment, you must *establish the stage of dentition development for your patient*. This is best done by panoramic radiography. The goal here is to determine if the patient is advanced or delayed in dentition development compared to chronologic

averages, allowing you to gauge the timeline of anticipated maxillary permanent canine eruption, and aiding your plan for clinical supervision.

2) *Establish the spatial position of the maxillary canines relative to the permanent maxillary lateral incisors.* This is determined by palpation for the developing maxillary permanent canine crowns in the buccal alveolar plate and estimating maxillary permanent canine position radiographically (using periapical radiography and Clark's rule, or panoramic and cephalometric images, or 3-D cephalometry) [5–7]. This allows an assessment of potential impaction or damage to adjacent teeth due to malposition of the maxillary canines and supports the decision to apply treatment early or opt for continued clinical supervision.

3) *Determine if other factors may have a negative impact on continuing eruption of the maxillary permanent canines* (e.g. crowding of developing permanent teeth, ectopic eruption of adjacent permanent teeth, abnormal sequence of permanent tooth development, maxillary anteroposterior or transverse deficiency, or hypodontia).

Q: Why is palpation of the developing maxillary permanent canine crowns in a patient being evaluated for early treatment important?

A: Using a large sample of children in the mixed dentition, and following them longitudinally, Ericson and Kurol [2, 8] observed that a palpable bulge of the buccal alveolar plate in the area apical to the primary canine and permanent lateral incisor roots was generally predictive of normal maxillary permanent canine eruption. In cases of delayed dental age, a palpable bulge was not always present, and early radiography in these cases did not always reveal abnormal position or predict ectopic eruption. However, during continued clinical supervision, if the developing canines became palpable to the buccal, they erupted without impaction. Furthermore, children who did not display palpable maxillary permanent canines after age eleven had a higher incidence of later canine impaction, prompting the recommendation for further radiographic investigation if this finding occurs during clinical supervision.

This supports our three important principles noted earlier: During early treatment diagnosis, considering the maxillary permanent canines, you must establish:

- *The stage of dentition development*
- *The spatial position of the maxillary permanent canines*
- *If other factors may have a negative impact on continued eruption*

Q: You are viewing a panoramic radiograph for a patient in the mixed dentition. Does the amount of overlap (i.e. superimposition of structures on the image) seen between the maxillary permanent canine crown and root of the adjacent maxillary permanent lateral incisor predict palatal displacement of the canine (Figures 3.2a–3.2c)?

A: Yes, as seen on a panoramic image, the more the maxillary permanent canine crown overlaps the lateral incisor root, the greater the chance that the canine will become palatally displaced [9]. For example, look at the panoramic image of a patient in the late mixed dentition shown in Figure 3.3. The erupting maxillary *left* permanent canine crown is not overlapping the left lateral incisor root, and we can predict that it will most likely erupt normally if adequate space is present. However, the maxillary right canine crown *is* overlapping the right lateral incisor root, so we can predict that it may become palatally displaced and impacted. The greater the overlap, the greater the likelihood of impaction.

Q: Based upon the principles of ectopic eruption treatment we just presented, what early treatment options would you consider that will increase the likelihood of the maxillary right permanent canine shown in Figure 3.3 erupting?

A: The principle we should apply is to *create a path for the ectopically erupting tooth to follow*. One way to create a path [10, 11] is to extract the maxillary right primary canine, but the success of primary canine extraction *alone* has proven equivocal [12, 13]. Instead, the benefit of primary canine extraction appears to be enhanced when it is performed in conjunction with space opening procedures [12–26], including:

- Using fixed orthodontic appliances to trap a compressed open coil spring between the posterior teeth and the lateral incisor. The spring force should be kept light during space opening, and the lateral incisor bracket should be positioned to tip the lateral incisor root away from the erupting permanent canine crown (and not drive the lateral incisor root into the canine crown).

Important note: this approach will *create space between the crowns of the teeth and between coronal portions of the roots but less space at the root apices where the space is needed if the canine crown is located there.* For this approach to create space at the root apices, you must assure that appropriate root tip results at the root apices to diverge the roots away from the erupting tooth.

- RME (to create space both between maxillary central incisor crowns and between root apices) [27] followed by a TPA

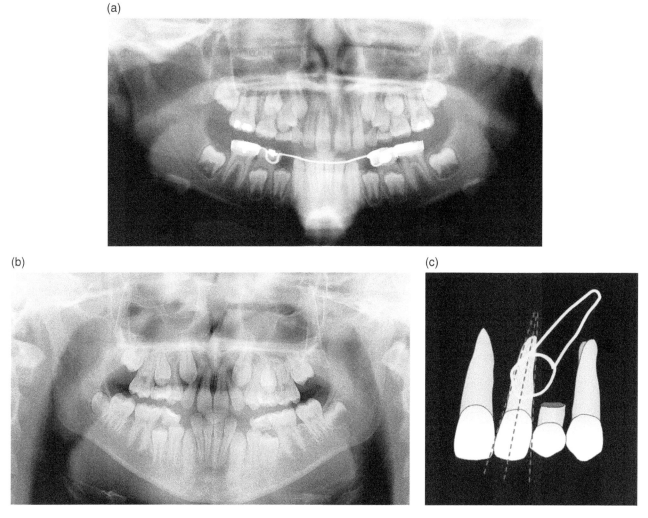

Figure 3.2 Erupting maxillary permanent canines: (a) normal eruption with the canine crowns erupting along the distal of the maxillary lateral incisor roots, (b) ectopic eruption with the canine crowns partially overlapping the maxillary lateral incisor roots, (c) schematic illustration showing the degree of canine crown overlap relative to the lateral incisor midline.

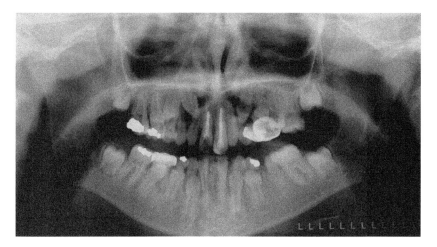

Figure 3.3 Panoramic image of a patient in the late mixed dentition who presents with the maxillary right permanent canine crown overlapping the right lateral incisor root at its apex.

- Distal movement of the posterior teeth using headgear
- Extraction of the maxillary primary first molar in addition to extraction of the primary canine
- Permanent tooth extractions

If the maxillary primary first molar is extracted in addition to the primary canine (Figures 3.4a and 3.4b), then the first premolar can erupt down and out of the way of the canine crown (assuming that the premolar root is at least at least 1/2 developed) [28]. This accelerated eruption provides space for the permanent canine and encourages its eruption. Or, if the maxillary arch can afford to be expanded (Figure 3.4c), then RME can create additional space for the maxillary permanent canine to erupt.

For the patient in Figure 3.3, we chose to extract the maxillary right primary canine and right primary first molar. The maxillary right permanent canine (and left permanent canine) then erupted uneventfully (Figure 3.4d).

Q: Regarding treatment of ectopically erupting maxillary permanent canines, can you compare concomitant extraction of maxillary primary canines plus primary first molars to extraction of primary canines alone?

A: Study results are mixed. Bonetti et al. [24] reported concomitant primary canine and first molar extractions more effective at promoting eruption of ectopically erupting permanent canines positioned palatally or centrally. Although the study found equivalent clinical success over an 18-month postextraction observation period, the authors' conclusions are based on significant differences in spatial positioning of maxillary permanent canines in response to simultaneous primary canine and primary first molar extractions compared to primary canine extractions alone. Hadler-Olsen et al. [29] reported the two methods are equivalent in promoting normal eruption of palatally displaced maxillary canines, but did not see a significant

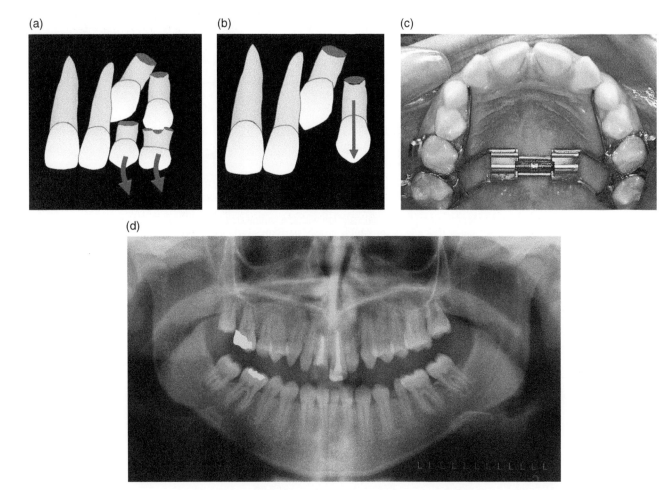

Figure 3.4 Early treatments to increase the likelihood that ectopically erupting maxillary permanent canines will erupt normally are based upon the principle of *creating a path for the ectopically erupting tooth to follow:* (a and b) extraction of the primary canine may be of benefit, especially if other space creation is performed such as extracting the primary first molar. Doing so can result in accelerated eruption of the first premolar if the first premolar root is at least half developed, which creates space for the canine to erupt; (c) RME can create additional anterior space for the permanent canine to erupt; (d) as an example, the ectopically erupting maxillary right canine of the patient in Figure 3.3 erupted uneventfully following extraction of the maxillary right primary canine and primary first molar.

(a)

(b)

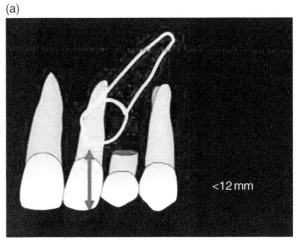
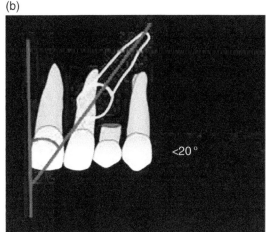

Figure 3.5 Position factors affecting spontaneous eruption of ectopic maxillary canines: (a) a vertical position of <12 mm appears to be important; (b) an inclination of <20° is important for labially displaced permanent canines.

improvement of maxillary canine spatial position using different measurement criteria.

In our clinical experience, *concomitant primary canine and first molar extractions are more effective at promoting eruption of ectopically erupting maxillary canines when the maxillary first premolar roots are ≥1/2 developed.* Why? Eruption of the first premolar is accelerated. The first premolar erupts down and away from the permanent canine crown, providing a path and additional space for the canine to erupt.

Q: Let's assume that you extract a maxillary primary canine and make space for the ectopically erupting permanent canine. What positional factors influence whether the permanent canine will erupt spontaneously?

A: The *further apically* the vertical position of the canine cusp tip (relative to the occlusal plane) and the more *horizontally tipped* the canine crown, the more likely the canine will be impacted [30] (and in our clinical opinion, the more difficult it will be to erupt it orthodontically).

One study found that a vertical position <12 mm is important for spontaneous canine eruption (Figure 3.5a). An inclination of <20° (Figure 3.5b) is important for spontaneous eruption of *labially* displaced canines but appears to have no impact on palatally displaced canines [31]. Finally, the more *mesial* the permanent canine crown position relative to the incisor roots, the worse the prognosis for spontaneous eruption [11, 32].

Q: So, what is the "take home" message regarding early treatment of ectopically erupting maxillary permanent canines?

A: Use our three principles to establish your *timeline* for canine eruption, the *spatial position* of the canine, and *other factors* that may impede normal eruption (e.g. crowding). If you decide treatment to improve canine eruption is warranted, you cannot guarantee spontaneous eruption of the canine. However, extraction of the primary canine *in conjunction with space creation* can be a reasonable early treatment.

Q: You make a panoramic image (Figure 3.6) of a nine-year-old. What do you observe?

A: The maxillary right first premolar is erupting ectopically and is blocking eruption of the maxillary right permanent canine. The maxillary left permanent canine is erupting normally.

Q: Would you recommend early treatment for the patient shown in Figure 3.6? If yes, what treatment would you recommend?

A: Yes, we would recommend early treatment for this patient. Otherwise, the maxillary right permanent canine and first premolar could remain impacted with potential future root resorption of the maxillary right lateral incisor.

This condition is challenging. We reasoned that because of its near horizontal angulation, the maxillary right first premolar would never erupt even if we cleared a path for it. However, we decided that the least invasive early treatment would be to extract the maxillary right primary canine and both maxillary right primary molars – and recall the patient in six months (note that the premolar roots have developed to at least 1/2 of their final length). If, at the six-month recall appointment, the position of the maxillary right first premolar and canine improved on a panoramic

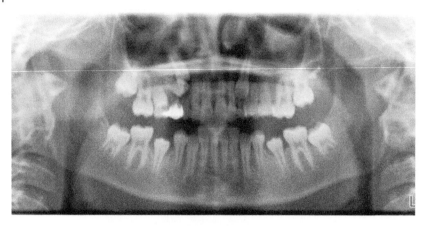

Figure 3.6 Initial panoramic image of a nine-year-old.

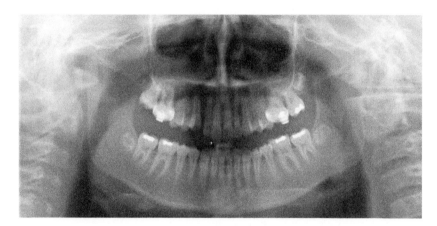

Figure 3.7 Progress panoramic image of the patient shown in Figure 3.6, six months after primary tooth extraction and headgear wear. Note spontaneous eruption of the maxillary right first premolar and canine.

image, then we would continue monitoring. However, if the position of the maxillary right premolar and canine did not improve, then we would refer for surgical exposure of the maxillary right first premolar and use fixed orthodontic appliances to erupt it into the arch.

We extracted the maxillary right primary canine and both primary molars. We also placed the patient, who exhibited a Class II molar relationship, on a high-pull headgear (preventing maxillary right first permanent molar mesial drift). We made another panoramic radiograph six months later (Figure 3.7). Remarkably, the maxillary right premolar had erupted normally along with all other permanent teeth.

How/why did this ectopic eruption pattern self-correct? We can't be certain, but the ectopic eruption of the maxillary right first premolar was a significant "*other factor*" influencing eruption of the right canine. Normalizing the ectopic eruption of the right first premolar created space for continued eruption of the right canine.

Q: Look at the ectopically erupting mandibular permanent canines in Figure 3.8. Would you recommend early treatment? If yes, what treatment would you recommend?

A: We would recommend early treatment for the ectopically erupting mandibular permanent canines. Otherwise, they may remain impacted and/or resorb the mandibular permanent lateral incisor roots. Treatment consisted of mandibular primary canine extractions. The mandibular permanent canines then erupted spontaneously (Figure 3.9a and b).

In addition to extraction of the mandibular primary canines, extraction of the mandibular primary first molars (Figure 3.8) may have been beneficial to encourage eruption of the mandibular first premolars and thereby make room for the mandibular permanent canines (mandibular first premolar root development was >1/2).

Q: An ectopically erupting permanent canine fails to erupt, and you decide to surgically expose it. Do you have any suggestions for this surgery and subsequent tooth movement?

A: Suggestions include the following:

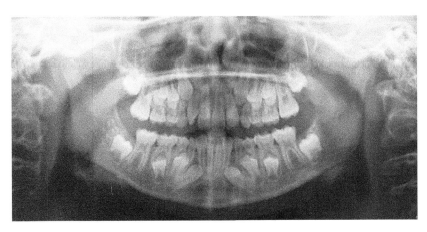

Figure 3.8 Radiograph illustrating ectopically erupting mandibular canines (*Source:* Courtesy of Drs. Herb and Justin Hughes).

(a)

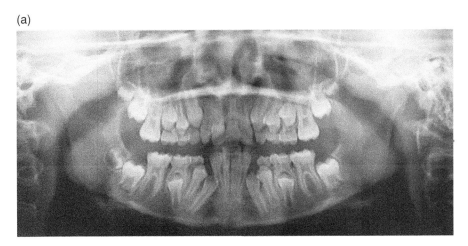

(b)

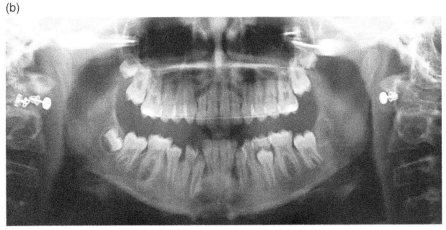

Figure 3.9 Progress records of the patient shown in Figure 3.8 following extraction of mandibular primary canines. (a) Early mixed dentition. (b) Late mixed dentition. The ectopically erupting mandibular permanent canines erupted spontaneously during the transition to the late mixed dentition.

- Direct your surgeon to *remove all bone covering the impacted canine crown in the direction you intend to move it* (Figure 3.10). Why? Once the dental follicle is disrupted during surgery, there are no cells to remove bone [33]. Bone is then be removed only, and slowly, by pressure necrosis.

- Direct the surgeon to check mobility of the unerupted canine using an elevator (Figure 3.11). If the canine is non-mobile (ankylosed), then a decision must be made either to attempt breaking the ankyloses (immediately applying an eruptive force before ankylosis recurs) or to extract the canine.

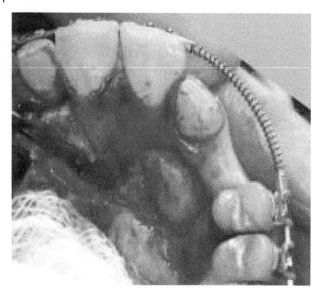

Figure 3.10 Surgical exposure of an ectopically erupting maxillary left permanent canine that did not erupt following early treatment. Note that the surgeon has removed all bone off the canine crown *in the direction of the intended crown movement* (distally).

- *Initially move the canine crown away from adjacent tooth roots.* Do not drag the canine crown across adjacent tooth roots. *Dragging the canine crown across adjacent tooth roots* can result in resorption of adjacent roots [34]. Once the canine crown is clear of neighboring roots, then move it toward its future position in the arch.

Look at Figure 3.12a. Here, the elastomeric chain from the premolars is pulling the surgically exposed maxillary left canine crown *across the root* of the lateral incisor, possibly resorbing the lateral incisor root. To make matters worse, we bonded the left lateral incisor. Bonding the lateral incisor makes it hard for the canine to push the lateral incisor out of the way. A better approach is to first move the surgically exposed canine crown *away* from the incisor roots (Figure 3.12b, TPA helping to direct the elastic force) before moving the canine laterally into the arch (Figure 3.12c).

These same suggestions apply to labially impacted maxillary canines (Figure 3.13a–d) and impacted mandibular canines (Figure 3.14a–d). That is, *first move the surgically exposed canine crowns away from adjacent roots before moving the canines into the arch.*

Q: Another technique has been suggested for treating palatally impacted maxillary canines in the mixed dentition, as follows:
- Ask your surgeon to elevate a full-thickness mucoperiosteal palatal flap over the impacted canine crown
- Remove all palatal bone covering the canine crown to the level of the cementoenamel junction

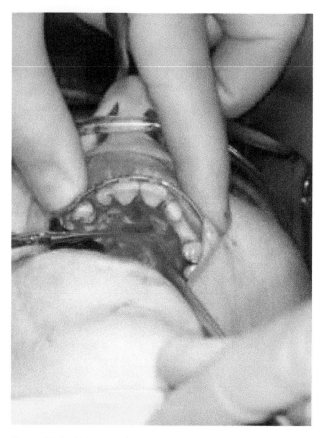

Figure 3.11 Using an elevator to check mobility of the impacted maxillary canine.

- Place a hole in the palatal flap over the canine crown
- Suture the flap back in place [33, 35].

The canine should erupt without orthodontic force. What are your thoughts of this technique?

A: If the impacted canine is not ankylosed, then this technique should be successful in providing a path for the canine to spontaneously erupt. However, once the patient has this surgical procedure, an argument can be made for proceeding with forced (orthodontic) eruption of the exposed canine – instead of hoping for spontaneous eruption.

Q: We discussed ectopically erupting maxillary *molars,* and regaining space lost by such ectopic eruption, in our chapter on Crowding. Referring again to Figure 3.1a (intraoral photos of the same patient are shown in Figure 3.15), what treatment options would you consider for the ectopically erupting maxillary right first permanent molar?

A: Options include:
- *Monitoring (self-correction), which is possible between 6 and 7 years of age.* However, early treatment to bring the ectopically erupting permanent first molar into occlusion should begin as soon as it is realized that self-correction will not occur [36].

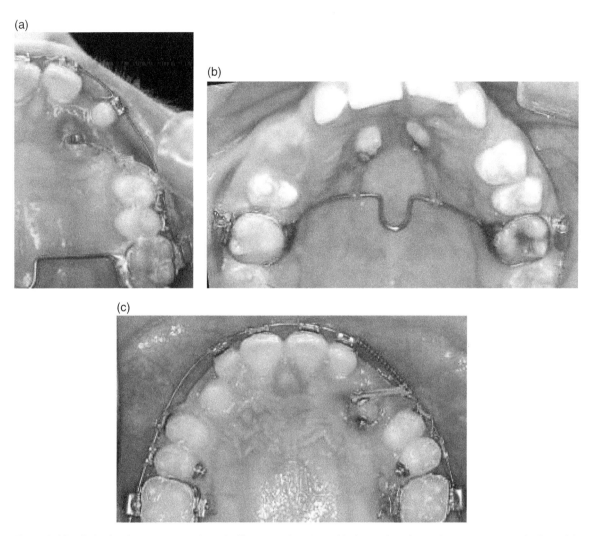

Figure 3.12 Orthodontic movement of surgically exposed canines: (a) *do not* drag the canine crown across the lateral incisor root (as shown here) because the canine crown can resorb the lateral incisor root; instead (b), initially move the canine crown *palatally* away from the incisor root; (c) later, move the canine crown into the arch.

- *Insertion of an elastomeric separator* (or twisted brass wire) between the maxillary right primary second molar and maxillary right permanent first molar to release the trapped permanent molar. In this patient, we were unable to gain access to place a separator.
- *Extraction of the maxillary right primary second molar* to free the maxillary right permanent first molar and allow it to erupt. We chose this option because the maxillary right primary second molar was very mobile and would exfoliate soon. After we extracted the primary second molar, the maxillary right permanent first molar erupted in a mesial position (Figure 3.16a). We next considered three options: (i) placing fixed appliances and inserting a compressed spring between the maxillary right primary first molar and permanent first molar – to move the maxillary right permanent first molar distally and regain space for the maxillary right second premolar, (ii) fabricating a removable maxillary spring appliance to move the maxillary first

permanent molar distally, and (iii) banding the maxillary permanent first molars and using a headgear to move the maxillary right permanent molar distally.

We chose to band the maxillary first permanent molars (Figure 3.16b) and use a headgear to move the maxillary right permanent molar distally. We also placed an LLHA. Once all permanent teeth had erupted, we bonded both arches with fixed orthodontic appliances, leveled and aligned the arches, and finished treatment (Figure 3.16c).

- If the maxillary right primary second molar had been nonmobile (an anchor) instead of mobile, then you could have *bonded brackets and placed a segmental archwire* to free the permanent first molar and move it distally (Figure 3.17). A compressed open coil spring could be trapped between the permanent first molar and the primary second molar to help push the permanent first molar distally.

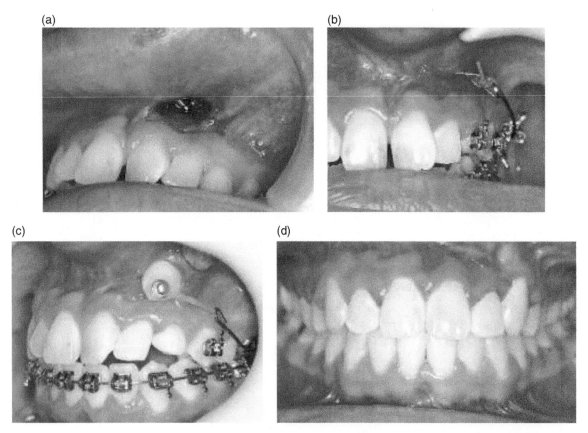

Figure 3.13 Orthodontic movement of surgically exposed, labially impacted, maxillary canines: (a and b) first move the canine crown *labially,* away from the incisor root; (c and d) before moving the canine into the arch. Note that the maxillary left primary canine was not extracted until we were reasonably confident that the maxillary left permanent canine could be brought into the arch. Why? If the maxillary permanent canine was ankylosed, then we may have chosen to extract the permanent canine and retain the primary canine.

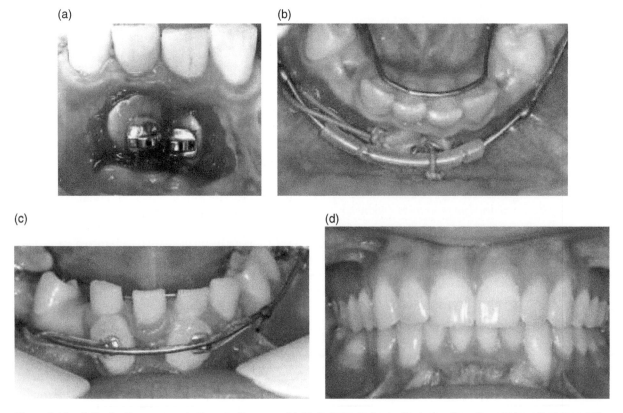

Figure 3.14 Orthodontic movement of surgically exposed, labially impacted, mandibular canines: (a and b) we first moved the canine crowns *labially,* toward a lip bumper and away from the incisor roots; (c and d) before we moved the canines into the arch, distally.

(a)
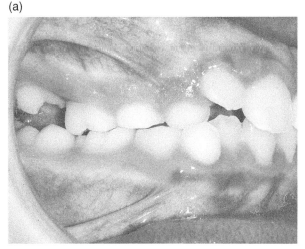

(b)
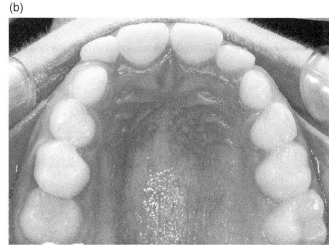

Figure 3.15   (a and b) Intraoral photos of a patient presenting with ectopic eruption of the maxillary right permanent first molar (panoramic image shown in Figure 3.1a).

- Use of a *Halterman appliance* which consists of a metal hook soldered to a maxillary right primary second molar band. The hook extends to the tuberosity area. A button is bonded to the maxillary right permanent first molar, and an elastomeric power chain stretched to apply tension between the hook and the button to move the permanent first molar distally. Since the maxillary right primary second molar was mobile, this approach was not employed.

Q: Can you offer treatment options to correct ectopically erupting *mandibular* permanent molars?
A: Similar to early treatment of ectopically erupting maxillary molars, options include (Figure 3.18):
  - *Insertion of an elastomeric separator* (or twisted brass wire) between the ectopically erupting mandibular permanent molar and primary second molar.
  - *Extraction of the mandibular primary second molar* to free the mandibular permanent first molar and allow it to erupt. Figure 3.18a illustrates an ectopically erupting mandibular left permanent first molar. The problem is that if we extract the primary second molar and allow the permanent first molar to erupt, then the erupting molar will drift mesially and arch perimeter will be lost. To avoid this problem, place a distal shoe (Figures 3.18b and 3.18c), which allows the permanent first molar to erupt but prevents it from drifting mesially.

Once the mandibular first permanent molar erupts, you can either place an LLHA (the distal shoe will fall out when the primary first molar exfoliates) or regain space by moving the permanent first molar distally using fixed orthodontic appliances or a removable appliance. Neither was done in this patient, and the mandibular left second premolar erupted uneventfully (Figure 3.18d).

- If the mandibular primary second molar is nonmobile (useful as anchorage), and if you have access to the crown of the ectopically erupting mandibular permanent first molar Figure 3.18e, mandibular right permanent first molar), then you can *bond brackets and place a segmental archwire* to free the permanent first molar and move it distally (Figures 3.18f–3.18g). A compressed open-coil spring can be trapped between the permanent first molar and the primary second molar to help move the permanent first molar distally.
- Use of a *Halterman appliance* (Figure 3.19, shown here erupting second molars).
- Surgical luxation, elevation, and immobilization of second molars (Figure 3.20) [37, 38].

Q: Look at the panoramic radiograph of the late mixed dentition patient in Figure 3.21a. Specifically, compare the *alveolar crest bone levels* of the mandibular primary second molars to the alveolar crest bone levels of their respective permanent first molars. What do you observe? Next, look at the panoramic radiograph of the early mixed dentition patient in Figure 3.21b. Specifically, compare the alveolar crest bone levels of the mandibular primary second molars to that of their respective permanent first molars. What do you observe?
A: In Figure 3.21a, the alveolar bone crest levels of both mandibular primary second molars are at the same level as the alveolar bone crest levels of their respective permanent first molars. This relationship is seen during normal tooth eruption (Figure 3.22a, red lines represent normal alveolar bone crest levels).
In Figure 3.22b, a large step is seen between the alveolar bone crest level of the right mandibular primary second molar and the alveolar bone crest level of the right

(a)

(b)

(c)

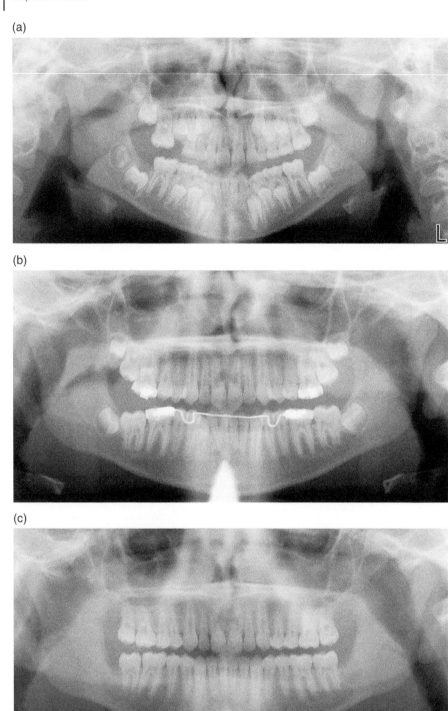

Figure 3.16 Treatment of the patient shown in Figure 3.15: (a) following extraction of the mobile maxillary right primary second molar, the maxillary right permanent first molar erupted – blocking eruption/impacting the maxillary right second premolar; (b) the maxillary first permanent molars were banded, high-pull headgear treatment was initiated to move the maxillary right permanent first molar distally, and the maxillary right second premolar erupted. Early treatment was completed at this point; (c) deband radiograph following comprehensive treatment.

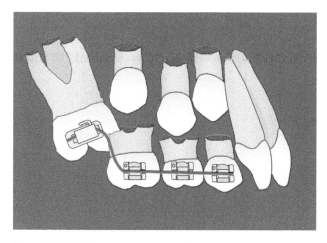

Figure 3.17 If the maxillary right primary second molar had been nonmobile, then the maxillary right quadrant could have been bonded and a segmental archwire placed to correct the permanent first molar's ectopic eruption.

mandibular permanent first molar. This relationship (Figure 3.22b) is indicative of primary second molar ankylosis.

Q: Why do we judge primary tooth ankylosis based upon (radiographic) alveolar bone crest heights? Why can't we simply look (clinically) for an occlusal step between the suspect primary tooth and the adjacent teeth?

A: Primary second molars often have naturally shorter clinical crowns than permanent first molars. Therefore, a patient *without ankylosis* could exhibit a clinical occlusal step between the shorter primary second molar crown and the taller permanent first molar crown. A clinical occlusal step is not a reliable indicator of primary tooth ankylosis.

On the other hand, a (radiographic) discrepancy in alveolar bone crest heights indicates that eruption of the normal tooth has continued while eruption of the ankylosed tooth has halted. The earlier the onset of ankylosis, the greater will be the alveolar bone crest height discrepancy.

The best way to confirm ankylosis of a tooth is to look for an alveolar bone crest height discrepancy between it and adjacent teeth. Of course, you can always check its mobility. If a primary tooth is mobile, then it is not ankylosed.

Some clinicians advocate identifying ankylosis by listening for a difference in sound between the suspect tooth and adjacent teeth when the teeth are tapped with the end of an intraoral mirror handle. We do not feel comfortable using this method. Perhaps others have better hearing than we do.

Q: In Figure 3.21b, notice that the mandibular right permanent first molar and primary first molar have both tipped into the depressed mandibular right primary second molar space. Why does this happen?

A: Transeptal fibers from the depressed, ankylosed primary second molar pull vertically on both teeth, causing them to tip [39, 40].

Q: How would you deal with the ankylosed mandibular right primary second molar shown in Figure 3.21b?

A: We elected to have the mandibular right primary second molar and primary first molar extracted. We also placed an LLHA. Let us explain:

If the mandibular right second premolar was in a normal position, and if the mandibular right permanent first molar was upright, then we would recommend monitoring only (recalling the patient in nine to twelve months). If this were the case, then exfoliation of the ankylosed primary second molar would be delayed by about six months, but the alveolar bone crest level at that site would eventually be normal after the second premolar erupted [41, 42].

However, the progressive infraocclusion of the mandibular right primary second molar in Figure 3.21b has resulted in severe mesial tipping of the mandibular right permanent first molar. This mesial tipping could worsen if we do nothing. Therefore, we elected to place an LLHA now. Also, we were concerned that the very low position of the mandibular right primary second molar could hinder root development of the mandibular right second premolar. Therefore, we asked a surgeon to extract the mandibular right primary second molar and right primary first molar.

Q: When else would you consider extracting a mandibular primary second molar having a permanent second premolar successor?

A: If over a period of a year we do not see radiographic evidence of *continuing primary second molar root resorption* by an erupting second premolar (with > 1/2 second premolar root development), then we will extract the primary second molar.

Q: The roots of the mandibular right first and second premolars in Figure 3.22b are barely developed. Isn't it true that extracting primary molars when their successor (premolar) roots are minimally developed can actually *delay* premolar eruption?

A: Yes, it is true that early primary tooth extraction can cause delayed eruption and emergence of its successor, probably as a result of scar tissue forming a mechanical

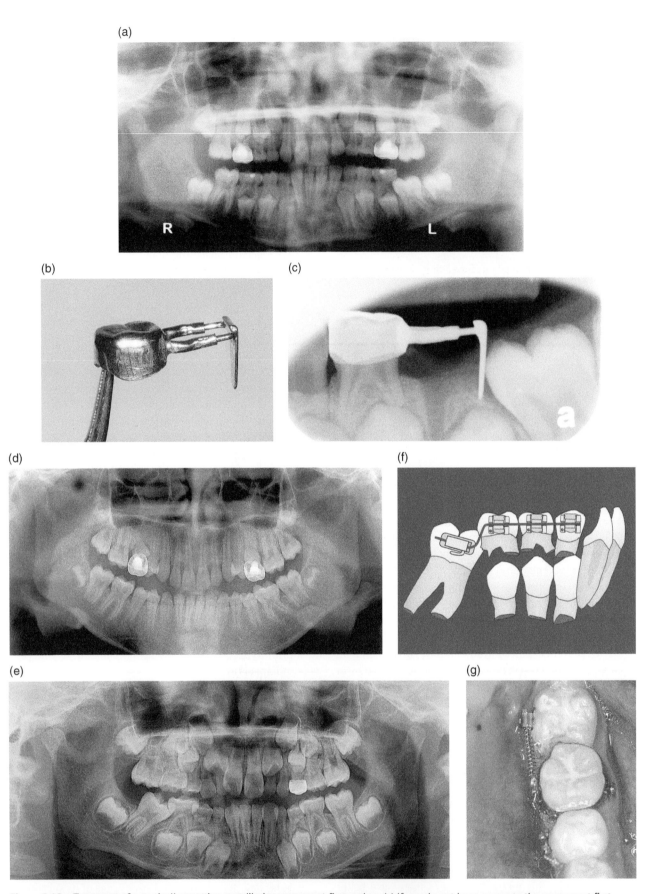

Figure 3.18 Treatment of ectopically erupting mandibular permanent first molars. (a) If you do not have access to the permanent first molar crown (mandibular left permanent first molar), then consider extracting the primary second molar and placing a (b and c) distal shoe, which maintains space for the erupting mandibular left second premolar but allows the molar to erupt (d). (e) If the mandibular primary second molar is nonmobile, and if you have access to the crown of the ectopically erupting mandibular permanent first molar mandibular right permanent first molar), then (f) the mandibular right quadrant can be bonded and a segmental archwire placed to correct the permanent molar's ectopic eruption. (g) An open-coil spring can be trapped to aid freeing of the permanent molar (shown here freeing a second molar).

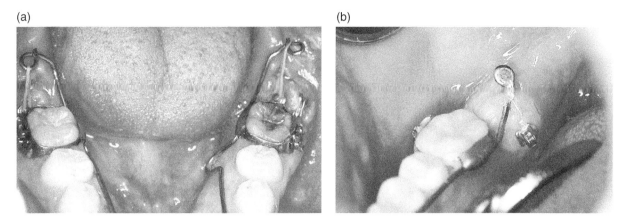

Figure 3.19 Halterman appliances used to (a) free ectopically erupting mandibular permanent second molars by moving them distally, (b) uprighting a lingually tipped molar.

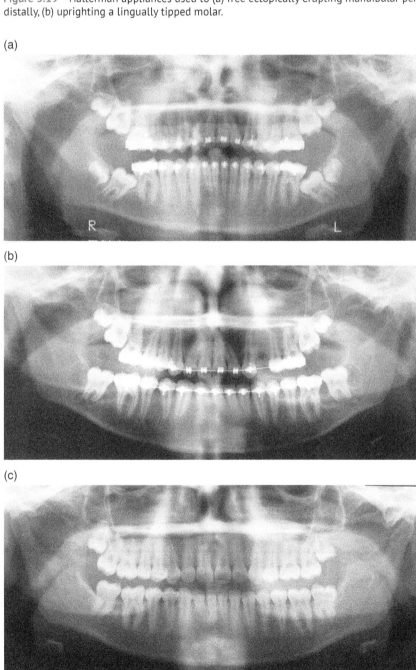

Figure 3.20 Surgical luxation and elevation of ectopically erupting mandibular permanent second molars: (a) impacted mandibular second molars prior to surgery, (b) following mandibular second molar surgical luxation/elevation and third molar extraction, (c) deband panoramic radiograph. Note improvement in mandibular second molar alveolar bone crest level.

(a)

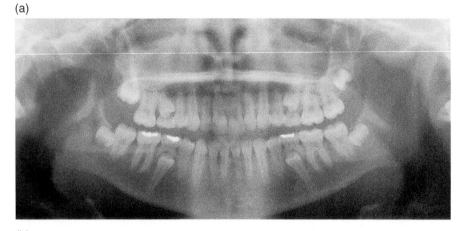

(b)

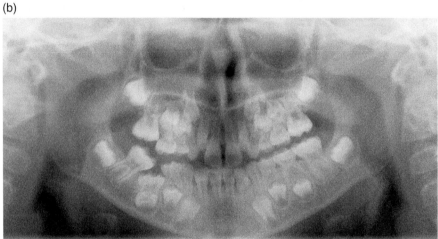

Figure 3.21 Panoramic images of two mixed dentition patients. Take note of the alveolar bone crest levels of the mandibular primary second molars.

(a)   (b)

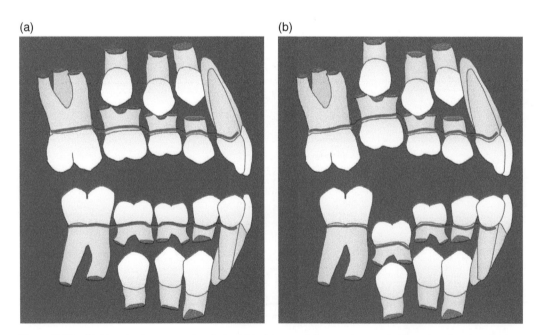

Figure 3.22 (a) Alveolar bone crest levels (red lines) in normally erupting teeth. Note that the alveolar bone crest levels follow a relatively straight line; (b) ankylosis of mandibular and maxillary primary second molars. Note the discrepancy in alveolar bone crest levels between the ankylosed primary second molars and their adjacent teeth. This discrepancy is seen because the ankylosed teeth stop erupting while the adjacent teeth continue erupting.

barrier [28]. As a general rule, *a primary tooth should not be removed until its permanent successor has an appropriate amount of root formation – at least 1/2 of its root length.*

However, in this patient (Figure 3.21b), we were concerned that if the ankylosed mandibular primary second molar remained, then the mandibular right second premolar root could not develop. Therefore, we extracted the ankylosed mandibular right primary second molar. The mandibular right primary first molar had to be extracted in order for the surgeon to gain access to the primary second molar.

Q: The patient in Figure 3.21b returned 1 1/2 years later (Figure 3.23a). What do you observe in the mandibular right quadrant? How would you proceed?

A: The mandibular right second premolar is showing signs of root development and eruption away from the lower border of the mandible. We planned to remove the LLHA and upright the mandibular right permanent first molar (space regaining) using fixed orthodontic appliances or a removable appliance. We would then fabricate a new LLHA to maintain the permanent first molar in its upright position while the remaining permanent teeth erupted.

The patient did not return to our clinic for five years (Figure 3.23b). Our LLHA had been removed, but no other treatment had been performed. Note the full root development of both mandibular right premolars and significant uprighting of the mandibular right permanent first molar. Did eruptive force from the impacted mandibular right second premolar cause the permanent first molar to upright? We do not know. The patient is now in adult dentition and entering comprehensive treatment.

Q: Why did we not upright the mandibular right permanent first molar (Figure 3.21b) when we extracted the mandibular right primary second molar?

A: Our reasoning was as follows: if the mandibular right second premolar did not form a root and begin to erupt, then we would have extracted it and attempted to move the mandibular right permanent first molar mesially (closing the space). Because the mandibular right permanent first molar crown was already tipped forward,

(a)

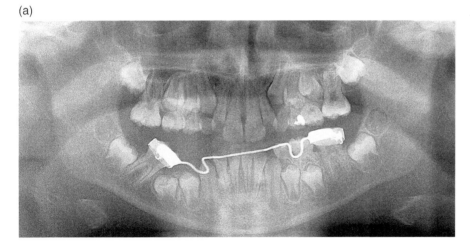

(b)

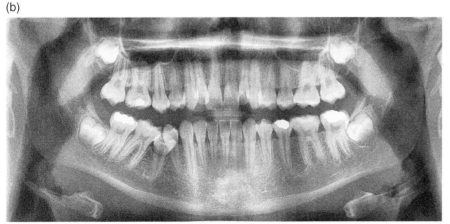

Figure 3.23 Progress panoramic images of the patient shown in Figure 3.21b. (a) 1½ years later; (b) 6½ years later.

we would have left it tipped forward and rotated the roots forward with fixed appliances.

Therefore, we decided to leave the first permanent molar tipped forward until we could determine whether the second premolar root was developing and the tooth erupting.

Q: A seven-year-old girl is referred to you specifically for evaluation of her maxillary permanent molars (Figure 3.24). What do you observe?

A: Her maxillary right permanent first molar exhibits normal root development and has erupted to the occlusal plane. Her maxillary left permanent molar lacks root development and has failed to erupt.

Q: Can you suggest at least three possible reasons why her maxillary left permanent molar (Figure 3.24) has not erupted?

A: Possible reasons include:
- Ankylosis
- Eruption blocked by the maxillary left primary second molar root
- Systemic factors found in patients with certain syndromes, such as cleidocranial dysplasia, ectodermal dysplasia, Gardner syndrome, and Apert syndrome.
- Delayed eruption
- Primary failure of eruption (PFE).

Q: Is there another, simple explanation for the maxillary left condition?

A: Yes, a simple explanation is that the maxillary left permanent first molar was extracted and that the molar we see is the maxillary permanent *second* molar (whose development matches that of the maxillary right permanent second molar). However, the parent stated that the maxillary left permanent first molar had never been extracted. Did the left first permanent molar never develop? We cannot be sure whether it is the first or second permanent molar.

Q: What is PFE? Are there specific signs that the patient in Figure 3.24 could be exhibiting PFE? If this is an example of PFE, what treatments can be considered in dealing with it?

A: Primary failure of eruption (PFE) refers to failure of a non-ankylosed tooth to erupt due to a disturbance of the eruption mechanism [43]. A wide range of clinical variability exists, thought to be the result of variation in the timing and intensity of the dysregulation [44]. The following characteristic signs of PFE could apply to the patient in Figure 3.24 [45–48]:
- Permanent first molars are always involved and present with no apparent barrier to eruption (100% for genetically confirmed PFE).
- Posterior teeth are more frequently affected.

Other signs of PFE that do *not* specifically apply to the patient in Figure 3.24 include:
- *If a tooth in a more anterior position is affected, then teeth more distal to that tooth are usually affected as well* (i.e. when premolars are affected then molars are also likely to be affected).
- Both primary and permanent teeth can be affected.
- The condition is often bilateral (50/50 for PFE patients, versus 80/20 unilateral/bilateral for molar ankylosis).
- Teeth in both arches are often affected (91% for patients with genetically confirmed PFE).

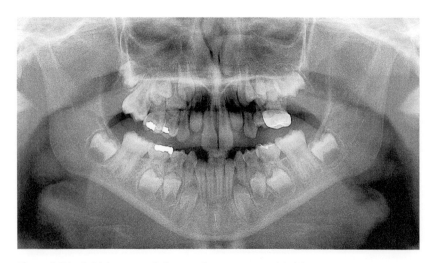

Figure 3.24 Initial panoramic image of a seven-year-old girl.

- Affected teeth resorb the alveolar bone above the crown, may erupt into initial occlusion and then cease to erupt further, or may fail to erupt entirely.
- Affected teeth may be displaced back and forth with manual pressure (indicating that they are not initially ankylosed). However, affected teeth tend to become ankylosed as soon as orthodontic eruptive forces are applied.
- If a small area of ankylosis is broken by luxating the ankylosed tooth, it might be possible to move the tooth for a short time, but re-ankylosis is inevitable.
- Other concurrent skeletal problems (Class III malocclusion for 63% of genetically confirmed PFE patients) and dental anomalies (tooth agenesis, microdontia of maxillary lateral incisors, anomalous root morphology) may be present.

Possible treatment options for posterior open bites resulting from PFE include:
- Restoring the involved erupted teeth with buildups or crowns after vertical growth is complete.
- Extraction of the involved teeth and replacement with bone grafts/implants.
- With first and second molar involvement, leaving the affected teeth in place and accepting a premolar occlusion.
- A segmental osteotomy or distraction osteogenesis to close the posterior open bite.
- A removable prosthetic (overlay) partial denture to provide posterior occlusion.

Q: How do you recommend dealing with the unerupted maxillary left first (or second) permanent molar shown in Figure 3.24?

A: Since we were uncertain as to whether this condition resulted from PFE, ankylosis, delayed eruption of the first permanent molar, or normal development of the second permanent molar, we decided to monitor the maxillary left permanent molar. Also, we placed an LLHA and corrected an anterior crossbite with fixed appliances (Figure 3.25).

Q: Figure 3.26a shows the same patient one year later. Regarding the maxillary left permanent molar, what do you observe?

A: The maxillary left molar was erupting. Clinically, it had pierced the gingiva. Why did this happen? We suspect that this represents normal development of the maxillary left *second* molar (with first molar agenesis). Or, perhaps bonding the maxillary left primary second molar freed the permanent first molar, allowing it to erupt. We decided to monitor its eruption longer. Eventually, the molar erupted (Figure 3.26b).

Q: An early mixed dentition patient presents to you (Figure 3.27). Regarding permanent tooth eruption, what do you observe?

A: Permanent tooth eruption appears normal.

Q: Three years later (Figure 3.28), you make another panoramic image. What do you notice regarding second premolar eruption?

A: The maxillary second premolars are erupting symmetrically. The mandibular right second premolar has erupted. The mandibular left second premolar eruption is relatively delayed. The roots of the mandibular left primary second molar do not appear to be resorbing appreciably.

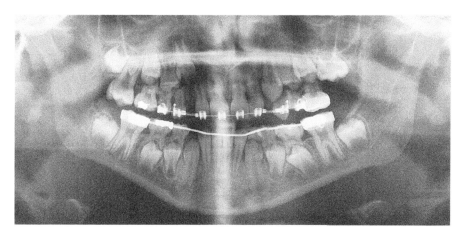

Figure 3.25 Progress panoramic radiograph of the patient in Figure 3.24.

(a)

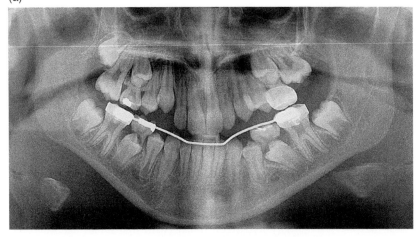

(b)

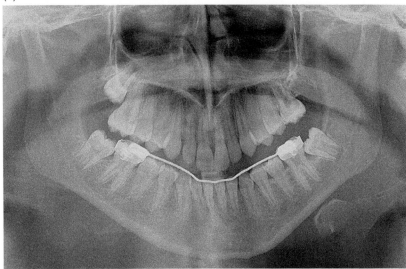

Figure 3.26 Progress radiograph of the patient in Figure 3.24 (a) 1 year later, and (b) 2½ years later. The maxillary left molar erupted spontaneously.

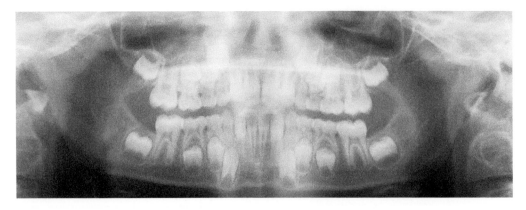

Figure 3.27 Initial panoramic image of an early mixed dentition patient.

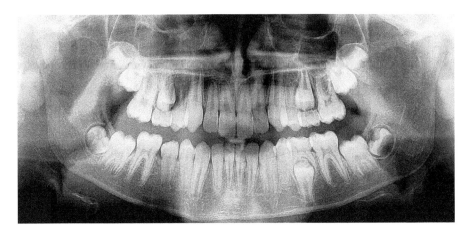

Figure 3.28 Progress record of the patient in Figure 3.27 three years later.

Q: What could be the causes for the relatively delayed mandibular left second premolar eruption (Figure 3.28)? How might you proceed?

A: Possible causes include:
- Normal variation in eruption timing
- Recent ankylosis of the mandibular left primary second molar
- Mandibular left primary second molar roots failing to resorb

  Treatment options include continuing to monitor eruption of the mandiblar left second premolar or extracting the mandibular left primary second molar (since root development of the mandibular left second premolar > 1/2 complete).

Q: A decision was made to extract the mandibular left primary second molar in order to accelerate eruption of the mandibular left second premolar. Six months later, the mandibular left second premolar still had not erupted. How would you proceed?

A: We decided to take a periapical radiographic of the mandibular left second premolar.

Q: A periapical radiograph was made (Figure 3.29a). What do you see? How would you proceed?

A: A supernumerary tooth is present, which may be blocking eruption of the mandibular left second premolar. We requested surgical extraction of the supernumerary tooth. We will continue to monitor eruption of the mandibular left second premolar.

  Occasionally (Figure 3.29b), ectopically erupting premolars will resorb mainly one primary molar root, leaving the other primary root essentially intact. The primary molar will remain nonmobile. How should

you proceed in a case such as this? We waited six more months, noted that the condition was unchanged, and extracted the primary second molar.

Q: Excluding wisdom teeth, what are the most common *missing* permanent teeth?

A: Second premolars [49–51].

Q: A patient presents to you with the parent's chief complaint, "We do not like the spaces between our daughter's front teeth." You make a panoramic image and complete mouth survey of the girl (Figure 3.30). What do you observe?

A: Oligodontia is noted (congenitally missing more than five permanent teeth), including her missing maxillary right second premolar, mandibular right second premolar, and mandibular left second premolar. In place of the three missing second premolars are the retained primary second molars. A developing maxillary left second premolar, with minimal root development, is also present. Other permanent teeth are missing.

Q: Can you state general recommendations for dealing with a retained primary tooth lacking a permanent successor?

A: Our recommendations are as follows:
- For non-extraction cases – *if the retained primary tooth has a good crown, good root, and good bone (not ankylosed), then consider maintaining it for the long term.* However, always have a contingency plan prepared in case the retained primary tooth is eventually lost. Such a contingency or "fallback" plan could include implant replacement.

(a)

(b)

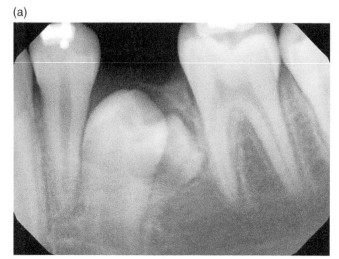
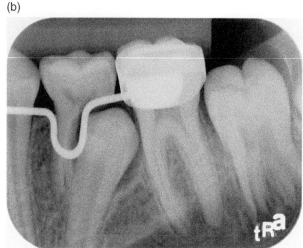

Figure 3.29 Two possible reasons for a delayed eruption of a permanent second premolar: (a) supernumerary tooth. This is a periapical radiograph of the mandibular left second premolar of the patient shown in Figure 3.28. (b) Ectopically erupting mandibular second premolar mainly resorbing the primary second molar distal root.

- Whenever possible, *avoid bonding (placing brackets on) retained primary teeth* in order to reduce the risk that their roots will resorb. If you must bond (place brackets on) retained primary teeth, then try to *avoid moving them*.
- For non-extraction cases – if the retained primary tooth does *not* have a good crown, root, or bone, then seriously consider extracting it.
- For extraction cases (e.g. cases involving severe anterior crowding) – consider extracting the retained primary tooth as one of your extraction treatment options.

Q: Based upon her dental spacing, we concluded that the patient in Figure 3.30 was to be treated non-extraction. Knowing this, and following our above guidelines, how would you deal with her three retained primary second molars lacking permanent successors?

A: Because all three retained primary second molars have *excellent crowns, roots, and alveolar bone heights* (*not ankylosed*), we chose to keep them. However, we informed the patient and parents that they may need to be replaced at some future date with implants.

Q: How would you deal with the underdeveloped maxillary left second premolar?

A: You have only two choices, either you can extract the underdeveloped premolar or you can give it some time to develop. We chose to monitor it, and we gave it one year to develop. If it developed, then we would maintain space for it and allow it to erupt. If it did not develop, then we would extract it and replace it with an implant or FPD.

Q: Some months later, we placed fixed orthodontic appliances and began leveling and aligning both arches. The maxillary left second premolar developed and erupted. Looking at the progress image in Figure 3.31, we feel that we did something foolish. Can you guess what that was?

A: It was foolish to place fixed appliances on the retained primary second molars. If we were to retreat this treatment today, we would *avoid bonding the retained primary teeth* in the hope that their roots would be less likely to resorb. Also, we would *avoid moving them*.

Q: After completion of orthodontic and prosthodontic treatment, a radiograph was made (Figure 3.32), followed by a final radiograph 10 years later (Figure 3.33). What do you observe?

A: The retained primary molars are intact. If root resorption of the primary molars has occurred, then it is not noticeable – even though they were bonded. The maxillary left second premolar developed, and erupted, beautifully.

   The maxillary right second permanent molar has super-erupted because it lacks an antagonist. If we could retreat this patient today, then we would place a right distal acrylic extension on the mandibular Hawley retainer to act as an antagonist for the maxillary right second molar (to prevent super-eruption).

Q: Can you suggest "take home pearls" regarding this patient's treatment (Figures 3.20–3.23)?

A: "Pearls" include the following:

(a)

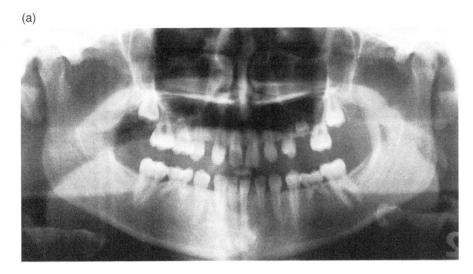

(b)

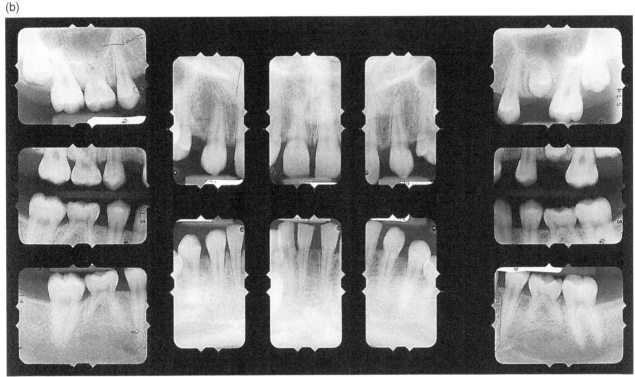

Figure 3.30 (a and b) Initial radiographs of a 15-year-old girl.

- Retaining this patient's primary second molars was a reasonable option because she was a non-extraction case, and because each primary second molar had *good crown, good root, and good bone*.
- Whenever possible, *avoid bonding and moving retained primary teeth*.
- The decision to monitor the underdeveloped maxillary left second premolar was prudent. One of the hardest things for orthodontists to do is to *wait* and give nature time to act.

- When you leave a tooth (e.g. the maxillary right permanent second molar) unopposed, retain the patient so that the unopposed tooth does not super-erupt. We neglected to do this here because the unopposed maxillary right second molar had not erupted at deband (Figure 3.32).

Q: There are two options for dealing with a retained primary tooth lacking a successor. You can extract the primary tooth or you can maintain it. In what cases

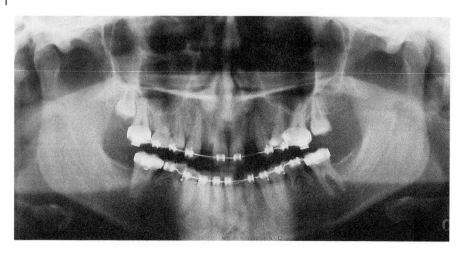

Figure 3.31 Progress image of the patient shown in Figure 3.30.

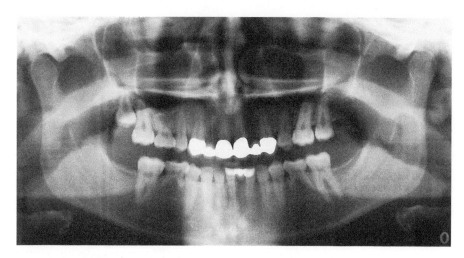

Figure 3.32 Radiograph of the same patient in Figure 3.30 following completion of all treatment.

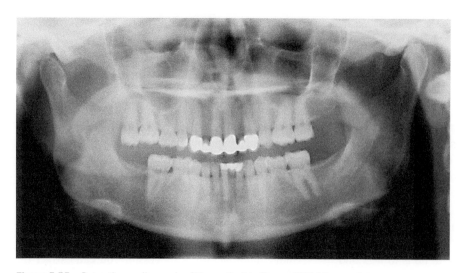

Figure 3.33 Retention radiograph of the patient in Figure 3.30 10 years later.

should you *extract* primary second molars lacking successors?

A: Extraction should be considered in:
- *Extraction* cases (e.g. patients with severe anterior crowding)
- Instances where caries, crown restoration, periodontal breakdown, or root resorption (Figure 3.34a) compromise the primary tooth's longevity – that is, where the primary molar exhibits *poor crown, poor root, or poor bone*.
- Instances where ankylosis/infraocclusion disturb occlusal development or bone level (Figure 3.34b, *poor bone*).

Q: If you decide to *extract* a retained primary second molar lacking a successor, what treatment options do you have for the extraction space?

A: Options include:
- Closing the extraction space entirely (Figure 3.35).
- Not closing the extraction space or closing it partially (e.g. closing it to the size of the missing second premolar for prosthetic replacement). Following primary second molar extraction (Figure 3.36), the edentulous ridge bucco-lingual *width* decreases by 25% within three years (30% within six years), while the edentulous ridge *height* decreases minimally by less than 2% [52].
- Restoring the extraction space using an implant when the patient reaches adulthood (Figure 3.37) or restoring with a fixed partial denture or removable partial denture.
- Autotransplantation using an extracted donor tooth from another site [53].

Q: Compare the left and right mandibular second premolar regions in Figure 3.38. What do you observe in this 12-year-old girl? What treatment, if any, would you recommend regarding these regions?

A: Her mandibular right second premolar is underdeveloped, erupting ectopically, and appears to be resorbing only the distal root of the mandibular right primary second molar. Her mandibular left premolar appears to be absent, but the mandibular left primary second molar appears to have a good crown, reasonable roots, and good bone level.

A decision was made to monitor eruption of the mandibular right second premolar and to maintain the retained mandibular left primary second molar. Comprehensive, non-extraction, orthodontic treatment was begun with space being maintained for both mandibular primary second molars.

Q: One year later, a progress radiograph was made (Figure 3.39). What do you now observe in the mandibular second premolar regions?

A: The mandibular right second premolar has resorbed the mandibular right primary second molar distal root and threatens to resorb the mandibular right permanent first molar mesial root. A clear step exists between both mandibular primary second molar alveolar bone crests and the alveolar bone crests of their adjacent teeth. That is, both mandibular primary second molars are *ankylosed*.

Q: How would you proceed with the patient in Figure 3.39?

A: Both mandibular primary second molars were extracted. Orthodontic treatment commenced and was completed before the mandibular right second premolar had erupted. The patient was placed in retention and followed periodically.

(a)

(b)

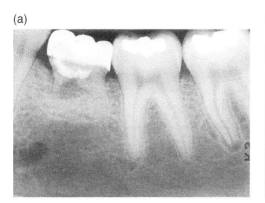
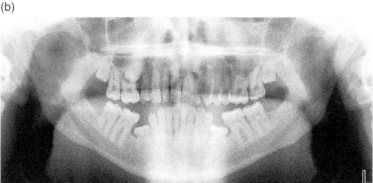

Figure 3.34 Examples where the retained primary second molar (lacking a successor) should be extracted: (a) significant restoration, caries, and root resorption threaten this primary tooth's longevity (*poor crown, poor root, poor bone*); (b) ankylosis/infraocclusion disturb occlusal development and inability to clean (*poor bone*).

(a)

(b)

(c)

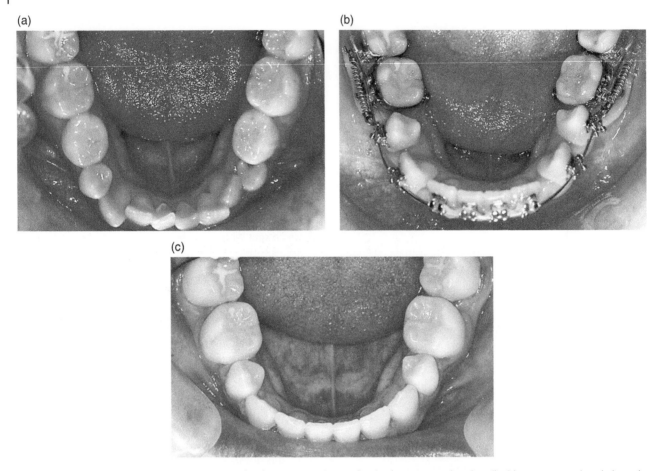

Figure 3.35 (a–c) For extraction cases, one option is to extract the retained primary second molars (lacking successors) and close the extraction space completely. Since nearly a centimeter of extraction space will need to be closed, the possibility of root resorption during tooth translation through bone must be discussed with the patient and parents.

Q: The patient returned at age of 16 years for a retention check (Figure 3.40). What do you observe in the mandibular second premolar regions?

A: The mandibular right second premolar erupted spontaneously, without surgical exposure, into a normal position with a normal alveolar crestal bone height. Extraction of the ankylosed mandibular right primary second molar followed our principle for ectopic tooth eruption treatment – *create a path and space for eruption!* The mandibular right permanent first molar mesial root appears to have suffered root resorption. The mandibular left edentulous area alveolar crest bone height appears to be normal.

Q: The favorable eruption of the mandibular right second premolar (Figures 3.28–3.30), following extraction of the mandibular right primary second molar, was not too surprising. However, the change in alveolar bone crest level of the mandibular left primary second molar region is fascinating. Can you state *what*

happened to the mandibular left crestal bone level during this time? Can you explain *why* this happened?

A: Look at the magnified images of the mandibular left primary second molar area during these years (Figure 3.41). At age 12 (Figure 3.41a), the alveolar bone crest of the mandibular left primary second molar (red arrow) appears to be at approximately the same level as the alveolar bone crest of the first permanent molar (yellow arrow).

By age 13 (Figure 3.41b), a large alveolar bone crest *step* exists between the mandibular left primary second molar and permanent first molar. How did this happen? Eruption of the mandibular left primary second molar had halted (ankylosed), while eruption of the mandibular left permanent first molar continued. At this time, a decision was made to extract the mandibular left primary second molar.

By age 16 (Figure 3.41c), the alveolar crest step between these teeth had disappeared (note the ghost image of the mandibular left primary second molar roots). What

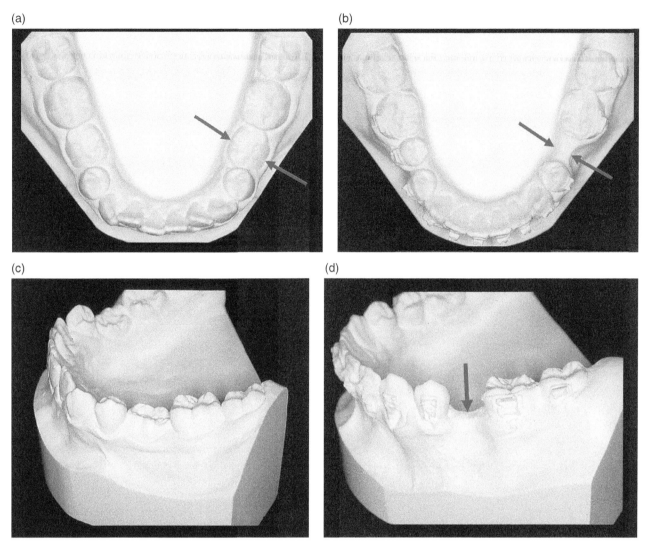

Figure 3.36 Following extraction of a retained primary second molar lacking a successor, (a and b) the bucco-lingual width of the edentulous ridge decreases into an hour-glass shape, but (c and d) the ridge height decreases minimally.

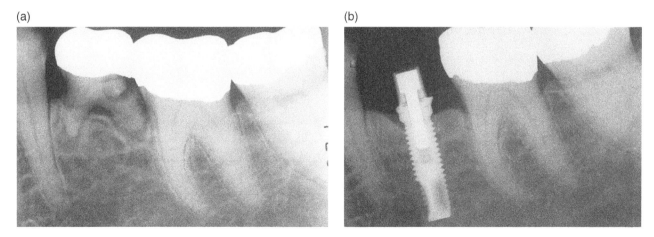

Figure 3.37 (a) Following extraction of a hopeless mandibular primary second molar in an adult, (b) the extraction space was restored with an implant.

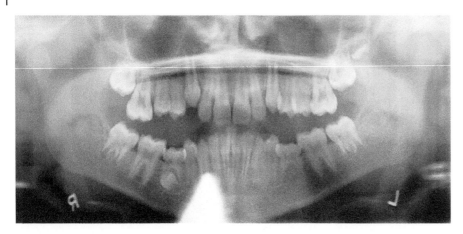

Figure 3.38 Initial panoramic image of a 12-year-old girl.

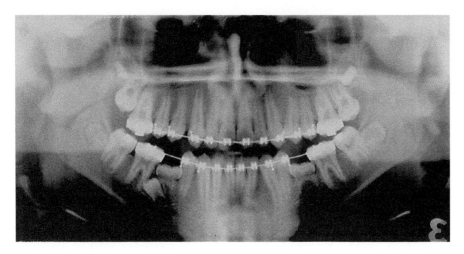

Figure 3.39 Progress radiograph of the same patient in Figure 3.38 at age 13 years.

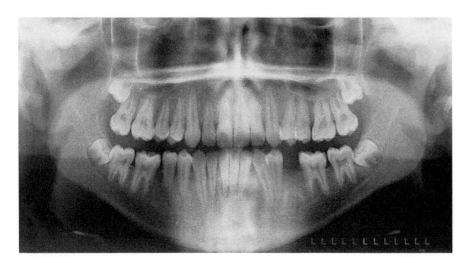

Figure 3.40 Panoramic image of the patient in Figure 3.38 at age 16 years.

(a) (b) (c)

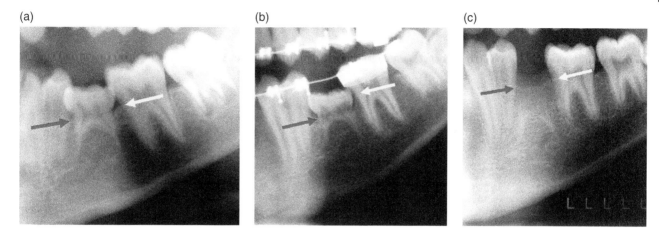

Figure 3.41 Magnified images of the mandibular left primary second molar region shown in Figure 3.39. Red arrows indicate alveolar bone crest level of the primary second molar, and yellow arrows indicate alveolar bone crest level of the permanent first molar at (a) age 12 years, (b) 13 years, and (c) 16 years.

happened? Following extraction of the mandibular left primary second molar, transeptal fibers from the mandibular left first premolar and mandibular left permanent first molar pulled vertically on the edentulous site crestal bone and elevated it [52].

Q: Why was elevation of the mandibular left alveolar bone crest to a normal level (Figures 3.41b and 3.41c) following extraction of the ankylosed mandibular left primary second molar so important?

A: Elevation of this crestal bone to a normal level is important for future bone grafting. In other words, grafting bone *vertically* can be very challenging while grafting bone bucco-lingually can be less so. Therefore, the fact that the bone elevated spontaneously can be of significant benefit when we wish to graft for implant placement later.

Q: What point can be drawn from Figure 3.41 regarding extraction of ankylosed primary second molars (without successors) in growing patients?

A: In patients having significant anticipated future growth, *it is prudent to extract ankylosed primary second molars as early as ankylosis is detected – so that normal vertical bone height of the edentulous area can be achieved.*

Q: But what if ankylosis of a primary second molar occurs later during growth. Should you extract the ankylosed primary second molar?

A: If the alveolar bone crest step is small between the ankylosed tooth and adjacent permanent teeth, if the ankylosed tooth exhibits good crown and root, if minimal future growth is anticipated (minimal future eruption of normal adjacent teeth/minimal worsening of the step), and if the patient can cleanse the ankylosed tooth,

then you could consider *maintaining* the ankylosed tooth. Note: you may wish to place an occlusal composite buildup on the ankylosed tooth to prevent the permanent first molar from tipping over it and to prevent teeth in the opposing arch from super-erupting.

Q: Can ankylosed mandibular primary second molars be used as anchorage to protract mandibular first permanent molars?

A: Yes, you can hemi-sect ankylosed primary second molars (Figures 3.42a and 3.42b), extract the distal roots (Figures 3.42c and 3.42d), and use the mesial roots as anchors for permanent molar protraction (Figure 3.42e). Of course, only one-half of the primary second molar space can be closed this way, and a second surgical procedure is required to remove the primary molars' mesial roots (unless they resorb). As an alternative option, the primary second molar can be extracted and a temporary anchorage device (TAD) inserted for protraction anchorage.

Q: Can any ankylosed primary tooth be used as anchorage?

A: Yes. Assuming their roots do not resorb, any ankylosed primary tooth can be used as a TAD. Your biomechanical creativity is the only limit to their usefulness.

Q: Some authors have suggested *early extraction* of primary second molars lacking permanent successors – in order to achieve bodily space closure with minimal therapy. However, there exists a danger in performing such early extractions [54, 55]. What is that danger?

A: The danger arises from *late tooth germ development*. As an example, compare the left and right mandibular second premolar regions in the eight-year-old shown

(a)　　　　　　　　　　(b)　　　　　　　　　　(c)

(d)　　　　　　　　　　(e)

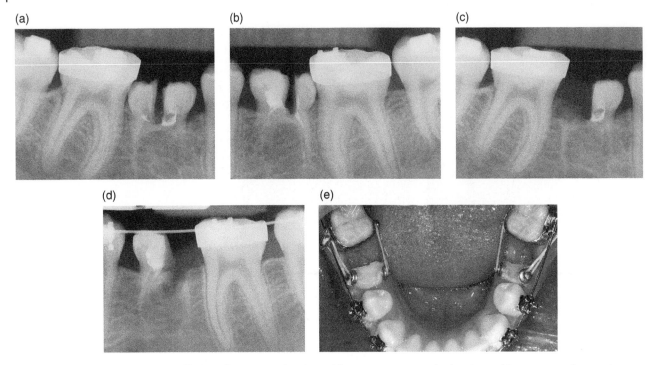

Figure 3.42 (a–e) Ankylosed mandibular primary second molars without successors can be hemisected for use as anchorage to protract mandibular molars.

below (Figure 3.43a). Compared to development of the mandibular left second premolar, agenesis of the mandibular right second premolar is suspected. However, it would be a mistake to extract the mandibular right primary second molar at this time (to expedite space closure). Why? Look at Figures 3.43b and 3.43c. What do you see? Crown development of the mandibular right second premolar is delayed but beginning to form. The point is this: avoid rushing to extract primary teeth lacking permanent successors. Give teeth time to develop. *When in doubt, wait it out.*

Q: What is "controlled slicing"?

A: Controlled slicing (Figure 3.44) of primary second molars (lacking permanent successors) is a technique used to produce bodily mesial movement of first permanent molars [56]. We are not advocates of this treatment due to the number of operative and surgical procedures required, including surgical hemi-section of the primary tooth.

Q: In what cases should you *maintain* primary second molars lacking successors?

A: Consider *maintaining* primary second molars in non-extraction cases (e.g. patients with minimal anterior crowding) where the primary second molars have *good crowns, good roots, and good bone.*

Q: If you decide to *maintain* a retained primary second molar, what treatment options are available for it?

A: Options include:

- Reducing the primary second molar mesiodistal width (~9.9 mm) to the width of a mandibular second premolar (~7 mm). This is termed "slenderizing" (Figures 3.45a–3.45c). It is done with the intent of eventually replacing the primary second molar with an implant crown the size of a second premolar. The reduced primary second molar maintains both mesiodistal space and alveolar process bone [52].

  This mesiodistal width reduction also permits the mandibular permanent first molar to be moved mesially into an ideal Class I molar relationship (Figure 3.45b). However, because the primary second molar roots diverge, its roots will resorb as the permanent teeth are brought into contact with them (Figure 3.45c).

- Maintaining the primary tooth intact, and restoring it with a composite (veneer) buildup to prevent super-eruption of opposing teeth and tipping of adjacent teeth (Figure 3.46a–c) [57].

Q: Which of these two maintenance options do you recommend: slenderizing the retained primary second molar lacking a successor or leaving the primary second molar intact?

(a)

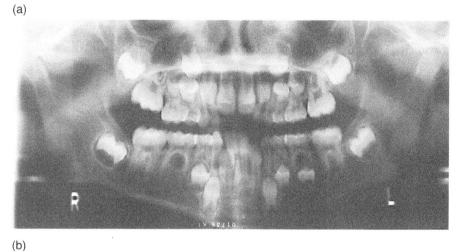

(b)

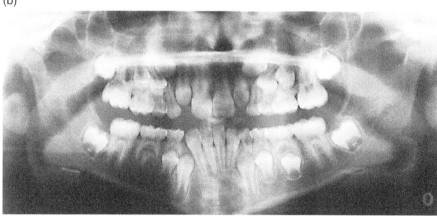

(c)

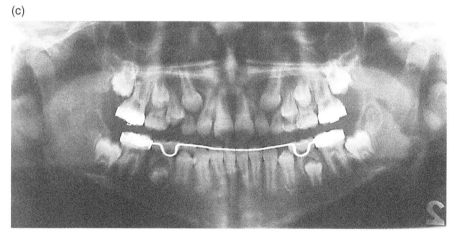

Figure 3.43 Late premolar crown development. (a) When comparing development of this patient's mandibular left second premolar to the right, agenesis of the right was suspected (b and c). However, the mandibular right second premolar was not missing, its development was merely delayed. It would have been a mistake to extract the mandibular right second primary molar early in order to expedite space closure.

A: We recommend leaving the retained primary second molar intact, not slenderizing it. Why? Although slenderizing creates space for the mandibular first permanent molar to be brought forward into an ideal Class I relationship, slenderizing can initiate root resorption of the primary second molar's bell-shaped roots – condeming the primary second molar and forcing future prosthetic replacement.

Leaving the retained primary second molar intact avoids initiating root resorption and increases the likelihood that

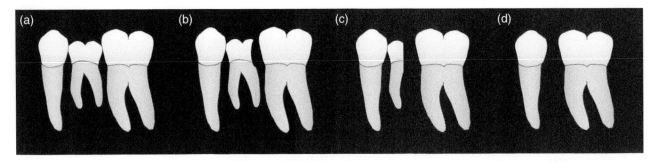

Figure 3.44 (a–d) Controlled slicing is a technique to achieve bodily first permanent molar mesial movement in the presence of retained primary second molars (lacking permanent successors).

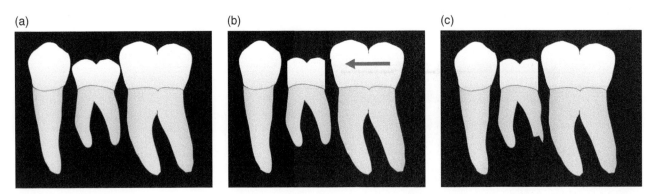

Figure 3.45 (a–c) Reducing the mesiodistal width of a primary second molar to the size of a missing mandiublar second premolar, or "slenderizing."

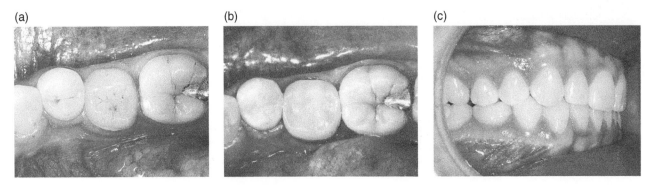

Figure 3.46 (a) If you keep a retained mandibular primary second molar lacking a successor, then (b) restoring it with a composite veneer buildup can prevent mesial tipping of the first permanent molar over the primary second molar and can prevent super-eruption of the opposing maxillary teeth. (c) Because of the large mesiodistal width of the retained primary second molar, the permanent first molar will be finished in an "end-on" relationship (Class II by 2–3 mm) when canines are Class I.

the primary second molar can be maintained long-term. The resulting "end-on" permanent first molar relationship is a small price to pay for leaving the primary second molar intact.

Q: But if a primary second molar is maintained intact, will it eventually be lost? What does the literature tell us about the longevity of retained primary second molars lacking permanent successors?

A: The literature reveals that:

- In children followed until their mid- to late 20s, ~90% of retained primary second molars lacking permanent successors survive [58, 59].
- In adults followed from a mean age of 36 years to a mean age of 49 years, 86% of retained primary second molars lacking permanent successors survive. Further, we discovered that even the primary second molars that were lost survived an average of more than a decade beyond the initial examination, which approximates the lifespan of some prosthetic appliances [60, 61].

- The above findings support the recommendation that if a retained primary second molar has a good crown, root, and bone in a non-extraction case, maintaining it intact is worthwhile (with a "fallback" plan in case it is eventually lost).

Q: Again, when do you recommend maintaining an *ankylosed* primary second molar lacking a permanent successor (step in alveolar bone crest level between anklylosed primary tooth and adjacent teeth)?

A: If the ankylosed primary second molar has good crown and root, if little or no future growth is anticipated, and if the patient can keep it clean, then consider maintaining it (Figure 3.47).

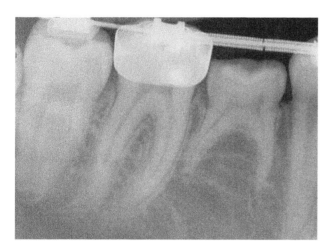

Figure 3.47 Maintaining an *ankylosed* mandibular primary second molar lacking a successor. Because minimal future growth of this patient was anticipated, because only a small alveolar bone crest step existed between the primary second molar and adjacent permanent teeth, because the patient could readily floss the ankylosed primary second molar, and because the primary second molar exhibited good crown and root, a decision was made to maintain the primary second molar in spite of it being ankylosed.

Q: Assume that you have a primary tooth lacking a successor that you hope to maintain. Should you band/bond or move the primary tooth?

A: If you can avoid doing so, *do not bond the primary tooth, do not band the primary tooth, and do not move the primary tooth* (Figure 3.48). Any of these actions increases the likelihood that the primary tooth roots will resorb and your chances of maintaining it will diminish.

Q: We have focused on retained primary second molars because second premolars are frequently missing. But can similar treatment planning and treatment options be applied to other retained primary teeth lacking permanent successors?

A: Yes. If a patient presents with any retained primary tooth lacking a permanent successor, then you should consider extracting the primary tooth if it is an extraction case and/or if the primary tooth has poor crown, poor root, or poor bone. If a patient presents with a retained primary tooth lacking a permanent successor, then you should consider maintaining the primary tooth if it is a non-extraction case and the primary tooth has good crown, good root, and good bone. If you maintain it, always have a contingency plan in place for the patient in case the primary tooth is eventually lost.

Q: A child presents to you in the late mixed dentition with a retained mandibular left primary lateral incisor (lacking a successor) together with a missing mandibular right permanent lateral incisor (Figure 3.49a, magnified view Figure 3.49b). You plan to treat the patient without extracting permanent teeth and with prosthetic replacement of the missing right permanent lateral incisor. Look closely at the mandibular left primary lateral incisor. Would you recommend extracting the mandibular left primary lateral incisor or maintaining it?

(a)

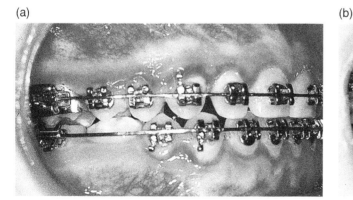

(b)

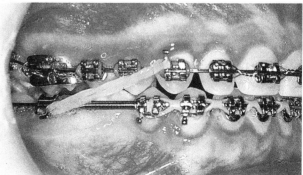

Figure 3.48 (a) If you wish to maintain a primary tooth, avoid bonding it, banding it, or moving it – any of which actions could initiate root resorption. (b) To maintain space for the primary tooth trap a closed coil spring along the archwire. Even with the trapped closed coil spring shown here, the primary second molar roots could resorb as Class II elastic force pulls the permanent first molar and primary second molar forward.

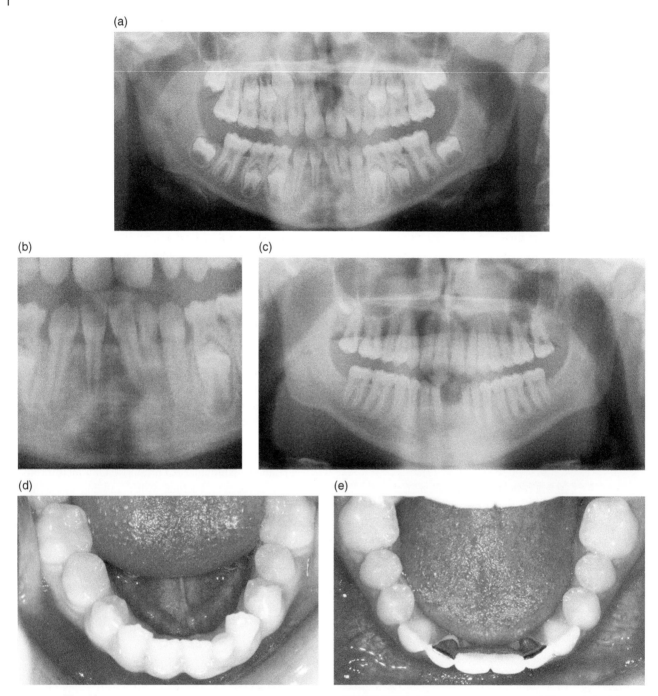

Figure 3.49 (a and b) Child in the late mixed dentition with a retained mandibular left primary lateral incisor lacking a successor and missing a mandibular right permanent lateral incisor Because the bone level of the mandibular left primary lateral incisor was poor (enveloping only one half to two thirds of the root), a decision was made to extract it and open space for two prosthetic central incisors (Figure 3.49c). Before and after intraoral photos of the mandibular arch (Figures 3.49d and 3.49e).

A: Close radiographic examination of the retained mandibular left primary lateral incisor reveals a *poor bone level*, only one half to two thirds of its root is embedded within bone. For this reason, we recommended extracting it. Following extraction, space was created (Figure 3.49c) for a bonded FPD. Intraoral photos (Figures 3.49d and 3.49e) illustrate before and after treatment.

An argument could have been made for maintaining the mandibular left primary lateral incisor, or at least its root (decoronation), in order to maintain the alveolar process bone for as long as possible. If this were done, then the patient would need to be informed that eventual prosthetic replacement (implant, FPD) would be anticipated.

Q: Consider a more complicated example. A child presents to you with retained mandibular primary second molars, retained maxillary primary lateral incisors, and retained maxillary primary canines. None of the retained primary teeth have successors (Figure 3.50a). For the purpose of this example, assume that the patient would normally be treated as an extraction case (four first premolar teeth extracted). Examining Figure 3.50a closely, would you recommend extracting or maintaining the six retained primary teeth?

A: Start with the mandible. The retained primary second molars have good crowns, *poor (resorbed) roots*, and good bone levels. Although in a non-extraction case we might argue for maintaining the mandibular primary second molars in order to maintain bone, extracting these primary teeth makes sense here in order to avoid extracting first premolars.

If we extract the mandibular primary second molars, then the patient and parent must be informed of potential root resorption during space closure. If significant root resorption occurs (as seen on a progress panoramic image made after six to nine months of space closure), then we may need to terminate space closure and treat the remaining space with prostheses.

Now consider the maxilla. Here, we have four retained primary teeth without successors. Their roots and bone levels appear poor, and their long-term survival is questionable. So, in this extraction case we chose to keep all maxillary premolars and extract the maxillary primary teeth. We extracted maxillary primary canines, substituted maxillary first premolars as canines, and maintained the maxillary primary lateral incisors for as long as possible in order to keep bone. We planned to eventually extract the maxillary primary lateral incisors and replace them with prostheses.

Figure 3.50b is a progress radiograph following extraction of mandibular primary second molars, extraction of maxillary primary canines, fixed appliance placement, leveling and aligning of both arches, and mandibular space closure. Significant mandibular posterior tooth root resorption is noted. The patient and parents were informed of this, and a decision was made to complete treatment as soon as possible. The maxillary primary lateral incisors were very mobile and extracted at deband (Figure 3.50c). Bonded fixed partial dentures were placed to maintain space for eventual implants (Figure 3.50d), and wisdom teeth were extracted.

Q: Can you suggest "take home pearls" for retained primary teeth lacking permanent successors?

A: "Take home pearls" include the following:
- There are only two options for dealing with retained primary teeth lacking successors. You can either *extract* the retained primary teeth or you can attempt to *maintain* them.
- For non-extraction cases – *if the retained primary tooth has a good crown, good root, and good bone, then consider maintaining it for the long term* (Figure 3.51). But, be sure to have a contingency plan prepared in case the retained primary tooth is eventually lost.
- Whenever possible, *avoid bonding/banding retained primary teeth* in order to reduce the risk that their roots will resorb. If you must bond/band retained primary teeth, try to *avoid moving them*.
- Consider extracting retained primary teeth lacking successors: (i) in extraction cases (e.g. patients with severe anterior crowding); (ii) in instances where caries, crown restoration, periodontal breakdown, or root resorption compromise the primary tooth's longevity; and (iii) and in instances where ankylosis/infraocclusion disturb occlusal development/bone level.
- Even in non-extraction cases – if the retained primary tooth does *not* have a good crown, root, or bone, seriously consider extracting it.
- If you *extract* a retained primary tooth lacking a successor, then treatment options for the extraction space include not closing the space at all; closing the space partially; closing the space entirely; restoring the extraction space with an implant, fixed partial denture, or removable partial denture; or autotransplanting a tooth donated from another site into the space.
- In patients having significant anticipated future growth, it is prudent to extract ankylosed primary teeth as soon as ankylosis is detected – so that normal *vertical* crestal bone height of the edentulous site can be achieved.
- If you decide to *maintain* a retained mandibular primary second molar lacking a successor, then treatment options include reducing the mesiodistal width of the primary second molar to the size of a missing mandibular second premolar ("slenderizing") with the intent of eventually replacing the narrower primary second molar with an implant; or maintaining the primary tooth intact, and restoring it with a composite (veneer) buildup to prevent super-eruption of opposing teeth or tipping of adjacent teeth. We recommend the latter option.
- In all orthodontic treatments, always have a "fallback plan" in case your primary plan (e.g. maintaining a primary tooth) fails.

Q: Let's finish this section by introducing the concept of early treatment permanent first molar extractions. Suppose a pediatric dentist forwards a panoramic

(a)

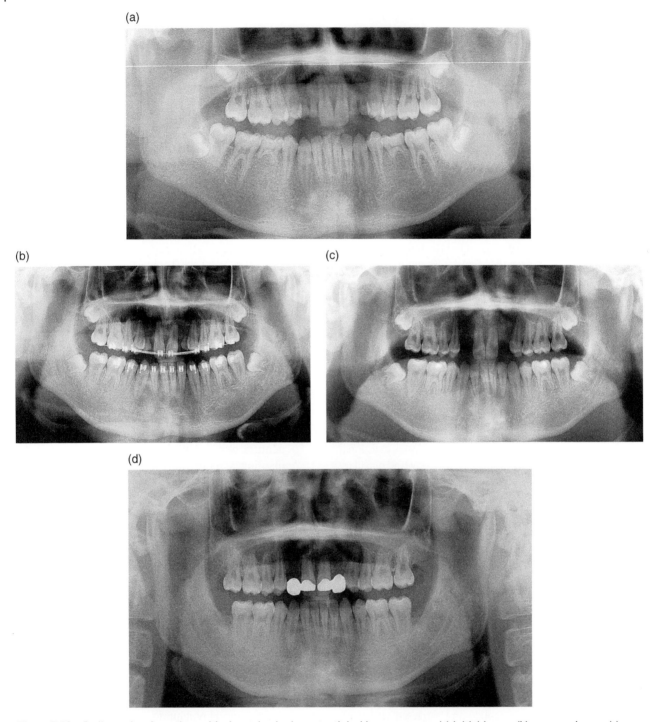

(b)

(c)

(d)

Figure 3.50 Radiographs of a patient with six retained primary teeth lacking successors: (a) initial image, (b) progress image, (c) deband image (note the mucous retention cyst in the left maxillary sinus which will be monitored), (d) after placement of bonded maxillary bridges to maintain lateral incisor space until future implants are provided.

radiograph of a 10-year-old girl to you (Figure 3.52). Due to severe decay/severe hypocalcification, he recommends extraction of all four permanent first molars. He hopes that the permanent second molars will erupt to replace the extracted permanent first molars. He

asks your opinion. What factors should you consider that will influence your opinion?

A: Extraction of *any* tooth is a surgical procedure and should never be taken lightly. A decision to extract compromised permanent first molars in a developing

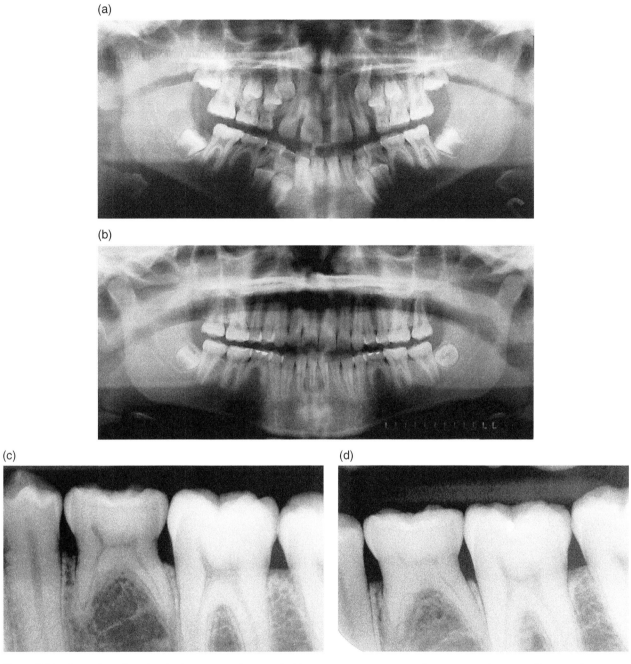

Figure 3.51 Examples of retained primary second molars lacking permanent successors in non-extraction cases. Because the mandibular primary second molars presented with good crowns, good roots, and good bone levels, decisions were made to maintain the primary second molars with treatment in (a and b) an adolescent, and (c and d) in an adult (21 years of age and 45 years of age, respectively).

occlusion must be arrived at after an exhaustive review of the patient's circumstances, malocclusion, and the feasibility of successful orthodontic treatment in the future. Key factors in the decision include [62]:

- Underlying malocclusion
- Presence and stage of development of second molars

- Potential cooperation of the child with restorative or orthodontic treatment
- Likely future preventive practice within the family
- Fact that spontaneous space closure is more difficult to achieve in the mandible than in the maxilla following first permanent molar extractions [63].

If the pediatric dentist deems the permanent first molars to be non-restorable and hopeless, then there is no choice. The permanent first molars should be extracted to prevent infection. However, if any of the permanent first molars are questionable, then you should examine the patient, make records, and perform a complete diagnosis and treatment plan. Communication with the pediatric dentist, parents, and child will be of paramount importance. In the case of the girl shown in Figure 3.52, an examination was conducted, discussions held, and a decision was made to remove all permanent first molars except the mandibular left permanent first molar.

Q: The panoramic image of a 10-year-old boy is sent to you by his family dentist (Figure 3.53). The dentist noted severe caries of all four permanent first molars and says, "The boy's four permanent first molars are hopeless and I need to extract them. But if I extract them, will the second molars (including the ectopically-erupting mandibular left second molar) erupt into acceptable positions?" How do you respond?

A: Never guarantee the future eruption of any tooth. However, eruption of the boy's maxillary second molars and mandibular right second molar is likely. The dentist and parents were informed that eruption of the mandibular left second molar would be monitored, that surgical exposure of it may be necessary, and that future comprehensive orthodontic treatment should be anticipated. The dentist first extracted the maxillary right permanent first molar (Figure 3.54) and then the remaining permanent first molars. Fortunately, all four second molars erupted (Figure 3.55).

Case Brody

Q: Brody is 10 years and 9 months old (Figure 3.56). He has been referred to you by his pediatric dentist because his maxillary left central incisor remains unerupted. All other incisors display normal eruption. His PMH, PDH, periodontal evaluation, and TMJ evaluations are WRN. CR = CO. Compile your diagnostic findings and problem list for Brody. Also, state your diagnosis.

A:

Table 3.1 Diagnostic findings and problems list for Brody.

Full face and profile	*Frontal view*
	Face is symmetric
	Long soft tissue LAFH (soft tissue Glabella – Subnasale < Subnasale – soft tissue Menton)
	Lip competence
	Lack of eruption of maxillary left central incisor
	Profile view
	Convex profile
	Obtuse NLA
	Obtuse lip-chin-throat angle
	Retrusive chin projection

(*Continued*)

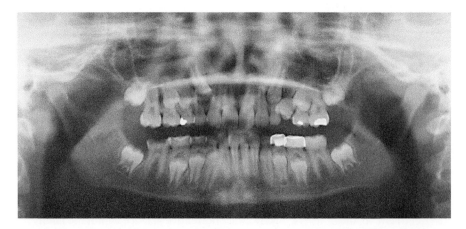

Figure 3.52 Panoramic image of a 10-year-old girl having severe decay/severe hypocalcification of all four permanent molars.

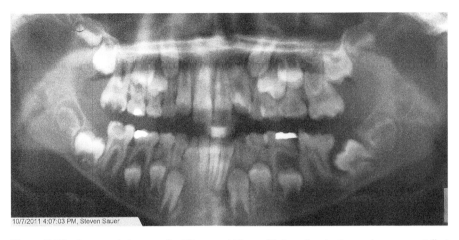

Figure 3.53 Panoramic image of a 10-year-old boy with hopelessly decayed permanent first molars and ectopic eruption of a mandibular left second molar.

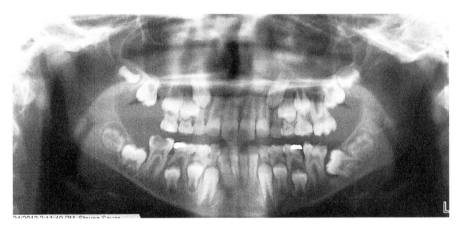

Figure 3.54 Patient shown in Figure 3.53 six months later following extraction of his maxillary right permanent first molar.

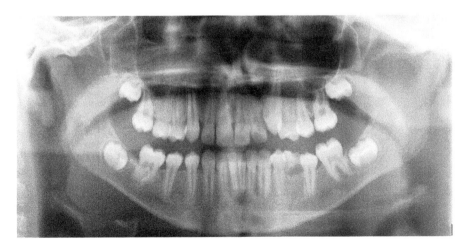

Figure 3.55 Patient shown in Figure 3.53 three years later following extraction of all four permanent first molars. All four permanent second molars erupted.

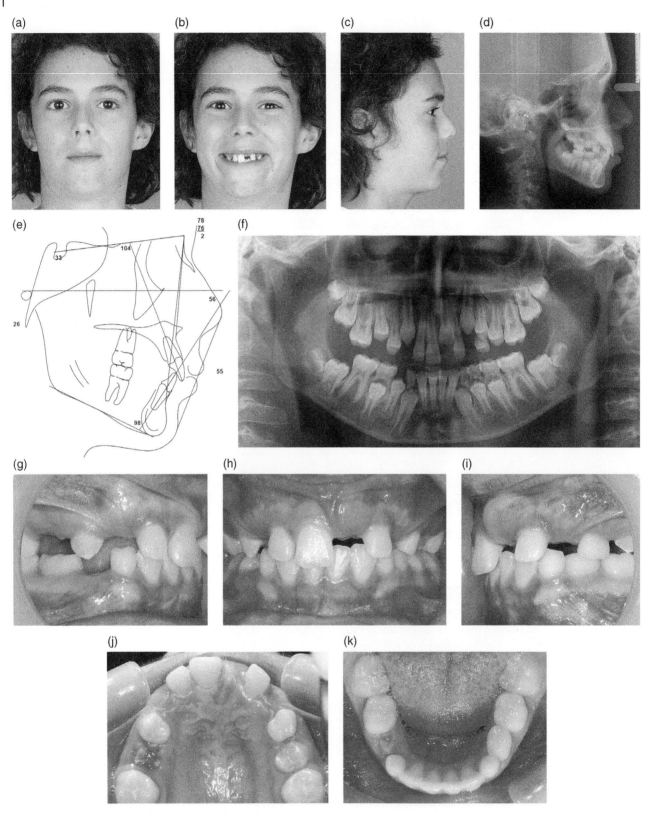

(a)

(b)

(c)

(d)

(e)

78
76
2

104

33

56

26

55

98

(f)

(g)

(h)

(i)

(j)

(k)

Figure 3.56 Initial records of Brody: (a–c) facial photographs, (d and e) lateral cephalometric radiograph and tracing, (f) pantomograph, (g–k) intraoral photographs, (l–p) models.

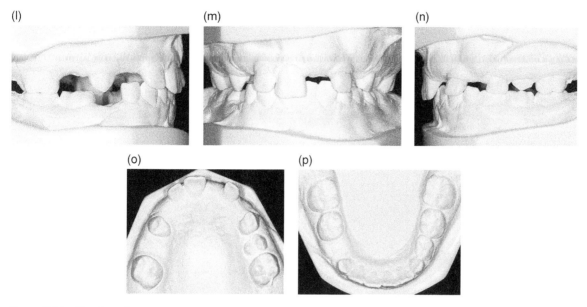

(l) **(m)** **(n)**

(o) **(p)**

Figure 3.56 (Continued)

Table 3.1 (Continued)

Ceph analysis	***Skeletal***
	Deficient maxillary anteroposterior position (A-Point lies behind Nasion-perpendicular line)
	Deficient mandibular anteroposterior position (ANB angle = 2° but maxilla is deficient anteroposteriorly)
	Skeletal LAFH WRN (ANS-Menton/ Nasion-Menton X 100% = 55%)
	Mandibular plane angle WRN (FMA = 26°; SNMP = 33°)
	Effective bony Pogonion (Pogonion lies ahead of a line extended from Nasion through B-point)
	Dental
	Maxillary incisor inclination WRN (U1 to SN = 104°)
	Proclined mandibular incisor inclination (FMIA = 56°)
Radiographs	Late mixed dentition
	Delayed eruption of maxillary left central incisor
	The facial surface of the maxillary left central incisor is prominent in the labial alveolar cortical plate (Figure 3.56d)
Intraoral Photos and Models	Angle Class II division 1
	Iowa Classification: II (2–3mm) X (canine missing) X (canine missing) II (2–3 mm)
	OJ ~1 mm
	OB 60% (based upon maxillary right central incisor)
	Unerupted maxillary left central incisor (open bite)
	4.0 mm maxillary anterior crowding currently present (difference between space available for unerupted maxillary permanent canines and left central incisor versus their anticipated widths)
	2.5 mm maxillary crowding is anticipated if space maintenance is employed
	0.0 mm mandibular incisor crowding is currently present
	0.6 mm mandibular spacing is anticipated if proper space maintenance is employed
	Maxillary and mandibular dental arches are symmetric
Other	None
Diagnosis	Class II malocclusion with unerupted maxillary left central incisor

Q: How can Brody have a convex profile and a deficient mandible when his ANB angle is normal (2 degrees)?

A: The answer lies in the fact that *both* his mandible and maxilla are retrusive. In other words, draw a line vertically down from Nasion (Figure 3.57a, green line) passing perpendicular to FH (blue line). This line is called the Nasion perpendicular line (see Appendix). An *ideal maxillary anteroposterior position is one in which A-Point lies on the Nasion perpendicular line* [64, 65].

Brody's A-Point lies significantly behind Nasion perpendicular, indicating that his maxilla is deficient anteroposteriorly. With A-Point being deficient, we cannot use ANB angle to judge mandibular position.

(a)

(b)

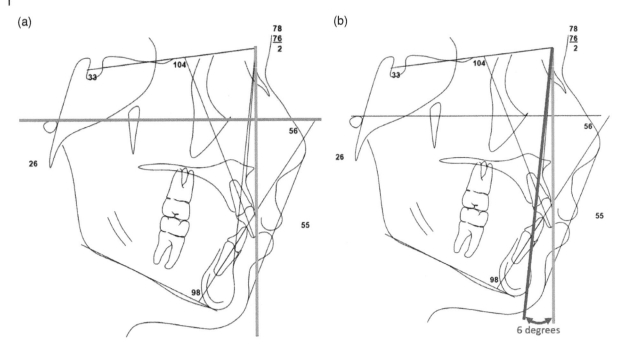

Figure 3.57 Judging mandibular skeletal position when the maxillary anteroposterior position is not ideal. (a) Brody's maxilla is deficient, as illustrated by the fact that A-Point lies behind Nasion-perpendicular line (green line); (b) because Brody's maxilla is deficient, we cannot use ANB angle to judge his mandibular anteroposterior skeletal position. Instead, we use the angle formed between Nasion-perpendicular and Nasion-B Point lines.

Instead, we relate his mandibular position *to* Nasion perpendicular, measuring the angle formed between Nasion perpendicular and the N-B line (Figure 3.57b, red line). In Brody's case, this angle equals 6 degrees, indicating a deficient mandible, which corroborates our clinical impression of a convex profile and retrusive chin position.

Q: Provide a detailed space analysis for Brody's maxillary and mandibular arches. How were the 2.5 mm of maxillary arch crowding and 0.6 mm of mandibular arch spacing calculated (if space maintenance is employed)?

A:

Below are space estimates:
Average mesiodistal widths of permanent teeth (mm) [66]:

Maxillary Central Incisor	8.5	Mandibular Central Incisor	5.0
Maxillary Lateral Incisor	6.5	Mandibular Lateral Incisor	5.5
Maxillary Canine	7.5	Mandibular Canine	7.0
Maxillary First Premolar	7.0	Mandibular First Premolar	7.0
Maxillary Second Premolar	7.0	Mandibular Second Premolar	7.0
Maxillary First Molar	10.0	Mandibular First Molar	11.0
Maxillary Second Molar	9.0	Mandibular Second Molar	10.5

Average mesiodistal widths of *primary* teeth (mm) [66]:

Maxillary Central Incisor	6.5	Mandibular Central Incisor	4.2
Maxillary Lateral Incisor	5.1	Mandibular Lateral Incisor	4.1
Maxillary Canine	7.0	Mandibular Canine	5.0
Maxillary First Molar	7.3	Mandibular First Molar	7.7
Maxillary Second Molar	8.2	Mandibular Second Molar	9.9

Maxillary Arch

+8.2 mm space available for maxillary right second premolar

−7.0 mm anticipated width of maxillary right second premolar

+6.8 mm space available for maxillary right permanent canine

−7.5 mm anticipated width of maxillary right permanent canine

+6.8 mm space available for maxillary left permanent central incisor

−8.5 mm anticipated width of maxillary left central incisor

+5.9 mm space available for maxillary left permanent canine

−7.5 mm anticipated width of maxillary left permanent canine

+7.3 mm width of maxillary left primary first molar

−7.0 mm anticipated width of maxillary left first premolar

+1.0 mm space mesial to maxillary left second premolar

Balance = +8.2 mm −7.0 mm + 6.8 mm −7.5 mm +6.8 mm −8.5 mm +5.9mm −7.5 mm +7.3 mm −7.0 mm +1.0 mm = −2.5 mm

Mandibular Arch (since the mandibular right primary first molar is missing, we cannot use right leeway space)

0 mm of mandibular anterior crowding

+20 mm arch perimeter length from mesial of right permanent first molar to mesial of right primary canine

−7.0 mm anticipated width of mandibular right permanent canine

−7.0 mm anticipated width of mandibular right first premolar

−7.0 mm anticipated width of mandibular right second premolar

+1.6 mm of anticipated left leeway space (1.6 mm/side)

Balance = 0 mm +20 mm −7.0 mm −7.0 mm −7.0 mm +1.6 mm = +0.6 mm

That is, *2.5 mm of maxillary arch crowding and 0.6 mm of mandibular arch spacing is anticipated following eruption of all permanent teeth (if proper space maintenance is employed).*

Q: What are Brody's *primary* problems in each dimension – plus other problems that you must stay focused on?

A:

Table 3.2 Primary problems list for Brody.

	Angle Class II Iowa Classification: II (2–3 mm) X X II (2–3 mm)
AP	
Vertical	OB 60%
Transverse	—
Other	Unerupted maxillary left central incisor

Q: Are you concerned with the maxillary left central incisor's lack of eruption? Is the eruption timing of Brody's other permanent teeth normal?

A: Average ages of permanent tooth eruption (emergence through gingival tissue) are listed below [67]. At ten years and nine months of age, Brody exhibits delayed eruption of his maxillary left central incisor – *by almost three years.* We should be concerned that it has not erupted.

Eruption of his mandibular permanent canines appears delayed by about one year, but they will erupt soon. Eruption of all other permanent teeth appears to be on-track.

	Maxillary	Mandibular
Central Incisor	7–8	6–7
Lateral Incisor	8–9	7–8
Canine	11–12	9–10
First Premolar	10–11	10–12
Second Premolar	10–12	11–12
First Molar	6–7	6–7
Second Molar	12–13	11–13

Q: Can you list possible etiologies for Brody's maxillary left central incisor's delayed eruption (open bite)?

A: Possible eruption etiologies include:

- *Delayed tooth development* – looking at Figure 3.56f, the root apex of the maxillary left central incisor appears to have a more open apex than the right central incisor (delayed development). Although difficult to tell from this radiographic view, if an open apex is suspected, additional periapical radiographs can confirm (or deny) the diagnosis. This was not done.
- *Thick keratinized tissue blocking eruption* – looking at Figures 3.56h and 3.56j, we feel that a thick band of gingival tissue is present, which could delay eruption.
- *Lack of space (tooth impaction)* – is probably not the cause. There appears to be a small amount of space (Figure 3.56f) between the mesial of the unerupted maxillary left central incisor crown and the root of the maxillary right central incisor. Furthermore, even though there appears to be inadequate space for the maxillary left central incisor crown to erupt aligned (Figure 3.56j), it could still erupt into a rotated position.
- *Tongue interposition habit or digit-sucking habit* – are not likely causes since the maxillary right central incisor erupted normally and since the maxillary left central incisor has not even pierced the gingiva (where a habit could prevent its eruption).
- *Temporary open bite occurring after normal exfoliation of the primary left central incisor* – is not a likely cause since the pediatric dentist has been concerned with this problem for many months.
- *Ankylosis of the maxillary left central incisor* – is a possible cause. However, we could not locate previous dental radiographs, so we are unsure whether the maxillary left central incisor has ceased erupting or is simply erupting slowly.
- *Premature loss of maxillary left primary central incisor* – is a possible cause since scar tissue could have filled in

over the permanent incisor crown following premature loss of the primary tooth. However, Brody's mother states that the maxillary left primary central incisor was not lost early.

Q: *When* should Brody's Class II relationship be addressed? *How* would you address it?

A: *Now* is the appropriate time to address Brody's Class II problem because he is entering the late mixed dentition stage of development. There is no advantage in treating Class II relationships in the early mixed dentition except possibly a reduction in incisal trauma [68–74] (unless the patient shows good statural growth). However, if we wait until all of Brody's permanent teeth erupt to begin Class II treatment, then we will miss useful jaw growth.

Of the three options for treating a Class II skeletal discrepancy (orthopedics, camouflage, and surgery), orthopedics is the most reasonable option at Brody's stage of development. Class II skeletal orthopedics consists of either restricting maxillary forward growth (while permitting the mandible to continue growing forward) and/or accelerating mandibular growth. Class II orthopedic options include headgear and functional appliance treatment.

- High-pull headgears work in growing individuals by restricting maxillary forward growth, distalizing maxillary molars, possibly reducing maxillary corpus descent and maxillary molar eruption, and allowing the mandible to continue growing forward. Cervical-pull headgears restrict maxillary forward growth, distalize maxillary first molars, create anterior palatal plane downward rotation, and erupt maxillary first molars by less than 1 mm [75–78].
- Class II functional appliances (e.g. Herbst appliance) work in growing individuals by restricting maxillary forward growth, distalizing maxillary posterior teeth, advancing mandibular posterior teeth, accelerating condylar growth, and displacing the glenoid fossae anteriorly. Functional appliances do *not* enhance mandibular horizontal growth beyond that found in control subjects [79–84].

Q: Brody has a *retrusive* maxilla. Why would you recommend applying a headgear force to a maxilla which is already deficient?

A: This is an excellent question. We investigated profile esthetic changes resulting from headgear use in growing Class II patients with protrusive, normal, and *retrusive* maxillae [85]. Based upon the results of our study, we concluded that in growing Class II patients, headgear treatment in conjunction with fixed orthodontic appliances is effective in improving facial profile esthetics for everyone, including Class II patients with *retrusive* maxillae.

Q: Brody has proclined mandibular incisors. Would you recommend Class II functional appliance treatment in patients with proclined mandibular incisors?

A: The answer to this question is based upon the *magnitude* of the incisor proclination. Mandibular incisor proclination (or uprightness) depends not only upon the angulation of the incisors relative to the mandible itself (IMPA) but also upon the steepness of the mandible plane (MPA), and is reflected in the FMIA angle. An ideal FMIA is approximately 65–68°.

If a skeletal Class II adolescent presents with mild mandibular incisor proclination (e.g. FMIA = 64–60°), then we would look upon Class II functional appliance treatment more favorably than if the adolescent presents with severe incisor proclination (e.g. FMIA = 50–45°). Why? Class II functional appliance treatment will increase mandibular incisor proclination. Since Brody's FMIA = 56°, in our clinical opinion he is borderline for Class II functional appliance treatment.

Q: Discuss Brody in the context of three principles applied to every early treatment patient.

A: Principles include:

1) The goal of early treatment is to correct developing problems – get the patient *back to normal for their stage of development* (including preventing complications such as resorption of adjacent tooth roots, reducing later treatment complexity, or eliminating unknowns). Correcting Brody's unerupted maxillary left permanent central incisor, Class II relationship, and 60% OB would get Brody back on track.

2) Early treatment should address *very specific problems with a clearly defined end point*, usually within six to nine months. Surgical exposure and forced eruption of his maxillary left central incisor could bring it into the arch in less than nine months (assuming that it is not ankylosed). Since he has entered the late mixed dentition stage of development, and since his Class II relationship is mild (2–3 mm), correction of his Class II relationship could probably be completed in less than one year if he cooperated. OB correction could be achieved in less than nine months using fixed orthodontic appliances to level his arches.

3) Always ask: Is it necessary that I treat the patient now? *What harm will come if I choose to do nothing*

now? There would be no harm in waiting a year to surgically expose and erupt Brody's maxillary left central incisor, *unless it is ankylosed* and a vertical bony defect worsens as adjacent teeth continue to erupt. We anticipate no harm in waiting one year to address Brody's mild Class II relationship. Finally, since no pain or tissue damage is resulting from his 60% OB, there is no need to address this problem now.

Q: What unknowns will you face in treating Brody?

A: Unknowns include jaw growth magnitude and direction, the possibility that his maxillary left central incisor is ankylosed, an undetected CR-CO shift, cooperation, and hygiene.

Q: Should space maintenance be employed?

A: An LLHA is recommended in order to use the 1.6 mm left leeway space to eliminate the 1 mm anticipated crowding on the right side (+20 mm arch perimeter length from mesial of right permanent first molar to mesial of right primary canine, −7.0 mm anticipated width of mandibular right permanent canine, −7.0 mm anticipated width of mandibular right first premolar, −7.0 mm anticipated width of mandibular right second premolar = −1 mm). A Nance holding arch would be useful in the maxilla unless a headgear or Herbst appliance was employed to retract the maxillary first permanent molars distally.

Q: What options can you suggest for dealing with his unerupted maxillary left central incisor?

A: Options include:
- *Recall* (no treatment, monitor only) – reevaluate in six months. This option is reasonable if Brody does not object to having a large space in his smile. If the maxillary left central incisor has not pierced the gingiva in six months, then a radiograph should be made to determine whether it is slowly erupting. If it is erupting, then a decision to continue monitoring would be reasonable. If it is not erupting, then more aggressive treatment should be considered.
- *Space regaining* – to open approximately 2 mm additional space for the maxillary left central incisor crown (8.5 mm total space, Figure 3.56j) using fixed orthodontic appliances. This option is reasonable while you monitor the central incisor's eruption.
- *Surgical exposure of the maxillary left central incisor's incisal edge (gingivectomy)* – is reasonable in the hope that creating a pathway through the thick gingival band will aid the central incisor's eruption.
- *Surgical exposure of maxillary left central incisor's entire crown with apically repositioned flap followed by forced orthodontic eruption* – would be a viable option once we are certain that the central incisor is not going to erupt spontaneously. If we request surgical expose of the entire crown, then we should ask the surgeon to determine (using gentle elevator luxation) whether the left central incisor is mobile or ankylosed. If it is ankylosed, then a decision must be made either to break the ankylosis and quickly erupt the tooth orthodontically, or to extract it.

Two points should be mentioned regarding apically repositioned flaps with high (very apical) tooth exposures. First, it may be impossible for the surgeon to place a very high apically repositioned flap successfully. Second, as the tooth is erupted, soft tissue will stretch – leading to potential posttreatment intrusion (relapse). In cases of high exposures, it is often best to first erupt the tooth into the arch without an apically repositioned flap and then to request a soft-tissue grafting procedure later to provide keratinized attached gingival tissue [86, 87].

Q: What is your recommended treatment? How would you proceed?

A: We banded Brody's maxillary and mandibular first permanent molars, placed him on a high-pull headgear which he wore at night and delivered an LLHA. Brody did not care about having the missing maxillary left central incisor space for another six months, and we decided to monitor its eruption.

If it did not erupt, then we would make a new radiograph to determine whether it was erupting slowly. At that time, we also planned to make a decision whether to expose the maxillary left central incisor incisal edge with a laser (removing the thick band of gingiva which we suspected was preventing it from erupting) or to surgically expose the entire crown, determine whether it was ankylosed, and either orthodontically erupt it or extract it.

Q: During the next six months, Brody corrected his Class II relationship with headgear wear and the maxillary left central incisor's incisal edge pierced the gingiva. Intraoral photographs (Figure 3.58) were made at the age of eleven years and six months. What do you note? How would you proceed at this time?

A: Brody's maxillary left central incisor erupted into labioversion. He is Class I, all permanent teeth are nearly erupted, and *early treatment is complete.* Comprehensive treatment will commence as soon as the remaining permanent teeth are fully erupted. Teeth will be banded/bonded, arches leveled and aligned, and remaining spaces closed.

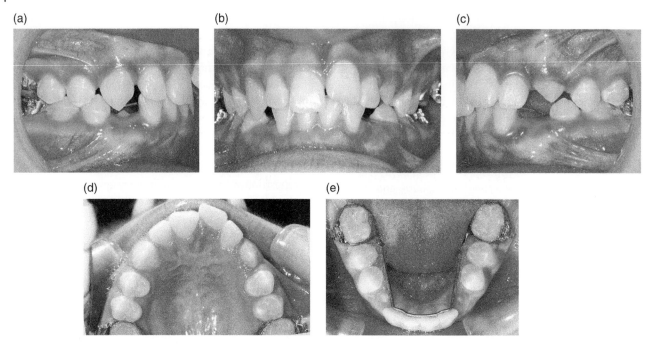

Figure 3.58 (a–e) Progress photos of Brody.

Q: Can you suggest "take-home pearls" regarding Brody's treatment?

A: "Take-home pearls" include the following:

- Brody was 10 years and 9 months old when he presented in the late mixed dentition as Class II (2-3mm) with delayed eruption of the maxillary left permanent central incisor.
- Possible etiologies of this delayed eruption included delayed dental development, thick keratinized gingival tissue blocking/slowing eruption, lack of space (tooth impaction), tongue interposition or digit interposition habit, temporary open bite occurring after normal exfoliation of the primary left central incisor, ankylosis of the maxillary left permanent central incisor, and premature loss of the maxillary left primary central incisor. In retrospect, the etiology was probably thick gingiva covering the incisor or delayed dental development.
- If Brody's maxillary left incisor had not erupted spontaneously, then our next step would have been to *clear a path* for it by performing laser gingivectomy of the thick band of gingival tissue at its incisal edge. We have witnessed instances where such a gingivectomy resulted in rapid spontaneous tooth eruption toward the occlusal plane. It gingivectomy was unsuccessful, then we would have performed a full crown surgical exposure of the incisor and attempted orthodontic eruption.

Case Rebecca

Q: Rebecca is ten years and two months old (Figure 3.59). She is being followed by her general dentist for "delayed eruption of teeth." Her PMH, PDH, periodontal evaluation, and TMJ evaluations are WRN. CR=CO. Compile your diagnostic findings and problem list for Rebecca. Also, state your diagnosis.

A:

Table 3.3 Diagnostic findings and problems list for Rebecca.

Full face and profile	*Frontal view*
	Face is symmetric
	Long soft-tissue LAFH (soft-tissue Glabella – Subnasale < Subnasale – soft-tissue Menton)
	Lip competence
	Missing central incisors in smile
	Profile view
	Relatively straight profile
	Obtuse NLA
	Chin projection WRN
	Lip-chin-throat angle WRN
Ceph analysis	*Skeletal*
	Maxillary anteroposterior position WRN (A-Point lies on Nasion-perpendicular line)

Mandibular anteroposterior position WRN (ANB angle = 3° with maxilla WRN)

Long skeletal LAFH (ANS-Menton/Nasion-Menton X 100% = 58%; however, Rebecca is slightly open on her lateral cephalometric radiograph)

Mandibular plane angle WRN (FMA = 27°; SNMP = 33°)

Effective bony Pogonion (Pogonion lies on or ahead of a line extended from Nasion through B-point)

Dental

Proclined maxillary incisor inclination (unerupted maxillary central incisor to SN = 114°)

Proclined mandibular incisor inclination (FMIA = 57°)

Radiographs

Permanent dentition

Unerupted maxillary right central incisor

Ectopic eruption (possible impaction) of maxillary left central incisor

Intraoral photos and models

Angle Class I

Iowa Classification: I I I I

OJ ~0 mm (based upon maxillary lateral incisors)

Anterior open bite

Erupting maxillary right central incisor is beginning to pierce the gingiva

Missing maxillary left central incisor

OB 10–20% (based upon maxillary lateral incisors)

2 mm of future maxillary arch crowding anticipated (15 mm space currently present but 8.5 mm required for two erupting central incisors)

2.0 mm mandibular incisor crowding currently present

Maxillary right permanent canine facial composite resin over-contoured (Figure 3.59j)

Maxillary and mandibular dental arches are symmetric

Other

None

Diagnosis

Class I malocclusion with anterior open bite due to partially erupted maxillary right central incisor and possibly impacted ectopically erupting maxillary left central incisor

Q: Were we correct in classifying Rebecca's profile as relatively *straight* (Figure 3.59c)? Could her profile be classified as mildly convex?

A: This is a good question, and we had difficulty choosing her classification. On the one hand, her profile does curve down and back from her nose and maxillary lip (convex). On the other hand, soft-tissue Pogonion sits slightly ahead of her zero-meridian line (vertical line drawn down from soft tissue Nasion and perpendicular to Frankfort horizontal) indicating adequate chin projection. Considering both aspects of her profile, we chose to classify it as relatively straight, especially since her maxillary and mandibular anteroposterior skeletal positions are both normal.

Q: Is our "A-Point" location correct?

A: We were forced to *estimate* where to place A-Point (Figure 3.59d). Why? A-Point is the most concave point of the anterior maxilla and should be located approximately 1–2 mm ahead of the maxillary central incisor roots (1–2 mm being the presumed thickness of the alveolar process bone over the central incisor roots). In Rebecca's cephalometric radiograph, it was difficult to determine this location because of the unerupted central incisors.

Q: What are Rebecca's *primary* problems in each dimension, plus other problems?

A:

Table 3.4 Primary problems list for Rebecca.

AP	—
Vertical	Anterior open bite
Transverse	—
Other	Partially erupted maxillary right central incisor
	Ectopically erupting (possibly impacted) maxillary left central incisor

Q: The timing of Rebecca's permanent tooth eruption is unusual (Figure 3.59f). Why?

A: She exhibits both delayed *and* early eruption. Average ages of permanent tooth eruption (emergence through gingival tissue) are listed below [67]. At 10 years of age, Rebecca exhibits delayed eruption of her maxillary central incisors by at least two years but *early* eruption of her maxillary canines, maxillary second molars, mandibular second premolars, and mandibular second molars.

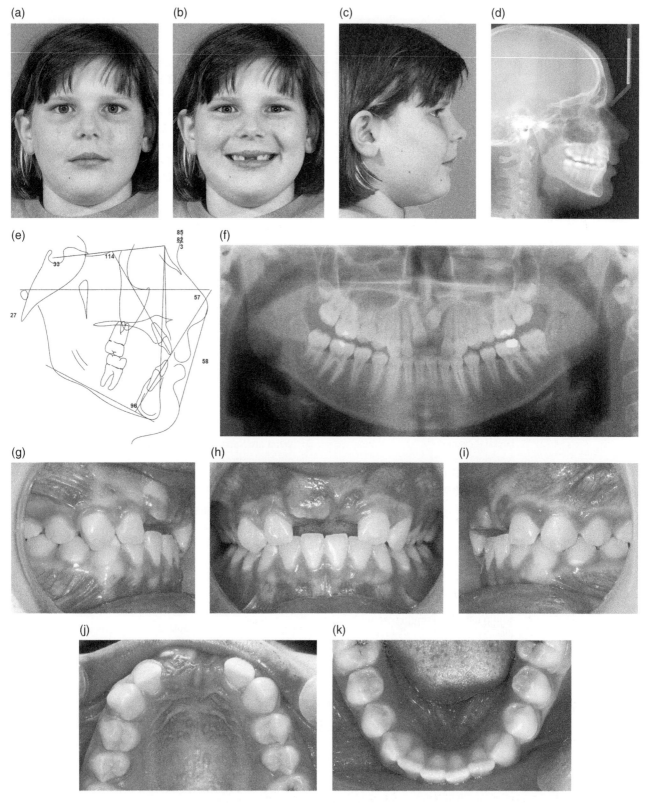

Figure 3.59 Initial records of Rebecca: (a–c) facial photographs, (d and e) lateral cephalometric radiograph and tracing, (f) pantomograph, (g–k) intraoral photographs. Note that Rebecca's posterior teeth are slightly separated in her lateral cephalometric radiograph.

	Maxillary	Mandibular
Central Incisor	7–8	6–7
Lateral Incisor	8–9	7–8
Canine	11–12	9–10
First Premolar	10–11	10–12
Second Premolar	10–12	11–12
First Molar	6–7	6–7
Second Molar	12–13	11–13

Q: What is the etiology of her maxillary central incisors delayed eruption?

A: Both maxillary central incisors appear to have dilacerations which could delay their eruption [88]. The maxillary right central incisor appears to be impacting the ectopically erupting maxillary left central incisor. Is the maxillary left central incisor pushing against the right central incisor and preventing its full eruption?

There are other possible causes of this delayed eruption, including ankylosis, blockage from other developing structures (supernumerary teeth, odontomas), blockage from surgical/traumatic scaring, premature loss of primary teeth (scarring/bone formation), and thick keratinized gingival tissue blocking eruption of the right central incisor.

Q: Is there anyone you should contact who might help determine the delayed eruption etiology?

A: Yes, ask Rebecca's general dentist for any history he/she could provide.

Q: Her dentist sends you the panoramic image made two years earlier (Figure 3.60). What do you observe in the region of her maxillary central incisors?

A: Rebecca's maxillary primary central incisors are retained (her maxillary permanent lateral incisors have already erupted). There appears to be two supernumerary teeth apical to the primary central incisors with the permanent central incisors apical to the two supernumeraries.

Q: How would you have dealt with the central incisor situation shown in Figure 3.60?

A: We would have recommended proceeding in the same way that the general dentist did – by *creating a pathway and space* for the permanent central incisors to erupt. The general dentist extracted the primary central incisors and both supernumeraries, and then she monitored eruption of the permanent incisors.

Q: Your treatment goal is to get Rebecca back on track for her stage of development. Thankfully, she is normal in the anteroposterior, vertical, and transverse dimensions (Figure 3.59), but her remaining problem is her maxillary central incisors, which have erupted a limited amount during the previous two years.

Should you continue to monitor maxillary central incisor eruption or recall Rebecca? If you start treatment, what treatment options would you consider?

A: Your options include the following:
- *Recall* (monitor only) – reevaluate in one year. Since the maxillary right central incisor's distal incisal edge is piercing the gingiva (Figure 3.59h), it would be reasonable to recommend monitoring it. If it continues to erupt, then it could make room for the maxillary left

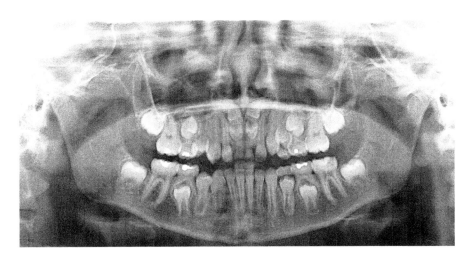

Figure 3.60 Panoramic image of Rebecca made at age eight.

central incisor to erupt. However, we feel that spontaneous eruption of the left central incisor is unlikely.

- *Surgical exposure of maxillary central incisor crowns* – then, monitor eruption. Since the maxillary right central incisor is nearly erupted, and since it is piercing the gingiva, it will most likely erupt without additional treatment. Removing additional attached tissue from the maxillary right central incisor crown could accelerate its eruption. Exposing the maxillary left central incisor may, or may not, aid its eruption.
- *Surgical exposure of maxillary central incisor crowns followed by forced eruption* – could bring both incisors into the arch (unless either is ankylosed).

Q: Always ask: Is it necessary that I treat the patient now? *What harm will come if I choose to do nothing now?*

A: Possible risks of monitoring only include:
- A vertical bony defect worsening if the maxillary central incisors are ankylosed and adjacent teeth continue to erupt
- The ectopically erupting maxillary left central incisor continuing to erupt ectopically and resorbing the root of the maxillary right central incisor
- Concern that Rebecca could be teased about her missing incisors.

Q: What unknowns do you face?

A: An undetected CR-CO shift, ankylosis of the maxillary central incisors, and cooperation.

Q: What is your recommended treatment? How would you proceed?

A: At her case presentation appointment, Rebecca's Class I relationship was confirmed. Always check the bite, and check for the presence of a CR-CO shift, at every appointment. If you do not, and if an undetected CR-CO shift exists, then it could radically impact your treatment outcome.

Rebecca did not want us to monitor her maxillary incisor eruption any longer. She wanted treatment. We consulted her dentist – who removed the composite veneer covering Rebecca's maxillary right permanent canine labial surface. We fabricated, and placed, a Nance holding arch. Why? The acrylic button of the Nance holding arch would resist reactive intrusive and crown tipping forces on the maxillary (anchorage) teeth when an *extrusive* eruptive force was applied to the maxillary central incisors.

The maxillary teeth (excluding the maxillary left central incisor) were bonded. As the maxillary arch was leveled, the maxillary right central incisor erupted (Figure 3.61). Next, the maxillary left central incisor was surgically exposed with an apically positioned flap (Figure 3.62)

to provide a band of keratinized gingival tissue. The surgeon gently luxated the left central incisor with an elevator and reported that the left central incisor was mobile, not ankylosed. Elastic traction was applied (Figures 3.62d and 3.62e), the left central incisor was erupted into the arch, the mandibular arch was bonded, and both arches were leveled, aligned, and finished (Figure 3.62f).

Q: Rebecca's deband records were made at age twelve (Figure 3.63). What changes do you note?

A: Changes include the following:
- Rebecca's smile has improved dramatically with eruption of her permanent maxillary central incisors. However, there appears to be excessive mesial crown tip of her maxillary right central incisor (Figure 3.63b), which is distracting. This tip is not apparent on her intraoral frontal view (Figure 3.63f). If the tip is noticed again during a retention visit, then it may be corrected using simple incisal edge enameloplasty.
- Increased chin projection (compare Figures 3.63c–3.59c).
- All permanent teeth have erupted with good root alignment (Figure 3.63d).
- Dilacerations are seen in the roots of both maxillary central incisors, but their root lengths appear normal and no root resorption is noticeable.
- Maxillary and mandibular midlines are coincident (Figure 3.63f).
- Poor oral hygiene has resulted in inflamed and hypertrophied gingiva.
- Minimal OB (10%) and minimal OJ (0 mm) are noted.
- Development/eruption of her wisdom teeth will be monitored.

Q: Was the amount of deband OB adequate?

A: In our opinion, no. Orthodontic eruption of teeth can be unstable, especially orthodontic eruption following an apically repositioned flap procedure where the attached keratinized tissue is stretched during eruption. If we could retreat Rebecca, then we would increase her OB at deband to 30%, hold her in that position for months, and then closely monitor her for openbite relapse.

Q: What retention protocol would you recommend for Rebecca?

A: Rebecca was placed in removable Hawley retainers and asked to wear them at night, for life. Lifelong retention is the only guarantee that alignment of teeth can be guaranteed.

In retrospect, Rebecca should be retained as an *openbite patient*. In other words, she should be placed in

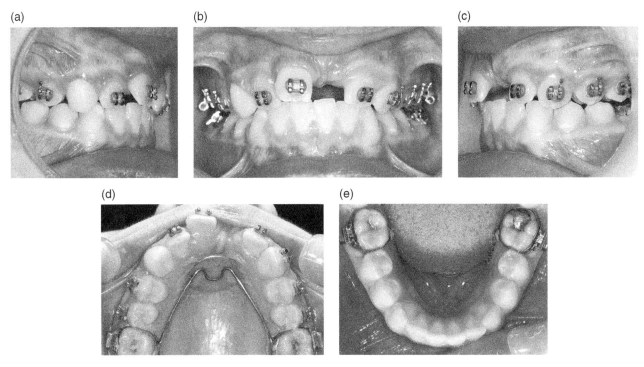

Figure 3.61 (a–e) Progress records of Rebecca.

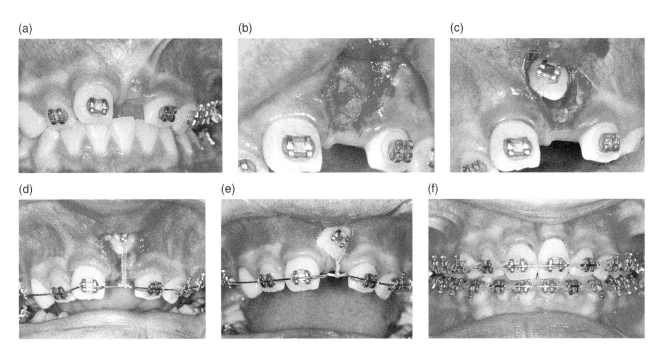

Figure 3.62 (a–f) Progress records of Rebecca.

clear, vacuum-formed retainers with small tooth-colored blebs of composite bonded onto the labial surfaces of her maxillary incisors. The clear retainers would *snap* over the blebs and prevent her central incisors from relapsing apically. Also, the clear retainer material covering the posterior occlusal surfaces would act as a bite plate to reduce posterior tooth eruption during further growth. We would ask her to wear these clear retainers full time, except when eating, for a year or more.

Q: Can you suggest "take-home pearls" regarding Rebecca's treatment?

A: "Take-home pearls" include the following:

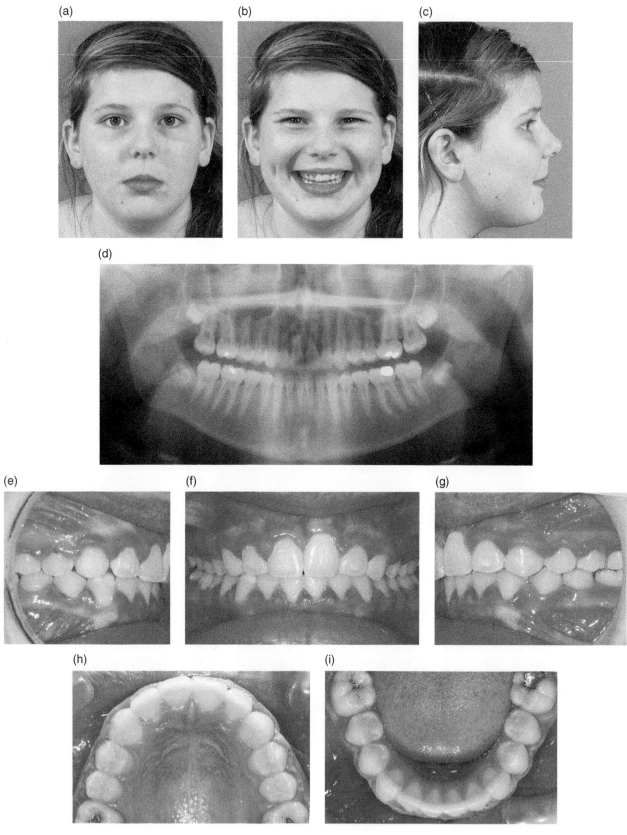

Figure 3.63 (a–i) Deband records of Rebecca.

- Rebecca presented when she was ten years old. She was developing normally except for delayed maxillary permanent central incisor eruption. Two years earlier her maxillary primary central incisors and two supernumerary central incisors had been extracted. Her maxillary right permanent central incisor was partially erupted, but her left central incisor was ectopically erupting/possibly impacted. Rebecca was successfully treated with surgical exposure of her left central incisor and orthodontic eruption of both maxillary central incisors.

- Rebecca highlights the importance of taking thorough dental (and medical) histories of patients at the consultation/records appointment. We initially failed to ask Rebecca's parents for information about her delayed central incisor eruption. It was not until after we examined her records that we sought counsel from her family dentist and discovered the history.

- Her delayed maxillary permanent central incisor eruption resulted from the presence of supernumerary teeth (and retained primary central incisors) that blocked the permanent central incisor eruption and probably contributed to their dilaceration development.

- Rebecca was treated by her family dentist appropriately. In other words, the doctor *cleared a path for the unerupted central incisors to follow*. Surgical exposure, and orthodontic eruption, was performed because Rebecca was no longer willing to wait for further eruption. Also, we suspect that the maxillary left central incisor may never have erupted unaided.

- If we could treat Rebecca again, then we would recommend exposure of the maxillary left central incisor without an apically repositioned flap. Why? It was a *high* exposure (Figure 3.62c). As the maxillary left central incisor is erupted, the apically repositioned keratinized tissue will be stretched – increasing the likelihood of relapse (posttreatment apical movement of the incisor). Instead, we would recommend exposing the maxillary left central incisor enamel with a small window at its incisal edge, erupting the incisor with orthodontics, and then having the surgeon place a keratinized gingival graft later, if needed.

- We are always concerned with long-term retention of teeth that are orthodontically erupted. We should have retained Rebecca using clear vacuumed-formed retainers (with small composite blebs bonded on the labial surface of the maxillary central incisors). However, Rebecca failed to return for follow-up retention visits so we could do this.

Case Alicia

Q: Alicia is nine years and seven months old (Figure 3.64). She presents to you with the chief complaint, "My teeth are crooked." Her PMH, PDH, periodontal, and TMJ evaluations are WRN. CR=CO. Compile your problem list and make a diagnosis.

A:

Table 3.5 Diagnostic findings and problems list for Alicia.

Full face and profile	***Frontal view***
	Face is symmetric
	3–4 mm interlabial gap
	Mildly exaggerated cupid's bow
	Soft-tissue LAFH WRN (soft-tissue Glabella – Subnasale approximately equal to Subnasale – soft-tissue Menton)
	UDML WRN
	Excessive gingival display in posed smile (maxillary central incisor gingival margins 3–4 mm below the maxillary lip)
	Profile view
	Straight profile
	Chin projection WRN
	Obtuse NLA
	Lip-chin-throat angle WRN
	Chin-throat length WRN
Ceph analysis	***Skeletal***
	Maxillary anteroposterior position WRN (A-Point lies approximately on Nasion-perpendicular line)
	Mandibular anteroposterior position WRN (ANB angle = 2° with maxillary anteroposterior position WRN)
	Long skeletal LAFH (LAFH/TAFH X 100% = 58%; normal = 55% with sd = 2%)
	Normal FMA (27°) but steep SNMP (39°)
	Effective bony Pogonion (Pogonion lies forward of extended Nasion-B Point line)
	Dental
	Upright maxillary central incisors (U1 to SN = 96°)
	Upright mandibular incisors (FMIA = 82°)
Radiographs	Early mixed dentition
	Ectopic eruption of mandibular lateral incisors
	Blocked and potentially impacted mandibular permanent canines and first premolars
	Delayed eruption of maxillary right central incisor
	Premature loss of mandibular right primary first molar (Figure 3.64g)

(Continued)

Table 3.5 (Continued)

Intraoral Photos and Models	Angle Class I Iowa Classification: I I I I 10–20% OB of left central incisors Anterior open bite of right central incisors Left anterior crossbite of maxillary central and mandibular lateral incisors 7.8 mm maxillary anterior crowding is currently present (5 mm of incisor crowding with 1.4 mm of additional space needed for right and left permanent lateral incisors) 5.8mm maxillary arch crowding is anticipated following eruption of all permanent teeth (if proper space maintenance is employed) 6.8mm mandibular anterior crowding is currently present (4mm of incisor crowding with 1.4mm of additional space needed for right and left permanent lateral incisors) 3.6mm mandibular arch crowding is anticipated following eruption of all permanent teeth (if proper space maintenance is employed) Premature loss of mandibular right primary first molar *without space loss* Ectopic eruption of mandibular lateral incisors Midlines are coincident Minimal posterior OJ of right permanent first molars Maxillary and mandibular dental arches display symmetric arch forms Thick periodontal biotype labial to the mandibular anterior teeth
Other	
Diagnosis	Class I malocclusion with moderate anterior crowding and ectopically erupting mandibular lateral incisors

Q: Why did we state that the eruption of Alicia's maxillary right permanent central incisor is delayed?

A: Average ages of permanent tooth eruption (emergence through gingival tissue) are listed below [67]. At the age of nine years and seven months, the emergence of her maxillary right central incisor is delayed by nearly two years.

	Maxillary	Mandibular
Central Incisor	7–8	6–7
Lateral Incisor	8–9	7–8
Canine	11–12	9–10
First Premolar	10–11	10–12
Second Premolar	10–12	11–12
First Molar	6–7	6–7
Second Molar	12–13	11–13

Q: What is the cause of the delayed eruption of Alicia's maxillary right permanent central incisor?

A: We cannot be sure. An excellent review of delayed tooth eruption is provided by Suri et al. [88] wherein a range of possible causes is provided, including ankylosis, blockage from other developing structures (supernumerary teeth, odontomas), blockage from surgical/traumatic scaring, premature loss of primary teeth (scarring/bone formation), arch-length deficiency, thick keratinized gingival tissue blocking eruption, and many others.

Q: Is there anything you wish to check for or ask Alicia regarding her open bite? Is her open bite a *dental* open bite? Is her open bite a *skeletal* open bite?

A: We checked for an anterior interpositional tongue habit that was absent. We asked Alicia if she had a thumb-sucking habit or other habit. She denied having any habits. Her *dental* open-bite features include the fact that her:

- Anterior open bite is limited to her right incisors.
- Maxillary right central incisor is stepped up compared to her posterior teeth.
- Maxillary right central incisor's eruption is delayed, but the incisor is erupting.

Next, consider each feature of a skeletal open bite and see if it exists in Alicia:

- Long *soft-tissue* LAFH (soft-tissue Glabella – Subnasale < Subnasale – soft tissue Menton) – Alicia does *not* exhibit this feature. Her soft-tissue LAFH is approximately equal to her midface height.
- ILG ≥ 2 mm without a short upper lip (suggesting that vertical soft tissue facial growth has not kept pace with vertical skeletal growth) – Alicia does *not* exhibit this feature. While she exhibits a 3–4 mm ILG, that ILG is partially due to an exaggerated cupid's bow.
- Long *skeletal* LAFH – Alicia *does* exhibit this feature (LAFH/TAFH $\times$ 100% = 58%).
- Cant of the palatal plane (PNS much lower than ANS due to excess maxillary posterior vertical growth compared to anterior maxilla) – Alicia does *not* exhibit this feature.
- Lack of posterior face height development – Alicia does *not* exhibit this feature. If her posterior face height was short, then we would expect to see a steep FMA. Instead, Alicia exhibits a normal FMA (27°).
- Steep MPA – Alicia *does* (SNMP = 39°) and does *not* (FMA = 27°) exhibit this feature. SNMP is probably steep due to a low sella.
- Anterior open bite extending posteriorly beyond the canines – Alicia does *not* exhibit this feature.

In summary, Alicia exhibits a long skeletal LAFH but lacks other features commonly found in skeletal open bites. We believe that Alicia's limited anterior open bite is a *dental* open bite due to a delayed transition from primary to permanent dentition. However, we recommend monitoring her future vertical facial growth closely.

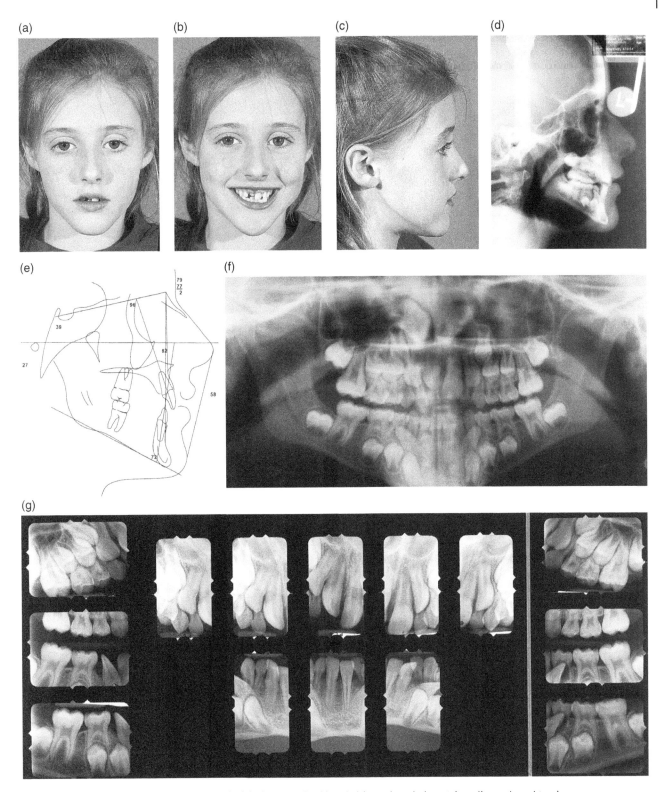

Figure 3.64 Initial records of Alicia: (a–c) facial photographs, (d and e) lateral cephalometric radiograph and tracing, (f) pantomograph, (g) full mouth series of radiographs, (h–l) intraoral photographs, (m–q) model photographs. Note: her panoramic image was made before the mandibular right primary first molar exfoliated.

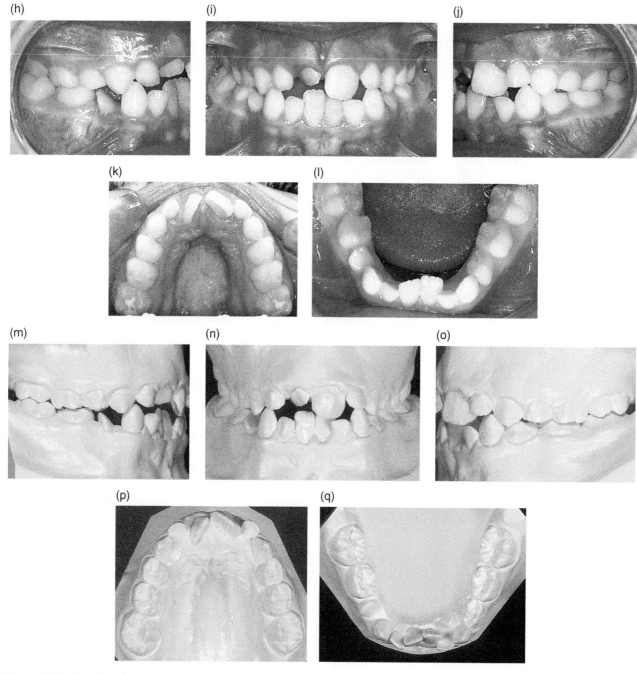

Figure 3.64 (Continued)

Q: Provide a detailed space analysis for Alicia's maxillary and mandibular arches. In other words, how were the anticipated 5.8 mm maxillary arch crowding and 3.6 mm mandibular arch crowding calculated (*if proper space maintenance is employed*)?

A:

Average mesiodistal widths of permanent teeth (mm) [66]:

Maxillary Central Incisor	8.5	Mandibular Central Incisor	5.0
Maxillary Lateral Incisor	6.5	Mandibular Lateral Incisor	5.5
Maxillary Canine	7.5	Mandibular Canine	7.0
Maxillary First Premolar	7.0	Mandibular First Premolar	7.0

Maxillary Second Premolar	7.0	Mandibular Second Premolar	7.0
Maxillary First Molar	10.0	Mandibular First Molar	11.0
Maxillary Second Molar	9.0	Mandibular Second Molar	10.5

Average mesiodistal widths of *primary* teeth (mm) [66]:

Maxillary Central Incisor	6.5	Mandibular Central Incisor	4.2
Maxillary Lateral Incisor	5.1	Mandibular Lateral Incisor	4.1
Maxillary Canine	7.0	Mandibular Canine	5.0
Maxillary First Molar	7.3	Mandibular First Molar	7.7
Maxillary Second Molar	8.2	Mandibular Second Molar	9.9

Maxillary Arch

−5.0 mm of maxillary anterior crowding is currently present (Figures 3.64k and 3.64p)
+5.1 mm width of right primary lateral incisor
−6.5 mm anticipated width of right permanent lateral incisor
+5.1 mm width of left primary lateral incisor
−6.5 mm anticipated width of left permanent lateral incisor
+2 mm of anticipated leeway space (1 mm/side)
Balance = −5 mm +5.1 mm −6.5 mm +5.1 mm −6.5 mm +2 mm = −5.8 mm

Mandibular Arch (right "D space" has *not* been lost, so we can use right and left leeway spaces in our calculations)

−4.0 mm of mandibular incisor crowding is currently present (Figures 3.64l and 3.64q)
+4.1 mm width of right primary lateral incisor
−5.5 mm anticipated width of right permanent lateral incisor
+4.1 mm width of left primary lateral incisor
−5.5 mm anticipated width of left permanent lateral incisor
+3.2 mm of anticipated leeway space (1.6 mm/side)
Balance = −4 mm +4.1 mm −5.5 mm +4.1 mm −5.5 mm +3.2 mm = −3.6 mm

That is, *5.8 mm of maxillary arch crowding and 3.6 mm of mandibular arch crowding is anticipated following eruption of all permanent teeth (if proper space maintenance is employed).*

Q: With every orthodontic patient, focus on the patient's *primary* problems in each dimension, plus other problems, at every appointment. What are Alicia's primary problems?

A: Alicia's primary problems are:

Table 3.6 Primary problems list for Alicia.

AP	—
Vertical	Anterior open bite
Transverse	Minimal OJ of right permanent first molars
Other	Delayed eruption of maxillary right permanent central incisor
	Ectopic eruption of mandibular permanent lateral incisors
	Blockage and possible impaction of mandibular permanent canines and first premolars
	Moderate anterior crowding
	Anterior crossbite

Q: What principle should you follow when treating Alicia's ectopically erupting mandibular lateral incisors?

A: *Clear a path and provide adequate space for their eruption.* This may involve extraction of teeth and orthodontics to move the lateral incisors into their correct positions.

Q: If we move Alicia's mandibular permanent lateral incisors into their correct positions, then what will this be an example of?

A: *Space regaining.* Why? Posterior space has been lost by the ectopic eruption of her mandibular lateral incisors if we leave the lateral incisors in their current positions. Moving the lateral incisors mesially will regain this lost space.

Q: What three principles apply to every early treatment patient, and how do these principles apply to Alicia?

A: The three principles are as follows:
1) The goal of early treatment is to correct developing problems with the intent of getting the patient *back to normal for their stage of development* including preventing complications such as resorption of adjacent teeth roots, reducing later treatment complexity, or reducing/eliminating unknowns. For Alicia, this means moving her mandibular permanent lateral incisors into a normal position to allow eruption of mandibular permanent canines and premolars (eliminate potential impactions). In addition,

eruption of her maxillary right central incisor, anterior crossbite correction, and elimination of anterior crowding are necessary to get her back on a normal track.

2) Early treatment should address *specific problems with a clearly defined end point*, usually within six to nine months (except for some orthopedic problems). Alicia's ectopically erupting mandibular permanent lateral incisors, delayed maxillary incisor eruption, and anterior crossbite are specific problems with clearly defined end points which could be treated in a relatively short time. Correction of her moderate crowding will take longer – depending upon eruption of her permanent teeth.

3) Always ask: Is it necessary that I treat the patient now? *What harm will come from not doing anything now?* It is necessary to treat Alicia now. Otherwise, her mandibular permanent canines and first premolars could remain potentially impacted, and they could resorb the mandibular permanent lateral incisor roots. If the crowding is not addressed, then the maxillary lateral incisors could block maxillary permanent canine eruption, maxillary lateral incisors could erupt ectopically, or maxillary lateral incisors could suffer root resorption as the maxillary permanent canines erupt. Damage to the left permanent incisors may occur if the anterior crossbite is not corrected. It is necessary to treat Alicia now.

Q: Can you list features that would, or would not, make Alicia an ideal serial extraction candidate? Is she a candidate for serial extraction?

A: The ideal serial extraction patient is in the early mixed dentition and exhibits the following:

- *Normal anteroposterior relationship* (Class I): Alicia exhibits this feature.
- *Normal vertical relationship* (minimal OB) *or possibly a mild open bite but not a deep bite:* Alicia exhibits this feature.
- *Normal transverse relationship*: Alicia exhibits this feature although she has minimal OJ of her right permanent first molars.
- *Normal incisor angulation or proclined incisors (protrusive lips), but not upright incisors:* Alicia does not exhibit this feature.
- *Severe anterior crowding* (≥ 9 mm per arch): Alicia does not exhibit this feature.

Based upon the fact that Alicia has only moderate (6.8–7.8 mm) anterior crowding and upright incisors, she is not an ideal candidate for serial extraction.

Q: Should you start early treatment now or recall Alicia? Exhaustively discuss all options.

A: Options include the following:

- *Recall* (no treatment, monitor only, reevaluate in one year) – is not recommended. Early treatment is justified because the complexity of Alicia's later treatment, and the likelihood of future complications, will be dramatically reduced with early treatment.

  The ectopic eruption of her mandibular permanent lateral incisors causes the most concern. Not only are her mandibular permanent canines and first premolars potentially impacted by the lateral incisors, the roots of the lateral incisors could be resorbed by these teeth if treatment is delayed.

  Also, we are concerned with potential tooth damage if the left anterior crossbite is not corrected. Early treatment is justified.

- *Space maintenance* (placement of an LLHA and Nance holding arch) – is not recommended. While it is true that space maintenance could reduce her anterior crowding, space maintenance will not address her ectopic eruption, potentially impacted teeth, potential root resorption, delayed eruption, and potential dental damage from her crossbite.

- *Space regaining* (advancing mandibular permanent lateral incisors into their correct positions) – is strongly recommended. Extracting mandibular primary lateral incisors, mandibular primary canines, and mandibular left primary first molar would create a pathway/space for mandibular permanent lateral incisor mesial movement. Fixed orthodontic appliances could be used to advance the mandibular permanent lateral incisors into their correct positions, regaining lost posterior space for eruption of the mandibular permanent canines and first premolars. Space maintenance could then be employed.

- *Serial extraction* – is not recommended. Alicia has only moderate anterior crowding and upright incisors.

- *Extraction of maxillary primary lateral incisors and primary canines* (to create eruption space for maxillary permanent lateral incisors) – is a reasonable option.

- *Fixed orthodontic appliance treatment to erupt the maxillary right permanent central incisor and correct the left anterior crossbite* – is reasonable. However, since no damage appears to have occurred to the left incisors, it would also be reasonable to wait until the maxillary permanent lateral incisors erupt to correct the left crossbite. Finally, there is no harm in monitoring eruption of the maxillary right permanent central incisor.

Q: What unknowns will you face if you treat Alicia?

A: The most significant unknown is Alicia's future vertical facial growth. You must monitor development of a skeletal open bite. Other unknowns include an undetected CR-CO shift and potential non-eruption of maxillary incisors, mandibular canines, and mandibular premolars.

Q: What is your recommended treatment? How would you proceed?

A: Alicia's mandibular primary lateral incisors, mandibular primary canines, mandibular left primarily first molar, maxillary primary lateral incisors, and maxillary primary canines were extracted. Her mandibular permanent first molars were banded, permanent mandibular incisors were bonded, and mandibular lateral incisors were brought forward into alignment effecting mandibular *space regaining* (Figure 3.65).

An LLHA (with spurs soldered distal to the lateral incisors) was delivered to prevent lateral incisor distal drift. Later, the mandibular second primary molars were extracted, and the erupted mandibular right first premolar was retracted to create space for eruption of the mandibular right permanent canine (Figure 3.65e).

The maxillary right central incisor and lateral incisors erupted uneventfully (Figure 3.66a). Maxillary teeth, including primary teeth, were bonded (Figure 3.66b). The upright maxillary incisors were aligned, and space for the maxillary permanent canines was opened using compressed open coil springs placed between the maxillary lateral incisors and maxillary primary first molars.

Primary teeth exfoliated were extracted as they became loose (Figure 3.66c). Maxillary teeth were debanded, and a maxillary Hawley retainer was delivered to be worn nightly (the maxillary Hawley retainer did not cover erupting maxillary canines or premolars). *This completed early treatment.*

Alicia was placed on recall until her remaining permanent teeth erupted. At that time, records were made. We decided that Alicia should be treated non-extraction, with comprehensive, fixed orthodontic appliances (Figure 3.67):

- Air rotor stripping (interproximal reduction, IPR) was performed in all four quadrants to help alleviate crowding.
- Arches were bonded, leveled, aligned, detailed, and finished.
- Maxillary and mandibular Hawley retainers were delivered, which she was asked to wear every night for her lifetime.

Q: Alicia's deband records are illustrated in Figure 3.68. What changes do you note?

A: Changes include the following:
- Alicia's smile esthetics were dramatically improved.

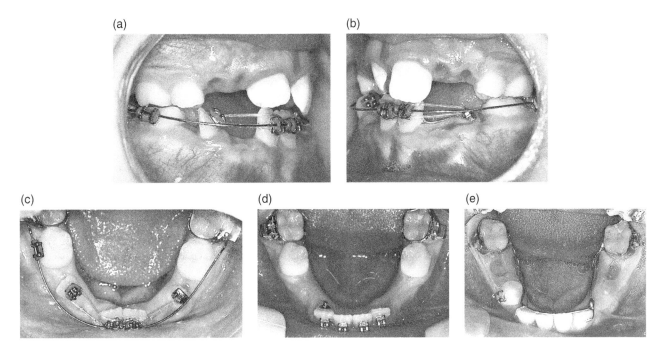

(a)　　(b)

(c)　　(d)　　(e)

Figure 3.65 (a–e) Progress records of Alicia.

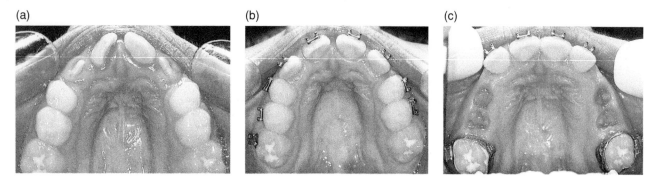

Figure 3.66 (a–c) Progress records of Alicia.

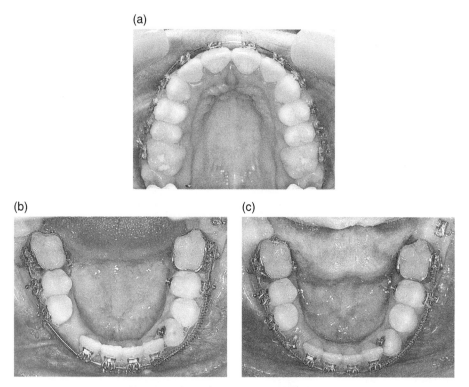

Figure 3.67 (a–c) Progress records of Alicia during comprehensive treatment.

- Lip competence was achieved (although she may be exhibiting mentalis strain in Figure 3.68a).
- Alicia exhibited significant vertical skeletal facial growth (Figure 3.68f, A-Point and B-Point descended, but horizontally their positions appear unchanged). Her skeletal LAFH remains excessively long (LAFH/ TAFH × 100% = 59%; normal = 55%, sd = 2%).
- In spite of significant mandibular growth, her mandibular plane rotated down and back slightly (Figure 3.68f). Why? The amount of maxillary corpus descent plus molar eruption prevented B-point from advancing.
- Following correction of her ectopically erupting mandibular lateral incisors, advancement of her maxillary incisors to make room for her maxillary permanent canines, and comprehensive orthodontic

treatment, her permanent teeth erupted uneventfully into a very nice occlusion.
- Class I canine and molar relationships were maintained.
- Open bite closure (10% deband OB), correction of anterior crossbite, elimination of crowding, and coincidence of midlines was achieved.
- Maxillary incisors proclined (U1 to SN increased from 96° to 104°).
- Mandibular incisors proclined (FMIA increased from a very upright 82° to an ideal 67°, IMPA increased from 72° to 82°).
- Developing wisdom teeth will be monitored.

Q: Alicia was finished with minimal OB. Was this ideal?

A: No. Considering her initial vertical skeletal growth pattern, her right incisor open bite, and her left incisor

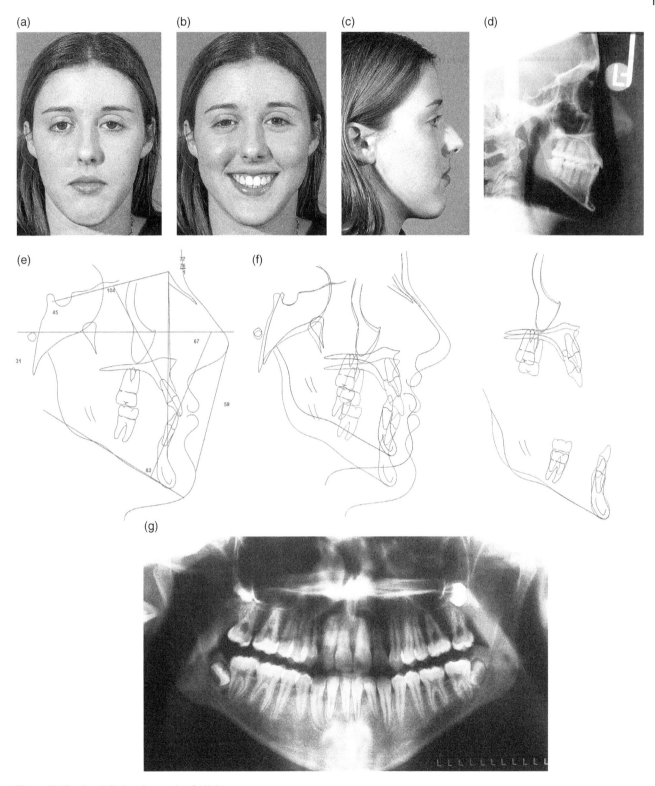

Figure 3.68 (a–q) Deband records of Alicia.

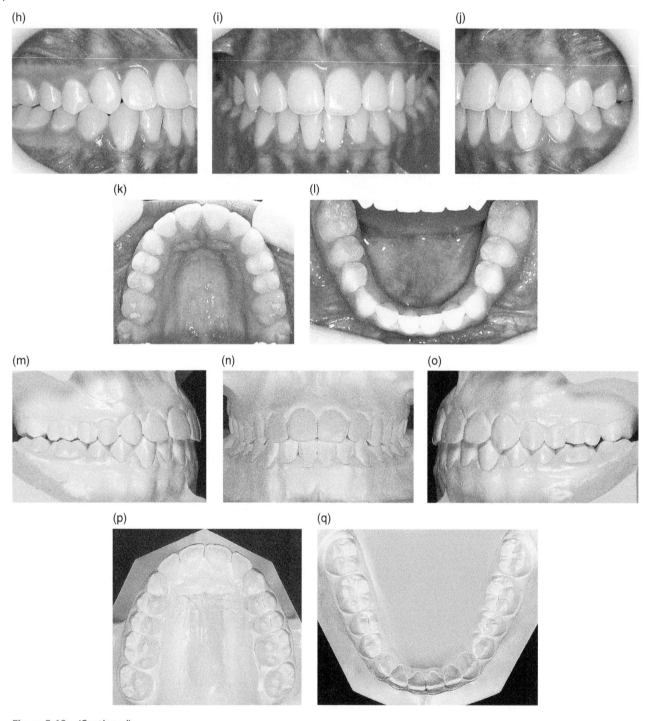

(h) (i) (j)

(k) (l)

(m) (n) (o)

(p) (q)

Figure 3.68 (Continued)

shallow OB, we probably should have *over-corrected* her to a deeper OB than normal, say 30–40%. Why? Some posttreatment bite opening should be anticipated.

Q: Alicia had excessive vertical facial growth (Figure 3.68f) but did not develop an anterior open bite. Why?

A: She had significant incisor eruption, which *compensated* for the vertical facial growth.

Q: Should Alicia have worn a vertical pull chin cup in order to reduce her vertical facial growth? Or, should TAD anchors have been placed to intrude posterior teeth and reduce her vertical facial growth?

A: Neither. We monitored Alicia's vertical relationships carefully throughout treatment. If she had started to develop a skeletal open bite, then we would have aggressively attempted to control it. However, she had an excellent result without application of either a vertical pull chin cup or TAD intrusion.

Q: Alicia initially presented with minimal right permanent first molar overjet. Should she have been treated with RME?

A: Possibly. However, she did not present with either a posterior crossbite or with significant posterior transverse dental compensations for an underlying constricted maxilla (maxillary molar buccal crown tip, mandibular molar lingual crown tip). Her transverse treatment consisted of maxillary and mandibular arch wire coordination, which provided excellent final occlusal interdigitation and minimal buccal corridors.

Q: Was early treatment validated?

A: Absolutely. By treating Alicia's mandibular lateral incisor ectopic eruption early, we simplified later comprehensive treatment and eliminated the possibility that her mandibular lateral incisor roots would be resorbed by her erupting mandibular canines. In addition, space creation (incisor proclination) in the maxillary arch provided room for canine eruption.

Q: What retention protocol would you recommend for Alicia?

A: She was placed in removable Hawley retainers and asked to wear them at night for life. Lifelong retention is the only guarantee that alignment of teeth can be maintained. A mandibular fixed canine-to-canine retainer could also have been used instead of a mandibular Hawley retainer. Clear vacuum-formed retainers also suffice for many patients.

Q: Can you suggest "take-home pearls" regarding Alicia's treatment?

A: "Take-home pearls" include the following:
  - Alicia presented at nine years and seven months of age with a Class I dental relationship, excessive vertical facial skeletal development, and ectopic eruption of permanent mandibular lateral incisors. She was treated with *space regaining* by extracting primary teeth and moving mandibular lateral incisors into their proper position. In addition, space was created in the maxillary arch by proclining upright incisors in order to make room for maxillary canine eruption.
  - Principles for treating ectopic tooth eruption include: *clearing a path/making space for the ectopically erupting tooth to follow, space regaining to move the permanent tooth back to its correct position* (especially if arch perimeter has been lost), and *considering all possible anterior and posterior extraction patterns* if the patient is clearly an extraction case or in instances of severe root resorption. Surgical exposure of ectopically erupting teeth may also be required.
  - Even though Alicia's early treatment centered on moving mandibular lateral incisors into their correct positions, additional treatments were also necessary (e.g. mandibular primary second molar extractions and retraction of the erupted mandibular right first premolar to make room for the mandibular right permanent canine, Figure 3.65e). Our point is that focused, early treatment plans often evolve into more complicated treatments. You must keep a fresh eye at every patient appointment and constantly look for developing problems.
  - In cases of early crowding, options of monitoring, space maintenance, space regaining, and permanent tooth extraction must all be considered. Alicia is an example of space regaining, combined with interproximal reduction (IPR) in both arches.

Case Trista

Q: Trista is nine years and ten months old (Figure 3.69). She presents to you with her parents' chief complaint, "Trista needs braces." Her PMH, PDH, periodontal evaluation, and TMJ evaluations are WRN. CR=CO. Compile your diagnostic findings and problem list for Trista. Also, state your diagnosis.

A:

Table 3.7 Diagnostic findings and problems list for Trista.

Full face and profile	Frontal view
	Face is symmetric
	Long soft-tissue LAFH (soft-tissue Glabella – Subnasale < Subnasale – soft-tissue Menton)
	Lip competence (but lip incompetence on lateral cephalometric radiograph)
	UDML WRN
	Excessive gingival display in posed smile (maxillary central incisor gingival margins below the maxillary lip)
	Profile view
	Mildly convex profile
	Obtuse NLA
	Chin projection WRN (soft-tissue Pogonion lies on Zero Meridian line)
	Lip-chin-throat angle WRN

(Continued)

Table 3.7 (Continued)

Ceph analysis	***Skeletal***
	Maxilla protrusive (A-Point lies ahead of Nasion-perpendicular line)
	Mandible deficient relative to the maxilla but normal relative to Nasion-perpendicular line
	Skeletal LAFH WRN (ANS-Menton/ Nasion-Menton X 100% = 54%)
	Mandibular plane angle WRN (FMA = 24°; SNMP = 38°)
	Effective bony Pogonion (Pogonion lies along line extended from Nasion through B-point)
	Dental
	Maxillary incisor inclination WRN (maxillary central incisor to SN = 102°)
	Proclined mandibular incisors (FMIA = 59°)
Radiographs	Early mixed dentition
	Premature loss of mandibular left primary canine
	Blocked and potentially impacted mandibular left permanent canine
	Ectopically erupting maxillary right permanent canine crown overlaps maxillary lateral incisor root by >½
	Ectopically erupting maxillary left permanent canine crown overlaps maxillary lateral incisor root by <½
	Roots of permanent canines and first premolars ≥ ½ developed
Intraoral photos and models	Angle Class II division 1
	Iowa Classification: II (5 mm) II (5 mm) II (4 mm) II (3 mm)
	OJ 4–5 mm
	OB 50% (note that Trista is slightly open in 3.69h while a more accurate OB assessment is found on her models in 3.69m)
	Maxillary midline diastema with significant distal crown tip of maxillary permanent central incisors
	6.0 mm maxillary anterior crowding is currently present
	4.0 mm of maxillary crowding is anticipated following eruption of all permanent teeth (if proper space maintenance is employed)
	9.0 mm of mandibular anterior crowding is currently present (3.0 mm of mandibular incisor crowding, 1 mm of space distal to the mandibular left lateral incisor, 7.0 mm anticipated width of mandibular left permanent canine)
	3.8 mm of mandibular crowding is anticipated following eruption of all permanent teeth (if proper space maintenance is employed)

	Maxillary right lateral incisor is in crossbite
	LDML has shifted to the left of maxillary midline diastema center by ~2 mm
	Maxillary and mandibular dental arches are symmetric
	Thin periodontal biotype (note thin tissue labial to mandibular central incisors)
	Significant posterior transverse compensations (3.69q and 3.69r), buccal crown torque of maxillary permanent first molars and lingual crown torque of mandibular permanent first molars)
Other	None
Diagnosis	Class II division 1 malocclusion with moderate maxillary and severe mandibular anterior crowding, ectopic eruption of maxillary permanent canines, and significant posterior transverse compensations

Q: We stated that Trista's mandible was deficient relative to her maxilla but normal relative to her Nasion-perpendicular line. Can you explain why?

A: Trista's ANB angle = 6°, which would normally indicate that her mandible was deficient *if her maxilla was in a normal anteroposterior position* (please see Appendix). However, because her maxilla is protrusive, we cannot use her ANB angle to judge her mandibular position. Instead, we should use the angle made between Nasion-perpendicular line and Nasion-B Point line (Figure 3.69t), which is 3°. We feel that her mandible is relatively normal.

Q: In Figure 3.69g you can see a slight posterior open bite on Trista's right side which is absent in her articulated models (Figure 3.69l). What is the likely cause of this open bite?

A: One explanation is that Trista has a slight (undetected) CR-CO shift due to her maxillary right lateral incisor, which is in crossbite. As she shifts back into CR, she may contact the maxillary right lateral incisor and open slightly (Figure 3.69g).

This underscores an important point with respect to unknowns: always check carefully for CR-CO shift in a patient when maxillary lateral incisors are in crossbite occlusion. Why? In a child with excessive overjet of the central incisors, if the maxillary lateral incisors erupt in linguoversion, then their lingual position may create an occlusal interference with the mandibular incisors prompting the patient to posture forward into lateral incisor crossbite in order to avoid the interference. This will mask the excessive overjet and a more severe underlying

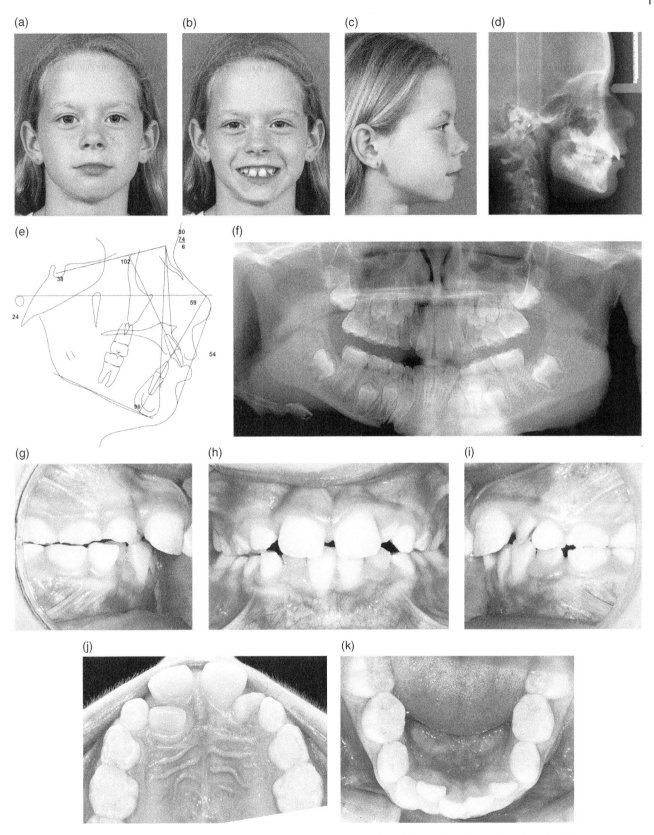

Figure 3.69   Initial records of Trista: (a–c) facial photographs, (d and e) lateral cephalometric radiograph and tracing, (f) pantomograph, (g–k) intraoral photographs, (l–s) model photographs, (t) lateral cephalometric radiograph tracing with Nasion perpendicular line drawn in red.

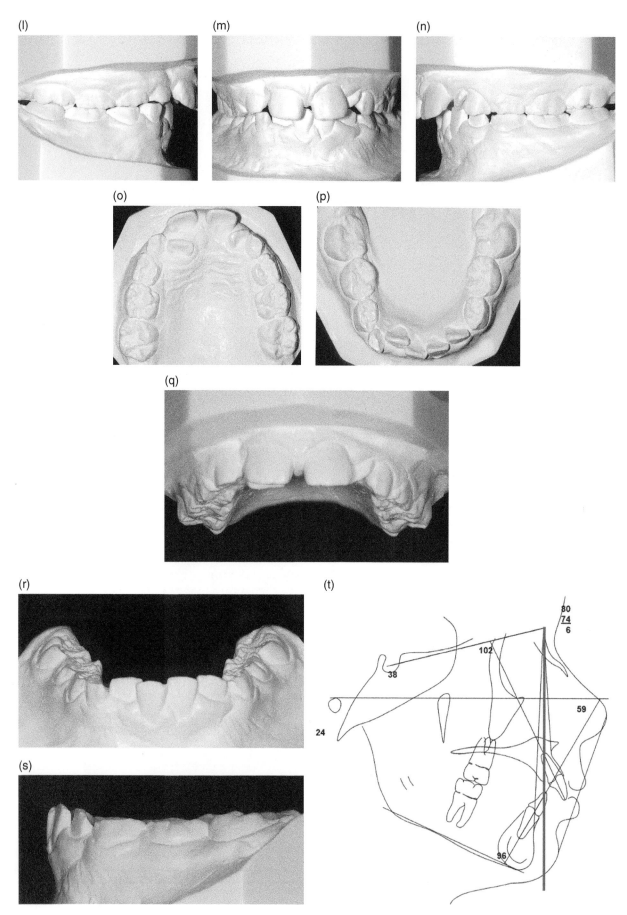

Figure 3.69   (Continued)

Class II relationship. It is better to detect this early rather than to have a more severe Class II relationship suddenly "appear" after correcting a maxillary lateral incisor crossbite during early treatment.

Q: Trista's maxillary right permanent canine crown overlaps her maxillary right lateral incisor root much more than her maxillary left permanent canine crown overlaps her maxillary left lateral incisor root (Figure 3.69f). How do these positions affect the chances that each canine will erupt or not erupt?

A: The more a maxillary permanent canine crown overlaps a lateral incisor root on a panoramic image, the greater the chance that the canine will become impacted [89]. Therefore, the maxillary right permanent canine has a greater chance of becoming impacted.

Q: What early treatment principle, and early treatment options, would you consider in order to increase the chances that the ectopically erupting maxillary permanent canines will erupt?

A: Principle: *clear a path (and make space) for the ectopically erupting teeth to follow.* Treatment options include:

- Placing fixed maxillary orthodontic appliances, trapping a compressed open coil spring between the primary canines and the central incisors to create space for the lateral incisors and permanent canines. *Note: opening space this way creates space at the level of the gingiva and coronal portion of the root and less at the apices of the teeth where the space is needed by the canine crowns.*
- RME to create maxillary anterior space, including space at the teeth apicies [27], followed by a TPA to maintain the expansion.
- Distal translation of the maxillary posterior teeth using headgear or Herbst appliances.
- Extraction of the maxillary primary canines and primary first molars in order to accelerate first premolar eruption and thereby make room for the permanent maxillary canine crowns (note: the maxillary first premolar roots are at least ½ developed).
- Permanent tooth extractions, as needed.
- Surgical exposure of the permanent canine crowns followed by their orthodontic eruption.

Q: Trista's mandible is normal relative to Nasion-perpendicular line, but it is deficient relative to her maxilla. In addition, she exhibits a mildly convex profile and a 3–5 mm Class II molar relationship. Because of these features, Class II orthopedics should be considered. If you attempt Class II orthopedics, then *when* would you begin?

A: Trista is in the early mixed dentition, but she is very close to entering the late mixed dentition (Figure 3.69f). Also, she is almost ten years old. *Now* is a good time to initiate Class II orthopedics.

The strongest scientific evidence finds no advantage to beginning Class II treatment in the early mixed dentition (except for a possible decrease in incisal trauma as a result of excess overjet) [68–71, 90–92]. We subscribe to this guideline unless the patient shows good statural growth in which case we will begin Class II treatment in the early mixed dentition.

Since Trista will soon enter the late mixed dentition, we would rather begin Class II treatment now as opposed to waiting to begin and possibly missing good mandibular growth.

Q: Trista lacks a posterior crossbite. So, what is the significance of her transverse dental *compensations* (maxillary first permanent molar buccal crown torque and mandibular first permanent molar lingual crown torque)?

A: Her large transverse dental compensations reflect a significant difference between her maxillary and mandibular transverse skeletal widths. As recently reported, there is a large variation in transverse skeletal widths (and transverse dental compensations) between subjects lacking crossbites [93].

Think of it this way – our goal will be to eventually upright Trista's posterior teeth. If we uprighted her posterior teeth now, her maxillary first permanent molar crowns would move lingually, her mandibular first permanent molar crowns would move buccally, and a bilateral lingual crossbite would result. This indicates that Trista's maxillary transverse skeletal width is too narrow for her mandibular transverse skeletal width – and her *first permanent molars have erupted with compensations which reflect this underlying skeletal discrepancy.*

Q: Provide a detailed space analysis for Trista's maxillary and mandibular arches. In other words, how were the anticipated 4.0 mm maxillary dental arch crowding and 3.8 mm mandibular dental arch crowding calculated (*if proper space maintenance is employed*)?

A:

Average mesiodistal widths of permanent teeth (mm) [66]:

Maxillary Central Incisor	8.5	Mandibular Central Incisor	5.0
Maxillary Lateral Incisor	6.5	Mandibular Lateral Incisor	5.5
Maxillary Canine	7.5	Mandibular Canine	7.0

Maxillary First Premolar	7.0	Mandibular First Premolar	7.0
Maxillary Second Premolar	7.0	Mandibular Second Premolar	7.0
Maxillary First Molar	10.0	Mandibular First Molar	11.0
Maxillary Second Molar	9.0	Mandibular Second Molar	10.5

Average mesiodistal widths of *primary* teeth (mm) [66]:

Maxillary Central Incisor	6.5	Mandibular Central Incisor	4.2
Maxillary Lateral Incisor	5.1	Mandibular Lateral Incisor	4.1
Maxillary Canine	7.0	Mandibular Canine	5.0
Maxillary First Molar	7.3	Mandibular First Molar	7.7
Maxillary Second Molar	8.2	Mandibular Second Molar	9.9

Maxillary Arch

−6.0 mm of incisor crowding currently present (Figure 3.69j)
+2 mm of anticipated leeway space (1 mm/side)
Balance = −6.0 mm +2 mm = −4.0 mm

Mandibular Arch (could not use leeway space on left because primary canine is exfoliated)

−3.0 mm of incisor crowding currently present (Figure 3.69k)
+9.9 mm mesiodistal width of left primary second molar
−7.0 mm anticipated width of left second premolar
+7.7 mm width of left primary first molar
−7.0 mm anticipated width of left first premolar
+1.0 mm of space between the mandibular left lateral incisor and mandibular left primary first molar
−7.0 mm anticipated width of left permanent canine
+1.6 mm anticipate leeway space right side
Balance = −3.0 mm +9.9 mm −7.0 mm +7.7 mm −7.0 mm +1.0 mm −7.0 mm +1.6 mm = −3.8 mm

That is, *4.0 mm of maxillary dental arch crowding and 3.8 mm of mandibular dental arch crowding is anticipated following eruption of all permanent teeth (if proper space maintenance is employed).*

Q: What are Trista's *primary* problems in each dimension, plus other problems that we must focus on?

A:

Table 3.8 Primary problems list for Trista.

AP	Class II division 1 malocclusion
	Iowa Classification: II (5 mm) II (5 mm) II (4 mm) II (3 mm)
	Crossbite of the maxillary right lateral incisor
Vertical	OB 50%
Transverse	Significant transverse compensations (buccal crown torque of maxillary permanent first molars and lingual crown torque of mandibular permanent first molars)
Other	Maxillary permanent canines ectopically-erupting (right and left canine crowns overlap maxillary lateral incisor roots on panoramic radiograph)
	Potential impaction of mandibular left canine
	Moderate maxillary (6 mm) and severe mandibular (9 mm) anterior crowding currently Present

Q: Discuss Trista in the context of three principles applied to every early treatment patient.

A:

1) The goal of early treatment is to correct developing problems – get the patient *back to normal for their stage of development* (including preventing complications, reducing later treatment complexity, or reducing/eliminating unknowns). Correcting the following problems will get Trista back on track:
   - Class II relationship
   - Maxillary right lateral incisor crossbite
   - 50% OB
   - Transverse compensations
   - Ectopic eruption of maxillary permanent canines
   - Potential impaction of mandibular left permanent canine
   - Moderate to severe crowding.

2) Early treatment should address *very specific problems with a clearly defined end point*, usually within six to nine months. Let's consider this principle applied to each of the aforementioned problems:
   - Class II relationship – correction could take longer than a year, depending upon Trista's jaw growth magnitude and direction.
   - Maxillary right lateral incisor crossbite – could be corrected in less than nine months with limited maxillary fixed appliances (e.g. a maxillary 2×4 appliance) if space was first created for the lateral incisors.
   - 50% OB – could be corrected in nine months if arches were leveled with fixed orthodontic appliances.

- Transverse compensations – could be corrected in less than nine months by expanding Trista's maxilla with RME and using excess posterior OJ to upright her mandibular permanent first molars. Crossbite elastics could be worn between buttons bonded on the lingual of mandibular permanent first molars and buccal hooks on the RME appliance to upright mandibular molars, or an expanded LLHA could be used to upright mandibular molars. Excess buccal overjet could be used later to upright the buccally inclined maxillary permanent first molars.
- Ectopic eruption of maxillary permanent canines – is a focused problem but may take longer than six to nine months to correct if space is created for the canines and the canines are permitted to erupt.
- Potential impaction of mandibular left permanent canine – this could be improved in six to nine months via space regaining with fixed orthodontic appliances. However, recession of the thin mandibular labial periodontal biotype is a concern if the incisors are proclined during space regaining.
- Anterior crowding – may take longer than nine months to correct (if space maintenance is employed), depending upon how soon Trista's permanent canines and premolars erupt. Residual crowding could be dealt with later, during comprehensive treatment, after all permanent teeth have erupted.

3) Always ask: Is it necessary that I treat the patient now? *What harm can result if I choose to do nothing now?* Again, let's consider this principle applied to each of the aforementioned problems:
- Class II relationship – if you do not to begin Class II orthopedics now, then you could miss valuable growth.
- Maxillary right lateral incisor crossbite – because no tissue damage is apparent, we do not anticipate harm in waiting to make this correction.
- 50% OB – because there is no pain or tissue damage resulting from the deep bite, we do not anticipate any harm in waiting to treat it.
- Transverse compensations – no harm will result from waiting to treat these compensations. However, if you intend to use RME to widen the maxilla in order to create posterior overjet for uprighting molars, then RME should be done before puberty. *The most marked RME skeletal effect occurs before/during the pubertal growth spurt,* and expansion after the pubertal growth spurt is mainly dentoalveolar (not orthopedic/skeletal) [94–100].
- Ectopically erupting maxillary permanent canines – could resorb maxillary lateral incisor roots, or could erupt into even worse positions, if not corrected now.
- Potential impaction of mandibular left permanent canine – the canine could become impacted or resorb the mandibular left lateral incisor root.
- Moderate to severe anterior crowding – if not corrected could result in root resorption of the lateral incisor roots by the ectopically erupting/impacted permanent canines; or worsening of the canine positions.

Q: Can you list three factors that qualify Trista as a candidate for serial extraction? Can you list three factors that disqualify Trista as a candidate? Is Trista a candidate for serial extraction?

A: Factors that would qualify Trista as a candidate for serial extraction include the fact that she:
- Is in the early mixed dentition stage of development
- Has proclined mandibular incisors – which will tend to upright to a normal inclination if permanent teeth are extracted and incisors retracted
- Presents with severe (9 mm) mandibular anterior crowding

Factors that would disqualify Trista as a candidate for serial extraction include the fact that she:
- Presents with a Class II molar relationship which could worsen if four first premolars are extracted, spaces are closed reciprocally, and maxillary molars move forward more than mandibular molars.
- Has normally inclined maxillary incisors which will tend to upright too much if permanent teeth are extracted and incisors retracted.
- Presents with only moderate (6 mm), not severe, maxillary anterior crowding.
- Has a 50% OB, which will tend to deepen if first premolars are extracted and incisors are retracted/uprighted around their apices.
- Has significant posterior transverse compensations (she has maxillary skeletal transverse deficiency).

The ideal serial extraction patient is in the *early mixed dentition and is normal in every way except has severe anterior crowding (≥ 9 mm anterior crowding in both arches).* Based upon the above, Trista is not an ideal candidate for serial extraction.

Q: Should you start early treatment or recall Trista? If you start treatment, what treatment options would you consider?

A: Your treatment options include the following:
- *Recall* (no treatment, monitor only) – reevaluate in one year. We do not recommend this option. Why? We could miss out on valuable mandibular growth for Class II orthopedic correction, crowns of ectopically

erupting maxillary canines could resorb maxillary permanent lateral incisor roots, ectopically erupting maxillary canines could erupt into worse positions, or the potentially impacted mandibular left permanent canine could remain impacted or resorb the lateral incisor root.

- *RME* – is recommended in order to create posterior overjet and permit uprighting of lingually inclined mandibular first permanent molars and buccally inclined maxillary first permanent molars. RME will also create space at the level of the crowns and *at the apices* of the maxillary anterior teeth – improving chances that the maxillary permanent canines could erupt normally.

- *Space maintenance* – an LLHA would be recommended once Trista's lingually inclined mandibular first permanent molars are uprighted (3.8 mm of mandibular arch crowding is anticipated following eruption of all permanent teeth if an LLHA is employed). An expanded LLHA could be used to upright the lingually inclined molars.

Of course, the precise amount of final crowding will depend upon the actual size of the erupted mandibular permanent canines and premolars. A Nance holding arch is not recommended at this time if Class II orthopedics is used to distalize Trista's maxillary first permanent molars.

- *Space regaining* – opening space for Trista's maxillary permanent lateral incisors and mandibular left permanent canine (due to loss of the corresponding primary teeth) is not recommended. Why? Her proclined mandibular incisors would be proclined even more as space is opened; and advancing her maxillary lateral incisor crowns will tend to reciprocally distalize the lateral incisor root apices – potentially driving them into the ectopically erupting maxillary permanent canine crowns.

- *Extraction of maxillary primary canines* – would provide space for alignment of permanent lateral incisors but could result in arch perimeter loss (less space for permanent canines and premolars) if mesial drift of the maxillary posterior teeth is not prevented. Extraction of maxillary primary canines alone will not provide enough space for eruption of the maxillary permanent canines.

- *Extraction of maxillary primary canines and maxillary primary first molars* – is recommended. Following these extractions, accelerated maxillary first premolar eruption should occur (their roots appear to be ≥½ developed). Eruption of the first premolars will provide space at their apices for eruption of the permanent canines.

- *Extraction of the mandibular right primary canine* – is not recommended. Nothing will be gained by extraction of this tooth except some spontaneous incisor alignment and midline shift to the right. Further, unless an LLHA is placed, arch perimeter could be lost as the mandibular right posterior teeth drift mesially.

- *Serial extraction* – is not recommended. Trista has a Class II relationship, 50% OB, and significant posterior transverse compensations. She is not an ideal candidate for serial extraction.

- *Class II orthopedics* – is recommended. Trista is nearly ten years old and close to entering the late mixed dentition stage of development. Now it is an appropriate time to begin Class II orthopedics.

Q: What is your recommended treatment? How would you proceed?

A: As should be done at every appointment, the presence of a CR-CO shift was assessed at her case presentation. Trista's Class II occlusal relationship in CR was verified. RME was initiated with the maxillary first permanent molars banded as anchors and with soldered arms extended mesially to the maxillary lateral incisors. The maxillary primary second molar lingual surfaces were bonded to the soldered arms in order to increase RME anchorage.

As soon as posterior OJ was created with RME, Trista's lingually inclined mandibular permanent first molars were uprighted using an expanded LLHA. Class II orthopedic treatment (high-pull headgear) was initiated during RME. Height was measured at each appointment in order to monitor statural growth. Once active RME was complete, Trista's maxillary primary canines and primary first molars were extracted (Figure 3.70). Months later, the metal arms soldered mesial to the maxillary permanent first molar bands were removed, with the remaining Hyrax appliance used as a TPA.

We informed Trista and her parents that this early treatment would continue as Trista grew and her permanent teeth erupted. We told them that early treatment would be followed by re-evaluation using new records to assess Trista's growth magnitude and direction, her treatment compliance, and the need for possible extraction of permanent teeth. They were also informed of the possible need for a fixed maxillary lingual retainer between Trista's central incisors (following comprehensive treatment) if the diastema did not close with permanent canine eruption.

Q: Trista was placed on a high-pull headgear for Class II orthopedics. Could she have been treated with a Herbst appliance instead?

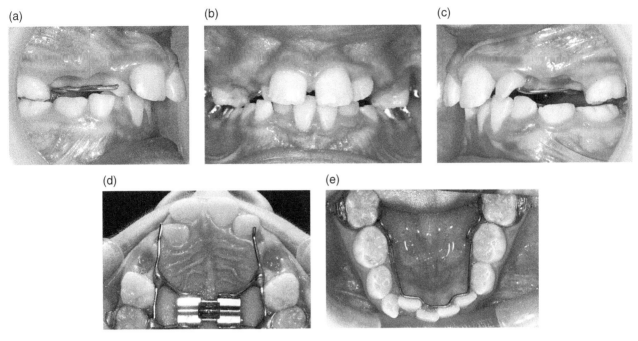

Figure 3.70 (a–e) Progress records of Trista at 10 years and 3 months of age.

A: Compare and contrast the effects of both to answer this question. *Headgears and Class II functional appliances are equally effective in correcting Class II malocclusions in children* (before comprehensive treatment*)* [101]. Headgears and functional appliances (used *in conjunction* with fixed orthodontic appliances) can effectively correct Class II malocclusions, but higher levels of evidence to answer the question of whether their effects are equal is missing.

The effects of a high-pull headgear in correcting Trista's Class II include [75–78]:

- Restricting maxillary forward growth
- Distalization of maxillary molars
- Reducing descent of the maxillary corpus
- Reducing maxillary first molar eruption (permitting mandibular upward and forward rotation).

The effects of a Herbst appliance in correcting Trista's Class II include [79]:

- Inhibition of maxillary growth
- Distal movement of maxillary teeth
- Intrusion of maxillary molars in the majority of patients
- Acceleration of mandibular growth
- Mesial movement of mandibular teeth (including mandibular incisor proclination).

Note that Class II functional appliances, including Herbst appliances, *do accelerate* mandibular growth in growing individuals. However, functional appliances *do not enhance* mandibular horizontal growth beyond that found in control subjects [81]. In other words, slower than normal growth *after* Class II functional appliance therapy reduces or eliminates any long-term increase in mandibular size compared to controls.

Also note that the *direction* of condylar growth from functional appliance wear may not correct mandibular skeletal anteroposterior deficiency or improve chin projection [82, 83, 102]. In hyperdivergent individuals, backward mandibular rotation and increases in LAFH are seen with Herbst treatment [102]. Trista has a normal FMA (24°) but SNMP = 38°. She may be considered borderline hyperdivergent, which may be an issue for her and result in a poor response to Herbst treatment.

In summary, a high-pull headgear was employed for Trista's Class II orthopedics in order to reduce her maxillary forward growth while allowing continued mandibular forward growth, retract maxillary first permanent molars, and restrict eruption of maxillary first permanent molars. A Herbst appliance could have provided a similar high-pull headgear effect but would have increased Trista's mandibular incisor protrusion and possibly increased her LAFH.

Q: LLHAs reduce mandibular anterior crowding (maintaining leeway space) during the transition from mixed to permanent dentition. However, by maintaining leeway space, LLHAs prevent Class II molar correction because mandibular permanent first molar mesial drift is reduced [103]. Can LLHA's offer any benefit to Class II molar correction?

A: Yes. LLHAs *reduce mandibular permanent first molar eruption by 1–2 mm over a 1–2 year period*, compared to controls [104]. In growing patients, this reduction of mandibular first molar eruption can reduce downward and backward mandibular plane rotation, thereby tending to reduce LAFH, increase chin projection, and improve Class II relationships.

Q: Why is reduction of mandibular first permanent molar eruption with an LLHA especially important during high-pull headgear Class II orthopedic treatment?

A: If a high-pull headgear inhibits maxillary first permanent molar eruption, then the mandibular first permanent molars may over-erupt to fill the interocclusal space. This is termed *compensatory molar eruption*, and it negates the beneficial vertical effects of HPHG. By reducing mandibular first permanent molar eruption, LLHAs secure the beneficial vertical effects of HPHG on B-Point forward rotation.

Q: Records were made of Trista at age of thirteen years and seven months (Figure 3.71). What changes do you note?

A: Changes include:
- Trista is now in the permanent dentition.
- Her ectopically erupting maxillary permanent canines erupted.
- A significant amount of facial growth (Figures 3.71e–3.71f) occurred. Her nose, lips, chin, and mandible have all grown downward and significantly forward. Her maxilla has grown downward, but A-Point has grown forward only minimally. Her mandible has undergone significant CCW and forward growth, resulting in a decrease in ANB angle from 6° to 5°, a decrease in mandibular plane angle from FMA = 24° to 21°, and a decrease in SN-MP angle from 38° to 34°. Her skeletal LAFH has decreased from 54 to 52%. Her maxillary molars, mandibular molars, and incisors have erupted. Her molars have moved to the mesial slightly.
- Trista's profile is now straight and her labiomental sulcus is more obtuse (Figure 3.71c).
- Right Class II molar relationship has improved from 5 to 2 mm Class II. Left has improved from 3 mm Class II to Class I.
- Maxillary right lateral incisor crossbite corrected, and alignment of maxillary lateral incisors has improved.
- Maxillary anterior crowding has reduced to ~4 mm (Figure 3.71k).
- LLHA was removed, impacted mandibular left canine erupted, and mandibular anterior crowding is ~5 mm (Figure 3.71l).

- Expansion at the RME appliance screw has collapsed significantly (compare Figures 3.60d and 3.61k). Only a 3-mm maxillary intermolar width increase has been achieved at this time.
- Wisdom teeth are developing.

Q: FMIA increased from 59° to 64° (compare Figures 3.59e and 3.61e) indicating that Trista's mandibular incisors *uprighted*. But IMPA remained 96° indicating that Trista's mandibular incisor inclination was unchanged. Can you explain this contradiction?

A: This is an excellent question and underscores the importance of using FMIA (not IMPA) to judge mandibular incisor inclination. IMPA relates incisor inclination relative *only* to the mandible. FMIA relates incisor inclination *relative to the face*, which is a combination of incisor inclination relative to the mandible and mandibular plane inclination. Trista's mandibular plane rotated CCW improving the mandibular incisor inclination relative to the face.

Q: We anticipated 3.8 mm of mandibular dental arch crowding after permanent teeth erupted if an LLHA was used. However, mandibular dental arch crowding is now ~5 mm. What accounts for the difference?

A: The difference is small, only 1.2 mm. Estimates of future anterior crowding are based upon *average* mesiodistal tooth widths. Final crowding depends upon actual tooth sizes.

Q: Was early treatment successful?

A: Yes and no. On the one hand:
- Trista was cooperative, and headgear treatment was clearly beneficial – her maxilla (A-Point) grew forward minimally while B-Point grew forward significantly. That is, headgear wear restricted maxillary forward growth while allowing continued mandibular forward growth. This *differential jaw growth* improved her anteroposterior jaw relationships.
- Her maxillary right lateral incisor crossbite corrected spontaneously with RME and the transition to permanent dentition.
- Ectopically erupting maxillary permanent canines erupted.
- Blocked out/potentially impacted mandibular left permanent canine erupted.

On the other hand:
- Her Class II relationship was not fully corrected. Ideally, we would *over-correct* Trista to a mildly Class III (1–2 mm) molar relationship and then slowly reduce headgear wear while monitoring her response.
- Transverse dental compensations remain.
- Moderate anterior crowding still exists in both arches.

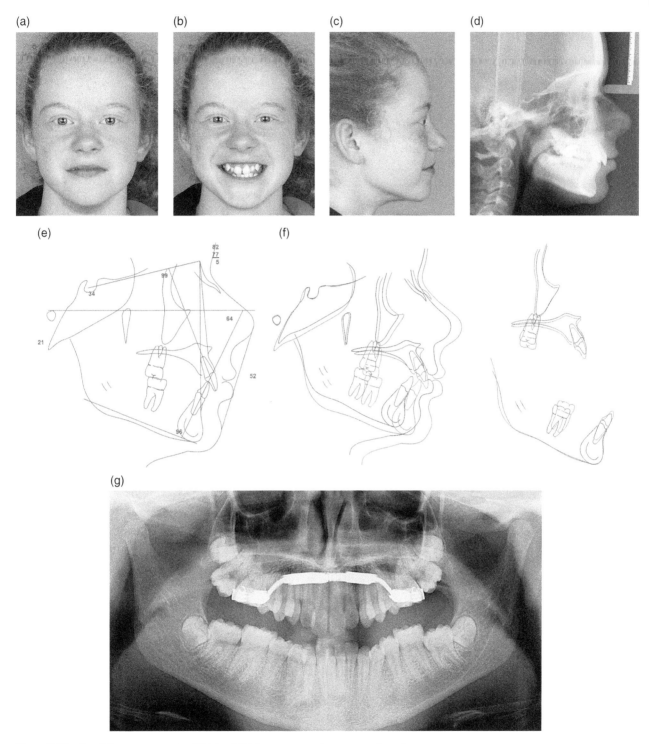

Figure 3.71 (a–q) Progress records of Trista at thirteen years and seven months of age.

Q: We noted the partial collapse of transverse (Hyrax appliance) expansion between ages ten and thirteen years. We speculate that the appliance expansion screw reversed during this period. What mistake did we make after expansion was complete (Figure 3.70d)?

A: We should have inserted a stainless-steel ligature wire through the expansion key hole and around the appliance

framework to "tie off" the screw so that it could not reverse. Alternatively, we could have replaced the RME with a banded TPA cemented to the maxillary first molars.

Q: Trista is now in the permanent dentition, and further treatment will no longer be *early* treatment. Comprehensive orthodontic treatment is not the focus

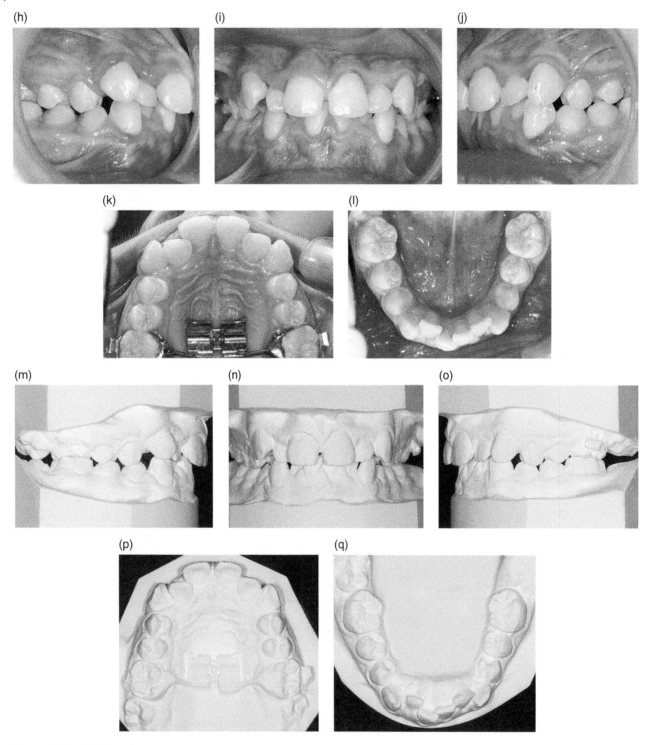

Figure 3.71 (Continued)

of this textbook (we cover many important comprehensive treatment principles in another textbook) [105]. However, can you suggest some possible comprehensive treatment options for Trista?

A: As with any comprehensive treatment patient, we re-established Trista's chief complaint, carefully reviewed

her PMH and PDH, discussed airway/breathing issues, conducted a head and neck exam, evaluated her TMJs/ periodontal tissues, confirmed the absence of a CR-CO shift, studied all current orthodontic records, and established a problem list. Trista's current primary problems include:

Table 3.9   Primary problems list for Trista as she enters comprehensive treatment.

AP	Angle Class II division 1
	Iowa Classification: II (2 mm) II (6 mm)
	II (4 mm) I
Vertical	OB 50%
Transverse	Significant transverse compensations
Other	Maxillary anterior crowding ~4 mm
	Mandibular anterior crowding ~5 mm

Next, we *exhaustively* consider all reasonable treatment options, including:

- *Continued HPHG wear* – to correct (over-correct) her Class II relationship through a combination of maxillary forward growth restriction, mandibular forward growth, and maxillary posterior teeth distalization. Of course, any further orthopedic improvement is dependent upon Trista's remaining growth magnitude and direction. We need to verify that Trista is still growing and ask if she has achieved menarche (reached puberty).
- *Maxillary dentition retraction using TADs* – with TAD anchorage placement on the palate, in the infrazygomatic crest, or buccally between teeth roots, her remaining Class II correction could be achieved.
- *Use of Class II correctors* (Forsus, Class II elastics, Powerscope, etc.) – to retract maxillary teeth and protract mandibular teeth into a Class I relationship. The negative consequence of these *inter-arch* mechanics would be increased mandibular incisor proclination.
- *Continued use of this RME appliance or of a replacement RME appliance* – to separate the two hemi-maxillae at the mid-palatal suture and increase posterior OJ. This would permit uprighting of maxillary and mandibular molars. To maximize skeletal width increase, we should do this *now* before/during puberty.
- *Non-extraction treatment* – is possible. However, we are concerned that Trista has only 1 mm of keratinized attached tissue labial to her mandibular central incisors (Figure 3.71i). If we align her mandibular arch by proclining her mandibular incisors, then we will stress this gingiva and possibly cause recession.
- *Mandibular central incisor extraction* – would provide the 5 mm of space needed to align the mandibular incisors without proclining them. However, the maxillary anterior teeth are not narrow and extracting a mandibular central incisor will lead to an anterior Bolton tooth-size discrepancy, excess anterior OJ, and lack of permanent canine coordination/coupling.

- *Mandibular interproximal reduction (IPR)* – would provide 2.5 mm of space if we remove 0.5 mm of enamel from between each anterior tooth contact from the mesial of the mandibular right canine to the mesial of the mandibular left canine. Since about 5 mm of mandibular anterior crowding exists, 2.5 mm of IPR would reduce the amount of mandibular incisor proclination by about one-half of non-extraction treatment without IPR. However, we could still end with an anterior Bolton tooth-size discrepancy.
- *Extraction of a mandibular central incisor and both maxillary first premolars* – and resulting space closure could eliminate anterior crowding in both arches and permit bilateral maxillary canine retraction to Class I (the maxillary molars would move reciprocally forward into a 6 mm Class II relationship). However, with mandibular incisor extraction there would be an anterior Bolton tooth-size discrepancy, leading to excess anterior OJ and lack of permanent canine coordination/coupling. Furthermore, reciprocal closure of the 7 mm first premolar spaces would result in over-retraction of the maxillary permanent canines – leading to a Class III canine relationship (Class III elastics, or Class III springs, could be used to correct this relationship to Class I). Instead of extracting maxillary first premolars, maxillary second premolars could be extracted – reducing the amount of maxillary canine over-retraction since the molars would move further to the mesial.
- *Extraction of maxillary and mandibular first premolars (four first premolars)* – resulting space closure could eliminate anterior crowding in both arches without stressing mandibular labial periodontium. However, Trista would need to continue wearing headgear as anchorage during retraction of maxillary anterior teeth (or TADs could be placed as anchors). If headgear or TADs were not used as anchorage, then maxillary posterior teeth would probably move to the mesial more than mandibular posterior teeth during space closure – resulting in a Class II molar relationship.
- *Extraction of maxillary first premolars and mandibular second premolars* – would result in *less* mandibular canine and incisor retraction and *more* mandibular first permanent molar mesial movement during reciprocal space closure than if we extracted mandibular first premolars. Extracting mandibular second premolars improves our chances of achieving a Class I molar relationship in molar "end-on" Class II cases but provides less space to unravel crowded anterior teeth. Overcorrection of Class I canines would be reduced with this extraction pattern – versus extracting four first premolars.

• Mandibular advancement surgery (with or without mandibular premolar extractions) – is not recommended because Trista has a very nice profile (Figure 3.71c).

Q: Which of these comprehensive treatment options would you recommend?

A: We decided to extract Trista's maxillary first premolars and mandibular second premolars. We asked Trista to continue wearing her headgear. Following extractions, fixed orthodontic appliances will be bonded, arches will be leveled and aligned, and extraction spaces closed with the goal of achieving Class I molars, Class I canines, minimal OJ and OB, and ideal occlusal interdigitation, tissue health, function.

Q: Can you suggest "take home pearls" regarding Trista's treatment?

A: "Take home pearls" include the following:

• Trista presented at nine years and ten months of age with her parents' chief complaint, "Trista needs braces." She was Angle Class II division 1, Iowa Classification: II (5 mm) II (5 mm) II (4 mm) II (3 mm) with a crossbite of her maxillary right lateral incisor, 50% OB, significant transverse compensations, maxillary permanent canines ectopically erupting, potentially impacted mandibular left canine, moderate maxillary anterior crowding, and severe mandibular anterior crowding. Her early treatment included RME, high-pull headgear wear, extraction of maxillary primary canines and primary first molars, and an LLHA.

• The *more* maxillary canine crowns overlap maxillary lateral incisal roots on a panoramic image, the *less* likely the canines will erupt unassisted. We were very concerned that Trista's maxillary canines would remain impacted, would continue to erupt ectopically, or would resorb the maxillary lateral incisor roots. We began early treatment by making space for her ectopically erupting maxillary canines with RME, attempting distal movement of the maxillary posterior teeth using headgear, and extraction of her maxillary primary canines/primary first molars. Thankfully, this treatment was effective, and her maxillary canines erupted.

• Treatment for ectopically erupting teeth may include:

a) *Clearing a path for the ectopically erupting teeth to follow* – removing primary teeth, removing permanent teeth, or creating space for the ectopically erupting teeth using headgear, RME, fixed orthodontic appliances, or a removable appliance;

b) *Space regaining to move the ectopically erupting permanent tooth back to its correct position*, especially if arch perimeter has been lost. Surgical exposure may be required to place an orthodontic bracket on an ectopically erupting tooth so that space regaining forces can be applied;

c) *Considering all possible anterior and posterior extraction patterns* (if extractions are indicated).

• Because Trista was ten years old, and because she was close to transitioning into her late mixed dentition, we decided to proceed with Class II orthopedics. High-pull headgear treatment restricted maxillary growth while permitting the mandible to grow forward. As the mandible grew forward, the Class II molar relationship on the left corrected to Class I and the Class II molar relationship on the right was significantly improved.

• *Even if a patient is in the early mixed dentition but has good statural growth velocity (is growing continuously or is in their adolescent growth spurt), you should consider initiating Class II orthopedic treatment.*

• Patients lacking posterior crossbites may present with significant transverse dental compensations (usually maxillary permanent molar buccal crown torque and mandibular permanent molar lingual crown torque) and benefit from RME to create posterior OJ and permit molar uprighting.

• LLHAs are typically used to convert leeway space (or "E space") into improved spontaneous mandibular anterior tooth alignment during the transition from mixed dentition to permanent dentition. LLHAs can also reduce mandibular first permanent molar eruption during growth, thereby helping to rotate the mandible closed, advance B-Point, and correct Class II molar relationships.

• We included Trista in this book as an example of early treatment of ectopic maxillary permanent canine eruption. However, we wish to emphasize another point with Trista – rarely will you encounter patients whose care begins, and ends, with early treatment. It is far more common for a patient to undergo specific early treatments (to prevent complications, reduce later treatment complexity, or reduce unknowns) and then to finish with later comprehensive treatment in the adult dentition. Finally, whether during early treatment or comprehensive treatment, always make your best treatment decision at each step with the aim of providing the patient the finest possible treatment outcome.

Case Melissa

Q: Melissa is eight years and four months of age (Figure 3.72). She was referred by her general dentist for "ectopic eruption of maxillary right lateral incisor."

Her PMH, PDH, periodontal evaluation, and TMJ evaluation are WRN. CR=CO. Compile your diagnostic findings and problem list for Melissa. Also, state your diagnosis.

A:

Table 3.10 Diagnostic findings and problems list for Melissa.

Full face and profile	**Frontal** *view*
	Face is symmetric
	Soft-tissue LAFH WRN (soft-tissue Glabella – Subnasale = Subnasale – soft-tissue Menton)
	Lip competence
	UDML 1 mm right of facial midline
	Profile view
	Straight profile
	Chin projection WRN
	Obtuse NLA
	Lip-chin-throat angle WRN
Radiographs	Early mixed dentition
	Ectopic eruption of maxillary permanent canines and maxillary left first premolar
Intraoral photos and models	Angle Class I
	Iowa Classification: I I I I
	OJ ~0 mm
	OB 60%
	UDML to right of LDML by 1–2 mm due to right shift of maxillary centrals incisors
	3.0 mm maxillary anterior crowding currently present (blocked right lateral incisor)
	1.0 mm maxillary dental arch crowding anticipated after all permanent teeth erupt (if space maintenance is employed)
	2.0 mm mandibular incisor crowding currently present
	1.2 mm mandibular dental arch spacing anticipated after all permanent teeth erupt (if space maintenance is employed)
	Maxillary and mandibular dental arches are symmetric (Figures 3.72h and 3.72i)
Other	None
Diagnosis	Class I malocclusion with ectopic eruption of maxillary permanent canines and maxillary left first premolar

Q: Are you concerned that Melissa's maxillary right lateral incisor has not erupted?

A: Yes and no. On the one hand, inadequate space exists for it to erupt into alignment (Figure 3.72h), and we are concerned that it will either remain blocked from erupting or that it will erupt in torsiversion. Further, her maxillary left lateral incisor has already erupted.

On the other hand, according to the eruption timing values below [67], emergence of the maxillary right lateral incisor is on track, and its incisal edge appears to be nearly piercing the gingiva (Figure 3.72e).

	Maxillary permanent tooth eruption (years)	Mandibular
Central Incisor	7–8	6–7
Lateral Incisor	8–9	7–8
Canine	11–12	9–10
First Premolar	10–11	10–12
Second Premolar	10–12	11–12
First Molar	6–7	6–7
Second Molar	12–13	11–13

Q: Provide a detailed space analysis for Melissa's maxillary and mandibular arches. In other words, how were the anticipated 1.0 mm maxillary dental arch crowding and 1.2 mm mandibular dental arch spacing calculated (*if proper space maintenance is employed*)?

A:

Average mesiodistal widths of permanent teeth (mm) [66]:

Maxillary Central Incisor	8.5	Mandibular Central Incisor	5.0
Maxillary Lateral Incisor	6.5	Mandibular Lateral Incisor	5.5
Maxillary Canine	7.5	Mandibular Canine	7.0
Maxillary First Premolar	7.0	Mandibular First Premolar	7.0
Maxillary Second Premolar	7.0	Mandibular Second Premolar	7.0
Maxillary First Molar	10.0	Mandibular First Molar	11.0
Maxillary Second Molar	9.0	Mandibular Second Molar	10.5

Average mesiodistal widths of *primary* teeth (mm) [66]:

Maxillary Central Incisor	6.5	Mandibular Central Incisor	4.2
Maxillary Lateral Incisor	5.1	Mandibular Lateral Incisor	4.1
Maxillary Canine	7.0	Mandibular Canine	5.0
Maxillary First Molar	7.3	Mandibular First Molar	7.7
Maxillary Second Molar	8.2	Mandibular Second Molar	9.9

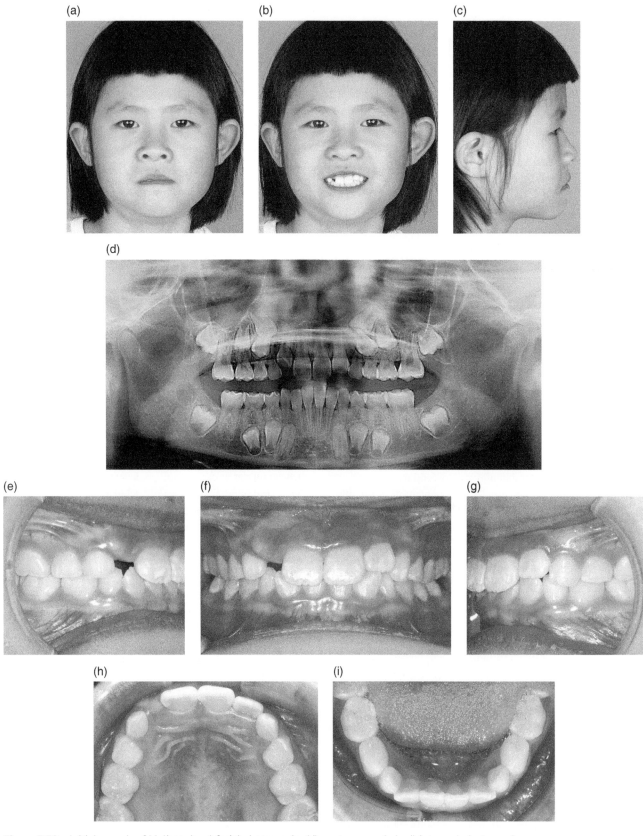

Figure 3.72 Initial records of Melissa: (a–c) facial photographs, (d) pantomograph, (e–i) intraoral photographs.

Maxillary Arch

+4.5 mm space present for maxillary right permanent lateral incisor (Figure 3.72h)

−6.5 mm space needed for unerupted maxillary right permanent lateral incisor

−1 mm of crowding at distal of maxillary left lateral incisor

+2 mm of anticipated leeway space (1 mm/side)

Balance = +4.5 mm −6.5 mm −1 mm +2 mm = −1.0 mm

Mandibular Arch

−2 mm of incisor crowding currently present (Figure 3.72i)

+3.2 mm of anticipated leeway space (1.6 mm/side)

Balance = −2 mm +3.2 mm = +1.2 mm

That is, *1.0 mm of maxillary dental arch crowding and 1.2 mm of mandibular dental arch spacing is anticipated following eruption of all permanent teeth (if proper space maintenance is employed).*

Q: What are Melissa's *primary* problems in each dimension, plus other problems?

A:

Table 3.11 Primary problems list for Melissa.

AP	—
Vertical	60% OB
Transverse	—
Other	Ectopic eruption of maxillary permanent canines and maxillary left first premolar
	Mild maxillary (3 mm) and mandibular (2 mm) anterior crowding currently present

Q: Should you contact Melissa's general dentist regarding her present findings?

A: Yes, it would be a good idea to contact her general dentist to discuss the ectopic eruption of Melissa's maxillary permanent canines and maxillary left first premolar. Our primary concern is these ectopic eruptions and *not* the blocked out maxillary right lateral incisor.

Q: You contact Melissa's general dentist. He is delighted that you have diagnosed the ectopic canine and premolar eruptions. He sends you a panoramic image he made eighteen months earlier. What changes have occurred since he exposed this radiograph?

A: During the past eighteen months (compare Figures 3.62d and 3.63), Melissa's permanent mandibular lateral incisors, permanent maxillary central incisors, and permanent maxillary left lateral incisor have emerged. Permanent canine and premolar root development has begun. *Ectopic maxillary permanent canine and maxillary left first premolar eruption was evident as early as six years and ten months of age.*

Q: Discuss Melissa in the context of three principles applied to every early treatment patient.

A:

1) The goal of early treatment is to correct developing problems – get the patient *back to normal for their stage of development* (including preventing complications, reducing later treatment complexity, or reducing/eliminating unknowns). Correcting ectopic eruption of her maxillary permanent canines and left first premolar, alleviating her mild anterior crowding, and correcting her deep bite would get her back on track.

2) Early treatment should address *very specific problems with a clearly defined end point*, usually within six to nine months (except for some orthopedic treatments). Extraction of Melissa's maxillary primary canines and maxillary primary first molars, combined with placement of a Nance holding arch to prevent permanent first molar mesial drift/arch perimeter loss, could create a path/space for eruption of her maxillary permanent canines and first premolars. However, we are concerned that the roots of her maxillary permanent canines and first premolars are <½ developed, and extracting these primary teeth could *delay* eruption of the maxillary permanent canines and first premolars [28].

   Placement of an LLHA could reduce mandibular anterior crowding using leeway space as the permanent teeth erupt. However, the mandibular permanent canines and premolars are not close to erupting. Limited fixed orthodontic appliances (e.g. maxillary 2×4 appliance) could intrude her maxillary incisors and reduce her OB in six to nine months.

3) Always ask: Is it necessary that I treat the patient now? *What harm will come if I choose to do nothing now?* If we do nothing, then the ectopic eruption of Melissa's maxillary permanent canines and left first premolar could worsen, and the permanent canines could resorb the maxillary first premolar roots. We do not anticipate any harm if LLHA placement is delayed for at least a year. Finally, because no pain or tissue damage is resulting from her deep bite, we anticipate no harm in delaying correction of Melissa's deep bite until comprehensive treatment in the permanent dentition.

Q: Can you summarize treatment guidelines to follow when correcting ectopic eruption of permanent teeth?

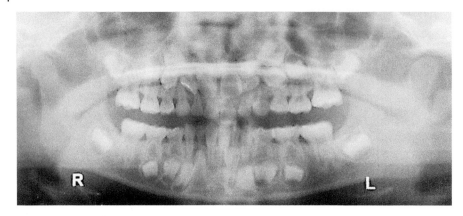

Figure 3.73 Panoramic image of Melissa made at age 6 years and 10 months.

A: Guidelines include:
- *Clearing a path (making space) for the ectopically erupting tooth to follow.*
- *Space regaining to move the ectopically erupting permanent tooth back to its correct position*, especially if arch perimeter has been lost. Surgical exposure of the ectopically erupting tooth may be necessary.
- *Consider all possible anterior and posterior extraction patterns* if the patient is clearly an extraction case or in instances of severe root resorption.

Q: Should you start treatment now or recall Melissa? What options would you consider?

A: Options include the following:
- *Recall* (monitor only, reevaluate in one year) – is not recommended. The complexity of later comprehensive treatment and the likelihood of future complications could be dramatically reduced with early treatment. Specifically, the ectopic eruption of her maxillary permanent canines and left first premolar should be addressed. Not only are her maxillary permanent canines potentially impacted, but the roots of her maxillary first premolars could be resorbed by the canines if treatment is delayed.
- *Extraction of maxillary primary canines and primary first molars* (to create space and provide an eruption path for maxillary permanent canines and first premolars) – is recommended. Even though the maxillary permanent canine and premolar roots are <1/2 developed, and even though their delayed eruption could result if we extract the primary teeth, the risk of *not* extracting primary teeth is worse (potential impaction of maxillary permanent canines and/or resorption of the first premolar roots).
- *Maxillary space maintenance* (Nance holding arch) – is recommended to prevent mesial drift of the maxillary permanent first molars (arch perimeter loss) if the

maxillary primary canines and primary first molars are extracted.
- *Mandibular space maintenance* (placement of an LLHA) – is not recommended at this time because exfoliation of the mandibular primary canines and primary molars is not anticipated during the next year.
- *Space regaining* (opening space for the maxillary right lateral incisor) – is not recommended because only minimal (1.0 mm) maxillary anterior crowding is anticipated if maxillary space maintenance is employed.
- *Serial extraction* – is not recommended because only mild maxillary (3 mm) and mandibular (2 mm) crowding is present.

Q: What is your recommended treatment? How would you proceed?

A: We recommended bilateral extraction of Melissa's maxillary primary canines and primary first molars in order to create space for maxillary first premolar and right lateral incisor eruption. Eruption of the first premolar roots away from the canine crowns would, hopefully, make space to encourage eruption of the canines. We also recommended placement of a Nance holding arch to prevent mesial drift of the maxillary first permanent molars.

Along with primary teeth extractions, we asked the surgeon to remove bone covering the maxillary first premolar occlusal surfaces in the hope of freeing those teeth to erupt. We explained to Melissa's parents that additional early treatment may be necessary (surgical exposure and forced orthodontic eruption of maxillary permanent teeth), that the ectopically erupting teeth may be ankylosed and not erupt, and that root resorption of the maxillary first premolars may have already occurred.

Q: One year and four months later, we made another panoramic image of Melissa (Figure 3.74). What do you observe and what additional early treatment (if any) do you recommend?

A: Her maxillary first premolars have not erupted, but the maxillary right lateral incisor did erupt. All permanent canine and premolar roots are developing, and eruption of the mandibular permanent canines is imminent. The maxillary first premolars direction of eruption is *into the roots* of the maxillary second primary molars.

We next recommended extraction of the maxillary primary *second* molars, followed by a period of observation to see if the first premolars would erupt. If the first premolars did not erupt, then we would consider surgical exposure of the first premolars.

Q: Due to the COVID-19 pandemic, Melissa did not return to our clinic until she was ten years and ten months of age. Progress records were made (Figure 3.75). Can you describe her primary problems at this time?

A:

Table 3.12 Primary problems list for Melissa.

AP	Angle Class II division 1
	Iowa Classification: II (3 mm) X X II (3 mm)
Vertical	50% OB (noted in Figure 3.75d and m)
	Flat MPA (FMA = 19°, SNMP = 21°)
Transverse	—
Other	Upright mandibular incisors (FMIA = 72°)
	Ectopic eruption of maxillary left permanent canine
	Inadequate space for eruption of maxillary second premolars (blocked out)

Q: Do you recommend additional early treatment? If you do, then what treatment would you recommend?

A: We removed the Nance holding arch, fitted bands to the maxillary first permanent molars, and placed Melissa on a HPHG to retract her maxillary first permanent molars into a mild Class III (1 mm) molar relationship. This movement would provide additional space for her maxillary second premolars to erupt. An LLHA was also fabricated and placed.

We plan to monitor eruption of all permanent teeth, and her parents have been informed of the need for eventual comprehensive treatment in the adult dentition. Although the erupting maxillary right permanent canine position has improved, the possible need to surgically expose both canines was discussed.

Q: Can you suggest "take home pearls" regarding Melissa's treatment?

A: "Take home pearls" include:
- Melissa was eight years of age when she presented for treatment of right lateral incisor ectopic eruption. Since the general dentist did not make a current panoramic image, he was unable to observe that ectopic eruption of Melissa's maxillary permanent canines and left first premolar were the more serious problems. Also, the maxillary right permanent lateral incisor was blocked out – not erupting ectopically.
- Following our recommended guideline for treatment of ectopically erupting teeth – we *cleared a path (made space) for the ectopically erupting teeth to follow*. We extracted Melissa's maxillary primary canines and maxillary primary first molars in the hope that space creation would allow the maxillary first premolars to erupt. The maxillary first premolars did not erupt, and

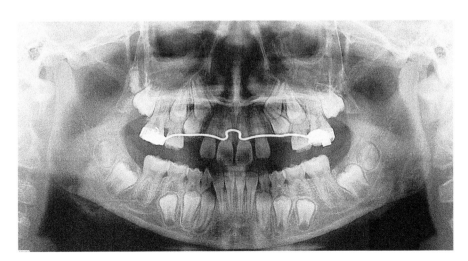

Figure 3.74 Progress panoramic image of Melissa at age nine years and eight months.

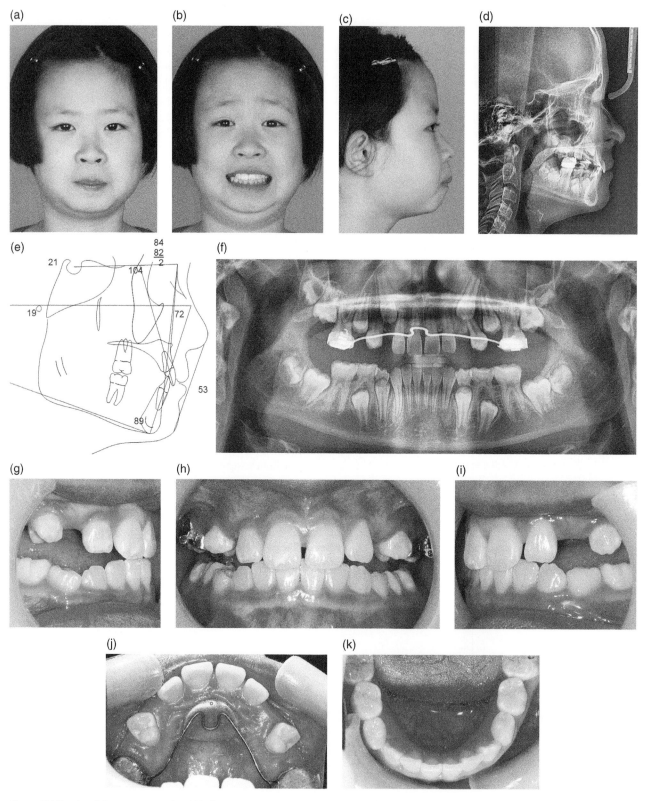

Figure 3.75 (a–p) Progress records of Melissa at ten years and ten months of age. Note in (a) and (c) that her lips are pursed and that she appears slightly open in her intraoral photographs.

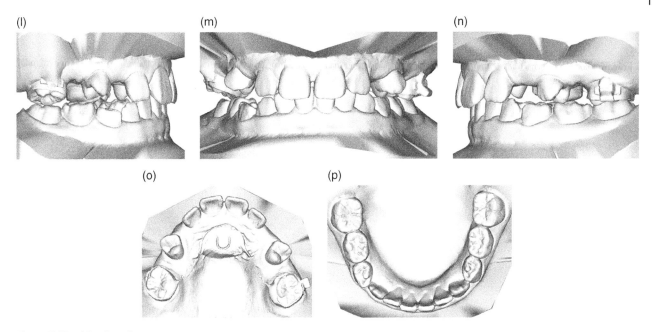

Figure 3.75 (Continued)

it appeared that they were blocked by the maxillary primary second molars. Extraction of the maxillary primary second molars resulted in the maxillary first premolars erupting and the maxillary right permanent canine appearing to be in better position.

- Should we have extracted the maxillary primary *second* molars when we extracted the maxillary primary canines and primary first molars? Examining Figure 3.72d, our decision to extract *only* the maxillary primary canines and primary first molars seemed reasonable.
- Melissa's case underscores the following: early orthodontic treatment requires a clear initial assessment of the problem(s) followed by focused treatment to address the problem(s) followed by monitoring and reassessment.

Case Cara

Q: Cara is ten years old (Figure 3.76). She presents to you with her parents' question, "Does Cara need braces?" They state that Cara has seen another doctor who recently graduated, and they would like a second opinion. Cara's PMH, PDH, periodontal evaluation, and TMJ evaluations are WRN. CR=CO. Her mandibular right primary canine is very mobile. Compile your diagnostic findings and problem list for Cara. Also, state your diagnosis.

A:

Table 3.13 Diagnostic findings and problems list for Cara.

Full face and profile	*Frontal view*
	Face is symmetric
	Soft-tissue LAFH WRN (soft-tissue Glabella – Subnasale > Subnasale – soft-tissue Menton in frontal view, but Cara appears tipped down compared to profile view)
	Lip competence
	UDML WRN
	Profile view
	Convex profile
	Obtuse NLA
	Mildly deep labiomental sulcus
	Retrusive chin projection
	Lip-chin-throat angle WRN
Radiographs	Early mixed dentition (eruption of mandibular left permanent canine is imminent)
	Large occlusal steps between mandibular first permanent molars and primary second molars
Intraoral Photos and Models	Angle Class II
	Iowa Classification: II (3 mm) II (3 mm) II (3 mm) II (3 mm)
	OJ ~ 2–3 mm
	OB 50%

(Continued)

Table 3.13 (Continued)

	Right posterior open bite at primary first and second molars
	Large occlusal steps between mandibular first permanent molars and primary second molars (Figures 3.76e and 3.76g)
	0.0 mm maxillary anterior crowding currently present
	2.0 mm maxillary arch spacing is anticipated following eruption of all permanent teeth (if proper space maintenance is employed)
	1.0 mm mandibular anterior spacing currently present
	4.2 mm mandibular arch spacing is anticipated following eruption of all permanent teeth (if proper space maintenance is employed)
	Maxillary and mandibular dental arches are symmetric
	Maxillary incisors are over-erupted relative to posterior teeth (Figures 3.76e and 3.76g)
Other	None
Diagnosis	Class II malocclusion in the early mixed dentition with posterior open bite

Q: Provide a detailed space analysis for Cara's maxillary and mandibular arches. In other words, how were the anticipated 2.0 mm maxillary arch spacing and 4.2 mm mandibular arch spacing calculated (*if proper space maintenance is employed*)?

A:

Average mesiodistal widths of permanent teeth (mm) [66]:

Maxillary Central Incisor	8.5	Mandibular Central Incisor	5.0
Maxillary Lateral Incisor	6.5	Mandibular Lateral Incisor	5.5
Maxillary Canine	7.5	Mandibular Canine	7.0
Maxillary First Premolar	7.0	Mandibular First Premolar	7.0
Maxillary Second Premolar	7.0	Mandibular Second Premolar	7.0
Maxillary First Molar	10.0	Mandibular First Molar	11.0
Maxillary Second Molar	9.0	Mandibular Second Molar	10.5

Average mesiodistal widths of *primary* teeth (mm) [66]:

Maxillary Central Incisor	6.5	Mandibular Central Incisor	4.2
Maxillary Lateral Incisor	5.1	Mandibular Lateral Incisor	4.1
Maxillary Canine	7.0	Mandibular Canine	5.0
Maxillary First Molar	7.3	Mandibular First Molar	7.7
Maxillary Second Molar	8.2	Mandibular Second Molar	9.9

Maxillary Arch

0.0 mm maxillary anterior crowding currently present (Figure 3.76h)

+2.0 mm of anticipated leeway space (1 mm/side)

Balance = 0.0 mm +2.0 mm = +2.0 mm

Mandibular Arch

+1.0 mm mandibular anterior spacing currently present (Figure 3.76i)

+3.2 mm of anticipated leeway space (1.6 mm/side)

Balance = +1.0 mm +3.2 mm = +4.2 mm

That is, *2.0 mm of maxillary spacing and 4.2 mm of mandibular spacing is anticipated following eruption of all permanent teeth (if proper space maintenance is employed).*

Q: Always focus on the patient's *primary* problems in each dimension, plus other problems, at each appointment. What are Cara's primary problems?

A:

Table 3.14 Primary problems list for Cara.

AP	Angle Class II Iowa Classification: II (3 mm) II (3 mm) II (3 mm) II (3 mm)
Vertical	50% OB Right posterior open bite
Transverse	—
Other	—

Q: Can you list probable causes of Cara's right posterior open bite?

A: Probable causes include:
- Ankylosis of primary mandibular molars
- Tongue interposition habit
- Digit or other interposition habit

Q: What three principles apply to every early treatment patient, and how do these apply to Cara?

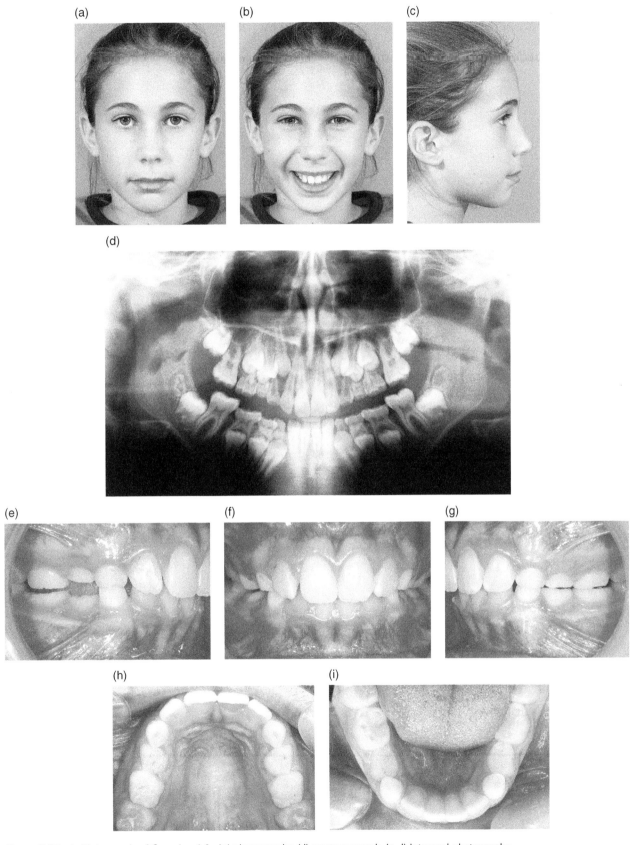

Figure 3.76 Initial records of Cara: (a–c) facial photographs, (d) pantomograph, (e–i) intraoral photographs.

A: The three principles are:
1) The goal of early treatment is to correct developing problems with the intent of getting the patient *back to normal for that stage of development*. Corrections include preventing complications such as adjacent tooth root resorption, reducing later treatment complexity, and reducing/eliminating unknowns. Cara's problems include her Class II relationship (3 mm bilaterally), deep bite (50%), and right posterior open bite.
2) Early treatment should address *very specific problems with a clearly defined end point*, usually within six to nine months (not drag on for years except for some orthopedic treatments). Class II orthopedics would address a focused problem but could take years depending upon growth and compliance. The deep bite is a specific problem that could be treated in six to nine months with fixed orthodontic appliances by intruding over-erupted incisors. Her right posterior open bite may take longer to correct, depending upon its etiology (ankylosis of primary molars or tongue interposition habit).
3) Always ask: Is it necessary that I treat the patient now? *What harm will come from not doing anything now?* If we do not begin Class II orthopedics as Cara enters her late mixed dentition stage of development, or as she exhibits good statural growth in the early mixed dentition, then we may miss helpful jaw growth. Since she exhibits neither mandibular incisor palatal impingement nor pain/tissue damage, there is no need to correct her deep bite now. Lastly, no harm will come from monitoring her posterior open bite.

Q: Cara's parents state that the other doctor recommended beginning Class II orthopedic treatment now. What do you think?

A: We feel that beginning Class II orthopedics is reasonable since Cara will be entering the late mixed dentition stage of development soon (note in Figure 3.76d that the mandibular left permanent canine is near eruption.

Q: Cara and her parents thank you for your opinion. One year later, you receive a call from the Cara's (other) doctor. He says that Cara has been compliant wearing a headgear and asks you to look at the panoramic image he just made (Figure 3.77). What do you observe?

A: Space has opened between the maxillary first permanent molars and primary second molars as headgear retracted the maxillary first molars. Permanent tooth eruption is proceeding.

Q: We missed it! Did you miss it? Look closely and compare the magnified panoramic images of Cara's mandibular right primary second molar (Figure 3.78a at age ten, Figure 3.78b at age eleven) and magnified images of her left primary second molar (Figure 3.78c at age ten, Figure 3.78d at age eleven). What do you now observe?

A: Close examination of her mandibular right reveals that the occlusal step between the primary second molar and permanent first molar increased during the past year and that the alveolar bone crest slants downward (is not horizontal) from the permanent first molar to the right primary second molar. Her mandibular left images also reveal a downward slant of the alveolar bone crest from the mandibular left permanent first molar to the mandibular left primary second molar.

Q: What do these observations mean?

A: The mandibular right primary second molar is ankylosed. As the mandibular right permanent first molar continued to erupt and the primary second molar

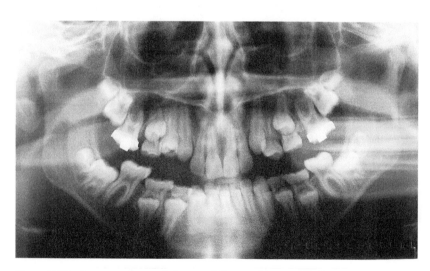

Figure 3.77 Progress panoramic image of Cara at eleven years of age.

(a) (b) (c) (d)

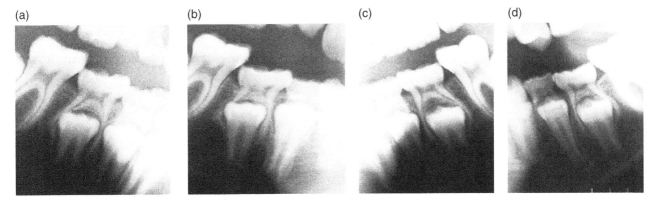

Figure 3.78 Magnified panoramic images of Cara's mandibular right primary second molar (a) at age ten, (b) at age eleven. Magnified images of her mandibular left primary second molar (c) at age ten, (d) at age eleven.

stopped erupting, the alveolar bone crest level of the ankylosed right primary second molar was left behind at a more apical level. Although less pronounced, the mandibular left primary second molar is also ankylosed. This is what the younger doctor thought, and you confirm his suspicions.

Q: Could these primary second molar ankyloses have been initially diagnosed based upon their *occlusal* steps with the permanent first molars (Figure 3.76d)?

A: No, it is unwise to diagnose ankylosis based upon an occlusal step between primary second molars and permanent first molars. Why? The primary second molar crown heights are short relative to the permanent first molar crown heights. Because of this difference, *an occlusal (clinical) step between the primary second molar and permanent first molar is not unusual – even without ankylosis.* An occlusal step is not a reliable indicator of primary tooth ankylosis.

On the other hand, a radiographic discrepancy in alveolar crest bone heights indicates that eruption of the ankylosed tooth has halted while eruption of the non-ankylosed tooth has continued. The earlier the onset of ankylosis, the greater will be the alveolar crest bone height discrepancy. *The best way to confirm ankylosis of a tooth in growing individuals is to look for an alveolar crest bone height discrepancy between the suspect tooth and adjacent teeth.* Of course, you can always check mobility. If a primary tooth is mobile, then it is not ankylosed or close to exfoliation.

Q: What options can you suggest for dealing with Cara's ankylosed mandibular primary second molars?

A: Options include:
- *Monitor only (recall)* – is reasonable since Cara's mandibular permanent first molars (and erupting second premolars) are in reasonably good positions (Figures 3.78b–3.78d). Eruption of the second premolars may be

delayed by six months because of the ankylosed primary second molars, but the final bone (levels) will be normal after the second premolars erupt [36, 41, 106].
- *Space maintenance* – is reasonable. Placement of an LLHA would prevent further permanent first molar mesial tip (space loss, arch perimeter loss) over the ankylosed primary second molars as the first molars erupt.
- *Space regaining* – is not recommend in Cara's case – at least not now. However, in cases where a mandibular permanent first molar has erupted and tipped significantly to the mesial [39] *over* the ankylosed primary second molar (Figure 3.79), it is prudent to first tip the mandibular first molar to the distal before placing an LLHA. Such space regaining prevents the mandibular permanent first molar from impacting the second premolar.
- *Extraction of mandibular primary second molars* – would accelerate eruption of second premolars whose

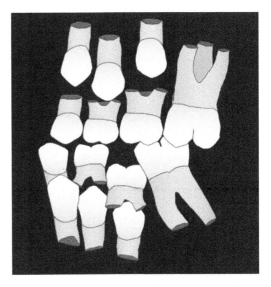

Figure 3.79 An erupting mandibular permanent first molar tipping to the mesial over an ankylosed mandibular primary second molar. Space loss from this movement can impact the second premolar.

roots are >1/2 developed [28]. However, extraction of ankylosed primary second molars would require a significant surgery. Furthermore, the mandibular second premolars are erupting (Figures 3.78a–3.78d), and second primary molar extraction is therefore unnecessary.

Q: You discuss the above options with the other doctor. How do *you* recommend dealing with Cara's anklyosed mandibular primary second molars?

A: **A.** We recommended placement of an LLHA and monitoring, but Cara's mandibular primary second molars were extracted instead. As her mandibular second premolars erupted, he noted that inadequate space was available for them (Figure 3.80). In fact, if you compare Figures 3.67–3.70, you will notice that significant space has been lost following second primary molar extractions. At this time, Cara's early treatment ended as she was now in adult dentition. We recommended beginning comprehensive treatment, and he placed fixed orthodontic appliances in both arches.

Arches were leveled and aligned, and additional space was opened for the mandibular second premolars using compressed open coil springs placed along the archwire between the mandibular permanent first molars and mandibular first premolars. Once the mandibular second premolars erupted, they were bonded, leveled and aligned, and treatment finished. He sent you the deband panoramic image shown in Figure 3.81.

Q: Can you suggest "take home pearls" regarding Cara's treatment?

A: "Take home pearls" include the following:

- Cara presented to us for a second opinion at age ten. She was Class II by 3 mm bilaterally with a 50% OB. She

was placed on a headgear to correct her Class II molar relationship. One year later, ankylosis of both mandibular primary second molars was observed, they were extracted, and space was created for her mandibular second premolars during comprehensive treatment.

- *The best way to confirm ankylosis of a tooth in a growing individual is to look for an alveolar crest bone height discrepancy between it and adjacent (erupting) teeth.*
- Even if you do not suspect ankylosis in initial radiographic images, continue to look for developing ankylosis in progress images of all children.
- Because there appeared to be adequate space for eruption of her mandibular second premolars (Figure 3.77), an LLHA was not placed at the time of primary second molar extractions. However, space was lost following primary second molar extractions, and this space needed to be regained during comprehensive treatment.
- Instead of primary second molar extractions, we recommended placement of an LLHA and waiting for (delayed) eruption of her mandibular second premolars. As expected, the final alveolar crestal bone heights of erupted mandibular second premolars were normal (Figure 3.81).

Case Easton

Q: Easton is eight years and three months of age (Figure 3.82). He was referred by his family dentist for "ectopic eruption of maxillary left permanent first molar following premature loss of maxillary left primary second molar." His PMH, PDH, periodontal evaluation, and TMJ evaluations are WRN. CR=CO. Compile your diagnostic findings and problem list for Easton. Also, state your diagnosis.

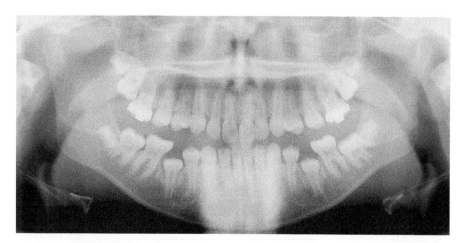

Figure 3.80 Progress panoramic image of Cara made sometime after extraction of her ankylosed mandibular primary second molars. Note that inadequate space is available for her erupting mandibular second premolars.

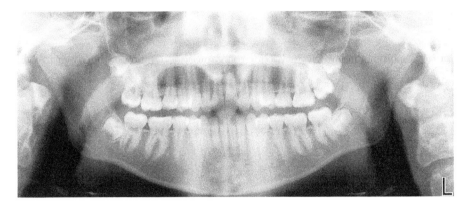

Figure 3.81 Deband panoramic image of Cara.

A:

Table 3.15 Diagnostic findings and problems list for Easton.

Full face and Profile	***Frontal view*** Face is symmetric Long soft-tissue LAFH (soft-tissue Glabella – Subnasale < Subnasale – soft-tissue Menton) Lip competence UDML WRN	**Intraoral Photos and Models**	Ectopically erupting and potentially impacted maxillary left second premolar Maxillary left permanent first molar is tipped to the mesial Angle Class II subdivision left Iowa Classification: I I III (1 mm) II (6 mm) OB 30% (left central incisors) OJ ~1 mm Maxillary right central incisor just emerging 7.8 mm of *total* maxillary arch crowding is currently present (anterior plus posterior) 6.8 mm anticipated future maxillary arch crowding (if proper space maintenance is employed. Space regaining by distalizing the maxillary left permanent first molar could significantly reduce future crowding) 3.8 mm of mandibular incisor crowding is currently present (permanent lateral incisors have not erupted but are included in this calculation) 0.6 mm anticipated future mandibular arch crowding – if proper space maintenance is employed UDML left of LDML by ~0.5 mm Maxillary dental arch asymmetry – maxillary left permanent first molar is positioned *ahead* of the maxillary right permanent first molar. Also, the maxillary left primary canine is positioned *behind* the maxillary right primary canine. Mandibular dental arch is symmetric
	Profile view Convex profile Obtuse NLA Retrusive chin projection Obtuse lip-chin-throat angle		
Ceph Analysis	***Skeletal*** Maxillary anteroposterior position WRN (A-Point lies on Nasion-perpendicular line) Mandibular anteroposterior position WRN (ANB angle = 1° with maxilla WRN) Long skeletal LAFH (ANS-Menton/Nasion-Menton X 100% = 58%; normal = 55%, s.d. = 2%) Mandibular plane angle WRN (FMA = 24°; SNMP = 38°) Effective bony Pogonion (bony Pogonion lies slightly ahead of a line extended from Nasion through B-point)		
	Dental Maxillary incisor inclination WRN (U1 to SN – 104°; normal U1to SN – 101–104°) Mandibular incisor inclination WRN (FMIA = 68°, normal FMIA = 65°–68°)	**Other**	None
Radiographs	Early mixed dentition Maxillary right central incisor just emerging Unerupted maxillary and mandibular lateral incisors	**Diagnosis**	Class II subdivision left malocclusion in the early mixed dentition with mesial drift of maxillary left permanent first molar, moderate maxillary and mild mandibular arch crowding, ectopic and potentially impacted maxillary left second premolar

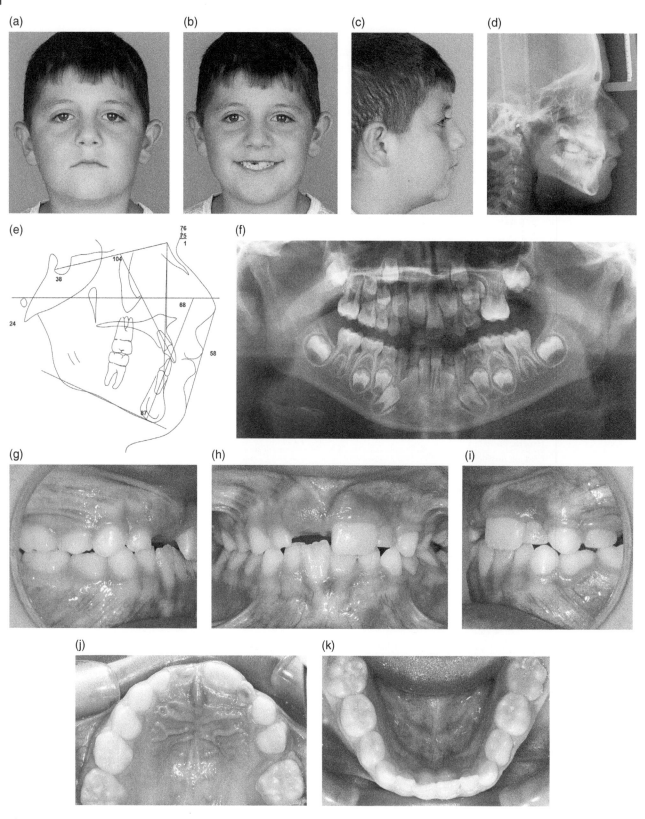

Figure 3.82 Initial records of Easton: (a–c) facial photographs, (d and e) cephalometric radiograph and tracing, (f) pantomograph, (g–k) intraoral photographs, (l–p) model photographs.

(l)   (m)   (n)

(o)   (p)

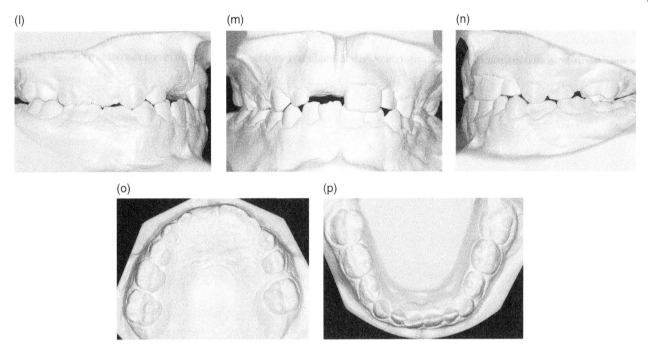

Figure 3.82   (Continued)

Q: How can Easton's profile be convex (Figure 3.82c) when his maxillary and mandibular anteroposterior positions are normal (Figure 3.82e)?

A: Although Easton's bony chin projection is effective, it is *minimally* effective. If his bony Pogonion was more effective, then he would have greater soft tissue chin projection and a straighter profile.

Q: How can Easton's mandibular plane angle be WRN when SN-MP = 38° (normal SN-MP =32°)?

A: You need to consider SN-MP *and* FMA when judging MPA. We consider his MPA to be WRN because his FMA (24°) is *less* than the average FMA (25°) and because Nasion appears high/Sella appears low making SM-MP greater than average. In other words, ~7° is the normal upward inclination of the S-N line relative to Frankfort horizontal. Easton's S-N line is ~14° divergent from Frankfort horizontal due to a high Nasion or low Sella.

Finally, it is not necessary for any cephalometric measurement to be the exact average value for it to be considered WRN. For instance, an FMA in the range of 21–29 degrees would be considered normal.

Q: Easton is an excellent example of unfavorable changes accompanying premature loss of a maxillary primary second molar. Can you list his unfavorable changes?

A: His unfavorable changes include:
Mesial drift of the adjacent permanent first molar
Distal drift of the adjacent primary first molar and ipsilateral primary canine

Impaction of the second premolar due to mesial drift of the maxillary permanent first molar
Maxillary dental arch asymmetry in cases of unilateral primary second molar loss

Q: What are Easton's *primary* problems in each dimension, plus other problems?

A:

Table 3.16   Primary problems list for Easton.

AP	Angle Class II subdivision left
	Iowa Classification: I I III (1 mm) II (6 mm)
Vertical	Anterior open bite
Transverse	—
Other	Mesial drift of maxillary left permanent first molar
	Distal drift of maxillary left primary canine and primary first molar
	Ectopic eruption and potential impaction of maxillary left second premolar
	Moderate maxillary and mild mandibular arch crowding

Q: Are you concerned that eruption of Easton's maxillary right permanent central incisor (and lateral incisors) is delayed?

A: Compared to the *average* permanent tooth eruption times shown below [67], eruption of Easton's maxillary right permanent central incisor is (slightly) delayed. Eruption of his maxillary lateral incisors appears to be on track (Figure 3.82f). We are not concerned.

	Maxillary	**Mandibular**
Central Incisor	7–8	6–7
Lateral Incisor	8–9	7–8
Canine	11–12	9–10
First Premolar	10–11	10–12
Second Premolar	10–12	11–12
First Molar	6–7	6–7
Second Molar	12–13	11–13

Q: You contact Easton's dentist to obtain more information regarding the missing maxillary left primary second molar. He sends you a panoramic image made two years earlier (Figure 3.83). What do you observe?

A: At six years of age, Easton was in the primary dentition. Contrasted with his maxillary right primary second molar, maxillary primary canines, and maxillary primary first molars, Easton's *maxillary left primary second molar is not erupting*. The dentist states that he extracted the maxillary left primary second molar because he thought it was ankylosed.

Q: What should have been placed at the time Easton's maxillary left primary second molar was extracted?

A: Early extraction of a maxillary second primary molar, whether due to caries or ankylosis, will result in mesial drift of the adjacent permanent first molar. In Easton's case, a space maintainer should have been placed to lessen maxillary left permanent first molar mesial drift. A distal shoe appliance could have been cemented to the maxillary left primary first molar to engage the mesial surface of the developing permanent first molar and guide its eruption [107]. Remember, such a space maintainer will be lost when the primary first molar exfoliates.

Alternatively, as soon as the maxillary first permanent molars erupt, the distal shoe can be removed and a Nance holding arch cemented to the permanent first molars. Or, a clear thermoplastic retainer could have been worn. *A space maintainer should be placed following premature loss of primary second molars, primary first molars, or primary canines if arch perimeter loss due to tooth drift is a concern.*

Q: Provide a detailed space analysis for Easton's maxillary and mandibular arches. How were the anticipated 6.8 mm maxillary arch crowding and 0.6 mm mandibular arch crowding calculated (if we employ proper space maintenance)?

A:

Average mesiodistal widths of permanent teeth (mm) [66]:

Maxillary Central Incisor	8.5	Mandibular Central Incisor	5.0
Maxillary Lateral Incisor	6.5	Mandibular Lateral Incisor	5.5
Maxillary Canine	7.5	Mandibular Canine	7.0
Maxillary First Premolar	7.0	Mandibular First Premolar	7.0
Maxillary Second Premolar	7.0	Mandibular Second Premolar	7.0
Maxillary First Molar	10.0	Mandibular First Molar	11.0
Maxillary Second Molar	9.0	Mandibular Second Molar	10.5

Average mesiodistal widths of *primary* teeth (mm) [66]:

Maxillary Central Incisor	6.5	Mandibular Central Incisor	4.2
Maxillary Lateral Incisor	5.1	Mandibular Lateral Incisor	4.1
Maxillary Canine	7.0	Mandibular Canine	5.0
Maxillary First Molar	7.3	Mandibular First Molar	7.7
Maxillary Second Molar	8.2	Mandibular Second Molar	9.9

Maxillary Arch (we cannot use maxillary left leeway space because the maxillary left primary second molar exfoliated)

+1.0 mm of anticipated right leeway space (Figure 3.82j)

+5.1 mm mesiodistal width of maxillary right primary lateral incisor

−6.5 mm of space needed for maxillary right permanent lateral incisor

+8.0 mm of maxillary right central incisor space present

−8.5 mm of space needed for maxillary right permanent central incisor

+5.1 mm mesiodistal width of maxillary left primary lateral incisor

−6.5 mm of space needed for maxillary left permanent lateral incisor

+17 mm distance from mesial of maxillary left primary canine to mesial of maxillary left permanent first molar

−7.5 mm of space needed for maxillary left permanent canine

−7 mm of space needed for maxillary left first premolar

−7 mm of space needed for maxillary left second premolar

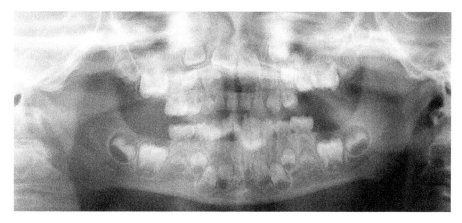

Figure 3.83 Panoramic image of Easton made at six years of age.

Balance = +1.0 mm +5.1 mm −6.5 mm +8.0 mm −8.5 mm +5.1 mm −6.5 mm +17.0 mm −7.5 mm −7.0 mm −7.0 mm = −6.8 mm

Mandibular Arch (mandibular permanent lateral incisors have not erupted)

−1 mm of incisor crowding currently present (Figure 3.82k)
+4.1 mm mesiodistal width of mandibular left primary lateral incisor
−5.5 mm of space needed for mandibular left permanent lateral incisor
+4.1 mm mesiodistal width of mandibular right primary lateral incisor
−5.5 mm of space needed for mandibular right permanent lateral incisor
+3.2 mm of anticipated leeway space (1.6 mm/side)
Balance = −1 mm +4.1 mm −5.5 mm +4.1 mm −5.5 mm +3.2 mm = −0.6 mm

That is, *6.8 mm of maxillary arch crowding and 0.6 mm of mandibular arch crowding are anticipated following eruption of all permanent teeth (if proper space maintenance is employed).*

Q: What guidelines should you follow in dealing with the ectopically erupting (and potentially impacted) maxillary left second premolar (Figure 3.82f)?

A: Guidelines include:
- *Clear a path (make space) for it to follow/erupt*
- Employ *space regaining to move the maxillary left permanent first molar distally to its correct position*, especially since arch perimeter has been lost. Surgical exposure, and orthodontic forced eruption, of the maxillary left second premolar may be necessary.
- If you conclude that Easton is an extraction case (or if you determine that the ectopically-erupting second premolar is causing severe root resorption of the

permanent first molar), then *consider all possible anterior and posterior extraction patterns* including extraction of the second premolar or permanent first molar.

Q: Discuss Easton in the context of three principles applied to every early treatment patient.

A:

1) The goal of early treatment is to correct developing problems – get the patient *back to normal for their stage of development* (including preventing complications, reducing later treatment complexity, or reducing/eliminating unknowns). Facilitating eruption of Easton's maxillary left premolars and maxillary right central incisor, eliminating his crowding, and correcting his left Class II molar relationship would get him back on track for his stage of development.

2) Early treatment should address *very specific problems with a clearly defined end point*, usually within six to nine months (except for some orthopedic problems). Space regaining by retracting his maxillary left permanent first molar into a Class I relationship will probably take less than nine months, but subsequent eruption of his maxillary left premolars may take longer. Eruption of his maxillary right permanent central incisor should take less than six months. Crowding reduction will take years because space lost because of maxillary left permanent first molar mesial drift must first be regained and because permanent canine and premolar roots are only beginning to develop (assuming that space maintenance will be employed to use leeway space for crowding reduction).

3) Always ask: Is it necessary that I treat the patient now? *What harm will come if I choose to do nothing now?* If we chose to do nothing:
   - The ectopically erupting maxillary left second premolar could resorb roots of the maxillary left permanent first molar.

- Maxillary left premolars and maxillary left permanent canine could remain impacted.
- The anterior open bite could possibly remain, or the maxillary right permanent central incisor could erupt into a malaligned position.

Q: Should you start treatment or recall Easton? If you start treatment, what treatment options would you consider?

A: Treatment options include the following:

- *Recall* (monitor only, reevaluate in one year) – is not recommended. Why? Correcting the ectopically erupting maxillary left second premolar and maxillary left Class II molar relationship could dramatically reduce later (comprehensive) treatment complexity. In addition, if the ectopically erupting maxillary left second premolar remains in its current position, then it could resorb the maxillary left permanent first molar roots. Monitoring eruption of the maxillary right central incisor *is* a viable option.

- *Maxillary space maintenance* (Nance holding arch) – is not recommended because it would not address the maxillary left second premolar ectopic eruption nor would it address the left Class II molar relationship. We *would* recommend placement of a Nance holding arch or other retainer once the maxillary left permanent first molar was retracted to the distal into a Class I relationship.

- *Mandibular space maintenance* (placement of an LLHA) – is not recommended yet because exfoliation of the mandibular primary canines and primary molars is not anticipated during the next year.

- *Space regaining* (opening space for the maxillary left second premolar by moving the maxillary left permanent first molar to the distal into a Class I relationship) – is strongly recommended and could result in normal eruption of the maxillary left premolars.

- *Extraction of maxillary left primary lateral incisor, primary canine and primary first molar* – in order to create space for eruption of the maxillary left permanent lateral incisor and first premolar. This could eventually be a good option because subsequent eruption of the maxillary left lateral incisor and first premolar could provide room for eruption of the maxillary left permanent canine and second premolar. However, we would not recommend this option yet because roots of the maxillary premolars and maxillary permanent canine are <1/2 developed, and extracting the primary teeth now could result in *delayed* eruption of the permanent canine and first premolar [28].

- *Serial extraction* – is not recommended because only mild to moderate crowding is found in both arches and because maxillary space regaining could reduce maxillary crowding significantly.

Q: What is your recommended treatment? How would you proceed?

A: We examined mobility of Easton's maxillary left primary canine and primary first molar. They were immobile and could be used as anchor teeth during space regaining. Following discussion of options with Easton and his mother, we proceeded with space regaining using a removable molar screw distalizer appliance (Figure 3.84, 0.5 mm opening per week). We also monitored eruption of the maxillary right central incisor. An LLHA would be placed when mandibular primary canines or primary first molars became mobile.

Another option for space regaining involves placing fixed orthodontic appliances (bonded to the maxillary left primary canine, primary first molar, and permanent first molar) and trapping a compressed open coil spring between the primary first molar and permanent first molar.

Q: When Easton reaches nine years of age, you make intraoral photographs and a panoramic radiograph (Figure 3.85). What do you observe?

A: Changes include:

- Easton's maxillary right central incisor erupted spontaneously.
- We regained 7 mm of maxillary left posterior space using the distalizer appliance.
- Left Class I canine and permanent molar relationships were achieved.
- The maxillary left permanent first molar uprighted (Figure 3.85f).
- Easton continued to wear his appliance as a retainer without further activation.

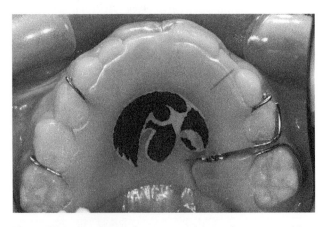

Figure 3.84 Maxillary left space regaining using a removable screw distalizer appliance.

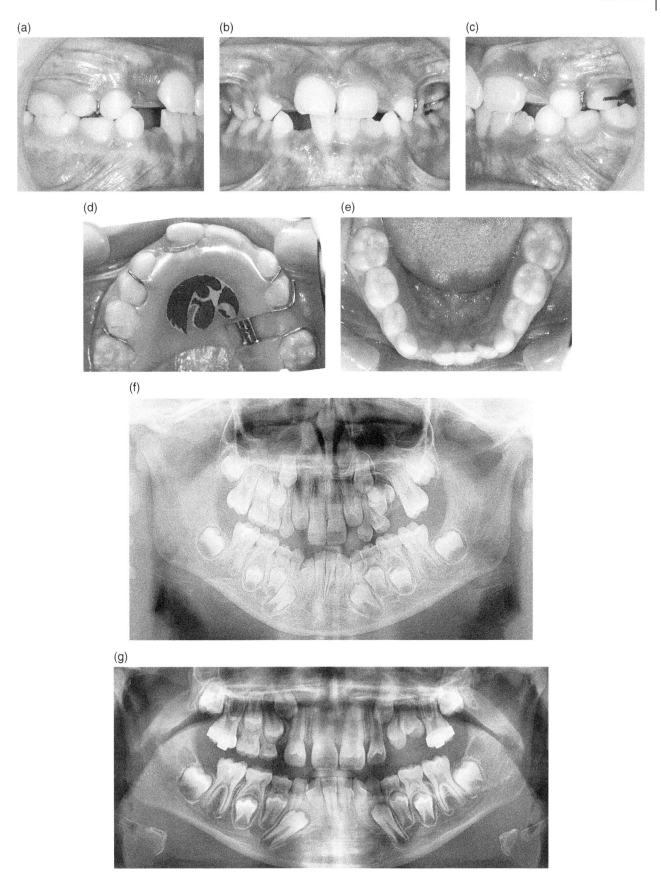

Figure 3.85 (a–f) Progress records of Easton at nine years of age. (g) Progress panoramic image of Easton at ten years and ten months of age.

Q: Are the maxillary left premolars *fused*?

A: We cannot determine the answer from Figure 3.85f. We could make a CBCT image, but there is no guarantee that it would reveal the answer either, and a CBCT would expose Easton to additional radiation. Since ankylosis of the maxillary left primary second molar and mesial drift/tip of the maxillary left permanent first molar presumably played a role in the ectopic eruption of the maxillary left second premolar, fusion as the cause of the premolar positions is unlikely.

Q: Would you recommend any additional early treatment at this time?

A: Yes. We followed the same principle we apply in all cases of ectopic eruption – create space, clear an eruption path, apply surgical exposure and orthodontic eruptive force when needed. Lastly, we hope to avoid permanent tooth extractions.

We referred Easton for extraction of maxillary primary canines and maxillary left primary first molar. We hoped the maxillary lateral incisors would erupt (making room at their apices for the maxillary permanent canines to erupt) and that the maxillary left first premolar would erupt (making room for the maxillary left permanent canine and second premolar to erupt). We informed Easton's mother that eventual surgical exposure (and orthodontic forced eruption) of the maxillary left permanent premolars may be necessary.

Easton failed to wear his space regaining appliance for a while, and his maxillary left permanent first molar drifted mesially. We placed him on a high-pull headgear to move his maxillary permanent first molars distally. A panoramic image was made when he was ten years and ten months old (Figure 3.85g). Thankfully, his maxillary lateral incisors erupted, and his maxillary premolars appear to be erupting. At this time, we extracted his maxillary left primary first molar and mandibular canines. We are concerned with the overlap of his maxillary permanent canine crowns over the roots of the maxillary lateral incisors. We will monitor creation of maxillary space by distal movement of the first molars with headgear, and we will make our final decision to proceed non-extraction or with extraction of premolars once the premolars erupt. Finally, at this time we will place an LLHA.

Q: Can you suggest "take home pearls" regarding Easton's treatment?

A: "Take home pearls" include:

- Easton was eight years old when he presented to us with a 6-mm left Class II molar relationship due to mesial drift of the maxillary left permanent first molar. His maxillary left second premolar was erupting ectopically and potentially impacted as a result of this mesial molar drift.

- Treatment included *clearing a path (creating space) for the ectopically erupting premolar to follow*. We did this by *regaining space* lost during mesial drift of the maxillary left permanent first molar.

- Easton's early treatment is still in progress. We continue to monitor eruption of his permanent canines and premolars. Easton underscores the importance of frequent monitoring of early treatment patients. Adjustments to plans are made as you deem appropriate.

Case Katie

Q: Katie is seven years and eleven months old (Figure 3.86). Her parents state, "Katie's dentist sent us here." Her PMH, PDH, periodontal, and TMJ evaluations are WRN. CR=CO. Compile your problem list and make a diagnosis.

A:

Table 3.17 Diagnostic findings and problems list for Katie.

Full face and profile	***Frontal view***
	Face is symmetric
	Soft-tissue LAFH WRN (soft-tissue Glabella – Subnasale = Subnasale – soft tissue Menton)
	UDML 1 mm to right of facial midline
	Excess gingival display in posed smile (maxillary central incisor gingival margins extend below the maxillary lip)
	Profile view
	Convex profile
	Obtuse NLA
	Retrusive chin
	Lip-chin-throat angle WRN
	Chin-throat length WRN
Ceph analysis	***Skeletal***
	Maxillary anteroposterior position WRN (A-Point lies approximately on Nasion-perpendicular line)
	Mandibular anteroposterior position is *deficient* (ANB angle = 5° with maxillary anteroposterior position WRN)
	Skeletal LAFH WRN (LAFH/TAFH X 100% = 56%; normal = 55% with s.d.= 2%)
	Steep MPA (FMA=32°, SNMP=40°)
	Ineffective bony Pogonion (Pogonion lies behind Nasion-B Point line extended)
	Dental
	Upright maxillary central incisors (U1 to SN=99°)
	Mandibular incisor inclination WRN (FMIA=62°)

Table 3.17 (Continued)

Radiographs	Early mixed dentition
	Blocked and potentially impacted maxillary right lateral incisor
	Impacted maxillary left permanent first molar (impacted under maxillary left primary second molar stainless steel crown)
	Missing mandibular left primary second molar with distal shoe space maintainer
	Maxillary permanent canines do not appear to have bilateral symmetry
Intraoral photos and models	Angle Class I
	Iowa Classification: I I I I
	20 % OB
	~1 mm OJ
	UDML 1mm to right of LDML
	4.0 mm maxillary anterior crowding is currently present (9.0 mm of space but 13.0 mm of space needed for both maxillary lateral permanent incisors)
	2.0 mm of maxillary dental arch crowding is anticipated following eruption of all permanent teeth (if proper space maintenance is employed)
	3.0 mm mandibular incisor crowding currently present
	0.2 mm of mandibular dental arch spacing is anticipated following eruption of all permanent teeth (if proper space maintenance is employed)
	Premature loss of mandibular left primary second molar (*space has been maintained*)
	Maxillary dental arch is symmetric (Figure 3.86o)
	Mandibular dental arch is symmetric (Figure 3.86p)
	Maxillary midline diastema
Other	
Diagnosis	Class I malocclusion in the early mixed dentition with moderate maxillary and mild mandibular anterior crowding, blocked and potentially impacted maxillary right permanent lateral incisor, and impacted maxillary left first permanent molar

Q: Who should you contact and why?

A: Contact her dentist and ask if there is a specific problem he observed (chief complaint). He says that he is concerned that her maxillary left molar is impacted.

Q: Is Katie's maxillary left permanent first molar *ectopically erupting*?

A: No. Ectopic eruption is *eruption where the tooth is not following its normal path*. The maxillary left permanent first molar appears to be erupting along a normal path but impacted under the distal margin of the maxillary left primary second molar stainless steel crown.

Q: Examine the space maintainer extending from Katie's mandibular left primary first molar to her mandibular

left permanent first molar (Figures 3.86f and 3.86k). What is the name of this space maintainer? What is a potential problem in using it this way?

A: The space maintainer is a *distal shoe appliance*. Her dentist delivered it following premature exfoliation of the mandibular left primary second molar but before complete eruption of the mandibular left permanent first molar. Its vertical arm at the mesial of the mandibular left permanent first molar allowed eruption of the permanent first molar and prevented mesial drift of the permanent first molar.

The potential problem with this distal shoe is evident. If Katie's mandibular left primary first molar exfoliates before the mandibular second premolar erupts, then the mandibular left permanent first molar will drift/tip to the mesial – potentially impacting the mandibular left second premolar and reducing arch perimeter.

Q: What is a solution to this potential problem?

A: Now that the mandibular left permanent first molar has erupted, an LLHA (bands on mandibular permanent first molars) should be delivered, and the distal shoe should be removed.

Q: Provide a detailed space analysis for Katie's maxillary and mandibular arches. In other words, how did we calculate 2.0 mm maxillary dental arch crowding and 0.2 mm mandibular dental arch spacing (*if we employ proper space maintenance*)?

A:

Average mesiodistal widths of permanent teeth (mm) [66]:

Maxillary Central Incisor	8.5	Mandibular Central Incisor	5.0
Maxillary Lateral Incisor	6.5	Mandibular Lateral Incisor	5.5
Maxillary Canine	7.5	Mandibular Canine	7.0
Maxillary First Premolar	7.0	Mandibular First Premolar	7.0
Maxillary Second Premolar	7.0	Mandibular Second Premolar	7.0
Maxillary First Molar	10.0	Mandibular First Molar	11.0
Maxillary Second Molar	9.0	Mandibular Second Molar	10.5

Average mesiodistal widths of *primary* teeth (mm) [66]:

Maxillary Central Incisor	6.5	Mandibular Central Incisor	4.2
Maxillary Lateral Incisor	5.1	Mandibular Lateral Incisor	4.1
Maxillary Canine	7.0	Mandibular Canine	5.0
Maxillary First Molar	7.3	Mandibular First Molar	7.7
Maxillary Second Molar	8.2	Mandibular Second Molar	9.9

Maxillary Arch

+3.0 mm right lateral incisor space (Figure 3.86j)

−6.5 mm anticipated width of maxillary right permanent lateral incisor

+1.0 mm midline diastema

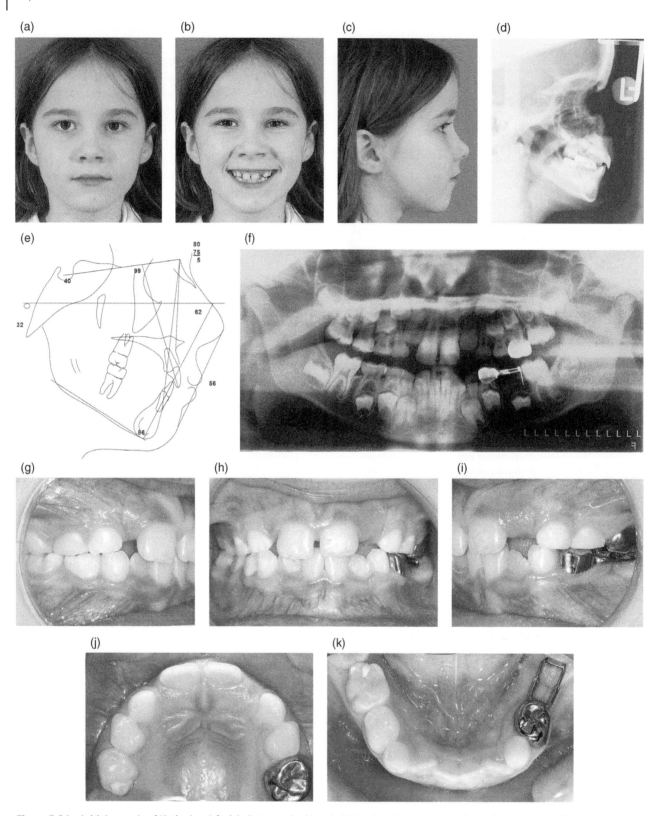

Figure 3.86 Initial records of Katie: (a–c) facial photographs, (d and e) lateral cephalometric radiograph and tracing, (f) pantomograph, (g–k) intraoral photographs, (l–p) models.

(l)   (m)   (n)

(o)   (p)

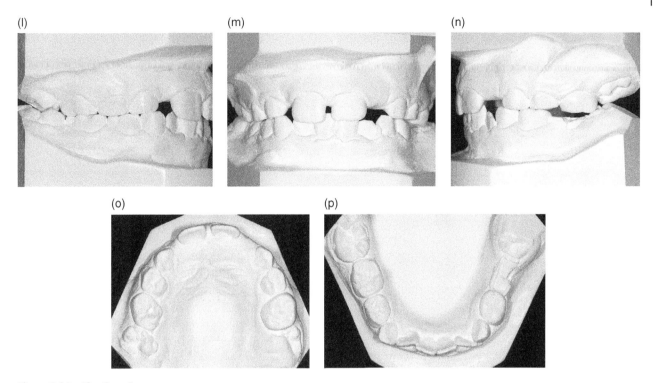

Figure 3.86 (Continued)

+5.0 mm left lateral incisor space
−6.5 mm anticipated width of maxillary left permanent lateral incisor
+2 mm anticipated leeway space (1 mm/side)
Balance = +3.0 mm −6.5 mm +1.0 mm +5.0 mm −6.5 mm +2.0 mm = −2.0 mm

Mandibular Arch (because space for mandibular left primary second molar was maintained, we can use right and left leeway spaces)

−3.0 mm mandibular incisor crowding is currently present (Figure 3.86k)
+3.2 mm of anticipated leeway space (1.6 mm/side)
Balance = −3.0 mm +3.2 mm = +0.2 mm

That is, *we anticipate 2.0 mm of maxillary dental arch crowding and 0.2 mm of mandibular dental arch spacing following eruption of all permanent teeth (if we employ proper space maintenance).*

Q: What is suggested by the fact that Katie's maxillary incisors are upright (U1 to SN = 99°), her UDML is to the right of her facial midline and LDML by 1 mm, and her maxillary right permanent lateral incisor space is smaller than the left? How may these features impact you approach to correcting her maxillary anterior crowding?

A: These features suggest that Katie's maxillary right primary lateral incisor was lost prematurely and that her maxillary

central incisors drifted to the right and uprighted. These features also suggest that one treatment option will be to *regain lost maxillary right lateral incisor space* by opening space for the right lateral incisor – proclining the incisors and shifting the UDML to the left. Space regaining may be a better approach than space maintenance because 2.0 mm of maxillary anterior crowding is anticipated if we use space maintenance alone.

Q: Focus on the patient's *primary* problems in each dimension, plus other problems, at every appointment. What are Katie's primary problems?

A:

Table 3.18 Primary problems list for Katie.

AP	—
Vertical	—
Transverse	—
Other	Moderate maxillary anterior crowding
	Blocked and potentially impacted maxillary right permanent lateral incisor
	Impacted maxillary left first permanent molar

Q: What three principles apply to every early treatment patient, and how do these principles apply to Katie?

A: The three principles are as follows:

1) The goal of early treatment is to correct developing problems with the intent of getting the patient *back to normal for that stage of development*, including preventing complications such as resorption of adjacent teeth roots, reducing later treatment complexity, or reducing/eliminating unknowns. Freeing the maxillary left permanent first molar from impaction, regaining maxillary space lost from the molar impaction, freeing the maxillary right lateral incisor from impaction, and alleviating moderate maxillary anterior crowding will put Katie back on track. An LLHA should be placed to prevent drifting/tipping of the mandibular left first permanent molar before the mandibular left primary first molar exfoliates.

2) Early treatment should address *very specific problems with a clearly defined end point*, usually within six to nine months (except for some orthopedic problems). Freeing the impacted maxillary molar, regaining any space lost as a result of the impaction, creating space for the impacted maxillary right permanent lateral incisor, and placing an LLHA could be readily accomplished in a few months.

3) Always ask: Is it necessary that I treat the patient now? *What harm will come from not doing anything?* It is not necessary to treat Katie for the next six to twelve months *so long as the distal shoe appliance remains in place*. Also, if we choose to recall Katie, then her maxillary left permanent first molar will likely remain impacted under the stainless steel crown, and her maxillary right permanent lateral incisor will likely remain impacted or erupt malaligned.

Q: Should you start treatment now or recall Katie? Please discuss options.

A: Options include the following:

- *Recall* (monitor only, reevaluate in one year) – is not recommended. Her mandibular left primary first molar may possibly exfoliate. Her mandibular left permanent first molar will then drift forward – losing arch perimeter and impacting her mandibular left second premolar. Katie's maxillary left permanent first molar will likely remain impacted until the second primary molar exfoliates, and it may decay if Katie cannot clean it. Finally, her maxillary right lateral incisor will remain impacted (preventing eruption of her maxillary right permanent canine) or erupt malaligned.

- *Space maintenance* (LLHA with banded permanent first molars) – is recommended before the remaining primary teeth become mobile – especially before the mandibular left primary first molar (with distal shoe) becomes mobile.

- *Space maintenance* (Nance holding arch) – is recommended once Katie's maxillary left permanent first molar erupts and before the maxillary primary canines and primary molars exfoliate.

- *Space regaining to move the impacted maxillary left permanent first molar slightly posterior (de-impact it)* – is strongly recommended. If the maxillary left primary second molar is nonmobile, then it could be used as anchorage to push the maxillary left permanent first molar distally with fixed orthodontic appliances and a trapped open coil spring or with a Halterman appliance. Furthermore, once the maxillary left permanent first molar has been moved distally, then the nonmobile maxillary left primary second molar could be used as a space maintainer to hold the permanent first molar distally. If the maxillary left primary second molar is mobile, then a removable appliance (palatal coverage) should be fabricated with a spring to push the maxillary left permanent first molar distally while all other maxillary teeth act as anchorage.

Where access permits, simply placing an elastomeric separator or twisted brass wire between the primary second molar and permanent first molar contact can de-impact the first permanent fist molar (Figure 3.87).

- *Replacement of the maxillary left primary second molar stainless steel crown* – is a viable option if the distal margin of the new crown can be seated below (de-impacting) the maxillary left permanent first molar mesial contact.

- *Extraction of the maxillary left primary second molar* – could be a viable option if the maxillary left permanent first molar was distalized following eruption (space regaining) and if a Nance holding arch was then placed to maintain its corrected position. Since the root of the maxillary left second premolar is <1/2 complete, its eruption could be delayed if the primary second molar is extracted [28].

- *Fixed orthodontic treatment to open space (regain space) for the maxillary lateral incisors* – is recommended. In addition to creating space for the lateral incisors, this treatment would procline the maxillary central incisors to a more normal angulation.

- *Extraction of maxillary primary canines to create space for lateral incisor eruption* – is a reasonable option. As the lateral incisors erupt, space will be created at their apices for eruption of the maxillary permanent canines. If this option is selected, then placement of a Nance holding arch is recommended to prevent maxillary permanent first molar mesial drift and arch perimeter loss.

- *Serial extraction* – is not recommended because the magnitude of dental crowding in both arches is only mild to moderate – not severe.

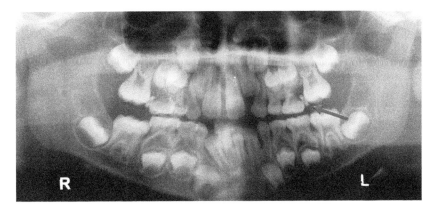

Figure 3.87 An elastomeric separator (or twisted brass wire) can be inserted between the primary second molar and permanent first molar to de-impact the permanent first molar (*Source:* Courtesy of Dr. Karin Weber-Gasparoni.)

Q: What unknowns will you face in treating Katie?

A: Unknowns exist in treating any patient. The most significant unknowns for Katie include future jaw growth magnitude and direction, treatment compliance, an undetected CR-CO shift, and possible tooth eruption problems.

Q: What is your recommended treatment? How would you proceed?

A: Mobility of the maxillary left primary second molar was evaluated. It was found to be nonmobile.

Katie was placed in maxillary fixed orthodontic appliances (Figure 3.88). Impaction of her maxillary left permanent first molar was corrected by trapping a compressed open-coil spring between the maxillary left permanent first molar and maxillary left primary first molar. This approach avoided the need to band the maxillary left primary second molar stainless steel crown.

Space was created for the maxillary right lateral incisor by trapping a compressed open coil spring between the maxillary right primary canine and maxillary right permanent central incisor. Closed coil springs were then placed to maintain this correction. Katie was debanded and a clear maxillary vacuum-formed retainer (with openings to permit maxillary lateral incisor eruption) was worn by her nightly.

Q: Figure 3.89 shows progress records of Katie following eruption of her maxillary permanent lateral incisors. What changes do you observe?

A: Changes include the following:
- Maxillary left permanent first molar has erupted (Figure 3.89d).
- Maxillary left primary second molar (non-mobile) is acting as a space maintainer.
- Maxillary *right* permanent first molar has drifted to the mesial into the distal of the maxillary right primary second molar (Figure 3.89f, the distal of the maxillary right primary second molar appears decayed).
- Maxillary lateral incisors have erupted to the labial.
- Maxillary left permanent canine is erupting ectopically (Figure 3.89f, maxillary left permanent canine crown is overlapping the root of the maxillary left lateral incisor). This position increases the likelihood that the maxillary left permanent canine will not erupt spontaneously.
- Inadequate space exists for eruption of the mandibular permanent canines (Figure 3.89e).
- The distal shoe *will be lost soon* due to imminent exfoliation of the mandibular left primary first molar.

Q: Would you recommend additional early treatment?

A: Yes, we recommend the following:
- *Removal of the mandibular left primary first molar/distal shoe* and placement of an LLHA – so that Katie does not swallow or aspirate the distal shoe. Placement of an LLHA will prevent mesial drift of the mandibular left permanent first molar and provide "E-space" when the mandibular right primary second molar exfoliates and the second premolars erupt. This space will help improve mandibular anterior crowding.
- *Space regaining* – distal movement of maxillary right permanent first molar (followed by restoration of the maxillary right primary second molar distal surface).
- *Extraction of maxillary primary canines and maxillary primary first molars* – to encourage accelerated eruption of maxillary first premolars whose roots appear to be 1/2 developed. As the maxillary first premolars erupt, space is provided at their apices for eruption of the maxillary permanent canines. A Nance holding arch should be placed before the extractions in order to prevent first permanent molar mesial drift and arch perimeter loss.

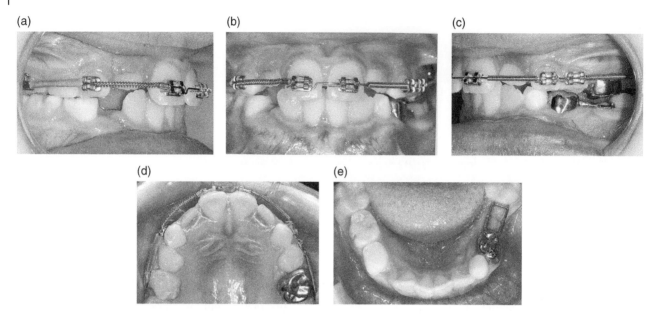

(a)　(b)　(c)

(d)　(e)

Figure 3.88 (a–e) Early treatment progress images of Katie.

Q: There appeared to be adequate space created for Katie's maxillary permanent lateral incisors to erupt (Figure 3.88d). Why are they now malaligned (Figure 3.89d)?

A: There was an early indication that the maxillary permanent canine crowns were labial to the maxillary permanent lateral incisor roots (Figure 3.86d). As space regaining commenced and her permanent lateral incisors descended, her maxillary permanent canines also descended, maintaining a forward position relative to the lateral incisor roots (canine bulge above right lateral incisor in Figure 3.89a, and labial canine overlap of left lateral incisor root in Figure 3.89f). This spatial relationship between developing maxillary canine crowns and lateral incisor roots promoted a labial inclination of the lateral incisor crowns (Figures 3.89a–3.89c).

There is an important take home message here. We were wise *not to bracket the maxillary permanent lateral incisors*. Why? Moving them may have forced their roots to the labial, forcing contact with the developing permanent canines and risking lateral incisor root resorption. Waiting for later comprehensive treatment to adjust maxillary lateral incisor position reduces this risk.

Q: Should we have extracted Katie's maxillary primary canines – initially?

A: If we could treat Katie again, then we would probably extract her maxillary primary canines to allow the maxillary permanent lateral incisors to erupt – creating space at their apices for the maxillary permanent canines to erupt. On the other hand, the maxillary lateral incisors did erupt as space was orthodontically

created for them, obviating the need for an extraction procedure.

Q: Katie moved away from the area. Can you suggest "take home pearls"?

A: "Take home pearls"
- Katie was nearly eight years old when she was referred to us because her maxillary left permanent first molar was trapped under the primary second molar stainless steel crown. She had a Class I dental relationship, normal vertical relationship, normal transverse relationship, and mild to moderate anterior crowding. She was treated with space regaining using fixed orthodontic appliances in order to:
  1) De-impact her maxillary left permanent first molar and move it slightly distal
  2) Open space for her impacted maxillary right permanent lateral incisor to erupt
- We were able to create space for Katie's maxillary permanent lateral incisors using fixed orthodontic appliances and compressed springs because her lateral incisors had erupted to a coronal position. If the lateral incisors had been apical, then braces alone may not have created adequate apical space to allow them to erupt. You can create apical space using braces, but you must generate adequate root torque to diverge roots. In contrast to braces, RMEs create maxillary space coronally *and* apically.
- Initial early treatment was justified and successful. Later, the need for additional early treatment became evident.

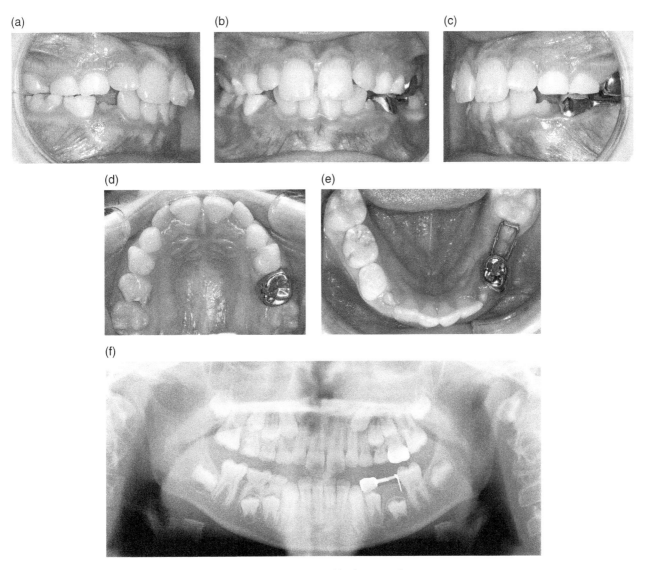

Figure 3.89 Records of Katie following maxillary permanent lateral incisor eruption.

The need for an LLHA to replace the mandibular left distal shoe had always been anticipated. But the need to regain space lost through maxillary right permanent first molar mesial drift was not anticipated, and the need to address ectopic eruption of the maxillary left permanent canine was not anticipated.

We wish that early treatments were always of short duration and would always proceed as planned. However, the reality of our specialty is that you must constantly monitor patient treatment progress. At every appointment, you must carefully assess all problems, make progress records as you deem appropriate, and modify your treatment plan to suit changing conditions. Short-term treatment plans can evolve into long-term treatment delivery. Ultimately, your care for a patient is not complete until that patient has a healthy and stable permanent occlusion. Even then, you must monitor the patient in retention.

Case Erin

Q: Erin is eleven years and six months old (Figure 3.90). She presents to you with her parents' chief complaint, "Erin has crooked teeth." Her PMH, PDH, TMJ evaluation, and periodontal evaluation are WRN. She exhibits thin mandibular periodontal biotype labial to central incisors. CR=CO. Compile your diagnostic findings and problem list. Also, state your diagnosis.

A:

Table 3.19 Diagnostic findings and problem list for Erin.

Full face and profile	**Frontal view**
	Face is symmetric
	Long soft-tissue LAFH (soft-tissue Glabella – Subnasale < Subnasale – soft-tissue Menton)
	Mentalis strain appears necessary to achieve lip competence (Figure 3.90a), but she does not exhibit an ILG in any image including lateral cephalometric radiograph
	UDML WRN
	Inadequate gingival display in posed smile (maxillary central incisor gingival margins ~2 mm apical to maxillary lip)
	Moderate buccal corridors in posed smile
	Profile view
	Mildly convex profile
	Inadequate chin projection (soft tissue Pogonion positioned 4–5 mm behind zero meridian line)
	Obtuse NLA (upturned nose)
	Lip-chin-throat angle WRN
Ceph analysis	**Skeletal**
	Maxillary anteroposterior position WRN (A-Point lies on Nasion-perpendicular line, 3.90e)
	Mandibular anteroposterior position WRN (ANB angle = 3° with normal maxillary position)
	Skeletal LAFH WRN (ANS-Menton/Nasion-Menton x 100% = 56%)
	Mandibular plane angle WRN (FMA = 28°; SNMP = 39°)
	Effective bony Pogonion (Pogonion lies ahead of the line extended from Nasion through B-point)
Radiographs	**Dental**
	Upright maxillary incisors (U1 to SN = 94°)
	Mandibular incisor inclination WRN (FMIA = 66°)
	Late mixed dentition (Figure 3.90f)
	Retained mandibular right primary second molar
	Congenital absence of mandibular right second premolar
Intraoral photos and models	Angle Class I
	Iowa Classification: I X III(3 mm) I
	Maxillary and mandibular midlines are coincident
	5.0 mm maxillary arch crowding currently exists
	5.0 mm maxillary arch crowding is anticipated following eruption of all permanent teeth
	8.5 mm mandibular anterior crowding currently exists
	4.2 mm mandibular arch crowding is anticipated if an LLHA is placed and if the mandibular right primary second molar is maintained
	Symmetric maxillary and mandibular arches
	Maxillary right permanent first molar is rotated to the mesial
	Thin mandibular periodontal biotype labial to central incisors (Figures 3.90h and 3.90m)
	OB 10%
	OJ 1 mm
	Minimal overjet maxillary left primary canine and both permanent first molars (Figures 3.90o and 3.90p)
	Left primary second molars are in crossbite
	Anterior crossbite of maxillary left permanent lateral incisor
	Transverse posterior compensations (Figures 3.90s and 3.90t); significant buccal crown torque of maxillary first permanent molars, lingual crown torque of mandibular first permanent molars)
	Retained mandibular right primary second molar (without successor) which is not aligned with the mandibular right permanent first molar (Figures 3.90k and 3.90r)
	Blocked out maxillary left first premolar (Figures 3.90j and 3.90q)
Other	—
Diagnosis	Class I malocclusion with 5.0 mm maxillary arch crowding, 8.5 mm mandibular anterior crowding, retained mandibular right primary second molar lacking a successor, anterior crossbite of maxillary left permanent lateral incisor, lingual crossbite of left primary second molars, and posterior transverse compensations.

Q: How can Erin have inadequate chin projection/convex profile when her maxilla and mandible are WRN with an effective bony Pogonion?

A: Soft-tissue chin projection is judged using the "zero meridian line" – a line visualized perpendicular to the Frankfort horizontal, passing through soft-tissue Nasion, and extending vertically down to the chin. *Ideal chin projection exists when the chin lies on the zero meridian line or just short of it* [108]. Erin's chin sits back 4–5 mm from the zero meridian line, which makes her profile convex.

Soft-tissue chin projection is based upon mandible anteroposterior position relative to the maxilla/face, bony Pogonion anteroposterior position, and soft-tissue thickness overlying bony Pogonion. Erin's mandibular position

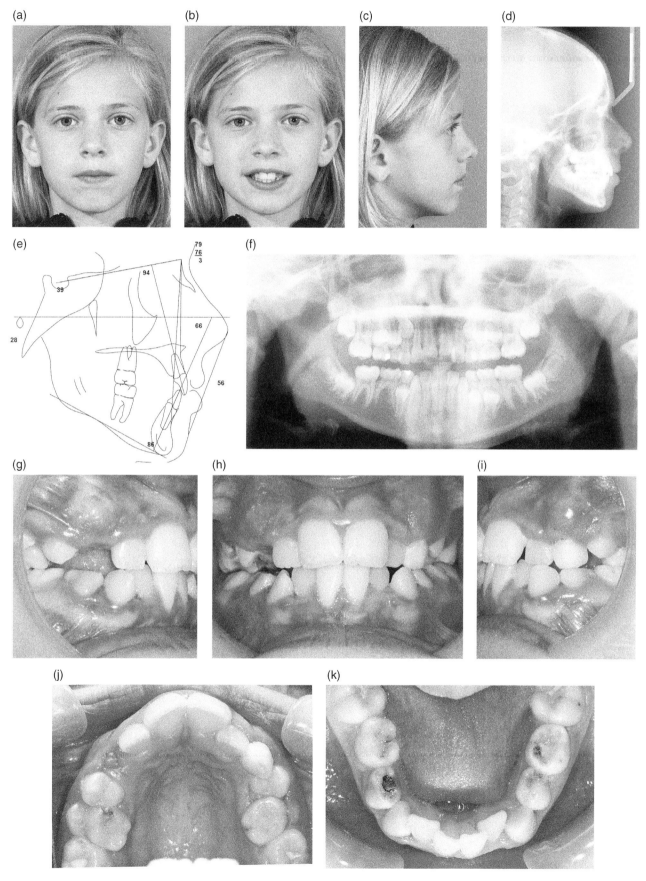

Figure 3.90 Initial records of Erin: (a–c) facial photographs, (d and e) lateral cephalogram and tracing, (f) pantomograph, (g–k) intraoral photographs, (l–u) photographs of models. Note: The pantomograph was taken a number of months earlier than lateral cephalometric radiograph, photographs and models.

(l)   (m)   (n)

(o)   (p)

(q)   (r)

(s)   (t)   (u)

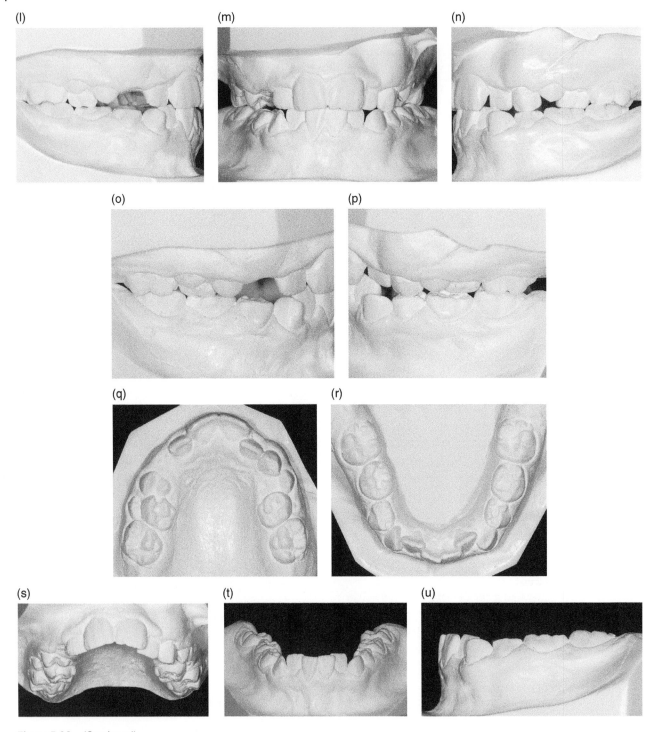

Figure 3.90 (Continued)

is WRN and bony Pogonion is effective, but soft-tissue thickness overlying bony Pogonion is relatively thin (Figure 3.90d) – leading to inadequate chin projection and a convex profile.

Q: We noted that Erin's maxillary right permanent first molar is rotated mesially (Figure 3.90q). How can this rotation affect her molar relationship when viewed from the buccal? From what direction should you also check the molar relationship?

A: When a maxillary molar rotates to the mesial, the molar will appear more Class II from the buccal than it really is. When you see a rotated maxillary molar, check it *from the lingual* (models or scans) to confirm its true anteroposterior relationship. Fortunately, when we check Erin's permanent molars from the lingual

(a) (b)

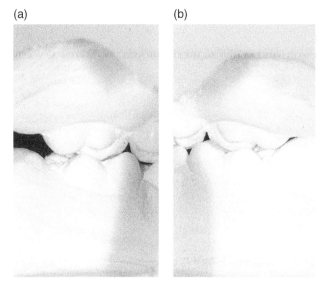

Figure 3.91 Erin's permanent molar relationships as seen from the lingual. (a) Left molars and (b) right molars are Class I.

(Figures 3.91a and 3.91b), we see that she has a solid Class I molar relationship – bilaterally.

Q: How would you manage Erin's thin periodontal biotype covering the labial aspect of her mandibular central incisors?

A: Let's review two important points before making a recommendation:

- A wide zone of keratinized attached gingiva is considered more desirable than either a narrow zone or total absence because a wide zone withstands gingival inflammation, trauma from mastication, toothbrushing, forces from muscle pull, and orthodontic procedures better [109–111].
- Less than 1 mm of attached keratinized gingiva may be compatible with gingival health [111–114].

  Because Erin has *some* keratinized attached gingiva labial to her mandibular central incisors, and because the underlying alveolar process bone is not thin (mandibular incisor roots are not palpable), we recommend monitoring her mandibular anterior gingiva. However, her parents were informed that the need for a future gingival graft exists if recession occurs in this area.

Q: Provide a detailed space analysis for Erin's maxillary and mandibular arches. In other words, how was the 5.0 mm anticipated maxillary arch crowding calculated? How was the anticipated 4.2 mm mandibular crowding calculated (if an LLHA is placed and if the mandibular right primary second molar is maintained).

A:

Average mesiodistal widths of permanent teeth (mm) [66]:

Maxillary Central Incisor	8.5	Mandibular Central Incisor	5.0
Maxillary Lateral Incisor	6.5	Mandibular Lateral Incisor	5.5
Maxillary Canine	7.5	Mandibular Canine	7.0
Maxillary First Premolar	7.0	Mandibular First Premolar	7.0
Maxillary Second Premolar	7.0	Mandibular Second Premolar	7.0
Maxillary First Molar	10.0	Mandibular First Molar	11.0
Maxillary Second Molar	9.0	Mandibular Second Molar	10.5

Average mesiodistal widths of *primary* teeth (mm) [66]:

Maxillary Central Incisor	6.5	Mandibular Central Incisor	4.2
Maxillary Lateral Incisor	5.1	Mandibular Lateral Incisor	4.1
Maxillary Canine	7.0	Mandibular Canine	5.0
Maxillary First Molar	7.3	Mandibular First Molar	7.7
Maxillary Second Molar	8.2	Mandibular Second Molar	9.9

Maxillary Arch (Figure 3.90j, leeway space cannot be used because primary first molars and primary canines are absent. "E-space" cannot be used because primary second molars are exfoliating and space appears to have been lost)

+7.0 mm space held by exfoliating maxillary right primary second molar

−7.0 mm anticipated space needed for maxillary right second premolar

+6.0 mm space available for maxillary right permanent canine

−7.5 mm anticipated width of maxillary right permanent canine

−1.5 mm crowding mesial of maxillary left permanent lateral incisor

+7.0 mm width of maxillary left primary canine

−7.5 mm anticipated width of maxillary left permanent canine

−1.5 mm crowding distal of maxillary left primary canine

+7.0 mm space held by exfoliating maxillary left primary second molar

−7.0 mm anticipated space needed for maxillary right second premolar

Balance = +7.0 mm −7.0 mm +6.0 mm −7.5 mm −1.5 mm +7.0 mm −7.5 mm −1.5 mm +7.0 mm −7.0 mm = −5.0 mm

Mandibular Arch (Figure 3.90k), leeway space cannot be used because the permanent canines are present.

"E-space" cannot be used on the right if the retained mandibular primary second molar is maintained)

+9.9 mm width of mandibular left primary second molar
−7.0 mm anticipated width of mandibular left second premolar
+7.7 mm width of mandibular left primary first molar
−7.0 mm anticipated width of mandibular left first premolar
−3.0 mm crowding mesial of mandibular left canine
−1.5 mm crowding mesial of mandibular left lateral incisor
−0.5 mm crowding mesial of mandibular right central incisor
−0.5 mm crowding mesial of mandibular right lateral incisor
−3.0 mm crowding mesial of mandibular right canine
+7.7 mm width of mandibular right primary first molar
−7.0 mm anticipated width of mandibular right first premolar
Balance = +9.9 mm −7.0 mm +7.7 mm −7.0 mm −3.0 mm −1.5 mm −0.5 mm −0.5 mm −3.0 mm +7.7 mm −7.0 mm = −4.2 mm

That is, 5.0 mm of maxillary arch crowding currently exists, and 5.0 mm of maxillary arch crowding is anticipated following eruption of all permanent teeth; 8.5 mm mandibular arch crowding currently exists, and 4.2mm of mandibular crowding is anticipated if an LLHA is placed and if the mandibular right primary second molar is maintained.

Q: What are Erin's *primary* problems in each dimension, plus other problems?

A:

Table 3.20 Primary problems list for Erin.

AP	—
Vertical	—
Transverse	Minimal posterior overjet of maxillary left primary canine and both permanent first molars, lingual crossbite of left primary second molars, and posterior transverse compensations (buccal crown torque of maxillary first permanent molars, lingual crown torque of mandibular first permanent molars)
Other	5.0 mm maxillary arch crowding currently exists, 8.5 mm mandibular arch crowding currently exists, retained mandibular right primary second molar lacks a successor, and anterior crossbite of maxillary left permanent lateral incisor

Q: Can you think of additional records we should have made of Erin?

A: To more clearly assess her mandibular right primary second molar's crown, root, and bone level, a periapical radiograph is necessary. We failed to make a periapical radiograph.

Q: Erin has a retained mandibular right primary second molar lacking a permanent successor. Can you state our recommendations made in the Introduction to this chapter regarding the treatment of retained primary teeth lacking successors? Can you apply these recommendations to Erin's retained primary molar?

A: Our recommendations, and their application to Erin, are as follows:
- Recommendation: for non-extraction cases (non-extraction of permanent teeth), *if the retained primary tooth has a good crown, good root, and good bone level, then consider maintaining it for the long term.* However, always have a "fallback" plan (contingency plan, such as implant or FPD), if the retained primary tooth is lost.
Erin's mandibular right primary second molar (Figure 3.90f) appears to have a good crown, good root, and good bone level. If Erin is treated non-extraction, then we would recommend attempting to retain the mandibular right primary second molar.
- Recommendation: whenever possible *avoid bonding orthodontic brackets, and avoid applying orthodontic forces, to retained primary teeth in order to reduce the risk that their roots will resorb.* If you must bond brackets to retained primary teeth, then try to *avoid moving them.*
If we treat Erin non-extraction, then we should avoid bonding a bracket to the mandibular right primary second molar. If we bond a bracket to it, then we should apply orthodontic force to it for *only a short period of time and move the primary molar only a short distance.*
- Recommendation: for non-extraction cases, *if the retained primary tooth has a poor crown, root, or bone level, then seriously consider extracting it.*
- Recommendation: *for extraction cases, consider extracting the retained primary tooth.* If we determine that Erin is an extraction case, then we should consider options which include extracting her mandibular right primary second molar instead of a premolar in that quadrant.

Q: Can you suggest and discuss specific treatment options for Erin's retained mandibular right primary second molar?

A: Options include the following:

1) Maintain the mandibular right primary second molar, *intact*. With Class I canines and non-extraction treatment, the right permanent first molars will finish in an "end-on" relationship with this approach (Class II by 2–3 mm). However, there is no evidence that leaving molars Class II by 2–3 mm causes harm. Further, leaving the mandibular right primary second molar intact provides the greatest chance of maintaining it, long-term. Even if the primary molar is eventually lost, we will have maintained its bone for implant placement.

2) Maintain the mandibular right primary second molar *but reduce its mesiodistal width to 7 mm*. Assuming non-extraction treatment, the advantage of this option is that the mandibular right permanent first molar can be moved to the mesial and finished Class I. The disadvantage of this option is that the bell-shaped roots of the mandibular right primary second molar will resorb as roots of adjacent teeth are brought into them – diminishing chances of maintaining the mandibular right primary second molar long-term.

3) Extract the mandibular right primary second molar and replace it with either an implant or FPD. If we replace it with an implant, then we will need to wait until growth is complete in order to prevent the implant from submerging relative to the erupting adjacent teeth. Also, as soon as the mandibular primary second molar is extracted, the alveolar process bone at the extraction site will begin to resorb and a bone graft may be required to place an implant at a future date.

4) Extract the mandibular right primary second molar and close the extraction space orthodontically. This will be the ideal treatment if we decide Erin is an extraction patient (e.g. extraction of four premolars with reciprocal space closure). Or, we could extract only the mandibular right primary second molar and close the entire extraction space by advancing both mandibular right permanent molars (using TAD anchorage). However, this approach would leave the maxillary right permanent second molar unopposed, and possibly without a vertical stop to prevent supra-eruption.

Q: Discuss Erin in the context of three principles applied to every early treatment patient.

A:

1) The goal of early treatment is to correct developing problems – get the patient *back to normal for their stage of development* (including preventing complications, reducing later treatment complexity, or reducing/eliminating unknowns). Eliminating Erin's maxillary and mandibular crowding, anterior crossbite, primary molar crossbite, posterior transverse compensations, and addressing her retained mandibular right primary second molar would get her back on track for her stage of development.

2) Early treatment should address *very specific problems with a clearly defined end point*, usually within six to nine months (except for some orthopedic problems). RME plus expanded LLHA are focused treatments, which could reduce crowding and permit transverse compensation removal. These treatments could be performed in less than one year. Maxillary lateral incisor crossbite correction may occur spontaneously with RME or may require additional treatment of less than nine months duration. Addressing her retained mandibular right primary molar could take longer than nine months depending upon the treatment chosen.

3) Always ask: Is it necessary that I treat the patient now? *What harm may come if I choose to do nothing now?* The most marked RME skeletal effect occurs before/during the pubertal growth spurt, and expansion after the pubertal growth spurt is mainly dentoalveolar (not orthopedic/skeletal) [94–100]. At age of 11 years and 6 months, Erin may enter puberty soon, so the RME skeletal effect could diminish if we wait too long. Also, many of her permanent canines and premolars are close to eruption, so mandibular space maintenance should begin now in order to prevent permanent first molar mesial drift (arch perimeter loss). The maxillary left lateral incisor does not appear to be damaged, but damage could occur at any time if the crossbite is not corrected. Finally, we anticipate no harm to the retained mandibular right primary second molar if we wait.

Q: Can you briefly describe the ideal serial extraction patient? What factors suggest that Erin is, or is not, an ideal serial extraction candidate? Would you recommend serial extraction for Erin?

A: The ideal serial extraction patient is in the *early mixed dentition stage of development and is normal in every way except has severe anterior crowding (≥9 mm anterior crowding in each arch)*.

Factors suggesting that Erin is a candidate for serial extraction include the fact that she:

• Presents with a Class I molar relationship.
• Is normal vertically (long soft tissue LAFH, but normal skeletal LAFH) with minimal OB of 10%. If we

perform serial extraction, then her bite will deepen after first premolars are extracted and incisors are retracted/uprighted around their apices.

- Presents with nearly severe (8.5 mm) mandibular anterior crowding

Factors suggesting that Erin is not a candidate for serial extraction include the fact that she:

- Is in the late mixed dentition stage of development.
- Presents with only moderate (5 mm) maxillary arch crowding.
- Has normal mandibular incisor inclination (FMIA = 66°) but *upright* maxillary incisors (U1 to SN = 94°). Her maxillary incisors will tend to upright more with premolar extractions/incisor retraction.
- Lacks a normal transverse relationship (posterior crossbite of left primary second molars, minimum overjet of maxillary left primary canine and both permanent first molars, and posterior transverse compensations).

Based upon the above factors, Erin is *not* an ideal candidate for serial extraction.

Q: What unknowns do you face in treating Erin? Specifically, *what unknowns should you eliminate before performing any irreversible procedure* (e.g. extracting permanent teeth)?

A: The greatest unknown is the longevity of Erin's retained mandibular right primary second molar. However, because it has a good crown, good root, and good bone, we have a good chance of maintaining it long term (assuming we do not apply orthodontic force to it and/ or move it, and assuming that we treat Erin nonextraction). Other unknowns include an undetected CR-CO shift, magnitude and direction of future jaw growth, and patient cooperation.

Q: Should you start early treatment now or recall Erin? If you start treatment, then what treatment options would you consider?

A: Treatment options include the following:

- *Recall* (monitor only, reevaluate in one year) – is not recommended. At age of eleven years and six months, Erin may soon enter puberty. So, RME skeletal effects could diminish if we wait too long. Also, many of her permanent canines and premolars are close to eruption, so mandibular space maintenance should begin now in order to prevent permanent first molar mesial drift (arch perimeter loss). The maxillary left lateral incisor does not appear to be damaged, but damage could occur at any time if the crossbite is not corrected.
- *RME* – is recommended. RME will increase Erin's maxillary skeletal width, reduce buccal corridors,

increase posterior overjet (which can be used to upright first permanent molars), and increase maxillary arch perimeter (which can be used to reduce maxillary crowding).

- *Space maintenance* – placement of an LLHA is recommended in order to spontaneously reduce Erin's mandibular crowding during the transition to adult dentition. The LLHA could be expanded and its bands flexed labially before cementation in order to upright her mandibular permanent first molars (once posterior overjet is created with RME). We do not recommend placement of a Nance holding arch because the maxillary primary second molars are exfoliating, and the maxillary second premolars are nearly erupted.
- *Space regaining* – is a possible option in the maxilla. Why? Space has been lost following exfoliation of the maxillary left primary first molar (Figure 3.90j), space is being lost during exfoliation of both maxillary primary second molars, and upright maxillary incisors could afford to be proclined as posterior spaces are opened.
- *Serial extraction* – is not recommended because Erin exhibits only moderate (5 mm) maxillary arch crowding, has *upright* maxillary incisors (U1 to SN = 94°), and lacks a normal transverse relationship. She is not an ideal candidate for serial extraction.
- *Correcting her anterior crossbite* – is recommended in order to prevent trauma/wear of her left lateral incisors and to determine whether an undetected CR-CO shift exists.
- *Retention of the mandibular right primary second molar* – is recommended if Erin is treated nonextraction. In order to increase the primary second molar's chances of being maintained long term, we recommend leaving the primary second molar *intact* and not moving it (or moving it minimally).
- *Extraction of maxillary left primary canine* to ensure eruption of the permanent canine – is not recommended since her maxillary permanent canines appear to be erupting normally. This recommendation is especially true if RME is employed since RME will create additional anterior maxillary space for canine eruption.

Q: Erin's mandibular right primary second molar is not perfectly aligned in the arch (Figures 3.90k and 3.90r). If you choose to maintain the mandibular right primary second molar, should you move it into alignment?

A: Orthodontists are perfectionists. If the mandibular right primary second molar is maintained, then we would like to align it with the rest of the arch. However, this alignment should be done using very *light force and for as short a time as possible* (at the end of treatment).

Any orthodontic movement of the primary second molar increases the likelihood that its roots will resorb, and this fact should be explained to Erin and her parents. If you chose to maintain the mandibular right primary second molar, then another option is not to move it but instead to leave it slightly malaligned.

Q: If you maintain Erin's mandibular right primary second molar, what "fallback," or contingency, plan would you recommend if it is eventually lost?

A: If Erin is treated non-extraction, and if the retained mandibular right primary second molar is lost *before Erin is an adult*, then we would recommend maintaining the edentulous space with a Hawley retainer or with a bonded fixed partial denture (FPD). Maintaining the space with a bonded FPD is preferred because roots of the adjacent first premolar and first permanent molar could not tip into the space. When Erin reaches adulthood, we would recommend placing an implant in the space.

If Erin is treated non-extraction, and if the retained mandibular right primary second molar is lost *when Erin is an adult*, then we would recommend replacing it with an implant to maintain bone.

If Erin is treated with extraction of permanent teeth, then we would probably recommend extraction of the retained primary second molar and space closure.

Q: What early treatment(s), if any, do you recommend for Erin?

A: We performed RME and uprighted her mandibular first permanent molars using an expanded LLHA. Crossbite of her maxillary left lateral incisor corrected spontaneously with RME. As we monitored growth and tooth eruption, we noted that her maxillary first permanent molars drifted mesially into a slight Class II (1 mm) relationship following exfoliation of the maxillary primary second molars. We prescribed high-pull headgear wear (expanded inner bow to maintain maxillary intermolar width) when her RME appliance was removed. She corrected her molar relationship to Class I with the headgear. Once Erin's permanent teeth erupted, *early treatment was complete*.

After confirming that Erin's mandibular right primary second molar was nonmobile, we decided to treat Erin non-extraction. We bonded fixed orthodontic appliances to all teeth *except* her mandibular right primary second molar. We maintained space for the mandibular right primary second molar by trapping a tight closed coil spring between the mandibular right first premolar and mandibular right permanent first molar. We leveled and aligned both arches. A few months before the end of treatment, we bonded a bracket to the mandibular right primary second molar and aligned it with the arch. Erin was debonded and placed in removable clear (vacuum-formed) retainers at night.

Q: Final records are shown in Figure 3.92. What changes occurred with Erin's treatment, and what "take home pearls" can you suggest?

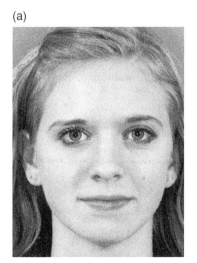
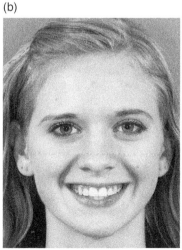
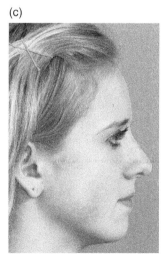

(a) (b) (c)

Figure 3.92 Final records of Erin at age fourteen years.

(d)

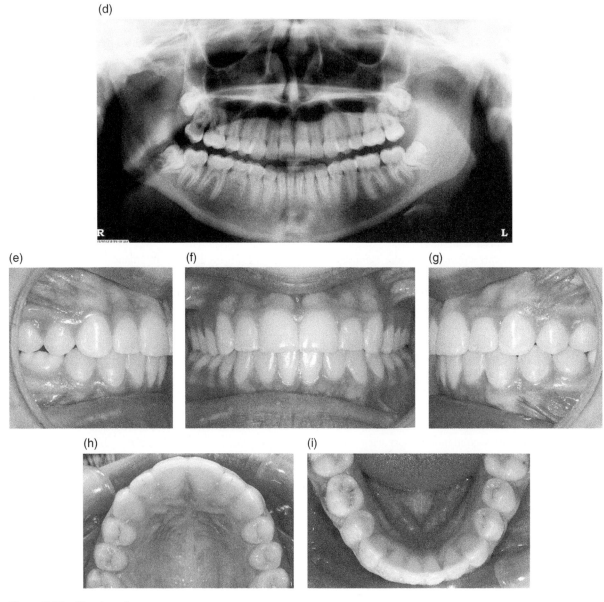

(e) (f) (g)

(h) (i)

Figure 3.92 (Continued)

A: Changes and "take home pearls" include the following:

- Erin was eleven years and six months old when she presented with her parents' chief complaint, "Erin has crooked teeth." Her permanent first molars were Class I. She displayed moderate maxillary arch crowding (5.0 mm), nearly severe mandibular anterior crowding (8.5 mm), a retained mandibular right primary second molar lacking a successor, an anterior crossbite of the maxillary left permanent lateral incisor, posterior crossbite of the left primary second molars, and significant posterior transverse compensations. CR and CO were coincident. She was treated early with:

a) Maintenance of the mandibular right primary second molar;

b) RME to create posterior overjet, correct the left primary second molar crossbite, and eliminate posterior transverse compensations;

c) Placement of an expanded LLHA to upright her mandibular first permanent molars and to utilize mandibular left "*E space*."

Early treatment ended once her remaining permanent teeth erupted. Non-extraction comprehensive treatment began, but we did not place a bracket on her retained mandibular right primary second molar until near the end of treatment. Her wisdom teeth were developing, and she was referred to an oral surgeon to have them removed following orthodontic appliance removal.

We were delighted with Erin's outcome and the improvement in her smile esthetics (compare Figures 3.80b and 3.82b). Her maxillary and mandibular midlines are coincident, maxillary lip is coincident with maxillary central incisor gingival margins, her smile is broad with minimal buccal corridors, and her mild smile arc is relatively congruent with her lower lip. Her profile remains slightly convex, and her nasal tip has descended (Figure 3.92c). Her permanent teeth roots are relatively parallel (Figure 3.92d), and her canines have erupted into an ideal Class I relationship (Figures 3.92e and 3.92g). Note the mandibular left-to-right permanent first molar asymmetry (left permanent first molars are ahead of right) due to retention of the mandibular right primary second molar. Her mandibular anterior gingiva appears healthy (Figure 3.92f), overbite and overjet are minimal, and both arches are aligned (including the retained mandibular right primary second molar).

- Since we decided to treat Erin non-extraction (non-extraction of permanent teeth), it was reasonable to attempt maintaining the retained mandibular right primary second molar. Why? It had *a good crown, good root, and good bone level.*

- If you attempt to maintain a primary tooth lacking a permanent successor, then *avoid bonding an orthodontic bracket to it and avoid moving it orthodontically – to reduce the risk that its roots will resorb.* If you must move the primary tooth, then *apply light orthodontic force to it for only a short period of time and move it to the minimal possible distance.*

- In accordance with the above guidelines, we did not bond Erin's mandibular right primary second molar to align it until late in treatment. But even using light forces for only a few months, Erin's mandibular right primary second molar had significant resorption of its distal root (Figure 3.93).

- *Another viable option would have been to not move the mandibular right primary second molar but to leave it slightly malaligned instead.*

- A question that must be answered now (Figure 3.93b) is whether to continue maintaining the mandibular right primary second molar. What do you recommend? A discussion of options was held with Erin and her parents. Because it still has a good crown, good bone level, and reasonable roots, a decision was made to continue maintaining the primary second molar for as long as possible. A fallback plan will be to replace it with an FPD if it exfoliates while she is a child or to replace it with an implant if it exfoliates when she is an adult.

(a) 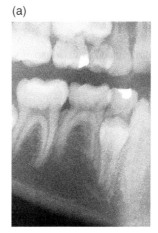 (b)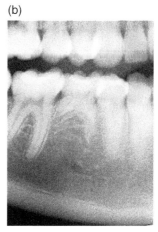

Figure 3.93 Erin's retained mandibular right primary second molar (a) before and (b) after orthodontic alignment. Note resorption of its roots. Resorption of the mesial root may have resulted during eruption of the first premolar. Resorption of the distal root occurred during orthodontic alignment.

- We were initially concerned with possible mentalis strain to achieve lip closure (Figure 3.90a). But in her final photographs (Figures 3.92a–3.92c), lip strain is absent.

- Because Erin had *some* keratinized attached gingiva labial to her mandibular central incisors, and because the alveolar process bone labial to her mandibular incisors was not thin (mandibular incisor roots were not palpable), we recommended monitoring her mandibular anterior gingiva. Thankfully, at the end of treatment, her mandibular anterior periodontal tissues appeared healthy.

However, in orthodontics and in life, *expect the unexpected.* We were careful to monitor these tissues throughout treatment and informed Erin and her parents that the need for a future gingival graft existed if recession occurred. If you have any concerns with a patient's periodontal tissues, seek consultation with a board-certified periodontist.

Case Brian

Q: Brian is thirteen years old (Figure 3.94) and presents to you with his parents' chief complaint, "Brian needs braces." He was in the late mixed dentition when his consultation panoramic image was made (Figure 3.94f). His PMH is WRN, PDH includes a unilateral left cleft lip and incomplete cleft alveolus, periodontal evaluation is WRN, and TMJ evaluation is WRN. *What was not evaluated?*

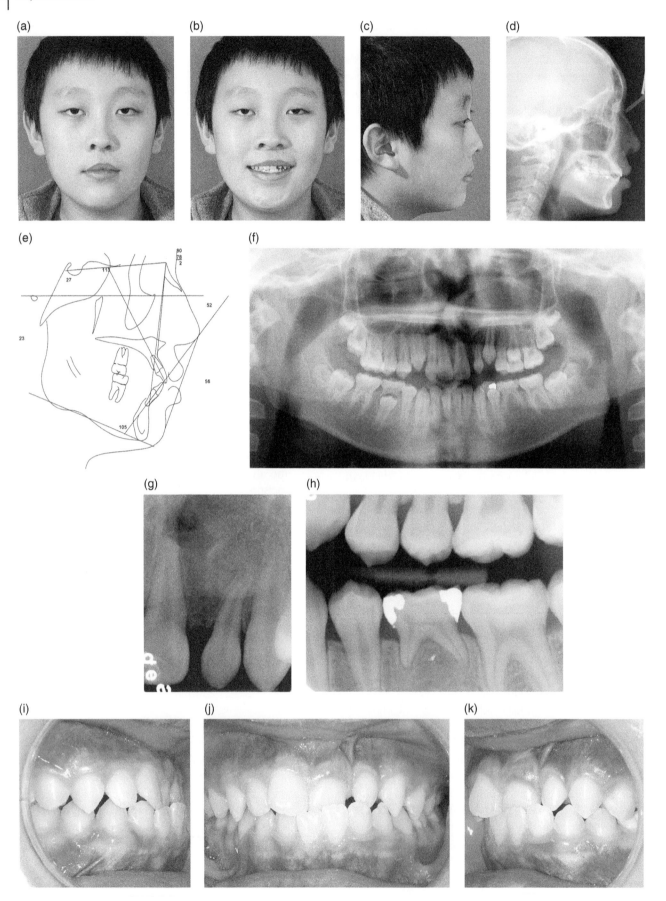

Figure 3.94 Initial records of Brian: (a–c) facial photographs, (d and e) lateral cephalogram and tracing, (f) pantomograph (a consultation image made before remaining records), (g–h) dental radiographs, (i–m) intraoral photographs.

(l)

(m)

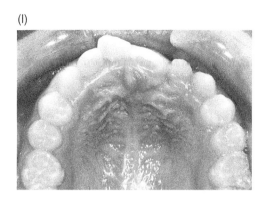
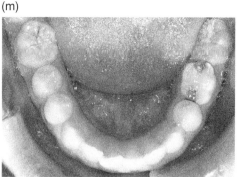

Figure 3.94 (Continued)

(a)

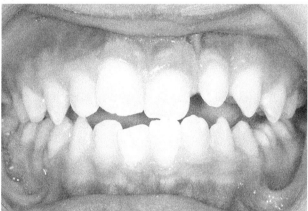

(b)

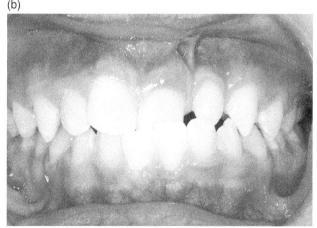

Figure 3.95 Frontal photograph of Brian (a) in CR and (b) shifting forward by 1–2 mm and to the left by 2 mm into CO.

A: We failed to examine Brian for a CR-CO shift. *You must check for a CR-CO shift in every orthodontic patient at every appointment.* Otherwise, you cannot establish existing dental and skeletal relationships. This was done at Brian's case presentation (Figures 3.95a and 3.95b). As shown, Brian presents with "edge-to-edge" left central incisors in CR (Figure 3.95a). However, as he closes

into CO (Figure 3.95b), he shifts to the left (note change in midlines) and slightly forward on the right. The result? In CO, he is Class III by 1–2 mm on the right but Class I on the left, and in anterior crossbite.

Q: Compile your diagnostic findings and problem list for Brian. Also, state your diagnosis.

A:

Table 3.21 Diagnostic findings and problems list for Brian.

Full face and profile	**Frontal view**
	Face is symmetric
	Soft-tissue LAFH WRN (soft-tissue Glabella – Subnasale approximately equal to Subnasale – soft-tissue Menton)
	Repaired unilateral left cleft lip
	Lip competence
	UDML 1mm to right of facial midline
	Inadequate gingival display in posed smile (maxillary central incisor gingival margins ~3 mm apical to maxillary lip)
	Profile view
	Convex profile
	Obtuse NLA (upturned nose)
	Chin projection deficient
	Obtuse lip-chin-throat angle
Ceph analysis	**Skeletal**
	Retrusive maxillary anteroposterior position (A-Point lies behind the Nasion-perpendicular line, Figure 3.94e).
	Retrusive mandibular anteroposterior position (ANB angle = 2° but maxilla is retrusive)
	Normal LAFH (ANS-Menton/Nasion-Menton X 100% = 56%)
	Mandibular plane angle WRN (FMA = 23°; SNMP = 27°)
	Effective bony Pogonion (Pogonion lies slightly ahead of a line extended from Nasion through B-point)

(Continued)

Table 3.21 (Continued)

Radiographs	***Dental*** Proclined maxillary incisors (U1 to SN = 113°) Proclined mandibular incisors (FMIA = 52°)
Intraoral Photos and Models	Late mixed dentition (Figure 3.94f) Diminutive maxillary left permanent lateral incisor Retained mandibular left primary second molar (note that this tooth has been restored in Figure 3.94h) Congenital absence of mandibular left second premolar Angle Class I in CR (Class III by ~1–2 mm on right in CO) Iowa Classification: I I I I in CR Mandibular midline to the left of maxillary midline by ~1 mm in CR (Figure 3.95a) but to the left of the maxillary midline by ~3mm in CO (Figure 3.95b) Anterior crossbite of central incisors and left maxillary lateral incisor in CO OB of 30% Unilateral left incomplete cleft alveolus 1.0 mm of maxillary incisor spacing is currently present (i.e. 1.0 of crowding combined with 2.0mm of spacing) 1.0 mm of maxillary crowding is anticipated if the diminutive maxillary left lateral incisor is cosmetically enlarged or is extracted and prosthetically replaced to make it 6.5 mm in mesiodistal width 1.0 mm of mandibular incisor crowding is currently present 1.9 mm of mandibular arch spacing is anticipated if the retained mandibular left primary second molar is extracted and replaced with a 7 mm second premolar (implant or fixed partial denture) Maxillary left and right permanent first molars are symmetric Mandibular left first premolar and canine are ahead of right Thin labial periodontal biotype covering mandibular central incisors (some keratinized attached gingiva is present)
Other	Maxillary incisal wear/damage due to the anterior crossbite (Figure 3.95a)
Diagnosis	Class I malocclusion in CR with forward and left lateral shift into CO resulting in anterior crossbite and right Class III relationship. Diminutive maxillary left permanent lateral incisor, missing mandibular left second premolar, and retained mandibular left primary second molar

Q: How can we conclude that Brian's mandible is *retrusive* when his ANB angle = 2° (normal ANB angle = 1° to 3°)?

A: As discussed in the Appendix, when the maxilla is retrusive you should relate mandibular position to *Nasion-perpendicular line* (maxillary A-point would lie on this line if the maxilla was normal). In Brian's case, the angle formed between Nasion-perpendicular line and Nasion-B point line is 7°, which indicates that his mandible is skeletally retrusive.

Q: Provide a detailed space analysis for Brian's maxillary and mandibular arches. In other words, how were the anticipated *1.0 mm of maxillary arch crowding (assuming a 6.5 mm maxillary left lateral incisor is achieved restoratively)* and *1.9 mm of mandibular arch spacing (if the retained mandibular left primary second molar is extracted and replaced with a 7 mm second premolar)* calculated?

A:

Average mesiodistal widths of permanent teeth (mm) [66]:

Maxillary Central Incisor	8.5	Mandibular Central Incisor	5.0
Maxillary Lateral Incisor	6.5	Mandibular Lateral Incisor	5.5
Maxillary Canine	7.5	Mandibular Canine	7.0
Maxillary First Premolar	7.0	Mandibular First Premolar	7.0
Maxillary Second Premolar	7.0	Mandibular Second Premolar	7.0
Maxillary First Molar	10.0	Mandibular First Molar	11.0
Maxillary Second Molar	9.0	Mandibular Second Molar	10.5

Average mesiodistal widths of *primary* teeth (mm) [66]:

Maxillary Central Incisor	6.5	Mandibular Central Incisor	4.2
Maxillary Lateral Incisor	5.1	Mandibular Lateral Incisor	4.1
Maxillary Canine	7.0	Mandibular Canine	5.0
Maxillary First Molar	7.3	Mandibular First Molar	7.7
Maxillary Second Molar	8.2	Mandibular Second Molar	9.9

Maxillary Arch

−1.0 mm crowding (Figure 3.94l, distal of right central incisor overlaps right lateral incisor)

+6.5 mm distance between distal of maxillary left central incisor and mesial of maxillary left permanent canine

−6.5 mm space required for average maxillary left permanent lateral incisor

Balance = −1.0 mm +6.5 mm −6.5 mm = −1.0 mm

Mandibular Arch

−1.0 mm of incisor crowding currently present (Figure 3.94m)

+9.9 mm mesiodistal width of retained left primary second molar

−7.0 mm of space is needed for mandibular left second premolar (if replaced prosthetically)

Balance = −1.0 mm +9.9 mm −7.0 mm = +1.9 mm

That is, *1.0 mm of maxillary crowding is anticipated if a 6.5 mm maxillary left lateral incisor is achieved restoratively, and 1.9 mm of mandibular spacing is anticipated if the retained mandibular left primary second molar is extracted and replaced with a 7 mm second premolar (implant or fixed partial denture).*

Q: What are Brian's *primary* problems in each dimension, plus other problems?

A:

Table 3.22   Primary problems list for Brian.

AP	Anterior crossbite in CO (anterior and left lateral CR-CO shift)
	Class III by 1–2 mm on right in CO
Vertical	—
Transverse	Left lateral CR-CO shift
Other	Retained mandibular left second primary molar without successor
	Diminutive maxillary left permanent lateral incisor

Q: Brian has a retained primary second molar. Can you restate our recommendations from the Introduction regarding treatment of retained primary teeth lacking successors? Can you apply these recommendations to Brian's retained primary tooth?

A: Our recommendations and their application to Brian are as follows:

- Recommendation: *for non-extraction cases, if the retained primary tooth has a good crown, good root, and good bone level, then consider maintaining it for the long term.* However, always have a contingency plan in case the retained primary tooth is lost. Such a contingency, or "fallback," plan could include implant replacement or replacement with an FPD.

Brian's mandibular left primary second molar (Figure 3.94h) is heavily restored and has partially resorbed roots. Long-term retention of this primary second molar is not recommended.

- Recommendation: *whenever possible, avoid bonding orthodontic brackets to and avoid applying orthodontic force against retained primary teeth – in order to reduce the risk that their roots will resorb.* If you must bond brackets to retained primary teeth, then try to *avoid moving them.*

This recommendation applies to Brian. If we choose to maintain his mandibular left primary second molar, then we should not bond an orthodontic bracket to it. If we do bond a bracket to it, then we should *apply light orthodontic force to it for only a short period of time and move it to the minimal possible distance.*

- Recommendation: *for non-extraction cases, if the retained primary tooth does not have a good crown, root, or bone level, then seriously consider extracting it.* Because Brian's mandibular left primary second molar is heavily restored with partially resorbed roots, we do not recommend maintaining it, long term. But a follow-up question is *when* to extract it? If we plan to replace it with an implant, then we should keep it for as long as possible in order to maintain the alveolar process bone level (avoiding the need for a bone graft).

- Recommendation: *for extraction cases, consider extracting the retained primary tooth.*

If we determine that Brian is an extraction case, then we should consider all tooth extraction options including extraction of his mandibular left primary second molar and extraction of his diminutive maxillary left lateral incisor.

Q: Can you suggest three specific treatment options for Brian's diminutive maxillary left lateral incisor?

A: Options include:
1) Maintain it.
2) Extract it and replace it with a lateral incisor implant or FPD.
3) Extract it and substitute the left permanent canine as the lateral incisor (canine substitution). This would involve moving the maxillary left permanent canine forward if Brian is treated non-extraction (opening a space distal to the permanent canine for an implant) or moving the maxillary left permanent canine, premolars, and molars mesial by an entire premolar width. Or, this would involve substituting the maxillary left first premolar as a canine (if a mandibular left first premolar was extracted and the space closed by retracting the mandibular left canine).

Q: Let's consider option 3 of the previous question in more detail (maxillary left canine substitution for a lateral incisor). What makes an ideal canine substitution case? Can you list characteristics that define such a case? Can you apply each of these characteristics to Brian? Would you recommend treating Brain as a canine substitution case?

A: Principle: The ideal canine substitution case (canines replacing missing lateral incisors) is a case where the maxillary permanent canines look exactly like missing lateral incisors and are already positioned precisely in the correct maxillary lateral incisor positions, the maxillary first premolars look exactly like maxillary canines and are positioned exactly in the correct maxillary canine positions, and the rest of the dentition is properly interdigitated, healthy, and aligned without spacing. In other words, *the ideal canine substitution case is a case where there is nothing for the orthodontist or restorative dentist to do.* All other cases are compromises to some degree. Generally, the less ideal the patient would be for canine substitution, the more ideal the patient would be for prosthetic replacement of the missing lateral incisors.

Let's list each ideal canine substitution feature and see if Brain exhibits it:

- *Both* maxillary lateral incisors are missing. Why is this feature important? It is difficult to esthetically match right and left sides if only one permanent canine is substituted for a lateral incisor.

  Brian *does not* exhibit this feature. He has only one diminutive maxillary lateral incisor we would consider extracting.

- *Maxillary* incisors have good inclination, and there is adequate lip support. Why? There would be no need to increase lip support via incisor proclination during opening of a lateral incisor space for prosthetic replacement.

  Brian *does* exhibit this feature. His maxillary incisors exhibit good inclination, and he exhibits adequate lip support.

- Assuming that the mandibular arch will be treated non-extraction, maxillary posterior teeth are already a full step Class II (6–7 mm) without spacing. Why? There is no need to protract maxillary posterior teeth.

  Brian *does not* exhibit this feature. He is Class I on the left, and his maxillary left canine and maxillary posterior teeth would need to be advanced 7 mm (a full premolar width) in order to place the maxillary left permanent canine in the lateral incisor position (assuming his mandibular arch is treated non-extraction). Of course, his maxillary left permanent canine alone could be advanced 7 mm, opening space distal to it for an implant.

- If the mandibular arch will be treated with premolar extractions, then there exists a Class I molar relationship. Why? With missing lateral incisors (or with extraction of diminutive maxillary lateral incisors), and with the extraction of mandibular premolars, the canine substitution patient is essentially treated as a four premolar extraction case.

  Brian is not missing maxillary lateral incisors. He has one normal lateral incisor (right) and one diminutive lateral incisor (left). We have not yet determined whether Brian will be treated with, or without, mandibular premolar extractions.

- The maxillary permanent canines look just like lateral incisors: color, shape (flat bucco-lingually so that the restorative dentist can build up the facial surface for color match), and narrow gingival margin width (emergence profile, like that of a lateral incisor).

  Brian *does not* exhibit this feature. His maxillary left permanent canine does not look like a lateral incisor.

- The maxillary permanent canines are already positioned exactly in the lateral incisor locations.

  Brian *does not* exhibit this feature. His maxillary left canine is not located in the lateral incisor position.

- Maxillary first premolars look exactly like maxillary canines (when the first premolar lingual cusps are reduced). Note: rotating the maxillary first premolars to the mesial slightly can improve their cuspid-like appearance).

  Brian *does* exhibit this feature. His maxillary left first premolar looks (reasonably) like a canine from the buccal (Figure 3.94k).

In summary, Brian is *not* an ideal candidate for maxillary left canine substitution (extraction of the maxillary left diminutive lateral incisor) if he is treated non-extraction (replacement of the mandibular left second primary molar with implant or FPD). Also, he is not a good candidate for maxillary left canine substitution if we extract *only* his mandibular left primary second molar and close that space reciprocally. Why? Left side only maxillary and mandibular space closure would shift his midlines dramatically to the left of facial center.

Brian would be a candidate for maxillary left canine substitution if we extracted his maxillary left lateral incisor and advanced only his maxillary left permanent canine into the lateral incisor space (opening a space distal to the permanent canine for an implant). This is assuming that the restorative dentist felt that the maxillary left canine could be cosmetically altered to look like a lateral incisor.

Brian would be a candidate for bilateral maxillary canine substitution (extraction of the maxillary left diminutive lateral incisor and maxillary right lateral incisor) if we also extracted his mandibular left primary second molar and a mandibular right premolar (leaving right and left permanent first molars in a Class I relationship). Again, this assumes that a restorative dentist feels that both maxillary permanent canines could be made to look like maxillary lateral incisors.

Q: In maxillary canine substitution cases, should an anterior Bolton tooth-size discrepancy be anticipated?

A: Yes, and the anterior Bolton tooth-size discrepancy should be dealt with using veneers to add structure to teeth or IPR to remove structure from teeth.

Q: What unknowns do you face in treating Brian? Specifically, *what unknowns should you eliminate before performing any irreversible procedure* (e.g. extracting permanent teeth)?

A: Elimination of Brian's CR-CO shift is critical *before* you establish a final treatment plan. If you do not know where you are starting from, then you cannot plan a route to take you to where you want to end up.

Future growth is an unknown, but since Brian is Class I (in CR) at thirteen years of age, it is much less of a concern than if he were only seven years old. Brian's compliance during treatment is an unknown, but his mother says that he is a cooperative child.

Q: What are your overall treatment goals for Brian?

A: We wish to provide Brian a healthy and esthetic smile, occlusion, and function. We want to correct his CR-CO shift, eliminate his anterior crossbite, deal intelligently with his retained primary molar and diminutive lateral incisor, and finish with Class I canines plus minimal OB and OJ.

Q: Although Brian was in the late mixed dentition when his panoramic image was made (Figure 3.94f), he is now in the permanent dentition. Further treatment will no longer be *early treatment,* but rather *comprehensive* treatment. The focus of this textbook is on early treatment, but can you suggest comprehensive treatment options for Brian?

A: As we emphasize in our earlier textbook [105], in addition to eliminating unknowns prior to instituting irreversible treatments, consider *all treatment options before deciding upon a final plan.* Ask yourself – should comprehensive treatment include orthognathic surgery, non-extraction treatment, extraction of anterior teeth, or extraction of posterior teeth?

Comprehensive treatment options for Brian include the following:

- *Monitor only* – we do not recommend this option. Brian's maxillary central incisor damage could worsen. Furthermore, if his lateral CR-CO shift remains untreated, then there is the possibility that mandibular asymmetric growth could result.
- *Orthognathic surgery* – is not recommended since Brian looks normal.
- *Non-extraction treatment (of permanent teeth)* – is reasonable. Brian's incisors are proclined according to European cephalometric standards but satisfactory according to Chinese standards [115]. Furthermore, Brian has attractive facial, and profile, esthetics. Although he exhibits a thin periodontal biotype labial to his mandibular incisors, he has *some* attached keratinized gingiva. We anticipate this tissue remaining stable during leveling and aligning of his mild mandibular arch crowding.
- *Extraction of maxillary anterior teeth (right permanent lateral incisor, left permanent diminutive lateral incisor) performed in conjunction with bilateral mandibular posterior extractions* would set Brian up as a maxillary canine substitution case, permit uprighting of anterior teeth (something Brian and his parents may want or may not want), and allow a Class I molar finish. This option would be considered only if a restorative dentist felt that the maxillary canines can be restored to look like maxillary lateral incisors. The mandibular extractions would most likely include the right second premolar and left primary second molar (symmetric mandibular extractions).
- *Extraction of a mandibular central incisor or mandibular anterior IPR* – would create space to align the mandibular anterior teeth without additional incisor proclination. Either treatment would require a careful anterior Bolton tooth-size analysis to determine if excess overjet would result.
- *Extraction of posterior teeth only (two maxillary premolars, a mandibular right premolar, and the mandibular left primary second molar)* – is not recommended as severe root resorption of the maxillary left permanent diminutive lateral incisor would likely occur during its retraction (space closure). Loss of this tooth due to root resorption during incisor retraction is feared.
- *Correcting his anterior crossbite* – is *essential* and must be performed to eliminate Brian's CR-CO shift before we can establish a final, definitive treatment plan. Correcting the anterior crossbite would also eliminate further central incisor trauma. The anterior crossbite could be corrected using either fixed orthodontic appliances or a removable appliance.
- *Retention of the maxillary left permanent diminutive lateral incisor* – would be considered only if Brian was

treated non-extraction (no permanent posterior teeth extracted), without moving the maxillary left lateral incisor (to avoid root resorption) or moving it minimally, and only if a restorative dentist felt that she/he could alter the lateral incisor crown to look like a normal maxillary lateral incisor crown form. If the maxillary left lateral incisor was retained, then a "fallback" or contingency plan (prosthetic replacement) must be discussed with Brian's parents in case the lateral incisor is eventually lost.

- *Retention of the mandibular left primary second molar* – is considered reasonable only over the short term. Why? Its crown and roots are less than ideal, and we would not expect it to be retained long term. Certainly, the primary second molar could be retained for as long as possible to maintain alveolar process bone if Brian is treated non-extraction in the mandibular arch. If he is treated with mandibular posterior extractions, then the primary second molar would be the extraction tooth of choice on the left side.

Q: If we chose non-extraction treatment but the maxillary left permanent lateral incisor is lost, then why would we replace it with a *bonded FPD* instead of a pontic on a *removable* maxillary Hawley retainer?

A: A bonded FPD would hold the roots of the left central incisor and permanent canine precisely in position until an implant could be placed when Brian is an adult. Moved roots may relapse with a Hawley retainer making implant placement difficult. Of course, if Brian is an adult when the maxillary left lateral incisor is lost, then we would recommend immediate placement with implant and crown.

Q: What treatment do you recommend for Brian?

A: We discussed options with Brian and his parents exhaustively. They did not want permanent teeth extracted. We consulted with a dentist who felt that the maxillary left permanent lateral incisor could be restored to normal maxillary permanent lateral incisor crown form. We consulted with a prosthodontist who advised that the mandibular left primary second molar be retained *intact* for as long as possible before replacement with a dental implant.

We placed fixed orthodontic appliances on Brian's maxillary teeth (Figure 3.96), aligned his maxillary arch, and corrected his anterior crossbite, which eliminated his CR-CO shift. Thankfully, we confirmed Brian was Class I, *bilaterally*. At this time a non-extraction treatment approach was definitively chosen. Note: we bonded Brian's maxillary left lateral incisor and moved it slightly. Brian's mandibular arch was bonded, leveled, and aligned (his mandibular left primary second molar was not bonded). We noted that the distal amalgam restoration of the mandibular left primary second molar had been lost and that the primary molar roots were continuing to resorb (Figure 3.97). The prosthodontist was consulted and recommended leaving the primary molar unrestored since the tooth was not sensitive and since adequate space remained for eventual implant placement. Following detailing, consultations were held with the dentist and the prosthodontist. To maximize esthetics, including midline coincidence, it was suggested that space be placed at the distal of the maxillary right lateral incisor and at the mesial of the maxillary left lateral incisor for composite veneers. This was done. Brian was debanded, the maxillary lateral incisors were restored with composite veneers (Figure 3.98), and he was placed in maxillary and mandibular Hawley retainers, which he was instructed to wear nightly. Years later, when Brian was in his 20s, his mandibular left primary second molar

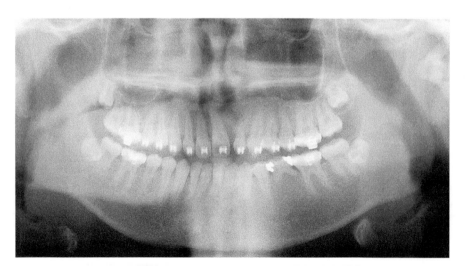

Figure 3.96 Progress panoramic image of Brian following alignment of his maxillary teeth, correction of his anterior crossbite, and correction of his CR-CO shift.

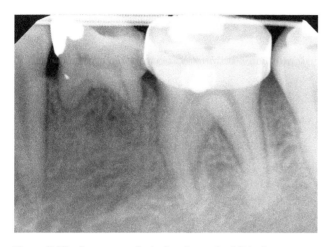

Figure 3.97 Progress periapical radiograph of Brian's mandibular left primary second molar.

was extracted and replaced with an implant (Figure 3.99) and crown. A new mandibular Hawley retainer was provided to fit with the new crown.

Q: What changes occurred with Brian's treatment and what "take home pearls" can you suggest?

A: Changes with treatment and "take home pearls" include the following:

- Brian presented when he was thirteen years old with his parents' chief complaint, "Brian needs braces." PDH included unilateral left cleft lip and incomplete cleft alveolus. He was Angle Class I in CR but shifted forward and to the left in CO into Angle Class III on the right side. He presented with an anterior crossbite, 30% OB, diminutive maxillary permanent left lateral incisor, retained mandibular left second primary molar, and missing mandibular left second premolar.

(a)

(b)

(c)

(d)

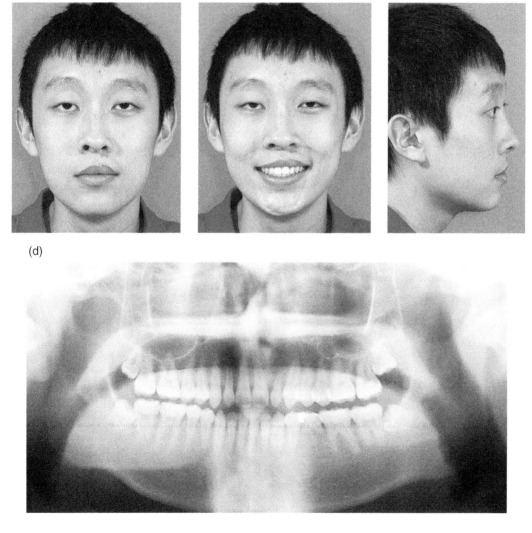

Figure 3.98 (a–i) Deband records of Brian.

(e)   (f)   (g)

(h)   (i)

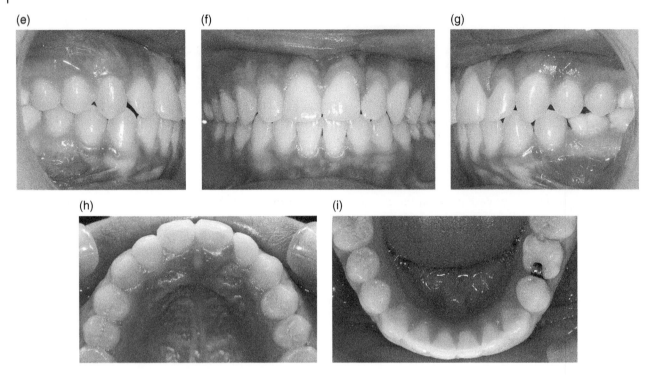

Figure 3.98   (Continued)

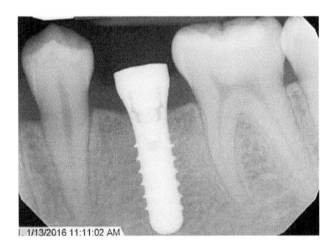

Figure 3.99   Brian's mandibular left primary second molar was extracted, and replaced with an implant and crown, when Brian was in his early 20s.

He was treated non-extraction, with retention of the primary molar and the diminutive lateral incisor. Composite veneers were placed on his maxillary lateral incisors just after deband, and his mandibular left primary second molar was eventually extracted and replaced with an implant and crown.

- Brian's smile improved dramatically with treatment (compare Figures 3.84b and 3.88b), and his parents noted that he now smiles more. His lower lip protrusion and labiomental sulcus depth increased. The anterior crossbite was corrected, and Brian now has an excellent Class I occlusion with minimal overbite/ overjet and well-aligned arches. His third molars developed (Figure 3.98d), and he was referred to an oral and maxillofacial surgeon for their extraction.

- It was prudent to *correct Brian's CR-CO anterior and lateral shift before a final treatment plan was definitively established.* The importance of eliminating CR-CO shifts before finalizing treatment plans (especially before doing anything irreversible) has been underscored throughout this textbook and cannot be overemphasized. You must examine every patient for a CR-CO shift at every appointment. Thankfully, Brian was bilaterally Class I after the shift was eliminated.

- Retaining Brian's maxillary left diminutive lateral incisor was reasonable because he was treated non-extraction, the lateral incisor was moved minimally, and the dentist was confident he could restore the diminutive lateral incisor to resemble a normal lateral incisor.

- Whenever possible, *avoid bonding orthodontic brackets to, and moving, retained primary teeth or diminutive incisor teeth with short roots.* We were fortunate that Brian's lateral incisor root did not resorb although it was moved.

- It was prudent to plan for eventual loss of the mandibular left primary second molar. Why? It had a poor crown (restored, Figure 3.94h) and poor roots (resorbed). It was also prudent to retain this primary molar for as long as possible in order to maintain mandibular alveolar process bone.

- Whenever a primary tooth (lacking a successor) is maintained, establish a "fallback" or contingency plan if the primary tooth is eventually lost.
- Brian was not an ideal canine substitution case (maxillary canines substituting for missing/extracted maxillary lateral incisors). An ideal canine substitution case is one where: the maxillary permanent canines look exactly like missing lateral incisors and are positioned exactly in the maxillary lateral incisor spots; the maxillary first premolars look exactly like maxillary canines and are positioned exactly in the maxillary canine spots; and the rest of the dentition is properly interdigitated, healthy, and aligned without spacing. In other words, *the ideal canine substitution case is one where there is nothing for the orthodontist or restorative dentist to do.* All other cases are compromises in some way.

Generally, the less ideal the patient would be for canine substitution, the more ideal the patient would be for prosthetic replacement of the missing maxillary lateral incisors.

- We discussed with Brian and his parents the fact that gingival recession, and the need for a gingival graft, was a distinct possibility during mandibular arch alignment (mandibular incisor proclination). Fortunately, his mandibular labial tissue did not recede (note: Brian initially had *some* keratinized attached gingival tissue). Ideally, every patient presents with a thick periodontal biotype, everywhere. If you have any concerns regarding your treatment plan and the patient's periodontal tissues, seek consultation with a board-certified periodontist.
- Brian was a multidisciplinary case. In all multidisciplinary cases, the key to success is "communication, communication, communication" with the other doctors.

References

1 Thilander, B. and Myrberg, N. (1973). The prevalence of malocclusion in Swedish schoolchildren. *Scand. J. Dent. Res.* 81 (1): 12–21.

2 Ericson, S. and Kurol, J. (1986). Longitudinal study and analysis of clinical supervision of maxillary canine eruption. *Community Dent. Oral Epidemiol.* 14 (3): 172–176.

3 Rutledge, M.S. and Hartsfield, J.K. Jr. (2010). Genetic factors in the etiology of palatally displaced canines. *Semin. Orthod.* 16 (3): 165–171.

4 Peck, S., Peck, L., and Kataja, M. (1994). The palatally displaced canine as a dental anomaly of genetic origin. *Angle Orthod.* 64 (4): 249–256.

5 Clark, C.A. (1910). A method of ascertaining the relative position of unerupted teeth by means of film radiographs. *Proc. R. Soc. Med.* 3 (Odontol Sect): 87–90.

6 Richards, A.G. (1952 Oct). Roentgenographic localization of the mandibular canal. *J. Oral. Surg. (Chic).* 10 (4): 325–329.

7 Richards, A.G. (1953). The buccal object rule. *J. Tenn. State Dent. Assoc.* 33: 263–268.

8 Ericson, S. and Kurol, J. (1987). Radiographic examination of ectopically erupting maxillary canines. *Am. J. Orthod. Dentofac. Orthop.* 91 (6): 483–492.

9 Lindauer, S., Rubenstein, L., Hang, W. et al. (1992). Canine impaction identified early with panoramic radiographs. *J. Am. Dent. Assoc.* 123 (3): 91–92. 95-7.

10 Buchner, H.J. (1936). Root resorption caused by ectopic eruption of maxillary cuspid. *Int. J. Orthod. Oral. Surg.* 22 (12): 1236–1238.

11 Ericson, S. and Kurol, J. (1988). Early treatment of palatally erupting maxillary canines by extraction of the primary canines. *Eur. J. Orthod.* 10 (4): 283–295.

12 Parkin, N., Benson, P.E., Shah, A. et al. (2009). Extraction of primary (baby) teeth for unerupted palatally displaced permanent canine teeth in children. *Cochrane Database Syst. Rev.* 2: CD004621.

13 Naoumova, J., Kurol, J., and Kjellberg, H. (2011 Apr). A systematic review of the interceptive treatment of palatally displaced maxillary canines. *Eur. J. Orthod.* 33 (2): 143–149.

14 Power, S.M. and Short, M.B. (1993). An investigation into the response of palatally displaced canines to the removal of deciduous canines and an assessment of factors contributing to favourable eruption. *Br. J. Orthod.* 20 (3): 215–223.

15 Kettle, M.A. (1958). Treatment of the unerupted maxillary canine. *Dent. Pract. Dent. Rec.* 8: 245–255.

16 Jacobs, S.G. (1994 Aug). Palatally impacted canines: aetiology of impaction and scope for impaction. Report of cases outside the guidelines of interception. *Aust. Dent. J.* 39 (4): 206–211.

17 Olive, R.J. (2002). Orthodontic treatment of palatally impacted maxillary canines. *Aust Orthod J.* 18 (2): 64–70.

18 Leonardi, M., Armi, P., Franchi, L., and Baccetti, T. (2004 Oct). Two interceptive approaches to palatally displaced canines: a prospective longitudinal study. *Angle Orthod.* 74 (5): 581–586.

19 Baccetti, T., Leonardi, M., and Armi, P. (2008). A randomized clinical study of two interceptive approaches to palatally displaced canines. *Eur. J. Orthod.* 30 (4): 381–385.

20 Baccetti, T., Mucedero, M., Leonardi, M., and Cozza, P. (2009). Interceptive treatment of palatal impaction of maxillary canines with rapid maxillary expansion: A randomized clinical trial. *Am. J. Orthod. Dentofac. Orthop.* 136 (5): 657–661.

21 Giulio, A.B., Serena, I.P., Matteo, Z., and Ida, M. (2010 Sep-Oct). Double vs single primary teeth extraction approach as prevention of permanent maxillary canines ectopic eruption. *Pediatr. Dent.* 32 (5): 407–412.

22 Armi, P., Cozza, P., and Baccetti, T. (2011). Effect of RME and headgear treatment on the eruption of palatally displaced canines: a randomized clinical study. *Angle Orthod.* 81 (3): 370–374.

23 Sigler, L., Baccetti, T., and McNamara, J. (2011). Effect of rapid maxillary expansion and transpalatal arch treatment associated with deciduous canine extraction on the eruption of palatally displaced canines: a 2-center prospective study. *Am. J. Orthod. Dentofac. Orthop.* 139 (3): e235–e244.

24 Bonetti, G.A., Zanarini, M., Parenti, S.I. et al. (2011). Preventive treatment of ectopically erupting maxillary permanent canines by extraction of deciduous canines and first molars: a randomized clinical trial. *Am. J. Orthod. Dentofac. Orthop.* 139 (3): 316–323.

25 Baccetti, T., Sigler, L.M., and McNamara, J.A. Jr. (2011). An RCT on treatment of palatally displaced canines with RME and/or transpalatal arch. *Eur. J. Orthod.* 33 (6): 601–607.

26 Naoumova, J., Kurol, J., and Kjelberg, H. (2015 Apr). Extraction of the deciduous canine as an interceptive treatment in children with palatal displaced canines – part I: shall we extract the deciduous canine or not? *Eur. J. Orthod.* 37 (2): 209–218.

27 Barros, S.E., Hoffelder, L., Araújo, F. et al. (2018). Short-term impact of rapid maxillary expansion on ectopically and normally erupting canines. *Am. J. Orthod. Dentofac. Orthop.* 154 (4): 524–534.

28 Fanning, E.A. (1962). Effect of extraction of deciduous molars on the formation and eruption of their successors. *Angle Orthod.* 32 (1): 44–53.

29 Hadler-Olsen, S., Sjögren, A., Steinnes, J. et al. (2020). Double vs single primary tooth extraction in interceptive treatment of palatally displaced canines: a randomized controlled trial. *Angle Orthod.* 90 (6): 751–757.

30 Alqerban, A., Storms, A., Voet, M. et al. (2016). Early prediction of maxillary canine impaction. *Dentomaxillofac Radiol.* 45 (3): 20150232.

31 Smailienė, D., Sidlauskas, A., Lopatienė, K. et al. (2011). Factors affecting self-eruption of displaced permanent maxillary canines. *Medicina (Kaunas)* 47 (3): 163–169.

32 Naoumova, J. and Kjellberg, H. (2018). The use of panoramic radiographs to decide when interceptive extraction is beneficial in children with palatally displaced canines based on a randomized clinical trial. *Eur. J. Orthod.* 40: 565–574.

33 Kokich, V. (2004). Surgical and orthodontic management of impacted maxillary canines. Am. *J. Orthod. Dentofac. Orthop.* 126: 278–283.

34 Woloshyn, H., Årtun, J., Kennedy, D.B., and Joondeph, D.R. (1994). Pulpal and periodontal reactions to orthodontic alignment of palatally impacted canines. *Angle Orthod.* 64: 257–264.

35 Schmidt, A. and Kokich, V. (2007 Apr). Periodontal response to early uncovering, autonomous eruption, and orthodontic alignment of palatally impacted maxillary canines. *Am. J. Orthod. Dentofac. Orthop.* 131 (4): 449–455.

36 Kurol, J. (2002 Jun). Early treatment of tooth-eruption disturbances. *Am. J. Orthod. Dentofac. Orthop.* 121 (6): 588–591.

37 Lygidakis, N.A., Bafis, S., and Vidaki, E. (2009 Nov). Case report: surgical luxation and elevation as treatment approach for secondary eruption failure of permanent molars. *Eur. Arch. Paediatr. Dent.* 10 (Suppl 1): 46–48.

38 Kravitz, N.D., Yanosky, M., Cope, J.B. et al. (2016 Jan). Surgical uprighting of lower second molars. *J. Clin. Orthod.* 50 (1): 33–40.

39 Becker, A. and Karnei-R'em, R.M. (1992 Sep). The effects of infraocclusion: Part 1. Tilting of the adjacent teeth and local space loss. *Am. J. Orthod. Dentofac. Orthop.* 102 (3): 256–264.

40 Becker, A. and Karnei-R'em, R.M. (1992 Oct). The effects of infraocclusion: Part 2. The type of movement of the adjacent teeth and their vertical development. *Am. J. Orthod. Dentofac. Orthop.* 102 (4): 302–309.

41 Kurol, J. and Thilander, B. (1984 Nov). Infraocclusion of primary molars and the effect on occlusal development: a longitudinal study. *Eur. J. Orthod.* 6 (4): 277–293.

42 Kurol, J. and Olson, L. (1991 Oct). Ankylosis of primary molars – a future periodontal threat to the first permanent molars? *Eur. J. Orthod.* 13 (5): 404–409.

43 Proffit, W.R. and Vig, K.W. (1981 Aug). Primary failure of eruption: a possible cause of posterior open-bite. *Am. J. Orthod.* 80 (2): 173–190.

44 Frazier-Bowers, S.A., Puranik, C.P., and Mahaney, M.C. (2010 Sep). The etiology of disruption disorders – further evidence of a genetic paradigm. *Semin. Orthod.* 16 (3): 180–185.

45 Stellzig-Eisenhauer, A., Decker, E., Meyer-Marcotty, P. et al. (2010 Jan). Primary failure of eruption

(PFE) – clinical and molecular genetics analysis. *J. Orofac. Orthop.* 71 (1): 6–16.

46 Ahmad, S., Bister, D., and Cobourne, M.T. (2006 Dec). The clinical features and aetiological basis of primary eruption failure. *Eur. J. Orthod.* 28 (6): 535–540.

47 Rhoads, S.G., Hendricks, H.M., and Frazier-Bowers, S.A. (2013 Aug). Establishing the diagnostic criteria for eruption disorders based on genetic and clinical data. *Am. J. Orthod. Dentofac. Orthop.* 144 (2): 194–202.

48 Frazier-Bowers, S.A., Koehler, K.E., Ackerman, J.L., and Proffit, W.R. (2007 May). Primary failure of eruption: further characterization of a rare eruption disorder. *Am. J. Orthod. Dentofac. Orthop.* 131 (5): 578.e1–e11.

49 Rølling, S. (1980 Oct). Hypodontia of permanent teeth in Danish school children. *Scand. J. Dent. Res.* 88 (5): 365–369.

50 Brook, A.H., Jernvall, J., Smith, R.N. et al. (2014 June). The dentition: the outcomes of morphogenesis leading to variations of tooth number, size and shape. *Aust. Dent. J.* 59 (Suppl 1): 131–142.

51 Kreiborg, S. and Jensen, B.L. (2018 Oct). Tooth formation and eruption – lessons learnt from cleidocranial dysplasia. *Eur. J. Oral Sci.* 126 (Suppl 1): 72–80.

52 Ostler, M.S. and Kokich, V.G. (1994 Feb). Alveolar ridge changes in patients congenitally missing mandibular second premolars. *J. Prosthet. Dent.* 71 (2): 144–149.

53 Slagsvold, O. and Bjerke, B. (1978). Indications for autotransplantation in cases of missing premolars. *Am. J. Orthod.* 74 (3): 241–257.

54 Joondeph, D.R. and McNeill, R.W. (1971 Jan). Congenitally absent second premolars: an interceptive approach. *Am. J. Orthod.* 59 (1): 50–66.

55 Bergstrom, K. (1977). An orthopantomographic study of hypodontia, supernumeraries and other anomalies in school children between the ages of 8-9 years. An epidemiological study. *Swed. Dent. J.* 1 (4): 145–157.

56 Valencia, R., Saadia, M., and Ginberg, G. (2004 May). Controlled slicing in the management of congenitally missing second premolars. *Am. J. Orthod. Dentofac. Orthop.* 125 (5): 537–543.

57 Bonin, M. (1976 May-Jun). Simplified and rapid treatment of ankylosed primary molars with an amalgam and composite resin. *ASDC J. Dent. Child.* 43 (3): 159–162.

58 Bjerklin, K., Al-Najjar, M., Kårestedt, H., and Andrén, A. (2008 Jun). Agenesis of mandibular second premolars with retained primary molars: a longitudinal radiographic study of 99 subjects from 12 years of age to adulthood. *Eur. J. Orthod.* 30 (3): 254–261.

59 Ith-Hansen, K. and Kjaer, I. (2000 Jun). Persistence of deciduous molars in subjects with agenesis of the second premolars. *Eur. J. Orthod.* 22 (3): 239–243.

60 Sletten, D.W., Smith, B.M., Southard, K.A. et al. (2003 Dec). Retained deciduous mandibular molars in adults: a radiographic study of long-term changes. *Am. J. Orthod. Dentofac. Orthop.* 124 (6): 625–630.

61 Scurria, M.S., Bader, J.D., and Shugars, D.A. (1998 Apr). Meta-analysis of fixed partial denture survival: prostheses and abutments. *J. Prosthet. Dent.* 79 (4): 459–464.

62 Cobourne, M.T., Williams, A., and Harrison, M. (2014 Dec 5). National clinical guidelines for the extraction of first permanent molars in children. *Br. Dent. J.* 217 (11): 643–648.

63 Saber, A.M., Altoukhi, D.H., Horaib, M.F. et al. (2018 Apr 5). Consequences of early extraction of compromised first permanent molar: a systematic review. *BMC Oral Health.* 18 (1): 59.

64 Riedel, R.A. (1948). A cephalometric roentgenographic study of the relation of the maxilla and associated parts to the cranial base in normal and malocclusion of the teeth [M.S.D. thesis]. Evanston (IL): Northwestern University.

65 McNamara, J.A. Jr. (1984 Dec). A method of cephalometric evaluation. *Am. J. Orthod.* 86 (6): 449–469.

66 Wheeler, R.C. (1974). *Dental Anatomy, Physiology, and Occlusion*, 5ee. Philadelphia: W.B. Saunders.

67 ADA Division of Communications. For the dental patient (2006 Jan). Tooth eruption: the permanent teeth. *J. Am. Dent. Assoc.* 137 (1): 127.

68 Proffit, W.R. and Tulloch, J.F. (2002 Jun). Preadolescent Class II problems: treat now or wait? *Am. J. Orthod. Dentofac. Orthop.* 121 (6): 560–562.

69 Tulloch, J.F.C., Proffit, W.R., and Phillips, C. (2004 Jun). Outcomes in a 2-phase randomized clinical trial of early Class II treatment. *Am. J. Orthod. Dentofac. Orthop.* 125 (6): 657–667.

70 Ghafari, J., Shofer, F.S., Jacobsson-Hunt, U. et al. (1998 Jan). Headgear versus function regulator in the early treatment of Class II division 1 malocclusion: a randomized clinical trial. *Am. J. Orthod. Dentofac. Orthop.* 113 (1): 51–61.

71 Keeling, S.D., Wheeler, T.T., King, G.J. et al. (1998 Jan). Anteroposterior skeletal and dental changes after early Class II treatment with bionators and headgear. *Am. J. Orthod. Dentofac. Orthop.* 113 (1): 40–50.

72 Ghafari, J., King, G.J., and Tulloch, J.F. (1998 Nov). Early treatment of Class II, division 1 malocclusion – comparison of alternative treatment modalities. *Clin. Orthod. Res.* 1 (2): 107–117.

73 Thiruvenkatachari, B., Harrison, J., Worthington, H., and O'Brien, K. (2015 Jul). Early orthodontic treatment for Class II malocclusion reduces the chance of incisal trauma: results of a Cochrane systematic review. *Am. J. Orthod. Dentofac. Orthop.* 148 (1): 47–59.

74 Thiruvenkatachari, B., Harrison, J.E., Worthington, H.V., and O'Brien, K.D. (2013, Nov. 13). Orthodontic treatment

for prominent upper front teeth (Class II malocclusion) in children. *Cochrane Database Syst. Rev.* 11: CD003452.

75 Firouz, M., Zernik, J., and Nanda, R. (1992 Sep). Dental and orthopedic effects of high-pull headgear in treatment of Class II, Division 1 malocclusion. *Am. J. Orthod. Dentofac. Orthop.* 102 (3): 197–205.

76 Baumrind, S., Korn, E.L., Isaacson, R.J. et al. (1983 Nov). Quantitative analysis of the orthodontic and orthopedic effects of maxillary traction. *Am. J. Orthod.* 84 (5): 384–398.

77 Elder, J.R. and Tuenge, R.H. (1974 Dec). Cephalometric and histologic changes produced by extraoral high-pull traction to the maxilla in Macaca mulatta. *Am. J. Orthod.* 66 (6): 599–617.

78 Kirjavainen, M., Kirjavainen, T., Hurmerinta, K., and Haavikko, K. (2000 Aug). Orthopedic cervical headgear with an expanded inner bow in Class II correction. *Angle Orthod.* 70 (4): 317–325.

79 Pancherz, H. (1997 Dec). The effects, limitations, and long-term dentofacial adaptations to treatment with the Herbst appliance. *Semin. Orthod.* 3 (4): 232–243.

80 Le Cornu, M., Cevidanes, L.H.S., Zhu, H. et al. (2013 Dec). Three-dimensional treatment outcomes in Class II patients treated with the Herbst appliance: a pilot study. *Am. J. Orthod. Dentofac. Orthop.* 144 (6): 818–830.

81 2005 AAO Council on Scientific Affairs (COSA) (2005 Sept). Ask us – functional appliances and long-term effects on mandibular growth. *Am. J. Orthod. Dentofac. Orthop.* 128 (3): 271–272.

82 Pancherz, H., Ruf, S., and Kohlhas, P. (1998 Oct). "Effective condylar growth" and chin position changes in Herbst treatment: a cephalometric roentgenographic long-term study. *Am. J. Orthod. Dentofac. Orthop.* 114 (4): 437–446.

83 Araujo, A.M., Buschang, P.H., and Melo, A.C.M. (2004 Oct). Adaptive condylar growth and mandibular remodeling changes with bionator therapy – an implant study. *Eur. J. Orthod.* 26 (5): 515–522.

84 Ruf, S., Baltromejus, S., and Pancherz, H. (2001 Feb). Effective condylar growth and chin position changes in activator treatment: a cephalometric roentgenographic study. *Angle Orthod.* 71 (1): 4–11.

85 Mann, K.R., Marshall, S.D., Qian, F. et al. (2011 Feb). Effect of maxillary anteroposterior position on profile esthetics in headgear-treated patients. *Am. J. Orthod. Dentofac. Orthop.* 139 (2): 228–234.

86 Vermette, M.E., Kokich, V.G., and Kennedy, D.B. (1995). Uncovering labially impacted teeth: apically positioned flap and closed-eruption techniques. *Angle Orthod.* 65 (1): 23–33.

87 Kokich, V.G. and Mathews, D.P. (1993 Apr). Surgical and orthodontic management of impacted teeth. *Dent. Clin. N. Am.* 37 (2): 181–204.

88 Suri, L., Gagari, E., and Vastardis, H. (2004 Oct). Delayed tooth eruption: pathogenesis, diagnosis, and treatment. A literature review. *Am. J. Orthod. Dentofac. Orthop.* 126 (4): 432–445.

89 Lindauer, S.J., Rubenstein, K.L., Hang, W.M. et al. (1992). Canine impaction identified early with panoramic radiographs. *J. Am. Dent. Assoc.* 123 (3): 91–97.

90 Dolce, C., McGorray, S.P., Brazeau, L. et al. (2007 Oct). Timing of Class II treatment: skeletal changes comparing 1-phase and 2-phase treatment. *Am. J. Orthod. Dentofac. Orthop.* 132 (4): 481–489.

91 O'Brien, K. (2006). Is early treatment for Class II malocclusions effective? Results of a randomized controlled trial. *Am. J. Orthod. Dentofac. Orthop.* 129 (4 Suppl): S64–S65.

92 O'Brien, K., Wright, J., Conboy, F. et al. (2009 May). Early treatment for Class II Division 1 malocclusion with the Twin-block appliance: a multi-center, randomized, controlled trial. *Am. J. Orthod. Dentofac. Orthop.* 135 (5): 573–579.

93 Miner, R.M., Al Qabandi, S., Rigali, P.H., and Will, L.A. (2012 Sept). Cone-beam computed tomography transverse analysis. Part I: Normative data. *Am. J. Orthod. Dentofac. Orthop.* 142 (3): 300–307.

94 Krebs, A. (1964). Mid-palatal expansion studies by the implant method over a seven-year period. *Rep. Congr. Eur. Orthod. Soc.* 40: 131–142.

95 Krebs, A. (1959). Expansion of the midpalatal suture studied by means of metallic implants. *Acta Odontol. Scand.* 17: 491–501.

96 Hicks, E.P. (1978 Feb). Slow maxillary expansion: a clinical study of the skeletal versus dental response to low-magnitude force. *Am. J. Orthod.* 73 (2): 121–141.

97 Wertz, R. and Dreskin, M. (1977 Apr). Midpalatal suture opening: a normative study. *Am. J. Orthod.* 71 (4): 367–381.

98 Baccetti, T., Franchi, L., Cameron, C.G., and McNamara, J.A. Jr. (2001 Oct). Treatment timing for rapid maxillary expansion. *Angle Orthod.* 71 (5): 343–350.

99 Betts, N.J., Vanarsdall, R.L., Barber, H.D. et al. (1995). Diagnosis and treatment of transverse maxillary deficiency. *Int. J. Adult Orthodon. Orthognath. Surg.* 10 (2): 75–96.

100 Shetty, V., Caridid, J.M., Caputo, A.A., and Chaconas, S.J. (1994 Jul). Biomechanical rationale for surgical-orthodontic expansion in the adult maxilla. *J. Oral Maxillofac. Surg.* 52 (7): 742–751.

101 Southard, T.E., Marshall, S.D., Allareddy, V. et al. (2013 Sep). An evidence-based comparison of headgear and functional appliance therapy for the correction of class II malocclusions. *Semin. Orthod.* 19 (3): 174–195.

102 Rogers, K., Campbell, P.M., Tadlock, L. et al. (2018 Jan). Treatment changes of hypo- and hyperdivergent Class II Herbst patients. *Angle Orthod.* 88 (1): 3–9.

103 Rebellato, J., Lindauer, S.J., Rubenstein, L.K. et al. (1997 Oct). Lower arch perimeter preservation using the lingual arch. *Am. J. Orthod. Dentofac. Orthop.* 112 (4): 449–456.

104 Villalobos, F.J., Sinha, P.K., and Nanda, R.S. (2000 Oct). Longitudinal assessment of vertical and sagittal control in the mandibular arch by the mandibular fixed lingual arch. *Am. J. Orthod. Dentofac. Orthop.* 118 (4): 366–370.

105 Southard, T.E., Bonner, L.L., and Marshall, S.D. (2015). *Orthodontics in the Vertical Dimension: A Case-Based Review*. Hoboken, N.J: Wiley Blackwell.

106 Kurol, J. and Koch, G. (1985 Jan). The effect of extraction of infraoccluded deciduous molars: a longitudinal study. *Am. J. Orthod.* 87 (1): 46–55.

107 Soxman JA, Wunsch PB, Haberland CM. Anomalies of tooth eruption. In: Soxman JA, Wunsch PB, Haberland CM. Anomalies of the Developing Dentition. 1e. New York: Springer; 58–61; 2019.

108 González-Ulloa, M. and Stevens, E. (1968 May). The role of chin correction in profileplasty. *Plast. Reconstr. Surg.* 41 (5): 477–486.

109 Maynard, J.G. and Ochsenbein, C. (1975 Sept). Mucogingival problems, prevalence and therapy in children. *J. Periodontol.* 46 (9): 543–552.

110 Maynard, J.G. Jr. and Wilson, R.D. (1980). Diagnosis and management of mucogingival problems in children. *Dent Clin North Ame* 24 (4): 683–703.

111 Andlin-Sobocki, A. (1993 Mar). Changes of facial gingival dimensions in children. A 2-year longitudinal study. *J. Clin. Periodontol.* 20 (3): 212–218.

112 Wennström, J., Lindhe, J., and Nyman, S. (1982 Jan). The role of keratinized gingiva in plaque-associated gingivitis in dogs. *J. Clin. Periodontol.* 9 (1): 75–85.

113 Dorfman, H.S., Kennedy, J.E., and Bird, W.C. (1982 Jun). Longitudinal evaluation of free autogenous gingivai grafts. A 4-year report. *J. Periodontol.* 53 (6): 349–359.

114 Miyasato, M., Crigger, M., and Egelberg, J. (1977 Aug). Gingival condition in areas of minimal and appreciable width of keratinized gingiva. *J. Clin. Periodontol.* 4 (3): 200–209.

115 Cooke, M.S. and Wei, S.H. (1989 Summer). A comparative study of southern Chinese and British Caucasian cephalometric standards. *Angle Orthod.* 59 (2): 131–138.

4

Anteroposterior Problems

Introduction

Anteroposterior treatment has probably received more attention in the orthodontic literature than any other treatment. This chapter provides a review of the etiology, diagnosis, and early management of anteroposterior problems ranging from excessive anterior overjet (OJ) and Class II dental/skeletal relationships to anterior crossbites and Class III dental/skeletal relationships.

Q: What is OJ? What is the ideal amount of OJ?

A: OJ is the measure of horizontal (anteroposterior) distance between the maxillary and mandibular incisors (Figure 4.1a, left). Ideal OJ is minimal, or zero OJ (Figures 4.1a, right and 4.1b–d). Ideal OJ is found when the mandibular incisal edges contact the maxillary incisor lingual surfaces with about 10–20% (1–2 mm) overbite (OB).

Q: What factors influence the magnitude of OJ that is present?

A: Factors influencing the magnitude of OJ include:
- Canine anteroposterior relationship (Class I, Class II, or Class III)
- Maxillary and mandibular incisor inclinations in the sagittal plane
- Maxillary and mandibular incisor alignments, spacing, crowding, and rotations
- Sum of the mesiodistal widths of the maxillary anterior teeth compared to the sum of the mesiodistal widths of the mandibular anterior teeth (presence or absence of an anterior Bolton discrepancy)

Q: When does *excessive* OJ occur?

A: Excessive OJ results when:
- Canines are in a Class II relationship (Figure 4.2a) due to an underlying *skeletal* Class II discrepancy –

either mandibular anteroposterior deficiency and/or maxillary anteroposterior excess
- *Dentally*, maxillary incisors are proclined too far labially and/or mandibular incisors are too upright (Figure 4.2b)
- Maxillary anterior teeth are severely spaced or mandibular anterior teeth are severely crowded
- A severe maxillary anterior Bolton tooth size excess exists or a severe mandibular anterior Bolton deficiency exists
- Discrepant maxillary and mandibular arches form; maxillary arch forms narrow and tapering toward the anterior ("V-shaped") and mandibular arch forms square anteriorly

Q: A seven-year-old girl presents to you with excessive OJ (Figure 4.3). Is there an increased risk of traumatic dental injuries in patients with excessive OJ?

A: Yes, children with OJ exceeding 3 mm have twice the risk for dental injuries as children with OJ less than 3 mm [1, 2].

Q: This girl's parents are concerned that she is at an increased risk for dental injuries. In addition to her OJ exceeding 3 mm, can you list other variables which could affect her susceptibility to injury?

A: Other variables include:
- Presence or absence of lip incompetence (exposed maxillary incisor crowns are more likely to suffer trauma than incisors with lip coverage)
- History of dental trauma
- History of risk-taking behavior
- Sports participation
- Attention deficit hyperactivity disorder (ADHD)
- Cognitive psychomotor issues
- Teasing
- Family values

Practical Early Orthodontic Treatment: A Case-Based Review, First Edition. Thomas E. Southard, Steven D. Marshall, Laura L. Bonner, and Kyungsup Shin.
© 2023 John Wiley & Sons, Inc. Published 2023 by John Wiley & Sons, Inc.
Companion website: www.wiley.com/go/southard/practical

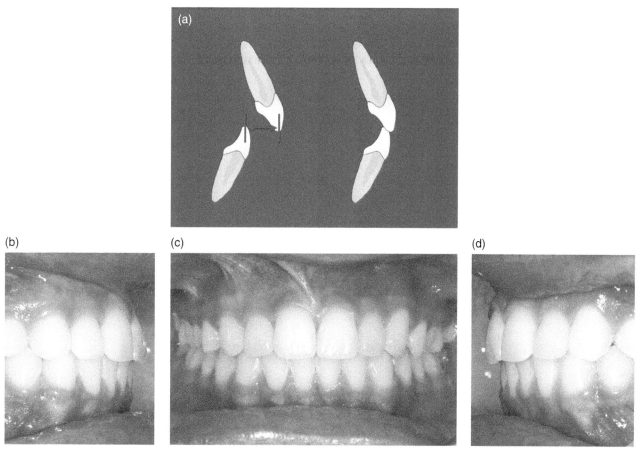

Figure 4.1 (a, left) Measure of overjet and (a, right) ideal OJ. (b–d) Example of ideal OJ.

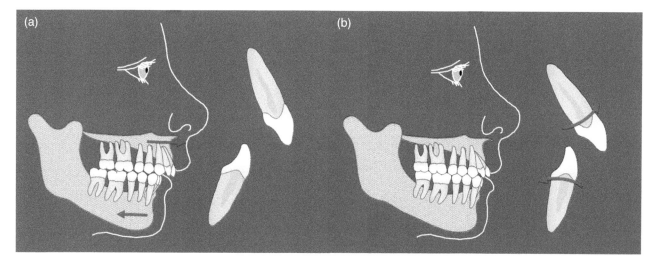

Figure 4.2 Excessive OJ can result from: (a) a skeletal discrepancy between the jaws – a mandibular anteroposterior deficiency and/ or maxillary anteroposterior excess; or (b) excessive maxillary incisor proclination/excessive mandibular incisor retroclination.

Q: Can excessive OJ lead to soft tissue injuries?

A: Yes. In cases of excessive OJ, mandibular incisors can erupt, bite into, and damage lingual periodontal or palatal soft tissues.

Q: Assume that you and this girl's parents decide to proceed with early treatment to reduce her OJ. What other discussions should you have with her parents?

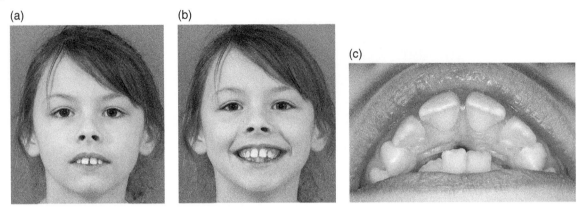

Figure 4.3 (a–c) A 7-year-old girl with excessive OJ.

A: Discuss:
- Treatment options
- Confidence in reducing her OJ with each option
- Other (nontreatment) options to reduce the likelihood of dental trauma (e.g. wearing a mouthguard when playing sports)

Q: Examine the maxillary anterior spacing in Figure 4.3c. What treatment could reduce her OJ?

A: One option to reduce her OJ is to close interdental spaces between her maxillary anterior teeth (Figure 4.4). This reduces the length of the arc described by the incisal and cuspal edges of the anterior teeth (Figures 4.4a and 4.4b). However, this procedure is not without risk if fixed edgewise brackets are used to accomplish the incisor retraction. Why? Look at a similar case of severe OJ in Figures 4.4e–4.4g. Note that the developing maxillary permanent canine crowns are in the proximity of the maxillary lateral incisor roots (Figure 4.4g). When presented with this scenario, you must be careful

not to cause root resorption by driving the maxillary permanent lateral incisor roots into the canine crowns. When you place fixed appliances on the maxillary lateral incisors in such cases, consider positioning the brackets in such a way that the lateral incisor roots are tipped *mesially* and not driven into the canine crowns. Also, proceed slowly and keep your forces light.

Another option to reduce her OJ would be to place her on a removable Class II functional appliance (e.g. a twin-block, bionator, mandibular anterior repositioning appliance (MARA), or activator appliance). Her OJ would diminish through a combination of maxillary incisor uprighting and mandibular incisor proclination. Of course, we must consider other factors before placing her on a Class II functional appliance, including her lower anterior face height (LAFH), her mandibular incisor inclination, and her periodontal biotype. Ideal patient characteristics for treatment with Class II functional appliances are presented in detail in our next patient, Alana.

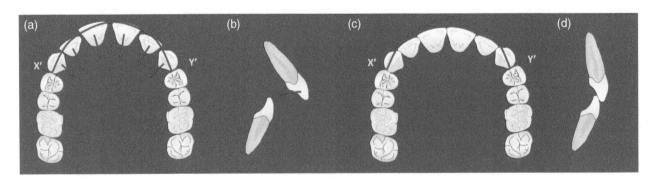

Figure 4.4 (a–d) Diagram illustrating the fact that closing maxillary anterior spaces retracts the maxillary anterior teeth, reduces their protrusion, and reduces OJ. (e–f) intraoral images, (g) panoramic image. The arc described by the anterior teeth (X' to Y' in a) is reduced in length by anterior tooth retraction (compare a and c). In patients where the developing maxillary permanent canine crowns are in proximity to the maxillary lateral incisor roots (shown in g for a patient with a similar maxillary anterior spacing problem depicted in e and f), you must be careful not to drive the maxillary permanent lateral incisor roots into the canine crowns during space closure. Doing so may result in lateral incisor root resorption.

(e)　　　　　　　　　　　　　　　　　　(f)

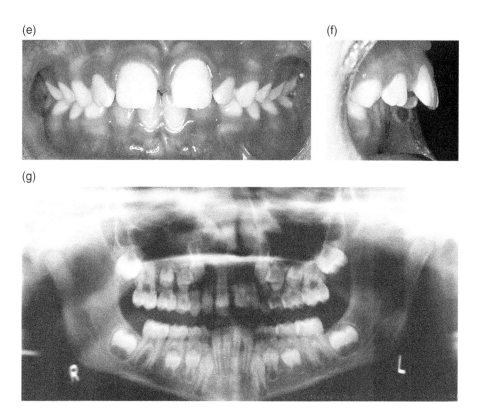

(g)

Figure 4.4　(Continued)

Q: A nine-year-old girl, Alana, presents to you (Figures 4.5a–4.5q) entering the late mixed dentition stage of development with her parents' chief complaint, "Alana's top teeth stick out, and our family dentist is worried that she may break them if she falls." Past medical history (PMH) and past dental history (PDH) are within the range of normal (WRN). Centric relation (CR) = centric occlusion (CO). Temporomandibular joint (TMJ)s, periodontal tissues, and mucogingival tissues are WRN. Can you list her *primary* problems in each dimension (plus other)?

(a)　　　　　　　　　　(b)　　　　　　　　　　(c)

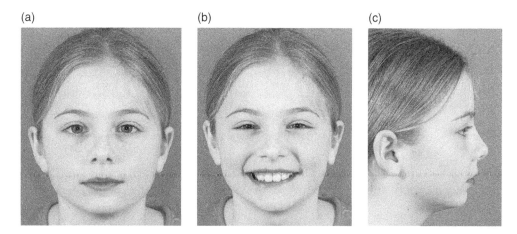

Figure 4.5　Initial records of Alana. (a–c) facial photographs, (d–e) lateral cephalometric radiograph and tracing, (f) panoramic image, (g–k) intraoral images, (l–q) model images.

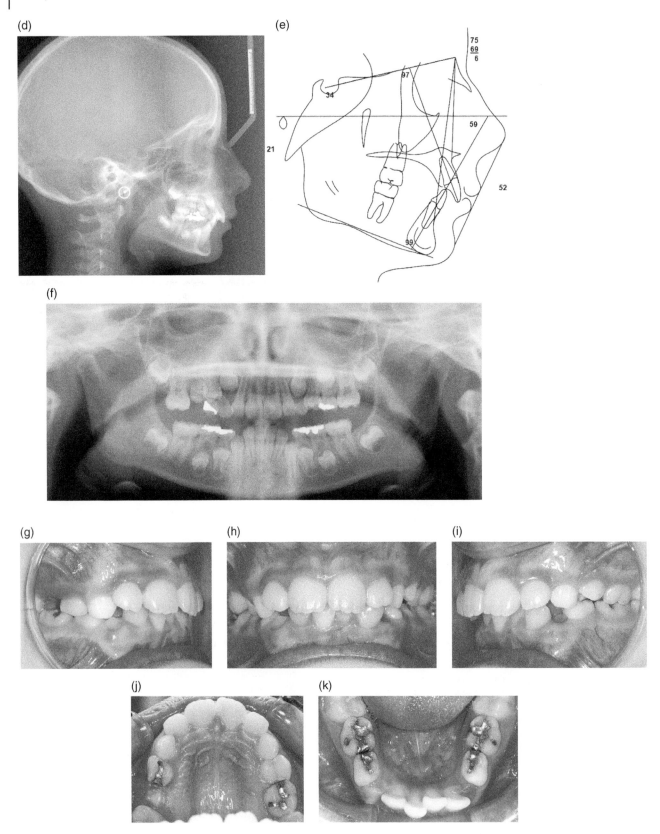

Figure 4.5 (Continued)

(l) (m) (n)

(o) (p) (q)

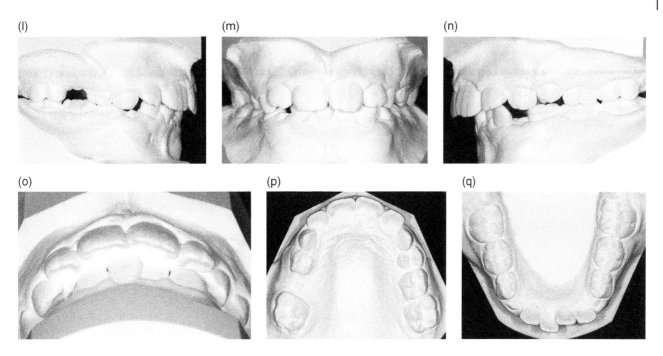

Figure 4.5 (Continued)

A:

Table 4.1 Primary problem list for Alana.

AP	Maxillary skeletal anteroposterior deficiency (A-point lies slightly behind Nasion-perpendicular line)
	Mandibular skeletal anteroposterior deficiency (ANB = 6° with maxillary deficiency)
	Bilateral Class II (3–4 mm) molar relationship secondary to mandibular skeletal anteroposterior deficiency
Vertical	Short skeletal LAFH (LAFH/ TAFH×100% = 52%)
	OB 60%
Transverse	–
Other diagnosis	Proclined mandibular incisors (FMIA = 59°)
	4–5 mm OJ (Figure 4.5o)
	~2 mm of maxillary incisor crowding currently present
	~7 mm of mandibular anterior crowding currently present
	Blocked out mandibular permanent canines

Q: Are Alana's maxillary incisors upright (U1 to Sella–Nasion [SN] = 97°, Figure 4.5e)?

A: No, we feel that her maxillary incisor angulation is WRN. Although it is true that the measured U1 to SN is less than the normal range of 101–104°, Sella appears low which reduces this angle.

An alternative estimate is to compare, on the cephalometric tracing, the line describing the long axis of the maxillary central incisors with the most posterior aspect of the lateral margin of the orbit. As an approximation, if the extended long axis line is significantly posterior to the lateral orbital margin, then the maxillary incisors are proclined. Conversely, if the extended long axis is significantly anterior to the lateral orbital margin, then the maxillary incisors are retroclined. In Alana's case, her maxillary central incisor-extended long axis lies just in front of the traced lateral orbital margin (Figure 4.5e), suggesting a maxillary central incisor angulation WRN.

Q: Alana has a 4–5 mm OJ. What is the cause of this OJ?

A: Alana's OJ resulted from the skeletal Class II discrepancy between her jaws. Her maxilla is mildly deficient anteroposteriorly, but her mandible is severely *deficient*.

Q: How does Alana's mandibular incisor inclination affect her OJ?

A: Alana's OJ is less than what it would be with normal mandibular incisal inclination. Why? Her mandibular incisors are proclined – which reduces her OJ.
Alana's proclined mandibular incisors are *dental compensations* reflecting her underlying Class II skeletal discrepancy. In other words, with her severely deficient mandible, her tongue proclined her mandibular incisors during eruption.

Q: Alana lacks maxillary anterior spacing, so you cannot reduce her OJ with maxillary anterior space closure.

Instead, her excessive OJ has an underlying skeletal etiology. Can you discuss three *general* ways to reduce Alana's OJ by correcting her Class II skeletal relationship?

A: There are three general ways to address *any* skeletal discrepancy – whether in the anteroposterior, vertical, or transverse dimensions. These include orthopedics, masking (camouflage), and surgery. For a skeletally deficient mandible resulting in a Class II relationship, we can consider:

- *Orthopedics* – which seeks to restrict forward maxillary growth while the mandible continues to grow forward (Figure 4.6a) or to accelerate forward mandibular growth (Figure 4.6b). Examples include the use of headgears or Class II functional appliances.

- *Masking or camouflage* – seeks to correct Class II dental relationships by *masking* the underlying skeletal discrepancy without changing jaw relationships. Generally, we consider masking only during comprehensive treatment in adult dentition.

Class II masking involves moving maxillary teeth distally and/or moving mandibular teeth mesially (Figure 4.6c). Examples of masking include the use of various Class II correctors (e.g. Powerscope™,

Forsus™), Class II elastics (Figures 4.6d–4.6e), headgears to retract maxillary teeth, Class II functional appliances to retract maxillary teeth and advance mandibular teeth, temporary anchorage devices (TADs) to help move maxillary teeth distally or mandibular teeth mesially, or various combinations of permanent tooth extractions (e.g. extracting maxillary first premolars to create space in order to retract maxillary canines into a Class I canine relationship).

Note: Class II elastic effects are mainly dentoalveolar – maxillary incisors are erupted and tipped lingually, mandibular molars are moved mesially and erupted, and mandibular incisors are proclined [3]. Most orthodontists use Class II elastics at some time during Class II treatment, but be wary of using heavy Class II elastics in patients with steep mandibular plane angle (MPA)s for extended periods of time. Why? As mandibular molars erupt with Class II elastic wear, the mandible is rotated down and back – worsening the convex profile.

Principle of Class II correction: avoid treatments that rotate the mandible down and back (worsening the convex profile).

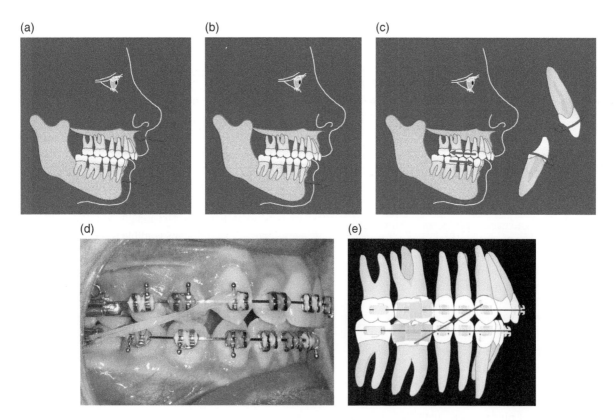

(a) (b) (c)

(d) (e)

Figure 4.6 Options for correcting Class II skeletal relationships may include: (a–b) orthopedics, (c) masking/camouflage such as Class II elastics (d–e), or (f–j) mandibular advancement surgery. (f–j) This adult was treated with mandibular first premolar extractions followed by space closure and mandibular advancement surgery. Note the surgical fixation screws placed in the ramus of the mandible (g).

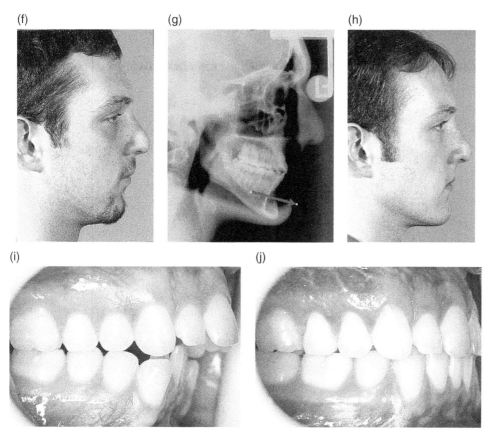

(f) (g) (h)

(i) (j)

Figure 4.6 (Continued)

Note: The effects of Class II-compressed spring correctors (e.g. a Forsus™ appliance) include: distal movement of maxillary molars, mesial movement of mandibular molars, maxillary incisor retrusion, mandibular incisor proclination, and mandibular incisor intrusion [4, 5]. Restriction of maxillary growth has also been reported, but these appliances are generally not used for long enough periods of time for this effect to be significant.

Principle of Class II correction: you must have anterior OJ. Without anterior OJ, either the anterior teeth will be traumatized as Class II correction drives the mandibular incisors into the maxillary incisors, or the patient will be thrown into an anterior crossbite.

- *Surgery* – Other than some patients with airway problems or craniofacial anomalies, Class II surgery (Bilateral Sagittal Split Osteotomy [BSSO] advancement) would generally not be considered in the mixed dentition. However, a mandibular advancement osteotomy would be a possible future option for Alana depending upon her growth, treatment compliance, and profile concerns. Figures 4.6f–4.6j illustrate profile and occlusal changes as a result of a mandibular advancement osteotomy in an adult.

Q: Orthopedics to address Alana's Class II skeletal discrepancy (mandibular deficiency) could include the use of headgears or Class II functional appliances. Let's consider each starting with headgears. Can you state the skeletal and dental effects of *high-pull* headgears in Class II growing children?

A: High-pull headgear effects during growth include (Figure 4.7a): [6, 7]
- Distalization of maxillary molars (correcting the Class II molar relationship *dentally* and creating space mesial to the maxillary molars for distalization/alignment of more anterior teeth)
- Restricting maxillary forward growth (correcting the Class II relationship *skeletally* as the mandible continues to grow forward)
- Reducing descent of the maxillary corpus. High-pull headgear application in monkeys demonstrated maxillary corpus displacement posteriorly and superiorly [8]. This effect, theoretically, permits the mandible to rotate upward and forward, helping correct the Class II relationship.
- Reducing maxillary first molar eruption. This effect, theoretically, permits the mandible to rotate upward and forward, helping correct the Class II relationship.

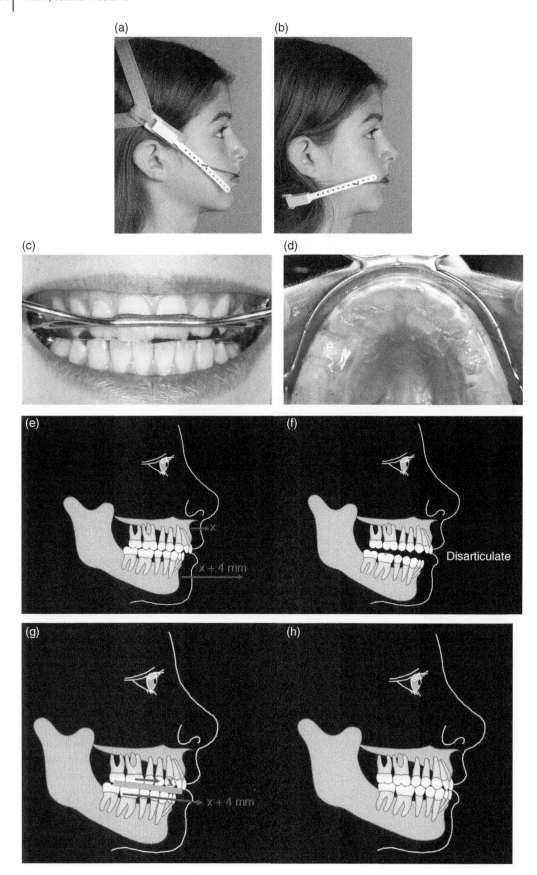

Figure 4.7 (a) High-pull headgear; (b) cervical-pull headgear; (c–d) full coverage occlusal bite plate used in conjunction with a facebow headgear; (e–h) effect of occlusal disarticulation using a full coverage bite plate.

High-pull headgear effects, combined with favorable mandibular growth, facilitate correction of a Class II skeletal discrepancy, correction of Class II dental relationship, straightening of a convex profile, and increased chin projection.

Q: What is *compensatory* molar eruption? How can you reduce it?

A: A benefit of high-pull headgear wear in growing patients is the reduction in maxillary first molar eruption – which permits the mandible to rotate upward and forward helping correct the Class II relationship. However, if the maxillary first molar eruption is impeded, then the mandibular first molar may overerupt (*compensatory molar eruption),* negating the beneficial high-pull headgear vertical effect. To reduce mandibular first molar eruption by 1–2 mm over a one- to two-year period (compared to controls), a lower lingual holding arch (LLHA) may be placed in a mixed dentition child [9].

Q: What are the *long-term* skeletal effects of high-pull headgear wear followed by fixed appliances for the treatment of Class II malocclusions. Are the effects stable?

A: We reported that one-phase treatment for Class II malocclusions with high-pull headgear followed by fixed orthodontic appliances resulted in correction to Class I molar through *restriction of maxillary horizontal growth with continued mandibular horizontal growth.* The anteroposterior molar correction and skeletal effects of this treatment were stable long term [10].

Q: Can you state the skeletal and dental effects of cervical-pull headgears in Class II growing children?

A: Cervical-pull headgear effects in growing children include (Figure 4.7b): [3, 11]

- Distalization of maxillary molars (correcting the Class II molar relationship *dentally* and creating space mesial to the maxillary molars for distalization/alignment of more anterior teeth)
- Restricting maxillary forward growth (correcting the Class II relationship *skeletally* as the mandible continues to grow forward)
- Anterior palatal plane is tipped down
- Increasing maxillary first molar eruption slightly (compared to controls, less than 1 mm of additional maxillary first molar eruption).

  Cervical pull-headgear effects, combined with favorable mandibular growth, will facilitate correction of Class II skeletal discrepancy, correction of Class II dental relationship, straightening of a convex profile, and increased chin projection.

We use high-pull and cervical-pull headgears interchangeably, whichever the patient is most comfortable wearing, with the understanding that *maxillary molar eruption is restricted with a high-pull headgear but increased very slightly with a cervical-pull headgear.* Furthermore, because the anterior palatal plane is tipped down with a cervical-pull headgear, we would generally *not* recommend using a cervical-pull headgear in a patient who exhibits excess maxillary anterior gingival display.

Finally, a *straight-pull headgear* consists of wearing a high-pull and cervical-pull headgear together. Consequently, the skeletal and dental effects of a straight-pull headgear lie somewhere between the effects of a high-pull and a cervical-pull headgear (depending upon the resultant force vector magnitude and direction of each).

Q: A full-coverage occlusal bite plate (Figures 4.7c–4.7d) can be beneficial when worn in conjunction with a headgear. Alternatively, the inner bow of the facebow can be embedded in the occlusal bite plate – which is a Thurow appliance [12]. How can occlusal coverage be helpful in correcting a Class II relationship?

A: Benefits of using an occlusal bite plate for Class II correction include:

- *Bite plate effect* – the thick plastic between the maxillary and mandibular posterior teeth stretches the masseter/medial pterygoid musculature resulting in a reactive occlusal force that tends to reduce posterior tooth eruption. The result is a *relative intrusion* of posterior teeth compared to controls, and it aids mandibular upward and forward growth and Class II correction.
- *Occlusal disarticulation* – during adolescence, the mandible grows forward an average of 4 mm more than the maxilla (Figure 4.7e) [13]. However, because of interocclusal locking, the mandibular molars are held back by the maxillary molars – maintaining the Class II molar relationship. By *disarticulating the dentition* during growth (Figure 4.7f), for example with a flat bite plate (Figure 4.7g), the *mandibular molars can move forward with the mandible* instead of being held back by the maxillary molars – which helps correct the Class II molar relationship to Class I (Figure 4.7h).

Q: *When* each day should your patient wear a headgear? How much force should the headgear apply?

A: In our opinion, start the patient wearing a headgear for only two–three hours each evening with a very light force (the lightest force possible to keep the headgear on). After one week, increase wear to four hours in the evening. The goal is to develop a habit of nightly wear. Then, have the patient begin wearing the headgear *from 7–8 pm each evening until the next morning (when most growth is thought to occur)*. After the first few weeks, gradually increase the force to 250 gm per side.

Q: Next, let's consider Class II functional appliances. Numerous ones exist including the Herbst appliance (Figures 4.8a and 4.8b) and bionator (Figure 4.8c). The application and effects of Class II functional appliance wear in growing individuals are fundamentally the

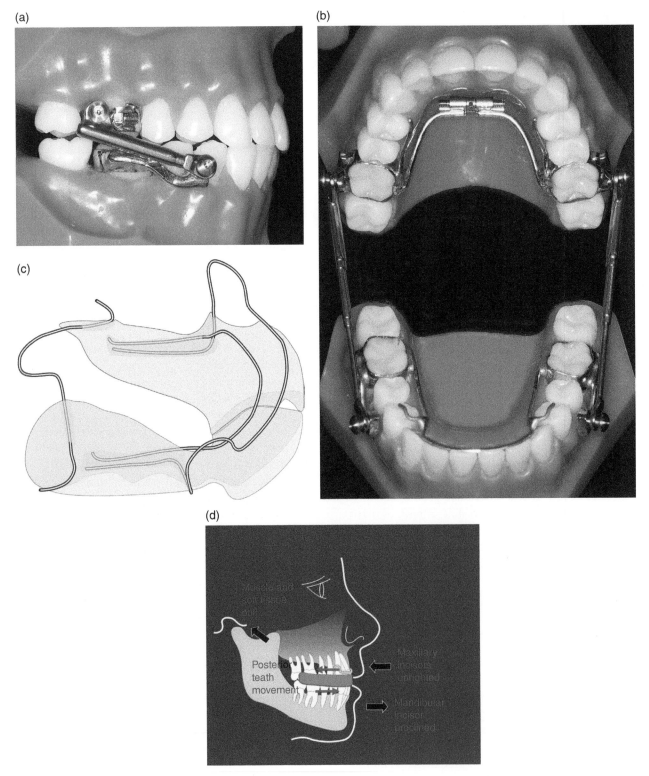

(a)

(b)

(c)

(d)

Figure 4.8 Class II functional appliances. (a–b) Herbst appliance; (c) bionator; (d) dentoalveolar effects.

same – they force the patient to posture the mandible forward (Figure 4.8d), distracting the condylar head out of the glenoid fossa. As the mandible is held forward, the stretched musculature and other soft tissues tend to retract the mandible. Because the maxillary and mandibular teeth are locked together by the functional appliance, the soft tissue retraction force is translated into a tendency for restriction of maxillary forward growth, retraction of maxillary posterior teeth, uprighting of maxillary incisors, mesial movement of mandibular posterior teeth, proclination of mandibular incisors, and acceleration of condylar growth/anterior displacement of the glenoid fossae [14, 15].

Care must be taken to minimize posterior tooth eruption with functional appliance wear. Why? As the mandible is postured forward in deep bite patients, the mandibular incisors slide down along the maxillary incisor lingual surfaces, a posterior open bite may result, posterior teeth may erupt, and the mandible may undergo backward rotation – reducing Class II correction. To minimize posterior tooth eruption with Class II functional appliances, maxillary fixed appliances can first be placed to advance the maxillary incisors and create OJ, permitting the mandible to be postured forward while maintaining posterior occlusal contacts. Or, the posterior teeth in one jaw can be capped with the functional appliance acrylic to prevent their eruption.

The Herbst appliance is cemented in the mouth – requiring minimal patient compliance. Because of this fact, and because the Herbst appliance is worn 24 hours per day, we prefer using the Herbst appliance to other Class II functional appliances. Can you state the skeletal and dental effects of a Herbst appliance in Class II growing children?

A: Below are the effects of a Herbst functional appliance in a growing Class II patient:

- Inhibition of maxillary growth (restraint of maxillary growth occurs to some degree with all Class II functional appliances) [14].
- Distal movement of maxillary teeth.
- Intrusion of maxillary molars in most patients.
- Anterior occlusal plane tipping downward in most patients.
- Acceleration of mandibular growth.
- Mesial movement of mandibular teeth (including mandibular incisor proclination).

Note: Class II functional appliances *do accelerate* mandibular growth in growing individuals. However, long-term Class II functional appliances *do not enhance* mandibular horizontal growth beyond that found in control subjects [16]. Why? Slower-than-normal growth after Class II functional appliance use reduces or eliminates increases in mandibular size compared to control

subjects. Also, the *direction* of condylar growth with functional appliance wear may not correct the mandibular skeletal anteroposterior deficiency or improve chin projection [17–19]. In fact, *hyperdivergent* patients experience a deleterious backward mandibular rotation and increases in face height with Herbst treatment [19].

Q: In which stage of dental development should the Herbst appliance be used?

A: Disagreement exists regarding the answer to this question. On the one hand, it has been suggested that the Herbst appliance is *not* recommended in the deciduous or mixed dentition stages. Why? Because a stable dental intercuspation is difficult to achieve during these stages and because the desired orthopedic effects are maximized only when a stable intercuspation is achieved. Instead, it has been suggested that the Herbst appliance is indicated in the permanent dentition at, or just after, the pubertal peak of growth [14, 20]. On the other hand, another study reported that a significant Class II correction with Herbst therapy *was* maintained throughout the transitional dental period [21]. So, disagreement exists regarding what stage of dental development is best to use a Herbst appliance.

Q: What characteristics would define an *ideal* Herbst appliance candidate (or other Class II functional appliance candidate)?

A: Ideal candidate characteristics include:

- Class II *growing* child.
- *Short* lower anterior face height (hypodivergent, vertical skeletal deficiency with mandibular condyles growing more vertically). Why? As the Herbst appliance postures the mandible forward, condylar growth will be directed into a more normal posterior-superior direction). In a hyperdivergent patient, condylar growth may be directed into an excessively posterior-superior direction.
- *Deep bite* (not open bite).
- *Proclined* maxillary incisors (because they will tend to be uprighted).
- *Upright* mandibular incisors (because they will be proclined).
- *Thick mandibular anterior labial periodontal biotype* (because the mandibular incisors will be proclined, stressing the anterior periodontal tissue).

Q: The ideal candidate for Herbst appliance treatment presents with a short lower anterior face height (hypodivergent). But what are the effects of treating a *hyperdivergent* Class II growing child with a Herbst appliance?

A: *Hyperdivergent Herbst patients experience a deleterious backward true mandibular rotation.* The primary maxillomandibular correction effect of the Herbst appliance is a *headgear effect* – maxillary growth restriction. Mandibular treatment changes depend upon divergence. Hypodivergent Herbst patients, untreated hypodivergent controls, and hyperdivergent controls, all undergo forward true mandibular rotation.

However, hypodivergent Herbst patient chins do not advance any more than expected for hypodivergent controls. While the mandibular growth of hypodivergent Herbst patients overcome the negative rotational effects of the Herbst appliance, *hyperdivergent Herbst patients undergo a deleterious backward mandibular rotation and increases in face height* [19]. Again, the ideal Class II functional appliance patient has a short lower anterior face height – they are hypodivergent and not hyperdivergent.

Q: Are headgears and functional appliances equally effective in correcting Class II malocclusions in children *before comprehensive treatment*? Are headgears and functional appliances, followed by fixed orthodontic appliances, equally effective?

A: *Headgears and functional appliances are equally effective in correcting Class II malocclusions before comprehensive orthodontic treatment* [22–33]. Short-term skeletal effects include a small restriction in forward maxillary growth with headgears (SNA decreases 0.5–3°) and a small forward positioning of B-Point with functional appliances (1–2°), resulting in an A-point – Nasion – B-point angle (ANB) improvement in Class II patients of about 1° with headgears or functional appliances. A significant portion of the Class II correction is a distal maxillary molar movement with headgears and mesial mandibular molar movement (along with mandibular incisor proclination) with functional appliances. Higher levels of evidence are needed to answer the question of whether headgear and functional appliance effects *following* comprehensive treatment are equal.

Q: How does profile improvement in growing Class II patients treated with headgears versus Herbst appliances compare? Are profiles improved with activator or Twin-block functional appliances?

A: *We found that headgear and Herbst treatments result in significantly improved profiles that are judged to be similarly attractive* [34]. Treatment with activators or Twin-block appliances (followed by fixed orthodontic appliances) led to slight improvements in patients' convex profiles – a difference that was relatively small and clinically questionable [35].

Q: How would the initial presence of skeletal Class II dental compensations (proclined mandibular incisors) influence your decision to use, or not use, a Class II functional appliance?

A: Since Class II functional appliances *procline mandibular incisors*, using a Class II functional appliance may not be desirable if the incisors are already proclined (dental compensations frequently observed in skeletal Class II patients). The initial presence of proclined mandibular incisors is one reason we often choose to treat a Class II patient with headgear (no mandibular incisor effects) versus a Class II functional appliance (additional mandibular incisor proclination).

Q: When treating a Class II patient, do you recommend correcting only to Class I, or do you recommend *overcorrecting* slightly to Class III?

A: We recommend *overcorrecting*. If you are using headgears/functional appliances to treat a Class II skeletal discrepancy, don't just treat to Class I molars and stop. Instead, *overcorrect* slightly to Class III (1–2 mm). Then, *slowly* taper off the headgear or functional appliance wear over a period of months while you *monitor* stability.

Q: In Class II division 2 children (upright maxillary central incisors, deep bite, minimal or no OJ), should you first procline maxillary incisors/create OJ before treating the patient with a headgear or Herbst appliance?

A: In our clinical opinion, yes – *first create OJ before treating a child using headgear*. Why? We recommend first creating OJ under the assumption that upright maxillary incisors could restrict forward mandibular growth. Proclining upright maxillary incisors first may permit forward mandibular growth. Of course, with a Herbst appliance, you must either create OJ before activating the appliance or place the child in an anterior crossbite with the appliance.

Q: What you are talking about in the previous question is *unlocking the bite*. Does unlocking the bite in Class II division 2 children result in mandibular anterior positioning and improvement in the Class II relationship? Does unlocking the bite enhance future mandibular forward growth?

A: Proclining maxillary incisors (unlocking the bite) plus correcting the deep bite with a removable plate does *not* result in mandibular anterior positioning [36]. However, the effect of unlocking the bite on future mandibular growth is unknown. We did find a recent case report of SNB increase after deep bite correction [37], but future research is needed to fully answer this question. Until then, *we recommend unlocking the bite in Class II division*

2 children prior to orthopedic treatment for its potential benefit on future mandibular forward growth.

Q: Based upon the above, do you recommend using headgears or Class II functional appliances to treat skeletally Class II growing children?

A: Neither appliance is ideal. We love the effects of headgears and have had many amazing outcomes using them. However, patient compliance can be a real problem. If you attempt headgear treatment, then try using it for a fixed test period (three or four months). If the patient is not cooperating fully, then consider other options.

We love cemented Herbst appliances because, in large measure, you remove patient compliance. However, the ideal Herbst patient (Class II growing child, short lower anterior face height/hypodivergent, deep-bite, proclined maxillary incisors, upright mandibular incisors, thick mandibular anterior labial periodontal biotype) is somewhat uncommon which limits their ideal application. Furthermore, most skeletal Class II patients present with proclined mandibular incisors (dental compensations), and all Class II functional appliances procline mandibular incisors even further. Finally, using a Herbst appliance in a hyperdivergent patient results in the chin position *worsening* (rotating down and back) which is just the opposite effect from what we desire.

In summary, neither headgears nor Class II functional appliances are a panacea for Class II skeletal correction. We discuss both options with parent and child. If a child will wear a headgear, then we will usually first attempt treatment with a headgear (it is inexpensive). If a child is an ideal Herbst patient, or nearly ideal, then we will use a Herbst appliance if the child would prefer that option.

Q: Let's return to our patient, Alana. Can you suggest principles to follow in deciding *whether* to treat her Class II skeletal discrepancy orthopedically? If you decide to treat her orthopedically, then *when* would you initiate Class II orthopedic treatment?

A: First, let's decide *whether* to attempt orthopedic correction. This decision is based upon two factors: the *magnitude* of her skeletal discrepancy and the *time* remaining to correct it orthopedically. Looking at Alana's lateral cephalometric tracing (Figure 4.5e), we see that her anteroposterior skeletal discrepancy is severe (ANB angle of 6° with a retrusive mandible and maxilla), but her dental Class II molar relationship is moderate (only 3–4 mm Class II). Further, she is only nine years old, so you should have years of adolescent growth left to attempt Class II correction. Therefore, if Alana is cooperative, we have a good chance to fully correct her to a Class I molar relationship (or overcorrect to a slight Class III) plus a good chance to improve

her skeletal discrepancy and chin projection. Even if Alana does not fully correct her skeletal discrepancy, at least she may be able to improve it to the point where we can acceptably mask it (camouflage). We conclude that we should attempt Class II orthopedic treatment for Alana. On the other hand, if Alana had been older (had reached puberty years earlier), then we would not attempt orthopedics to correct her severe Class II skeletal discrepancy because we would not anticipate much remaining growth.

Second, let's decide *when* to begin Class II orthopedic treatment. Alana is just entering her late mixed dentition stage of development, so now is a good time to start. Starting sooner, in the early mixed dentition, is generally ill-advised. Why? The strongest scientific evidence finds no advantage to beginning Class II treatment in the *early* mixed dentition (except for a possible decrease in incisal trauma as a result of excess OJ) [22–24, 29, 38–40]. However, this is a general guideline and not a fixed rule. The dental stage is poorly correlated with skeletal growth – so use your judgment in deciding when to initiate orthopedic treatment. The average onset of statural growth spurt is a little more than nine years of age for girls and a little less than twelve years for boys; peak statural growth spurt is about one and a half to two years later; facial skeletal growth peaks later; and there is considerable variation in these times [41]. If Alana had been in the early mixed dentition, but her parents told you she had *good statural growth (regular incremental change in stature)*, then we would recommend initiating Class II orthopedic treatment immediately.

To summarize, considering her severe skeletal Class II discrepancy, moderate dental Class II discrepancy, age, and stage of dental development, Alana is a good candidate for initiating orthopedic treatment now. Even if Alana had been in the early mixed dentition stage of development, *if her parents told you she had good statural growth (regular incremental change in stature), then we would recommend initiating Class II orthopedic treatment.*

By way of review, the term "good statural growth" or "regular incremental change in stature" refers to a relatively constant growth velocity in stature over time, as opposed to mildly declining growth velocity, which is often seen in advance of the pubertal period of growth acceleration. Remember, some individuals, particularly females, may not experience a true acceleration during puberty, but rather show good, relatively constant growth velocity during their years of growth in stature.

Q: Some clinicians would dispute the science and logic of our statements in the previous question. In fact, a recent prospective cohort study [1] reported that 65 Class II *five-year-old children* treated for three years with eruption guidance therapy corrected 86% of their initial Class II molar or canine relationships. What is myofunctional/eruption guidance therapy, and should we be using this approach to treat Class II malocclusions in the early mixed dentition?

A: Myofunctional/eruption guidance therapy consists of a series of exercises and the use of preformed positioner-like appliances. Dr. Kevin O'Brien conducted a thorough review of the Keski-Nisula et al. report [42], expressed concerns regarding it, suggested that potential for this form of treatment may exist, but concluded that further research is necessary before such treatment is generally adopted [43].

Q: The strongest scientific evidence finds no advantage to beginning Class II treatment in the early mixed dentition. As we stated, we generally follow this guideline but will begin Class II orthopedics if the early mixed dentition patient shows good statural growth (regular incremental change in stature).

But what about the incidence of incisal trauma, specifically? Should we institute Class II treatment in the early mixed dentition if the child is experiencing incisor trauma?

A: The evidence suggests that early orthodontic treatment for children seven–eleven years old with prominent upper front teeth is more effective in reducing incisal trauma than later orthodontic treatment. Early treatment reduces the risk of trauma by 33% and 41% when patients are treated with functional appliances and headgears, respectively. However, these data should be interpreted with caution because of the high degree of uncertainty. Further, the authors concluded that there are no other advantages in providing two-phase treatment compared with one-phase in early adolescence [44, 45], and they have subsequently reported that the only effect of early Class II treatment was a 12% reduction in the incidence of incisal trauma. At the end of all treatment, 19% of the early treatment group had experienced trauma. Whereas, 31% of those that did not have early treatment had trauma [2]. Finally, *the dental injuries tend to be minor, and the cost of incisor trauma treatment small, compared with the expected additional cost of a two-phase orthodontic intervention* [46].

So, should we institute Class II treatment in the early mixed dentition patient with a history of incisal trauma and prominent maxillary incisors? We feel that this decision must be made on a case-by-case basis. It must be made after considering the following factors:
- OJ magnitude
- Lip competence or lip incompetence

- History of incisal trauma (frequency/severity)
- History of risk-taking behavior
- Sports participation
- ADHD
- Cognitive psychomotor issues

Based upon these factors, we will consider early Class II treatment or other, simpler, treatments (e.g. sports mouthguard wear).

Q: What is one important observation you need to make regarding Alana's 4–5 mm OJ (Figure 4.5o)?

A: Check for lip competence (Figure 4.1a). Thankfully, Alana exhibits lip competence – her incisors are covered by soft tissue which should act as a cushion and reduce any likelihood of dental trauma.

Q: Are there any questions you wish to ask Alana's parents about her excess OJ? If they ask about incisal trauma, what discussions should you have with them regarding her excess OJ?

A: You need to inquire about the following (all of which her parents deny): history of dental trauma, risk-taking behavior, participation in sports, ADHD, cognitive psychomotor issues, and teasing. Further, they are not overly concerned with her appearance at this age. Discussions with her parents should include:
- Treatment options – tell them that orthopedic treatment to correct Alana's Class II relationship may reduce the possibility of incisal trauma, but that dental injuries resulting from excess OJ tend to be minor. Tell them that Alana could still have incisal trauma even with treatment, or that she may not have incisal trauma without treatment. Finally, explain that Alana is entering the late mixed dentition stage of development, and now is a good time to begin orthopedic treatment.
- Your confidence in reducing OJ with each orthopedic option – tell them that, with Alana's cooperation, treatment with either headgear or a Class II functional appliance will reduce her OJ.
- Other (nontreatment) options to reduce the likelihood of dental trauma (e.g. Alana wearing a sports mouthguard, as needed).

Q: Should you start early treatment now or recall Alana? If you start now, then what treatment(s) would you recommend?

A: We decided to place Alana on an LLHA and an high pull headgear (HPHG). The LLHA would utilize mandibular "E-space" (not leeway space since the mandibular primary canines were exfoliated) to help align incisors spontaneously. The LLHA would also reduce/prevent mandibular permanent first molar mesial drift and force Class II molar correction to be made with the HPHG.

Finally, an LLHA would reduce mandibular first permanent molar eruption (and compensatory mandibular first permanent molar eruption) – thereby helping the mandible to rotate forward-aiding Class II correction.

Q: We attempted orthopedic treatment using an HPHG. It makes sense that we did not treat Alana with jaw surgery at eight years of age, but why not treat her with masking instead?

A: *Masking (camouflage)* is an attempt to improve a malocclusion with *dental movements only* – not by addressing an underlying skeletal discrepancy. With masking, you are trying to get the teeth together without orthopedics or surgery. Masking (e.g. use of Class II elastics or extraction of maxillary first premolars to permit canine relationship improvement, etc.) would be considered a *fallback* option or contingency plan if Alana does not respond to orthopedic treatment.

Q: Alana responded well to early treatment. After all mandibular premolars and canines had erupted (Figure 4.9a), a discussion was held with her parents regarding premolar extraction vs. non-extraction comprehensive treatment. They were emphatic and wanted Alana treated without extractions. Comprehensive treatment began, fixed appliances were placed, her arches were leveled and aligned, and all spaces closed. Alana's deband photographs are shown in Figures 4.9b–4.9i. Radiographs were not taken at that time. At a subsequent recall visit, a cephalometric radiograph was taken (Figures 4.9j–4.9l). What changes due to growth and treatment do you observe?

A: Changes include the following:
- Facial and smile esthetic improvement – Alana is now a beautiful young woman with a beautiful smile.
- Straighter profile with good chin projection.
- Maxilla grew downward but not forward (Figure 4.9l).
- Mandible grew downward *and forward*.
- *Differential jaw growth* as a result of the HPHG restraining maxillary forward growth but permitting mandibular forward growth (ANB angle decreased from 6° to 3°).
- Increase in skeletal LAFH (LAFH/total anterior face height [TAFH] × 100% increased from 52 to 55%).
- Maxillary and mandibular molars erupted and moved mesially, lower incisors proclined.
- Class I occlusion has been achieved.
- Mandibular left permanent canine and second premolar are rotated (Figure 4.9i).
- *OJ has been reduced from 4–5 mm to minimal*, and Alana has been free of maxillary incisor trauma.

(a)

(b) (c) (d)

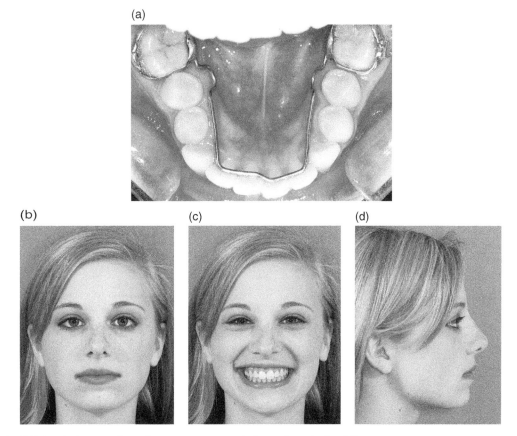

Figure 4.9 (a–l) Deband photographs and post-treatment cephalometric analysis of Alana.

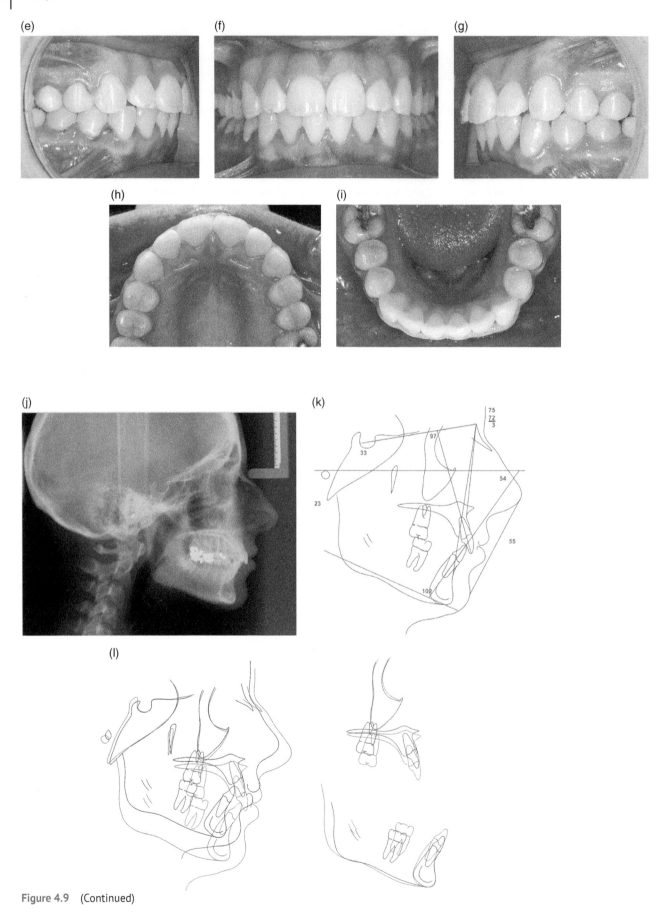

Figure 4.9 (Continued)

Q: Do you have any "*take-home pearls*" regarding Alana's treatment?

A: "Take-home pearls" include the following:

- Alana presented when she was nine years old and entering the late mixed dentition stage of development. Her parents were concerned that her top teeth stuck out (4–5 mm OJ), and that she might break them if she fell. Her first permanent molars were Class II bilaterally by 3–4 mm secondary-to-mandibular skeletal anteroposterior deficiency (ANB = 6° with maxillary anteroposterior deficiency). She was successfully treated non-extraction to Class I molars with minimal OJ via HPHG orthopedics in conjunction with an LLHA and fixed orthodontic appliances.

- Children with an OJ exceeding 3 mm are at twice the risk for dental injuries as children with an OJ less than 3 mm. However, the dental injuries tend to be minor.

- Early treatment to reduce OJ can reduce the possibility of incisal trauma, but research supporting this decision should be interpreted with caution, and there are no other advantages to early Class II treatment.

- In addition to the presence of an interlabial gap (ILG) (exposed maxillary incisor crowns), other factors that weigh into your decision to treat excessive OJ early include a history of past dental trauma, history of risk-taking, participation in sports, ADHD, cognitive psychomotor issues, and teasing.

- Before deciding to treat or not treat, you and the parents should discuss options, your confidence in each option to reduce the child's OJ, and other (nontreatment) options to reduce the likelihood of dental trauma.

- Parents should be informed that their child may still have incisal trauma even with treatment, or that their child may not have incisal trauma without treatment.

- Excessive OJ in children can be reduced by closing spaces between maxillary anterior teeth (retracting maxillary incisors), proclining mandibular incisors, moving all maxillary teeth distally, moving all mandibular teeth mesially, or via Class II orthopedic treatment resulting in differential jaw growth (mandible growing forward more than the maxilla).

- In our opinion, neither headgears nor Class II functional appliances are a panacea for early Class II skeletal correction. Headgears can be effective, but patient cooperation can be problematic. Class II functional appliances can be effective, especially Herbst appliances, but lower incisors are proclined and functional appliance use in hyperdivergent patients can be problematic.

- Class II orthopedic treatment (headgear or functional appliance treatment) should generally begin no earlier than the late mixed dentition stage of development *unless the patient demonstrates good statural growth in the early mixed dentition* (displaying regular incremental change in stature).

Q: Finally, Alana's parents ask you, "How do Class II molar relationships develop?" What is your answer?

A: In general terms, Class II molar relationships can be of *dental* origin (e.g. early loss of maxillary primary second molars with mesial drift of maxillary first permanent molars) or of *skeletal* origin (inadequate mandibular forward growth and/or excessive maxillary forward growth).

Q: Now, let's consider the other end of the anteroposterior spectrum. When does *inadequate* anterior OJ/anterior crossbite/underbite occur?

A: Inadequate anterior OJ/anterior crossbite/underbite occurs when:

- A *skeletal* Class III discrepancy (Class III apical base discrepancy, Figure 4.10a) exists between the jaws – either mandibular anteroposterior excess and/or maxillary anteroposterior deficiency. Such a skeletal discrepancy places the molars and canines in a Class III relationship.

- *Dentally*, maxillary incisors are too upright and/or mandibular incisors are too proclined (Figure 4.10b). Such a situation can exist with severe maxillary anterior crowding, severe mandibular anterior spacing, severe mandibular anterior Bolton excess, or severe maxillary anterior Bolton deficiency.

- A combination of both.

Q: What is a pseudo Class III malocclusion?

A: A pseudo Class III malocclusion (Figures 4.11a and 4.11b) exists when a child has a Class I molar relationship in CR but, because of premature occlusal contacts, shifts forward into a Class III molar relationship in CO. The child's posterior teeth occlude in CO but usually do not occlude in CR because the incisors are in edge-to-edge contact.

Q: List the etiologic factors in pseudo Class III malocclusions.

A: Nakasima [47] reported the following etiologic factors:

- Dental factors – ectopic eruption of maxillary central incisors and premature deciduous molar loss.

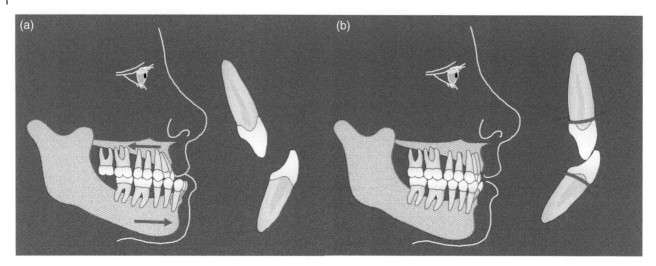

Figure 4.10 (a) Inadeqate OJ/anterior crossbite usually results: *skeletally*, from mandibular anteroposterior excess and/or maxillary anteroposterior deficiency; and (b) *dentally* from maxillary incisor retroclination/mandibular incisor proclination.

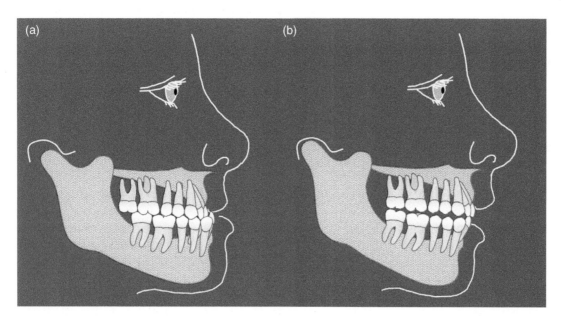

Figure 4.11 Pseudo Class III malocclusion (a) with anterior crossbite in CO due to a functional mandibular forward shift (note the forward displaced position of the mandibular condylar head in the glenoid fossa). (b) When the patient is positioned back into CR, the posterior teeth are out of occlusion because the incisors usually occlude edge-to-edge, but the molar relationship is Class I.

- Functional factors – anomalies in tongue position, neuromuscular features, and airway problems.
- Skeletal factors – minor transverse maxillary discrepancies.

Q: A six-year-old boy in the primary dentition presents to you with a Class III (1 mm) malocclusion and anterior crossbite in CO (Figure 4.12a). He can shift his jaw back 1 mm to CR at which time his molars and canines are Class I and his incisors are edge-to-edge (Figure 4.12b). What do you call his malocclusion?

A: The patient has a pseudo Class III malocclusion. He is really Class I but presents as Class III when his mandible shifts forward into CO. According to one study, pseudo Class III patients usually have a mesial step (in CO) that is less than 3 mm, retroclined maxillary incisors, and mandibular incisors that are proclined and spaced [48].

(a)　　　　　　　　　　　　　　　　(b)

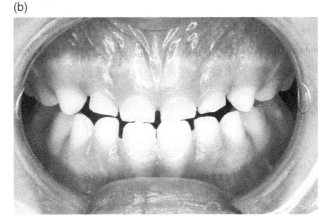

Figure 4.12　Malocclusion due to a 1 mm CR-CO shift in the primary dentition: (a) in CO the patient is Class III (1 mm); (b) in CR the patient has a Class I molar and canine relationship with incisors edge-to-edge.

Q: Why is it important to differentiate between pseudo Class III malocclusions and true *skeletal* Class III malocclusions?

A: Once the anterior crossbite (CR-CO shift) has been corrected in pseudo Class III children, they become Class I and can complete orthodontic treatment as Class I patients. Future anteroposterior growth is usually not a concern.

However, even after an anterior crossbite has been corrected in *skeletal* Class III children, they will probably remain Class III and their *future Class III growth pattern (excessive mandibular growth and/or deficient maxillary growth) is a major concern that impacts future treatment success*. Our point is that you must carefully differentiate whether you are dealing with a pseudo Class III or skeletal Class III malocclusion.

Q: Should you correct anterior crossbites like that of the six-year-old child (Figure 4.12a) in the *primary* dentition? Or, should you wait until the permanent incisors erupt?

A: Some authors feel that anterior crossbites resulting from CR-CO shifts should be treated very early [49], but *we generally recommend waiting at least until the permanent incisors erupt*. We suggest that you make this decision on a case-by-case basis. Let's examine the factors which will influence your decision:

- *Presence of an underlying skeletal discrepancy* – determining whether the patient is truly Class I in CR (skeletally normal) or is skeletally Class III. If you correct an anterior crossbite in a child with normal skeletal growth by advancing the maxillary primary incisors with a removable appliance or fixed appliances, then the crossbite should remain corrected. However, if you correct an anterior crossbite in a child with a Class III *skeletal* discrepancy (maxillary anteroposterior deficiency and/or mandibular anteroposterior excess), then you need to begin orthopedic treatment to address the skeletal discrepancy (e.g. high-pull chin cup, reverse pull headgear (RPHG), TAD-supported Class III elastics) – or, you will end up chasing a recurring anterior crossbite as the child continues the same Class III growth pattern.

- *Permanent incisor eruption status* – if the maxillary permanent incisors are close to erupting, then anterior crossbite correction should probably be postponed. As the primary central incisors exfoliate, the CR-CO shift may disappear, and the permanent incisors may erupt normally and resolve the crossbite. Also, advancing the primary incisor crowns out of crossbite could result in their roots being tipped distally into the crowns of the erupting permanent incisors causing primary incisor root resorption and premature primary incisor exfoliation. Note: Algorithms to predict permanent incisor crossbites based upon primary incisor crossbites have been formulated [50] but are unproven.

- *Damage to permanent incisors or to soft tissue* – ongoing trauma to permanent anterior teeth is a compelling reason to correct anterior crossbites due to functional shifts. This could be either hard tissue (enamel) trauma or soft tissue (gingival) trauma.

- *Compliance* or lack of compliance – at what age will a child take an interest in correcting an anterior crossbite? The answer depends upon their maturity and desire.

- *Psychosocial issues* – is the patient being teased because of the crossbite?

- *Magnitude of CR-CO shift* – a child shifting the mandible forward into an anterior crossbite is analogous to a child wearing a Class II functional appliance. The result should be analogous – accelerated mandibular growth, maxillary forward growth restriction, uprighting of maxillary incisors, and proclination of mandibular incisors. The greater the magnitude of the CR-CO shift, the more pronounced these changes should be. This notion, originally put forward by Charles Tweed [51], is intuitively plausible, but is unproven.

Based upon the above factors, and after benefit/risk discussions with parents, a mutual decision can be made to correct the primary incisor anterior crossbite or to recall the child until permanent incisors erupt. *We generally recommend waiting to correct the anterior crossbite until the permanent incisors erupt.* However, we will correct an anterior crossbite in the primary dentition if we wish to proceed with Class III orthopedics.

Q: What if a child presents with a Class I occlusion, an anterior crossbite, but *no CR-CO shift*? Must the crossbite be corrected early?

A: Not necessarily. In the absence of a CR-CO shift, tissue damage, or esthetic concerns, you may decide to monitor the anterior crossbite until later comprehensive orthodontic treatment. Figures 4.13a–4.13f illustrate an example of such an occlusion – where a decision was made to monitor the crossbite until comprehensive treatment. And Figure 4.13g–4.13h illustrates a sixteen-year-old girl who waited until comprehensive treatment to correct her anterior crossbite without any harmful effects.

On the other hand, Figure 4.13i–4.13o illustrates an eight-year-old boy who complained of repeated trauma to his maxillary left central incisor as he bit into anterior crossbite. In this patient, we recommended early crossbite correction. Figure 4.13p shows another child with developing gingival recession labial to her mandibular central incisors presumably due to trauma from the anterior crossbite. We noted fremitus of the

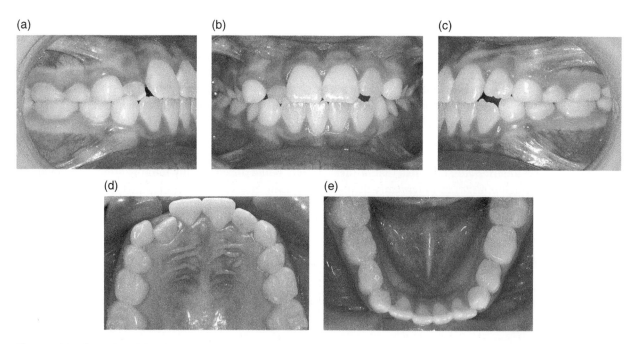

Figure 4.13 Examples of decisions to either correct anterior crossbites or not to correct anterior crossbites: (a–f), an eight-year-old girl in the early mixed dentition who presented with a Class I occlusion, CR = CO, right lateral incisor crossbite, and no hard/soft tissue trauma. Following discussions with the patient and parent, we decided to monitor the crossbite; (g–h), a sixteen-year-old girl with an anterior crossbite which was left uncorrected until all permanent teeth erupted – no damage resulted from the crossbite and she will now begin comprehensive orthodontic treatment; (i–o) an eight-year-old boy who complained of repeated trauma to his maxillary left central incisor when he closed into anterior crossbite. We recommended immediate early treatment to correct his anterior crossbite and prevent further trauma; (p), a child with fremitus of the mandibular central incisors during closure into anterior crossbite. The child was also developing mandibular central incisor gingival recession, presumably due to the crossbite. We elected to begin early treatment to correct the crossbite.

(f)

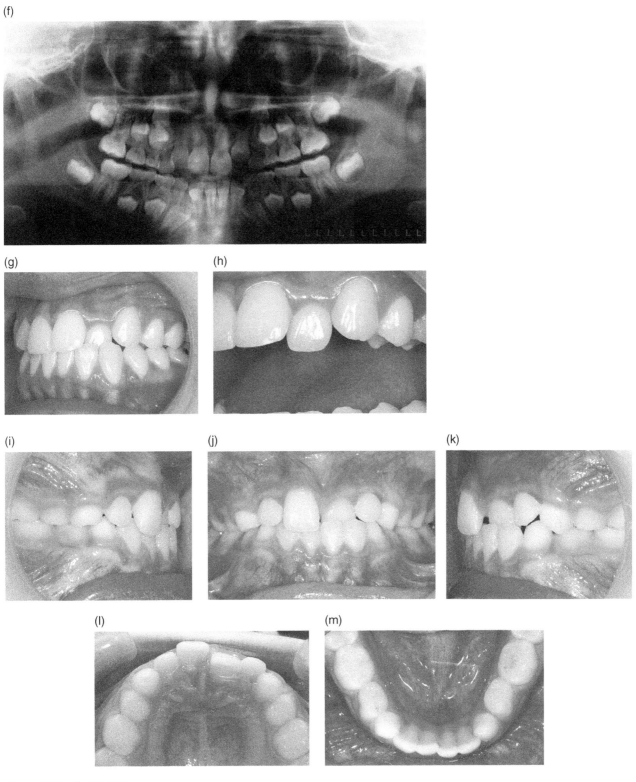

(g)

(h)

(i)

(j)

(k)

(l)

(m)

Figure 4.13   (Continued)

(o)

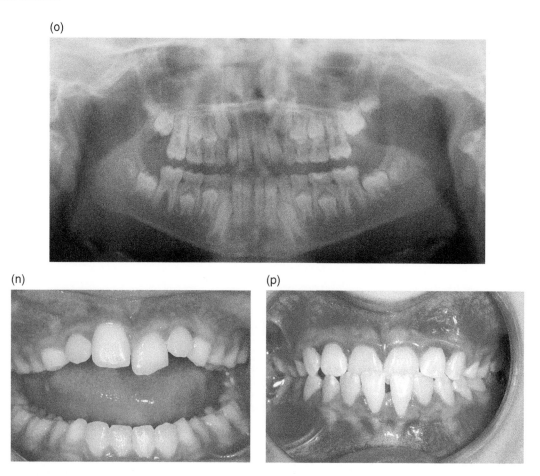

(n)

(p)

Figure 4.13 (Continued)

mandibular central incisors during closure and recommended early correction of this crossbite.

Q: Tomas is a seven-year-old boy (Figure 4.14) who presents to you for a consultation with his parents' chief complaint, "We were referred to by our dentist." PMH is WRN, periodontal and TMJ examinations are WRN, CR = CO, and he is in the early mixed dentition stage of development. What other problems do you note?

A: Although he has a slightly convex profile (Figure 4.14c), Tomas is dentally Class I and has an anterior crossbite of his primary incisors. His mandibular permanent central incisors are erupting into the oral cavity.

Q: Should you correct Tomas' anterior crossbite now, or should you recall Tomas in one year?

A: We would *not* recommend correcting his crossbite now. Why? A CR-CO shift is absent, and no tissue damage has occurred.

Notice the proximity of the maxillary primary incisor root apices to the crowns of the erupting maxillary permanent incisors (Figure 4.14d). Proclining his maxillary primary incisor crowns out of crossbite could drive their roots reciprocally into the permanent incisor crowns – initiating primary root resorption.

We recommend monitoring Tomas for one year to see if his permanent incisors erupt normally or into an anterior crossbite. If the permanent incisors erupt into crossbite, then a decision can be made to correct the crossbite.

Q: Ramus is a seven-year-old boy who presents to you in the early mixed dentition (primary incisors present) for treatment of an anterior crossbite (Figure 4.15). PMH is WRN, and he has a slight CR-CO shift (CO in Figure 4.15d; CR in Figure 4.15e). What problems do you note?

A: Ramus has a mildly convex profile and Class I malocclusion. He has maxillary and mandibular anterior spacing with an anterior crossbite of his primary teeth.

Q: Do you need additional records to make a decision whether to treat his anterior crossbite now or recall?

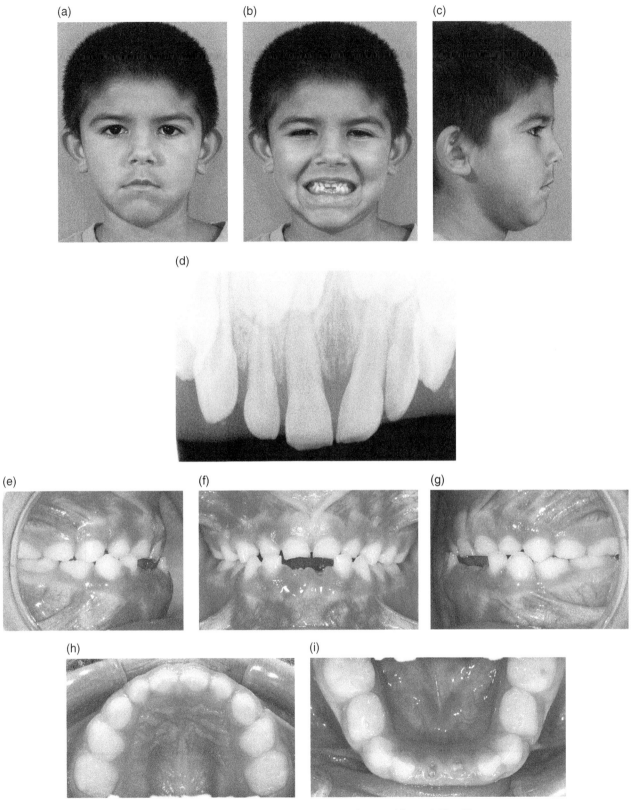

Figure 4.14 (a–i) Initial records of Tomas, a seven-year-old boy with anterior crossbite and CR = CO.

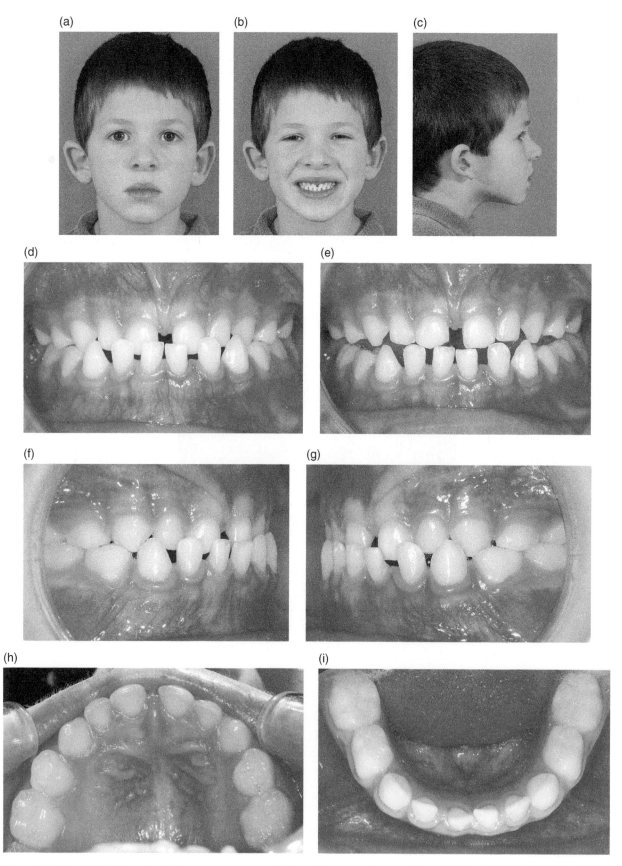

Figure 4.15 (a–i) Initial records of Ramus, a seven-year-old boy with an anterior crossbite and slight CR-CO shift: (d) CO; (e) CR.

A: Yes. A panoramic image would have been helpful to check his permanent tooth eruption status. A panoramic image was not made.

Q: Can you list factors that will help you decide whether to treat Ramus' anterior crossbite now or recall him?

A: The factors include:

- *Presence of an underlying skeletal discrepancy* (i.e. will he grow Class III and develop recurring anterior crossbites?) – Ramus does not appear to have a Class III skeletal discrepancy. He is dentally Class I and has a mildly convex profile.
- *Permanent incisor eruption status* – without a radiograph, we do not know the eruption status of his permanent incisors.
- *Damage to hard or soft tissue* – the maxillary right primary central incisor appears worn/damaged (Figure 4.15e), but his permanent incisors have not

erupted. There does not appear to be damage to his soft tissue as a result of the crossbite.

- *Compliance* or lack of compliance – Ramus' parents state that he is compliant.
- *Psychosocial issues* – none noted.
- *CR-CO shift magnitude* – his CR-CO shift is slight.

Q: Based upon the above, how do you wish to proceed? Will you treat his anterior crossbite now, or recall Ramus?

A: We decided *not* to treat him at this time. We decided to wait until his permanent central incisors erupted.

Q: Ramus returned to our clinic when his permanent central incisors were erupting (Figures 4.16a–4.16e). At that time, a panoramic image was made (Figure 4.16f). What do you observe?

A: His maxillary permanent central incisors are erupting into crossbite, he has a large midline diastema with a

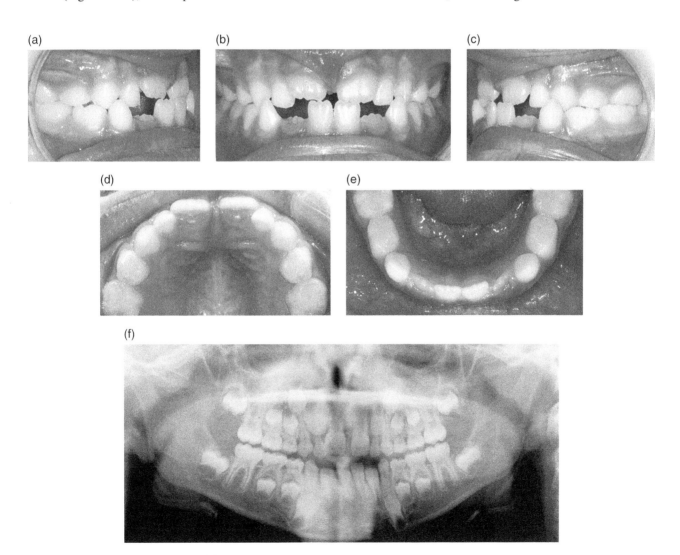

(a) (b) (c)

(d) (e)

(f)

Figure 4.16 (a–f) Progress records of Ramus.

low/thick maxillary labial frenum, and he is still Class I. His slight CR-CO shift disappeared.

Q: Should you begin treatment of his anterior crossbite now?

A: Since he lacks a CR-CO shift and tissue damage, you could monitor his anterior crossbite until comprehensive treatment begins. However, his parents stated that Ramus was being teased about his crossbite. They request that you begin treatment now.

Q: Can you suggest a simple and inexpensive way to treat his anterior crossbite?

A: Yes. Ramus was asked to bite firmly, but gently, on a wooden tongue blade covered with gauze as often as possible during the day (Figure 4.17).

Q: Progress records were made several months later (Figure 4.18). What do you observe? How would you proceed?

A: Repeated, and frequent, biting on the tongue blade corrected his anterior crossbite. However, the OB of his permanent central incisors was minimal, and it appears

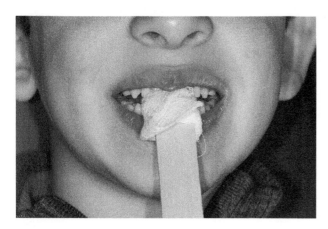

Figure 4.17 Ramus biting on a tongue blade.

that his maxillary lateral incisors may erupt into a crossbite. At this time, we decided to monitor for six months while his lateral incisors erupted. The patient never returned for follow-up.

Q: In addition to using a tongue blade, can you suggest other options which could have been used to correct Ramus' anterior crossbite?

A: Any number of appliances or techniques could be used, most of which require placement of a *posterior bite plate* to open the OB and permit the maxillary incisors to be advanced (Figures 4.19a–4.19d). Options include:

- Placement of orthodontic cement "bite plates" on the maxillary molars [52] to open the OB and allow the *tongue itself* to push/procline the maxillary incisors out of the crossbite. This technique is more successful if the maxillary incisor is tipped lingually in a single tooth crossbite with an adequate room for the incisor. Drs. Herb and Justin Hughes will also advise the patient to push the tooth forward with their thumb.
- Once the OB is opened with orthodontic cement (Figure 4.20c), fixed orthodontic appliances can be placed on maxillary teeth, and compressed open coil springs trapped between the primary canines and permanent central incisors to advance the incisors out of crossbite.
- Removable maxillary appliances (Figure 4.21) incorporate an acrylic posterior bite plate to open the OB plus springs, or screws, to advance the incisors.

Q: Marc (Figure 4.22) is a nine-year-old boy who presents to you in the late mixed dentition with his parents' concern, "Marc has a crossbite." PMH and PDH are WRN. CR = CO. TMJs, periodontal tissues, and mucogingival tissues are WRN. What *primary* problems do you observe in each dimension (plus other)?

(a)   (b)   (c)

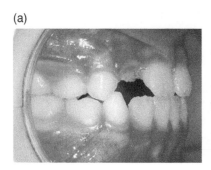
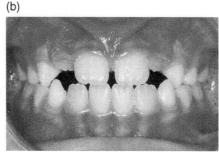
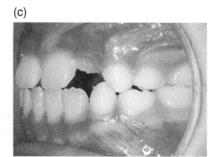

Figure 4.18 (a–c) Progress records of Ramus.

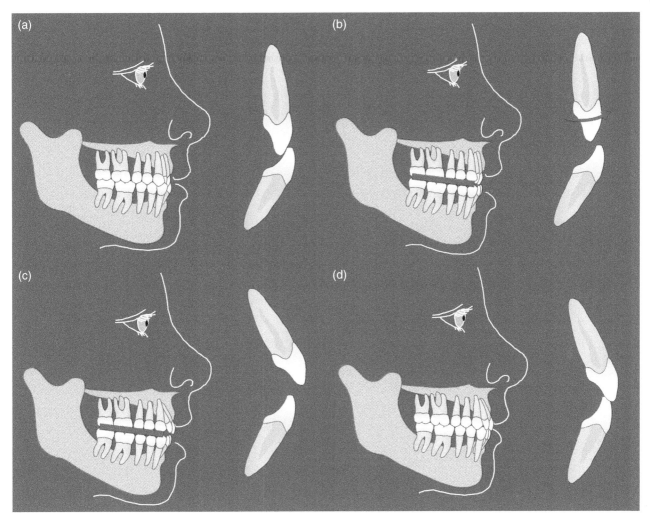

Figure 4.19 (a) Correcting an anterior crossbite (b) requires opening the OB with a posterior bite plate, then (c–d) advancing the maxillary incisors out of crossbite.

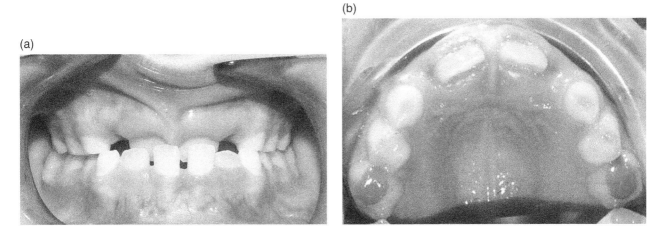

Figure 4.20 (a) Class I child with anterior crossbite. (b–c) Orthodontic cement was placed on the maxillary molars to open the bite. Tongue pressure alone advanced the incisors out of crossbite, and cement was gradually removed (d–e). Photographs courtesy of Drs. Herb and Justin Hughes.

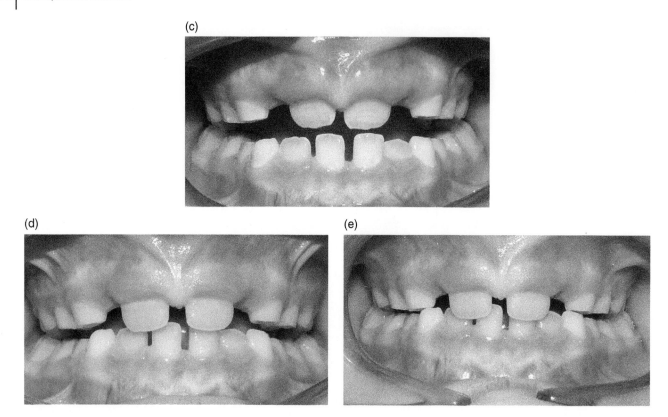

(c)

(d) (e)

Figure 4.20 (Continued)

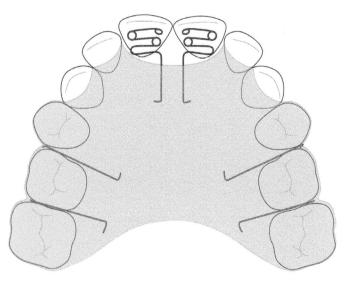

Figure 4.21 Removable maxillary appliances incorporate an acrylic posterior bite plate to open the OB plus springs, or a screw, to advance maxillary incisors out of crossbite.

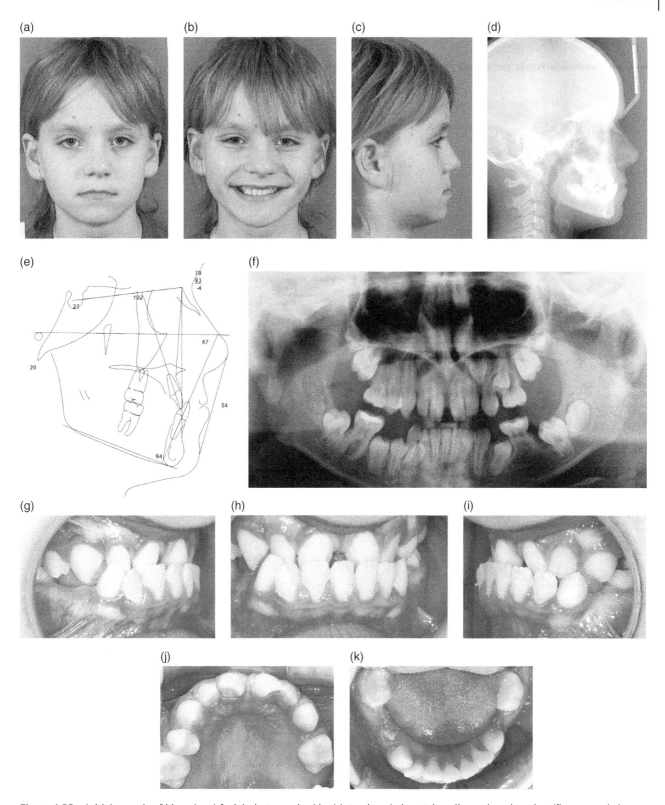

Figure 4.22 Initial records of Marc. (a–c) facial photographs, (d–e) lateral cephalometric radiograph and tracing, (f) panoramic image, (g–k) intraoral photographs.

A:

Table 4.2 Primary problems' list for Marc.

AP	Class III dental relationship (3 mm bilaterally) secondary to maxillary skeletal anteroposterior deficiency combined with mandibular skeletal anteroposterior excess
Vertical	–
Transverse	–
Other diagnosis	Anterior crossbite
	Large midline diastema
	Missing permanent teeth (maxillary right permanent first molar and second premolar; maxillary left first premolar and first permanent molar; mandibular left permanent first molar and second premolar)
	Ectopic eruption of maxillary left second premolar, mandibular left first premolar, and mandibular right permanent canine
	Numerous retained primary teeth (maxillary right primary second molar, maxillary left primary canine and primary second molar; mandibular left primary second molar, and mandibular right primary canine)
	Distal drifting of maxillary and mandibular left canines

Q: How did we determine that Marc's maxilla was *deficient* anteroposteriorly?

A: Marc's A-Point (Figure 4.22e) lies considerably behind the Nasion-perpendicular line. Therefore, as discussed in the Appendix, his maxilla is deficient (retrusive) anteroposteriorly.

Q: How did we determine that Marc's mandible was *excessive* anteroposteriorly?

A: B-Point should normally lie behind the Nasion-perpendicular line. Marc's B-Point lies slightly ahead of the Nasion-perpendicular line. Therefore, his mandible is excessive anteroposteriorly.

Q: What is the cause of Marc's anterior crossbite?

A: The cause is *skeletal* – a combination of maxillary anteroposterior deficiency (hypoplasia) combined with mandibular anteroposterior excess (hyperplasia).

Q: Can you correct Marc's anterior crossbite *dentally*, by proclining his maxillary incisors?

A: You can correct Marc's anterior crossbite *temporarily* by proclining his maxillary incisors, but the underlying cause is skeletal and not dental. So, even if you correct

his crossbite dentally, chances are that it will recur as he continues to grow.

Of course, once you correct his crossbite dentally, you could ask Marc to wear a high-pull chin cup to inhibit forward mandibular growth while permitting forward maxillary growth. If he cooperated with high-pull chin cup wear, then his anterior crossbite would not return.

Q: Incidentally, look at Marc's panoramic image (Figure 4.22f). What do you notice about his developing maxillary left permanent canine? How would the position of this tooth affect your decision to procline his maxillary left lateral incisor?

A: The root apex of his maxillary left lateral incisor appears to be superimposed on the erupting left permanent canine crown. Looking at the cephalometric radiograph, the developing maxillary permanent left canine appears to be posterior to the erupted maxillary permanent right canine (Figure 4.22d). Taken together, it appears that if you advance his maxillary left lateral incisor crown to eliminate the anterior crossbite, then you run the risk of reciprocally driving the lateral root tip into the canine crown – possibly resorbing the lateral incisor root. Before proceeding with this option, it would be best to take a 3-D radiograph to determine the spatial relationship between these two teeth. This was not done.

Q: If you advance Marc's maxillary incisors, do you have any suggestions for reducing the chances that the maxillary permanent left lateral incisor root tip will be resorbed by the erupting permanent canine crown?

A: Yes. If you advance the maxillary left lateral incisor crown, then *proceed slowly with light forces* and position the maxillary left lateral incisor bracket so that the lateral incisor root will be tipped mesially (Figure 4.23), away from the canine crown.

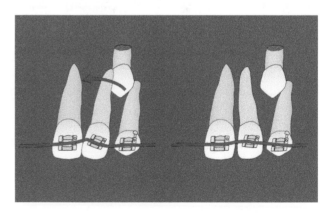

Figure 4.23 The maxillary lateral incisor bracket can be tipped (left) so that its root is moved away from the erupting canine crown (right).

Q: Can you discuss three *general* ways to correct Marc's Class III skeletal relationship?

A: Orthopedics, masking (camouflage), and surgery are the three general ways to address *any* skeletal discrepancy whether in the anteroposterior, vertical, or transverse dimension. Specifically, for a skeletally deficient maxilla and/or skeletally excessive mandible (Class III relationship):

- *Orthopedics* – seeks to enhance maxillary forward growth and/or restrict mandibular forward growth (Figure 4.24a). Examples include RPHG treatment, high-pull chin cup treatment, and Class III elastics worn between maxillary and mandibular TADs.
- *Masking or camouflage* – seeks to correct Class III dental relationships (Figure 4.24b) by *masking* the underlying skeletal discrepancy and not changing the jaws. Generally, we consider Class III masking

only during comprehensive treatment in the adult dentition with patients who have completed, or nearly completed, growth.

Class III masking involves moving maxillary teeth mesially and/or moving mandibular teeth distally. Options include the use of interarch Class III elastics or springs (Figure 4.24c), RPHG to move maxillary teeth mesially, TADs used as anchorage to help move maxillary teeth mesially or mandibular teeth distally, and various combinations of permanent teeth extractions followed by space closure (e.g. extraction of mandibular first premolars in order to create space for mandibular canine retraction into a Class I canine relationship).

Class III elastics or springs are generally worn between the maxillary first permanent molars and mandibular canines. In addition to their desirable

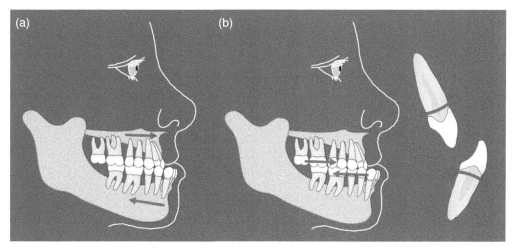

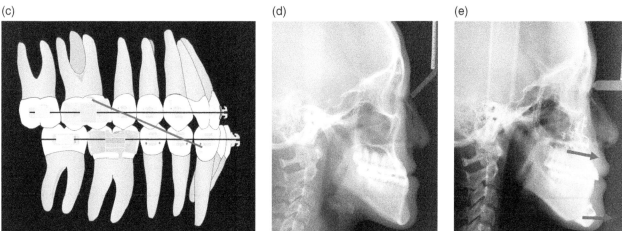

Figure 4.24 Marc's Class III relationship could be corrected with orthopedics (a) by enhancing maxillary forward growth and/or restricting mandibular forward growth. Or later, masking/camouflage could be employed during comprehensive treatment in the adult dentition (b) using dental movements alone to correct the occlusion. The use of Class III elastics or springs (c) is an example of masking. (d–e) illustrate surgical correction of a Class III skeletal relationship using a maxillary advancement osteotomy combined with a genioplasty advancement osteotomy in an adult patient presenting with maxillary anteroposterior deficiency.

effects of moving maxillary anterior teeth mesially and mandibular teeth distally, Class III elastics can have undesirable effects such as erupting maxillary molars and mandibular incisors, rotating the occlusal plane counterclockwise (CCW), and rotating the mandibular plane clockwise (CW).

- *Surgery* – surgery would generally not be considered in children, other than in cases of craniofacial anomalies and/or airway problems. Depending upon his growth and compliance, future surgery for Marc may include either a maxillary advancement osteotomy and/or a mandibular setback osteotomy. Figures 4.24d–4.24e illustrate skeletal changes as a result of maxillary and genioplasty advancement osteotomies in an adult.

Q: Orthopedics to address a Class III skeletal discrepancy may include the use of an RPHG, high-pull chin cup, or TAD-supported Class III elastics. RPHGs are often used during, or after, rapid maxillary expansion. Why? A maxilla that is small in the anteroposterior dimension is often small in the transverse dimension – and requires rapid maxillary expansion (RME). Consequently, elastics from the RPHG to the maxilla are often hooked to a tooth-borne RME. Can you state the skeletal and dental effects of an RPHG (Figure 4.25) in Class III growing children following RME?

A: The effects of RPHG [53, 54] wear (six months, 380 gm of force per side) following RME are, on average:
  - *1.8 mm forward maxillary growth.*
  - Labial movement of maxillary incisors (maxillary tooth movement is eliminated if miniplates are used for anchorage instead of maxillary teeth).

- Increased fullness of maxillary lip.
- 2.5 mm backward mandibular movement (chin cup effect).
- Downward and backward mandibular rotation (mandibular MPA increase of 1.5°).
- LAFH increase of 2.9 mm.
- Lingual movement of mandibular incisors.

Q: A child presents to you with maxillary anteroposterior deficiency which you treat using an RPHG. When is the best age to do this? Is there a difference in treatment effects between early and late maxillary RPHG protraction treatment?

A: Yes. A traditional guideline calls for RPHG treatment when a child's maxillary permanent incisors are erupting. *The skeletal effects of RPHGs are less in patients older than ten years of age* [55–57].

Q: Marc is nine years old. How does his age impact your decision to use RPHG to address his maxillary anteroposterior deficiency?

A: If you plan RPHG treatment on Marc, you should do it *now* to achieve maximal skeletal benefit.

Q: Does A-Point advance more with RPHG if circummaxillary sutures are loosened using RME?

A: Some studies report no difference in A-Point advancement with, or without, RME [58–60]. However, one study reported A-point advancing more if RPHG is applied (300–500 gm/side, twelve hours per day until the anterior crossbite is corrected) *during* RME, less after RME, and even less without RME [60]. W*hen using RPHG to advance a child's maxilla, we recommend*

(a)

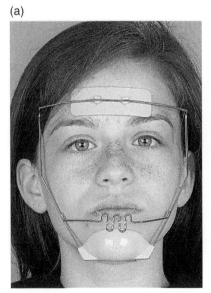

(b)

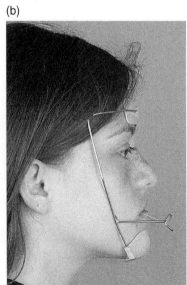

Figure 4.25 (a–b) Reverse-pull facemask or headgear.

applying RPHG during RME (assuming transverse correction is needed) because there is no disadvantage in doing so.

Q: Compare the effectiveness of early Class III treatment (maxillary anteroposterior deficiency) using RPHG in conjunction with RME – and using RPHG in conjunction with *alternating* rapid maxillary expansion and constriction.

A: Alternating rapid maxillary expansion and constriction protocol (Alt-RAMEC) was designed to maintain sutural stimulation over a longer period of time than RME alone, thus achieving greater maxillary protraction during RPHG treatment [61]. What is the protocol? The RME appliance is opened 1 mm per day (four turns per day), alternating one week of expansion with one week of constriction for seven to nine weeks.

In a recent study [62], Alt-RAMEC with RPHG was shown to be more effective in advancing the maxilla when compared to RME with RPHG. No significant differences were noted regarding mandibular projection, length, and vertical skeletal relationships. In another study [63] comparing the effects of facemask protraction combined with alternating rapid palatal expansion and constriction – the authors found only statistically significant differences (*not clinically significant differences*) when compared to RME with RPHG.

At this time, we feel that findings regarding the effectiveness of alternating rapid maxillary expansion and constriction during RPHG treatment are inconclusive.

Q: Marc does not have any erupted maxillary left permanent teeth, and his maxillary left primary second molar has nearly exfoliated (Figure 4.22f). In other words, there are no maxillary left teeth suitable for RPHG anchorage. Can you offer a solution to this problem?

A: Consider placing TADs in the maxilla [64]. Elastics can be worn directly from the RPHG to the TADs.

Q: How does RPHG protraction using miniplate (TAD) anchorage compare to conventional facemask (tooth-borne) protraction – where both groups of patients first undergo rapid maxillary expansion using a bonded appliance?

A: Compared to conventional RPHG patients, miniplate anchorage RPHG patients had *more maxillary forward movement* (without significant anterior rotation), less mandibular posterior rotation, less face height increase, and no dental movement [65]. In a similar study [66], a miniplate anchorage RPHG group showed more forward maxillary movement, less Frankfort horizontal to

mandibular plane angle (FMA) opening, and less sagittal and extrusive maxillary molar movement compared to a bonded RME appliance anchorage RPHG group. A meta-analysis [67] concluded that approximately *3 mm of horizontal A-point movement is reliably attainable with skeletal (miniplate) anchorage maxillary protraction – which is 1 mm greater than that expected with tooth-borne maxillary protraction* [58].

Q: Other than tooth-borne RPHGs, or TAD-supported RPHGs, can you suggest another anchorage option for RPHGs?

A: Intact maxillary primary canines can be intentionally ankylosed to serve as anchors. Root canal treatment is performed on extracted primary canines (Figure 4.26a), and the periodontal ligament is scraped off. Wires are attached to the primary canines (Figure 4.26b). The canines are reinserted into their respective sockets and stabilized until they ankylose (Figures 4.26c and 4.26d). Elastics are worn from the primary canine wires to the RPHG (Figure 4.26e). We have used this anchorage technique but are not enthusiastic about it. We prefer miniplates as anchors instead.

Q: Is the purpose of jaw orthopedics to *normalize growth*? In other words, if Marc wears an RPHG and achieves correction of his Class III skeletal discrepancy, does that mean his future maxillary and mandibular jaw growth will remain in balance? Or, will he simply grow out of the correction once you stop orthopedics?

A: While it is true that early RPHG treatment achieves short-term positive skeletal and dental changes, there is a lack of evidence on its long-term benefits [68] – except for the fact that early Class III protraction facemask treatment reduces the need for orthognathic surgery from 66% (control group) to 36% (facemask group) [69]. We are left with the clinical observation that *once orthopedic forces are discontinued, the former Class III growth pattern returns – tending to recreate the same skeletal discrepancy.* Whether the patient will eventually outgrow the correction depends on how much growth remains after orthopedics is stopped and whether (how much) you overcorrect the patient (made them Class II).

Q: Does this mean that RPHG therapy is inherently unstable?

A: Any orthopedic treatment, including RPHG treatment, is unstable in the sense that the old growth pattern returns after treatment [57, 70, 71] – as long as the patient is growing. The A-point advancement you achieve may not be lost after RPHG treatment, but the

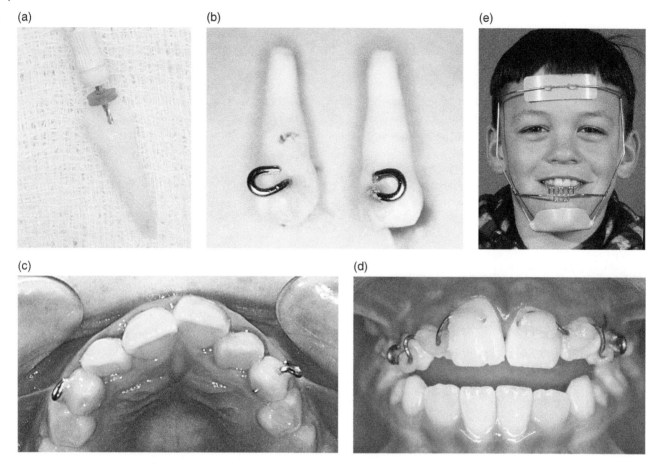

Figure 4.26 (a–e) Intentionally ankylosing maxillary primary canines for use as RPHG anchors.

Class III growth differential between the maxilla and mandibular will return. That is, Marc's excess mandibular growth will exceed his deficient maxillary growth.

Q: How do the above facts about stability and normalization of growth affect your RPHG protocol?

A: The key to using RPHG on growing, maxillary deficient, Class III children is *overcorrection*. Do not just correct the patient to a Class I molar relationship. Instead, overcorrect to a Class II molar relationship. Also, *monitor and maintain your correction until the patient is finished growing*. If the patient begins to grow Class III again, then decide whether to return to the RPHG, place the patient on a high-pull chin cup, or place the patient on TAD-supported Class III elastics.

Q: Once you have corrected a Class III skeletal relationship (deficient maxilla) with an RPHG, you need to maintain that correction until the patient has completed growth. A high-pull chin cup (Figure 4.27) can be worn to maintain the correction. What are the effects of high-pull chin cup wear in an adolescent?

A: *High-pull* chin cup effects (fourteen hours/day of wear for two years plus wear during sleep for three additional years) include: [72]
- ANB improvement
- Chin position improvement
- Inhibition of mandibular ramal height growth and inhibition of mandibular body length growth
- Backward rotation of mandible
- Closure of gonial angle
- Mandibular plane angle (FMA) flattened in high-pull chin cup patients but opened in controls
- Maxilla continues to grow forward
- *LAFH is not increased compared to controls* [73, 74]

   Note: Even in severe dolichofacial Class III patients who are compliant, long-term (>five years) high-pull chin cup therapy is effective [75]. However, wearing a chin cup (like wearing an RPHG) *does not normalize growth*. The changes listed above will not be

(a)

(b)

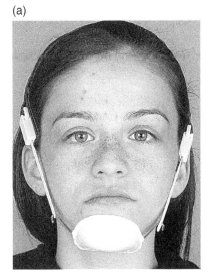
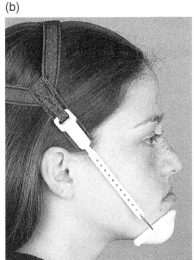

Figure 4.27 (a–b) High-pull chin cup.

maintained if chin cup wear is discontinued before facial growth is complete [72–76].

Q: Can an anterior crossbite due to a Class III skeletal discrepancy be treated with *only* a high-pull chin cup, and not with an RPHG first?

A: Yes. Anterior crossbites in skeletal Class III children result from:
- Deficient maxillary forward growth with normal mandibular forward growth
- Deficient maxillary forward growth with excessive mandibular forward growth
- Normal maxillary forward growth with excessive mandibular forward growth.

In every case, mandibular forward growth exceeds maxillary forward growth. So, restricting mandibular forward growth with a high-pull chin cup while allowing maxillary forward growth will improve the Class III relationship and tend to correct an anterior crossbite. Of course, the *magnitude* of the skeletal discrepancy, the amount of growth remaining (*time*), and the patient's compliance all play a role in determining success.

Q: But, how can you place a child on a high-pull chin cup if they are in anterior crossbite? In other words, wouldn't the high-pull chin cup drive the mandibular incisors back into the maxillary incisors – potentially traumatizing them?

A: Yes, that is correct – which brings us to our recommended protocol for treating anterior crossbites in Class III skeletal children (maxillary deficiency, mandibular excess, or a combination of both). We recommend *correcting the anterior crossbite first, dentally.*

Then, placing the child in a high-pull chin cup, or Class III elastics supported by TADs, until they finish growing.

To illustrate our protocol, examine Alex (Figure 4.28), a five-year- and six-month-old boy who presented with an anterior crossbite, Class I canine relationship, and negligible CR-CO shift. Alex could not get his incisors back to an edge-to-edge relationship. His pediatric dentist told his parents that Alex would need jaw surgery. Mom presented to our practice crying, and begging us to help Alex without surgery. Alex had a concave profile, an ANB angle of –2 degrees, and we felt that he was beginning to grow Class III (maxillary deficiency and mandibular excess).

We first corrected his anterior crossbite using a mandibular bite plate plus fixed appliances to advance his maxillary *primary* incisors (Figure 4.28l). We normally wait until maxillary permanent incisors erupt to correct anterior crossbites, but we were concerned about his unfavorable growth and decided to correct it in the primary dentition.

Following crossbite correction, Alex was placed on a high-pull chin cup (Figures 4.29a–4.29h). Alex wore the high-pull chin cup nightly until growth was complete. He had *no additional treatment.* He and his mom were delighted with his outcome and elected not to perfect the alignment of his teeth with braces (Figures 4.30a–4.30i). Our point is that this treatment protocol can be very effective with a compliant patient.

Some of our friends are gifted orthodontists who never use chin cups, and they only treat Class III growing patients with RPHGs. So, why do we recommend the above approach? Our reasons are as follows:
- *Jaw growth is not normalized* with orthopedics – when you stop orthopedic treatment, the

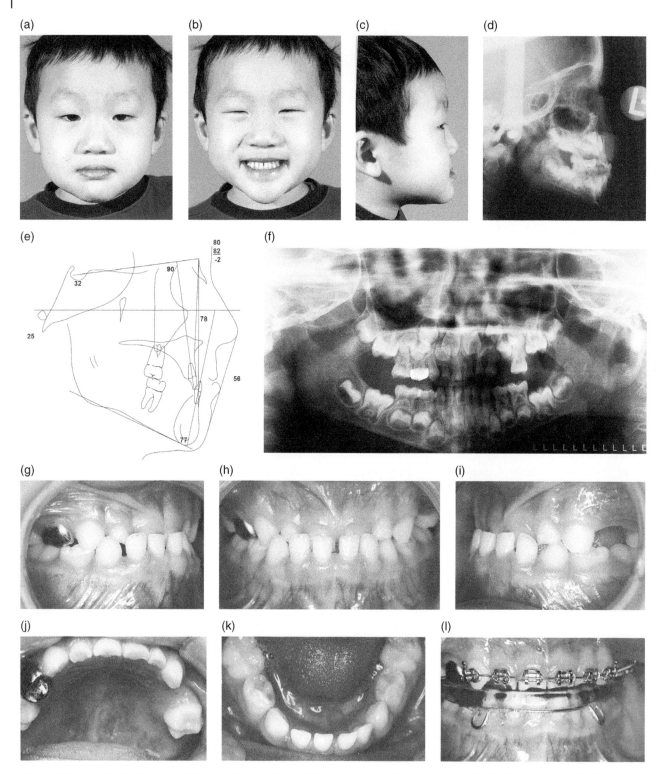

Figure 4.28 (a–k) Initial records of Alex and (l) correction of his anterior crossbite using a mandibular bite plate plus fixed appliances to advance his maxillary *primary* incisors. We normally wait until maxillary permanent incisors erupt before correcting an anterior crossbite, but we were concerned about his unfavorable growth and decided to correct his crossbite in the primary dentition.

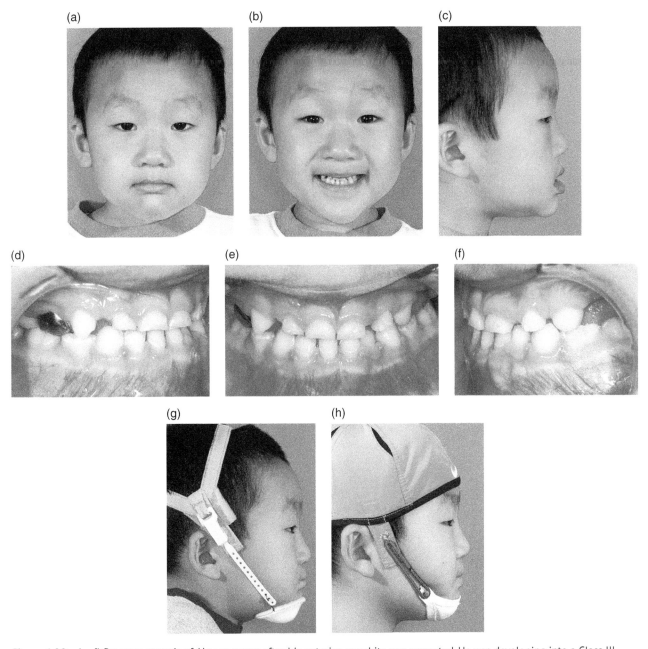

Figure 4.29 (a–f) Progress records of Alex one year after his anterior crossbite was corrected. He was developing into a Class III bilateral dental relationship (3 mm Class III on the right, 1 mm Class III on the left). (g) Alex was placed on a high-pull chin. (h) For reasons of comfort, this was switched to a high-pull chin cup fabricated from a cap.

underlying difference between maxillary and mandibular forward growth that caused the initial Class III relationship will return. With our approach, the *child and parents understand that they must be committed to wearing the chin cup every night until growth is complete.* Once you achieve Class III correction with a chin cup, you must hold that correction until growth is complete. The same is true for TAD-supported Class III elastic wear.

- RPHGs are not usually applied with the understanding that they must be worn until growth is complete. RPHGs are usually worn until the child's Class III relationship is corrected. Once RPHG wear is discontinued, the Class III skeletal growth pattern returns for as long as the child grows, and the child can grow out of your correction.
- For that reason, RPHG treatment usually includes overcorrection. But, deciding how much to

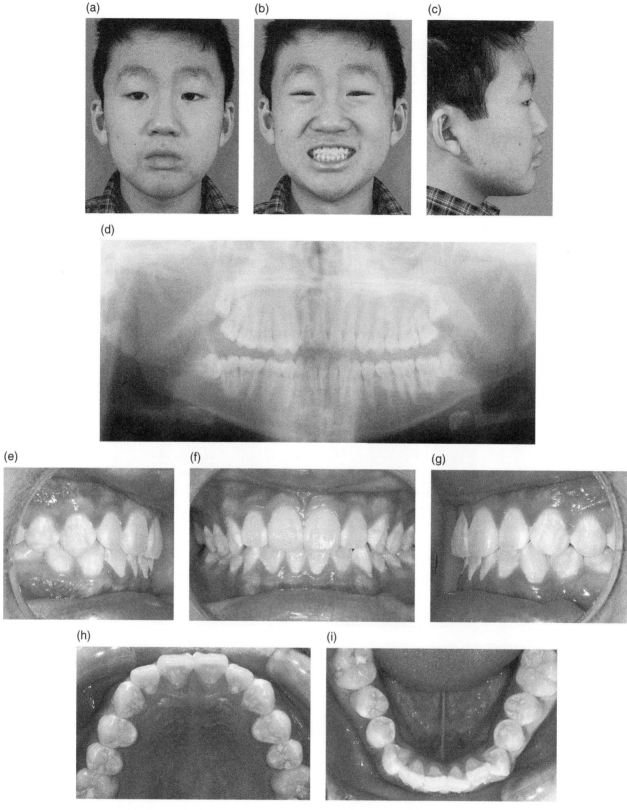

Figure 4.30 (a–i) Final records of Alex after growth was complete. Alex and his mother were delighted with the early treatment outcome and declined comprehensive treatment to align his teeth with braces. He was referred for third molar extractions.

overcorrect with RPHG is a gamble at a young age. If you overcorrect too much, the child may end Class II. If you overcorrect too little, the child will end Class III. Getting it just right is very, very difficult. And remember, the average additional forward maxillary growth with tooth-borne RPHG is limited, ranging from only 1–3 mm [58, 67].

- Overcorrection with RPHG can be a viable approach and it follows from our general principle for orthopedics, "*overcorrect and monitor until growth is complete.*" We ask only that you monitor the patient until growth is complete.
- With our approach (anterior crossbite correction – followed by high-pull chin cup or TAD-supported Class III elastic wear), the child is asked to comply with wearing only *one* orthopedic appliance (chin cup or Class III elastics). With RPHG, the child may be asked to switch over to a different appliance later (chin cup) and lose interest. Maintaining habits is generally easier than starting new habits.
- Finally, in cases of anterior crossbites due to Class III skeletal discrepancies, we suggest correcting the crossbite first, *even in the primary dentition*. If there was no skeletal discrepancy that needed to be addressed orthopedically, then we would generally not correct the anterior crossbite until permanent incisors erupted.

Q: *When* each day should your patient wear the chin cup? How much force should the chin cup apply?

A: In our opinion, start the patient wearing a high-pull chin cup for only two to three hours each evening with a very light force (the lightest force possible to keep the chin cup on). After one week, increase wear to four hours in the evening. The goal is to develop a habit of nightly wear. Then, have the patient begin wearing the high-pull chin cup *from 7–8 pm each evening until the next morning (when most growth is thought to occur)*.

After the first few weeks, gradually increase the force. The ideal force for chin cup therapy is unknown, but a force exceeding 125–250 gm, measured at the center of the chin cup, appears to be necessary. Why do we say this? In a recent study, fewer than 50% of patients treated with a light-force chin cup had favorable clinical outcomes [77]. Therefore, *we recommend an eventual chin cup force of 250 gm per side*, the same force recommended for TAD-anchored Class III elastic wear.

Q: High-pull chin cups apply pressure to the TMJ. Should you have concerns about the patient developing temporomandibular joint disorder (TMD) when wearing a chin cup?

A: You should always be concerned about loading the TMJs – whether with chin cups, Class III elastics, or

soft tissue stretching following BSSO advancements. However, there is no evidence that 500 gm or even 1000 gm orthopedic chin cup force, applied at the center of the chin, induces TMD. In a recent study of 250 chin cup-treated female subjects [75], 5% developed *transient* symptoms of TMD during or after active treatment (temporary muscular pain and difficulty achieving maximum mouth opening). Their TMDs were treated using conservative measures (e.g. splint therapy).

Here are our recommendations regarding chin cups and TMD:

- *Do not load TMJs using chin cups (or Class III elastics or Class III springs) in patients who initially present with TMJ pain or restricted function*
- *Inform patients of the possibility of transient symptoms developing during chin cup treatment*
- *In patients who develop TMD symptoms during chin cup treatment, discontinue chin cup wear.*

Q: Class III orthopedic effects can also be achieved by placing TADs in both jaws and having the patient wear Class III elastics between them (Figure 4.31). How does the growth of untreated Class III subjects compare to the growth of Class III patients treated with elastics worn between maxillary and mandibular TADs?

A: TAD-anchored Class III elastic patients have an average maxillary advancement of 4 mm, and B-Point improvement of 2 mm, compared to Class III control subjects [78].

Q: How dsswoes maxillary A-Point advancement in prepubertal patients compare between RME-RPHG and Class III elastics worn between infrazygomatic and anterior mandibular TADs (miniplates)?

A: *Class III elastics worn between miniplates resulted in over 2 mm more maxillary advancement than RME followed by RPHG* [79]. The Class III elastics were initially applied with a force of 150 gm but gradually increased to 250 gm after three months, and they were coupled with a bite plate to eliminate occlusal interference in the incisor region until anterior crossbite correction was achieved.

Q: Can you list advantages and disadvantages of TAD (bone anchored) Class III elastic orthopedic treatment?

A: Advantages include:

- Improved compliance - patients are more likely to wear intraoral elastics between maxillary and mandibular TADs than they are to wear a facemask or highpull chincup.
- The force from the Class III elastics is applied *all day and night*, not just at night when the patient wears a facemask or chincup.
- *Unilateral* mandibular hyperplasia can be treated with TAD-supported Class III elastics. The

(a)

(b)

(c)

(d)

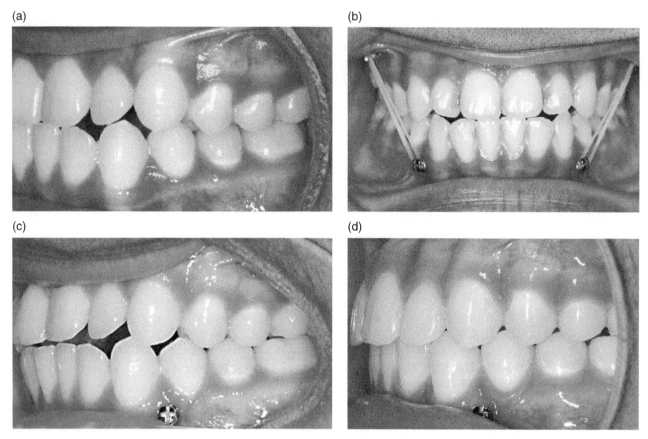

Figure 4.31 Orthopedic treatment using Class III elastics supported by TAD (screw) anchors: (a) initial Class III (2 mm) relationship; (b) Class III elastics supported by maxillary and mandibular TADs worn 24 hours per day except when eating; (c) orthopedic treatment resulted in a *Class II (1 mm) overcorrected* relationship; (d) five months following cessation of Class III elastic wear to TADs (the patient was seventeen years of age and growth had ended).

orthopedic forces generated by chincup or RPHG are *bilateral*.

- Vertical changes and retroclination of mandibular incisors are better controlled compared to skeletally anchored RPHGs [79].

Disadvantages include:

- Non-compliance can still be a problem. Even after repeatedly explaining the necessity of elastic wear, we have had patients refuse, or forget, to wear their Class III elastics.
- Depending upon the location of screw insertion, developing/unerupted teeth can be damaged by the screws.
- Screws may become loose or embedded in bone during growth with bony surface apposition.

Q: What is the advantage of placing an LLHA in a mixed dentition skeletal Class III patient?

A: When the mandibular primary canines and primary molars exfoliate, the LLHA prevents/reduces mesial drift of the permanent molars and worsening of the Class III relationship.

Q: Let's discuss the timing of Class III orthopedic treatment. We have already stated that the strongest scientific evidence finds no advantage to beginning Class II treatment in the *early* mixed dentition (except for a possible decrease in incisal trauma as a result of excess OJ) [22–24, 29, 38–40]. We have already stated that we subscribe to this guideline unless an early mixed dentition child shows *good statural growth (regular incremental change in stature)* in which case we will consider beginning Class II orthopedic treatment.

Further, we already stated that for *Class III* orthopedic treatment, the skeletal effects of RPHGs are greatest in patients 10 years of age or younger [55–57]. However, what about timing for Class III children treated with high-pull chin cups or Class III elastics supported by TADs? What does the evidence tell us?

A: Unlike Class II treatment, we lack prospective, randomized clinical trials for Class III patients using either high-pull chin cups or Class III elastics supported by TADs. Instead, we have weaker levels of evidence. As a recent systematic review of Class III orthopedic outcomes concluded: "high-quality investigations are still needed to perform a definitive assessment of the effectiveness of Class III treatment at the skeletal level." [80]

So, what recommendations do we suggest for the timing of high-pull chin cup or TAD-supported Class III elastic treatment?

- The greater the Class III skeletal discrepancy *magnitude*, the earlier we recommend you should start orthopedics (to take advantage of as much future growth as possible).
- Compliance is critical. All patients will eventually suffer "burnout." Informing them that excellent cooperation may eliminate the need for future orthognathic surgery will motivate some patients. For others, it will not. If the child does not cooperate within a few months of starting orthopedics, discontinue and monitor them until they complete growth. At that time, re-evaluate for masking or surgery.
- Class III orthopedic treatment (chin cup or TAD-supported Class III elastic wear) would ideally bracket the time when the patient is growing most. However, that precise time is difficult to predict, and Class III mandibular excess patients *grow longer*

than other patients (e.g. mandibular-deficiency patients).
- Long-term orthopedic use of Class III elastics supported by TADs (five to ten years until the patient has completed growth) has not been reported.

For Alex (Figure 4.28), we started orthopedics at six years and six months of age because his mother (a physician) feared that Alex would require jaw surgery someday if we did not intercede. In terms of compliance, Alex was outstanding. He wore a high-pull chin cup *for nine years* – probably as a result of his mother's influence. Most likely, she kept her son out of the operating room.

Q: Let's return to Marc (Figure 4.22). Based upon our previous questions and answers, what Class III orthopedic treatment (if any) do you recommend for him – RPHG, high-pull chin cup, or Class III elastics supported by TADs?

A: Because Marc was nine years old, presented with a deficient maxilla, and lacked maxillary left posterior permanent teeth, we placed him on a TAD-supported RPHG (Figure 4.32).

(a) (b)

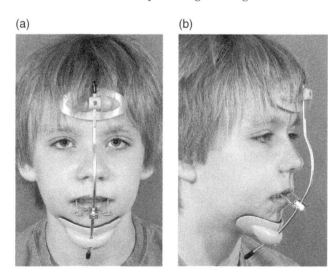

(c)

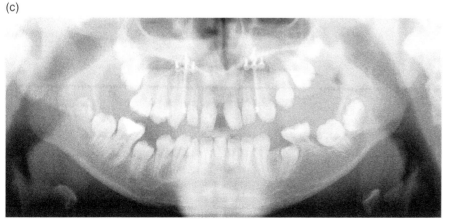

Figure 4.32 (a–c). Marc was treated with a TAD (miniplate)-supported RPHG.

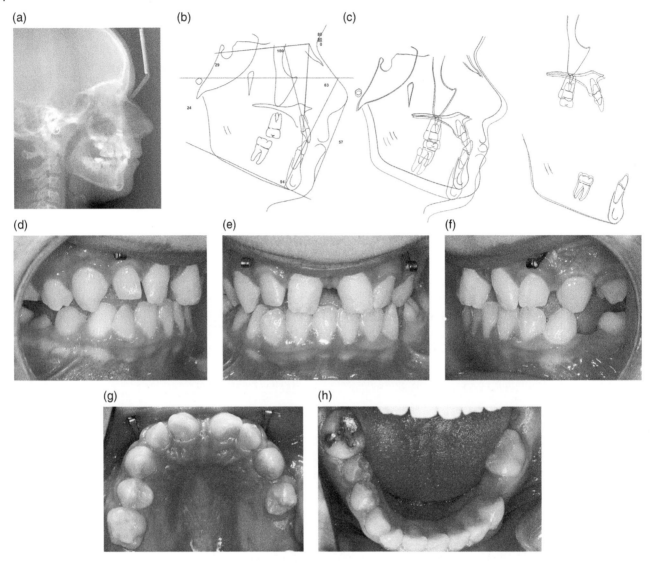

Figure 4.33 (a–h) Progress records of Marc. His anterior crossbite and Class III dental relationship were corrected using a TAD-supported RPHG.

This treatment alone corrected his anterior crossbite and Class III dental relationship (Figure 4.33). Note the orthopedic changes which occurred (Figure 4.33c):

- Maxilla grew downward and forward.
- Mandible rotated downward and backward (clockwise rotation) and exhibited slight condylar growth.
- Maxillary molar and incisors erupted.

Marc's anteroposterior relationship was monitored. We were prepared to maintain his anteroposterior correction using a high-pull chin cup if his Class III growth pattern returned, but he remained stable. His miniplates were removed, fixed orthodontic appliances were later placed, leveling/alignment of his arches attempted, and space closure attempted.

However, significant root resorption was noted on a routine panoramic image (Figure 4.34). Following

discussions with Marc and his parents, a decision was made to discontinue further treatment. Final records of Marc (Figure 4.35) were made years later after cosmetic veneers had been placed. Correction of his anterior crossbite via RPHG was stable, and ideal OJ has been achieved. Marc and his parents were very happy with the treatment he received, and he will be referred for extraction of his third molars.

Q: A parent asks you to explain in layman's terms how Class III molar relationships develop. What is your answer?

A: Class III molar relationships can be of *dental* origin (e.g. early loss of mandibular primary second molars with mesial drift of mandibular permanent first molars) or of *skeletal* origin (excessive forward growth of the mandible and/or inadequate forward growth of the maxilla).

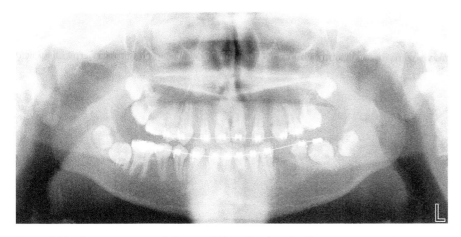

Figure 4.34 Progress panoramic image of Marc showing significant root resorption.

(a) (b) (c)

(d)

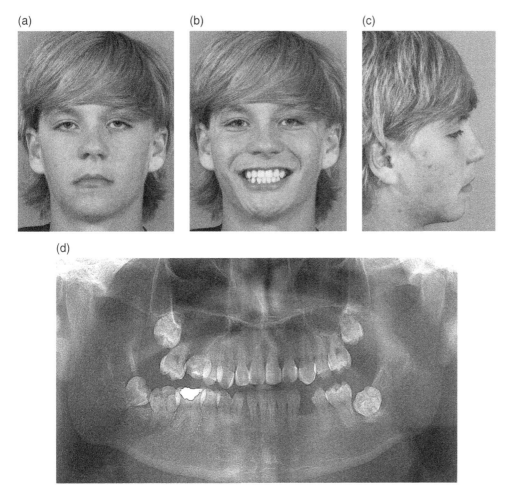

Figure 4.35 (a–i). Final records of Marc.

Q: Let's finish this introductory section by highlighting important "take-home pearls" about Marc and other early-treatment Class III and Class II patients.

A: "Take-home pearls" include the following:

- Marc was nine years old in the late mixed dentition when he presented with a 3 mm bilateral Class III relationship and anterior crossbite secondary to maxillary skeletal anteroposterior deficiency

(e) (f) (g)

(h) (i)

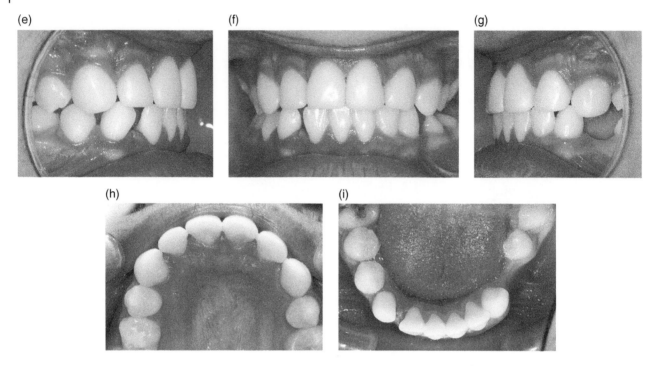

Figure 4.35 (Continued)

combined with mandibular skeletal anteroposterior excess. His crossbite was corrected, skeletally, using an RPHG and maxillary (miniplate) TADs.

- When you employ Class III or Class II orthopedics, you are *not normalizing growth*. You can alter anteroposterior jaw growth during orthopedic force application. But once you stop orthopedics, a growing patient will return to their previous growth pattern and may grow out of your correction. We were very fortunate that Marc's correction held without the need to place him on a high-pull chin cup (or Class III elastics to TADs) after the crossbite correction.

- For the above reason, you should *overcorrect and monitor* until growth is complete. If you are using RPHG/high-pull chin cup/Class III elastics supported by TADs to correct a Class III skeletal discrepancy, then don't just correct the patient to Class I and stop. Instead, overcorrect slightly to Class II (1–2 mm), and maintain/monitor your correction until the patient is finished growing.

  If you are using headgears or functional appliances to treat a Class II skeletal discrepancy, then don't just correct the patient to Class I and stop. Instead, overcorrect the patient slightly to Class III (1–2 mm), and *slowly* taper off the headgear or functional appliance wear over a period of months while you monitor the stability of your correction.

- In our experience, Class II orthopedic correction is more stable than Class III orthopedic correction. Why? Whereas Class II skeletal discrepancies usually result from deficient mandibular growth, Class III skeletal discrepancies usually result (at least partially) from excess mandibular growth, and excessively growing mandibles grow for longer periods of time than normal.

- A decision to employ Class III or Class II orthopedics is predicated upon two factors – the *magnitude* of the skeletal discrepancy and the *time* (growth) remaining to treat it. If you have a compliant child with a mild skeletal problem and years of growth ahead, then you have a reasonable chance of correction with orthopedics. If you have a moderate skeletal problem and years of growth ahead, you have less of a chance to achieve full correction with orthopedics. If you have a severe skeletal problem with minimal future growth, then your chances of full correction are greatly reduced. However, even in the latter case, you may still be able to improve the skeletal discrepancy with orthopedics to the point where you can successfully employ masking treatments.

- We generally recommend waiting to correct an anterior crossbite until the permanent incisors erupt. We will correct an anterior crossbite in the primary dentition if we wish to proceed with Class III orthopedics.

- Once an anterior crossbite (CR-CO shift) has been corrected in pseudo Class III children, the child becomes Class I and can complete orthodontic treatment as a Class I patient. Future anteroposterior growth is usually not a concern.

  However, even after an anterior crossbite has been corrected in *skeletal* Class III children, they will probably remain Class III and their *future Class III growth pattern will impact long-term treatment success.* You must remain vigilant in determining whether you are dealing with a pseudo Class III or a skeletal Class III. Your success will depend upon it.

- 3 mm of horizontal A-point movement is reliably attainable with skeletal (miniplate) anchorage maxillary RPHG protraction – which is 1 mm greater than what can be expected with tooth-borne maxillary RPHG protraction.

- For growing skeletal Class III patients, we recommend correcting the anterior crossbite first, dentally. Then, placing the child on a high-pull chin cup, or Class III elastics supported by TADs, until they finish growing.

- Principle of Class II correction: avoid treatments that rotate the mandible down and back – worsening a convex profile and worsening a Class II relationship.

- Principle of Class II correction: *you must have anterior OJ* in order to correct a Class II posterior relationship.

- Timing guidelines – You should wait to begin Class II orthopedic treatment until the late mixed dentition. However, *consider beginning in the early mixed dentition if the parent tells you that the child has good statural growth* (displaying regular incremental increases in stature).

  For Class III orthopedic correction – the more severe the anticipated Class III skeletal discrepancy, the earlier we recommend you start orthopedics (as early as six to seven years). As a rule, begin RPHG at the time the maxillary permanent central incisors are erupting, but before age ten. Begin high-pull chin cup or TAD-supported Class III elastics as early as the early mixed dentition.

- Compliance – if the compliance of a Class III patient wearing an RPHG or high-pull chin cup wanes, consider offering TAD-supported Class III elastics as an alternative. Some of our patients who refuse to wear an RPHG or chin cup successfully wear TAD-supported Class III elastics well.

No matter which appliance you use, patients must develop a habit of wear and stick to it, possibly for years.

- Whether Class III or Class II orthopedics, patients have only one cup of compliance. When it is gone, it is gone. When it is gone, consider other options. We are not here to make patients' lives, parents' lives, and our own lives miserable by forcing compliance.

- Although Class II and Class III masking can be performed in young children, masking is usually performed in the permanent dentition during comprehensive treatment and has not been discussed at length here. Likewise, we have only touched on maxillary or mandibular surgeries which are beyond the scope of this early treatment textbook.

  However, anytime orthopedics is attempted in a child, discussions of future "fallback" options (contingency plans including masking or surgery) should be discussed with parents in the event that orthopedics fails.

Case Jake

Q: Jake is eleven years old (Figure 4.36) and presents to you for a consultation. His parents' chief complaint is, "Jake needs braces." PMH, TMJ, and periodontal evaluations are WRN. CR = CO. *Compile your diagnostic findings and problem list.* State your *diagnosis.*

A:

Table 4.3 Diagnostic findings and problem list for Jake.

Full face and profile	**Frontal View**
	Face is symmetric
	LAFH WRN (soft tissue Glabella – Subnasale = Subnasale – soft tissue Menton)
	Lip competence
	UDML WRN
	Incisal display during smile inadequate (maxillary central incisor gingival margins apical to maxillary lip border)
	Large buccal corridors
	Profile View
	Convex profile
	Upturned nasal tip
	Obtuse NLA
	Retrusive chin
	Obtuse lip-chin-throat angle
	Short chin-throat length
Radiographs	Late mixed dentition

(Continued)

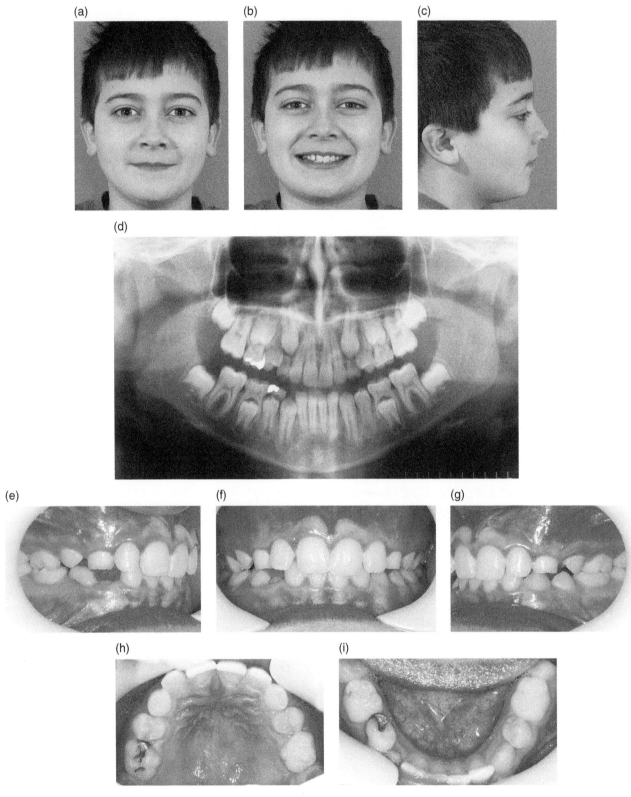

Figure 4.36 Initial records of Jake. (a–c) facial photographs, (d) pantomograph, (e–i) intraoral photographs.

Table 4.3 (Continued)

Intraoral photos	Angle Class I malocclusion in the mixed dentition
	Iowa classification: II (1 mm) x x II (1 mm) measured during his examination, but not clearly shown on the right and left intraoral photographs
	OJ 1 mm
	OB 50–60% (without palatal impingement)
	LDML 1 mm to right of UDML
	Mandibular labial anterior periodontal biotype WRN
	Plaque control inadequate
	0.0 mm of maxillary anterior crowding currently present
	3.4 mm of maxillary spacing is anticipated following the eruption of all permanent teeth (if appropriate space maintenance is employed)
	2.0 mm mandibular anterior crowding currently present (0 mm of incisor crowding,
	7 mm anticipated width of mandibular right permanent canine, but only 5 mm space available)
	4.5 mm of mandibular spacing is anticipated following the eruption of all permanent teeth (if appropriate space maintenance is employed)
	Maxillary and mandibular posterior arches are symmetric
Other	–
diagnosis	Angle Class I malocclusion in the mixed dentition with mild mandibular anterior crowding

Q: Provide a detailed space analysis for Jake's maxillary and mandibular arches. Can you describe how the 3.4 mm maxillary arch spacing and 4.5 mm mandibular arch spacing were calculated (if space maintenance is employed)?

A:

Average mesiodistal widths of permanent teeth (mm): [81]

Maxillary central incisor	8.5	Mandibular central incisor	5.0
Maxillary lateral incisor	6.5	Mandibular lateral incisor	5.5
Maxillary canine	7.5	Mandibular canine	7.0
Maxillary first premolar	7.0	Mandibular first premolar	7.0
Maxillary second premolar	7.0	Mandibular second premolar	7.0
Maxillary first molar	10.0	Mandibular first molar	11.0
Maxillary second molar	9.0	Mandibular second molar	10.5

Average mesiodistal widths of *primary* teeth (mm): [81]

Maxillary central incisor	6.5	Mandibular central incisor	4.2
Maxillary lateral incisor	5.1	Mandibular lateral incisor	4.1
Maxillary canine	7.0	Mandibular canine	5.0
Maxillary first molar	7.3	Mandibular first molar	7.7
Maxillary second molar	8.2	Mandibular second molar	9.9

MAXILLARY ARCH (leeway space cannot be used since maxillary first primary molars have exfoliated)

0.0 mm of maxillary anterior crowding currently present (Figure 4.36h)

+8.2 mm mesiodistal width of maxillary right primary second molar

−7.0 mm anticipated size of maxillary right second premolar

+1 mm space distal to maxillary right primary canine

+7.0 mm mesiodistal width of maxillary right primary canine

−7.5 mm anticipated width of maxillary right permanent canine

+7.0 mm mesiodistal width of maxillary left primary canine

−7.5 mm anticipated width of maxillary left permanent canine

+1 mm space distal to maxillary left primary canine

+8.2 mm mesiodistal width of maxillary left primary second molar

−7.0 mm anticipated size of maxillary left second premolar

Balance = 0 mm + 8.2 mm − 7.0 mm + 1 mm + 7.0 mm − 7.5 mm + 7.0 mm − 7.5 mm + 1 mm + 8.2 mm − 7.0 mm = +3.4 mm

MANDIBULAR ARCH (leeway space cannot be used since the primary canines and left primary first molar have exfoliated)

0 mm of mandibular incisor crowding currently present (Figure 4.36i)

+9.9 mm mesiodistal width of mandibular left primary second molar

−7 mm anticipated size of mandibular left second premolar

+5.0 mm space between mandibular right primary first molar and mandibular right lateral incisor

−7.0 mm anticipated size of mandibular right permanent canine

+7.7 mm mesiodistal width mandibular right primary first molar

−7.0 mm anticipated size of mandibular right first premolar

+9.9 mm mesiodistal width mandibular right primary second molar

−7 mm anticipated size of mandibular right second premolar

Balance = 0 mm + 9.9 mm − 7.0 mm + 5.0 mm − 7.0 mm + 7.7 mm − 7.0 mm + 9.9 mm

7.0 mm = +4.5 mm

That is, *3.4 mm of maxillary spacing and 4.5 mm of mandibular spacing is anticipated following the eruption of all permanent teeth (if proper space maintenance is employed).*

Q: As shown above, there is a discrepancy between the Angle molar classification (Class I) and the Iowa molar classification (Class II). Why?

A: Although both molar classification schemes are based on the mesiodistal relationship of the maxillary first molar mesiobuccal cusp and the mandibular first molar buccal groove, the Angle classification defines Class I molar occlusal relationship as a range of values, with the range determined by mandibular molar cusp width. The Iowa classification defines Class I molar occlusal relationship as a categorical discrete value, restricted to the ideal molar occlusal relationship. Any variation from this value is defined as "Class II" or "Class III" (see Appendix for a review of the Iowa classification method).

Edward H. Angle defined Class II molar occlusion when the mandibular molars are distal to the normal Class I position "to the extent of more than one-half the width of one cusp." [82] As mandibular molar buccal cusps are, on average, 4–5 mm in mesiodistal width, Angle Class II molar relationship occurs on average when mandibular molars are distal to ideal Class I position by more than 2–2.5 mm.

The Iowa classification simply measures the deviation from an ideal molar relationship. Mandibular molars deviating to the distal of the ideal position are classified as Class II by the millimeter deviation.

In Jake's case, his molar occlusal relationship is Angle Class I because he varies from ideal Class I by less than one-half mandibular buccal cusp width. His Iowa classification molar occlusal relationship is Class II by 1 mm.

Q: Why is the Iowa classification method an improvement?

A: The Iowa classification system gives a *quantitative* description of molar occlusal relationships. This is especially important in the mixed dentition, where diagnosis often includes an estimate of residual leeway space available for mesial movement of permanent first

molars after the loss of succedaneous teeth. Knowing the exact variation in the first permanent molar occlusal relationship allows for better treatment planning.

Q: What are Jake's *primary* problems that you must stay focused on?

A:

Table 4.4 Primary problem list for Jake.

AP	Probable mandibular skeletal deficiency as judged by his facial profile Angle Class I malocclusion Iowa Classification: II (1 mm) x x II (1 mm)
Vertical	50–60% dental deep bite (without palatal impingement)
Transverse	–
Other diagnosis	–

Q: Discuss Jake in the context of three principles applied to every early treatment patient.

A: In the context of the three principles:

1) The goal of early treatment is to correct developing problems – get the patient *back to normal for their stage of development* (including preventing complications such as resorption of adjacent tooth roots, reducing later treatment complexity, and reducing/eliminating unknowns). Obtaining bilateral Class I molar relationships, improving his convex profile/retrusive chin, and improving his deep bite would put Jake back on track.

2) Early treatment should address *very specific problems with a clearly defined end point.* An active treatment component should usually be completed within six to nine months (not protracted over many years, except for some orthopedic problems). Considering Jake's primary problems:

   - His minimal Class II molar relationship could be readily corrected now with Class II orthopedics or in the permanent dentition with any number of Class II correctors (e.g. Class II elastics).

   - His convex profile/retrusive chin may not be improved with orthopedic treatment because his molars are Class II by only 1 mm. Orthopedic treatment encouraging differential mandibular forward growth will likely result in an unacceptable Class III molar relationship. Further, his Class II (1 mm) molar relationship may self-improve with mandibular permanent first molar mesial drift when the mandibular primary second molars exfoliate.

   - His deep bite could be corrected now in six to nine months using fixed orthodontic appliances to level his arches.

3) Always ask yourself: Is it necessary that I treat the patient early? *What harm will come if I choose to do nothing now?* In our opinion, no harm will come if we place Jake on periodic recall. His permanent teeth should erupt normally, and his permanent mandibular molars should drift mesially (after exfoliation of his mandibular primary second molars) with his molars moving into a Class I relationship. In order to improve his chin projection with orthopedics, we would have to devise a treatment plan to provide a Class III molar occlusion.

Q: What reasons would compel you to correct Jake's deep bite now?

A: Reasons include palatal pain or tissue damage from incisor impingement. Jake exhibits neither pain nor tissue damage.

Q: Your associate recommends that you begin Class II orthopedics now to improve Jake's profile. What facts will influence your decision to follow this advice or not?

A: Key facts include the following:
- Jake has a convex profile. Laypersons prefer an orthognathic profile [83].
- The zero-meridian line is a vertical line drawn down from soft-tissue Nasion perpendicular to Frankfort horizontal (Figure 4.37). Ideally, *the chin should lie on the zero-meridian line or just short of it* [84]. Jake's chin is retrusive and sits back further than this.
- Jake is essentially Class I dentally with normal OJ. Using orthopedics to encourage forward growth of Jake's mandible relative to his maxilla would give him a Class III molar relationship and put him in anterior crossbite – unless our treatment plan included retraction of his mandibular anterior teeth. As we said previously, this is too risky and should

not be attempted. Alternatively, moving his maxillary teeth distally to retract his upper lip and reduce his profile convexity is not an option because it would cause his already obtuse nasolabial angle (NLA) to become more obtuse, worsening his nose-to-lip relationship.
- A range of attractiveness exists. We held a thoughtful, sensitive, discussion with Jake's parents – without Jake present. They felt that Jake was a good-looking young man with an acceptable chin position.

Q: Based upon everything we have discussed, what options would you suggest at the conclusion of Jake's consultation appointment?

A: Treatment options include the following:
- *Recall* (no early treatment, monitor only) – evaluate tooth eruption in one year. We feel that this is a reasonable option. Why?
  1) Jake's permanent first molars are Class II by only 1 mm. Our detailed space analysis tells us that his mandibular permanent first molars will have the space to drift to the mesial following exfoliation of his mandibular primary teeth. They will probably drift to the mesial into a bilateral Class I relationship.
  2) We anticipate that his permanent teeth will erupt uneventfully (Figure 4.36d).
  3) His parents are happy with Jake's facial esthetics – including his current profile.
- *Space maintenance* – place an LLHA and/or Nance holding arch before exfoliation of Jake's remaining primary canines and primary molars. We do not recommend this option. Jake currently has 0 mm of maxillary crowding and only mild (2 mm) mandibular anterior crowding. Space maintenance will provide us with *spacing* in both arches following the eruption of all permanent teeth, but an LLHA will greatly reduce/prevent the mandibular permanent first molars from drifting to the mesial into a Class I relationship.
- *Class II orthopedic treatment* – restriction of maxillary growth while allowing continued mandibular forward growth or attempting to accelerate mandibular forward growth. If you choose this option, then you should first make a lateral cephalometric radiograph/cone beam computed tomography (CBCT) to confirm that Jake has a Class II skeletal discrepancy – and not merely an ineffective Pogonion.

  However, we are not enthusiastic about this option. Why? While it is true that Jake has a convex profile/retrusive chin, and while it is true that *now* would be the appropriate time to apply Class II

(a) (b)

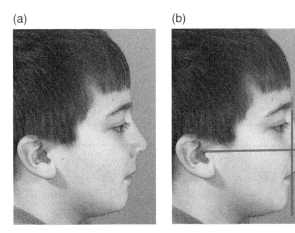

Figure 4.37 Evaluating Jake's chin projection. (a) profile, (b) ideally, the chin should lie on the zero-meridian line or just short of it.

orthopedic treatment (late mixed dentition), Jake is essentially Class I dentally with normal OJ, and his parents like his profile.

- *Extraction of maxillary primary canines* – to facilitate the eruption of Jake's maxillary permanent canines. We do not recommend this option since Jake's maxillary permanent canines appear to be erupting normally (Figure 4.36d).

Q: You present the above options to Jakes' parents at the consultation conclusion. They ask what *you* would do if Jake was your son. What treatment, if any, do you recommend?

A: We recommend *recalling Jake in one year* and treating him to a Class I molar relationship once his permanent teeth erupt. When he is an adult, Jake can decide whether he wants a stronger chin. If he does, then he could consider a genioplasty advancement.

Case Alexandra

Q: Alexandra is eight years old, and she presents to you for a consultation with her parents' chief complaint, "Our daughter's top teeth stick out." PMH and TMJ evaluations are WRN. CR = CO. *Compile your diagnostic findings and problem list*. State your *diagnosis*.

A:

Table 4.5 Diagnostic findings and problem list for Alexandra.

Full face and profile	Frontal View
	The face is symmetric (she appears slightly rotated toward her left in the frontal photo)
	LAFH WRN (soft tissue Glabella – Subnasale = Subnasale – soft tissue Menton)
	Lip competence
	UDML WRN
	Inadequate incisal display during posed smile (maxillary central incisor gingival margins apical to maxillary lip border)
	Large buccal corridors (narrow maxilla)
	Profile View
	Convex profile
	Upturned nasal tip
	NLA WRN (~ 90 degrees)
	Protrusive maxillary and mandibular lips
	Deep labiomental sulcus
	Retrusive chin (hypoplastic mandible)
	Obtuse lip-chin-throat angle
	Short chin-throat length
Radiographs	Early mixed dentition
Intraoral photos and models	Angle Class II division 1
	Iowa classification: II (6 mm) II (5 mm primary canine) II (5 mm primary canine) II (6 mm)
	Diastema between maxillary permanent central incisors
	OJ > 3 mm
	OB 100% (palatal impingement)
	Thin mandibular anterior periodontal biotype (apparent lack of keratinized attached tissue covering the roots of mandibular central incisors)
	Inadequate plaque control
	2 mm maxillary anterior spacing currently present
	1.2 mm of maxillary arch spacing is anticipated following the eruption of all permanent teeth (if appropriate space maintenance is employed)
	5 mm mandibular incisor crowding currently present
	1.8 mm mandibular arch crowding is anticipated following the eruption of all permanent teeth (if appropriate space maintenance is employed)
	Maxillary and mandibular dental arches are symmetric
Other	–
diagnosis	Class II division 1 malocclusion in the early mixed dentition secondary to a skeletally deficient mandible with moderate (5 mm) mandibular incisor crowding

Q: Do you need additional records of Alexandra at this consultation?

A: No additional records are needed in order to decide whether to recall or to initiate early treatment. However, we are certain that a lateral cephalometric radiograph would corroborate our finding of a hypoplastic mandible.

Q: Provide a detailed space analysis for Alexandra's maxillary and mandibular arches. How were the 1.2 mm of maxillary arch spacing and 1.8 mm of mandibular arch crowding calculated (if space maintenance is employed)?

A:

Below are space estimates:
Average mesiodistal widths of permanent teeth (mm): [81]

Maxillary central incisor	8.5	Mandibular central incisor	5.0
Maxillary lateral incisor	6.5	Mandibular lateral incisor	5.5

Maxillary canine	7.5	Mandibular canine	7.0
Maxillary first premolar	7.0	Mandibular first premolar	7.0
Maxillary second premolar	7.0	Mandibular second premolar	7.0
Maxillary first molar	10.0	Mandibular first molar	11.0
Maxillary second molar	9.0	Mandibular second molar	10.5

Average mesiodistal widths of *primary* teeth (mm): [81]

Maxillary central incisor	6.5	Mandibular central incisor	4.2
Maxillary lateral incisor	5.1	Mandibular lateral incisor	4.1
Maxillary canine	7.0	Mandibular canine	5.0
Maxillary first molar	7.3	Mandibular first molar	7.7
Maxillary second molar	8.2	Mandibular second molar	9.9

MAXILLARY ARCH

+2.0 mm of anterior spacing (Figure 4.38h, midline diastema plus small spaces distal to central incisors)
+5.1 mm width of the maxillary right primary lateral incisor
−6.5 mm space needed for maxillary right permanent lateral incisor
+5.1 mm width of maxillary left primary lateral incisor
−6.5 mm space needed for maxillary left permanent lateral incisor
+2.0 mm of anticipated leeway space (1 mm/side)
Balance = + 2 mm + 5.1 mm − 6.5 mm + 5.1 mm − 6.5 mm + 2 mm = +1.2 mm

MANDIBULAR ARCH

−5.0 mm of incisor crowding is currently present
+3.2 mm of anticipated leeway space (1.6 mm/side)
Balance = − 5.0 mm + 3.2 mm = − 1.8 mm

That is, *1.2 mm of maxillary arch spacing and 1.8 mm of mandibular arch crowding is anticipated following the eruption of all permanent teeth (if proper space maintenance is employed).*

Q: You must stay focused on the patient's most significant problems. What are Alexandra's *primary* problems in each dimension (plus other significant problems)?

A:

Table 4.6 Primary problem list for Alexandra.

AP	Angle Class II division 1
	Iowa classification: II (6 mm) II (5 mm primary canine) II (5 mm primary canine) II (6 mm)
	OJ > 3 mm (increasing the risk of dental trauma)
Vertical	100% dental deep bite (palatal impingement)
Transverse	Large buccal corridors (narrow maxilla)
Other diagnosis	Moderate (5 mm) mandibular anterior crowding
	Thin mandibular anterior periodontal biotype
	Inadequate plaque control

Q: Discuss Alexandra in the context of three principles applied to every early treatment patient.

A: In the context of the three principles:

1) The goal of early treatment is to correct developing problems – get the patient *back to normal for their stage of development* (including preventing complications such as resorption of adjacent tooth roots, reducing later treatment complexity, or reducing/eliminating unknowns). Addressing the following problems would put Alexandra back on track:

   - Class II (6 mm) anteroposterior molar relationship and excess incisor OJ (secondary to mandibular skeletal deficiency)
   - Deep bite (secondary to overeruption of mandibular permanent central incisors, Figures 4.38d and 4.38f)
   - Large buccal corridors (narrow maxilla)
   - Moderate mandibular anterior crowding (predicted mild mandibular arch crowding if proper space maintenance is employed)

2) Early treatment should address *very specific problems with a clearly defined end point*, with any active treatment component usually completed within 6 to 9 months and not protracted over years (except for some orthopedic problems). Evaluating Alexandra's problems with this in mind:

   - Her skeletal Class II relationship is a specific problem with a clearly defined end point, but it could take years to correct with orthopedics depending upon her mandibular and maxillary growth magnitude, direction, and timing.
   - Her deep bite could be corrected with fixed orthodontic appliances in six to nine months by leveling her lower arch. Mandibular incisor palatal impingement could be corrected immediately using a vacuum-formed clear maxillary retainer

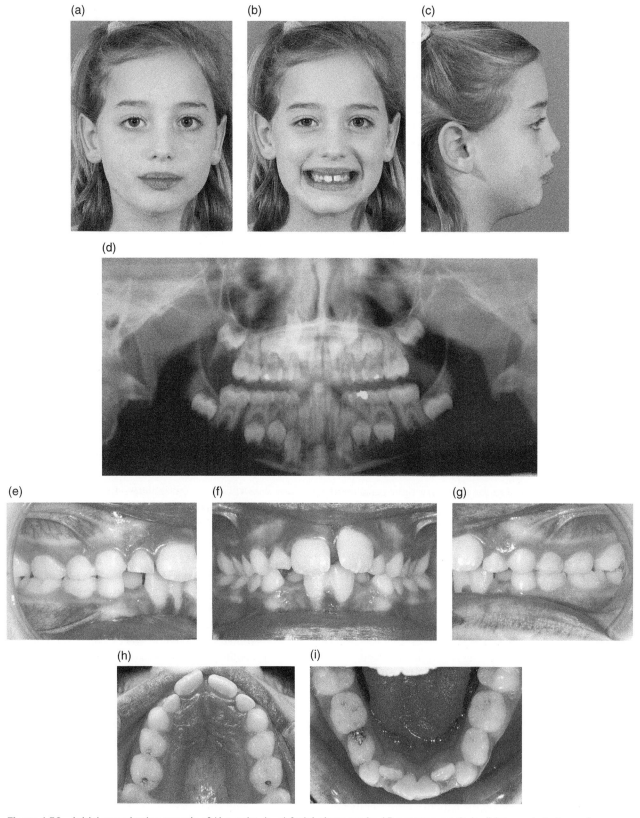

Figure 4.38 Initial consultation records of Alexandra. (a–c) facial photographs, (d) pantomograph, (e–i) intraoral photographs.

that covers only her palate and maxillary incisors (allowing her posterior teeth to erupt slightly).

- Her narrow maxilla could be readily expanded with RME.
- Her moderate (5 mm) mandibular anterior crowding could be reduced using leeway space with an LLHA, but eruption of her mandibular permanent canines and premolars could take years.

3) Always ask yourself: Is it necessary that I treat the patient early? *What harm may result if I choose to do nothing now?* If we do not begin Class II orthopedic treatment now, then we may miss the opportunity to maximize orthopedic treatment effects if she begins her growth acceleration soon. However, at the age of eight years, we anticipate she is about one and a half to two years in advance of beginning her facial growth acceleration, as the average age for female peak mandibular growth velocity is ~eleven and a half years [41]. Also, she is at increased risk for damage to her maxillary incisors if we do not reduce her OJ. Finally, if we do not place an LLHA for another year, or do not expand her maxilla with RME for another year, then we anticipate no harm will result.

Q: What would be a compelling reason to correct Alexandra's deep bite early?

A: A compelling reason would be *if pain or tissue damage resulted from mandibular incisor palatal impingement.* However, clinical examination and discussions with Alexandra reveal neither pain nor tissue damage is present.

Q: Her mom says, "Dad and I are concerned with Alexandra's crowded lower incisors. Shouldn't you take out some teeth?"

How do you respond? Should you extract her mandibular primary canines in order to align her mandibular incisors? Should you begin serial extraction? What do you recommend?

A: Let's consider our options and make a recommendation:

1) *Extraction of mandibular primary canines* – could reduce mandibular incisor crowding (improve incisor alignment) via transeptal fiber pull. However, by extracting mandibular primary canines, you incur the risk of primary and permanent molars drifting to the mesial resulting in arch perimeter loss. Further, we see no compelling reason to put the child through unnecessary surgical procedures. If you decide to extract mandibular primary canines, then we recommend placing an LLHA to *reduce* mesial molar drift and arch perimeter loss.

2) *Serial extraction* – Alexandra is not a good candidate for serial extraction. Why?

The ideal serial extraction patient is in the early mixed dentition and *normal in every way except severe anterior crowding (≥ 9 mm per arch).* Specifically, the ideal serial extraction patient presents with:

- *Class I permanent first molars.* Alexandra is severely Class II (6 mm) secondary to mandibular skeletal deficiency. This Class II relationship should be corrected to Class I *before* permanent tooth extractions. Why? If we follow a serial extraction protocol and eventually extract mandibular premolars in the presence of a Class II interarch relationship, then Alexandra's Class II canine relationship could worsen as her mandibular permanent canines move distally into the mandibular first premolar extraction spaces.
- *Vertically normal to slightly long soft tissue and skeletal LAFH, with minimal OB or possibly a mild open bite, but* not *a deep bite.* Alexandra has a 100% deep bite (palatal impingement). Retracting anterior teeth following premolar extractions could worsen her deep bite.
- *Normal incisor angulation or proclined incisors, but* not *upright incisors.* Without a cephalometric radiograph and analysis, we cannot state whether Alexandra exhibits this feature. However, based upon her intraoral photographs, we believe that her maxillary central incisors are proclined.
- *Normal posterior transverse relationship (normal intermolar arch widths with good posterior interdigitation; absence of posterior crossbites; and absence of significant transverse compensations).* Posterior crossbites are absent. However, Alexandra exhibits large buccal corridors, her maxilla appears narrow (Figure 4.38b), and we cannot rule out the presence of posterior transverse compensations from the records presented.
- *Severe (≥ 9 mm) anterior crowding:* Alexandra does not exhibit this feature because she has only moderate (5 mm) mandibular anterior crowding.

Based upon the above, Alexandra is *not* an ideal candidate for serial extraction. We recommend neither serial extraction nor extraction of mandibular primary canines.

Q: Alexandra has severe OJ (>3 mm) which doubles her risk of maxillary incisor trauma compared to patients without severe OJ. Are there any questions you wish to ask her parents regarding this OJ and trauma?

A: Yes, you should question them regarding: [1, 2]

- Past dental trauma
- Risk-taking behavior
- Participation in sports
- ADHD
- Cognitive psychomotor issues
- Teasing

Her parents deny all of these.

Q: Alexandra's lips cover her incisors (Figure 4.38a). How will this fact, coupled with her parents' negative responses in the previous question, influence your decision to treat early (or not to treat) her severe OJ?

A: Lip soft tissue coverage acts as an incisor cushion in the event of facial trauma. Lip soft tissue coverage and negative responses to the previous question will reduce the need for early OJ reduction treatment.

Q: Alexandra presents with significant mandibular skeletal deficiency (Figure 4.38c). There are three general ways to treat *any* skeletal discrepancy between the jaws. Can you briefly describe them in relation to Alexandra?

A: Skeletal discrepancies (apical base discrepancies) in the anteroposterior, vertical, or transverse dimensions can be treated using orthopedics, masking (camouflage), or surgery.
- *Class II orthopedics* would include restricting Alexandra's forward maxillary growth (while permitting the mandible to continue growing forward) or attempting to accelerate mandibular forward growth.
- *Masking or camouflage* seeks to achieve a Class I (canine) relationship, and excellent occlusion, *dentally* without addressing the underlying skeletal discrepancy. We generally consider masking during comprehensive treatment in adult dentition.
- *Surgery* would involve lengthening her mandible so that it relates properly to her maxilla. We generally consider surgery during comprehensive treatment in adult dentition.

Q: Most orthodontists would probably attempt Class II orthopedic treatment for Alexandra. But such a decision raises two important questions. Is her mandibular skeletal deficiency of prohibitive *magnitude* to attempt orthopedics? If you attempt orthopedics, *when* should you begin?

A: We lack a cephalometric analysis of Alexandra, so we are judging her mandibular skeletal deficiency based upon a very retrusive profile (Figure 4.38c) and 6 mm permanent first molar Class II relationship (Figures 4.38e and 4.38g). However, in our clinical opinion, her mandibular deficiency appears *severe*.

Alexandra is only eight years old, and we have her entire adolescent growth period to attempt correction. Even if we cannot achieve *full* orthopedic correction to Class I with an improved profile, with good compliance, we may be able to at least *improve* her skeletal discrepancy to the point where we can mask/camouflage her, acceptably.

In terms of *when* to attempt orthopedic treatment – there is no advantage in treating Class II relationships in the *early* mixed dentition (except for a possible decrease in incisal trauma as a result of excess OJ) [22–24, 29, 38–40]. However, *even if a patient is in the early mixed dentition – if he/she exhibits good statural growth, we recommend that you consider initiating Class II orthopedic treatment.* We spoke to Alexandra's parents who stated that she had not yet entered her growth spurt and did not appear to be growing continuously.

Q: In terms of growth, what should you ask Alexandra's parents to begin doing?

A: Ask them to begin recording her height, monthly, and to keep you informed of changes. Or, you can recall Alexandra bimonthly or trimonthly to record her change in height yourself.

Q: How else could Alexandra's OJ be reduced – without orthopedics?

A: Closing her maxillary anterior spaces with fixed appliances would retract her maxillary incisors and reduce her OJ. However, her diastema is only a few millimeters wide (Figure 4.38h), and its closure would reduce OJ *minimally*.

Q: What unknowns do you face with Alexandra's treatment?

A: Significant unknowns include future jaw growth magnitude and direction, an undetected CR-CO shift, and patient compliance.

Q: Based upon the above, would you expose and analyze a lateral cephalometric radiograph (or CBCT) of Alexandra and begin early treatment, or would you recall her? If you start early treatment, what options would you consider?

A: Treatment options include the following:
- *Recall* (no early treatment, monitor only) – recall Alexandra in one year to evaluate tooth eruption. This is an excellent option. Why? Alexandra's primary problems are her Class II molar relationship secondary to mandibular skeletal hypoplasia, dental deep bite, narrow maxilla, and moderate mandibular anterior crowding. These problems can all be corrected later.

The highest level of scientific evidence concludes that Class II correction in two stages (early initial treatment followed by later adolescent treatment) does not offer any advantages over one stage treatment (later adolescent) [85] – except possibly a reduction in incisal trauma. Alexandra has no history of incisor trauma, she is in the early mixed dentition, and her parents state that she does not appear to be growing.

Her dental deep bite can be corrected later (she lacks pain when biting and tissue trauma), her narrow maxilla can be corrected later (before puberty), and her moderate mandibular anterior crowding can be improved later using leeway space and placement of an LLHA.

- *Space maintenance* – placement of an LLHA before exfoliation of Alexandra's primary canines and primary molars. Space maintenance is reasonable at a future date because 1.8 mm of mandibular arch crowding is anticipated following the eruption of all permanent teeth if one is employed. However, there is no compelling need to place an LLHA now, since the emergence of her permanent canines and premolars is not imminent. We would not recommend a Nance holding arch since it will not improve Alexandra's Class II molar relationship.
- *Class II orthopedic treatment* – since Alexandra is in the early mixed dentition and a change in her statural height is not apparent, we recommend delaying initiation of Class II orthopedic treatment.
- *Mandibular space regaining* – opening space for Alexandra's mandibular permanent lateral incisors. Since we cannot say with certainty that Alexandra's mandibular primary lateral incisors were lost prematurely or that her deep bite forced her mandibular incisors lingually (reducing arch length), we cannot say with certainty that opening these spaces would be space regaining. Also, proclining her mandibular anterior teeth by opening lateral spaces would be ill-advised because of the very thin periodontal biotype labial to her mandibular central incisors (Figure 4.38f). Gingival recession could result if her mandibular central incisors are proclined. Finally, since we anticipate minimal mandibular arch crowding (1.8 mm) if we place an LLHA, there is no compelling reason to open space for the mandibular lateral incisors now.
- *RME* – to widen Alexandra's maxilla and reduce her large buccal corridors. If Alexandra exhibited a lateral CR-CO shift into a unilateral crossbite, then we would strongly recommend RME to reduce the likelihood of her growing into a mandibular skeletal asymmetry. However, she does not exhibit a lateral shift. RME may eventually be recommended, especially if Alexandra exhibits significant posterior dental compensations (maxillary molar buccal crown torque,

mandibular molar lingual crown torque). At that time, expanding her maxilla would increase her posterior OJ which could then be used to upright her mandibular posterior teeth transversely without putting her into posterior crossbite. Another reason to eventually consider RME would be to provide better arch coordination if differential jaw growth brings a wider part of her mandible forward relative to her maxilla.

- *Extraction of maxillary primary canines (and possibly maxillary primary first molars)* – to facilitate eruption of Alexandra's maxillary permanent canines. Although such treatment may eventually be considered, Alexandra's dental development is too early (Figure 4.38d) to consider primary tooth extractions now.
- *Extraction of mandibular primary canines* – to improve mandibular incisor alignment. Sometimes, parents insist on this treatment, but you must be careful about letting parents dictate treatment. It would be better to educate parents about leeway space and space maintenance which, in many cases, reduces or eliminates mandibular anterior crowding *spontaneously*. If you decide to extract mandibular primary canines, then place an LLHA to minimize potential arch perimeter loss due to mesial molar drift.
- *Serial extraction* – as discussed earlier, Alexandra is *not* an ideal candidate for serial extraction.

Q: What treatment do you recommend at the end of this consultation?

A: Since Alexandra was not exhibiting good statural growth velocity (was not growing continuously or entering her adolescent growth spurt), we decided to monitor only and recall her in one year. Her parents said they would measure her height each month and inform us of changes. We told her parents that Alexandra was at an increased risk of maxillary incisor trauma due to her OJ being >3 mm and recommended that she wear a mouthguard when playing sports.

Q: If Alexandra's parents later reported regular increases in her height, or when Alexandra enters the late mixed dentition, how will you proceed?

A: We would take new records, including a lateral cephalometric radiograph. Based upon our analysis at that time, we anticipate treating her with RME to widen her maxilla and reduce her buccal corridors, with an LLHA to reduce mandibular anterior crowding using leeway space and to reduce mandibular first permanent molar eruption (thereby helping B-point to rotate forward with mandibular growth), and with high-pull headgear to restrict forward maxillary growth while allowing her mandible to continue growing forward. High-pull headgear wear will also retract maxillary molars distally (helping to correct the Class II relationship) and reduce maxillary molar eruption (helping B-point to rotate forward with mandibular growth). We may also fabricate and ask her to wear a mandibular clear retainer to disarticulate her occlusion. We would not treat her with a Class II functional appliance because we do not want her mandibular incisors to procline and stress her mandibular labial periodontal tissue.

Note: Placement of an LLHA will force Class II correction through headgear effects – and not through mandibular permanent molar mesial drift.

Q: What will be your eventual goals (comprehensive treatment goals, not early treatment goals) for Alexandra?

A: Goals will include improving her profile and smile, increasing her chin projection, achieving a Class I canine relationship, achieving a Class I molar relationship if she is treated either non-extraction or with the extraction of two premolars in both arches, and achieving minimal OB and OJ.

Case Mark

Q: Mark is nine years and two months old (Figure 4.39). He presents to you with his parent's chief complaint, "Mark's top teeth stick out. We are afraid he may break them." His PMH, TMJ, and periodontal evaluations are WRN. CR = CO. *Compile your diagnostic findings and problem list.* State your *diagnosis.*

A:

Table 4.7 Diagnostic findings and problem list for Mark.

Full face and profile	**Frontal View**
	Face is asymmetric – right eye and ear are lower than left when nose and philtrum are vertical
	LAFH WRN (soft tissue Glabella – Subnasale = Subnasale – soft tissue Menton)
	ILG of 3 mm with maxillary incisor exposure
	UDML WRN
	Incisal display during posed smile WRN (maxillary central incisor gingival margins approximately coincident with maxillary lip border)
	Large buccal corridors
	Profile View
	Convex profile
	Protrusive maxillary lip
	Deep labiomental sulcus
	Retrusive chin position
	Lip-chin-throat angle WRN
	Chin-throat length WRN
Ceph analysis	**Skeletal**
	Maxilla-deficient anteroposteriorly (A-Point lies behind Nasion-perpendicular line)
	Mandible deficient anteroposteriorly (ANB angle = 5° with a maxillary deficiency)
	LAFH WRN (LAFH/TAFH × 100% = 55%)
	Steep MPA (FMA = 31°, SN-MP = 35°)
	Effective bony Pogonion (bony Pogonion ahead of line extended from Nasion through B-point)
	Dental
	Maxillary incisor inclination WRN (U1 to SN = 105° which is greater than a normal value of 101–103°, but Sella appears high)
	Proclined mandibular incisors (FMIA = 52°)
Radiographs	Mark is just entering the late mixed dentition stage of development
Intraoral photos and models	Angle Class II division 1
	Iowa Classification: II (6 mm) II (4 mm) II (4 mm) II (6 mm)
	OJ 8–9 mm (Figure 4.39r)
	OB 100% (palatal impingement, Figure 4.39q)
	0.0 mm of maxillary anterior crowding is currently present (1 mm midline diastema spacing and 1 mm of maxillary left lateral incisor crowding)
	2.0 mm maxillary spacing is anticipated following the eruption of all permanent teeth (if appropriate space maintenance is employed)
	4.0 mm mandibular anterior crowding is currently present
	3.2 mm mandibular spacing is anticipated following the eruption of all permanent teeth (if appropriate space maintenance is employed)
	Maxillary midline diastema with low frenum attachment (Figure 4.39h)
	Maxillary and mandibular dental arches are symmetric
	Maxillary and mandibular midlines are coincident
	Periodontal biotype labial to the mandibular central incisors WRN
	Palatal indentations due to mandibular incisor impingement (Figure 4.39j) but neither tissue trauma nor pain noted.
Other diagnosis	Class II division 1 malocclusion secondary to maxillary and mandibular skeletal hypoplasia with proclined and moderately crowded (4 mm) mandibular incisors

Q: Do you wish to make any additional records?

A: No additional records are needed in order to decide whether to recall Mark or begin early treatment.

Q: Provide a detailed space analysis for Mark's maxillary and mandibular arches. How were the 2.0 mm of maxillary spacing and 3.2 mm of mandibular spacing calculated (if space maintenance is employed)?

A:

Average mesiodistal widths of permanent teeth (mm): [81]

Maxillary central incisor	8.5	Mandibular central incisor	5.0
Maxillary lateral incisor	6.5	Mandibular lateral incisor	5.5

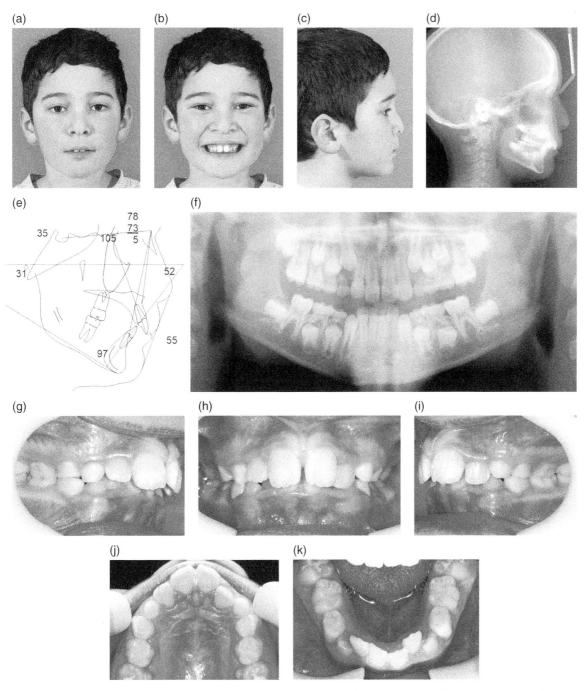

Figure 4.39 Initial records of Mark: (a–c) facial photographs, (d–e) lateral cephalometric radiograph and tracing, (f) pantomograph, (g–k) intraoral photographs, (l–r) models.

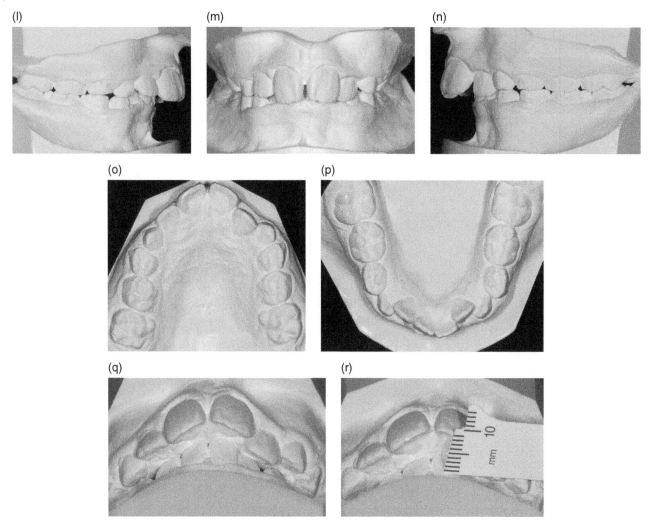

(l) (m) (n) (o) (p) (q) (r)

Figure 4.39 (Continued)

Maxillary canine	7.5	Mandibular canine	7.0	Maxillary first molar	7.3	Mandibular first molar	7.7
Maxillary first premolar	7.0	Mandibular first premolar	7.0	Maxillary second molar	8.2	Mandibular second molar	9.9
Maxillary second premolar	7.0	Mandibular second premolar	7.0				
Maxillary first molar	10.0	Mandibular first molar	11.0				
Maxillary second molar	9.0	Mandibular second molar	10.5				

Average mesiodistal widths of *primary* teeth (mm): [81]

Maxillary central incisor	6.5	Mandibular central incisor	4.2
Maxillary lateral incisor	5.1	Mandibular lateral incisor	4.1
Maxillary canine	7.0	Mandibular canine	5.0

MAXILLARY ARCH
+1.0 mm of anterior spacing (midline diastema, Figure 4.39j)
−1.0 mm of left lateral incisor crowding
+2.0 mm of anticipated leeway space (1.0 mm/side)
Balance = + 1.0 mm −1.0 mm + 2.0 mm = +2.0 mm

MANDIBULAR ARCH (leeway space cannot be included because mandibular permanent canines have already erupted)
+9.9 mm width mandibular left primary second molar
−7.0 mm anticipated width mandibular left second premolar
+7.7 mm width mandibular left primary first molar
−7.0 mm anticipated width mandibular left first premolar

−4.0 mm anterior crowding currently present

+7.7 mm width mandibular right primary first molar

−7.0 mm anticipated width mandibular right first premolar

+9.9 mm width mandibular right primary second molar

7.0 mm anticipated width mandibular right second premolar

Balance = +9.9 mm − 7.0 mm + 7.7 mm − 7.0 mm − 4.0 mm + 7.7 mm − 7.0 mm + 9.9 mm − 7.0 mm

= +3.2 mm

That is, *2 mm of maxillary spacing and 3.2 mm of mandibular spacing are anticipated following the eruption of all permanent teeth (if proper space maintenance is employed).*

Q: What is the first principle of all orthodontic treatment?

A: *First Principle: Define the patient's **primary** problems in each dimension (plus other major problems) and stay focused on these problems during treatment planning and throughout treatment delivery. At every appointment, check primary problems in CR.*

Q: What are Mark's primary problems?

A:

Table 4.8   Primary problem list for Mark.

AP	Maxillary and mandibular skeletal hypoplasia with relative mandibular deficiency
	(ANB angle = 5° with maxillary anteroposterior deficiency)
	Angle Class II division 1 molar (6 mm) relationship
	8–9 mm OJ
Vertical	Borderline hyperdivergent skeletal pattern (FMA = 31°; SN-MP = 35°, but high Sella position)
	100% dental deep bite (palatal impingement)
Transverse	–
Other diagnosis	Moderate (4 mm) mandibular anterior crowding
	Proclined mandibular incisors

Q: We lack a frontal intraoral photograph with Mark's teeth separated. Such a photograph would help evaluate his vertical dental relationship. However, we can separate his models to make this evaluation. What do you see in Figures 4.40a and 4.40b?

A: Mark's maxillary incisors are stepped down (overerupted) by 2–3 mm relative to his maxillary posterior teeth, and his mandibular incisors are stepped up (overerupted) 4 mm relative to his mandibular posterior teeth.

Q: What did this incisor overeruption cause?

A: Incisor overeruption caused Mark's dental deep bite and palatal impingement.

Q: Discuss Mark in the context of three principles applied to every early treatment patient.

A: In the context of the three principles:

1) The goal of early treatment is to correct developing problems – get the patient *back to normal for their stage of development* (including preventing complications such as resorption of adjacent tooth roots, reducing later treatment complexity, or reducing/eliminating unknowns). Correcting Mark's Class II skeletal and dental relationships, excessive OJ, and dental deep bite, alleviating his moderate mandibular anterior crowding, and uprighting his mandibular incisors would get Mark back on track for his stage of development.

2) Early treatment should address *very specific problems with a clearly defined end point*, with any active treatment component completed within six to nine months (except for some orthopedic problems). Orthopedic correction of Mark's Class II discrepancy and excessive OJ could take longer than six to nine months.

His deep bite could be corrected by leveling dental arches with fixed orthodontic appliances within six to nine months, but uprighting his mandibular incisors could take longer. His moderate (4 mm) mandibular crowding could be resolved by placing an LLHA, but this correction may take longer than nine months

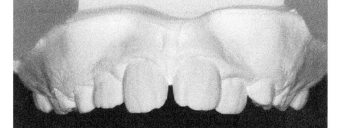

(a)

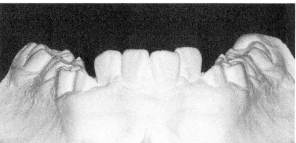

(b)

Figure 4.40   (a–b) Mark's models viewed from the front.

depending upon when Mark's permanent teeth erupt. Also, please remember that placement of an LLHA will not only prevent uprighting of his mandibular anterior teeth but will *procline* them slightly [86, 87].

3) Always ask yourself: Is it necessary that I treat the patient now? *What harm may occur if I choose to recall?* If we do not begin Class II orthopedics, then we may miss significant growth during the next year. If we do not place an LLHA, then the first permanent molar mesial drift will reduce the amount of leeway space available for incisor alignment as Mark transitions to the permanent dentition. Note the tradeoff – first molar mesial drift can improve Mark's Class II relationship but will reduce leeway space for incisor alignment. Finally, since neither pain nor tissue damage has resulted from mandibular incisor palatal impingement, we do not anticipate harm by postponing deep bite correction.

Q: What would be compelling reasons to correct Mark's dental deep bite now?

A: If Mark complained that biting the roof of his mouth hurt, or if we noted tissue damage, then these would be reasons to consider intruding his mandibular incisors early or providing a clear maxillary retainer with palatal coverage/anterior teeth coverage (promoting eruption of his posterior teeth to open his bite).

Q: Mark has moderate (4 mm) mandibular anterior crowding coupled with proclined mandibular incisors (Frankfort horizontal to mandibular incisor angle [FMIA] = 52°). To provide space to upright his proclined incisors, we could extract premolars. Let's discuss the possibility of treating him with premolar extractions. What features are found in an *ideal* serial extraction patient? Does Mark exhibit these features?

A: The ideal serial extraction patient is in the early mixed dentition stage of development and is *normal in every way except severe anterior crowding (≥ 9 mm per arch)*. Specifically, the patient should present with:

- *Class I first permanent molars.* Mark's first permanent molars are Class II by 6 mm secondary to mandibular deficiency. This relationship should be corrected to Class I *before* the thought of mandibular premolar extractions is entertained. If we extract mandibular premolars in the presence of a full-step Class II molar relationship, then Mark's Class II canine relationship could worsen as the canines are retracted distally into the premolar spaces.
- *Vertically normal to slightly long soft tissue and skeletal LAFH, with minimal OB or possibly a mild open bite, but* not *a deep bite.* Mark exhibits a normal skeletal LAFH but has a 100% OB. Depending upon the amount of crowding, when we extract premolars,

incisors are retracted by tipping the incisor crowns posteriorly along an arc viewed from the sagittal, with the incisor apices as the approximate center of rotation. If we employ premolar extraction treatment for Mark, then it may be difficult to improve his existing deep OB, or his deep OB could worsen. Mark's deep OB is not ideal for a serial extraction approach.

- *Normal incisor angulation or proclined incisors, but* not *upright incisors.* Mark exhibits this feature since he has proclined mandibular incisors and normally inclined maxillary incisors.
- *Normal posterior transverse relationship (normal intermolar arch widths with good posterior interdigitation; absence of posterior crossbites; and absence of significant transverse compensations).* Mark lacks a posterior crossbite, but his mandibular posterior teeth exhibit lingual crown torque (Figure 4.40b).
- *Severe (≥ 9 mm) anterior crowding*: Mark does not exhibit this feature.

Based upon the above, we conclude that Mark is *not* an ideal candidate for serial extraction.

Q: Mark has a midline diastema with low labial frenum attachment (Figure 4.39h). How do you deal with this condition? *When* do you deal with it?

A: Assuming that the midline diastema does not spontaneously close during maxillary permanent canine eruption, you can wait to close it orthodontically when Mark undergoes comprehensive orthodontic treatment. Of course, you can close it earlier if it is causing psychosocial problems (teasing).

If the diastema is closed orthodontically, then a bonded lingual retainer should be placed between the maxillary central incisors to keep it closed. To avoid Mark biting on a bonded maxillary lingual retainer, Mark's deep bite will first need to be reduced to a shallow OB. If the gingival tissues "bunch up" during space closure, then a gingivoplasty (frenectomy) should be performed – *after* diastema closure so the surgical scar tissue will aid in maintaining closure but not impede space closure [88].

Q: Mark has a significant Class II skeletal discrepancy (mandibular deficiency). Of the three general ways to deal with any skeletal discrepancy of the jaws, can you list specific treatments for each?

A: Skeletal discrepancies can be dealt with using orthopedics, masking (camouflage), or surgery.
Orthopedics (restriction of maxillary growth while permitting the mandible to continue growing or acceleration of mandibular growth). Options include:

- Headgears: High-pull, straight-pull, and cervical-pull headgears retract maxillary molars distally, restrict maxillary forward growth, but allow the mandible to grow forward. All three effects would help correct Mark's Class II molar relationship.

In addition, a high-pull headgear may reduce descent of the maxillary corpus and maxillary first molars, potentially further improving Class II correction by relative mandibular forward rotation [6–8]. A cervical-pull headgear rotates the palatal plane down and back slightly and erupts maxillary first molars (<1 mm) compared to controls [7, 8, 11] – but these effects will not help Mark. A straight-pull headgear (a combination of high-pull and cervical-pull headgears) will produce an effect somewhere between the effect of a high-pull and a cervical pull.

- Class II functional appliances: Tend to restrict maxillary forward growth, retract/distalize maxillary posterior teeth, upright maxillary incisors, move mandibular posterior teeth to the mesial, procline mandibular incisors, accelerate condylar growth, and displace the glenoid fossae mesially [14, 15].

Functional appliances *accelerate* mandibular growth in growing individuals but *do not enhance* mandibular horizontal growth beyond that found in control subjects [16]. Further, the *direction* of condylar growth when Class II functional appliances are employed (posterior superiorly) may not correct the mandibular skeletal deficiency or improve chin projection [17, 18]. Since Mark has a steep MPA and proclined mandibular incisors, he would not be an ideal candidate for a Herbst appliance or another functional appliance. Why? His MPA could steepen more, his mandibular incisors could procline more, and he may experience an undesirable increase in LAFH [19].

Masking or camouflage (achieving a Class I canine relationship and excellent occlusion without correcting the underlying skeletal discrepancy). Masking is generally an option in adult dentition during comprehensive orthodontic treatment when:

- The patient's response to orthopedics was unsatisfactory
- The patient's growth is complete or nearly complete (*avoid irreversible treatment, including extraction of premolars, until unknowns are reduced/eliminated*)
- Treating the patient dentally will not create unacceptable dental compensations or unfavorable esthetics
- *First Principle of Masking* – the smaller the skeletal discrepancy, more normal the patient esthetics, and smaller the dental compensations, the more successful masking (camouflage) will be; the greater the skeletal discrepancy, less normal the patient esthetics, and larger the dental compensations, the less successful masking (camouflage) will be.

Class II masking options in the permanent dentition include:

- Extraction of maxillary first premolars to permit retraction of maxillary canines and incisors – achieving a Class I canine relationship but leaving molars Class II. This is an example of intra-arch mechanics.
- Intra-arch mechanics employing TADs to distalize the entire maxillary arch into a Class I relationship. For example, using a Class II corrector such as a pendulum appliance supported by TADs attached to the palatal acrylic button. (Note: Such Class II correctors *without* TAD support are capable of distalizing molars but at the expense of reciprocal premolar-to-premolar mesial tooth movement).
- Interarch mechanics such as Class II elastics or Class II springs.

Surgery (mandibular advancement) is generally an option for more severe Class II skeletal discrepancies in the permanent dentition. If orthopedic treatment response is poor, and if the patient is a poor candidate for masking, then surgery may be our best option. Class II patients and their parents should be informed of this.

Q: If you choose to treat Mark's Class II skeletal discrepancy with orthopedics – *when* should you begin? Is the magnitude of his Class II discrepancy too large to attempt orthopedics?

A: Let's begin by considering the *magnitude* of his skeletal discrepancy. We see (Figures 4.39e, 4.39l, and 4.39n) that his Class II skeletal discrepancy is severe. He has an ANB angle of 5°, a retrusive mandible *and* retrusive maxilla, and he is 6 mm bilateral Class II at his molars.

However, he is only nine years old. So, we have his entire period of adolescent growth to attempt orthopedic correction. If Mark is cooperative, then we have a chance to at least improve his skeletal discrepancy with orthopedics. That is, even if he does not fully correct the Class II discrepancy, at least he may be able to improve it to the point where we could successfully mask it (camouflage).

Next, let's consider *when* to attempt orthopedic treatment. Generally, Class II correction should be delayed until the patient is in the late mixed dentition of development – as opposed to the early mixed dentition [22–24, 29, 38–40]. Since Mark is entering his late mixed dentition stage of development, now is a good time to attempt Class II orthopedic treatment. But remember: *even if a patient is in the early mixed dentition, if he/she has good statural growth velocity, then you should consider initiating Class II orthopedic treatment.*

Q: Not only is Mark's mandible deficient, his *maxilla* is deficient also. Should we be concerned about adverse profile effects if we restrain Mark's deficient maxilla with orthopedics – especially if he wears a headgear? In other words, will he end up with a "dished-in" profile if we use a headgear?

A: This is an excellent question, and the answer is surprising – no. Headgear treatment used in conjunction with fixed orthodontic appliances improves facial profile esthetics in growing Class II patients with protrusive, normally positioned, or *retrusive* maxillae [89].

Q: Mark has severe OJ (8 mm), and his maxillary incisors are only partially covered by his lip (Figure 4.39a). His severe OJ doubles the risk of maxillary incisor trauma compared to patients without severe OJ. Are there questions you should ask his parents in regards to this? How does his severe OJ affect your decision to begin Class II treatment?

A: You should ask Mark's parents about:
- Past dental trauma
- History of risk-taking behavior
- Participation in sports
- ADHD or cognitive psychomotor issues
- Teasing [1, 2].

His parents deny all of these. However, his severe OJ is one additional problem influencing your decision to begin orthopedic treatment.

Q: No compelling reason exists to correct Mark's 100% deep bite at the present time (no pain upon biting or tissue trauma). But, how will you eventually correct his deep bite?

A: Let's first clarify the above statement. You *could* open Mark's deep bite now by placing 2x4 fixed appliances in both arches (bonding first molars and incisors) to intrude overerupted incisors with archwires. However, Mark will eventually undergo comprehensive orthodontic treatment after all his permanent teeth erupt. So, waiting until then to correct his deep bite is reasonable.

How will you open Mark's deep bite after all permanent teeth erupt? We will place fixed appliances on all permanent teeth and level both arches with a series of increasingly stiffer archwires. The mechanics (Figure 4.41) that will open Mark's bite include:

- Intruding maxillary and mandibular incisors (0.26–1.88 mm and 0.19–2.84 mm, respectively) [90].
- Proclining maxillary and mandibular incisors (rotating incisal edges around apices).
- Erupting mandibular premolars by leveling the curve of Spee [91]. This premolar eruption will tend to

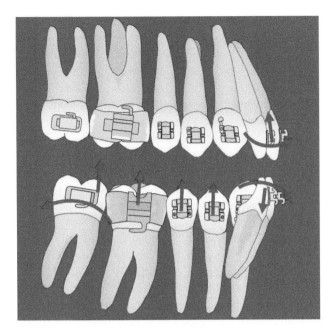

Figure 4.41 Effects of opening a deep overbite (OB) with fixed orthodontic appliances and archwires.

rotate Mark's mandible down and back – opening his OB but worsening his molar Class II relationship.
- Erupting mandibular molars. Because mandibular molars tip to the mesial as part of the curve of Spee, uprighting them will rotate their crowns around distal root tips causing their mesial roots to erupt, rotating the mandibular plane down and back, opening the OB, but worsening the molar Class II relationship.

Q: As noted earlier, Mark lacks a posterior crossbite, but his mandibular posterior teeth exhibit lingual crown torque. In addition, what do you observe regarding his *maxillary* posterior teeth (Figure 4.42a)?

A: Mark exhibits slight maxillary permanent first molar *lingual* crown torque in addition to his significant mandibular permanent first molar lingual crown torque.

Q: Is it necessary to upright Mark's permanent first molars by eliminating their lingual crown torque?

A: If our goal is to achieve an ideal occlusion, then we should upright Mark's permanent first molars. Why? Mandibular permanent first molars normally erupt with lingual torque, maxillary permanent first molars erupt with buccal crown torque, and all permanent first molars normally *upright* during adolescence [92]. So, it is normal for permanent first molars to upright, and ideal treatment should be directed at achieving upright molars.

On the other hand, leaving mandibular molars with some lingual crown torque, or maxillary molars with

(a)

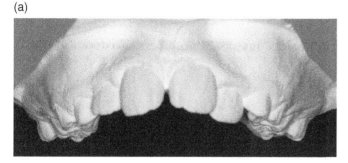

(b)

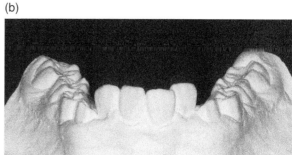

Figure 4.42 (a–b) Evaluation of Mark's maxillary and mandibular crown torque.

some buccal crown torque, is not detrimental to health. In fact, *posterior crown torques frequently act as compensation for transverse skeletal discrepancies in the absence of posterior crossbites.* One study reported a large range of transverse skeletal base relationships, with accompanying dental compensations, in Class I subjects without crossbites [93].

Q: How would you upright Mark's permanent first molars? When would you upright Mark's permanent first molars?

A: How? Like so many orthodontic problems, transverse treatment is based upon the *magnitude* of the problem. In Mark's case, the magnitude of this problem is not large, and we hope to be able to upright his first molars using archwires alone. In fact, Mark has slight maxillary first permanent molar *palatal* crown torque. So, his maxillary first permanent molars can be expanded labially (uprighted) with archwires to create OJ which will then allow some labial (uprighting) movement of his mandibular first permanent molars.

When? Since we do not anticipate using RME, there is no need to make this correction before/during puberty. Archwires can be used to address this problem during comprehensive treatment.

Q: What is the impact of Mark's full-step Class II molar relationship on his *transverse* relationship? In other words, if we incorporate orthopedics to achieve a Class I correction, then what impact will this have on Mark's transverse relationship?

A: Class II correction with orthopedics involves differential forward growth of the mandible relative to maxilla. As the mandible moves forward, a broader part of the mandibular arch moves forward relative to the maxillary arch. So, there is a tendency for a posterior *lingual* crossbite to develop.

Let's discuss this in more detail. Assuming normal maxillary lingual cusp-mandibular fossa occlusion, a full-step (6 mm) Class II molar relationship initially requires a reduction of the maxillary intermolar width, an expansion of mandibular intermolar width, or both, to accommodate maxillary molar occlusion in a narrower portion of the mandibular arch. That is, the cross-arch width at the distal fossa of the mandibular second premolar is less than the cross-arch width at the central fossa of the mandibular first molar and transverse molar positions must be modified to allow maxillary cusp-mandibular fossa occlusion. Studied longitudinally in mixed dentition subjects, it appears that the most common finding of Class II molar relationship is a narrowing of maxillary intermolar width by 1.5–2.5 mm [94].

Given this, during orthopedic correction from Class II molar relationship to Class I molar relationship, simultaneous expansion of maxillary first molar intermolar width may be required. This will accommodate maintenance of maxillary cusp-mandibular fossa occlusion during the differential forward growth of the mandible. Depending on initial transverse inclinations of the maxillary molars, the necessary expansion may be addressed via rapid maxillary expansion in combination with orthopedic Class II treatment, or simple headgear bow expansion to increase maxillary intermolar width during headgear treatment.

Q: What unknowns do you face with Mark?

A: Unknowns include amount and direction of maxillary and mandibular growth, compliance, and the presence of an undetected CR-CO shift.

Q: Based upon the above, would you start early treatment or recall Mark? If you start treatment, then what options would you consider?

A: Treatment options include the following:

- *Recall* (no early treatment, monitor only) – is not recommended. Why? Although Mark's age is nine years and two months which is younger than the average onset of growth acceleration for boys (~ 12 years of age [95]), Mark's parents state that he is *exhibiting statural growth now*. Further, his parents state that he would be very cooperative now. Finally, many of his canines and premolars may erupt before a twelve-month recall, and we may miss the opportunity to manage his leeway space if we wait. Based upon these facts, we recommend beginning early treatment and not waiting.

- *Space maintenance* – an LLHA is recommended before exfoliation of Mark's mandibular primary second molars in order to provide "E-space" for spontaneous incisor alignment. If RME is employed to create OJ, then we would recommend uprighting Mark's mandibular molars first – before LLHA placement. A Nance holding arch is not recommended if we attempt to move Mark's maxillary molars distally during Class II correction.
- *Mandibular space maintenance plus headgear orthopedics* – is recommended. Headgear wear will correct Mark's Class II relationship by moving his maxillary molars distally, restricting his maxillary forward growth, and allowing his mandible to continue growing forward.

Placement of an LLHA will reduce/prevent mandibular first permanent molar mesial drift as primary molars are lost – forcing Class II correction to occur through differential jaw growth or maxillary molar distal movement with headgear. An LLHA will also reduce mandibular first permanent molar eruption that often occurs as *compensation* for the restraint of maxillary molar eruption by HPHG. The combined effect fosters forward mandibular rotation and forward movement of B-point.

A high-pull headgear is the best option. It can reduce descent of the maxillary corpus and reduce eruption of maxillary molars which helps B-point rotate forward with mandibular growth. A cervical-pull headgear will tip Mark's anterior palatal plane down and erupt his maxillary first molars slightly – neither effect helping him.

- *Class II functional appliance orthopedics (Herbst treatment)* – is not recommended. Herbst treatment effects include:

Inhibition of maxillary growth

Distal movement of maxillary teeth

Intrusion of maxillary molars in the majority of patients

Occlusal plane tipping down in the anterior in the majority of patients

Acceleration of mandibular growth

Mesial movement of mandibular teeth (mandibular incisor proclination) [14]

The cost of using a Herbst appliance on Mark would be additional incisor proclination. His mandibular incisors are already proclined (FMIA = 52°). During Herbst treatment, lower incisors procline an average of 11°, and although post treatment, they rebound by an average of 8° [95], additional incisor proclination is still a fact. In addition, Mark has a steep MPA – *hyperdivergent Herbst patients undergo a deleterious backward mandibular rotation and increases in face height* [19]. Herbst appliance treatment is not the first choice for Mark.

- *Mandibular space regaining* (opening space for Mark's mandibular permanent canines) – is not recommended. First, we cannot term this *space regaining* because Mark's records do not show premature mandibular primary canine loss resulting in space loss. More importantly, opening space for Mark's mandibular permanent canines would procline his mandibular incisors more.
- *Extraction of maxillary primary canines (and possibly maxillary primary first molars)* – is not recommended. Extraction of maxillary primary teeth could be performed in order to create space for, and a pathway for the eruption of, Mark's maxillary permanent canines. Since there is no overlap of Mark's maxillary permanent canine crowns across the roots of his maxillary permanent lateral incisors (Figure 4.39f), and since his maxillary primary canine roots appear to be resorbing normally, there is no compelling reason to extract Mark's maxillary primary canines.
- *Mandibular anterior interproximal reduction (IPR)* – is not recommended. IPR could provide a few millimeters of space that could be used to upright proclined mandibular incisors. However, depending upon the amount of enamel removed, an anterior Bolton tooth size discrepancy could result (excess maxillary incisor OJ and excess canine OJ). Further, it is too early to perform this treatment. It would be better to reassess the need for IPR after all of the permanent teeth erupt.
- *RME* – would create posterior OJ and allow us to upright Mark's mandibular first permanent molars. However, Mark is not in posterior crossbite, and his maxillary molars are also tipped to the lingual. So, we think we can upright his mandibular molars using archwires alone after his maxillary incisors are uprighted.
- *Serial extraction* – is not recommended. As discussed earlier, Mark is *not* an ideal candidate for serial extraction.

Q: What treatment do you recommend?

A: A decision was made to *reduce unknowns* before making a final treatment decision, especially before making an irreversible treatment decision such as extracting permanent teeth. Mark was placed on an HPHG to correct his Class II relationship and reduce his profile convexity by promoting differential mandibular growth. Mark's parents were correct in their anticipation of Mark's compliance. Headgear was worn every day with approximately 300 gm of force per side from 8 pm until the next morning. Mark was very compliant. Once his molar relationship was slightly overcorrected to Class III (1 mm), he wore the headgear only to bed and only with minimum force to maintain the molar relationship. We monitored the correction during the remainder of the treatment.

Although Mark's deep bite correction could have been postponed until he was in the permanent dentition, a decision was made to correct it early. Mandibular *primary* second molars were bonded, a "tip-back" bend placed in the archwire mesial to the primary second molars, and incisors intruded (opening the bite). The advantage of using primary second molars, instead of permanent first molars, is that unfavorable reactive eruptive forces are applied against a primary tooth which will be later exfoliated.

The biomechanics of the tip-back bend are illustrated in Figures 4.43a and 4.43b. As shown, an intrusive force to the incisors results while a reactive extrusive force and CCW moment result against the primary molars. Once Mark's mandibular incisors were intruded, an LLHA was placed (Figure 4.43c).

Mark also wore a full-coverage maxillary occlusal bite plate to stretch his masseteric sling/reduce molar eruption and disarticulate his occlusion. Reducing molar eruption helps rotate the mandible forward during growth and thereby advances B-point. Occlusal disarticulation unlocks the bite and allows the mandibular teeth to move forward unimpeded with the growing mandible – thereby maximizing Class II correction.

Q: Following the eruption of all permanent teeth, early treatment was complete. Discussions were held with Mark and his parents regarding early treatment success

(a) (b)

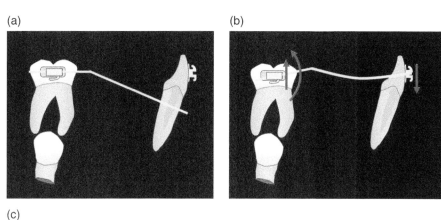

(c)

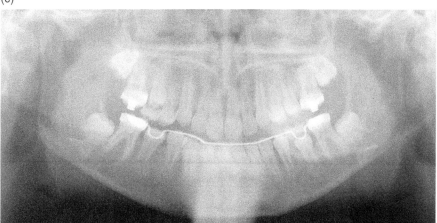

Figure 4.43 Mark's early mandibular arch treatment. (a and b) A 2x4 fixed appliance with "tip-back" bends placed in the archwire mesial to the mandibular primary second molars causes intrusion of mandibular incisors, the eruption of the primary molars, and opening of the bite. After his bite was opened, brackets were removed and an LLHA was placed (c).

and comprehensive treatment options – including extraction/non-extraction of premolars. Mark and his parents requested non-extraction treatment.

Fixed orthodontic appliances were placed. Arches were leveled, aligned, and finished. Mark was debanded and wore maxillary and mandibular Hawley retainers faithfully. Both retainers incorporated a band of labial acrylic across the incisors, and the maxillary retainer included an anterior bite plate to disclude the posterior teeth slightly and thereby reduce the recurrence of his deep bite. Deband records are shown in Figures 4.44a–4.44r. What treatment changes do you note?

A: Changes include the following:
- Facially, occlusally, and functionally Mark's treatment resulted in dramatic improvements.
- Lip competence was achieved (Figure 4.44a).
- Maxillary incisors are now covered by the maxillary lip.
- Large buccal corridors are still noted (Figure 4.44b).
- Mark's nasal tip descended with growth (Figure 4.44c).
- Ideal NLA achieved (90 degrees, Figure 4.44c) – maxillary lip is no longer protrusive.
- Labiomental sulcus has been favorably opened.
- Improved chin projection achieved (orthognathic profile).
- Significant mandibular growth (Figure 4.44f) and *differential* jaw growth – mandible grew forward more than maxilla.
- MPA decreased (FMA decreased from 31° to 27°, Sella–Nasion to mandibular plane angle (SNMP) decreased from 35° to 34° which indicates forward mandibular growth rotation).
- Lower incisor to mandibular plane angle (IMPA) increased slightly from 97° to 98°, but FMIA increased from 52° to 55° as a result of MPA decreasing. That is, relative to the mandible, the mandibular incisors proclined slightly, but relative to the face, the mandibular incisors uprighted.
- Maxillary first permanent molars were moved distally (Figure 4.44f, top right).
- Mandibular first permanent molars erupted and maintained their anteroposterior positions.
- Maxillary incisors intruded and uprighted.
- Mandibular incisors erupted.
- Mandibular anterior roots appear foreshortened (Figure 4.44g), probably due to their proclination.
- Correction to Class I canines and molars bilaterally (Figures 4.44h–4.44j).
- Reduction of severe OJ to ideal OJ (minimal, Figure 4.44r).
- OB reduction from 100% to ideal OB (minimal, 1–2 mm or 10%).

- Maxillary midline is approximately 1 mm to the right of the mandibular midline.
- Generalized bulbous interdental papilla present.
- Mark's total treatment time, from beginning early treatment with high-pull headgear until debanding of all fixed orthodontic appliances, was three years and ten months.

Mark returned for a recall appointment ten years later (Figure 4.45). Although he wore his retainers faithfully, his OB deepened to 20–30%.

Q: How was Mark's Class II relationship corrected?
A: Mark's Class II relationship was corrected with excellent high-pull headgear wear which restricted his maxilla's forward growth, retracted maxillary first permanent molars distally, and allowed his mandible to continue growing forward.

Q: Mark continued to wear his headgear (with reduced force and reduced time of wear) even after his molar relationship was overcorrected. What principle does this follow?
A: *Principle: Overcorrect and maintain!* Never correct a Class II relationship using a headgear to Class I molars and stop. Instead, overcorrect molars to slightly Class III (1 mm) and then slowly taper off headgear wear as you monitor the correction's stability and patient's growth.

This same concept applies whether using functional appliances (e.g. Herbst appliance) or Class II elastics. Don't just correct to Class I and stop. Instead, overcorrect and monitor as you reduce force level and time of wear. The same concept applies in the vertical dimension as well (overcorrect a deep bite to a shallow OB and overcorrect an open bite to a 20–40% deep bite).

Q: From the start of headgear wear until debanding, Mark was treated for nearly four years. Was it wise to begin Class II orthopedic treatment as Mark was just entering the late mixed dentition or should we have waited?
A: Mark's parents initially stated that he was *exhibiting statural growth* and would be very cooperative. These were the reasons we began Class II orthopedics, and Class II orthopedic treatment at that time was appropriate.

We subscribe to the concept of waiting until the late mixed dentition to begin Class II orthopedic treatment – which Mark was entering. Furthermore, even if a child is in the early mixed dentition, we will consider beginning Class II orthopedics if they exhibit *good statural growth velocity (are growing continuously or are in their adolescent growth spurt)*. We realize that length of

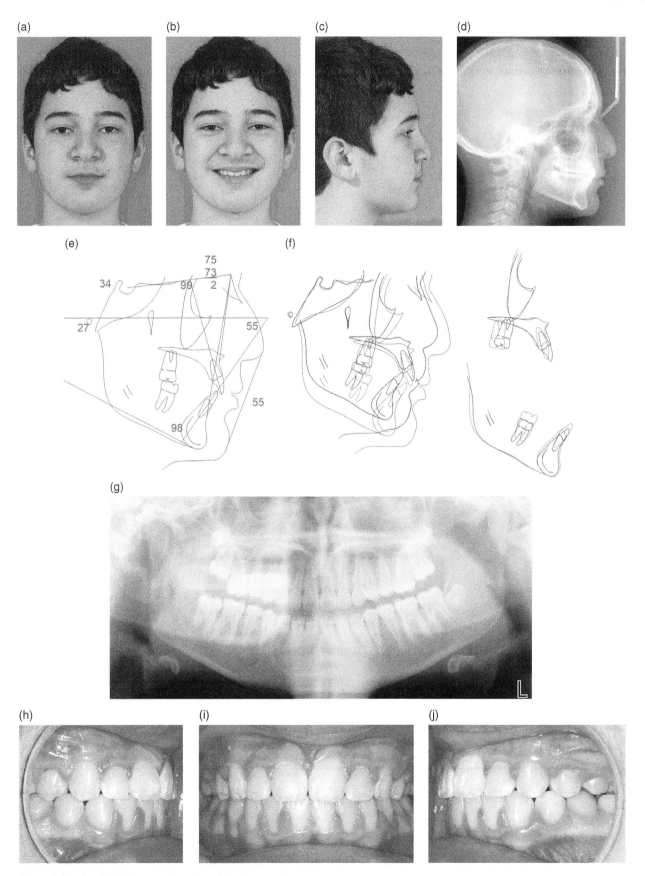

Figure 4.44 (a–r) Mark's comprehensive deband records.

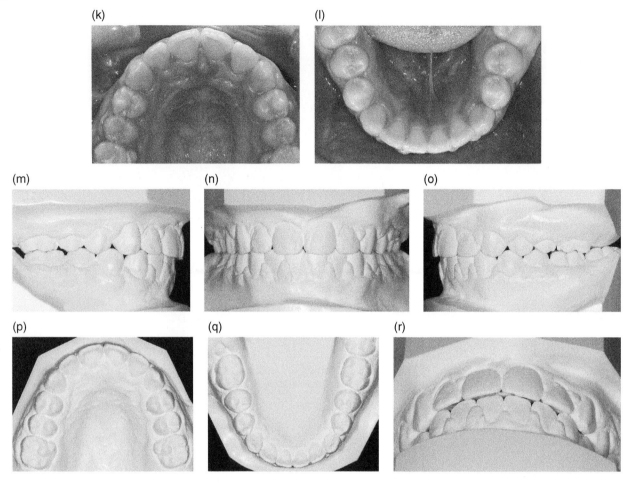

Figure 4.44 (Continued)

treatment time is a measure of treatment efficiency, but the most important metric of treatment outcome is result quality. Mark's treatment was long, but we feel his outcome was excellent.

Q: Mark began with large buccal corridors and ended with large buccal corridors. Should Mark have been treated with RME to reduce these?

A: Yes, in retrospect, Mark would have benefitted from RME. Not only would RME have reduced the size of his buccal corridors, RME would also have provided posterior OJ to permit uprighting of lingually torqued mandibular molars.

Q: Was it a mistake to treat Mark non-extraction?

A: No, we feel that non-extraction treatment was appropriate. The decision to treat patients with, or without, permanent teeth extractions is never to be taken lightly. We labor over these decisions, including our decision to treat Mark non-extraction. In an evidence-based orthodontic practice, each decision you make should be based upon the best science, your best clinical judgement, and the patient's desires. Mark and his parents strongly requested that Mark be treated non-extraction.

Relative to his mandible, Mark's mandibular incisors proclined by 1 degree during treatment (IMPA increased from 97° to 98°). However, relative to his face, Mark's mandibular incisors uprighted during treatment (FMIA increased from 52° to 55°) as a result of MPA decreasing. Furthermore, his profile esthetics improved dramatically with treatment (compare Figures 4.39c and 4.44c). Our goal is to achieve excellence in a patient's facial esthetics, occlusion, function, and tissue health – not necessarily to achieve ideal cephalometric numbers. Furthermore, Mark's maxillary incisors uprighted during non-extraction treatment, an ideal NLA was achieved (90 degrees, Figure 4.45c), and his maxillary lip is no longer protrusive. We would not have wanted his maxillary incisors and lip to retract more with maxillary premolar extractions. Finally, looking at Mark's profile 10 years after treatment (Figure 4.45c), we were very happy that we did not remove premolars.

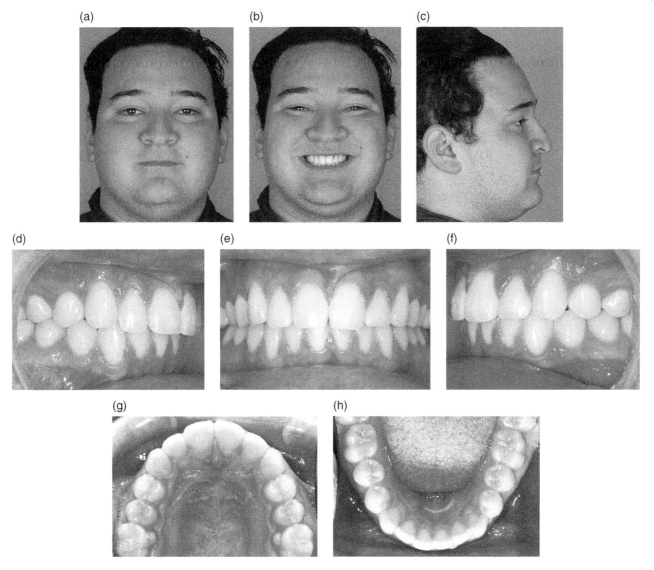

Figure 4.45 (a–h) 10-year recall records of Mark.

We *are* concerned about maintaining Mark's mandibular incisor alignment long-term. However, we are concerned about maintaining incisor alignment in every patient, whether treated with extractions or non-extraction. Mark has been very compliant wearing his Hawley retainers and understands that he must wear them at bedtime for as long as he wants to keep his teeth straight.

Q: Can you suggest "take-home pearls" for Mark?
A: "Take-home pearls" include the following:

- Mark presented at nine years of age. He was just entering the late mixed dentition with severe OJ (8 mm), a Class II (6 mm) molar relationship, maxillary skeletal deficiency, severe mandibular skeletal deficiency, a 100% deep bite, moderate (4 mm) mandibular anterior crowding, and proclined mandibular incisors. He was successfully treated non-extraction with high-pull headgear, LLHA, and fixed orthodontic appliances.

- Mark did not have a history of incisal trauma, but he was at increased risk for incisal trauma compared to someone without excess OJ. Children with OJ exceeding 3 mm are at twice the risk for dental injuries as children with OJ less than 3 mm [1, 2].

- Class II correction should be delayed until the patient is in the late mixed dentition, as opposed to the early mixed dentition. However, *even if a patient is in the early mixed dentition, if he/she has good statural growth velocity (is growing continuously or is in their adolescent growth spurt), you should consider initiating Class II orthopedic treatment.*

- As illustrated by this case (Figure 4.45f), the force of a high-pull headgear reduces forward maxillary growth while permitting the mandible to continue growing forward (differential jaw growth) and retracts maxillary molars distally. These effects corrected Mark's Class II relationship. His compliance was key.

- After overcorrection to a slight Class III (1 mm) molar relationship, Mark continued to wear his headgear to bed for months until we were sure that he was stable. Principle of orthodontic treatment: *overcorrect, maintain, monitor*!

- When using a headgear for Class II orthopedic treatment, consider having the patient also wear a full occlusal coverage splint. The splint disarticulates the occlusion, unlocks the bite, and allows the mandibular molars to move forward unimpeded as the mandible grows. The splint also stretches the masseter and medial pterygoid muscles which tends to reduce molar eruption and tends to rotate the mandible (B-point) up and forward.

- Headgear treatment used in conjunction with fixed orthodontic appliances improves facial profile esthetics in growing Class II patients with protrusive, normally positioned, or *retrusive* maxillae [89]. This concept was illustrated by Mark who had a deficient maxilla but improved facial esthetics with headgear treatment.

- Mark's mandibular arch was leveled early using his primary second molars as anchorage. The advantage of using primary second molars as 2x4 appliance intrusion arch anchorage is that the extrusive reactive force acts against them (exfoliated later) and not against permanent first molars.

- Mark is an example of what happens in many early orthopedic cases. You begin by treating a focused problem (skeletal Class II relationship) that drags on while the patient grows. By the time you achieve Class II correction, the permanent teeth erupt, and treatment is completed with fixed orthodontic appliances, total treatment time may take three to four years.

- Some friends will argue that Mark should have been treated with the extraction of four first premolars, and we are confident that they would have provided Mark with a superb outcome. We labor overextraction/non-extraction decisions with many patients, and we feel that Mark had an excellent esthetic and functional result with non-extraction treatment.

- Mark's maxillary midline diastema was closed orthodontically. He was never referred for a maxillary frenectomy, and a fixed maxillary retainer was never placed. Although the closure of the diastema has remained stable in retention for ten years, we generally recommend fixed lingual maxillary retention when we close diastemas orthodontically.

Case Cory

Q: Cory is 8 years old and presents to you (Figure 4.46) with his parents' chief complaint, "Please straighten Cory's teeth." His PMH, PDH, periodontal, and TMJ evaluations are WRN. He exhibits a CR-CO shift forward (1 mm) and to the right (2 mm). *Compile your diagnostic findings and problem list.* State your *diagnosis*.

A:

Table 4.9 Diagnostic findings and problem list for Cory.

Full face and profile	**Frontal View**
	Facial symmetry
	Soft tissue LAFH WRN (soft tissue Glabella – Subnasale = Subnasale – soft tissue Menton)
	ILG 8 mm
	UDML WRN
	Excess incisal display with relaxed lips (8 mm maxillary incisal display instead of an ideal 2–4 mm display)
	Excess gingival display in posed smile (maxillary lip border should be coincident with maxillary central incisor gingival margins)
	Maxillary midline diastema
	Profile View
	Convex profile
	Upturned nose
	90° NLA (upturned nose but maxillary lip protrusion)
	Mandibular lip protrusion (probable mandibular lip trapping by maxillary incisors)
	Retrusive chin
	Obtuse lip-chin-throat angle
	Chin-throat length WRN
	Deep labiomental sulcus
Ceph analysis	**Skeletal**
	Maxillary anteroposterior position WRN (A-Point lies along Nasion-perpendicular line)
	Mandibular anteroposterior position deficient (ANB angle = 5° with maxillary anteroposterior position WRN)
	Long skeletal LAFH (LAFH/ TAFH×100% = 58%, ideal = 55% with s.d. = 2%)
	Steep MPA (FMA = 32°, SN-MP = 37°)
	Effective bony Pogonion (Pogonion falls on the extension of N-B line)
	Dental
	Proclined maxillary incisors (U1 to SN = 111°)
	Proclined mandibular incisors (FMIA = 56°)

(Continued)

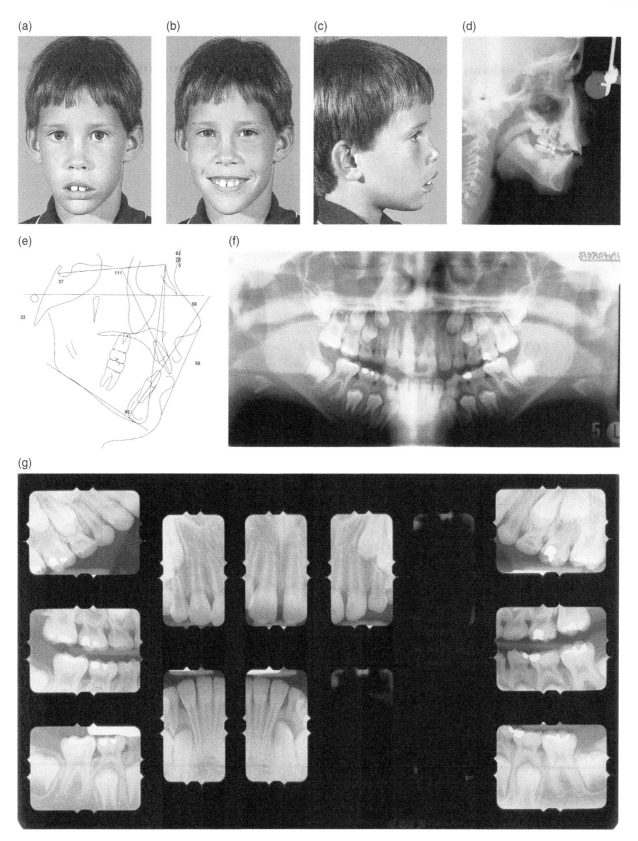

Figure 4.46 Initial records of Cory: (a–c) facial photographs, (d–e) lateral cephalometric radiograph and tracing, (f) pantomograph, (g) complete mouth series, (h–l) intraoral photographs, (m–s) models.

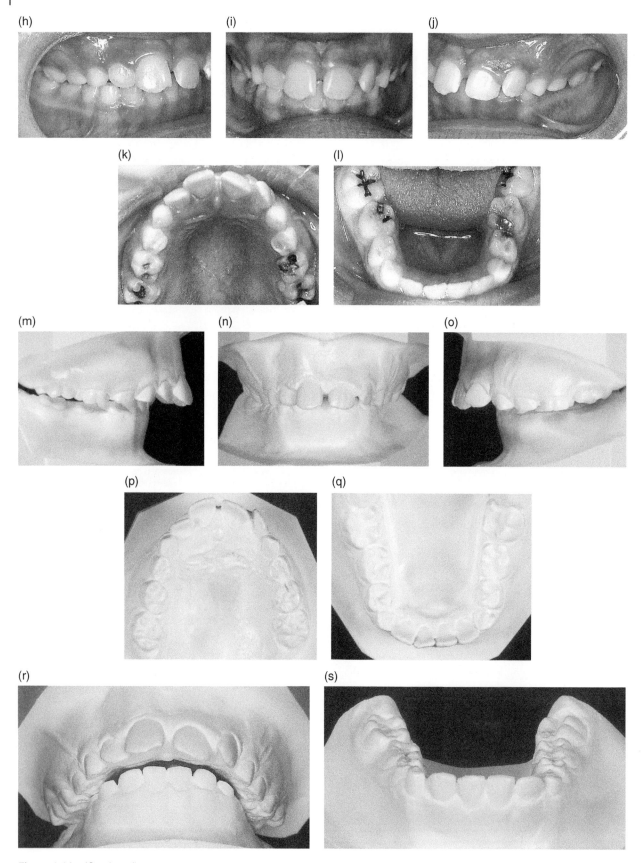

Figure 4.46 (Continued)

Table 4.9 (Continued)

Radiographs	Early mixed dentition
Intraoral photos and models	Angle Class II division 1
	Iowa Classification: II (6 mm) II (6 mm) II (6 mm) II (6 mm)
	OJ 9 mm (Figure 4.46r)
	60% OB without maxillary and mandibular incisor contact (Figure 4.46n)
	Excess right posterior OJ (Figure 4.46r)
	Complete left posterior buccal crossbite (scissors bite)
	Mandibular first permanent molars exhibit lingual crown torque (Figure 4.46s)
	Maxillary central incisor edges are level with posterior teeth (Figures 4.46m and 4.46o)
	0 mm maxillary anterior crowding currently present (sum of 2 mm midline diastema space and 2 mm maxillary lateral incisor crowding)
	2 mm maxillary space is anticipated following the eruption of all permanent teeth (if appropriate space maintenance is employed)
	0.5 mm mandibular anterior crowding is currently present
	2.7 mm mandibular spacing is anticipated following the eruption of all permanent teeth (if appropriate space maintenance is employed)
	Maxillary midline diastema with prominent labial frenum (Figure 4.46i)
	Symmetric maxillary and mandibular dental arches (Figures 4.46p and 4.46q)
	Thick periodontal biotype labial to mandibular anterior teeth (Figures 4.46h and 4.46j)
Other	
diagnosis	Class II division 1 malocclusion secondary to mandibular skeletal hypoplasia with a complete left buccal crossbite, a 1 mm forward and 2 mm right lateral CR-CO shift.

Q: In our estimation of OB, why did we specify that Cory lacks contact of his maxillary and mandibular incisors?

A: With the teeth in occlusion, OB is the amount of greatest vertical overlap measured from the incisal edges of the maxillary central incisors to the incisal edges of the mandibular central incisors, expressed as a percentage of overlap relative to the height of the clinical crown of the mandibular central incisors. That is, 100% OB is complete vertical overlap, 0% OB is no vertical overlap (maxillary and mandibular incisor incisal edges lie on the same transverse plane), and negative OB is defined as an anterior open bite.

When the maxillary and mandibular incisors make contact, with the teeth in occlusion, OB also implies the "depth" of the mandibular incisor incisal surface contact along the lingual surfaces of the maxillary incisor. Cory's 60% OB implies mandibular incisors contact more deeply along the maxillary incisors (more toward the maxillary incisor cingulum).

Although contact between maxillary and mandibular incisors in malocclusion is common, it is not always present even when vertical incisor overlap is evident. Such is the case with Cory. He has 60% vertical overlap of his mandibular incisor clinical crown, but his opposing incisors do not contact. Adding "without maxillary and mandibular incisor contact" as a qualifier to 60% OB gives more diagnostic information. For example, lack of incisor contact can be an indicator of a tongue interposition habit that impedes eruption of teeth.

Q: Do you wish to make any additional records?

A: No. No additional records are necessary to decide whether to treat Cory now or to recall him.

Q: Provide a detailed space analysis for Cory's maxillary and mandibular arches. In other words, how were the 2.0 mm maxillary arch spacing and 2.7 mm mandibular arch spacing calculated (if space maintenance is employed)?

A:

Average mesiodistal widths of permanent teeth (mm): [81]

Maxillary central incisor	8.5	Mandibular central incisor	5.0
Maxillary lateral incisor	6.5	Mandibular lateral incisor	5.5
Maxillary canine	7.5	Mandibular canine	7.0
Maxillary first premolar	7.0	Mandibular first premolar	7.0
Maxillary second premolar	7.0	Mandibular second premolar	7.0
Maxillary first molar	10.0	Mandibular first molar	11.0
Maxillary second molar	9.0	Mandibular second molar	10.5

Average mesiodistal widths of *primary* teeth (mm): [81]

Maxillary central incisor	6.5	Mandibular central incisor	4.2
Maxillary lateral incisor	5.1	Mandibular lateral incisor	4.1
Maxillary canine	7.0	Mandibular canine	5.0
Maxillary first molar	7.3	Mandibular first molar	7.7
Maxillary second molar	8.2	Mandibular second molar	9.9

MAXILLARY ARCH

0 mm of maxillary crowding is currently present
(2.0 mm midline diastema space and
2.0 mm lateral incisor crowding, Figure 4.46p)
+2.0 mm of anticipated leeway space (1 mm/side)
Balance = 0.0 mm + 2.0 mm = +2.0 mm

MANDIBULAR ARCH

−0.5 mm anterior crowding is currently present
+3.2 mm of anticipated leeway space (1.6 mm/side)
Balance = − 0.5 mm + 3.2 mm = +2.7 mm

That is, *2.0 mm maxillary arch spacing and 2.7 mm mandibular arch spacing is anticipated following the eruption of all permanent teeth (if proper space maintenance is employed).*

Q: What are Cory's primary problems in each dimension plus other problems (the main problems you must stay focused on)?

A:

Table 4.10 Primary problem list for Cory.

AP	Class II molar relationship of 6 mm secondary to mandibular skeletal deficiency
Vertical	60% OB without maxillary or mandibular incisor contact
Transverse	Complete left buccal crossbite with 2 mm right lateral shift
Other diagnosis	Bimaxillary incisor protrusion

Q: Discuss Cory in the context of three principles that apply to every early treatment patient.

A:
1) The goal of early treatment is to correct developing problems – get the patient *back to normal for their stage of development* (including preventing complications such as resorption of adjacent tooth roots, reducing later treatment complexity, or reducing/eliminating unknowns). Correcting Cory's Class II skeletal relationship, 60% OB, left complete buccal crossbite, right lateral CR-CO shift, and proclined incisors would put Cory back on track.
2) Early treatment should address *very specific problems with a clearly defined end point*, with any active treatment component usually completed within six to nine months (not protracted over many years except for some orthopedic problems). Cory's Class II skeletal discrepancy is a specific problem with a clearly defined end point, but depending upon his growth and cooperation, correcting it could take years.

His 60% OB could be readily corrected by leveling the mandibular arch with fixed orthodontic appliances. His complete left buccal crossbite, excess right posterior OJ, and right lateral CR-CO shift could be corrected in six to nine months by uprighting his mandibular posterior teeth and constricting his maxillary first permanent molars slightly. If premolar extractions are employed to create space to upright his proclined incisors, then incisor uprighting could take much longer than six to nine months.

3) Always ask: Is it necessary that I treat the patient now? *What harm could come if I choose to do nothing now?* If we choose not to begin Class II orthopedics now, then we anticipate years remaining to improve his Class II relationship because of his age – as he has ~three to four years prior to the onset of pubertal growth acceleration. If we do not correct his 60% OB now, then we do not anticipate harm.

However, if we do not correct his left complete buccal crossbite, then his left posterior teeth may supererupt, making it much harder to correct the crossbite in the future. Additionally, if we do not correct his right lateral CR-CO shift, then his mandible could grow asymmetrically.

Q: We estimated that Cory would have 2.7 mm of mandibular space following the eruption of all permanent teeth (if proper space maintenance is employed). Can you estimate the space needed to upright Cory's proclined mandibular incisors from the current FMIA = 56° to an ideal FMIA = 65°?

A: Tweed estimated that *0.8 mm of space was needed for every 1° FMIA lower incisors that were uprighted/retracted* [96]. Therefore, if you plan to upright Cory's incisors by 9 degrees (from FMIA = 56° to 65°), then you would need 7.2 mm of total space (9×0.8) or 4.5 mm of space beyond what space maintenance alone can provide.

Q: Is Cory an ideal candidate for serial extraction?

A: Let's answer this question by comparing the features of an ideal serial extraction patient to Cory's features. The ideal serial extraction patient is in the early mixed dentition and is *normal in every way except severe anterior crowding (≥ 9 mm per arch).* Specifically, the patient should present with:
- *Class I first permanent molars.* Cory does not exhibit this feature. Cory is skeletally Class II and has a full-step Class II molar occlusal relationship, a condition that should be corrected *before* permanent teeth extractions are considered. Extracting first premolars before Class II correction could worsen the Class II relationship. Why? During reciprocal space closure,

maxillary posterior teeth may move to the mesial more than mandibular posterior teeth.

- *Vertically normal to slightly long soft tissue and skeletal LAFH, with minimal OB or possibly a mild open bite, but* not *a deep bite.* Cory does not exhibit this feature. He has a 60% OB. Extracting his first premolars and closing extraction spaces would bring his maxillary and mandibular incisors into contact and could deepen his OB as his incisors retract and their protrusive angulations reduce.
- *Normal incisor angulation or proclined incisors, but* not *upright incisors.* Cory has proclined incisors – satisfying this feature.
- *Normal posterior transverse relationship (normal intermolar arch widths with good posterior interdigitation; absence of posterior crossbites; and absence of significant transverse compensations).* Cory does not exhibit this feature. He has a complete left buccal crossbite and excessive right posterior OJ.
- *Severe (≥ 9mm) anterior crowding*: Cory does not exhibit this feature.

Based upon the above, Cory is *not* an ideal candidate for serial extraction.

Q: Cory has a significant Class II skeletal discrepancy (mandibular skeletal deficiency). Can you list the three *general* ways to treat an anteroposterior, vertical, or transverse skeletal discrepancy and offer specific Class II treatments for each?

A: Class II skeletal discrepancies can be treated using: *Orthopedics* (restrict maxillary growth while the mandible continues growing forward or accelerate mandibular growth). Specific options include:

- Headgears: High-pull, straight-pull, or cervical-pull headgears restrict maxillary corpus forward growth, allow the mandible to continue growing forward, and move maxillary molars to the distal – all of which could correct Cory's Class II relationship. In addition, high-pull headgears may reduce descent of his maxillary corpus and maxillary first permanent molars – potentially improving Cory's anteroposterior correction by mandibular forward rotation [6–8]. On the other hand, cervical-pull headgears would tend to rotate Cory's anterior palatal plane down and back. This would increase (worsen) his maxillary incisor display. Further, a cervical-pull headgear would extrude maxillary first molars slightly (<1mm) [7, 8, 11, 14] which would tend to rotate his mandible down and back – potentially worsening his Class II relationship. Straight-pull headgears (a combination of high-pull and cervical-pull headgear) will produce an effect somewhere between that of a high-pull and a cervical pull.

- Class II functional appliances: As a classic Class II functional appliance, Herbst appliances restrict maxillary forward growth, retract maxillary posterior teeth, upright maxillary incisors, move mandibular posterior teeth to the mesial, *procline mandibular incisors*, accelerate condylar growth, and displace the glenoid fossae anteriorly [14, 15]. Class II functional appliances *accelerate* mandibular growth in growing individuals but *do not enhance* mandibular horizontal growth beyond that found in control subjects [16].

Further, the *direction* of condylar growth from Class II functional appliance wear (posterior superiorly) may not correct the mandibular skeletal deficiency or improve chin projection [17, 18]. In fact, *hyperdivergent* patients experience a deleterious backward mandibular rotation and increases in face height with Herbst treatment [19].

Since Cory is hyperdivergent with a steep MPA (FMA = 32°, SN-MP = 37°), a long skeletal LAFH (LAFH/TAFH × 100% = 58%), and proclined mandibular incisors (FMIA = 56°), he is *not* an ideal candidate for a Class II functional appliance. In contrast to Cory, the ideal Class II functional appliance patient has a short LAFH, flat MPA, and upright mandibular incisors (since they will be proclined during functional appliance treatment).

Masking or camouflage (achieving an ideal occlusion *dentally* without correcting the underlying skeletal discrepancy). We generally recommend masking later, during comprehensive treatment in the adult dentition when:

- The Class II orthopedic outcome is unsatisfactory.
- Growth is complete or nearly complete (i.e. *avoid doing anything irreversible such as extracting permanent teeth until unknowns such as growth are eliminated*).
- Obtaining Class I canines dentally is reasonable and will not result in unacceptable dental compensations or unfavorable esthetics.
- *First Principle of Masking – the smaller the skeletal discrepancy, the more normal the patient looks, and the smaller the dental compensations, the more successful masking (camouflage) will be; the larger the skeletal discrepancy, the less normal the patient looks; and the larger the dental compensations, the less successful masking (camouflage) will be.*

Class II masking options often include:

- Extraction of maxillary first premolars to permit retraction of the maxillary anterior teeth (achieving a Class I canine relationship but leaving molars Class II). This is an example of intra-arch mechanics.
- Using TADs as anchors to distalize the entire maxillary arch. For example, a pendulum appliance (Figures 4.47a and 4.47b) can be used to distalize

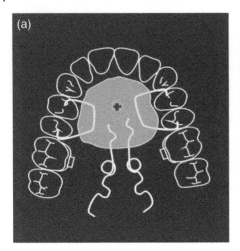 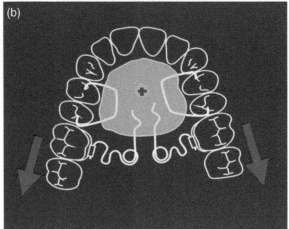

Figure 4.47 (a) Pendulum appliance supported with palatal TAD (green) in the center of the acrylic palatal button. When activated (b) the maxillary molars are distalized (red arrows) correcting the molar Class II relationship while the TAD prevents reciprocal forces from moving anterior teeth mesially.

maxillary posterior teeth if supported by a TAD attached to the palatal acrylic button. Without TAD anchorage, the molars will be distalized but at the expense of *reciprocal premolar-to-premolar mesial tooth movement* which must later be recaptured. This is another example of intra-arch mechanics.

- The use of Class II correctors such as Class II elastics or Class II springs. These are examples of interarch mechanics.

Surgery (mandibular advancement) is generally considered only during comprehensive treatment in the adult dentition. However, if the response to Class II orthopedics is unfavorable and masking unacceptable, then surgery may be our best option. Cory and his parents should be informed of this.

Q: Cory is eight years old and in the early mixed dentition. If you attempt Class II orthopedics – *when* would you begin?

A: All prospective, randomized clinical trials have consistently pointed to the same finding - there is no advantage in treating Class II relationships in the *early* mixed dentition (except for a possible decrease in incisal trauma as a result of excess OJ) [22–24, 29, 38–40]. We have always found this conclusion puzzling since dental development is not perfectly related to either chronological age or skeletal growth. Therefore, we teach Iowa orthodontic residents to follow a slight modification of this rule – generally wait until the patient enters the late mixed dentition to institute Class II orthopedic treatment, but consider beginning Class II orthopedic treatment in the early mixed dentition if the patient will be compliant with treatment and *has good statural growth.*

So, should you begin Class II orthopedic treatment now while Cory is in the early mixed dentition? Start by talking to Cory's parents – who state that he has grown very little lately. We therefore recommend waiting until he reaches the late mixed dentition – or earlier if his parents observe regular incremental increases in his height. We recommend that you ask his parents to measure Cory's height every month and report back to you. They should also monitor increasing mobility of his primary teeth as an indicator of imminent emergence of his succedaneous teeth and entry into the late mixed dentition.

Q: Is the *magnitude* of Cory's mandibular deficiency too large to attempt orthopedics?

A: No, it is not. Look at Cory's lateral cephalometric tracing (Figure 4.46e). He has a moderate-to-severe skeletal discrepancy (ANB = 5°, normal maxilla, deficient mandible). Also, he also has a severe bilateral Class II molar relationship (6 mm, Figures 4.46m and 4.46o).

However, he is only eight years old and is well in advance of entering pubertal growth acceleration, which is approximately age twelve to twelve and a half years old for males [41]. If Cory is cooperative, then we have a chance to correct his skeletal relationship with orthopedics or at least to improve it to the point where it can be acceptably masked (camouflaged).

Q: Cory has severe OJ (9 mm), and his maxillary incisors are exposed when in a relaxed lip position (Figure 4.46a). Is Cory at increased risk for dental injuries? Can you list other factors that you will want to discuss with his parents – factors that could increase his chances for incisor injury?

A: Since Cory's OJ exceeds 3 mm, he is at twice the risk for dental injuries as children with OJ less than 3 mm [97]. In addition to his severe OJ and exposed incisors (lip incompetence), you should also discuss the following with Cory's parents: [97, 98]

- History of dental trauma
- History of risk-taking behavior
- Participation in sports
- ADHD
- Cognitive psychomotor issues
- Teasing
- Family values related to excess OJ

Cory's parents deny any of these factors.

Q: Can you suggest reasons why Cory developed a complete left buccal crossbite?

A: Possible reasons include:

- His moderate-to-severe mandibular skeletal deficiency. A short mandible positions a narrow portion of its dental arch under the maxillary arch. We feel that this feature played a significant role in creating not only the left buccal crossbite but also in creating the excess right posterior OJ (Figure 4.46r).
- The 2 mm *right* lateral CR-CO shift. If the shift is eliminated, then maxillary right *and left* first permanent molar lingual cusps would oppose mandibular buccal cusps (increasing right posterior OJ but correcting the left buccal crossbite).
- Mandibular first permanent molar lingual crown torque (Figure 4.46s).

Q: If a posterior crossbite with a lateral shift is left *uncorrected*, what can result?

A: Development of a craniofacial asymmetry [97–99].

Q: If we can achieve Class II orthopedic correction, will the correction help or hurt Cory's *transverse* relationship?

A: It will help. Look at Figure 4.48a which depicts the hypothetical occlusal view of a patient, like Cory, with severe mandibular skeletal deficiency. In addition to excessive anterior OJ, this patient exhibits complete buccal crossbite at all premolars (Figure 4.48b). If differential jaw growth is achieved (Figure 4.48c, mandible growing forward more than maxilla), then a wider part of the mandibular dental arch is brought forward relative to the maxillary arch. The result is reduction, or elimination, of the buccal crossbites (Figure 4.48d).

Q: What is meant by a relative crossbite? What is meant by an absolute crossbite?

A: Consider the hypothetical patient in Figure 4.48. If by differential jaw growth or surgery the anteroposterior position of the mandibular arch is normalized to a Class I canine relationship with resulting *elimination of the posterior crossbite*, then the crossbite is considered *relative*. That is, the crossbite is relative to the anteroposterior interarch discrepancy. If under the same circumstances a posterior crossbite is not eliminated, then the crossbite is considered *absolute* – it is present regardless of the anteroposterior interarch relationship of the maxillary and mandibular dental arches.

Q: What unknowns do you face during the treatment of Cory?

A: Jaw growth (magnitude and direction), cooperation, hygiene, and the possibility of a larger (undetected) CR-CO shift.

Q: Based upon the above discussions, what *early* treatment options would you consider for Cory?

A: Early treatment options include:

- *Recall* (no early treatment, monitor only) – evaluate tooth eruption in nine to twelve months. We do not recommend this option. On the one hand, Cory just turned eight years of age, he is in the early mixed dentition, and his parents state that he does *not* exhibit good statural growth. For these reasons, we would not recommend beginning Class II orthopedics. This could change if his parents later report that he has begun to exhibit good statural growth velocity or if his primary teeth have begun to exhibit increased mobility (entering late mixed dentition).

  On the other hand, if we do not treat his left complete buccal crossbite and 2 mm CR-CO lateral shift, then his left posterior teeth may super-erupt, and his mandible may grow asymmetrically.
- *Mandibular space maintenance* – is recommended before Cory exfoliates mandibular primary canines and primary molars. Cory has mild (0.5 mm) mandibular anterior crowding, and an LLHA could provide 3.2 mm of leeway space, leaving him with 2.7 mm of space after all mandibular permanent teeth erupt. Three important points follow:

1) This small (2.7 mm) space could be used to upright his proclined mandibular incisors slightly.
2) LLHAs reduce, but do not eliminate, first molar mesial drift. As mandibular first permanent molars drift slightly to the mesial, the LLHA simultaneously drives the mandibular incisors forward [86, 87] adding to Cory's mandibular incisor proclination.
3) Reducing mandibular first permanent molar mesial drift will require more Class II correction via differential jaw growth (mandible growing forward more

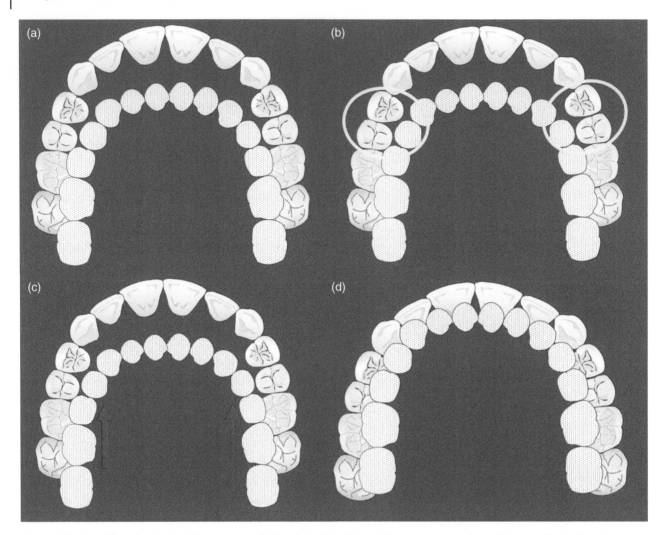

Figure 4.48 In a Class II patient with severe mandibular skeletal deficiency (a), a narrower portion of the mandibular dental arch articulates with the maxillary arch – resulting in excessive posterior OJ or even buccal crossbites (b). If orthopedic treatment results in more mandibular forward growth than maxillary forward growth (c, differential jaw growth), then a wider part of the mandibular dental arch is brought forward to articulate with the maxillary arch. In this way, buccal crossbites can be improved or eliminated (d). Of course, the same effect occurs if the mandible is *surgically* advanced after growth is complete.

than maxilla) or distal movement of maxillary first permanent molars.

- *Mandibular space maintenance with arch expansion* – is recommended. An expanded LLHA can widen the mandibular permanent first molars' intermolar width. The mandibular arch widening will help coordinate Cory's maxillary and mandibular arches, help eliminate the 2 mm right lateral CR-CO shift, help correct the complete left buccal crossbite, and help reduce the excess right posterior OJ.

If a removable appliance (e.g. a Schwarz appliance, Figure 4.49) is first used to expand the intermolar width (0.25–0.5 mm expansion per week), then we would recommend placing an LLHA after the expansion to maintain it. Whether an expanded LLHA or

Schwarz appliance is used to expand the intermolar width, the expansion will tend to upright lingually tipped molars (Figure 4.50).

- *Maxillary space maintenance* – is not recommended. Why? We want more than just holding maxillary first permanent molars in place with a Nance holding arch. We want a distal movement of maxillary first permanent molars to aid in Class II correction. Both headgears and functional appliances (e.g. Herbst appliance) will move maxillary molars to the distal.
- *Headgear Class II orthopedics* – is recommended when Cory enters the late mixed dentition or when he demonstrates good statural growth. High-pull and cervical-pull headgear wear will move Cory's maxillary molars distally, restrict his maxillary forward

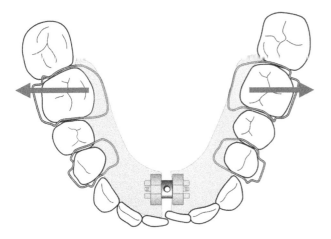

Figure 4.49 Schwarz appliance. As the midline screw is opened, posterior teeth move buccally (bilaterally) and upright.

growth, and allow his mandible to grow forward – all three effects improving his Class II molar relationship. In addition, a high-pull headgear could reduce descent of his maxillary corpus and reduce eruption of his maxillary molars – also helping B-point to rotate forward. We are less enthusiastic about using a cervical-pull headgear which will tip Cory's anterior palatal plane down (tending to increase maxillary incisal display) and erupt maxillary first molars slightly, neither effect helping him. Therefore, a high-pull headgear will be the best headgear option.

- *Functional appliance Class II orthopedics* – would be considered when Cory enters the late mixed dentition or demonstrates good statural growth velocity. Depending upon the specific appliance used, Class II functional appliances can move maxillary molars distally, inhibit maxillary forward growth, accelerate mandibular growth, move mandibular teeth mesially, and procline mandibular incisors [14, 19, 95, 100, 101].

However, Cory is hyperdivergent with a steep MPA (FMA = 32°, SN-MP = 37°), a long skeletal LAFH (LAFH/TAFH × 100% = 58%), and proclined mandibular incisors (FMIA = 56°). So, he is *not* an ideal candidate for a Class II functional appliance. With Class II functional appliance wear, we would expect a deleterious backward mandibular rotation, an increase in face height [19], and also an increase in mandibular incisor proclination. Functional appliance treatment will not be our first choice for orthopedics.

- *Extraction of maxillary primary canines (and possibly maxillary primary first molars)* – to create space and insure eruption of Cory's maxillary permanent canines. This treatment is not recommended because maxillary permanent canines appear to be erupting normally.
- *Maxillary 2x4 appliance to close the diastema and reduce OJ slightly* – is not recommended. Why? Cory currently has a 2 mm midline diastema space and 2 mm lateral incisor crowding which combine to give a net of 0 mm crowding – leaving no space for reducing OJ.
- *Correcting Cory's 60% OB* – is not recommended at this time because the mandibular incisors are not impinging on the palatal causing tissue damage or pain. The deep bite can be readily corrected later during comprehensive treatment.
- *Serial extraction* – as discussed previously, Cory is *not* an ideal candidate for serial extraction.

Q: What early treatment, if any, do you recommend?

A: A recommendation to begin early treatment was made by an attending orthodontist who supervised the case in our resident clinic. Some of his treatment decisions differed from our recommendations.

They initiated Cory's Class II orthopedic treatment immediately – in the early mixed dentition. We

(a)

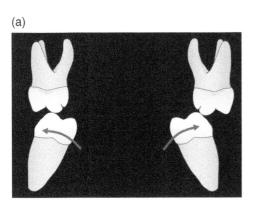

(b)

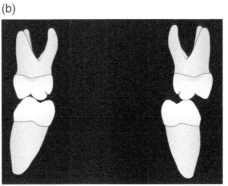

Figure 4.50 If an LLHA or Schwarz appliance is used to expand Cory's mandibular first permanent molars' intermolar width (a), then the molars will tend to upright. Expansion/uprighting of the molars will help eliminate his excess right posterior OJ and complete left posterior buccal crossbite (b).

recommended waiting until Cory entered the late mixed dentition or until his parents said he was growing.

Specifically, Cory was placed on a high-pull headgear which he wore every night from eight pm until the next morning. His growth and compliance were monitored. Reducing unknowns is almost always prudent.

His mandibular intermolar width was expanded using a Schwarz appliance to correct his left complete buccal crossbite (Figure 4.51) and eliminate his lateral shift. By eliminating his posterior crossbite occlusion and his lateral CR-CO shift, they reduced the potential for the development of mandibular skeletal asymmetry with growth and super-eruption of his maxillary left permanent first molar.

A 2x4 appliance was placed to align maxillary incisors which his parents specifically requested. As we have stated previously, we try to avoid allowing parents to dictate treatment. However, in our experience, diastemas between maxillary central incisors can be a source of emotional stress in certain children. We recommend ascertaining the importance of such concerns during your initial examination of the patient.

Following mandibular intermolar expansion with the Schwarz appliance, an expanded LLHA was placed to continue broadening the dental arch and reducing posterior OJ. Maxillary fixed appliances were removed, and a constricted transpalatal arch (TPA) was placed to decrease posterior OJ.

Headgear was discontinued (poor compliance), and Cory was asked to wear a removable Class II functional appliance (Frankel II appliance) for nine months. We disagree with this change of treatment. First, we were concerned that Cory was hyperdivergent and placing him on a Class II functional appliance would result in backward mandibular rotation, increase in face height, and increased mandibular incisor proclination. Second, in our experience, poor patient compliance with one removable appliance (headgear) does not improve through the use of another removable appliance (Frankel II).

(a)

(b)

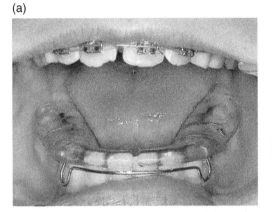
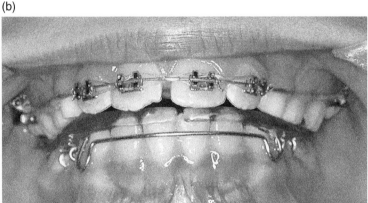

(c)

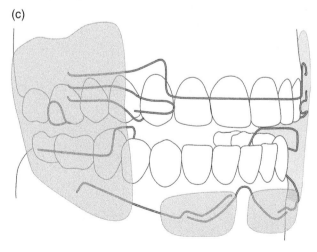

Figure 4.51 During early treatment, Cory wore a high-pull headgear for Class II orthopedic effect, a Schwarz appliance (a and b) to expand and upright his mandibular molars, a maxillary 2x4 appliance to align his maxillary incisors, and a Frankel II functional appliance (c) for Class II orthopedic effect.

At this time, all permanent teeth had erupted, and early treatment was complete. Comprehensive treatment began and consisted of placing fixed orthodontic appliances, leveling and aligning arches, and finishing. Cory was asked to wear high-pull headgear again along with Class II elastics. Cooperation was inconsistent. Cory was debanded and provided with Hawley retainers.

Q: Cory's deband records (age thirteen) are shown in Figure 4.52. What changes do you note?

A: Changes include:
- Facially, occlusally, and functionally, Cory had an excellent result.
- Although an ILG is not evident in Cory's facial photographs, we feel that he demonstrates mentalis strain to achieve lip closure (Figures 4.52a and 4.52c). Further, an ILG is present on his lateral cephalometric radiograph (Figure 4.52d). We, therefore, conclude that Cory still has a sizable ILG.
- Elimination of exaggerated cupid's bow (Figure 4.52a) because his maxillary lip grew downward (Figure 4.52f).
- Relative to his interpupillary line, Cory appears to have a mild right-to-left maxillary cant (Figure 4.52b).
- Reduction of maxillary and mandibular lip protrusion (compare Figures 4.46c and 4.52c).
- Ideal NLA achieved (90 degrees, Figure 4.52c).
- Labiomental sulcus has opened favorably.
- Improved chin projection.
- Differential jaw growth: B-point (Figure 4.52f) grew forward more than A-point. The mandible grew downward and forward. The maxilla descended with minimal forward growth.
- Differential jaw growth resulted in ANB angle reduction from 5 to 3° (Figures 4.46e and 4.52e) and aided dental correction to Class I molars and canines (Figure 4.52m and o).
- Maxillary incisors erupted and uprighted (Figure 4.52f, top right).
- Mandibular incisors erupted and proclined (Figure 4.52f, bottom right).
- Reduction of severe OJ (9 mm) to 1–2 mm.
- Reduction of 60% OB to 20% OB.
- Final maxillary midline approximately 1 mm to right of mandibular midline.
- Left complete buccal crossbite corrected.
- Excess right posterior OJ corrected.
- Total treatment time was five years.

Q: Can you state how Cory's 60% OB was reduced to 20%?

A: Looking at the initial-to-deband lateral cephalometric superimposition of the maxilla (Figure 4.52f, top right), we see that his maxillary molars and maxillary incisors erupted by approximately the same amount. However, looking at the superimposition of the mandible (Figure 4.52f, bottom right), we see mandibular molars erupted, but incisor edges were unchanged, probably due to their increased proclination as a result of treatment. (Remember, increasing incisor proclination tends to reduce OB). Therefore, we conclude that differential eruption between mandibular molars (~2 mm) and mandibular incisors (~0 mm) contributed to the reduction of Cory's initial 60% OB to 20% at deband.

Q: Was *early* treatment justified?

A: Early mandibular dental arch expansion with the Schwarz appliance was justified in order to upright posterior teeth, correct the left complete buccal crossbite, reduce posterior OJ, and eliminate the right lateral 2 mm CR-CO shift. We question whether treatment with a 2x4 appliance to close the diastema was justified.

We do not feel that Cory's Class II orthopedics was justified in the early mixed dentition. Why? Cody's parents stated that he was not growing. We would have recommended waiting to begin Class II orthopedics either until he reached the late mixed dentition or until his parents stated that he was growing.

This is the dilemma all orthodontists face with moderate-to-severe Class II patients in the early mixed dentition. We want to obtain as much orthopedic correction as possible which motivates us to start treatment earlier. However, the best science tells us to wait until the late mixed dentition to start treatment (unless the patient is growing).

Q: Can you suggest three reasons why Cory's mandibular incisors proclined during treatment?

A: Possible reasons include:
1) After mandibular expansion with a Schwarz appliance, Cory was placed in an LLHA. Although LLHAs substantially *reduce* mandibular first permanent molar mesial drift following primary teeth exfoliation, LLHAs *do not prevent* mandibular first molar mesial drift entirely. As a result, the LLHA simultaneously drives the mandibular incisors forward, proclining the incisors [86, 87].
2) Cory wore a Frankel appliance for nine months. Class II functional appliances cause mandibular incisor proclination.
3) Cory wore Class II elastics which cause mandibular incisor proclination.

Q: Extraction of mandibular premolars would have provided space to retract Cory's proclined mandibular incisors to a more ideal (upright) inclination. Should Cory have been treated with the extraction of four

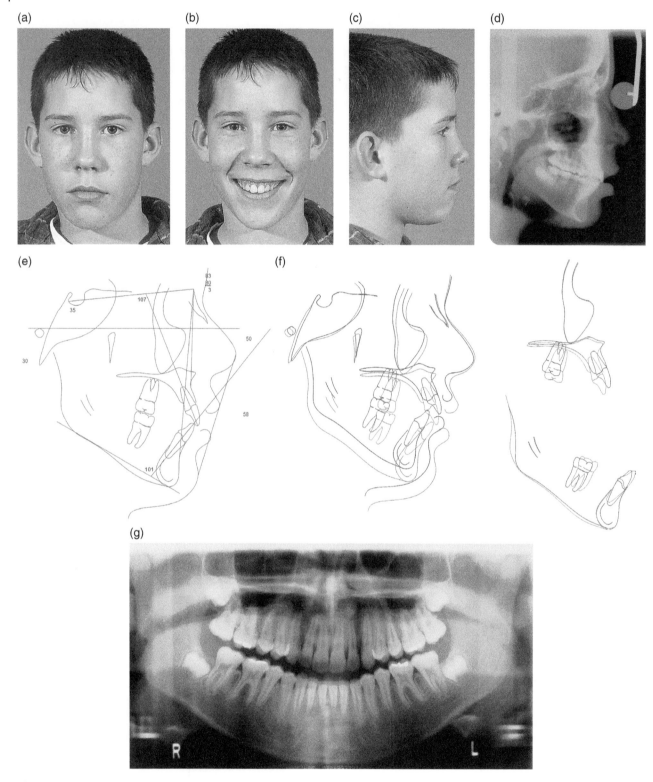

Figure 4.52 (a–r) Deband records for Cory.

(h)   (i)   (j)

(k)   (l)

(m)   (n)   (o)

(p)   (q)   (r)

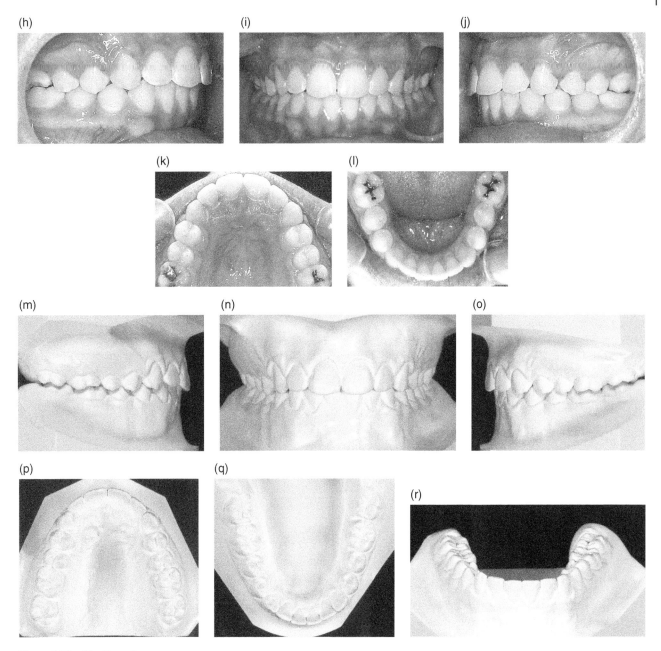

Figure 4.52   (Continued)

premolars to upright his incisors? Was it a mistake to treat Cory non-extraction?

A: You can make arguments either way – for extraction and for non-extraction. We have colleagues who would say, "four premolars should have been extracted," and we have colleagues who would say, "non-extraction treatment was the best option."

A reason to have treated Cory with the extraction of four premolars would have been to make space to upright his incisors and thereby retract his lips to reduce his ILG. We would *not* recommend extracting premolars for the sole purpose of ending with more ideal incisor inclination values. Cephalometric values are guidelines for orthodontists to use in making treatment decisions. They are not intended to be *must-haves* for any individual patient.

Reasons to have treated Cory non-extraction include the fact that he finished with excellent facial esthetics, profile esthetics, occlusion, function, and tissue health. Further, he finished with an ideal NLA which could have become obtuse following maxillary premolar extractions and space closure.

Q: Can you suggest any "take-home pearls" for Cory's early treatment?

A: "Take-home pearls" include the following:

- Cory was eight years old when he presented with a Class II (6 mm) permanent first molar relationship secondary to mandibular skeletal deficiency, 60% OB, a complete left buccal crossbite with 2 mm right lateral shift, and bimaxillary incisor protrusion. Early treatment consisted of a Schwarz appliance to expand his mandibular intermolar width, an LLHA, a maxillary 2x4 appliance to close his diastema, high-pull headgear/Frankel II appliances for Class II orthopedic correction, and a constricted TPA. He was treated non-extraction during comprehensive treatment.
- The attending orthodontist was wise to *reduce Cory's unknowns* (undetected CR-CO shift, growth, and compliance). Reduce unknowns *before* doing anything irreversible (e.g. extracting permanent teeth).
- The attending orthodontist was wise to *focus on Cory's primary problems* (complete left buccal crossbite and skeletal Class II relationship).
- Cory's complete left buccal crossbite was corrected by:
  - elimination of his 2 mm right CR-CO shift
  - uprighting/expanding his mandibular molars
  - TPA constriction of maxillary molars
  - differential jaw growth (advancement of a broader portion of his mandibular arch)
- When a child presents to you with a unilateral crossbite, it is imperative that you determine whether the crossbite is due to a CR-CO lateral shift or asymmetric mandibular growth. If the crossbite is due to a CR-CO lateral shift, then you must correct the shift in order to prevent asymmetric mandibular growth. However, the crossbite correction should then be stable. If the crossbite is due to asymmetric mandibular growth, then you must treat that asymmetric growth or the patient will grow out of your crossbite correction.
- Our highest levels of scientific evidence conclude that there is no advantage to initiating Class II treatment earlier than in the late mixed dentition (except perhaps to reduce incisal trauma) [22–24, 29, 38–40].

We generally subscribe to this principle, but we will consider beginning Class II orthopedic treatment if the child is in the early mixed dentition and *has good statural growth.*

- Cory suffered compliance *burnout* late in his five-year treatment. "Each patient gets one cup of compliance." (Dr. Mike Callan). When compliance is gone, it's gone. Patient burnout is one reason why initiating Class II treatment in the early mixed dentition is generally discouraged.
- *Principle of Class II orthopedic treatment: overcorrect, maintain correction, monitor!* No matter what Class II treatment you choose, we recommend slight overcorrection to Class III (1–2 mm) followed by a slow reduction of treatment while you monitor your correction.
- Because records were not made at each stage of Cory's treatment, we cannot separate the effects of headgear, Frankel II functional appliance wear, or Class II elastic wear. We can only note the cumulative changes that occurred, as we did earlier.
- Cory initially presented with severe OJ (9 mm) and without lip coverage of his maxillary incisors. He did not have a history of incisal trauma, but he was at increased risk for trauma compared to a person without excess OJ. With correction of excess OJ, he is no longer at increased risk for trauma, but he should be encouraged to wear a mouthguard when playing sports.
- To maintain post-treatment teeth alignment, Cory must wear retainers faithfully. He could wear maxillary and mandibular Hawley retainers every night when he goes to bed (with maxillary anterior bite plate to reduce chances of his deep bite returning and labial acrylic across maxillary and mandibular anterior teeth to prevent rotations/crowding). Because his mandibular arch was widened with a Schwarz appliance, we would not recommend a mandibular lingual fixed retainer only.
- If we were to treat Cory again, then we would begin by expanding/uprighting his mandibular first permanent molars to correct the left complete crossbite and eliminate the lateral shift. We would initiate high-pull headgear wear when he began to grow or reached the late mixed dentition. When his permanent canines and premolars erupted, we would make records and a final non-extraction/extraction decision. We would avoid using a Frankel II appliance in order to prevent further incisor proclination.
- Cory is an example of what can happen in early Class II orthopedic patients. Treatment time can be extended beyond what is reasonable. If Class II orthopedic treatment had been delayed for a year or two, perhaps Cory's total treatment time could have been reduced.

Case Mason

Q: Mason is nine years and eleven months old (Figure 4.53). He presents with his parents' chief complaint, "We were referred to by our dentist. We are concerned with Mason's jaw growth and crossbite." His PMH, PDH, periodontal, and TMJ evaluations are WRN. What is the first thing you need to check (with every patient)?

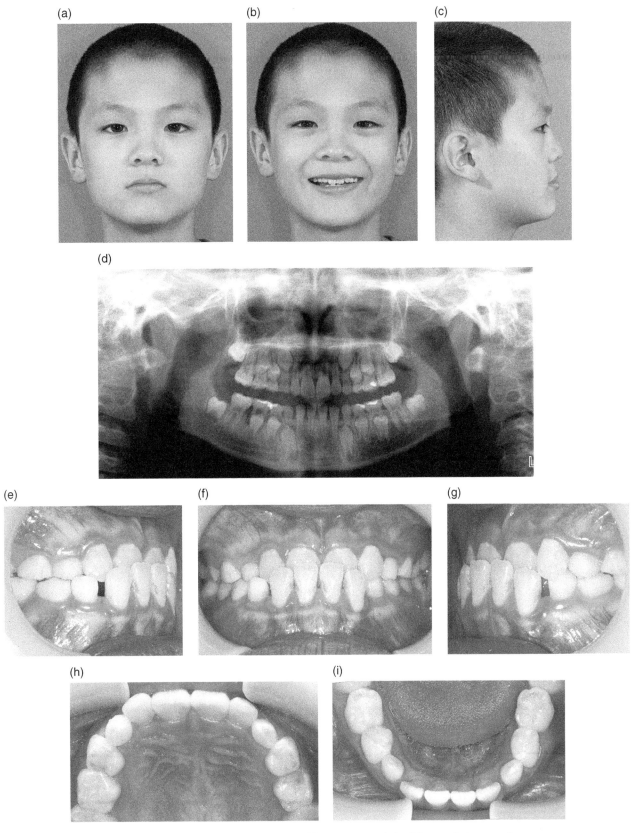

Figure 4.53   Initial records of Mason: (a–c) facial photographs, (d) pantomograph, (e–i) intraoral photographs.

A: Check for a CR-CO shift. *Always check for a shift in every patient at every appointment.* Compare Figures 4.53e–4.53g (made in CO) to Figures 4.54a–4.54c (made in CR). What do you see? Mason has a 1–2 mm CR-CO shift from edge-to-edge incisors into anterior crossbite.

Q: You decide to make a lateral cephalometric radiograph in CR (Figure 4.55). Using all records, *compile your diagnostic findings and problem list*. State your *diagnosis*.

A:

Table 4.11 Diagnostic findings and problem list for Mason.

Full face and profile	**Frontal View**
	Facial symmetry
	LAFH WRN (soft tissue Glabella – Subnasale = Subnasale - soft tissue Menton)
	Lip competence
	Maxillary incisal display inadequate during posed smile (maxillary incisor gingival margins are apical to maxillary lip border)
	UDML WRN
	Profile View
	Mildly concave profile in CO
	Strong chin projection in CO
	Nasal tip up
	NLA WRN (~90°)
	Protrusive mandibular lip
	Deep labiomental sulcus
	Lip-chin-throat angle WRN
	Chin-throat length WRN
Ceph analysis	**Skeletal**
	Maxillary anteroposterior deficiency (A-point significantly behind Nasion-perpendicular line)
	Mandibular skeletal deficiency (N-B line makes an angle of 5–6° with Nasion-perpendicular line)
	ANB = −2°
	Long skeletal LAFH in CR (LAFH/TAFH × 100% = 58%) – measurement in CO not available
	Effective bony Pogonion (Pogonion anterior to N-B line)
	Dental
	Maxillary incisor angulation appears WRN
	Mandibular incisors WRN (FMIA = 64°)
Radiographs	Early mixed dentition (approaching late mixed dentition)

Intraoral photos and models	Angle Class I in CO (Figures 4.53e–4.53g)
	Iowa Classification I I I I in CO
	60–70% OB in CO
	Anterior crossbite in CO
	Incisors edge-to-edge in CR
	LDML 1 mm to right of UDML in CO (Figure 4.53f)
	LDML coincident with UDML in CR (Figure 4.54b)
	Posterior transverse relationship WRN (Figures 4.53f and 4.54b)
	2.0 mm maxillary anterior crowding is currently present
	0 mm of maxillary crowding is anticipated following the eruption of all permanent teeth (if appropriate space maintenance is employed)
	3.0 mm mandibular anterior spacing is currently present
	6.2 mm of mandibular spacing is anticipated following the eruption of all permanent teeth (if appropriate space maintenance is employed)
	Maxillary and mandibular dental arches are symmetric (Figures 4.53h–4.53i)
	Thin periodontal biotype with reduced keratinized attachment labial to mandibular left primary canine
Other diagnosis	1–2 mm CR-CO shift
	Damage to the incisal edge of maxillary left central incisor (Figure 4.54b).
	Poor hygiene
Diagnosis	Class I malocclusion with CR-CO shift into anterior crossbite

Q: Mason's ANB = −2° which usually indicates a small maxilla relative to the mandible. Yet, we noted that Mason's *mandible is deficient*. Can you explain?

A: The answer lies in the fact that Mason's jaws are *both* deficient. His mandible is deficient (N-B line makes an angle of 5–6° with Nasion-perpendicular line) but his maxilla is even more deficient which leads to an ANB angle of –2°.

Q: Can we state with certainty Mason's true dental relationship?

A: We cannot because of his CR-CO shift and anterior crossbite. However, we can state that Mason is *not* Class III. Why? Because he is Class I in CO, he will either remain Class I when the shift is eliminated, or he will become (slightly) Class II. Examining Figures 4.54a and 4.54c, we anticipate Mason remaining Class I when his crossbite is corrected.

(a) (b) (c)

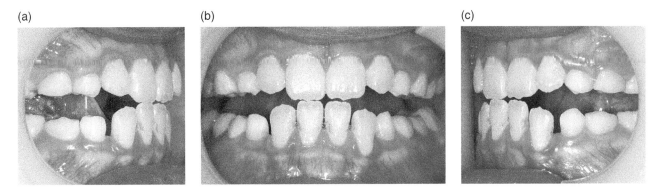

Figure 4.54 (a–c) Intraoral photographs of Mason in CR.

(a) (b)

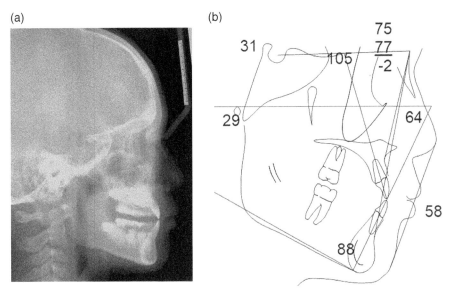

Figure 4.55 (a–b) Lateral cephalometric radiograph and tracing made in CR. Note that Mason's incisors contact edge-to-edge in CR resulting in a posterior open bite on the lateral cephalometric radiograph.

Q: We noted that Mason has a long skeletal LAFH (LAFH/ TAFH × 100% = 58%). But this measurement was calculated from a lateral cephalometric radiograph made in CR (central incisors edge-to-edge). Does Mason really have a long skeletal LAFH?

A: Probably not. As Mason shifted from CO into CR to make the lateral cephalometric radiograph, his mandible rotated down and back ~4 mm to where his incisors were edge-to-edge, lengthening his LAFH and creating a posterior open bite. Raising Menton ~4 mm would give a skeletal LAFH of ~55%, which is WRN, and matches our soft-tissue profile assessment of LAFH.

Q: An ideal U1-SN angle lies between 101 and 103°, but Mason's U1-SN angle = 105° which indicates that his maxillary incisors are proclined. We noted that the angulation of his maxillary incisors is not proclined but WRN. Are we wrong?

A: No, we are correct. Mason has a high Sella position (Figure 4.55b) which increases his U1-SN angle.

The average angular difference between Frankfort Horizontal line and S-N line is 7°, but Mason shows a difference between these lines of only 2°. To arrive at an estimate of his U1-SN, if Sella was in a normal position, we subtract 5° (7° – 2°) from 105° = 100°, an U1-SN slightly less than normal. This aligns with the expectation that his anterior crossbite occlusion would tend to upright his maxillary incisors due to posteriorly directed occlusal force against the crowns of his permanent maxillary incisors.

Q: Mason's mandibular midline is 1 mm to the right of his maxillary midline in CO (Figure 4.53f) but approximately congruent with his maxillary midline in CR (Figure 4.54b). What does this observation tell us about Mason's CR-CO shift?

A: It tells us that his CR-CO shift is not only forward but is also slightly to the right. He has a right lateral CR-CO shift but it is so subtle that an obvious chin deviation is not apparent (Figure 4.53a).

Q: Why is Mason's mandibular lip protruded?

A: His mandibular lip is held forward by his mandibular incisor crowns – which are positioned forward (note spacing distal to the mandibular permanent lateral incisors, Figure 4.53i). His mandibular lip could also be trapped forward by his maxillary lip upon closure in CO.

Q: Provide a detailed space analysis for Mason's maxillary and mandibular arches. In other words, how were the 0 mm of maxillary crowding and 6.2 mm of mandibular spacing calculated (if space maintenance is employed)?

A: Below are space estimates:

Average mesiodistal widths of permanent teeth (mm): [81]

Maxillary central incisor	8.5	Mandibular central incisor	5.0
Maxillary lateral incisor	6.5	Mandibular lateral incisor	5.5
Maxillary canine	7.5	Mandibular canine	7.0
Maxillary first premolar	7.0	Mandibular first premolar	7.0
Maxillary second premolar	7.0	Mandibular second premolar	7.0
Maxillary first molar	10.0	Mandibular first molar	11.0
Maxillary second molar	9.0	Mandibular second molar	10.5

Average mesiodistal widths of *primary* teeth (mm): [81]

Maxillary central incisor	6.5	Mandibular central incisor	4.2
Maxillary lateral incisor	5.1	Mandibular lateral incisor	4.1
Maxillary canine	7.0	Mandibular canine	5.0
Maxillary first molar	7.3	Mandibular first molar	7.7
Maxillary second molar	8.2	Mandibular second molar	9.9

MAXILLARY ARCH

−2.0 mm of maxillary anterior crowding currently present (Figure 4.53h)

+2.0 mm of anticipated leeway space (1 mm/side)

Balance = − 2.0 mm + 2.0 mm = 0 mm

MANDIBULAR ARCH

+3.0 mm of anterior spacing is currently present (Figure 4.53i)

+3.2 mm of anticipated leeway space (1.6 mm per side)

Balance = + 3.0 mm + 3.2 mm = +6.2 mm

That is, *0 mm of maxillary crowding and 6.2 mm of mandibular spacing is anticipated following the eruption of all permanent teeth (if proper space maintenance is employed).*

Q: What are your primary problems in each dimension (the main problems you must focus on)?

A:

Table 4.12   Primary problem list for Mason.

AP	Functional mandibular shift into anterior crossbite in CO (incisors are edge-to-edge in CR with estimated Class I molars)
Vertical	OB 60–70% in CO (vertical incisor overlap cannot be assessed in CR)
Transverse	–
Other diagnosis	Enamel damage to maxillary left permanent central incisor CR-CO anterior and lateral shift

Q: Mason has maxillary and mandibular skeletal deficiencies. Why are these deficiencies not listed as primary problems?

A: These deficiencies are not listed because Mason is a good-looking young man at nearly ten years of age because his mildly concave profile should improve when his anterior crossbite is corrected, and because we anticipate him being Class I dentally when his crossbite is corrected. In other words, we would not address these skeletal deficiencies if Mason was our son. We will certainly monitor Mason's growth to determine whether we need to address these skeletal problems later.

Q: Discuss Mason in the context of three principles applied to every early treatment patient.

A:

1) The goal of early treatment is to correct developing problems – get the patient *back to normal for their stage of development* (including preventing complications such as resorption of adjacent tooth roots, reducing later treatment complexity, or reducing/eliminating unknowns). For Mason, this would include:
   - Correcting his anterior crossbite (eliminating future damage to his maxillary left central incisor

- Eliminating his CR-CO shift
- Reducing his OB

2) Early treatment should address *very specific problems with a clearly defined end point*, usually begun and ended within six to nine months (not protracted over many years except for some orthopedic problems). Mason's anterior crossbite and CR-CO shift are focused problems that can be corrected in a short time with fixed orthodontic appliances by advancing maxillary anterior teeth and closing mandibular anterior spaces. If we close mandibular spaces, then we must be careful not to impact his mandibular permanent canines. His deep bite can be corrected with braces (2x4 appliance) by leveling his mandibular arch (erupting mandibular first permanent molars, intruding/proclining mandibular incisors). Mild maxillary crowding (2 mm) could be corrected while advancing/aligning maxillary incisors.

3) Always ask: Is it necessary that I treat the patient now? *What harm may come if I choose to do nothing now?* If Mason's anterior crossbite is not corrected, then:
   - Continued maxillary incisor damage is likely.
   - The 1–2 mm CR-CO shift could act as a Class II functional appliance, accelerating mandibular growth.
   - The CR-CO shift small *lateral* component could result in mandibular asymmetric growth.

Q: Do you recommend serial extraction for Mason?

A: No. The ideal serial extraction patient is in the early mixed dentition and is *normal in every way except severe anterior crowding (≥ 9 mm per arch).* Mason currently has only mild (2.0 mm) maxillary anterior crowding and 3.0 mm mandibular anterior spacing. With appropriate space maintenance, we anticipate that he will have 0 mm maxillary crowding and 6.2 mm mandibular spacing following the eruption of all permanent teeth. Mason is *not* a candidate for serial extraction.

Q: What unknowns do you face in treating Mason?

A: Future jaw growth (magnitude and direction), cooperation, hygiene, and a greater CR-CO shift than observed.

Q: Based upon the above discussions, what early treatment options would you consider for Mason?

A: Options include:
- *Recall* (no early treatment, monitor only) – evaluate tooth eruption in one year. We do not recommend this option because Mason could have additional damage to his maxillary incisors. Furthermore, his CR-CO shift into anterior crossbite could act as a

Class II functional appliance, accelerating mandibular growth, and the small *lateral* component of the shift could result in slight mandibular asymmetric growth.

- *Mandibular space maintenance* – placement of an LLHA before exfoliation of Mason's mandibular primary canines and primary molars. We do not recommend this option. Why? Mason currently has 3 mm mandibular anterior *spacing* with normal mandibular incisor angulation (FMIA = 64°). If an LLHA is placed, then we will not be able to close these anterior spaces to help correct his anterior crossbite.

- *Maxillary space maintenance* – placement of a Nance holding arch before exfoliation of Mason's maxillary primary canines and primary molars. We do not recommend this option. Why? Although Mason currently has 2 mm of maxillary crowding, normal maxillary incisor inclination, and 0 mm of anticipated maxillary crowding after all permanent teeth erupt if a Nance holding arch is placed – placing a Nance holding arch *alone* will not correct his anterior crossbite.

- *Space regaining* – opening space for Mason's maxillary permanent lateral incisors. Although Mason has 2 mm of maxillary anterior crowding and we could open space with fixed appliances to align the incisors, we cannot state with certainty that he lost space following premature primary incisor exfoliation. In other words, aligning his maxillary incisors may not be space regaining.

- *Extraction of primary canines and primary first molars* – to help ensure eruption of permanent canines is not necessary because Mason's permanent canines appear to be erupting normally.

- *Serial extraction* – Mason has minimal maxillary crowding, mandibular spacing, and is not a candidate for serial extraction.

- *Anterior crossbite correction* – would eliminate Mason's CR-CO shift, prevent further maxillary incisor crown damage, and permit us to evaluate his true anteroposterior dental relationship. This is a highly recommended early treatment option.

Q: Can you review each factor weighing into your decision to treat, or not treat, Mason's anterior crossbite early?

A: The factors include:
- *Presence of an underlying skeletal discrepancy* – If you correct an anterior crossbite in a child with *normal* skeletal growth, then the crossbite should remain corrected. However, if you correct an anterior crossbite in a child with a *Class III skeletal discrepancy,*

then you need to begin orthopedic treatment to address the skeletal discrepancy – or, you will end up chasing a recurring anterior crossbite as the child continues the same Class III growth pattern.

Mason has a Class III skeletal discrepancy (ANB = −2° in CR), and he has a mildly concave profile in CO. However, we anticipate that his mildly concave profile should improve when his anterior crossbite is corrected, and we anticipate him being Class I dentally when his crossbite is corrected. We will monitor his growth, but we are hopeful at this time that his Class III growth will not pose a problem.

- *Permanent incisor eruption status* – We usually recommend waiting until permanent incisors erupt before correcting anterior crossbites. Mason's permanent incisors are erupted.
- *Damage to permanent incisors or soft tissue* – his maxillary left permanent central incisor is damaged.
- *Compliance* or lack of compliance – Mason's parents state that he is a compliant boy.
- *Psychosocial issues* – none noted.
- *CR-CO shift magnitude* – 1–2 mm CR-CO shift.

Based upon the above factors, we recommend correcting Mason's anterior crossbite early.

Q: Would you begin early treatment or recall Mason? If you begin treatment, then what early treatment would you recommend?

A: You should correct Mason's anterior crossbite now in order to prevent further trauma to his maxillary incisors and in order to determine his true anteroposterior dental relationship.

Fixed appliances were placed (Figure 4.56a) to advance his maxillary incisors and retract his mandibular incisors. Based upon our space analysis, we were not worried about impacting his mandibular permanent canines. Orthodontic cement was placed on maxillary first permanent molar occlusal surfaces to act as a bite plate. This opened his bite and allowed maxillary incisors to advance beyond the mandibular incisors (Figures 4.56b and 4.56c).

Q: Do you have any concerns about advancing Mason's maxillary permanent lateral incisors?

(a)

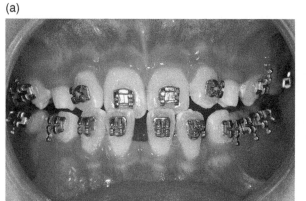

(b)

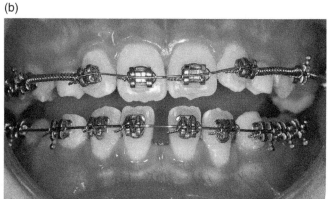

(c)

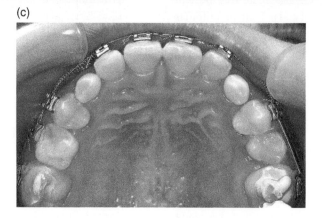

Figure 4.56 (a–c) Progress records of Mason. Fixed orthodontic appliances were placed to correct his anterior crossbite by advancing maxillary incisors and closing mandibular anterior spaces. Note orthodontic cement added on maxillary first permanent molar occlusal surfaces to act as a bite plate and allow anterior teeth to cross over each other. Looking ahead at Figure 4.57, we illustrate correction of Mason's anterior crossbite and correction of his CR-CO shift.

A: Changing the spatial position of permanent maxillary lateral incisors during the early treatment when developing maxillary permanent canine crowns are in the proximity of lateral incisor root apices *should always be a concern*. It is important to consider this spatial relationship *before* moving the permanent maxillary lateral incisors. Looking at Figures 4.53d and 4.55a, it appears the developing maxillary canine crowns are distal and labial to the root apices of the lateral incisors. The slight labial inclination of the maxillary lateral incisors in Figure 4.54 also suggests the lateral incisor roots are palatally inclined relative to the central incisors. Further confirmation of this can be made by digital palpation of the developing canine crowns in the vestibule, or by 3-D radiography. (This was not done.) To reduce the likelihood of moving the lateral incisor roots into the developing canine crowns, we tipped the maxillary lateral incisor brackets (Figures 4.57a and 4.57c) so that their root apices would move *mesially* – away from the erupting permanent canine crowns. Also, we informed Mason's parents of the potential for root resorption before treatment began, and the incisors were advanced slowly using light spring forces.

Q: Thankfully, at this time, Mason was Class I, and his CR-CO shift had disappeared. How would you proceed?

A: Fixed appliances were removed (except for the bracket on the mandibular right primary second molar which was exfoliating), and an LLHA was placed (Figure 4.58). Enameloplasty was performed on the maxillary left central incisor edge to smooth it. Mason was given a maxillary clear retainer to wear to bed at night (portions of the retainer were cut away to allow eruption of permanent teeth). Early treatment was complete, and we planned to monitor Mason while his remaining permanent teeth erupted.

Q: During a recall visit years later, Mason's mother stated that they were thrilled with his care. They requested that the LLHA be removed and that no further treatment be provided (Figures 4.59a–4.59i). What changes do you note?

A: Changes include the following:
- An esthetic smile and orthognathic profile (straight profile, no longer concave)
- A slight Class II (1–2 mm) dental relationship
- Iowa classification: II (1 mm) II (2 mm) II (2 mm) II (1 mm)
- Anterior crossbite correction is stable
- Slight maxillary and mandibular anterior spacing
- Mandibular second molars erupting
- Maxillary permanent canines nearly erupted

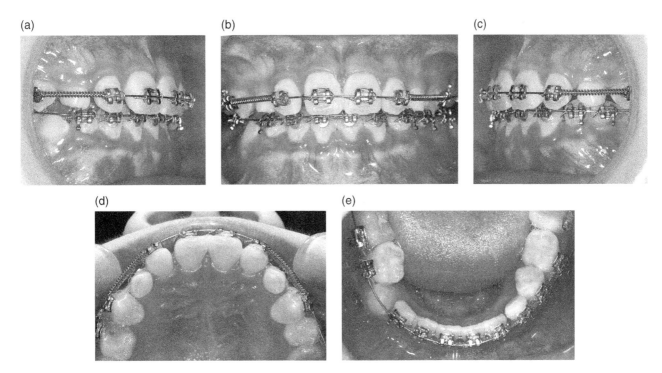

Figure 4.57 (a–e) Progress records after crossbite correction (orthodontic cement has been removed from the maxillary first permanent molars).

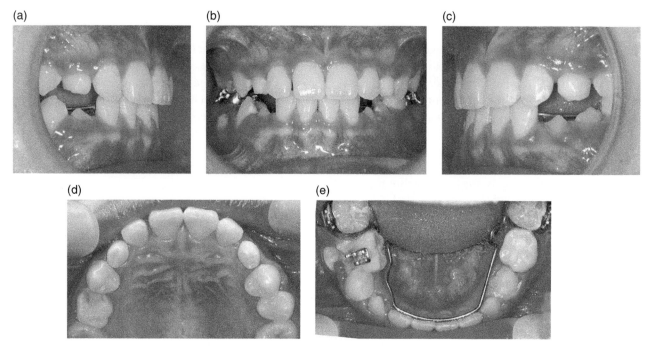

Figure 4.58 (a–e) Deband intraoral photos of Mason.

- OB 20%
- OJ 0 mm
- Attached keratinized tissue labial to maxillary and mandibular anterior teeth WRN
- Residual cement present on the maxillary right permanent first molar occlusal surface

Q: We were concerned that the maxillary lateral incisor roots could resorb as their crowns were advanced out of crossbite. Were they?

A: No, the maxillary lateral incisor roots did not resorb (Figure 4.59d). However, it is prudent to:
- Inform the patient and parents of this possibility
- Establish the spatial relationship of lateral incisor root apices and developing canine crowns
- Use light forces
- Advance incisor crowns slowly
- Bond lateral incisor brackets so that the archwire will tip the lateral incisor roots *away* from the erupting permanent canine crowns.

Q: As she is leaving, Mason's mother asks, "Will there be any harm in ending treatment at this point, and does Mason need to see you again?" What is your response?

A: Tell her that you do not anticipate any problems in discontinuing treatment at this point. However, we recommend that Mason be recalled every year and his growth monitored. If he begins to grow Class III, then the orthopedic option of high-pull chin cup wear (or TAD-supported Class III elastic wear) could be considered. To guarantee alignment of his teeth, Mason should be provided with retainers to wear every night once the permanent canines are fully erupted.

Q: When we considered early treatment options, we advised against placing an LLHA. However, later we placed an LLHA. Why?

A: We advised against placing an LLHA when Mason was in anterior crossbite with spaces mesial to primary canines. Why? We would have been unable to close these spaces to help correct the crossbite with an LLHA in place. But by the time his mandibular spaces closed and his anterior crossbite was corrected (Figure 4.57), we decided to maintain space for the erupting permanent teeth with an LLHA.

Q: Was *early* treatment justified?

A: Yes. Let's review our decision in the context of the three early treatment principles:
1) The goal of early treatment is to get the patient *back to normal for their stage of development*. Mason was brought back on track by correcting his anterior crossbite, eliminating his CR-CO shift, and leveling his arches (reducing his OB).
2) Early treatment should address *very specific problems with a clearly defined end point* – readily correcting

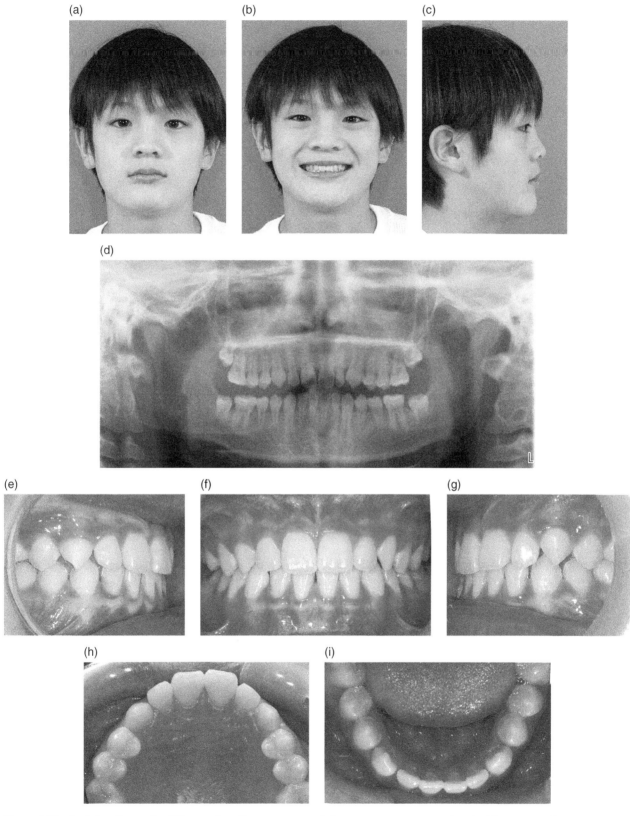

Figure 4.59 (a–i) Recall records of Mason after all permanent teeth (except permanent second molars) have erupted.

Mason's anterior crossbite, and eliminating his CR-CO shift, were focused problems with clearly defined end points.

3) Always ask, "*What harm may come if I choose to do nothing now?*" If we had not intervened, then additional damage to Mason's left central incisor may have occurred, and his CR-CO shift may have accelerated growth like a Class II functional appliance. Early treatment was justified.

Q: Can you suggest any "take-home pearls"?
A: "Take-home pearls" include the following:

- Mason was nine years and eleven months old when he was referred for correction of anterior crossbite and jaw growth. Mason's crossbite and CR-CO shift made the possibility of future jaw growth problems appear worse than they turned out to be. Early treatment consisted of crossbite correction which was warranted to prevent further enamel damage and to determine his true anteroposterior dental relationship.

- Treatment unknowns consisted of Mason's true anteroposterior dental relationship and future jaw growth. His true dental relationship was determined by correcting his anterior crossbite and eliminating his CR-CO shift.

- If you correct an anterior crossbite in a child with *normal* skeletal growth, then the crossbite should remain corrected. If you correct an anterior crossbite in a child with a *Class III skeletal discrepancy*, then you need to employ orthopedic treatment to address the skeletal discrepancy. If you do not, then you may end up chasing a recurring anterior crossbite as the child continues growing with the same Class III pattern.

- We are fortunate that Mason did not grow Class III after crossbite correction. If Mason had begun growing Class III, then Class III orthopedics would have been instituted. His growth will continue to be monitored.

- Early treatment eliminated the need for later comprehensive treatment.

Case Edward

Q: Edward is eight years old (Figure 4.60). He was referred to you by his pediatric dentist for crossbite correction. His PMH, PDH, and TMJ evaluations are WRN. The periodontium on the labial surface of his mandibular incisors appears thin, and the roots of the mandibular central incisors are noticeably prominent in the labial alveolar cortical plate. A 1–2 mm CR-CO shift exists, and you note fremitus of the mandibular central incisors

when he closes into CO. Figure 4.60e was made in CR. All other figures were made in CO. *Compile your diagnostic findings and problem list.* State your *diagnosis*.
A:

Table 4.13 Diagnostic findings and problem list for Edward.

Full face and profile	**Frontal View** Facial symmetry Soft tissue LAFH WRN Lip competence UDML right of the facial midline by ~1 mm Maxillary gingival display inadequate during posed smile (maxillary incisor gingival margins are apical to maxillary lip border) **Profile View** Mildly convex profile Nasal tip up NLA WRN Protrusive maxillary lip Protrusive mandibular lip Labiomental sulcus WRN Chin position slightly retrusive Lip-chin-throat angle obtuse
Radiographs	Early mixed dentition Bilateral overlap of maxillary permanent canine crowns over maxillary permanent lateral incisor roots
Intraoral photos and models	Angle Class III subdivision right (Figures 4.60f–4.60g, permanent molars not shown) Iowa Classification III (1 mm) III (1 mm) I I (using the relationship of primary second molars in CO) Anterior crossbite exists in CO *and* in CR (Figure 4.60e) 40% OB in CO (Figure 4.60g) LDML 1 mm left of UDML in CR and CO (Figures 4.60e and 4.60g) Thin gingival attachment labial to mandibular central incisors Maxillary permanent lateral incisors blocked out 6 mm maxillary anterior crowding currently present 4 mm maxillary crowding anticipated following the eruption of all permanent teeth (if appropriate space maintenance is employed) 3 mm mandibular anterior crowding currently present 0.2 mm mandibular spacing anticipated following the eruption of all permanent teeth (if appropriate space maintenance is employed)

(Continued)

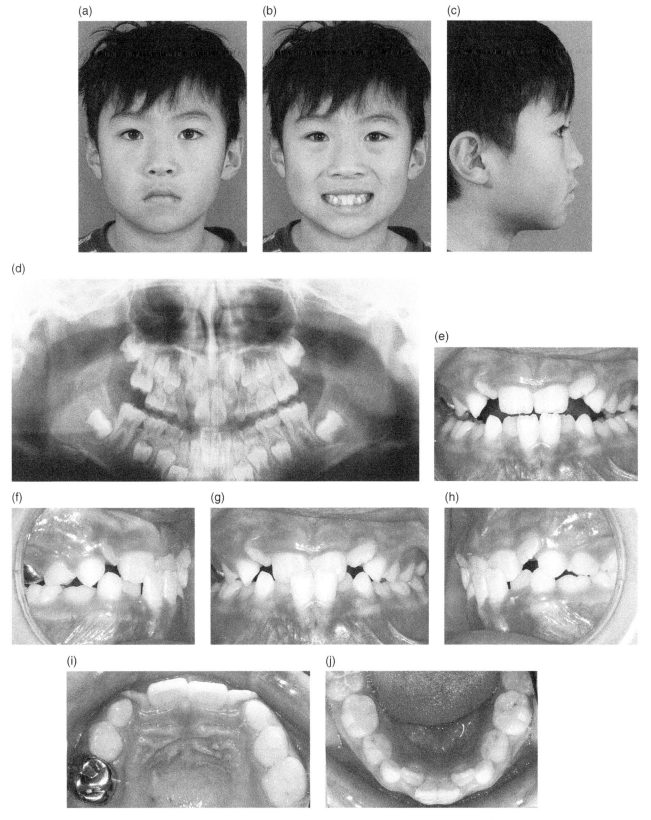

Figure 4.60 Initial records of Edward: (a–c) facial photographs in CO, (d) pantomograph, (e) intraoral frontal photograph in CR, (f–h) intraoral photographs in CO, (i–j) occlusal intraoral photographs.

Table 4.13 (Continued)

	Maxillary arch slightly asymmetric with right side ahead
	Mandibular dental arch symmetric
	Damage to incisal edge of maxillary right central incisor (Figure 4.60e)
Other	1–2 mm CR-CO anterior shift
diagnosis	Class I malocclusion in the early mixed dentition with 1–2 mm anterior CR-CO shift into Class III tendency for right permanent first molar relationship and right primary canine relationship

Q: Do you wish to make any additional records?

A: No additional records are necessary in order to decide whether to treat Edward early or to place him on observation recall.

Q: Provide a detailed space analysis for Edward's maxillary and mandibular arches. In other words, how were the 4 mm of maxillary anterior crowding and 0.2 mm of mandibular anterior spacing calculated (if space maintenance is employed)?

A:

Average mesiodistal widths of permanent teeth (mm): [81]

Maxillary central incisor	8.5	Mandibular central incisor	5.0
Maxillary lateral incisor	6.5	Mandibular lateral incisor	5.5
Maxillary canine	7.5	Mandibular canine	7.0
Maxillary first premolar	7.0	Mandibular first premolar	7.0
Maxillary second premolar	7.0	Mandibular second premolar	7.0
Maxillary first molar	10.0	Mandibular first molar	11.0
Maxillary second molar	9.0	Mandibular second molar	10.5

Average mesiodistal widths of *primary* teeth (mm): [81]

Maxillary central incisor	6.5	Mandibular central incisor	4.2
Maxillary lateral incisor	5.1	Mandibular lateral incisor	4.1
Maxillary canine	7.0	Mandibular canine	5.0
Maxillary first molar	7.3	Mandibular first molar	7.7
Maxillary second molar	8.2	Mandibular second molar	9.9

MAXILLARY ARCH

−6.0 mm anterior crowding currently present (Figure 4.60i)

+2.0 mm anticipated leeway space (1 mm/side)

Balance = − 6.0 mm + 2.0 mm = −4.0 mm

MANDIBULAR ARCH

−3.0 mm anterior crowding currently present

+3.2 mm anticipated leeway space (1.6 mm per side)

Balance = − 3 mm + 3.2 mm = + 0.2 mm

That is, *4 mm of maxillary crowding and 0.2 mm of mandibular spacing is anticipated following the eruption of all permanent teeth (if proper space maintenance is employed).*

Q: What are Edward's primary problems in each dimension (the main problems you must focus on)?

A:

Table 4.14 Primary problem list for Edward.

AP	Class III relationship tendency (right side) in CO
	Iowa Classification III (1 mm) III (1 mm) I I (using the relationship of primary second molars in CO)
	Anterior crossbite exists in CO *and* in CR
Vertical	40% OB in CO
Transverse	–
Other diagnosis	Traumatic damage to the incisal edge of the maxillary right central incisor

Q: Is Edward a pseudo Class III patient (Class III only as a result of his CR-CO shift)? Or, is Edward a *skeletal* Class III patient (Class III dental relationship resulting from growth)?

A: Although we lack a lateral cephalometric radiograph to better assess his skeletal relationships, Edward presents with a *convex* profile in CO (Figure 4.60c). Further, he is minimally Class III (1 mm) on his right side, Class I on his left side, and has a 1–2 mm CR-CO shift.

Based upon these observations, we conclude that Edward is a pseudo Class III patient. Of course, this conclusion could change depending upon future growth.

Q: Discuss Edward in the context of three principles applied to every early treatment patient.

A:

1) The goal of early treatment is to correct developing problems – get the patient *back to normal for their stage of development* (including preventing complications such as resorption of adjacent tooth roots,

reducing later treatment complexity, or reducing/eliminating unknowns). Addressing the following would get Edward back to normal:

- Correcting, and maintaining correction of, his anterior crossbite
- Eliminating his CR-CO shift
- Monitoring his anteroposterior relationship once his anterior crossbite is corrected
- Providing room for permanent teeth

2) Early treatment should address *very specific problems with a clearly defined end point*, usually begun and ended within six to nine months (not protracted over many years except for some orthopedic problems). The correction of Edward's anterior crossbite and CR-CO shift are focused problems that can be addressed in a short time. Reduction of maxillary anterior crowding can be addressed simultaneously while advancing permanent incisors out of crossbite plus later space maintenance. Correction of mandibular anterior crowding can be addressed with space maintenance but will require all permanent canines and premolars to erupt (longer than nine months).

3) Always ask: Is it necessary that I treat the patient now? *What harm may come if I choose to do nothing now?* If Edward's anterior crossbite is not corrected, then:

- Additional maxillary incisor damage is likely.
- Recession of mandibular labial periodontium could occur as a result of the crossbite occlusion stressing periodontal soft tissue.
- The 1–2 mm CR-CO shift could act as a Class II functional appliance – accelerating mandibular growth.
- If an LLHA is not placed in a timely manner, then the mandibular permanent first molars could drift mesially, worsening the mandibular right Class III relationship and reducing leeway space available for crowding.

Q: Should we consider serial extraction for Edward? Why or why not?

A: No, Edward is not a candidate for serial extraction. Let's examine the factors that determine whether a patient is a good candidate for serial extraction.

The ideal serial extraction patient is in the early mixed dentition and is *normal in every way except severe anterior crowding (≥ 9 mm per arch)*. Specifically, the patient should present with:

- *Class I first molars*. We cannot assess Edward's true permanent first molar relationship because he has a CR-CO shift. He may exhibit a Class I permanent molar relationship once his CR-CO shift is eliminated, but until this is accomplished, we cannot consider him a candidate for serial extraction based on this parameter. *We wish to stress that this is an important consideration for any patient for which you are considering serial extraction therapy and aligns with our principle of reducing unknowns.*
- *Vertically normal to slightly long soft tissue and skeletal LAFH, with minimal OB or possibly a mild open bite, but* not *a deep bite.* Although Edward presents with a soft tissue LAFH WRN, he has a 40% deep bite. Consequently, he does not satisfy this feature.
- *Normal incisor angulation or proclined incisors, but* not *upright incisors.* Without a lateral cephalometric radiograph, we cannot accurately evaluate this feature.
- *Normal posterior transverse relationship (normal intermolar arch widths with good posterior interdigitation; absence of posterior crossbites; and absence of significant transverse compensations).* Edward satisfies this feature.
- *Severe (≥ 9 mm) anterior crowding*: Edward presents with only moderate maxillary anterior crowding (6 mm) and mild mandibular anterior crowding (3 mm). He does not satisfy this feature.

Based upon the above, Edward is *not* a good candidate for serial extraction.

Q: What unknowns do you face in treating Edward?

A: Future jaw growth (direction and magnitude), cooperation, hygiene, and the possibility of a worse CR-CO shift than is currently detected.

Q: Can you review each factor that will help you decide whether to treat Edward's anterior crossbite early?

A: The factors include:

- *Presence of an underlying skeletal discrepancy* – Edward does not appear to have a Class III skeletal discrepancy. He appears to be a pseudo Class III, his anterior crossbite is probably not due to growth, and once we correct his crossbite, he will probably not require orthopedics.
- *Permanent incisor eruption status* – his permanent central incisors are erupted, and his permanent lateral incisors are partially erupted (we generally delay anterior crossbite correction until the permanent incisors erupt).
- *Damage to permanent incisors or soft tissue* – the maxillary right permanent central incisor is damaged, and the periodontium labial to the mandibular central incisors may be stressed during closure to CO (fremitus).
- *Compliance* – Edward's parents state that he is a compliant boy.

- *Psychosocial issues* – none noted.
- *CR-CO shift magnitude* – 1–2 mm CR-CO shift.

Q: Based upon the above discussions, what early treatment options would you consider for Edward?

A: Options include:

- *Recall* (no early treatment, monitor only) – recall Edward in one year to evaluate tooth eruption. We advise against this option because doing so could result in additional hard tissue or soft tissue damage. Furthermore, his 1–2 mm CR-CO shift into anterior crossbite could act as a Class II functional appliance – accelerating mandibular growth.
- *Mandibular space maintenance* – place an LLHA before exfoliation of Edward's mandibular primary canines and primary molars. Edward currently has 3 mm mandibular anterior crowding. If an LLHA is placed, we estimate that he will have 0.2 mm of mandibular spacing once all his permanent teeth erupt. As an added benefit, an LLHA will prevent/reduce right permanent first molar mesial drift into a worsened Class III relationship.

  However, Edward's mandibular permanent canine and first premolar roots are < ½ developed, their eruption is not imminent, and the need to place an LLHA is not immediate. On the other hand, it would be better to place an LLHA too early than to neglect to place one.
- *Maxillary space maintenance* – place a Nance holding arch before exfoliation of Edward's maxillary primary canines and primary molars. Edward currently has 6 mm of maxillary anterior crowding. If a Nance holding arch is placed, then he will have 4 mm of maxillary crowding following the eruption of all permanent teeth.

  Placing a Nance holding arch can limit mesial drift of maxillary permanent first molars during the transition from late mixed to permanent dentition. It is not possible to assess the consequences of limiting maxillary molar mesial drift with Edward's CR-CO shift. If a Nance holding arch is to be considered, then we would recommend correcting the anterior crossbite first – and then evaluating Nance holding arch advantages/disadvantages afterward (i.e. reduce unknowns).
- *Space regaining* – opening space lost following exfoliation of Edward's maxillary primary lateral incisors. Space regaining could be performed in conjunction with advancing his central incisors out of crossbite using fixed appliances.
- *Anterior crossbite correction* – to eliminate his CR-CO shift, limit further tissue damage, and permit evaluation of his true anteroposterior dental relationship. This option is highly recommended and a perfect example of *reducing unknowns* before making major treatment decisions – such as beginning orthopedic treatment.
- *Extraction of maxillary primary canines/primary first molars* – to help create space and a path for the eruption of maxillary permanent canines. Although this treatment may be recommended in the future, it would not be recommended yet. Why? If we advance Edward's maxillary incisors out of crossbite, then we may wish to use the primary canines as anchorage.
- *Serial extraction* – as discussed earlier, this option is not recommended for Edward.
- *Class III orthopedic treatment* – is not recommended. Edward has a convex profile and is Class III on the right side by only 1 mm in CO. Further, he has a 1–2 mm shift from CO back to CR. We recommend eliminating the shift first and then re-evaluating his anteroposterior relationship.

Q: Based on the above options, would you begin early treatment or recall Edward? If you treat, what early treatment would you recommend?

A: We decided to proceed with the following (Figure 4.61):

- Band maxillary first permanent molars, bond maxillary central incisors, bond maxillary primary canines and primary first molars, and place a cement bite plate on mandibular permanent first molars to open the bite and allow maxillary incisors to move forward, unimpeded.
- Place a 0.014-inch nitinol archwire and insert compressed open coil springs between maxillary primary canines and maxillary permanent *central* incisors to advance permanent central incisors.
- Insert closed coil springs between maxillary primary first molars and maxillary permanent first molars in order to prevent maxillary primary second molars from being displaced as a result of the compressed open coil spring reciprocal force.
- Another option would have been to fabricate a removable maxillary appliance to open the bite and advance the maxillary central incisors with springs or screws.

The anterior crossbite was corrected (Figure 4.62a), Edward was debanded (Figure 4.62b), and occlusal settling began to occur one month later (Figure 4.62c).

Q: No additional treatment was provided. Edward returned to our clinic seven years later. Records were made (Figure 4.63), but Edward and his parents stated that he was happy and not interested in additional (comprehensive) treatment. What changes do you observe compared to his initial records?

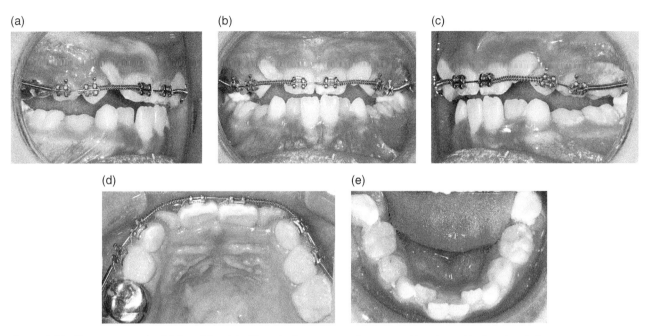

Figure 4.61 Progress records of Edward. (a–c) in CR occluding on posterior cement bite plates, (d–e) occlusal photos.

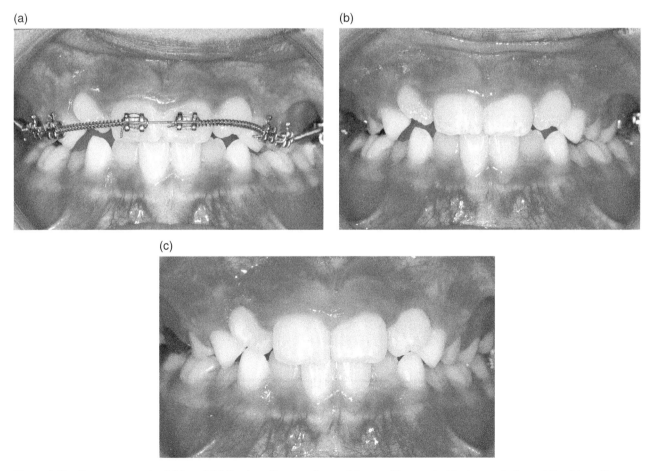

Figure 4.62 Progress records of Edward. (a) fixed appliances advanced the maxillary central incisors out of crossbite; (b) appliances removed; (c) one month after appliances were removed.

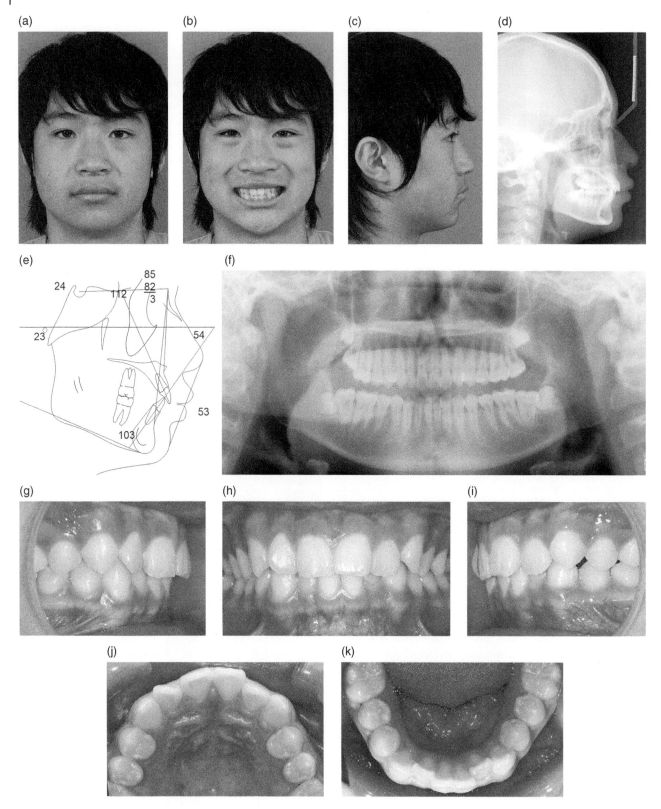

Figure 4.63 (a–k) Records of Edward made seven years after completion of early treatment.

A: Changes include:
- Edward is a handsome fifteen-year-old with noticeable maxillary anterior malalignment during posed smile.
- Convex profile.
- Maxillary anteroposterior deficiency (Figure 4.63e).
- Mandibular anteroposterior deficiency (ANB = 3° with deficient maxilla).
- Skeletal LAFH WRN (LAFH/TAFH×100% = 53% versus a normal value of 55%).
- FMA WRN (23°).
- Flat SNMP (24°, but Sella is high).
- Bimaxillary incisor protrusion (U1 to SN = 112°, FMIA = 54°).
- All permanent incisors, canines, and premolars have erupted.
- Mandibular second molars partially impacted (distal aspect of crowns unable to erupt) and crowns tipped distally.
- Angle Class II division 1 subdivision left.
- Iowa Classification: I I II (2 mm) II (2 mm).
- Anterior crossbite correction has remained stable.
- OB 30–40%.
- OJ 1–2 mm.
- 3 mm maxillary anterior crowding.
- 3 mm mandibular anterior crowding.
- Improved attached tissue labial to mandibular central incisors (compare Figures 4.60g and 4.63h).

Q: We were initially concerned with Edward's thin gingival biotype labial to his mandibular central incisors (Figure 4.60g). However, seven years later (Figure 4.63h), he exhibits an adequate band of keratinized attached tissue labial to all maxillary and mandibular anterior teeth. Can you explain this change?

A: Yes. In a two-year longitudinal study of children six to twelve years of age with well-aligned maxillary and mandibular teeth, increases in widths of facial keratinized and attached gingiva took place [102]. Why does this happen? We are not sure. But it is wonderful that it does.

Q: Should we have corrected Edward's anterior crossbite by bonding all *four* maxillary incisors instead of bonding only his maxillary central incisors?

A: No. We achieved anterior crossbite correction and CR-CO shift correction by bonding only the maxillary central incisors (Figure 4.62c). There was no need to bond the lateral incisors. Further, we had concerns regarding the proximity of the maxillary lateral incisor roots to the erupting maxillary permanent canine crowns (Figure 4.60d). To avoid resorbing the lateral incisor roots, we chose not to move these teeth during early treatment.

Q: Should we have placed an LLHA?

A: Yes. Edward initially presented with 3 mm mandibular anterior crowding, and we estimated that 0.2 mm of spacing would follow if we placed an LLHA. Instead, Edward ended with 2 mm mandibular anterior crowding because we failed to place an LLHA.

However, if mandibular first permanent molar mesial drift had been prevented/reduced with an LLHA, then Edward's anteroposterior molar relationship would have ended more Class II, and his mandibular second molars may have had even less eruption.

Q: Was *early* treatment justified?

A: Yes. Let's review this decision in the context of the three early treatment principles:
1) The goal of early treatment is to get the patient *back to normal for their stage of development* – correcting the anterior crossbite and CR-CO shift got Edward back to normal (except for his crowding).
2) Early treatment should address *very specific problems with a clearly defined end-point* – correcting the anterior crossbite, and eliminating the CR-CO shift, were focused problems with a clearly defined end point.
3) *"What harm may have come if we had chosen to do nothing?"* If we had only recalled Edward, then further incisal damage would probably have occurred.

Q: Can you suggest any "take-home pearls"?

A: "Take-home pearls" include the following:
- Edward was eight years old when he presented with damage to his maxillary right central incisor as a result of biting/shifting forward into an anterior crossbite. Also, his maxillary incisors were contacting his mandibular incisors on their lingual surfaces and forcing them labially during closure. We noted mandibular central incisor fremitus, suggesting regular undesirable forward pressure on these teeth. Early treatment to correct his anterior crossbite and shift was justified and successful.
- Edward was pseudo Class III. It is important to differentiate between pseudo Class III patients and *skeletal* Class III patients. Why? Once the anterior crossbite (CR-CO shift) is corrected in pseudo Class III children, they can complete orthodontic treatment as Class I patients. But once the anterior crossbite is corrected in *skeletal* Class III children, they must continue to be treated orthopedically as Class III growers. Otherwise, the crossbite will probably return as the Class III growth continues.

Edward was Class III on the right side by 1 mm in CO and Class I on the left side in CO, but he had a 1–2 mm CR-CO shift. By eliminating his crossbite and shift, we eliminated the Class III relationship. He was a pseudo Class III.

- A child shifting the mandible forward into an anterior crossbite is analogous to a child posturing forward when wearing a Class II functional appliance. The outcome should, theoretically, be the same – accelerated mandibular growth, maxillary forward growth restriction, uprighting of maxillary incisors, and proclination of mandibular incisors. The greater the magnitude of CR-CO shift into anterior crossbite, the more potential exists for these changes to occur. This notion is intuitively appealing but unproven.

- *An LLHA can prevent the worsening of a Class III molar relationship* by preventing/reducing the first permanent molar mesial drift into leeway space during the transition from mixed to permanent dentition. Please remember this "pearl" and incorporate it into your practice.

- Edward was referred for the extraction of wisdom teeth. If extraction of mandibular wisdom teeth does not result in the eruption of mandibular second molars, then comprehensive orthodontic treatment would be recommended (again).

Case Cooper

Q: Cooper is five years and one month old (Figure 4.64). He presents to you for a consultation with his parents' chief complaint, "Cooper's dentist says he has a jaw problem." His PMH, PDH, periodontal evaluation, and TMJ evaluation are WRN. CR = CO. Do you need any additional records in order to decide whether to recall Cooper or to perform the early treatment?

A: You do not need additional records in order to decide whether to recall Cooper or treat him now. If you decide to treat him, then you should make and analyze a lateral cephalometric radiograph or CBCT.

Q: Compile *your diagnostic findings/problem list* and state your *diagnosis.*

A:

Table 4.15 Diagnostic findings and problem list for Cooper.

Full face and profile	Frontal View
	Face is symmetric
	Soft tissue LAFH WRN (soft tissue Glabella – Subnasale approximately equal to Subnasale – soft tissue Menton)
	Lip competence
	Minimal buccal corridors (Figure 4.64b)
	UDML WRN
	Profile View
	Concave profile
	Obtuse NLA
	Mandibular lip protrusive
	Chin projection excessive
	Lip-chin-throat angle WRN
Radiographs	Primary dentition (mandibular first permanent molars will erupt soon)
Intraoral photos and models	Class III primary molar relationship (large mesial step)
	Iowa Classification: III (4 mm) III (4 mm) III (5 mm) III (5 mm)
	Anterior crossbite (underbite, no tissue damage or impingement)
	Posterior crossbite of the right primary first molar
	LDML to right of UDML by ~ 1 mm
	70% OB
	4 mm current maxillary anterior spacing
	3 mm current mandibular anterior spacing
	Maxillary and mandibular dental arches are symmetric
Other diagnosis	Class III malocclusion in the primary dentition with anterior and posterior crossbites

Q: We noted that Cooper has a concave profile with excessive chin projection. How do you judge chin projection?

A: Use the *zero-meridian line*. The zero-meridian line is a vertical line drawn from soft tissue Nasion perpendicular to the Frankfort horizontal line. Normal chin projection should lie on this line or just short of it [84, 103]. Cooper's chin (soft tissue Pogonion, Figure 4.65b) lies just anterior to the zero-meridian line. That is, his chin is mildly excessive.

Q: Can you discern from Figure 4.64d whether Cooper's maxillary first permanent molars are erupting normally or ectopically? If you cannot discern whether they are erupting normally, should you request additional imaging?

A: We cannot discern whether Cooper's maxillary first permanent molars are erupting normally or ectopically (resorbing the roots of his maxillary primary second molars). We feel that it is too early to make that determination. We could request additional imaging (periapical radiographs or a CBCT) but decided not to – in order to avoid additional radiation exposure to Cooper. His maxillary first permanent molars do not appear delayed relative to his mandibular first permanent molars (mesially directed maxillary first molars often experience delayed emergence). On average, maxillary first permanent molars emerge one to two months after

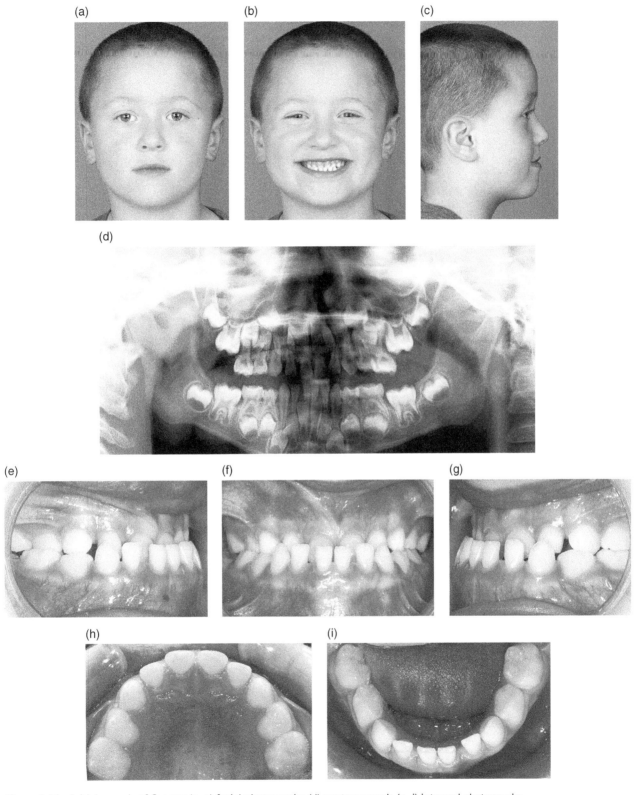

Figure 4.64   Initial records of Cooper: (a–c) facial photographs, (d) pantomograph, (e–i) intraoral photographs.

(a)

(b)

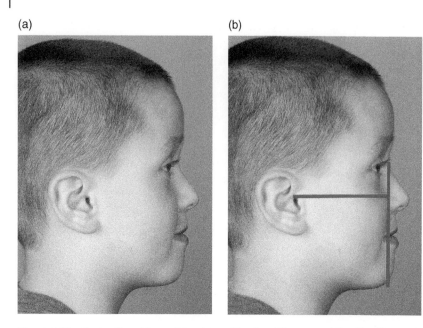

Figure 4.65 Evaluating chin position. (a) profile view, (b) zero meridian-line illustrating that Cooper has mildly excessive chin projection.

mandibular permanent first molars [104]. For now, we recommend monitoring the eruption of his maxillary first permanent molars.

Q: What are Cooper's *primary* problems in each dimension, plus other problems?

A:

Table 4.16 Primary problem list for Cooper.

AP	Class III primary molar relationship (large mesial step)
	Iowa Classification: III (4 mm) III (4 mm) III (5 mm) III (5 mm)
Vertical	70% OB
Transverse	Posterior crossbite of the right primary first molar
Other	Anterior crossbite (underbite)

Q: Is Cooper a pseudo Class III malocclusion patient, a *dental* Class III patient, or a *skeletal* Class III patient?

A: Cooper is *not* a pseudo Class III patient. He would be considered a pseudo Class III patient if he was Class I in CR but had a CR-CO shift into Class III. Cooper lacks a shift and is Class III by 4–5 mm in CR.

Cooper is *not* a dental Class III patient. He would be considered a dental Class III patient if he was skeletally normal but had mandibular teeth shifted forward into a Class III position relative to his maxillary teeth. This

situation could occur following the premature loss of mandibular primary canines or primary molars – and subsequent mesial drift of the permanent first molars.

Cooper *is* a skeletal Class III patient. His concave profile indicates this. He may have deficient maxillary growth (anteroposteriorly), excessive mandibular growth, or a combination of both. We will need to examine a lateral cephalometric radiograph of him to understand which jaw is at fault.

Q: Assume that Cooper is Class III due to excessive mandibular growth. Are there signs that he could be growing *asymmetrically* Class III?

A: Yes. With asymmetric mandibular growth (more growth on one side), you would expect to see (Figure 4.66):
- Chin deviation and lower dental midline (LDML) deviation *away* from the side with more growth.
- Greater Class III molar relationship *on* the side with more growth.
- A posterior crossbite on the side with less growth.

Of these features, Cooper does not demonstrate an overt chin deviation (Figure 4.64a), but his LDML is to the right of his upper dental midline (UDML). Further, he exhibits a slightly greater Class III relationship on his left than on his right and a primary molar right posterior crossbite. We conclude that Cooper could be growing with bilaterally excessive mandibular growth but with even more condylar growth on the left than on the right.

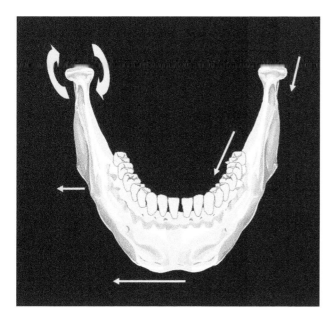

Figure 4.66 Left-side asymmetric excessive mandibular condylar growth. Note chin deviation and LDML deviation to the *right*, greater Class III molar relationship on the *left*, and tendency for posterior crossbite on the *right* as the mandible rotates around the right condyle.

Q: Discuss Cooper in the context of three principles applied to every early treatment patient.

A:

1) The goal of early treatment is to correct developing problems – get the patient *back to normal for their stage of development* (including preventing complications such as resorption of adjacent tooth roots, reducing later treatment complexity, or reducing/eliminating unknowns). Correcting the following problems would get Cooper back on track:
    - Class III relationship
    - Concave profile
    - Anterior crossbite
    - Right primary molar crossbite
    - 70% OB

2) Early treatment should address *very specific problems with a clearly defined end point*, usually within six to nine months. The problems we face with Cooper are specific. However, orthopedic treatment to correct his anteroposterior skeletal discrepancy (and anterior crossbite) could take many years. Correction of his right posterior crossbite and 70% OB could take six to nine months, but we would be moving primary teeth which could undergo premature root resorption and loss.

3) Always ask: Is it necessary that I treat the patient now? *What harm will come if I do nothing now?* If we do not attempt orthopedics to address Cooper's skeletal Class III relationship and anterior crossbite now, then we may miss some favorable growth. However, Cooper is only five years old and has many years of growth remaining. We do not see any harm in waiting to treat his posterior crossbite and OB.

Q: What unknowns do you face with treating Cooper?

A: Future jaw growth (direction and magnitude), cooperation, hygiene, and the possibility of an undetected CR-CO shift.

Q: Cooper has a 4–5 mm Class III skeletal discrepancy. Can you suggest specific orthopedic options to address it?

A: If we decide to attempt orthopedic correction, then we should first make a lateral cephalometric radiograph or CBCT to identify which jaw is at fault (deficient maxilla, excessive mandible, or combination). Orthopedic options include:

- RPHG (enhancing maxillary forward growth while inhibiting mandibular forward growth). We could use a *tooth-borne RPHG* which advances A-Point (1–2 mm), advances (proclines) maxillary incisors, restricts mandibular growth, increases MPA, and increases LAFH [53, 54]. We could use a *TAD-anchored RPHG* which advances A-Point (3 mm) but with less face height increase and no dental movement [65–67].
- High-pull chin cup (restricting mandibular forward growth while allowing maxillary forward growth to continue). If Cooper's anterior crossbite is corrected, or if he wears a bite plate to disclude his anterior teeth, then he could wear a high-pull chin cup. High-pull chin cup wear inhibits mandibular ramal height growth and mandibular body length growth while allowing the maxilla to continue growing forward – resulting in ANB improvement and improved chin position [58, 72, 73, 75, 76]. Note: The vertical force component of a high-pull chin cup appears to prevent LAFH increases compared to controls [74, 78].
- TAD-supported Class III elastic wear (enhancing maxillary forward growth while inhibiting mandibular forward growth). First, we would correct Cooper's anterior crossbite or place him on a bite plate to disclude his anterior teeth. Then, TADs are placed to which Class III elastics are worn. TAD-supported Class III elastic wear (250 gm force per side, the same force level we recommend for high-pull chin cup wear) would advance his maxilla (4 mm), and result in a B-Point improvement of 2 mm [74]. TADs must be placed carefully to avoid trauma to erupting teeth.

Q: In addition to potential improved patient compliance with TAD-supported Class III elastic wear, is there another potential benefit with this treatment?

A: Yes. TAD-supported Class III elastic wear offers the potential to treat *unilateral* mandibular asymmetric growth. In other words, RPHG or high-pull chin cup wear delivers a bilateral restrictive force to the mandible. TAD-supported Class III elastic wear can deliver *unilateral* orthopedic force to address unilateral asymmetric growth.

Q: Would you consider *masking/camouflage* (achieving an excellent dental relationship without addressing Cooper's underlying skeletal discrepancy) or *orthognathic surgery*?

A: No. Generally, we consider masking/camouflage and surgery during comprehensive treatment in the permanent dentition. In the mixed dentition, we would recommend attempting orthopedics.

However, you must talk to Cooper's parents about the possible future need for masking/surgery – depending upon Cooper's jaw growth magnitude, jaw growth direction, and his cooperation. Further, there are times when overriding medical concerns (e.g. a collapsed airway) may force early orthognathic surgery in some patients.

Q: We need to discuss treatment *timing*. As we stated, we would not recommend masking or surgical treatment for Cooper at five years of age. However, what are your thoughts about beginning Class III *orthopedic* treatment now?

A: Let's consider the facts regarding the timing of anteroposterior orthopedic treatment:

- Randomized, prospective clinical trials report no advantage gained by beginning *Class II* treatment in the early mixed dentition (except for a possible decrease in incisal trauma as a result of excess OJ) [22–24, 29, 38–40]. However, we will consider Class II orthopedics in the early mixed dentition if the patient is showing good statural growth velocity.
- For Class III skeletal correction, the effects of RPHGs are greatest in patients ≤ ten years old [55–57], and a rule of thumb is to begin RPHG treatment when the maxillary permanent central incisors are erupting (seven to eight years of age).
- Cooper's maxillary first permanent molars are unerupted. We need those molars for RPHG anchorage unless we use maxillary TADs for anchorage. We would not recommend placing TADs in a five-year-old child unless there was a medical necessity.

- The literature lacks randomized, prospective clinical trials of early Class III orthopedic treatment using high-pull chin cups or Class III elastics supported by TADs.
- We generally recommend that *the larger the Class III skeletal discrepancy, the earlier we will begin orthopedics* (to take advantage of as much future growth as possible). For some patients, this may be as early as five to six years of age. However, other important variables that will play a role in your decision to begin treatment include the maturity level of the patient, their interest in treatment, and the interest of the parents in treatment.
- If you are able to correct a Class III relationship orthopedically, then you must maintain the correction *until growth is complete*. This can take many years. Orthopedic treatment does not normalize growth. Once you achieve Class III correction, the patient will revert to their Class III growth pattern if you stop orthopedics before growth is complete. Some patients are capable of such long-term compliance, especially if it means they can avoid permanent tooth extractions or jaw surgery. Others are not.

Q: What discussions should you have with Cooper and his parents?

A: You should discuss the problems he presents with, treatment options for dealing with those problems, the parents' level of interest in beginning orthopedic treatment, his level of interest, and his level of maturity. Cooper's parents are interested in his care, but they state that they are very concerned about his potential lack of attention and cooperation.

Q: Should you start early treatment or recall Cooper? What treatment options would you consider?

A: Your treatment options include the following:

- *Recall* (no treatment, monitor only) – re-evaluate in one year. We anticipate no harm by monitoring Cooper for an additional year. He will still have many years of growth ahead of him. Based upon discussions we had with Cooper and his parents, we feel that delaying orthopedic treatment for at least a year is a viable option.
- *Mandibular space maintenance* – may be prudent someday, but not yet. Why? Someday, an LLHA will *prevent/reduce mandibular first permanent molar mesial drift*, and worsening of his Class III relationship, as his primary canines and primary molars exfoliate. However, it is far too early to consider placing an LLHA.

- *Extraction of primary canines or primary molars* – to help insure eruption of permanent teeth. This option is *not recommended* since Cooper's permanent canine and premolar roots are < ½ developed, their eruption is years away, and future extraction of these teeth may be unnecessary.
- *Primary teeth anterior crossbite correction* – in preparation for Class III skeletal orthopedics (e.g. high-pull chin cup). We generally prefer to wait until permanent incisors erupt before correcting anterior crossbites, but we will consider anterior crossbite correction of primary incisors if we decide to begin Class III orthopedics.

However, look closely at the maxillary and mandibular primary central incisor roots in Figure 4.64d. The roots are nearly two thirds resorbed by the erupting permanent central incisor crowns. If we attempt to move these primary teeth out of crossbite, then they may exfoliate. Instead, we recommend allowing these primary central incisors to exfoliate naturally, allowing the permanent central incisors to erupt naturally, and then possibly moving the permanent incisors forward out of crossbite.

- *Class III orthopedic treatment* – using an RPHG, high-pull chin cup, or TAD-supported Class III elastics. Cooper is certainly a candidate for Class III orthopedics, but the question is *when to start*? Based upon the Class III orthopedic timing facts we presented earlier, and considering our discussion with Cooper's parents, we do not recommend beginning Class III orthopedic treatment yet.

Q: After discussing the above options with Cooper and his parents, the consultation appointment is nearly over. Cooper's parents ask for your final recommendation. What do you recommend?

A: Based upon the magnitude of his Class III skeletal discrepancy, his age, his potential lack of cooperation, and the fact that his permanent incisors should be erupting during the next year, we decided to recall Cooper in one year. At that time, we will reassess his interest and maturity level. We may, or may not, make complete records (including a lateral cephalometric radiograph or CBCT) and begin Class III orthopedic treatment.

Case Allison

Q: Allison is seven years and ten months old (Figure 4.67). She presents to you with a chief complaint, "I want my crossbite fixed." Her PMH, PDH, periodontal evaluation, and TMJ evaluation are WRN. A 1–2 mm CR-CO shift forward and to the right is noted. Figures 4.67h–4.67i shows

her in CR. All other images are in CO. *Compile your diagnostic findings and problem list.* State your *diagnosis*.

A:

Table 4.17 Diagnostic findings and problem list for Allison.

Full face and profile	**Frontal View**
	Facial symmetry
	Long soft tissue LAFH but teeth appear separated
	2–3 mm incisal display in relaxed lip position (Figure 4.67a)
	ILG 3 mm but teeth appear separated
	UDML WRN
	Large buccal corridors (Figure 4.67b)
	Maxillary gingival display inadequate during posed smile (maxillary incisor gingival margins are apical to maxillary lip border)
	Profile View
	Straight profile
	NLA WRN
	Mildly protrusive lower lip
	Labiomental sulcus WRN
	Chin position WRN
	Lip-chin-throat angle WRN
	Chin-throat length WRN
Ceph analysis	**Skeletal (Figure 4.67e, lateral cephalometric radiograph made in CO)**
	Maxillary skeletal anteroposterior deficiency (A-point lies behind Nasion-perpendicular line)
	Mandibular skeletal position WRN
	LAFH WRN (LAFH/TAFH × 100% = 55%)
	MPA WRN (FMA = 22°, SNMP = 32°)
	Effective bony Pogonion (bony Pogonion lies on a line extending from Nasion through B-point)
	Dental
	Maxillary incisors proclined (U1-SN = 107° vs. ideal U1-SN between 101–104°)
	Mandibular incisor inclination WRN (FMIA = 67°)
Radiographs	Early mixed dentition
	Blocked and potentially impacted maxillary canines (note the absence of adequate space, Figure 4.67p)
Intraoral photos and models	Angle Class III malocclusion in CO
	Iowa Classification: III (2 mm) x x III (2 mm) in CO
	30–40% OB
	Moderate COS (Figures 4.67m and 4.67o)

(Continued)

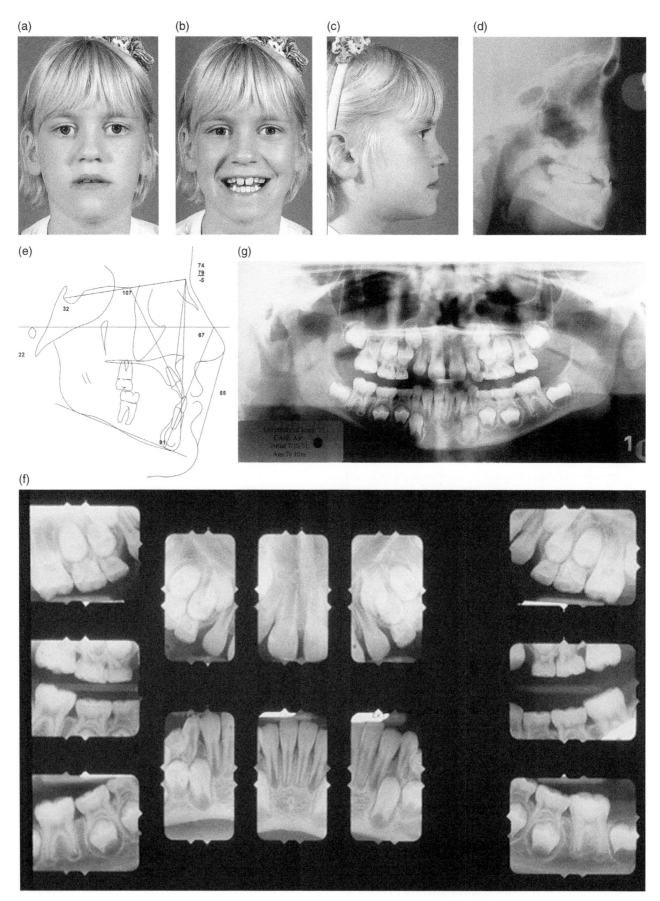

Figure 4.67 Initial records of Allison: (a–c) facial photographs, (d–e) lateral cephalometric radiograph and tracing in CO, (f) complete mouth radiographic survey, (g) pantomograph, (h–i) lateral cephalometric radiograph and frontal photograph in CR, (j–l) intraoral photographs – note posterior teeth slightly separated, (m–s) models.

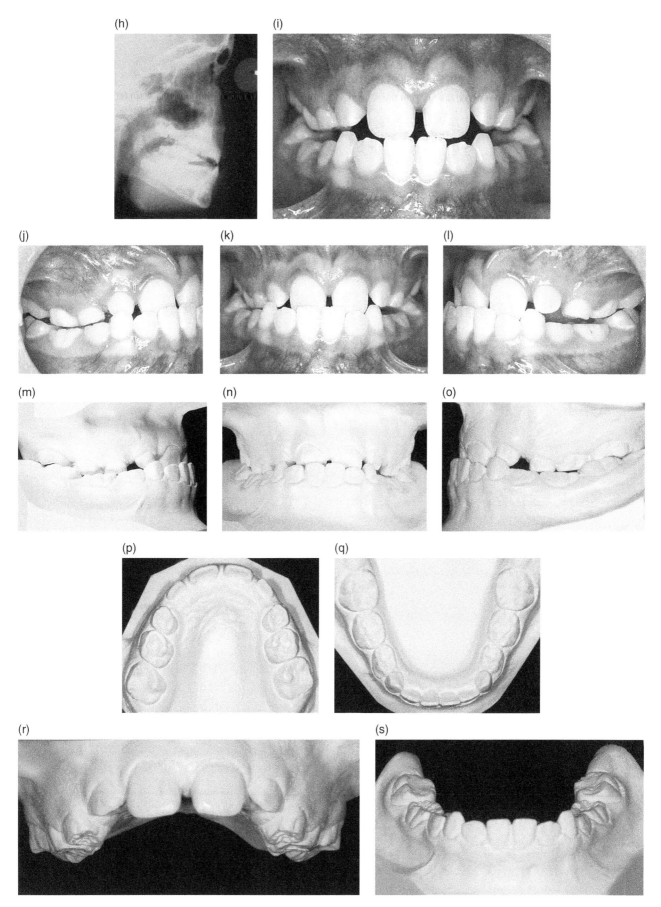

Figure 4.67 (Continued)

Table 4.17 (Continued)

	Anterior crossbite in CO
	Central incisors edge-to-edge in CR (Figures 4.67h–4.67i)
	No tissue damage noted due to anterior crossbite
	Mandibular midline to right of the maxillary midline by 1 mm in CR (Figure 4.67i) and 2 mm in CO (Figure 4.67k)
	Bilateral posterior lingual crossbite of primary molars and maxillary first permanent molar mesiobuccal cusps in CO (Figures 4.67m and 4.67o)
	Maxillary skeletal transverse deficiency: maxillary first permanent molar inter molar lingual cusp width = 47.3 mm; mandibular first permanent molar intermolar central fossa width = 51.9 mm
	Maxillary posterior transverse compensations – permanent first molars exhibit *labial* crown torque (Figure 4.67r)
	Mandibular posterior transverse compensations – permanent first molars exhibit *lingual* crown torque (Figure 4.67s)
	Thick periodontal biotype with adequate keratinized attached tissue labial to mandibular anterior teeth (Figure 4.67k)
	5 mm of maxillary anterior crowding currently present (10 mm of space with 15 mm of estimated space required for right and left permanent canines)
	2 mm of maxillary crowding anticipated following the eruption of all permanent teeth (if appropriate space maintenance is employed)
	0 mm of mandibular anterior crowding currently present
	3.2 mm of mandibular spacing is anticipated following the eruption of all permanent teeth (if appropriate space maintenance is employed)
	Maxillary midline diastema
	Maxillary and mandibular dental arches are symmetric (Figures 4.67p and 4.67q)
Other	–
diagnosis	Class III malocclusion secondary to maxillary skeletal anteroposterior (and transverse) hypoplasia, bilateral posterior lingual crossbite, anterior crossbite in CO, and 1–2 mm forward/right lateral CR-CO shift

Q: Do you wish to make any additional records?

A: No additional records are needed to decide whether to treat Allison now or recall her.

Q: Provide detailed space analysis for Allison's maxillary and mandibular arches. In other words, how were the 2 mm of maxillary crowding and 3.2 mm of mandibular spacing calculated (if space maintenance is employed)?

A:

Average mesiodistal widths of permanent teeth (mm): [81]

Maxillary central incisor	8.5	Mandibular central incisor	5.0
Maxillary lateral incisor	6.5	Mandibular lateral incisor	5.5
Maxillary canine	7.5	Mandibular canine	7.0
Maxillary first premolar	7.0	Mandibular first premolar	7.0
Maxillary second premolar	7.0	Mandibular second premolar	7.0
Maxillary first molar	10.0	Mandibular first molar	11.0
Maxillary second molar	9.0	Mandibular second molar	10.5

Average mesiodistal widths of *primary* teeth (mm): [81]

Maxillary central incisor	6.5	mandibular central incisor	4.2
Maxillary lateral incisor	5.1	Mandibular lateral incisor	4.1
Maxillary canine	7.0	Mandibular canine	5.0
Maxillary first molar	7.3	Mandibular first molar	7.7
Maxillary second molar	8.2	Mandibular second molar	9.9

MAXILLARY ARCH (leeway space cannot be used since primary canines are missing)

+8.2 mm width of maxillary right primary second molar Figure 4.67p)

−7.0 mm anticipated width of the maxillary right second premolar

+7.3 mm width of the maxillary right primary first molar

−7.0 mm anticipated width of the maxillary right first premolar

+10 mm of anterior spacing currently present

−7.5 mm anticipated width of the maxillary right permanent canine

−7.5 mm anticipated width of the maxillary left permanent canine

+7.3 mm width of the maxillary left primary first molar

−7.0 mm anticipated width of the maxillary left first premolar

+8.2 mm width of the maxillary left primary second molar

−7.0 mm anticipated width of the maxillary right second premolar

Balance = + 8.2 mm − 7.0 mm + 7.3 mm − 7.0 mm + 10 mm − 7.5 mm − 7.5 mm + 7.3 mm − 7.0 mm + 8.2 mm − 7.0 mm = −2.0 mm

MANDIBULAR ARCH

0 mm of anterior crowding currently present

+3.2 mm of anticipated leeway space (1.6 mm/side)

Balance = 0 mm + 3.2 mm = + 3.2 mm

That is, *2 mm of maxillary arch crowding and 3.2 mm of mandibular spacing is anticipated following the eruption of all permanent teeth (if proper space maintenance is employed).*

Q: What are your primary problems in each dimension (the main problems you must focus on)?

A:

Table 4.18   Primary problem list for Allison.

AP	Angle Class III malocclusion in CO
	Iowa Classification: III (2 mm) x x III (2 mm) in CO
	Maxillary skeletal anteroposterior deficiency
	Anterior crossbite in CO
Vertical	–
Transverse	Maxillary skeletal transverse deficiency
	Bilateral maxillary lingual posterior crossbite
	Transverse dental compensations of maxillary and mandibular posterior teeth
Other diagnosis	Blocked and potentially impacted maxillary canines
	1–2 mm forward/right lateral CR-CO shift

Q: Allison has proclined maxillary incisors (U1-SN = 107° versus ideal U1-SN between 101–104°) and ideal mandibular incisor inclination (FMIA = 67°). Can you speculate why?

A: The proclined maxillary incisor inclination is an example of Class III dental compensations. As teeth erupt, their path of eruption is dictated by the soft tissue trough between tongue and lips or tongue and cheeks. With a large mandible relative to maxilla, we assume that the tongue pushes the maxillary incisors forward resulting in proclined maxillary incisors.

Q: Is Allison a pseudo Class III patient? Is Allison a *dental* Class III patient? Or, should she be treated as a *skeletal* Class III patient?

A: Some features lead you to classify Allison as a pseudo Class III patient. Her 2 mm Class III molar relationship nearly disappears when she is shifted back 1–2 mm from CO to CR (incisors edge-to-edge).

However, she has a *significant* maxillary skeletal deficiency. In patients like Allison, it is prudent to assume the worst and begin treating her as a skeletal Class III patient. *Avoid doing anything irreversible (e.g. extracting permanent teeth) until she has finished growing or has minimal growth remaining.*

She is not a dental Class III patient. In other words, she is not skeletally normal and Class III due to premature loss of mandibular primary canines or primary molars with subsequent first permanent molar mesial drift into a Class III relationship.

Q: Discuss Allison in the context of three principles applied to every early treatment patient.

A:

1) The goal of early treatment is to correct developing problems – get the patient *back to normal for their stage of development* (including preventing complications such as resorption of adjacent tooth roots, reducing later treatment complexity, or reducing/eliminating unknows). Correcting Allison's following problems would get her back to normal:
   - Class III skeletal relationship (deficient maxilla)
   - Anterior crossbite
   - Bilateral posterior crossbite
   - CR-CO shift
   - Potentially impacted maxillary permanent canines
   - Proclined maxillary incisors

2) Early treatment should address *very specific problems with a clearly defined end point*, usually begun and ended within six to nine months (not protracted over many years except for some orthopedic problems). Allison's Class III skeletal discrepancy is a specific problem with a clearly defined end point. However, correcting (and maintaining correction of) this problem orthopedically may take years.

   Her maxillary transverse deficiency and bilateral posterior lingual crossbite could be corrected in a matter of weeks with RME – which would also create room for her maxillary permanent canines and expand her maxillary permanent lateral incisors out of crossbite (Figure 4.67i, Allison in CR). Her CR-CO shift could be readily corrected with RME followed by fixed appliance treatment to procline her maxillary central incisors out of crossbite.

3) Always ask: Is it necessary that I treat the patient now? *What harm could come if I chose to do nothing now?* If we decide to use RPHG Class III orthopedics, then we may miss out on favorable skeletal changes if we wait. A traditional guideline calls for RPHG orthopedics when a child's maxillary permanent incisors are erupting, and the skeletal effects of

RPHGs are less in patients older than 10 years of age [55–57]. If we decide to use high-pull chin cup or TAD-supported Class III elastic wear for orthopedics, then the Class III skeletal discrepancy could worsen if we wait – depending upon growth.

Postponing correction of her bilateral lingual crossbite with RME should not be a problem so long as we do not wait past puberty – after which time expansion will be more dental and less skeletal. If we do not correct Allison's anterior crossbite, then her CR-CO forward shift could act as a Class II functional appliance, accelerating mandibular growth and worsening her Class III relationship. Since her CR-CO shift includes a lateral component to the right, her mandible could also grow asymmetrically. Finally, if we do not make room for her maxillary permanent canines to erupt, then they may become impacted or possibly resorb her maxillary permanent lateral incisor roots.

Q: What will be your *long-term* (comprehensive, not early) treatment goals for Allison?

A: Long-term goals will include the following:
- Correcting and maintaining correction of her Class III skeletal discrepancy (achieving Class I canines and molars)
- Correcting her transverse skeletal discrepancy and removing posterior transverse compensations (uprighting posterior teeth)
- Avoiding extraction of permanent teeth and avoiding orthognathic surgery if possible
- Providing room for all permanent teeth
- Obtaining ideal OB, ideal OJ, alignment of teeth, and health of tissues.

Q: Which of the above long-term goals will be the most difficult to achieve?

A: The first goal – correcting (and maintaining correction of) her Class III skeletal discrepancy. Even if we correct her Class III skeletal relationship using RPHG, high-pull chin cup, or TAD-supported Class III elastics, *we cannot normalize her growth and must maintain the correction until she is finished growing.*

Q: Is Allison a candidate for serial extraction? Discuss five features that would (or would not) make her a candidate for serial extraction.

A: Allison is not a candidate for serial extraction. The ideal serial extraction patient is in the early mixed dentition and is *normal in every way except severe anterior crowding (≥ 9 mm per arch)*. Specifically, the patient should present with:

- *Class I first permanent molars.* Allison has Class III molars in CO and is growing Class III – a condition that should be corrected and maintained *before* extraction of permanent teeth. If you perform serial extractions to *mask* her underlying skeletal discrepancy (e.g. extraction of maxillary second premolars and mandibular first premolars), then she could grow out of your extraction treatment if the skeletal discrepancy is not addressed. *Eliminate unknowns, including growth, before extracting permanent teeth.*
- *Vertically normal to slightly long soft tissue and skeletal LAFH, with minimal OB or possibly a mild open bite, but* not *a deep bite.* Allison exhibits a 30–40% deep bite which is deeper than ideal.
- *Normal incisor angulation or proclined incisors, but not upright incisors.* Allison has proclined maxillary incisors and ideal mandibular incisor angulation, satisfying this feature.
- *Normal posterior transverse relationship (normal intermolar arch widths with good posterior interdigitation; absence of posterior crossbites; and absence of significant transverse compensations).* Allison has a bilateral lingual posterior crossbite with significant transverse compensations and does not satisfy this feature.
- *Severe (≥ 9 mm) anterior crowding* – Allison has 5 mm of maxillary anterior crowding currently present (10 mm of space with 15 mm of estimated space required for right and left permanent canines) and 0 mm of mandibular anterior crowding currently present. She does not satisfy this feature.

Based upon the above, Allison is *not* an ideal candidate for serial extraction.

Q: Allison has a significant Class III skeletal growth pattern (maxillary skeletal deficiency). There are three general ways to treat any skeletal discrepancy whether anteroposterior, vertical, or transverse. Can you list them and provide specific treatments for Allison?

A: Anteroposterior skeletal discrepancies can be treated using:

Orthopedics (enhancing Allison's maxillary forward growth and/or inhibiting mandibular forward growth). Options include:
- Tooth-borne RPHGs which advance A-Point by 1–2 mm, advance (procline) maxillary incisors, create downward and backward mandibular movement, increase MPA, and increase LAFH [53, 54]. TAD-anchored RPHGs which advance A-Point by 3 mm with less face height increase and no dental movement [65–67]. Note: Skeletal effects of RPHGs are less in patients greater than 10 years of age [55–57].

- High-pull chin cups, which inhibit mandibular ramal height growth, inhibit mandibular body length growth, and allow the maxilla to continue growing forward – resulting in ANB improvement (less Class III growth compared to controls) and improved chin position [72–76].

  Note: With high-pull chin cup wear, LAFH is *not* increased compared to controls [73, 74]. Also, to prevent Allison's maxillary anterior teeth from being traumatized by her mandibular teeth during chin cup wear, her anterior crossbite should be corrected first or she should be placed on a bite plate to disclude her anterior teeth.

- TAD-supported Class III elastic wear (250 gm force per side, the same force level we recommend for high-pull chin cup wear) which results in an average maxillary advancement of 4 mm, and B-Point improvement of 2 mm [78]. Note: Allison's anterior crossbite should be corrected first before placing her on TAD-supported Class III elastics or she should be placed on a bite plate to disclude her anterior teeth. Otherwise, her maxillary anterior teeth could be traumatized by her mandibular anterior teeth.

Masking or camouflage (achieving a Class I canine relationship using tooth movement alone without addressing the underlying Class III skeletal discrepancy). Masking would generally be considered later during comprehensive treatment in the adult dentition:

- If Allison's compliance/growth during Class III orthopedics is unsatisfactory.
- If her growth is complete or nearly complete (i.e. *avoid doing anything irreversible until unknowns, especially growth, are eliminated*).
- If obtaining Class I canines via dental movement alone appears reasonable and will not result in unacceptable dental compensations or unfavorable esthetics.
- *First Principle of Masking* – the smaller the skeletal discrepancy between the jaws, the more normal the patient looks, and the smaller the dental compensations, the more successful masking (camouflage) will be; the greater the skeletal discrepancy, less normal the patient looks, and the larger the dental compensations, the less successful masking (camouflage) will be.

Class III adult dentition masking options include:

- Extraction of mandibular first or second premolars in order to make space for retraction of mandibular anterior teeth (achieving a Class I canine relationship but leaving molars Class III). This is an example of intra-arch mechanics.
- Extraction of mandibular first premolars combined with extraction of maxillary second premolars in order to permit retraction of mandibular anterior teeth and protraction of maxillary molars (achieving Class I canine and Class I molar relationships). This is an example of intra-arch mechanics in both jaws.
- Using TADs inserted bilaterally into the ramus as anchors to distalize the entire mandibular dentition into a Class I canine relationship. This is an example of intra-arch mechanics.
- Using Class III correctors such as Class III elastics or Class III springs. These are examples of interarch mechanics.

Surgery (maxillary advancement osteotomy and/or mandibular setback osteotomy) would not be considered during early treatment. Surgery would be considered in the adult dentition if the patient desired surgery, was finished growing, and if masking was not a viable alternative. The possible need for future surgery should always be discussed with patients/parents if you think it may be a viable option.

Q: Allison is seven years and ten months old. What does the literature say about the *timing* of Class III orthopedic treatment compared to the timing of Class II orthopedic treatment?

A: Here is what we know:

- Prospective clinical trials consistently report no advantage in treating Class II relationships in the *early* mixed dentition (except for a possible decrease in incisal trauma as a result of excess OJ) [22–24, 29, 38–40]. We subscribe to this guideline unless the patient shows good statural growth in which case we will begin Class II treatment in the early mixed dentition. Encourage parents to measure their child's height every two months, to notify you of changes, and to provide you with this data.
- In contrast, we generally recommend beginning Class III orthopedic treatment earlier. First, the skeletal effects of RPHGs are reported to be greatest in patients ten years of age or younger [55–57], and a long-standing rule of thumb is to begin RPHG treatment when the maxillary permanent central incisors are erupting (seven to eight years of age).

Second, we lack randomized, prospective clinical trials of Class III treatment using either high-pull chin cups or Class III elastics supported by TADs. However, based upon our clinical experience, *we recommend that the larger the Class III skeletal discrepancy, the earlier you should begin orthopedics* (to take advantage of as much future growth as possible). For some patients, this may be as early as five to six years of age.

Q: Class III orthopedic treatment can be especially challenging. Why?

A: Because orthopedic treatment does not normalize growth, mandibular hyperplasia patients can grow for longer periods of time, and orthopedic treatment requires patient compliance. Even if you achieve a Class III to a Class I skeletal correction, once you stop orthopedics, the growing child can grow out of your correction.

As an illustrative example [105] groups of seven, nine, and eleven-year-old Class III girls were placed on chin cups for 4.5 years. The authors reported that anteroposterior control was excellent during treatment, but by age 17, all groups (including the control group) were equal – suggesting that profiles tended to return to their original shape once chin cups were no longer worn. When orthopedic treatment is discontinued before growth cessation, relapse can occur.

All Class III orthopedic correction must be monitored, and the correction maintained, until growth is complete – which can take years. But asking for this level of compliance can be challenging.

If the Class III correction was made with a chin cup or TAD-supported Class III elastics, then the patient will likely be asked to wear the chin cup or TAD-supported Class III elastics until growth is complete. If the Class III correction was made with an RPHG, then the child may be asked to maintain the correction with a chin cup or TAD-supported Class III elastics.

Q: If I use an RPHG to make a Class III skeletal correction, then why can't I simply *overcorrect* the patient to Class II in order to compensate for future Class III growth?

A: You could possibly do this, but it can be very difficult to estimate exactly how much overcorrection you need. Too little overcorrection and the child grows Class III again. Too much overcorrection, and the child is left Class II.

Q: Why do posterior *lingual* crossbites tend to develop in skeletal Class III patients?

A: Because dental arches taper anteriorly. In other words, if the maxilla is positioned posteriorly relative to the mandible (skeletal Class III), then a narrower part of the maxillary arch is located over a wider part of the mandibular arch. This relationship tends to place the maxillary molars *lingual* to the mandibular molars.

Q: What is the difference between a relative posterior crossbite and an absolute posterior crossbite?

A: If models of a Class III patient with a *relative* crossbite are positioned with canines Class I, then the posterior crossbite disappears. That is, the presence or absence of the crossbite is relative to the anteroposterior position of the dental arches. If models of a Class III patient with an *absolute* posterior crossbite are positioned with canines Class I, then the crossbite remains.

Q: Is Allison's posterior crossbite absolute or relative?

A: Absolute. Look at Figures 4.67m–4.67o. She has only a 1–2 mm CR-CO shift, and if that shift is eliminated (models positioned with canines Class I), the crossbite will remain.

Q: You position models so that the canines are Class I and note that a posterior crossbite still exists (absolute crossbite). How do you determine whether this is a *skeletal* posterior crossbite or a *dental* crossbite?

A: Ask what happens to the crossbite when you *upright the molars*. If uprighting the molars worsens the transverse discrepancy, then the crossbite is skeletal. If uprighting the molars improves or eliminates the transverse discrepancy, then the crossbite is dental.

For instance, in the lingual *skeletal* crossbite illustrated in Figure 4.68a, the transverse compensations are removed by uprighting the maxillary molars to the lingual and the mandibular molars to the buccal (red arrows). The result is a worsening of the crossbite (Figure 4.68b) revealing the full extent of the transverse skeletal (apical base) discrepancy.

In the lingual *dental* crossbite illustrated in Figure 4.68c, uprighting the molars (maxillary molars

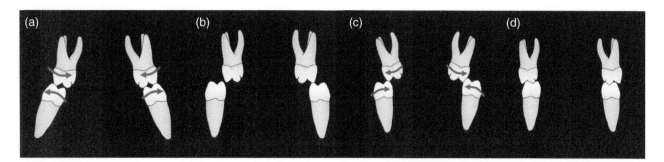

Figure 4.68 Determining whether a posterior crossbite is skeletal or dental. (a–b) If uprighting the molars worsens the transverse discrepancy, then the crossbite is skeletal. (c–d) If uprighting the molars improves or eliminates the transverse discrepancy, then the crossbite is dental.

uprighted to the lingual and mandibular molars uprighted to the buccal) eliminates the crossbite. This illustrates the fact that the apical bases are well related.

Q: Is Allison's posterior crossbite a dental or skeletal crossbite?

A: It is a skeletal crossbite.

- She exhibits inadequate maxillary first permanent molar intermolar width compared to mandibular first molar intermolar width. In other words, maxillary first molar intermolar lingual cusp width = 47.3 mm versus mandibular first molar intermolar central fossa width = 51.9 mm which is a deficit of 4.6 mm.
- She displays maxillary first permanent molar labial crown torque (Figure 4.67r) and mandibular first permanent molar lingual crown torque (Figure 4.67s). In other words, as her permanent molars are uprighted, her maxillary first molar intermolar lingual cusp width will decrease, her mandibular first molar intermolar central fossa width will increase, and the 4.6 mm linear discrepancy between arches will worsen.

Q: A posterior skeletal crossbite results from a discrepancy in the transverse dimension – typically a small maxillary width compared to a larger mandibular width. There are three general ways to treat skeletal discrepancies in the transverse, vertical, or anteroposterior dimensions. Can you list them and provide specific treatments for Allison's discrepancy in the transverse dimension?

A: The three general ways for treating any skeletal discrepancy are orthopedics, masking, and surgery. For Allison's transverse dimension:

Orthopedics – RME could provide maxillary skeletal expansion, create posterior OJ to permit molar uprighting/removal of transverse compensations, and increase maxillary arch perimeter to help eliminate crowding.

Masking or camouflage (correcting Allison's bilateral lingual posterior crossbite by increasing posterior compensations – that is, by increasing maxillary buccal crown torque or increasing mandibular lingual crown torque). Masking is usually performed in the adult dentition and will not correct her underlying transverse skeletal discrepancy. Possible treatments include:

- Crossbite elastic wear (elastics worn from the lingual of the maxillary molars to buccal of mandibular molars either unilaterally or bilaterally)
- Expanding maxillary archwires or constricting mandibular archwires (bilateral effect)
- Expanding a TPA or constricting an LLHA (bilateral effect)
- *Dental* expansion using an RME appliance, quad helix, or removable maxillary expansion appliance to increase maxillary intermolar width without achieving a mid-palatal suture separation (bilateral effect).

Surgery – would not be considered until Allison is an adult.

Q: What unknowns do you face in treating Allison?

A: Cooperation, future jaw growth (magnitude and direction), hygiene, and the possibility of a larger undetected CR-CO shift.

Q: Based upon the above discussions, what early treatment options would you consider for Allison?

A: Options include the following:

- *Recall* (no early treatment, monitor only) – evaluate tooth eruption in nine to twelve months. We advise against this option. Why? If we decide to use RPHG, high-pull chin cup, or TAD-supported Class III elastics for orthopedics, then we may miss out on favorable skeletal changes if we wait. In fact, her 1–2 mm CR-CO shift into anterior crossbite could act as a Class II functional appliance – accelerating mandibular growth and worsening her Class III relationship.

  Further, if we do not make room for her maxillary permanent canines to erupt, then they will remain blocked, potentially become impacted, and possibly resorb her maxillary permanent lateral incisor roots. Leaving her CR-CO shift to the right could foster asymmetric mandibular growth. On the other hand, waiting a year to correct her posterior crossbite should not be a problem.

- *Mandibular space maintenance* – place an LLHA before exfoliation of Allison's mandibular primary canines and primary molars. Allison currently has no mandibular anterior crowding, and 3.2 mm of mandibular spacing is anticipated following the eruption of all permanent teeth if an LLHA is placed. However, the *primary reason to place an LLHA in Allison is to prevent mandibular first permanent molar mesial drift* (worsening her Class III relationship).

- *Mandibular dental expansion followed by space maintenance* – place an expanded LLHA, upright her mandibular molars with crossbite elastics followed by an LLHA or employ a Schwarz expander appliance followed by an LLHA. This treatment would upright Allison's mandibular first permanent molars and prevent mandibular molar mesial drift, but it would need to be performed in conjunction with RME to avoid worsening her posterior crossbite.

- *Space regaining (anterior crossbite correction)* – opening space lost by premature exfoliation of maxillary primary canines. With fixed orthodontic appliances placed on the maxillary teeth, compressed open coil springs could be inserted between the maxillary lateral incisors and primary first molars to create space for the blocked and potentially impacted maxillary canines and correct her anterior crossbite. However, we anticipate three potential problems doing this:

1) Regaining space by advancing maxillary incisor crowns carries the risk of moving the maxillary permanent lateral incisor roots into the path of the developing maxillary permanent canines resulting in maxillary lateral incisor root resorption.

It is because Allison's maxillary central incisors are edge-to-edge in CR that advancing them out of crossbite could be readily accomplished. However, moving permanent maxillary lateral incisors during the early treatment when the crowns of the developing maxillary permanent canines are in proximity of lateral incisor root apices *should always be a concern*. Before moving the permanent maxillary lateral incisors, it is important to consider the spatial relationship of maxillary lateral incisor root apices and maxillary canine crowns using 3-D radiography, or a combination of panoramic and cephalometric radiography, periapical radiography, and digital palpation of the developing canine crowns. Looking at the panoramic and cephalometric radiography for Allison (Figures 4.67d and 4.67g), it appears the canine crowns are in the same coronal plane as the lateral incisor apices. Looking at the cephalometric radiograph in Figure 4.67h is not helpful in this assessment because the patient positioning for this cephalometric radiograph appears to be improper (note the bilateral asymmetry of the gonial angles and the permanent second molars and permanent canines in both maxillary and mandibular arches suggesting the patient's position was rotated on the vertical axis).

Looking at Allison's periapical radiographs (Figure 4.67f), and applying Clark's rule, we can see that the developing maxillary canine crowns are labial to the root apices of the lateral incisors. Both the panoramic radiograph and the periapical radiographs (Figures 4.67f–4.67g) suggest there is proximity between the distal aspect of the lateral incisor roots and the developing canine crowns. Given these findings, the relatively normal positions of the maxillary permanent incisors relative to the maxilla and the lack of maxillary incisor crowding, it may be prudent to move Allison's maxillary central incisors out of anterior crossbite *after* gaining transverse width (and moving the maxillary lateral incisors) using an RME. This action could decrease the tight proximity of the lateral incisor apices and the developing canines.

2) Advancing the maxillary incisors will procline them more.

3) This technique will create space primarily at the level of the maxillary arch and not at the level of the crowns of the developing maxillary canines where it is needed for their eruption.

- *Nance holding arch for maxillary space maintenance* – We are ambivalent about maxillary space maintenance. Currently, Allison has 5 mm of maxillary anterior crowding (10 mm of space with 15 mm of estimated space required for right and left permanent canines), and we anticipate 2 mm of maxillary crowding following the eruption of all permanent teeth if a Nance holding arch is employed. This reduction of maxillary arch crowding would be helpful.

However, placing a Nance holding arch would reduce maxillary first permanent molar mesial drift when maxillary primary molars exfoliate – negatively impacting an improvement in Class III molar relationship. Further, placing a Nance holding arch would inhibit posterior crossbite correction.

- *RME* – is recommended and would correct Allison's posterior crossbite, provide posterior OJ to permit uprighting maxillary and mandibular first permanent molars, and create anterior (coronal *and* apical) space for the blocked and potentially impacted maxillary permanent canines to erupt.

- *RPHG* – is a viable option and would advance A-Point by 1–2 mm if tooth-borne or by 3 mm if TAD-anchored. Tooth-borne RPHGs advance (procline) maxillary incisors, restrict mandibular growth, increase MPA, and increase LAFH. TAD-anchored RPHGs create less face height increase without dental movement (incisor proclination).

- *RPHG during RME* – studies are mixed regarding the advantage of combining these treatments. However, we recommend combining them (assuming transverse correction is needed) because there is no disadvantage in doing so. This would be the case with Allison.

- *High-pull chin cup wear* – is a viable option. High-pull chin cups inhibit mandibular ramal height growth, inhibit mandibular body length growth, permit the maxilla to continue growing forward, improve ANB [72–76], and do not increase LAFH compared to controls [73, 74]. If this Class III orthopedic approach is attempted, then we would recommend correcting Allison's anterior crossbite first in order to prevent incisor trauma. Discluding her anterior teeth with a bite plate (while wearing a high-pull chin cup) would offer the same benefit.

- *TAD-supported Class III elastic wear* – is a viable option. TAD-supported Class III elastic wear results in an average maxillary advancement of 4 mm and B-Point improvement of 2 mm [78]. If this Class III orthopedic approach is attempted, then we would recommend correcting Allison's anterior crossbite first in order to prevent incisor trauma. Discluding her anterior teeth with a bite plate (while wearing TAD-supported Class III elastics) would offer the same benefit.

- *Extraction of maxillary first primary molars* – to help provide space for the eruption of Allison's blocked and potentially impacted maxillary canines is not recommended since her maxillary first premolars and canine roots are < half developed, and since their eruption does not appear imminent.
- *Serial extraction* – as discussed in detail earlier, Allison is *not* an ideal candidate for serial extraction.

Q: Considering these options, what treatment (if any) would you recommend?

A: We began early treatment using tooth-borne RME in conjunction with RPHG (Figures 4.69a–4.69c). Beginning treatment at this age meant that Allison's total treatment will be protracted over many years. However, we justified this decision based upon our desire to maximize Allison's orthopedic correction (A-Point advancement and transverse expansion). We informed Allison and her parents that cooperation was of paramount importance and that high-pull chin cup wear, TAD-supported Class III elastic wear, permanent tooth extractions, or jaw surgery could eventually be required to provide an ideal result depending upon growth and compliance.

Allison's maxillary arch was expanded (bilateral posterior crossbite corrected) with RME while she wore the RPHG (500 gm per side for two months). Her lateral incisor crossbite and CR-CO shift corrected spontaneously with RME. Subsequent to RME activation, a maxillary 2x2 fixed appliance was used to advance her maxillary central incisors out of crossbite. Allison was very compliant. Her RME and 2x2 appliances were removed (Figures 4.70a–4.70d), and a TPA was inserted to maintain the transverse correction. With posterior and anterior crossbites corrected, and CR-CO shift corrected, active early treatment ended. Allison was placed on recall.

Q: What do you think of the posterior transverse correction (Figures 4.70a–4.70c)? Would you have done anything differently?

A: Yes. Although Allison's posterior crossbite was corrected with RME, her posterior OJ is minimal.

- Significantly more expansion should have been achieved. This would have provided more space for her blocked and potentially impacted maxillary permanent canines and more posterior OJ to upright permanent first molars.
- Her mandibular first permanent molars should have been uprighted (intermolar width expanded). In addition to achieving a better treatment outcome, uprighting mandibular molars would have required more maxillary transverse expansion to maintain posterior OJ and thereby created even more room for her blocked and potentially impacted maxillary canines.

Q: What do you think of her anteroposterior correction (Figures 4.70a and 4.70c)? Would you have done anything differently?

A: Allison appears Class I at the primary molars, but we should have overcorrected her to Class II with the RPHG. Why? Orthopedics does not normalize growth.

(a)   (b)   (c)

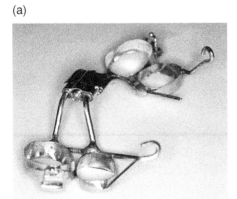 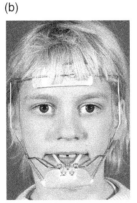 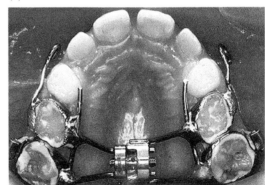

Figure 4.69 (a–c) Early treatment consisted of RME in conjunction with RPHG. RPHG elastics were attached to RME-soldered hooks.

(a)   (b)   (c)

(d)

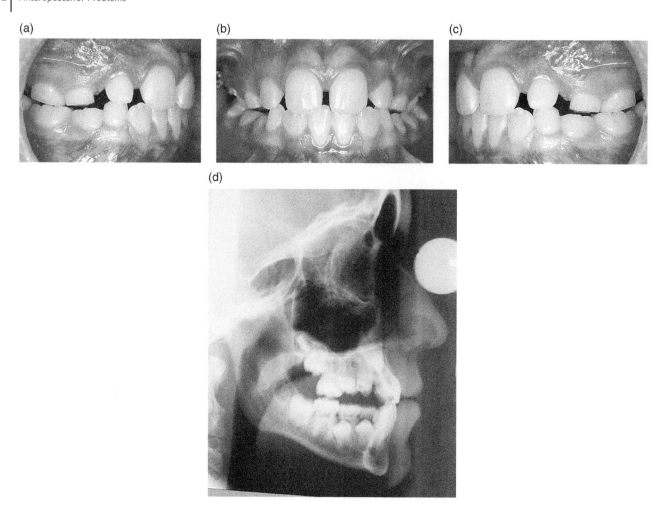

Figure 4.70 (a–d) Progress records of Allison following RME, RPHG, and maxillary 2x2 treatment.

Once her RPHG treatment ended, her Class III growth pattern returned (more forward mandibular growth relative to forward maxillary growth).

How much should we have overcorrected her? The answer to that question is unknown and always a gamble. If you overcorrect her too much, then she could remain Class II. If you overcorrect her too little, then she could outgrow your correction.

Q: At recall, we noted that Allison was entering the late mixed dentition and growing Class III. What treatment options, if any, would you recommend?

A: You could put her back on RPHG and overcorrect to Class II. Instead, since her anterior crossbite was corrected, we placed her on a high-pull chin cup. We asked her to wear it until she was done growing (TAD-supported Class III elastic wear was a third option).

Allison was very cooperative, and she wore the chin cup every night (eight pm–seven am, 250 gm per side). Figures 4.71a–4.71h shows Allison in the late mixed dentition stage of development after the Class III relationship had been corrected with the chin cup.

She wore the chin cup for one and a half years and was monitored closely until all permanent teeth erupted (except maxillary canines). Fixed appliances were placed, arches were leveled/aligned, and spaces were created between her maxillary lateral incisors and first premolars for erupting maxillary canines. When her maxillary canines erupted, they were bonded, leveled, and aligned.

Residual spaces were closed, and artistic bends were placed in final archwires to achieve final cusp seating. Unilateral Class III elastics were worn on her left side for several months during final cusp seating. Allison wore a tooth positioner for four weeks after debanding and then she began wearing Hawley retainers at

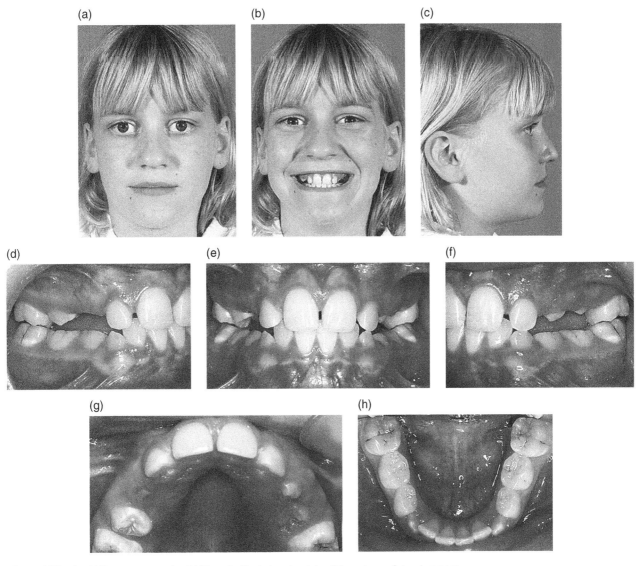

Figure 4.71   (a–h) Progress records of Allison in the late mixed dentition stage of development.

bedtime. Allison was asked to wear retainers at night for as long as she wanted to keep her teeth straight – a lifetime. Total active treatment time was six years and nine months.

Q: Allisons's deband records (age fourteen) are shown in Figure 4.72. What changes do you note?

A: Changes include:
- Excellent facial, occlusal, and functional outcome
- Straight profile maintained
- ILG reduced/eliminated
- Smile broadened and buccal corridors reduced
- Soft tissue LAFH WRN
- Maxilla descended (Figure 4.72f) but forward growth not observed

- Mandibular superimposition (Figure 4.72f, bottom right) shows significant mandibular ramal/condylar growth in a superior-posterior direction. This is associated with the movement of B-Point down and back during growth and treatment (Figure 4.72f, left)
- Skeletal LAFH lengthened (LAFH/TAFH×100% = 58%)
- MPAs increased (FMA from 22° to 26°; SNMP from 32° to 35°)
- Maxillary and mandibular molars erupted and moved mesially (Figure 4.72f)
- Maxillary and mandibular incisors erupted
- Bilateral Class I canine and molar relationships achieved
- Anterior and posterior crossbites corrected
- Ideal (minimal, 10%) OB achieved

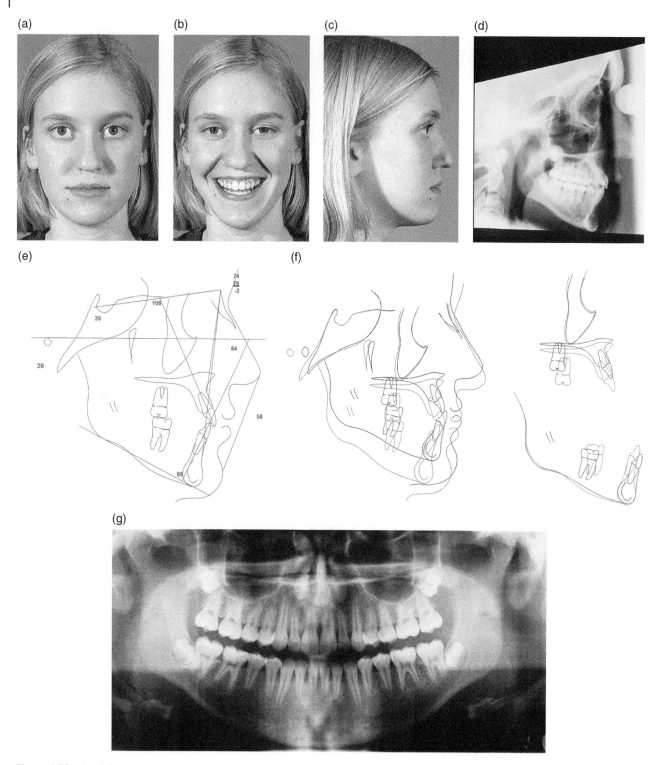

Figure 4.72 (a–p) Deband records for Allison.

(h)

(i)

(j)

(k)

(l)

(m)

(n)

(o)

(p)

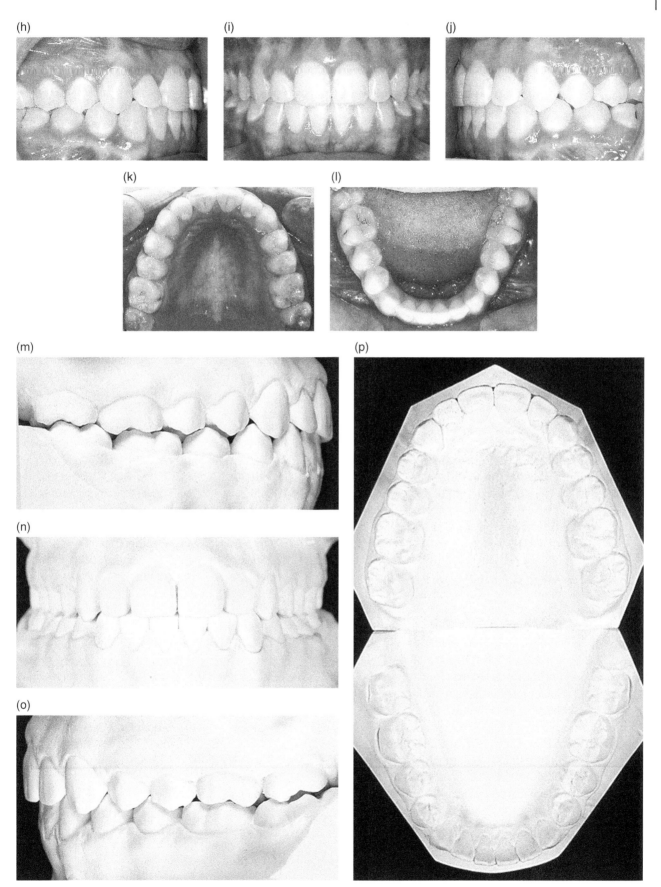

Figure 4.72 (Continued)

- Ideal (minimal, 0 mm) OJ achieved
- Coincidence of UDML and LDML achieved
- Maxillary crowding eliminated
- Anterior and lateral CR-CO shift eliminated

Q: Significant mandibular growth occurred, but ANB improved from –5° to –2°. Why?

A: It resulted because B-Point moved down and back. We cannot pinpoint when this clockwise mandibular rotation occurred because progress lateral cephalometric radiographs were not made at each stage of treatment. We can only state that it occurred through a combination of:

- CR-CO shift elimination. The initial lateral cephalometric radiograph was made in CO with Allison's mandible postured forward. The final lateral cephalometric radiograph was made in CR.
- RPHG wear
- High-pull chin cup wear
- Class III elastic wear
- Leveling and aligning of arches with fixed appliances
- Posterior growth rotation of her jaws. (Note in Figure 4.72f, the mandibular superimposition suggests her condylar growth was in a superior-posterior direction which is associated with clockwise rotation of the jaws [106]).

Q: Allison wore a high-pull chin cup after RPHG because she continued to grow Class III. In retrospect, could she have been treated without RPHG?

A: Yes, she could have been treated by first correcting her transverse relationship (and maxillary lateral incisor crossbite) with RME, then proclining her maxillary central incisors out of anterior crossbite, and then wearing either a high-pull chin cup or TAD-supported Class III elastics until growth was complete.

Q: What should have been placed in Allison's mandibular arch in the late mixed dentition (Figure 4.71h)?

A: An LLHA should have been placed to prevent mesial drift of mandibular first permanent molars (worsening her Class III molar relationship) and to make room for her mandibular permanent canines.

Q: Allison presented with a maxillary midline diastema (Figure 4.67b). In addition to wearing Hawley retainers at night, should we bond a fixed lingual retainer between her maxillary central incisors to prevent that space from returning?

A: No. She is stable, and we would not recommend bonding a fixed maxillary retainer between her central incisors. If a patient presents with a maxillary midline diastema after all permanent teeth are erupted, then we generally recommend bonding a fixed lingual retainer between their maxillary central incisors following space closure. However, Allison presented with her diastema long before her maxillary permanent canines erupted, and eruption of the permanent canines may have helped close the diastema [107].

In retention, we will monitor her. If a maxillary midline diastema begins to return, then we will close the space and retain it with a fixed lingual retainer. But, for now, she is stable.

Q: Was *early* treatment justified?

A: Yes. Let's review our decision to institute early treatment in the context of our three early treatment principles:

1) The goal of early treatment is to get the patient *back to normal for their stage of development*. Allison had a Class III skeletal growth pattern, as evidenced by the fact that she continued growing Class III even after RPHG wear ended and her anterior crossbite was eliminated. Correcting her anterior crossbite, posterior crossbite, CR-CO shift, and Class III relationship got her back to normal.

2) Early treatment should address *very specific problems with a clearly defined end point*. Correcting her crossbites and eliminating her shift were focused problems that could be completed in a matter of months. Allison and her parents considered her lengthy Class III orthopedics an acceptable trade-off to avoid extractions or surgery.

3) Always ask, "*What harm may come if I choose to do nothing early?*" By correcting her crossbites and eliminating her shift, acceleration of mandibular growth and possible asymmetric mandibular growth were avoided. By expanding her maxilla and creating anterior space, we diminished the crowding of her maxillary permanent canines – reducing the chance of their impaction and the possibility of lateral incisor root resorption associated with maxillary permanent canine crowding and ectopic eruption. Finally, Class III orthopedics eliminated the need for permanent tooth extractions or jaw surgery (treatment complexity reduced). Early treatment was justified.

Q: Can you suggest any "take-home pearls" regarding Allison's treatment?

A: "Take-home pearls" include:

- Allison was seven years and ten months old when she presented with significant skeletal discrepancies anteroposteriorly (deficient maxilla, anterior crossbite) and transversely (bilateral posterior lingual crossbite) with a forward and lateral CR-CO. Both skeletal discrepancies and CR-CO shift were successfully treated with orthopedics and without extraction of permanent teeth or orthognathic surgery.

- Even though Allison could shift back (incisors edge-to-edge) from Class III to nearly Class I (features of a pseudo Class III), she had a significant maxillary deficiency. It was prudent to treat her (orthopedically) as a skeletal Class III patient and not as a pseudo Class III.

- Decisions to treat skeletal discrepancies using orthopedics, masking (camouflage), or surgery depend upon the *age of the patient and the magnitude of the underlying skeletal discrepancy*. This is true in the anteroposterior, vertical, and transverse dimensions.

- Orthopedics can correct mild skeletal discrepancies if adequate growth potential remains and if the patient is compliant. Allison is a successful example of this.

- Orthopedics may improve moderate skeletal discrepancies to the point where they can be successfully treated with masking (e.g. permanent teeth extractions, increasing dental compensations).

- *First Principle of Masking* (dental correction without skeletal correction) – *the smaller the skeletal discrepancy between the jaws, the more normal the patient looks, and the smaller the dental compensations for the skeletal discrepancy – the more successful masking (camouflage) will be. However, the greater the skeletal discrepancy, the less normal the patient looks, and the larger the dental compensations, the less successful masking (camouflage) will be.*

- Surgery should be discussed with the patient/parent in all cases of moderate-to-severe skeletal discrepancies. Even if orthopedics is attempted, the patient and parents should understand that, depending upon growth and compliance, surgery may provide the best result.

- Class III orthopedic treatment restricted Allison's mandibular growth and led to a successful outcome but required Allison to be in treatment for over 6 years. Most patients are not as compliant as Allison. Remember, "each patient gets one cup of compliance." When compliance is gone, it's gone. Patient burnout is one reason why Class III orthopedic treatment in the early mixed dentition can be challenging. This fact needs to be discussed with the patient and parents before beginning. On the other hand, by being compliant, Allison avoided possible extraction of permanent teeth/jaw surgery and had an excellent outcome.

- The larger the Class III skeletal discrepancy *magnitude*, the earlier you should consider beginning orthopedics (to take advantage of as much future

growth as possible). For some patients, this may be as early as five to six years of age.

- *All orthopedic correction needs to be closely monitored and the correction maintained until growth is complete.*

- Skeletal effects of RPHGs are less in patients older than ten years of age.

- We should have overcorrected Allison to Class II with the RPHG because orthopedics does not normalize growth. Once her RPHG treatment ended, her Class III growth pattern returned (more forward mandibular growth relative to forward maxillary growth).

- Once her Class III growth pattern returned, we chose to place her on a high-pull chin cup (TAD-supported Class III elastic wear was another option). Thankfully, Allision wore her chin cup.

- Allison's RPHG was tooth-borne. If we were to repeat Allison's RPHG treatment today, we would have considered using a TAD-supported RPHG, or we would have considered treating her with TAD-supported Class III elastics.

- Removing a forward CR-CO shift will improve a Class III canine and molar relationship and improve a lingual posterior crossbite. Removing a forward CR-CO shift will worsen a buccal posterior crossbite.

- It was reasonable to expand Allison with RME while applying RPHG. Why? If a patient needs both, then there exists the possibility that expanding the maxilla while applying the RPHG will give the patient additional A-Point advancement.

- Although Allison's posterior crossbite was corrected with RME, her corrected posterior OJ was minimal. Significantly more RME should have been achieved. This would have provided more space for maxillary permanent canine eruption and more posterior OJ to upright permanent first molars.

- Skeletal effects of RME decrease after puberty.

- It is important to correct lateral shifts in growing patients in order to reduce the likelihood of mandibular growth asymmetry.

- *Reduce unknowns (e.g. jaw growth and patient compliance) before doing anything irreversible.* This principle is especially important when treating skeletal Class III patients. You want growth complete (or nearly complete but under control) before you consider permanent teeth extractions or surgery.

- Because skeletal Class III patients may have more growth for longer periods of time, it is especially important that you *monitor* your orthopedic correction until you are certain that their growth is complete. If you correct a patient to Class I and they begin to relapse and grow Class III again, then consider reinstituting Class III orthopedics (we will typically place them on a high-pull chin cup or TAD supported

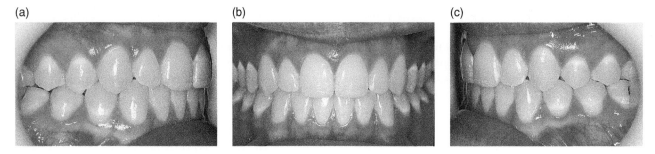

Figure 4.73 (a–c) Two-year post-treatment intraoral photographs of Allison.

Class III elastics until they have completed growth). Allison was followed closely for two more years after deband (Figures 4.73a–4.73c, age sixteen). As can be seen, she has remained stable.

- To guarantee continued alignment of anterior teeth, Allison must wear retainers faithfully every night.
- Allison is another example of what typically happens in early orthopedic treatment cases –treatment can take years.

Case Nathan

Q: Nathan is a boy eight years and three months old (Figures 4.74a - 4.74s), who transfers to your practice with the parents' chief complaint, "Nathan has a crossbite." His PMH, PDH, periodontal and TMJ evaluations are WRN. An anterior 1 mm CR-CO shift is noted. In Figure 4.74e, he is in CR. All other figures are in CO. *Compile your diagnostic findings and problem list. State your diagnosis.*

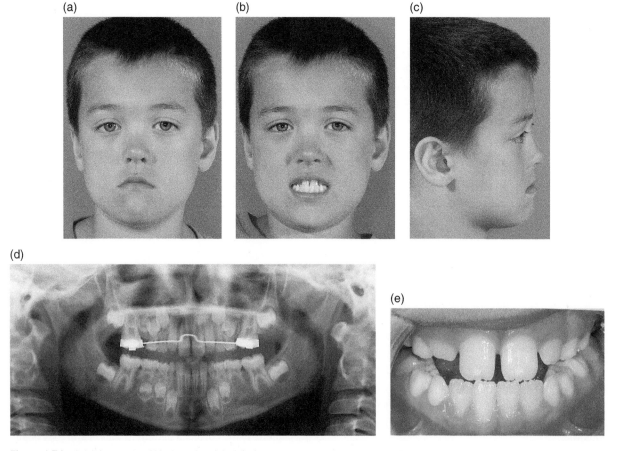

Figure 4.74 Initial records of Nathan: (a–c) facial photographs, (d) pantomograph, (e) intraoral frontal photograph in CR, (f–j) intraoral photographs in CO, (k–s) models.

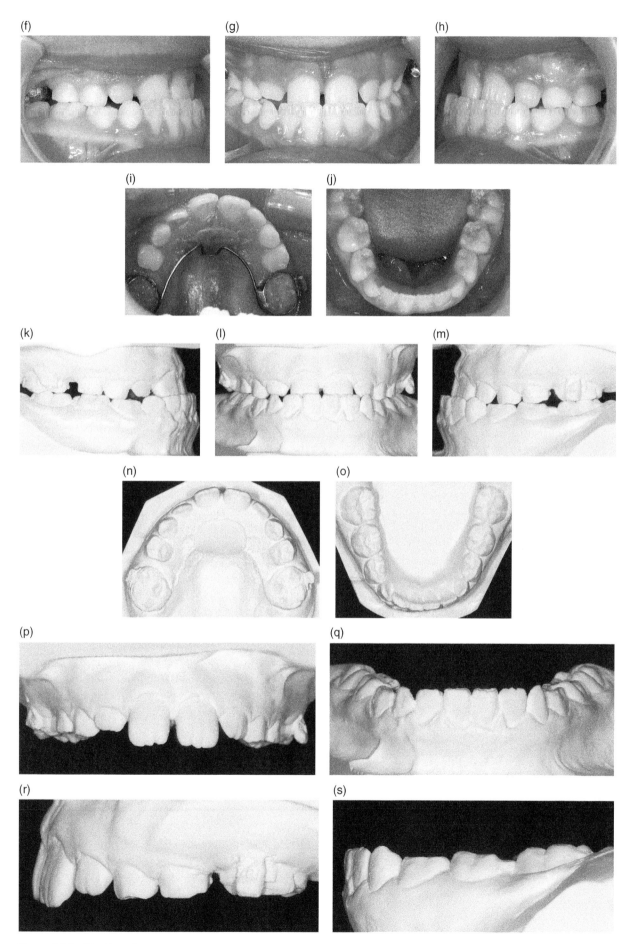

Figure 4.74 (Continued)

A:

Table 4.19 Diagnostic findings and problem list for Nathan.

Full face and profile	**Frontal View**
	Head appears rotated to the right on the frontal photograph
	Orbital asymmetry – right eye slightly lower than left
	Chin and philtrum of maxillary lip appear deviated to the right (head rotation)
	Soft tissue LAFH WRN
	Lip competence
	UDML WRN
	Smile is too narrow to judge buccal corridors
	Maxillary gingival display inadequate during posed smile (maxillary incisor gingival margins are apical to maxillary lip border)
	Profile View
	Slightly concave profile
	Nasal tip up
	Mildly obtuse NLA
	Labiomental sulcus WRN
	Chin position slightly forward
	Lip-chin-throat angle WRN
	Chin-throat length WRN
Radiographs	Early mixed dentition
	Probable absence of maxillary and mandibular left second premolars
	Anomalous shape of maxillary right second premolar (possibly be due to ectopic position or delayed development)
Intraoral photos and models	Angle Class I (molar) malocclusion
	Iowa Classification I III (6 mm) III (6 mm) I in CO
	Anterior crossbite exists in CO *and* in CR (Figure 4.74e)
	No posterior crossbite noted (Figures 4.74g and 4.74l)
	Missing maxillary primary second molars
	Blocked and potentially impacted maxillary right second premolar
	Nance holding arch in place
	20–30% OB in CO
	Dental midlines coincident
	Maxillary midline diastema
	Periodontal biotype WRN and thickness of mandibular anterior labial keratinized attached tissue WRN
	9.5 mm maxillary crowding currently present (4.5 mm of total maxillary spacing minus 14 mm of space required to allow for the eruption of two second premolars)
	9.9 mm of maxillary arch crowding is anticipated following the eruption of all permanent teeth, including second premolars (if appropriate space maintenance is employed)
	1.0 mm mandibular anterior crowding currently present (slipped contact between mandibular right primary canine and right lateral incisor)
	0.7 mm of mandibular arch crowding is anticipated following the eruption of all permanent teeth, assuming we maintain the left primary second molar (if appropriate space maintenance is employed)
	Maxillary and mandibular dental arches are symmetric (Figures 4.74i and 4.74j)
	1 mm CR-CO anterior shift
Other diagnosis	Class III malocclusion with anterior crossbite

Q: Nathan appears to be skeletally Class III (concave profile, anterior crossbite in CR), and his primary canines are Class III (6 mm). But his permanent first molars are Class I. How is this possible?

A: His maxillary primary second molars appear to have been lost prematurely (Figure 4.74i), and his maxillary permanent first molars appear to have drifted mesially into a Class I relationship with his mandibular permanent first molars. Note: His maxillary primary canines and primary second molars may also have drifted – distally.

Q: Nathan is a good example of why traditional Angle molar classification can mislead us in some cases. Can you explain?

A: If we state that Nathan is Class I, then another doctor would infer that Nathan has a normal anteroposterior jaw relationship. In fact, Nathan appears to be skeletally Class III. Instead of traditional Angle molar classification, we recommend using the Iowa Classification system which quantifies the molar *and canine* relationships. Please see the Appendix for a full explanation.

Q: What question(s) should you ask Nathan and his parents about his previous dental history?

A: Ask them what treatment was performed or suggested. They state that Nathan had baby teeth extracted and a Nance holding arch placed later.

Q: His parents give you records (Figures 4.75a–4.75d) which were made a year ago. Using these, can you list Nathan's cephalometric diagnostic findings?

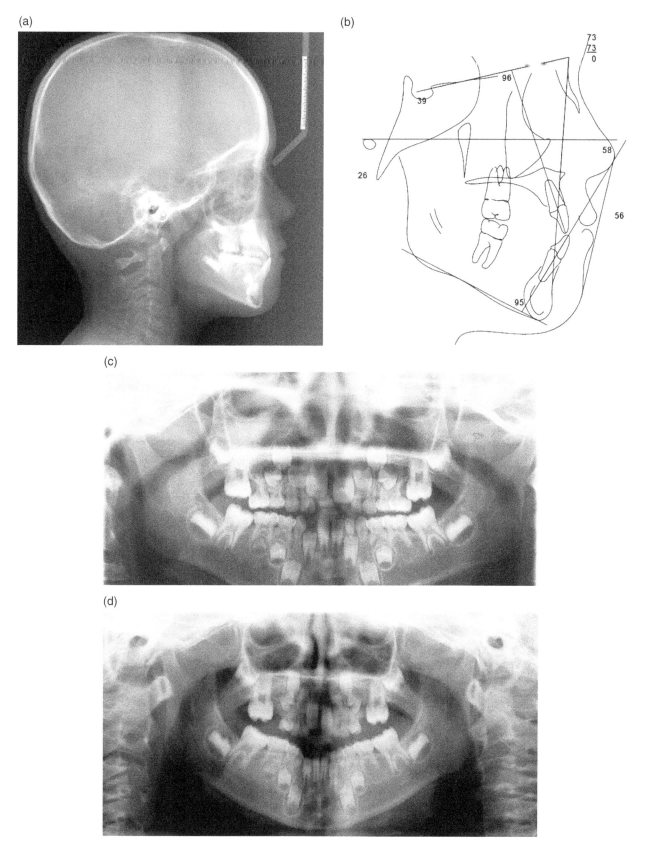

Figure 4.75 Records of Nathan made the previous year: (a–b) lateral cephalometric radiograph and tracing, (c) pantomograph, (d) pantomograph following extraction of maxillary primary second molars but prior to placement of Nance holding arch.

A:

Table 4.20 Cephalometric diagnostic findings and problem list for Nathan.

Ceph analysis	
	SKELETAL
	Maxillary skeletal anteroposterior deficiency (A-point lies behind Nasion-perpendicular line)
	Mandibular skeletal anteroposterior WRN (angle formed between Nasion-B point line and Nasion-perpendicular line = 3°)
	ANB = 0°
	LAFH WRN (LAFH/TAFH × 100% = 56%)
	MPA WRN (FMA = 26°, SNMP = 39° with Sella low relative to Nasion)
	Effective bony Pogonion (bony Pogonion lies on or ahead of Nasion-B point line)
	DENTAL
	Maxillary incisor angulation WRN (U1-SN = 96° versus ideal U1-SN angle between 101-104°)
	Mandibular incisors proclined (FMA = 58°)

Q: How can we conclude that Nathan's maxillary incisor angulation is WRN when U1-SN = 96°?

A: First, his low Sella position is influencing the value of U1-SN. Note that FH and SN diverge by $13°$ which is $6°$ greater than the average divergence of $7°$. Adding this $6°$–$96°$ gives $102°$, placing Nathan's maxillary incisor inclination WRN. Further, the U1 long axis extends through the distal of the orbit, which is WRN. Finally, in our clinical opinion the angulation of U1 just *looks* normal.

Q: What do Nathan's previous panoramic images tell you (Figure 4.75)?

A: The panoramic images illustrate the fact that Nathan's maxillary first permanent molars had been ectopically erupting and trapped under/resorbing his maxillary primary second molars (Figure 4.75c). The maxillary primary second molars were extracted, and the maxillary first permanent molars drifted mesially (Figure 4.75a compared to 4.75d).

Q: Do you wish to make any additional records?

A: No additional records are needed in order to decide whether to treat Nathan now, or recall him.

Q: For patients who present with Class III skeletal growth, we often see dental compensations for the underlying skeletal relationship – with maxillary incisors showing increased inclination (increased U1-SN) and mandibular incisors showing decreased inclination (increased FMIA). Why does Nathan display the opposite of this pattern?

A: His anterior crossbite occlusion promotes labially directed occlusal forces against (and labial inclination of) his mandibular incisors and lingually directed occlusal forces against (and lingual inclination) of his maxillary incisors. That is, his anterior crossbite occlusion is acting like a functional appliance that protrudes the lower jaw forward. Taken together, we speculate that Nathan's anterior crossbite occlusion has promoted proclination of his mandibular incisors and limited the increased proclination of his maxillary incisors, that is often seen in skeletal class III patients.

Q: Provide a detailed space analysis for Nathan's maxillary and mandibular arches. In other words, how were the 9.9 mm of maxillary arch crowding and 0.7 mm of mandibular arch crowding calculated (if space maintenance is employed)?

A:

Average mesiodistal widths of permanent teeth (mm): [81]

Maxillary central incisor	8.5	Mandibular central incisor	5.0
Maxillary lateral incisor	6.5	Mandibular lateral incisor	5.5
Maxillary canine	7.5	Mandibular canine	7.0
Maxillary first premolar	7.0	Mandibular first premolar	7.0
Maxillary second premolar	7.0	Mandibular second premolar	7.0
Maxillary first molar	10.0	Mandibular first molar	11.0
Maxillary second molar	9.0	Mandibular second molar	10.5

Average mesiodistal widths of *primary* teeth (mm): [81]

Maxillary central incisor	6.5	Mandibular central incisor	4.2
Maxillary lateral incisor	5.1	Mandibular lateral incisor	4.1
Maxillary canine	7.0	Mandibular canine	5.0
Maxillary first molar	7.3	Mandibular first molar	7.7
Maxillary second molar	8.2	Mandibular second molar	9.9

MAXILLARY ARCH (we cannot include leeway space since Nathan's maxillary primary second molars exfoliated; for this exercise, we will assume that both maxillary second premolars are present but developmentally delayed)

+4.5 mm of total maxillary spacing is currently present (Figure 4.74n, mesial of first permanent molars)

−7.0 mm space needed for the maxillary right second premolar

+7.3 mm width of the maxillary right primary first molar

−7.0 mm space needed for the maxillary right first premolar

+7.0 mm width of the maxillary right primary canine

−7.5 mm space needed for the maxillary right permanent canine

+7.0 mm width of the maxillary left primary canine

−7.5 mm space needed for the maxillary left permanent canine

+7.3 mm width of the maxillary left primary first molar

−7.0 mm space needed for the maxillary left first premolar

−7.0 mm space needed for the maxillary left second premolar

Balance = + 4.5 mm − 7.0 mm + 7.3 mm − 7.0 mm + 7.0 mm − 7.5 mm + 7.0 mm − 7.5 mm + 7.3 mm − 7.0 mm − 7.0 mm = − 9.9 mm

MANDIBULAR ARCH (we cannot use left leeway space since the left second premolar is missing; we will assume that we are retaining the mandibular left primary second molar)

−1.0 mm anterior crowding is currently present (note the slight overlap of the right primary canine and right lateral incisor)

+1.6 mm of anticipated right leeway space

+5.0 mm left primary canine width

−7.0 mm left anticipated permanent canine width

+7.7 mm left primary first molar width

−7.0 mm left anticipated permanent first premolar width

Balance = −1.0 mm + 1.6 mm + 5.0 mm − 7.0 mm + 7.7 mm − 7.0 mm = −0.7 mm

That is, 9.9 mm maxillary crowding and 0.7 mm mandibular crowding is anticipated following the eruption of all permanent teeth (if proper space maintenance is employed).

Q: What are your primary problems in each dimension plus other major problems (the main problems you must focus on)?

A:

Table 4.21 Primary problem list for Nathan.

AP	Maxillary skeletal deficiency Iowa Classification I III (6 mm) III (6 mm) I in CO
Vertical	–
Transverse	–
Other diagnosis	Severe maxillary arch crowding Anterior crossbite Blocked and potentially impacted maxillary right second premolar Possible missing maxillary left second premolar Missing mandibular left second premolar

Q: Is Nathan a pseudo Class III, a dental Class III, or a skeletal Class III patient?

A: He is not a pseudo Class III because he remains Class III even when he shifts back 1 mm into CR. He is not a dental Class III because he has not lost mandibular primary molars with subsequent mesial drift of his mandibular permanent molars into a Class III relationship.

Nathan is *skeletal Class III*. He has a maxillary skeletal deficiency as reflected in his concave profile and cephalometric radiograph. His primary canines are Class III (6 mm), and when he is shifted back into CR, his incisors are still in crossbite (Figure 4.74e). His permanent first molars are Class I only because his maxillary first permanent molars drifted forward during their ectopic eruption. *Nathan is a skeletal Class III patient.*

Q: Discuss Nathan in the context of three principles applied to every early treatment patient.

A:

1) The goal of early treatment is to correct developing problems – get the patient *back to normal for their stage of development* (including preventing complications such as resorption of adjacent tooth roots, reducing later treatment complexity, or reducing/eliminating unknowns). Correcting the following problems would get Nathan back to normal:

- Anteroposterior skeletal discrepancy (deficient maxilla, Class III skeletal relationship)
- Anterior crossbite
- CR-CO shift
- Severe maxillary crowding
- Blocked and potentially impacted maxillary right second premolar
- Missing left second premolars

2) Early treatment should address *very specific problems with a clearly defined end point*, usually begun and ended within 6 to 9 months (not protracted over many years except for some orthopedic problems). Nathan's skeletal discrepancy is a specific problem with a clearly defined end point, but correcting this problem orthopedically could take years.

Because Nathan's *central* incisors are nearly edge-to-edge in CR, fixed appliances could readily advance them out of crossbite. However, if we attempt to move his maxillary lateral incisors, then we must consider the proximity of the maxillary lateral incisor roots to the crowns of the developing permanent canines.

Space regaining by tipping the maxillary permanent first molars distally (Figure 4.74d) could provide room for the blocked and potentially impacted maxillary right second premolar. Correction of the missing left second premolars will be dependent upon the final extraction/non-extraction comprehensive treatment plan.

3) Ask yourself: Is it necessary that I treat the patient now? *What harm can come if I chose to do nothing now?* If orthopedics is not begun, then Nathan's Class III skeletal relationship may worsen with growth. If we do not correct Nathan's anterior crossbite, then his CR-CO shift (and forward posture) could act as a Class II functional appliance, accelerating mandibular growth and worsening his Class III relationship. Finally, if we do not make room for his maxillary right second premolar to erupt, then the premolar will remain blocked, possibly become impacted and possibly resorb adjacent tooth roots.

Q: With every early treatment patient, it is important to take the long view. What are your *long-term* goals for Nathan?

A: Long-term goals include the following:
- Correcting, and maintaining correction of, his anteroposterior skeletal discrepancy (achieving and maintaining Class I canines and molars)
- Correcting, and maintaining correction of, his anterior cross
- Eliminating his CR-CO shift
- Providing room for unerupted teeth (assuming he will be treated non-extraction)
- Obtaining ideal OB and OJ
- Providing room for all permanent teeth and addressing missing permanent teeth (prosthetic replacement or retention of the mandibular left primary second molar – assuming he will be treated non-extraction).
- Avoiding orthognathic surgery

Q: Which long-term goal(s) will be the most difficult to achieve?

A: The first goal will be the most difficult to achieve. Why? It is dependent upon Nathan's jaw growth magnitude, jaw growth direction, and his compliance. Even if we achieve Class III skeletal correction, *we cannot normalize Nathan's growth pattern with orthopedic treatment and must maintain the correction until Nathan has completed growth.* Superlative compliance will be required for many years.

Q: Depending upon Nathan's growth and compliance, he may require the extraction of permanent teeth. But is he a candidate for serial extraction? Discuss the five features which would (or would not) make him a candidate for serial extraction.

A: Nathan is not a good candidate for serial extraction. The ideal serial extraction patient is in the early mixed dentition and is *normal in every way except severe anterior crowding (≥ 9 mm per arch)*. Specifically, the patient should present with:
- *Class I first permanent molars.* Nathan does have Class I molars, but *only* because his ectopically erupting maxillary first permanent molars drifted mesially. His pattern of jaw growth is skeletal Class III, a condition that must be corrected and maintained *before* the extraction of permanent teeth. Nathan does not satisfy the feature of having Class I molars.
- *Vertically normal to slightly long soft tissue and skeletal LAFH, with minimal OB or possibly a mild open bite, but* not *a deep bite.* Nathan presents with normal soft tissue and skeletal LAFH, but he has a mild deep bite (20–30% OB) and does not satisfy this feature.
- *Normal incisor angulation or proclined incisors, but* not *upright incisors.* Nathan has proclined mandibular incisors (FMIA = 58°) but normal maxillary incisor inclination (U1-SN = 96° with low Sella). He satisfies this feature.
- *Normal posterior transverse relationship (normal intermolar arch widths with good posterior interdigitation; absence of posterior crossbites; and absence of significant transverse compensations).* Nathan satisfies this feature.
- *Severe (≥ 9 mm) anterior crowding.* Nathan has severe maxillary arch crowding (blocked maxillary right second premolar, and blocked left second premolar, if it develops) but only mild (1.0 mm) mandibular anterior crowding. He does not satisfy this feature.

Based upon the above, Nathan is *not* a good candidate for serial extraction.

Q: What unknowns do you face in treating Nathan?

A: Future jaw growth (direction and magnitude), cooperation, hygiene, and the possibility of an undetected CR-CO shift.

Q: Nathan has a Class III skeletal discrepancy (maxillary skeletal deficiency). There are three general ways to treat a skeletal discrepancy in the anteroposterior, vertical, or transverse dimensions. Can you list them and provide specific treatments for Nathan's Class III skeletal discrepancy?

A: Skeletal discrepancies can be treated in three general ways:

Orthopedics (enhancing Nathan's forward maxillary growth and/or inhibiting his mandibular forward growth). Options include:

- Either 1) a *tooth-borne RPHG* to advance A-Point (1–2 mm), advance (procline) maxillary incisors, restrict mandibular growth, increase MPA, and increase LAFH [53, 54] or 2) a *TAD-anchored RPHG* to advance A-Point (3 mm) – with less face height increase and no dental movement [65–67]. Since Nathan is 8 years old, an RPHG is a reasonable treatment option because the skeletal effects of RPHGs are greater in patients *10 years of age or less* [55–57].
- If Nathan's anterior crossbite is first corrected (or a bite plate is used to disclude anterior teeth), then a *high-pull* chin cup could be worn to inhibit mandibular ramal height growth, inhibit mandibular body length growth, and allow the maxilla to continue growing forward – resulting in ANB improvement and improved chin position [72–76]. The vertical force component of a high-pull chin cup appears to prevent LAFH increase compared to controls [73, 74].
- If Nathan's anterior crossbite is first corrected (or a bite plate is used to disclude the anterior teeth), then TAD-supported Class III elastic wear (250 gm force per side, the same force level we recommend for high-pull chin cup wear) would result in maxillary advancement (4 mm), and B-Point improvement of 2 mm [78].

Masking or camouflage (achieving a Class I canine relationship without addressing Nathan's underlying Class III skeletal discrepancy). We would not consider masking at this early age. We may consider masking later in the adult dentition during comprehensive orthodontic treatment:

- If Nathan's response to Class III orthopedics is poor (poor compliance, poor growth magnitude/direction)

- Once his growth is complete (*avoid doing anything irreversible such as permanent tooth extractions until unknowns, especially growth, are eliminated*).
- If obtaining Class I canines can be achieved with acceptable dental compensations and favorable esthetics.

Future masking options may include:

- Extraction of Nathan's mandibular first or second premolars to permit retraction of mandibular anterior teeth (finishing with a Class I canine and Class III molar relationship). This is an example of intra-arch mechanics.
- Extraction of mandibular first premolars to permit retraction of mandibular anterior teeth and extraction of maxillary second premolars to permit protraction of maxillary molars (achieving Class I canine and Class I molar relationship).
- Using TADs inserted bilaterally into the ramus to distalize the entire mandibular dentition. This is an example of intra-arch mechanics.
- Using Class III correctors such as Class III elastics or Class III springs. These are examples of interarch mechanics.

Surgery (maxillary advancement and/or mandibular setback osteotomies) would not be considered at Nathan's age. However, if his response to orthopedics is poor and if masking would create unacceptable dental compensations/esthetics, then surgery may be our best option. Nathan and her parents should be informed of this now.

Q: We would not consider masking now, but we may consider masking in the adult dentition. What is the First Principle of Masking in the anteroposterior, vertical, or transverse dimensions?

A: First Principle of Masking – *the smaller the skeletal discrepancy between the jaws, the more normal the patient looks, and the smaller the dental compensations, the more successful masking (camouflage) will be; the greater the skeletal discrepancy, less normal the patient looks, and the larger the dental compensations, the less successful masking (camouflage) will be.*

Q: Nathan is only eight years old and in the early mixed dentition. What are your thoughts about treatment timing if you institute *Class III* orthopedics?

A: All randomized, prospective clinical trials report no advantage in treating Class II relationships in the *early* mixed dentition (except for a possible decrease in incisal trauma as a result of excess OJ) [22–24, 29, 38–40], and we recommend waiting to begin Class II treatment until the late mixed dentition unless the early mixed dentition patient demonstrates good growth velocity.

We lack randomized, prospective clinical trials of Class III treatment using either high-pull chin cups or Class III elastics supported by TADs. However, we generally recommend beginning skeletal Class III treatment early. Further, the skeletal effects of RPHGs are reported to be greatest in patients ten years of age or younger [55–57], and a long-standing rule of thumb is to begin RPHG treatment when the maxillary permanent central incisors are erupting (seven to eight years of age).

We recommend that *the larger the Class III skeletal discrepancy, the earlier you should begin orthopedics* (to take advantage of as much future growth as possible). For some patients, this may be as early as 5–6 years of age.

Q: Assume that you orthopedically correct a skeletal Class III eight-year-old to Class I in one year. You discontinue treatment. What will happen?

A: The patient's Class III growth pattern will return, and your correction may be lost. Why? Orthopedic treatment does not normalize growth.

All Class III orthopedic correction must be monitored, and the correction maintained, until growth is complete. Once Class I correction is achieved, consider placing the patient on, or leaving them on, a high-pull chin cup or TAD-supported Class III elastics until growth is complete.

Another option is to *overcorrect* the patient from Class III to Class II and then discontinue treatment, but overcorrection requires you to gamble exactly *how much* overcorrection is needed to compensate for future growth. This gamble is difficult to win.

Q: Nathan has a maxillary midline diastema with a low labial frenum attachment (Figure 4.74g). How and when should you deal with this condition?

A: If the diastema does not close spontaneously during the maxillary permanent canine eruption, then you can wait to close it orthodontically when Nathan undergoes comprehensive orthodontic treatment. Of course, if he is self-conscious (teased) about it, then you can close it now orthodontically.

If the diastema is orthodontically closed, then a bonded lingual retainer should be placed between the maxillary central incisors to keep it closed (the OB will need to be shallow in order to have a room to bond a fixed retainer without the mandibular incisors hitting it). If gingival tissues "bunch up" during space closure, then a gingivoplasty (frenectomy) can be performed – *after* diastema closure so the resulting surgical scar tissue will aid in maintaining closure and not impede closure.

Q: Based upon the above discussions, what early treatment options would you consider for Nathan?

A: Options include:

- *Recall* (no early treatment, monitor only) – recall Nathan in one year to evaluate tooth eruption. We advise against this option because: (i) we will possibly miss out on favorable skeletal growth; (ii) the forward CR-CO shift into anterior crossbite could act as a Class II functional appliance, accelerating mandibular growth and worsening his Class III relationship; and (iii) his blocked and potentially impacted maxillary right second premolar might become impacted and possibly resorb adjacent roots.

- *Mandibular space maintenance* – place an LLHA before exfoliation of Nathan's mandibular primary canines and primary molars. Nathan currently has very mild (1 mm) mandibular anterior crowding, and 0.7 mm of mandibular anterior crowding is anticipated following the eruption of all permanent teeth if an LLHA is employed. However, the *primary reason to place an LLHA in a Class III patient is to prevent future permanent molar mesial drift and a worsening of the Class III relationship*. On the other hand, is no compelling reason to place an LLHA immediately, because the eruption of Nathan's mandibular permanent canines and premolars is not imminent.

- *Space regaining* – distalizing maxillary first permanent molars in order to regain space lost for the blocked right second premolar and in order to upright mesially tipped maxillary first permanent molars (Figure 4.74d). This is a reasonable option if you believe Nathan's maxillary arch will be treated non-extraction, but moving his maxillary first permanent molars distally will bring them into a Class III relationship.

- *Anterior crossbite correction* – to eliminate his CR-CO shift and permit us to evaluate Nathan's true anteroposterior relationship. This is a good option and a perfect example of *reducing unknowns*. Also, correcting the anterior crossbite will prevent incisor trauma if we later begin orthopedics.

- *RPHG* – could advance Nathan's deficient maxilla (A-Point) by 1–2 mm if tooth-borne or by 3 mm if TAD-anchored. TAD-anchored RPHGs create less face height increase without dental movement compared to tooth-borne RPHGs which advance (procline) maxillary incisors, restrict mandibular growth, increase MPA, and increase LAFH.

- *High-pull chin cup* – would inhibit mandibular ramal height growth, inhibit mandibular body length growth, and permit Nathan's maxilla to continue growing forward, thereby improving his ANB relationship – without increasing LAFH compared to controls. Again, if you decide to treat Nathan with a chin cup, then we recommend correcting his anterior crossbite first, or discluding his anterior teeth with a bite plate, in order to prevent incisor trauma.

- *TAD-supported Class III elastics* – could advance Nathan's deficient maxilla by 4 mm and aid B-Point improvement by 2 mm. Be sure to correct his anterior crossbite first (or disclude his anterior teeth with a bite plate first), and care must be taken to avoid screw placement near erupting teeth.
- *Extraction of primary canines or primary molars* – to help ensure eruption of permanent teeth *is not recommended* since Nathan's permanent canine and premolar roots are < half developed, and their eruption is not imminent.
- *Serial extraction* – as discussed earlier, Nathan is *not* an ideal candidate for serial extraction.

Q: Look at the mandibular left primary second molar in Figure 4.74d. Should you retain it or extract it?

A: *Attempt* to retain it – assuming that Nathan is a non-extraction case. Why? It has a *good crown*, *good root*, *and good bone* (alveolar bone level is even with the adjacent teeth). Furthermore, we are not certain that the mandibular left second premolar is absent.

Q: Based upon the options above, would you begin early treatment or recall Nathan? If you treat, what treatment would you recommend?

A: We decided to proceed with the following:
- Remove Nance holding arch
- Bond maxillary primary canines, primary first molars, and permanent central incisors. Band maxillary first permanent molars. Using compressed open coil springs, advance maxillary *central* incisors out of crossbite and open space for the maxillary right second premolar (space regaining)
- Fabricate a mandibular bite plate to disclude Nathan's anterior teeth and permit his anterior crossbite to be corrected
- After the anterior crossbite and CR-CO shift are corrected, re-evaluate Nathan's anterorposterior position and need for orthopedic treatment
- Maintain mandibular left primary second molar if possible
- Inform Nathan's parents that future permanent tooth extractions or jaw surgery may be necessary.

Q: At the start of treatment, we bonded Nathan's maxillary *central* incisors but avoided bonding his maxillary lateral incisors. Why was this prudent?

A: It was prudent because we could not confidently assess the proximity and spatial relationship of the maxillary permanent canine crowns and maxillary lateral incisor apices. Look at Figure 4.74d. Notice the proximity of the unerupted maxillary permanent canine crowns to the maxillary permanent lateral incisor roots. Looking at the cephalometric radiograph (Figure 4.75a) it was not possible to determine the canine anteroposterior position relative to the lateral incisor root apices.

However, the canines were palpable in the maxillary vestibule – indicating that they were buccal to the lateral incisor apices. This reduced our apprehension about moving the lateral incisor crowns labially, but some risk of causing lateral incisor root resorption by inadvertent contact of the lateral incisor apices with the crowns of the developing canines remained. We avoided this risk by beginning with labial movement of the maxillary *central* incisors only.

Q: We began early treatment. Five months after maxillary arch bonding and central incisor advancement out of crossbite, Nathan's maxillary canines were judged (by palpation of the maxillary vestibule) to be more favorably positioned. We decided to bond Nathan's maxillary *lateral* incisors in order to advance them out of crossbite. We attempted to position the lateral incisor brackets to favor mesial tipping of the lateral incisor roots away from the canine crowns. Nathan was debanded (Figure 4.76). What changes do you note?

A: Changes include the following:
- Profile remains concave
- Maxillary and mandibular lip protrusion
- Mentalis strain to achieve lip closure
- Maxillary skeletal anteroposterior deficiency
- ANB angle worsened from 0° to –3°
- Skeletal LAFH WRN (LAFH/TAFH × 100% = 56%)
- FMA WRN (26°)
- SNMP steep (38°, low Sella)
- Maxillary incisors proclined (U1-SN = 120°)
- Mandibular incisors WRN (FMIA = 64°)
- Anterior crossbite corrected
- CR-CO shift eliminated
- Inadequate space opened for maxillary right second premolar (Figures 4.76f and 4.76j)
- Primary canines Class III (8–9 mm)
- UDML coincident with facial midline
- LDML 2 mm right of UDML
- More mesial root tipping accomplished for maxillary right lateral incisor than for left (Figures 4.76f and 4.76h)
- No root resorption of maxillary lateral incisors noted

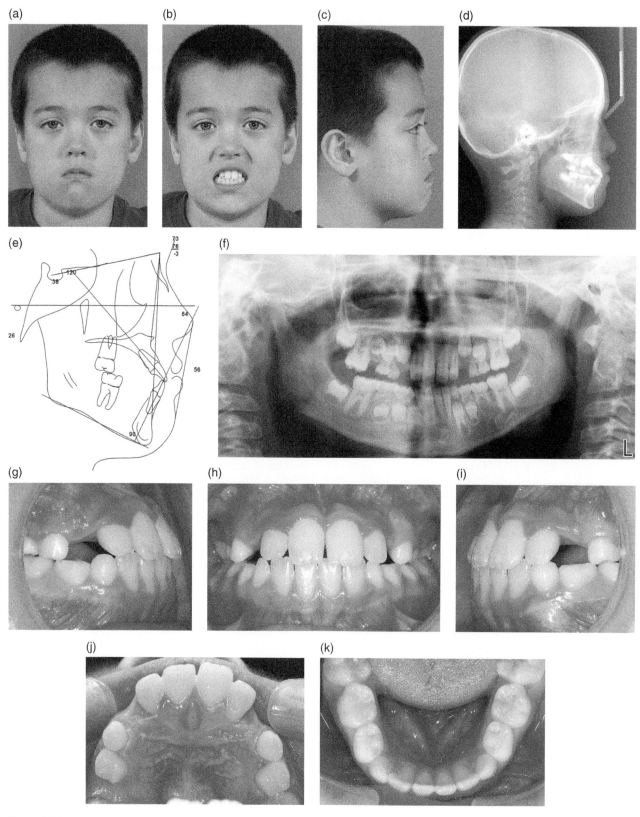

Figure 4.76 (a–k) Progress records of Nathan after advancing maxillary incisors out of crossbite.

Q: Nathan's ANB angle worsened from 0° to –3° with maxillary incisor proclination. Why?

A: As maxillary incisor crowns tipped forward, their roots tipped distally taking alveolar process bone (and A-Point) with them.

Q: Now that his anterior crossbite and CR-CO shift have been corrected, how would you recommend proceeding?

A: We began Class III orthopedics. Nathan was placed on a high-pull chin cup (250 gm per side, worn from 8 pm until 6 am).

Q: Nathan wore the high-pull chin cup for one year and four months, at which time a panoramic image was made (Figure 4.77). What do you note?

A: Nathan's permanent canines and premolars are erupting nicely – except for the maxillary right second premolar which remains blocked and now appears to be erupting ectopically in a horizontal direction.

Q: How would you proceed?

A: We asked Nathan to continue wearing the high-pull chin cup until he was finished growing. We placed brackets on his maxillary right permanent first molar, first premolar, and canine. A compressed open coil spring was inserted between his maxillary first permanent molar and first premolar to open space for the maxillary right second premolar. After the space was opened, we removed the fixed appliances and bonded a wire between the maxillary right first permanent molar and the first premolar to hold the space. In addition, an LLHA was fabricated and delivered to prevent mesial drift of the mandibular right first permanent molar when the right primary second molar exfoliated and to alleviate the mild anterior crowding via leeway space.

Q: Nine months later, we made a periapical radiograph of the maxillary right second premolar and bitewing radiographs (Figure 4.78). What do you observe?

A: There appears to be space around the crown of the maxillary right second premolar, but the premolar is erupting ectopically (transversely, not vertically). The mandibular right second premolar appears to be erupting normally, with plenty of "E space." A large occlusal step exists between the mandibular left primary second molar and the mandibular left permanent first molar. This occlusal step did not exist initially (Figure 4.74d), but is seen to be gradually developing (compare Figures 4.74d and 4.76f).

Q: What can you conclude about the mandibular left primary second molar based upon its occlusal step with the permanent first molar?

A: It is probably ankylosed since the occlusal step was initially absent. The mechanism promoting vertical drift of the primary tooth and alveolar bone is likely faulty [108, 109]. However, we must be cautious about concluding that a primary second molar is ankylosed because of an occlusal step. Why? Primary second molars typically have *shorter clinical crowns* which can present as an occlusal step between the mandibular permanent first molar and primary second molar – without ankylosis.

Q: If we cannot use an occlusal step as an indicator of primary second molar ankylosis, then how do we judge ankylosis?

A: By examining the *alveolar bone crest* of the primary second molar relative to the adjacent teeth. If a primary second molar is ankylosed, then it will cease erupting, and its bone level will submerge relative to (erupting) adjacent teeth.

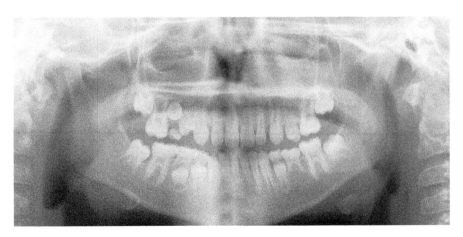

Figure 4.77 Progress panoramic image.

(a)

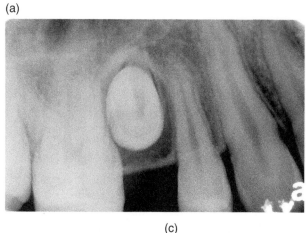

(b)

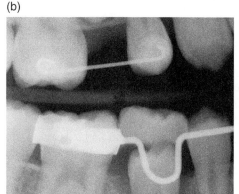

(c)

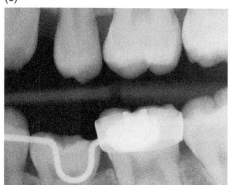

Figure 4.78 (a–c) Progress radiographs of Nathan.

Q: Does it appear, based upon alveolar crest bone levels, that Nathan's mandibular left primary second molar is ankylosed?

A: Quite possibly – because the mandibular left primary second molar mesial and distal bone crests appear to be lower relative to bone crests of adjacent teeth (Figure 4.78c). This fact suggests the primary second molar is not experiencing an equivalent upward vertical drift of tooth and alveolar socket.

Q: How would you recommend proceeding?

A: Nathan continued wearing his high-pull chin cup. We decided to monitor the ectopically erupting maxillary right second premolar to see if it would erupt spontaneously, without surgical exposure. We also decided to monitor the mandibular left primary second molar – to better judge whether it was ankylosed.

Q: Progress records were made at the age of thirteen years and eleven months (Figure 4.79). What do you note?

A: Changes include:
- Profile is now straight (Figure 4.79c).
- Mentalis strain absent.
- Lips do not appear protrusive.
- Maxillary anteroposterior position WRN.

- ANB angle has improved to –1°.
- MPA has flattened (FMA = 22°, SNMP = 35°).
- Maxillary incisors have uprighted (U1-SN = 109°).
- All permanent teeth have erupted – *including canines and maxillary right second premolar.*
- Mandibular left primary second molar is now clearly ankylosed (as shown by the dramatically lower alveolar crest bone level relative to adjacent teeth, Figure 4.790f).
- Canines are now Class III by only 1–2 mm.
- UDML 2 mm left of facial midline and LDML.
- Incisors are edge-to-edge.

Q: We were surprised that the ectopically erupting maxillary right second premolar erupted spontaneously. What principles did we follow in dealing with this ectopically erupting premolar?

A: We cleared a path for it to erupt by making space for it (Figure 4.78a).

Q: If the maxillary right second premolar had not erupted, then how would you have dealt with it?

A: If we decided that Nathan was to be treated non-extraction, then we would have surgically exposed it and erupted it orthodontically. If we decided that

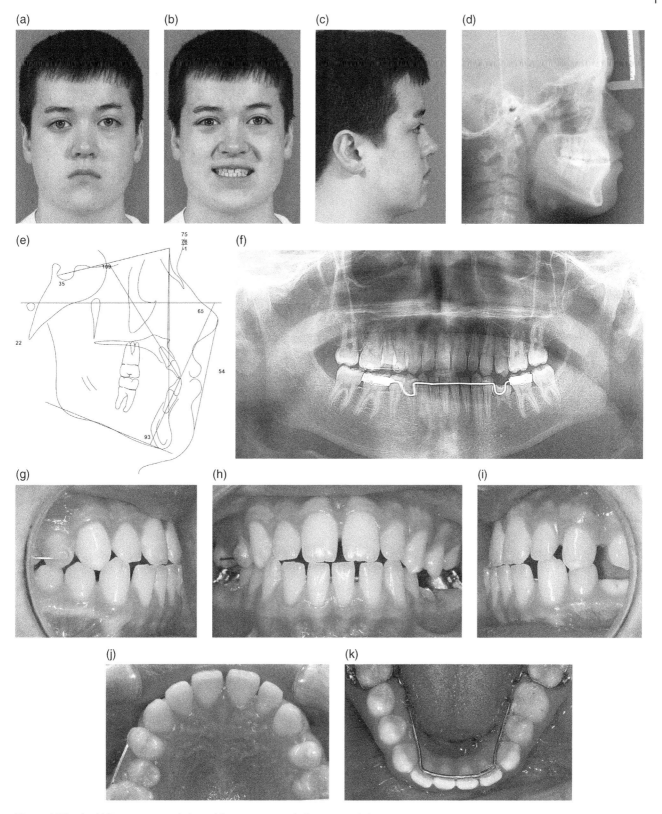

Figure 4.79 (a–k) Progress records (age thirteen years and eleven months).

Nathan was to be treated with premolar extractions, then we would have considered extracting it.

Q: Because the mandibular left primary second molar alveolar bone crest is below that of adjacent teeth (Figure 4.79f), we conclude that it is ankylosed and not erupting. That is, the adjacent teeth have continued to erupt bringing alveolar bone with them and leaving the ankylosed primary second molar bone submerged. Can you suggest three options for dealing with the mandibular left ankylosed primary second premolar?

A: Options include:
- *Do nothing; leave the ankylosed primary second molar.* This is a poor choice for Nathan because he has significant anticipated future growth, and the developing *vertical* bone defect will worsen as the adjacent teeth continue to erupt. This vertical bone defect could be very difficult to graft when Nathan is older.

  On the other hand, if Nathan had finished growing, if the primary second molar had a good crown (no caries, no large restorations), good roots (minimal or no root resorption), and *minimal* vertical bony discrepancy, and if the primary second molar was cleansable, then a viable alternative might be to retain it. If this were the case, then you would probably need to tip the permanent first molar distally in order to build up the primary second molar crown with composite material so the opposing permanent tooth would not super-erupt.
- *Extract the ankylosed primary second molar, leave the resulting edentulous space, and eventually replace the missing mandibular left second premolar with an implant or prosthesis.* This is a better choice. If you extract the ankylosed primary second molar, then you will develop a *buccal-lingual* narrowing of the edentulous site, but the alveolar crest *height* should improve as the adjacent permanent teeth transeptal fibers pull the edentulous site bone vertically. This vertical bone growth will improve the potential for successful bone grafting later. In other words, it is harder to achieve successful bone grafting vertically than buccolingually. So, it is better to get vertical bone growth now – at the expense of buccolingual bone loss.
- *Extract the ankylosed primary second molar and close the resulting edentulous space by protracting the left mandibular permanent molars using TADs or other anchorage techniques.* This could be a very satisfactory option, but there are two drawbacks: (i) you must protract both mandibular left permanent molars 10 mm (their roots could resorb), and (ii) the maxillary left permanent second molar would be

left unopposed and free to super-erupt (unless the maxillary left molars are also protracted).
- *Extract the ankylosed primary second molar and close the resulting space reciprocally.* This would be a poor option since the mandibular left permanent canine and the first premolar would retract distally into a Class II relationship and into an asymmetric relationship with the right permanent canine.
- *Extract the ankylosed primary second molar, close the resulting space reciprocally, and close the maxillary left space.* Even though you could finish with Class I canines bilaterally, this would be a poor option. Why? Left space closure in both arches would result in a significant arch asymmetry in both arches – leaving Nathan's midlines far to his left.
- *Extract the ankylosed primary second molar, close the resulting space reciprocally, close the maxillary left space reciprocally, extract maxillary and mandibular right premolars, and close the right spaces.* This is a viable option. However, Nathan's mandibular incisors are now at an ideal inclination, he has mandibular spacing, and this option could result in overly upright mandibular incisors.

Q: With the eruption of all permanent teeth, early treatment was finished. Let's discuss Nathan's comprehensive treatment. How do you recommend proceeding?

A: We discussed options with Nathan and his parents. Nathan said he was willing to continue wearing a high-pull chin cup until he finished growing, but Nathan and his parents did not want permanent teeth extracted or TADs placed to protract molars. They chose to have spaces opened on his left side for implants (a mandibular left second premolar implant and a maxillary left first premolar implant).

The LLHA was removed, mandibular left primary second molar was extracted, fixed orthodontic appliances placed (0.022 × 0.028-inch edgewise slots), arches leveled and aligned, and 7 mm spaces opened for eventual implants in his mandibular left primary second molar space and maxillary left first premolar space.

Q: Radiographs were made of the left edentulous sites once 0.18 × 0.025-inch stainless steel archwires had been placed and 7 mm spaces (for implants) opened between the tooth crowns (Figure 4.80). What do you observe?

A: Although 7 mm of edentulous space was measured between teeth crowns, the maxillary left canine and first premolar roots *converged* – leaving inadequate space for implant placement in bone. In contrast, the mandibular left first premolar and first molar roots diverged – leaving adequate space for an implant.

(a) 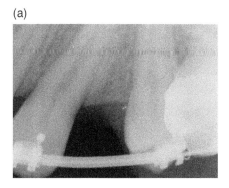 (b)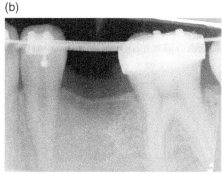

Figure 4.80 (a–b) Progress radiographs of edentulous sites (age fifteen years and two months).

Q: How would you address the converging maxillary left canine-first premolar roots?

A: By diverging the roots. The maxillary left canine and first premolar brackets were removed, and the teeth rebonded with new brackets so that archwires tipped their roots in a *diverging* manner. Both arches were level and aligned to 0.19 × 0.25-inch stainless steel wires. Additionally, artistic bends ("z-bends") were placed in the maxillary archwire across the canine and first premolar brackets to further diverge their roots.

Q: Radiographs were remade (Figure 4.81). What do you observe?

A: Adequate space now exists for implants at both sites. A prosthodontist was consulted and approved both sites for future implants. Nathan was debanded.

Q: Nathan's deband records are shown in Figure 4.82. What changes do you note?

A: Changes include the following:
- Excellent facial, occlusal, and functional result
- Orbital asymmetry still present – right eye lower than left
- Maxillary midline coincident with mandibular midline
- Broad smile with minimal buccal corridors
- Straight profile
- Downward and forward growth of both jaws (Figure 4.82f, left superimposition)
- Skeletal LAFH WRN (LAFH/TAFH × 100% = 55%)
- ANB angle has improved from –3° (Figure 4.76e) to –2° (Figure 4.82e)
- MPAs have flattened (FMA from 26° to 20°; SNMP from 38° to 33°)
- Mandibular incisors have uprighted to FMIA = 67°
- Maxillary molar has erupted and moved mesially (Figure 4.82f)
- Maxillary incisors have erupted and uprighted
- Mandibular molars and mandibular incisors have erupted
- Maxillary incisor roots have resorbed (blunting of maxillary incisor root apices, Figure 4.82g)
- Maxillary left lateral incisor has excessive distal root tip
- Bilateral Class I canine and molar relationships achieved
- Anterior crossbite corrected
- Ideal OB achieved (minimal, 10%)

(a) 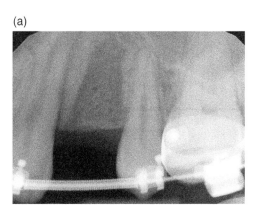 (b)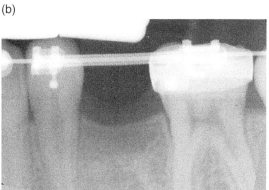

Figure 4.81 (a–b) Progress radiographs of edentulous sites (age fifteen years and ten months).

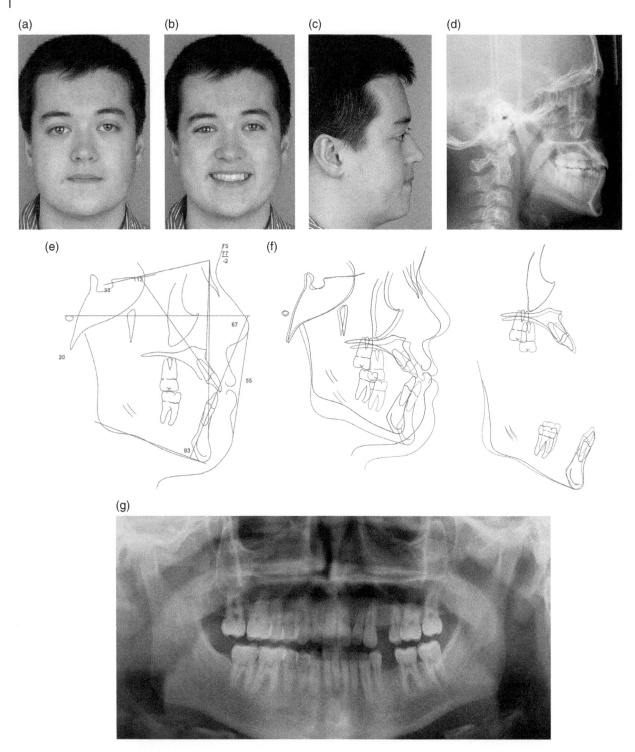

Figure 4.82 (a–l) Deband records of Nathan (age sixteen years and five months). (a) Note: Cephalometric superimposition is made from progress cephalometric tracing (Figure 4.76e) to deband tracing (Figure 4.82e).

(h) (i) (j)

(k) (l)

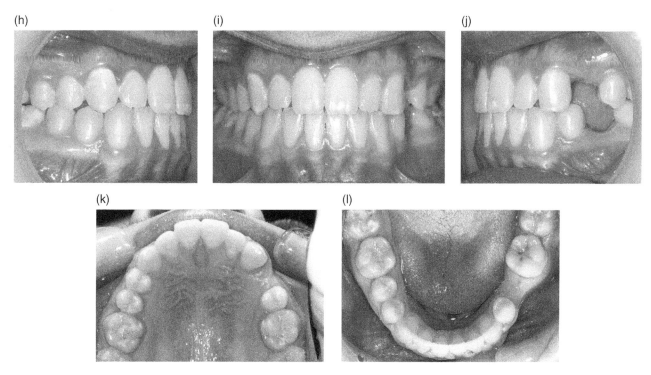

Figure 4.82 (Continued)

- Maxillary incisal embrasures present due to the minimal OB and incisor anatomy
- Minimal (0 mm) OJ
- Maxillary left permanent canine is rotated out on distal (Figures 4.82i and 4.82k)

Q: Nathan had significant mandibular growth (Figure 4.82f lower right superimposition – note increased ramus height and increased mandibular body length). Was this the result of treatment?

A: No. Nathan was treated for eight years in adolescence, and mandibular growth is expected over that time. In fact, Nathan demonstrated excellent chin cup wear compliance and, compared to controls, high-pull chin cups *inhibit* growth of mandibular ramal height and mandibular body length.

Q: Nathan experienced uprighting of his mandibular incisors relative to Frankfort Horizontal (FMIA increased from 65° to 67°), but showed no change in mandibular incisor angulation relative to his mandibular plane (IMPA remained 93°, compare Figures 4.79e and 4.82e). How did this occur?

A: Nathan's overall superimposition (Figure 4.82f) suggests he experienced true mandibular rotation during growth and treatment. His SN-MP decreased by 2°. This counterclockwise mandibular rotation effectively uprighted his mandibular incisors relative to maxillary and cranial base structures [110].

Q: Nathan will continue wearing his high-pull chin cup in retention (Figure 4.83) until we are sure he has finished growing. How can you be sure that he has finished growing?

A: Measure his height at each retention check appointment. Once we no longer detect a change in height, we

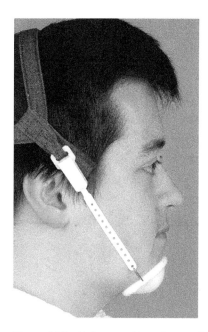

Figure 4.83 Nathan continues to wear his high-pull chin cup in retention until we are sure his growth has stopped.

will ask him to wear this chin cup for a few additional months.

Of course, the most ideal way to confirm jaw growth cessation is to examine serial cephalogram superimpositions made every nine to twelve months. However, you must weigh doing this against the additional radiation exposure.

Q: We are concerned that as we await implant placement years from now, Nathan's maxillary canine and first premolar roots will relapse – converging back into the edentulous space. How do you recommend retaining Nathan to prevent this?

A: The best way to maintain his maxillary canine and first premolar root parallelism is to place a bonded fixed partial denture. Maxillary and mandibular bonded fixed partial dentures were placed (Figure 4.84). In addition, Nathan wears Hawley retainers nightly.

Q: How would you deal with the incisal embrasures (Figure 4.82i)?

A: The ideal treatment would have been to finish Nathan deeper, say with 20% OB, which would have eliminated the incisal embrasures. Another option would be to have a restorative dentist close the embrasures with tooth-colored composite resin. Nathan and his parents were not concerned with the embrasures.

Q: Maxillary incisor root resorption was detected at deband (Figure 4.82g). How would you deal with this observation?

A: It was critical that Nathan and his parents were informed about the possibility of root resorption *before* treatment began. *Discuss the risks and benefits of orthodontic treatment with every patient before beginning treatment.* Document the fact that you discussed risks and benefits.

Also, a six to nine-month progress panoramic image should be made and examined for root resorption after comprehensive treatment begins on every patient. If root resorption is noted at nine months, then you need to reveal this fact to the patient and consider continuing or ending treatment. We failed to make a progress radiograph once comprehensive treatment began.

Nathan and his parents should be informed that apical root resorption was noted at deband, that it will not worsen in retention, and that it will not affect the longevity of his teeth (as long as he maintains excellent hygiene).

Q: Is there any way to predict future apical root resorption before treatment begins?

A: Not currently. *Radiographically examining tooth roots six to nine months after initiation of comprehensive orthodontic treatment appears to be useful in predicting severe resorption at the end of treatment* [111]. A risk of severe resorption at the end of treatment is absent in teeth lacking resorption after six to nine months of treatment. If resorption is found after six to nine months of active treatment, then a decision must be made to continue or discontinue treatment (knowing the risks).

Q: Was *early* treatment justified?

A: Yes. Let's review our decision to begin early treatment based on three early treatment principles:

1) The goal of early treatment is to get the patient *back to normal for their stage of development.* Correcting Nathan's Class III skeletal discrepancy, CR-CO shift, and anterior cross, plus creating room for eruption of his maxillary right second premolar, got him back on track.

2) Early treatment should address *very specific problems with a clearly defined end point.* All of Nathan's problems were focused, but Class III orthopedics took years.

3) Always ask, "*What harm can come if I choose to do nothing?*" If we had not begun early treatment, then Nathan may have required permanent tooth extractions and/or jaw surgery.

(a)

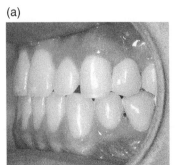

(b)

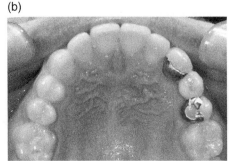

(c)

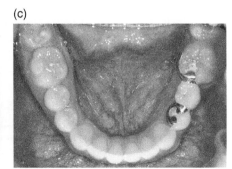

Figure 4.84 (a–c) Nathan's left maxillary and mandibular bonded bridges.

Q: Can you suggest "take-home pearls" from this patient?

A: "Take-home pearls" include the following:

- Nathan presented at eight years of age in the early mixed dentition with a significant Class III skeletal discrepancy (deficient maxilla, primary canines Class III by 6 mm, anterior crossbite). His skeletal discrepancy was successfully treated with orthopedics and without extraction of permanent teeth or orthognathic surgery.

- A decision to treat anteroposterior, vertical, or transverse skeletal discrepancies orthopedically depends upon two factors: *the age of the patient and the magnitude of the underlying skeletal discrepancy*.

- Mild skeletal discrepancies can be successfully corrected with orthopedics if adequate growth potential remains and if the patient is compliant. Nathan is an example.

- Moderate skeletal discrepancies can be corrected using orthopedics – with excellent growth magnitude, growth direction, and patient compliance. Or, they may at least be improved to the point where masking can be successful.

- When considering masking in the permanent dentition (dental correction only, not skeletal correction), always keep in mind the *First Principle* of masking – *the smaller the skeletal discrepancy between the jaws, the more normal the patient looks, and the smaller the dental compensations, the more successful masking (camouflage) will be; the greater the skeletal discrepancy, the less normal the patient looks, and the greater the dental compensations, the less successful masking (camouflage) will be.*

- Severe skeletal discrepancies can be challenging to correct with orthopedics. However, some parents may beg you to attempt orthopedics in the hope of avoiding surgery. Always *underpromise* what you can deliver. Yes, with excellent early treatment compliance and growth, you may be able to treat the child later with masking, but surgery may provide the best result.

- The possible need for surgery should be discussed for patients with moderate-to-severe skeletal discrepancies.

- It is critical to *reduce unknowns* (e.g. growth and compliance) *before doing anything irreversible* (e.g. extracting permanent teeth, jaw surgery). Nathan's response to high-pull chin cup wear was his most significant unknown. We evaluated this response before we finalized his comprehensive treatment plan.

- Nathan wore a high-pull chin cup for years – including during retention. The problem with Class III orthopedic treatment is that patients must remain compliant *until they are finished growing*. This fact must be explained to the patients/parents before you begin orthopedic treatment.

  On the other hand, Nathan probably avoided extraction of permanent teeth or jaw surgery, and he had an excellent result. Nathan and his parents were delighted with his outcome, and they considered the effort he expended well worth it.

- *Orthopedic correction must be closely monitored and the correction maintained until growth is complete.*

- For early Class II skeletal treatment, we recommend waiting to begin until the late mixed dentition – unless the early mixed dentition patient demonstrates good growth velocity. In contrast, with Class III skeletal treatment, we recommend beginning earlier. The larger the Class III skeletal discrepancy, the earlier you should consider beginning orthopedics to take advantage of as much future growth as possible.

- By preventing/reducing mandibular first permanent molar mesial drift, an LLHA can help a Class III molar relationship from worsening during the transition to permanent dentition.

- Nathan had anterior dental spacing in the permanent dentition (Figures 4.79g–4.79k). However, even with initial spacing, he must be compliant with retainer wear in order to prevent long-term dental crowding.

- The best retainer to prevent roots from tipping into an edentulous space (future implant site) is a bonded bridge or a wire bonded to teeth across the edentulous space. Do not assume that a removable retainer will prevent roots from tipping into an edentulous space.

- Tooth eruption is fascinating. We cannot explain how a transversely positioned maxillary right second premolar can rotate 90° and erupt (Figures 4.78a and 4.79f). However, this outcome was not unusual in our experience. With ectopic tooth eruption – make space, create a pathway for the tooth, and pray.

Case Carlie

Q: Carlie is nine years and three months old (Figure 4.85). She presents to you with her parent's chief complaint "Carlie has an underbite." PMH includes bilateral cleft lip and palate (complete on the right side and incomplete on the left side), and she previously underwent the following surgical procedures:

- Cleft lip repair at six months
- Palate repair at twelve months

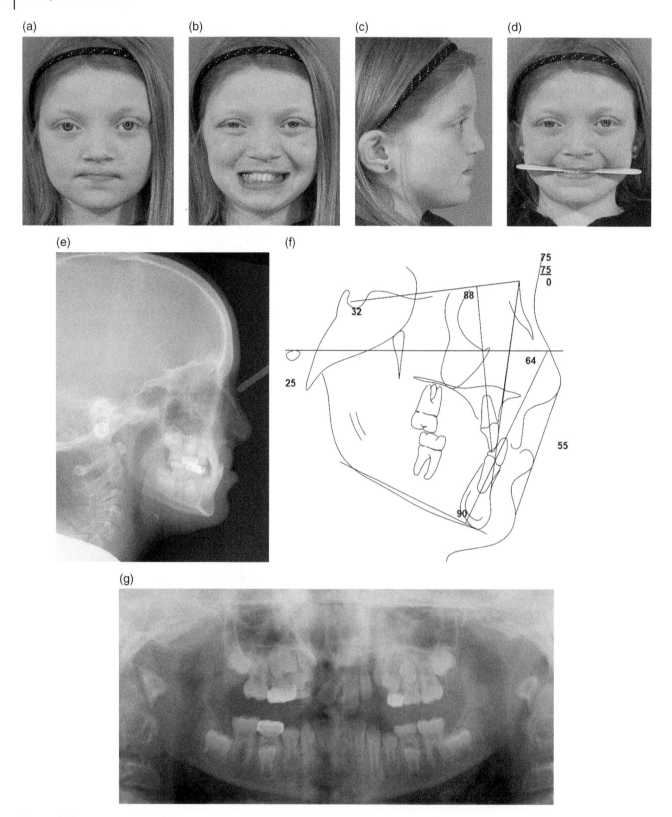

Figure 4.85 Initial records of Carlie: (a–c) facial photographs, (d) frontal photograph illustrating slight right-to-left posterior occlusal cant, (e–f) cephalometric radiograph and tracing, (g) panoramic radiograph, (h–l) intraoral photographs.

(h)　　　　　　　　　(i)　　　　　　　　　(j)

(k)　　　　　　　　　(l)

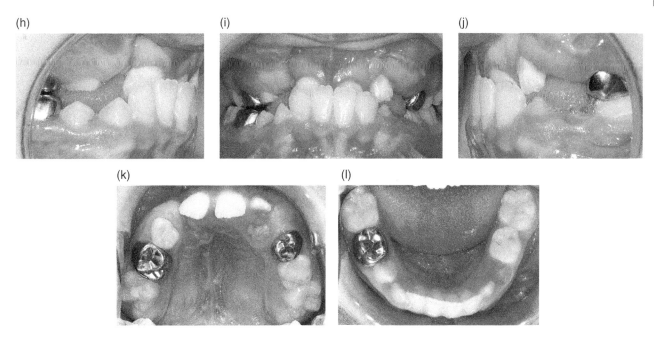

Figure 4.85　(Continued)

- Maxillary expansion at five years
- Alveolar bone grafting at six years

PDH, periodontal evaluation, and TMJ evaluation are WRN. CR = CO. Compile your diagnostic findings and problem list for Carlie. Also, state your diagnosis.

A:

Table 4.22　Diagnostic findings and problem list for Carlie.

Full face and profile	**Frontal View**
	Repaired cleft lip
	Deviation of the chin to the right
	Decreased upper lip length
	LAFH WRN
	Inadequate maxillary incisor display in the posed smile
	100% mandibular incisor display in posed smile
	Lip competence
	Large buccal corridors
	Right to left posterior occlusal cant
	Profile View
	Mildly concave profile
	Midface hypoplasia
	Obtuse NLA
	Mildly retrusive upper lip
	Protrusive lower lip
	Labiomental sulcus WRN
	Chin position WRN
	Lip-chin-throat angle WRN
	Chin-throat length WRN

Ceph analysis	**Skeletal**
	Maxillary skeletal anteroposterior deficiency (A-point lies behind Nasion-Perpendicular line)
	Mandibular skeletal anteroposterior deficiency
	Class III skeletal pattern (ANB = 0 degrees)
	LAFH WRN (LAFH/TAFH×100% = 55%)
	MPA WRN (FMA = 25°, SNMP = 32°)
	Dental
	Maxillary incisors retroclined (U1-SN = 88°)
	Mandibular incisors WRN (FMIA = 64°)
Radiographs	Late mixed dentition
	Grafted region of maxillary alveolar cleft is visible
	Maxillary right permanent canine erupting adjacent to the grafted area
	Root of the maxillary right central incisor is dilacerated
	Maxillary right lateral incisor is missing
Intraoral photos and models	Angle Class III malocclusion
	Iowa Classification: II (2 mm) x x III (3 mm)
	Anterior crossbite
	OB 90%
	Moderate curve of Spee
	Right posterior lingual crossbite
	Maxillary first permanent molar intermolar width at mesiolingual cusps = 41.5 mm
	Mandibular first permanent molar intermolar width at central fossae = 45.7 mm

(Continued)

Table 4.22 (Continued)

	Maxillary transverse skeletal deficiency
	Mandibular anterior periodontal biotype WRN (Figure 4.85i)
	Collapsed maxillary arch in right anterior segment adjacent to alveolar cleft (Figure 4.85k)
	Smaller mesiodistal width of maxillary right permanent central incisor compared
	to maxillary left permanent central incisor by ~1 mm
Other	Maxillary right alveolar bone grafted area
diagnosis	Class III malocclusion secondary to maxillary anteroposterior skeletal hypoplasia with bilateral clefting and unilateral right posterior crossbite

Q: We noted that Carlie has a Class III skeletal pattern (ANB = 0 degrees, deficient maxilla, mildly concave profile) but a *skeletally deficient mandible.* Can you explain this?

A: Because Carlie has maxillary skeletal anteroposterior deficiency (A-point lies behind Nasion-perpendicular line), we cannot use ANB angle to judge mandibular anteroposterior position. Instead, we must use the angle formed between Nasion-perpendicular line and Nasion-B point line to judge mandibular position. We estimate the angle formed between Carlie's Nasion-perpendicular line and Nasion-B point line to be nine degrees, which indicates mandibular deficiency. Carlie has both maxillary deficiency *and* mandibular deficiency. This analysis of skeletal anteroposterior deficiency is discussed in detail in the Appendix.

Q: Carlie's maxillary incisors are retroclined (upright). How do retroclined maxillary incisors influence the anteroposterior position of A-Point? What is the effect on the anteroposterior position of A-Point of applying lingual root torque to move the maxillary incisor roots toward the palatal?

A: Upright maxillary incisors have root apices positioned *forward* compared to normally inclined maxillary incisors. Because A-Point is measured at the cortical surface of the bone labial to the maxillary central incisor roots, the position of A-point is similarly forward.

If lingual root torque is applied to move maxillary incisor roots palatally, giving Carlie's incisors a normal inclination, then the labial bone covering the roots will follow palatally (posteriorly) [112], A-point will follow similarly, and her maxilla will be correctly judged as

having a more severe anteroposterior deficiency (i.e. a larger distance behind the Nasion-Perpendicular reference line).

Q: Would you recommend additional imaging for Carlie?

A: When compared to two-dimensional radiographs, three-dimensional radiographic images (e.g. CBCT, Figure 4.86) provide a better perspective of the cleft area, including the thickness of bone and proximity of teeth. This information can aid in treatment planning, such as helping us to decide if permanent teeth adjacent to the cleft area need to be extracted prior to, or at the time of, alveolar bone grafting. We did not feel a need for Carlie to have additional imaging.

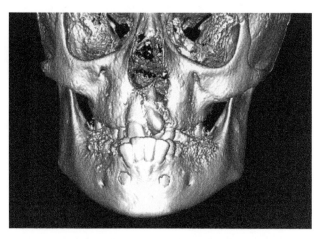

Figure 4.86 CBCT image of a patient with left unilateral complete cleft lip and palate. Note that the maxillary left permanent central incisor root is exposed to the alveolar cleft. Extraction of the left central incisor was recommended at the time of alveolar bone grafting.

Q: What are Carlie's primary problems in each dimension (the main problems you must focus on)?

A:

Table 4.23 Primary problem list for Carlie.

AP	Angle Class III malocclusion
	Iowa Classification II (2 mm) x x III (3 mm)
	Maxillary anteroposterior skeletal deficiency
	Anterior crossbite
Vertical	OB 90%
Transverse	Maxillary transverse skeletal deficiency
	Right posterior lingual crossbite
Other diagnosis	Questionable long-term viability of the alveolar bone graft area
	Missing maxillary right permanent lateral incisor

Q: Is Carlie a pseudo Class III, dental Class III, or skeletal Class III patient?

A: Carlie is a skeletal Class III patient. She would be considered a pseudo Class III patient if she shifted forward into a Class III relationship in CO but was Class I in CR. Carlie does not exhibit a CR-CO shift, is dentally Class III on her left by 3 mm in CR, and exhibits maxillary anteroposterior deficiency which will worsen when her maxillary incisors are inclined properly (as A-Point moves palatally). She is a true skeletal Class III patient with clinical manifestations typical of a patient with cleft lip and palate.

Q: Can you describe clinical features typical of patients with cleft lip and palate?

A: Patients with cleft lip and palate typically present with several of the following clinical features [113–118]:
- Maxillary hypoplasia
- Class III dental occlusion
- Anterior and posterior crossbites (the arch on the side of cleft is collapsed)
- Collapsed minor segment (anterior and superior autorotation of mandible, overclosure of vertical dimension, loss of face height, upward inclination of occlusal plane)
- Close to 25% of patients with cleft lip/palate need orthognathic surgery to correct their skeletal/dental malocclusions [116–118]

Q: What is the incidence rate of cleft lip and palate?

A: According to the World Health Organization, orofacial clefts are one of the most common head and neck congenital defects across the world [119]. In the United States, the estimated prevalence per 10 000 live births is 6.35 for cleft palate without cleft lip (with 2651 estimated annual number of cases nationally) and 10.63 for cleft lip with and without cleft palate (with 4437 estimated annual number of cases nationally) [120]. Note that clefts may involve lips, alveolus and hard/soft palate in various combinations and that several classifications are in vogue [121].

Q: Can you summarize typical interventions and intervention times for treating patients with cleft lip and palate?

A: Figure 4.87 illustrates the interventions, and intervention times, at the University of Iowa. Timelines of interventions and philosophy of treatment vary amongst craniofacial teams and institutes.

Q: What is *presurgical infant orthopedic treatment* and why is it used? Should presurgical infant orthopedic treatment have been performed on Carlie?

A: The earliest intervention that is performed on a cleft lip and palate patient is infant orthopedic treatment [122–124], and it is initiated prior to repairing the cleft lip.
- The goal of infant orthopedic treatment is to enhance the surgical repair of the lip and nose by establishing a good skeletal base and restoring skeletal, cartilaginous, and soft tissue anatomic relationships before the lip repair [124–127]. This is typically done in patients with a large cleft. The *major and minor segments of the maxillary arch are brought together in close proximity* prior to the lip repair.
- While several approaches are currently employed, by far the most widely used is the *Nasio Alveolar Molding* (NAM, Figures 4.88 and 4.89a and 4.89b) technique, which was developed by Dr. Grayson in the 1990s. In this technique, customized acrylic trays and nasal stents are adjusted to mold the alveolar processes and nasal alar cartilages [128]. The malleability of immature cartilage is used to establish and maintain a normalized maxillary arch form and position.
- Presurgical infant orthopedic treatment was not performed for Carlie since her initial cleft width was not considered severe enough to warrant this treatment.

Q: Are there any other infant orthopedic treatment techniques?

A: Yes, some centers elect to perform infant orthopedic treatment using the *Latham appliance protocol* [129–131]. The dento maxillary appliance (DMA) and the elastic chain premaxillary retraction (ECPR) appliance are used to treat patients with unilateral and bilateral cleft lip/palate, respectively (Figures 4.90a and 4.90b and 4.91a and 4.91b) [130, 131]. The typical infancy protocol is as follows:
- Impression for fabricating the DMA/ECPR using alginate with custom trays at three to four weeks of age.
- Placement of appliance (either DMA or ECPR) after five weeks of age. The appliances are placed under general anesthesia.
- Overnight hospitalization is typically required and the patients are discharged as soon as they are stabilized – able to feed. Prior to discharge, the airway should be patent.
- Three outpatient follow-up visits are required (at one week, three weeks, and five weeks post-placement of appliance).
- Parents activate the appliance daily for approximately five weeks.
- The appliance is removed under general anesthesia. During this operating time, either a nasolabial adhesion or lip repair procedure is conducted.

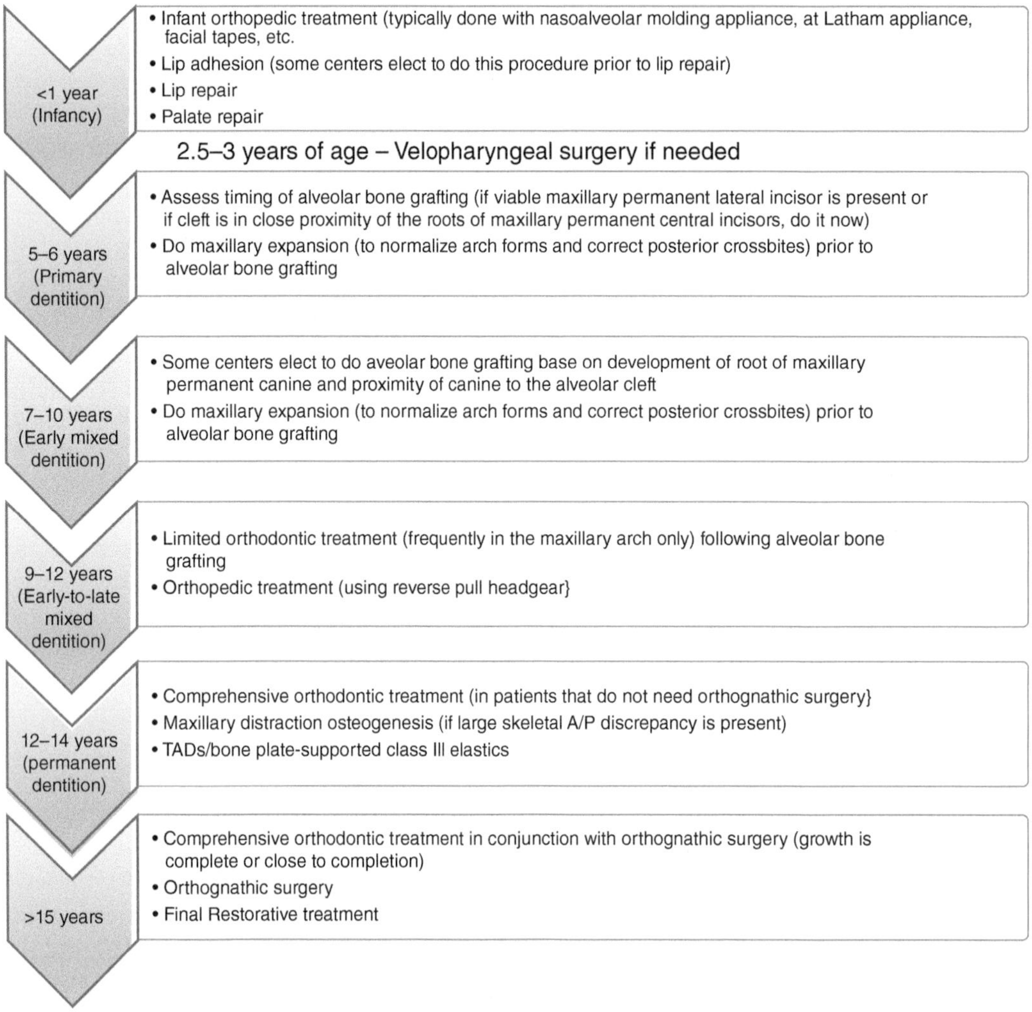

| <1 year (Infancy) | • Infant orthopedic treatment (typically done with nasoalveolar molding appliance, at Latham appliance, facial tapes, etc.
• Lip adhesion (some centers elect to do this procedure prior to lip repair)
• Lip repair
• Palate repair |

2.5–3 years of age – Velopharyngeal surgery if needed

| 5–6 years (Primary dentition) | • Assess timing of alveolar bone grafting (if viable maxillary permanent lateral incisor is present or if cleft is in close proximity of the roots of maxillary permanent central incisors, do it now)
• Do maxillary expansion (to normalize arch forms and correct posterior crossbites) prior to alveolar bone grafting |

| 7–10 years (Early mixed dentition) | • Some centers elect to do aveolar bone grafting base on development of root of maxillary permanent canine and proximity of canine to the alveolar cleft
• Do maxillary expansion (to normalize arch forms and correct posterior crossbites) prior to alveolar bone grafting |

| 9–12 years (Early-to-late mixed dentition) | • Limited orthodontic treatment (frequently in the maxillary arch only) following alveolar bone grafting
• Orthopedic treatment (using reverse pull headgear} |

| 12–14 years (permanent dentition) | • Comprehensive orthodontic treatment (in patients that do not need orthognathic surgery}
• Maxillary distraction osteogenesis (if large skeletal A/P discrepancy is present)
• TADs/bone plate-supported class III elastics |

| >15 years | • Comprehensive orthodontic treatment in conjunction with orthognathic surgery (growth is complete or close to completion)
• Orthognathic surgery
• Final Restorative treatment |

Figure 4.87 Timeline for cleft, lip, and palate interventions followed at the University of Iowa.

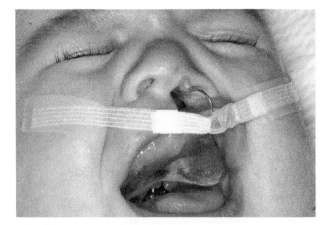

Figure 4.88 Nasio Alveolar Molding (NAM) appliance with nasal stent and facial tape in a patient with unilateral complete cleft lip and palate.

Q: Describe controversies associated with infant orthopedic treatment.

A: Multicenter studies originating from Europe have suggested that infant orthopedic treatment is not effective and that there is no uniform consensus on the treatment protocols [132–135]. The key findings from these studies are as follows:

- Benefits of the presurgical infant orthopedic treatment on maxillary arch dimensions are only temporary – not long term.
- Treatment is not cost-effective.
- A systematic review showed that treatment with passive infant orthopedic appliances has no positive effects on outcomes such as motherhood satisfaction, feeding, speech, facial growth, maxillary arch dimension, occlusion, and nasolabial appearance in patients with unilateral complete cleft lip/palate until the age of six years [134].

(a)

(b)

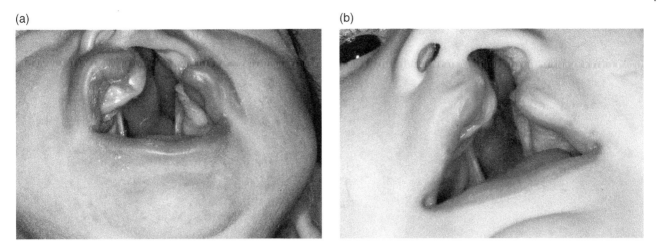

Figure 4.89 (a) Before and (b) after NAM treatment in a patient with left unilateral complete cleft lip and palate (observe the reduction in the width of alveolar cleft).

(a)

(b)

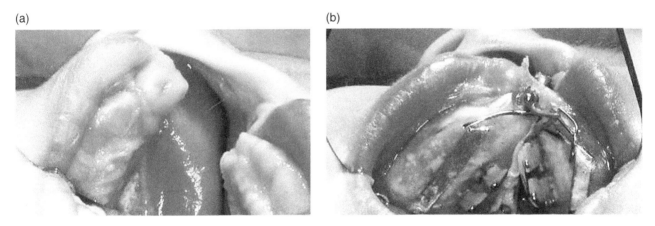

Figure 4.90 Before (a) and after (b) DMA treatment in a patient with left unilateral complete cleft lip and palate.

(a)

(b)

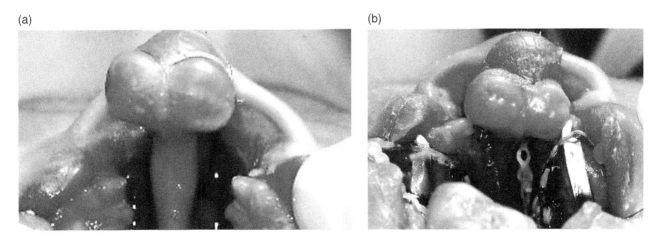

Figure 4.91 (a) Before and (b) after ECPR treatment in a patient with bilateral complete cleft lip and palate.

Q: When are lip and palate repairs typically performed?

A: Following infant orthopedic treatment, repair of the lip is performed between three and six months of age [122, 136]. A few craniofacial centers elect to do another surgery called the nasolabial adhesion procedure prior to repairing the cleft lip as it is purported to reduce the extent of undermining and minimize labial tension at the time of lip repair [137]. The cleft palate is typically repaired between ten and twelve months of age [136]. Carlie's lip was repaired at six months of age, her palate was repaired at twelve months of age, and no nasolabial adhesion procedure was performed.

Q: When is velopharyngeal surgery performed in cleft lip and palate patients?

A: Velopharyngeal surgery is performed between two and a half and three years of age [136] in cleft lip and palate patients to address speech development issues. Carlie did not have speech issues.

Q: Carlie had a right alveolar cleft. What procedure addresses this?

A: Patients with clefts of the alveolus require alveolar bone grafting to establish continuity of the maxillary arch and a pathway for permanent teeth to erupt [138–142].

Q: When is alveolar bone grafting performed? What are some graft sources?

A: The timing of alveolar bone grafting is dependent upon the development and position of the permanent dentition adjacent to the alveolar cleft area. If a viable permanent lateral incisor is present, or if the root of the developing maxillary central incisor is too close to the alveolar cleft, then alveolar bone grafting is recommended by 5 to 7 years of age. Some craniofacial centers perform alveolar bone grafting close to the time of the maxillary permanent canine eruption.

The most frequently used donor site for alveolar bone grafting is the iliac crest because of ease of access and abundance of bone. Other donor sites include mandibular symphysis, rib, cranial bones, and tibia. A few centers also use bone morphogenic proteins [138–142]. Carlie had her alveolar bone graft procedure at the age of 6 years. Bone was harvested from her iliac crest.

Q: Is maxillary expansion required prior to alveolar bone grafting?

A: Maxillary expansion should be performed prior to alveolar bone grafting in order to establish arch form, address transverse discrepancies, and facilitate better access for grafting. Depending upon the maxillary arch form, differential expansion or symmetric expansion is performed.

Q: What are some difficulties encountered with maxillary expansion prior to alveolar bone grafting?

A: Some commonly encountered problems include *overexpansion* (especially when we fail to anticipate future anteroposterior changes), *improper arch forms, difficulty placing the appliance* because of poorly formed teeth and/or delayed eruption of teeth, and *relapse* due to inadequate retention.

Carlie underwent maxillary expansion prior to alveolar bone grafting. Following expansion, we cemented a maxillary transpalatal arch (TPA, banded maxillary first permanent molars) with soldered mesial arms extending up to the first primary molars. The TPA prevented the arch from collapsing. Remember, *there is no continuity of palatal bone in patients with a cleft palate.* Consequently, there is a high tendency for the maxillary arch to collapse following expansion if it is not appropriately retained.

Unfortunately, two years after Carlie's transpalatal arch was cemented, it had to be removed and was never recemented. Her maxillary arch collapsed slightly on the right side, resulting in a right posterior crossbite.

Q: What is a reasonable protocol for cleft palate maxillary expansion?

A: Our recommended protocol includes:

- Banding four maxillary anchor teeth with adequate root structure. Frequently, the first primary molars/canines cannot be banded because of their shape or proximity to the cleft area. In such cases, we recommend cementing bands on maxillary first permanent molars and extending arms mesial to the primary canines/primary first molars.
- Determining the amount of expansion required in the anterior and posterior regions.
- Placing a fulcrum (using a fan-shaped expander) at an appropriate location for desired differential expansion (anterior expansion versus posterior expansion).
- Rapid expansion of 0.25 mm expansion/day until slightly overexpanded *if there is no risk of creating a fistula* (Figures 4.92a and 4.92b) or slow expansion (typically one turn every three to four days) if there is a risk for creating a fistula. The slow expansion provides an opportunity for the soft tissue to adapt to the expansion stresses generated by the appliance.
- Maintaining appliance for at least three months after expansion completed.

(a)

(b)

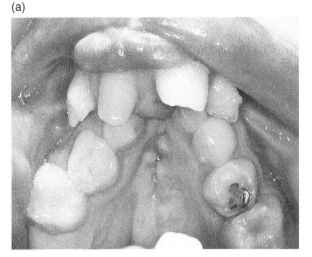
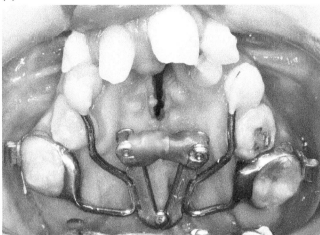

Figure 4.92   (a) Cleft palate where (b) RME using a fan-shaped expander resulted in a fistula.

- Retaining with the fixed appliance (transpalatal arch with mesial extension arms) or with fixed labial appliances.

Q: Is limited maxillary arch treatment *always* required after alveolar bone grafting?

A: While not an absolute requirement, there are instances when limited maxillary arch alignment will be required following alveolar bone grafting to facilitate the eruption of impacted teeth and to move teeth adjacent to (and into) the grafted area. It has been our experience that for grafted areas to survive, it is beneficial to place the grafted areas under mechanical stress, usually about four to six months following alveolar bone grafting. Moving teeth roots into the grafted area induces this stress.

Limited maxillary arch treatment following alveolar bone grafting was not required for Carlie. Her maxillary right permanent canine erupted into the grafted area – placing adequate stress on the grafted bone.

Q: What is the key factor to determine the timing of a comprehensive phase of orthodontic treatment for cleft patients?

A: The key factor is growth and development. During the early teen years, facial growth should be periodically assessed by the orthodontist. This assessment includes an eruption check of permanent teeth every six months. Depending upon growth, a comprehensive phase of orthodontic treatment, with or without orthognathic surgery (including possible maxillary distraction), can then be planned.

Q: What are your long-term treatment goals and objectives for Carlie?

A: Our long-term treatment goals and objectives include:
- Correcting, and maintaining correction of, her anteroposterior skeletal discrepancy (achieving and maintaining bilateral Class I molar and Class I canine relationships)
- Correcting anterior and posterior crossbites
- Obtaining ideal OJ and OB
- Providing room for all permanent teeth to erupt
- Creating space for restoring her missing maxillary right lateral incisor (implant or bonded fixed partial denture [FPD])
- Preparing ideal space to restore her maxillary left permanent lateral incisor to its ideal mesiodistal width

Q: What are possible orthopedic treatment options to address Carlie's anteroposterior relationship (maxillary skeletal anteroposterior deficiency and left dental Class III relationship)?

A: Orthopedic options include:
- Reverse-pull headgear
- High-pull chin cup wear (after correcting her anterior crossbite)
- Class III elastics worn between bone plates or TADs (after correcting her anterior crossbite)

Q: What unknowns do you face with Carlie's treatment?

A: Unknowns include:
- *Growth* – Carlie is certain to grow. At the time of initial presentation, she was nine years and three months of age and had not achieved menarche. If her future growth is favorable, Carlie could potentially be treated with orthodontics alone. However, if growth is unfavorable, surgical correction may be warranted.

- *Cooperation/compliance* – Oral hygiene is a critical factor. At the time of initial presentation, Carlie had only fair oral hygiene, and several teeth appeared to be hypocalcified. Poor compliance with oral hygiene could lead to dental white spot lesions and tooth decay. If orthopedics is instituted, then her cooperation will be instrumental to success.

- *Viability of alveolar bone-grafted area* – Carlie had a successful alveolar bone graft, and at this time, the grafted area appears good. In some instances, the grafted bone could become nonviable and another round of secondary alveolar bone grafting could be required. The risk of a poor outcome increases with repeated grafts, and the chance to successfully place an implant becomes tenuous in such cases (a bonded FPD may be required instead).

- *Long-term health of teeth roots adjacent to cleft area* – The long-term prognosis of her maxillary right central incisor root is guarded at best. This root is dilacerated and close to the maxillary left central incisor root. When we upright the root of the maxillary right central incisor, it will move nearly 5 mm to get close to the grafted area – which is a large movement to subject it to. Given the root dilaceration and the large root movement anticipated, we face the risk of increased root resorption.

Based upon her radiographs, there appears to be a bridge of bone in the cleft area following alveolar bone grafting, and the maxillary right permanent canine appears to be erupting close to this area. If the graft fails/recedes during the time that the maxillary right permanent canine is erupting, then the canine may never have adequate vertical bone on its mesial and mesiopalatal aspects.

Q: Based upon the foregoing discussions, how would you recommend treating Carlie now?

A: Treatment proceeded as follows:

- *Maxillary arch expansion* (Figure 4.93a, addressing the posterior crossbite and loosening the circummaxillary sutures in preparation for orthopedic advancement of the maxilla). The slow expansion was applied over a course of two months to minimize the risk of creating palatal fistulas. After three months, the maxillary expansion appliance was removed and a TPA with mesial extension arms was placed.

- *Class III orthopedics* – bone plates were surgically placed in the mandible (Figure 4.93b), and the TPA was anchored to a palatal TAD. Class III elastics were worn full time from the TAD-supported TPA to the mandibular bone plates with an elastic force of approximately 250 gm per side.

  Mandibular bone plates to support Class III elastic wear are not required. Miniscrews may also be used. In Carlie's case, the bone plates failed after one year and were removed. We then placed titanium miniscrews in the mandible ourselves and successfully ran Class III elastics to them for the duration of treatment (Figure 4.93c).

- *Fixed appliance orthodontic treatment* – we bonded mandibular teeth with fixed appliances to level the

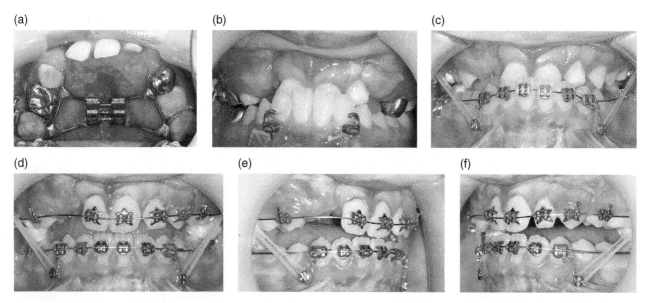

Figure 4.93 Progress photos of Carlie: (a) maxillary arch was slowly expanded; bone plates were placed by surgery in the mandible (b) as anchors for Class III elastic wear to a TAD-supported TPA; after mandibular bone plates failed, we placed titanium miniscrews in the mandible ourselves. These TADs successfully supported Class III elastic wear (c) for the duration of comprehensive treatment (d–f).

curve of Spee. We intruded mandibular incisors using the miniscrews as anchorage (Figure 4.93c). We bonded the maxillary arch (Figures 4.93d–4.93f), leveled and aligned both arches, created space for the maxillary right lateral incisor, corrected the anterior crossbite, placed artistic bends, debanded, and retained.

- *Restorative treatment* (bonded FPD to replace maxillary permanent right lateral incisor and composite veneer buildup of maxillary left lateral incisor).

Q: Carlie was debanded at twelve years and five months of age (Figures 4.94a–4.94l). What changes do you observe?

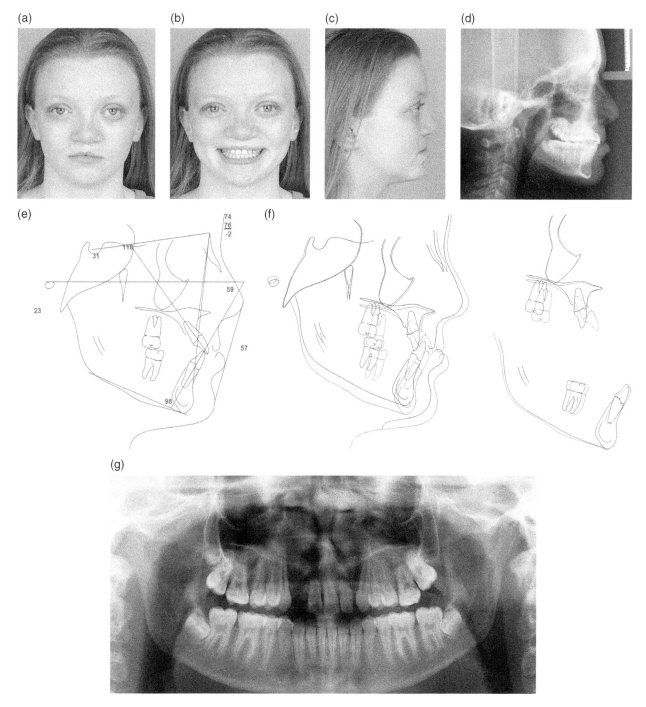

Figure 4.94 Deband records of Carlie. (a–c) Facial photos, (d–e) lateral cephalometric radiograph and tracing, (f) superimposition from nine years of age to twelve years of age, (g) panoramic radiograph, (h–l) intraoral photos.

(h) (i) (j)

(k) (l)

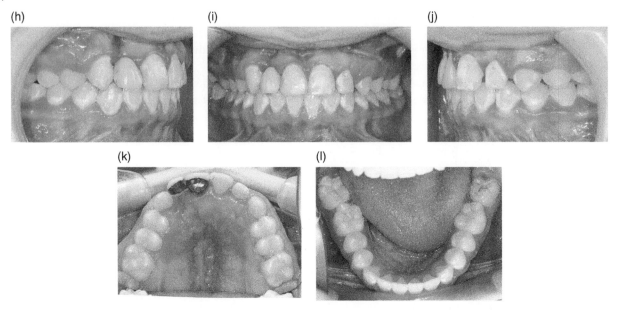

Figure 4.94 (Continued)

A: The following changes are noted:
- Carlie has undergone dramatic improvement in her smile esthetics. She now exhibits 70% maxillary incisor show during posed smiling compared to none initially. In addition, she exhibits a significant reduction in buccal corridor size, and her occlusal cant has been improved. However, her profile is unchanged. To realize improved lip esthetics, she could elect to undergo a lip-nose revision.
- Maxillary incisors proclined (U1-SN increased from 88° to 118°, compare Figures 4.85f to 4.94e).
- MPA flattened (FMA decreased from 25° to 23°, SN-MP decreased 32° to 31°).
- Mandibular incisors proclined (FMIA decreased from 64° to 59°).
- Carlie's nose, lips, and chin grew forward (Figure 4.94f). Her maxilla descended at posterior nasal spine with little descent at anterior nasal spine. A-point moved forward with growth and treatment. B-point moved downward and slightly forward. Maxillary molars descended. Maxillary molars moved forward and maxillary incisors proclined due to a treatment effect (more movement than anticipated with growth). Mandibular molars and incisors showed little change vertically.
- Final Angle classification: Angle Class III subdivision left.
- Final Iowa classification: I I III (1 mm) III (1 mm).
- OJ is 2 mm, OB is 20%, UDML is coincident with facial midline, and LDML is 1 mm to the right of the maxillary dental midline.

- Space was created for a composite veneer of the maxillary left lateral incisor.
- Space was created for a bonded FPD of the maxillary right lateral incisor. Recall that an implant was not chosen as a prosthetic solution as it would have required another bone grafting of the cleft area.
- Evaluation of the final panoramic radiograph (Figure 4.94g) reveals that the roots of the maxillary central incisors have undergone root resorption. This was anticipated. The roots of these teeth were dilacerated, had to be uprighted, and the maxillary right central incisor's roots were in close proximity to the cleft area.
- There are several teeth with white spot lesions. White spot lesions could have been minimized with better oral hygiene practice.

Q: Carlie was retained using wrap around Hawley retainers in both arches full time for one year. Then, clear retainers were delivered which she wears at nights only. She has been faithful with retainer wear. Two-year, post-deband records are presented in Figures 4.95a–4.95h. Her occlusion has settled nicely and shows excellent intercuspation of posterior teeth plus bilateral Class I canine and molar relationships. Can you suggest "take-home pearls" for Carlie's care?

A: "Take-home pearls" include the following:
- Carlie was nine years and three months old when she presented with her parent's chief complaint, "Carlie has an underbite." She had a bilateral cleft lip and palate and was successfully treated with

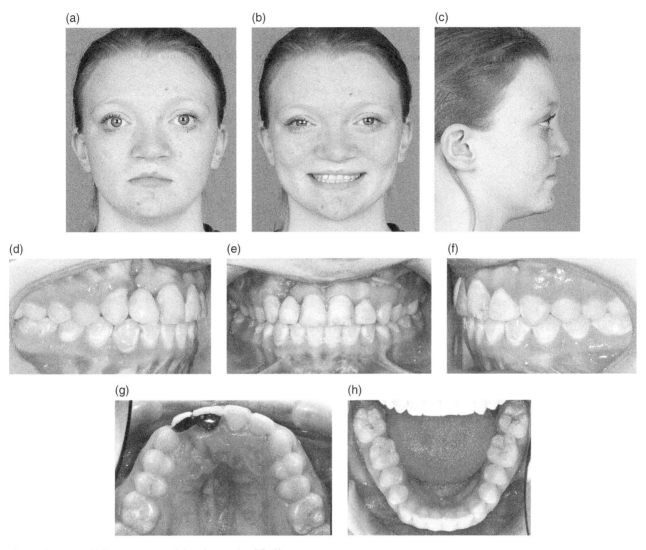

Figure 4.95 (a–h) Two-year post-deband records of Carlie.

maxillary expansion and TAD-supported Class III elastic wear.

- Growth is a key factor in any child's care. We initiated treatment prior to Carlie's peak growth spurt, and it worked in our favor.
- Following maxillary expansion in cleft palate patients – retain with a fixed appliance. We recommend the placement of a transpalatal arch with mesial extension arms. For Carlie, the expansion was not adequately retained. (Two years after Carlie's transpalatal arch was cemented, it had to be removed and was never recemented.) Consequently, there was a collapse of the maxillary right segment. This could have been avoided had the recommended post-expansion/alveolar bone graft retention protocol been followed.
- The long-term success of alveolar bone grafts is based on factors beyond the orthodontist's control. Carlie's

bone graft was successful. However, the grafted alveolus was too thin to place an osseointegrated implant.

- When teeth are moved, there is always a risk of root resorption. This is particularly true for teeth that are moved adjacent to cleft areas (e.g. Carlie's maxillary incisors).
- Oral surgery initially placed bone plates in Carlie's mandibular arch as Class III elastic anchors. These bone plates failed, and we replaced them with miniscrews (TADs) ourselves. The screws were stable for the duration of her treatment. More and more often, we are using miniscrews as Class III elastic anchors instead of bone plates as doing so eliminates the need for flap elevation.
- With better oral hygiene, white spot lesions could have been minimized or avoided entirely.
- Cleft and craniofacial care requires a team approach, involving many disciplines.

References

1 Nguyen, Q.V., Bezemer, P.D., Habets, L., and Prahl-Andersen, B. (1999). A systematic review of the relationship between overjet size and traumatic dental injuries. *Eur. J. Orthod.* 21 (5): 503–515.

2 K Bsl, B., Thiruvenkatachari, B., Harrison, J.E., and O'Brien, K.D. (2018). Orthodontic treatment for prominent upper front teeth (Class II malocclusion) in children and adolescents. *Cochrane Database Syst. Rev.* 3: CD003452. https://doi.org/10.1002/14651858. CD003452.pub4.

3 Janson, G., Sathler, R., Fernandes, T.M.F. et al. (2013). Correction of Class II malocclusion with Class II elastics: a systematic review. *Am. J. Orthod. Dentofac. Orthop.* 143 (3): 383–392.

4 Franchi, L., Alvetro, L., Giuntini, V. et al. (2011). Effectiveness of comprehensive fixed appliance treatment used with the Forsus Fatigue resistant device in Class II patients. *Angle Orthod.* 81 (4): 678–683.

5 Heinig, N. and Göz, G. (2001). Clinical application and effects of the Forsus spring. A study of a new Herbst hybrid. *J. Orofac. Orthop.* 62 (6): 436–450.

6 Firouz, M., Zernik, J., and Nanda, R. (1992). Dental and orthopedic effects of high pull headgear in treatment of Class II, division 1 malocclusion. *Am. J. Orthod. Dentofac. Orthop.* 102 (3): 197–205.

7 Baumrind, S., Korn, E.L., Isaacson, R.J. et al. (1983). Quantitative analysis of the orthodontic and orthopedic effects of maxillary traction. *Am. J. Orthod.* 84 (5): 384–398.

8 Elder, J.R. and Tuenge, R.H. (1974). Cephalometric and histologic changes produced by extraoral high pull traction to the maxilla in Macaca mulatta. *Am. J. Orthod.* 66 (6): 599–617.

9 Villalobos, F.J., Sinha, P.K., and Nanda, R.S. (2000). Longitudinal assessment of vertical and sagittal control in the mandibular arch by the mandibular fixed lingual arch. *Am. J. Orthod. Dentofac. Orthop.* 118 (4): 366–370.

10 Bilbo, E.E., Marshall, S.D., Southard, K.A. et al. (2018). Long-term skeletal effects of high pull headgear followed by fixed appliances for the treatment of Class II malocclusions. *Angle Orthod.* 88 (5): 530–537.

11 Kirjavainen, M., Kirjavainen, T., Hurmerinta, K., and Haavikko, K. (2000). Orthopedic cervical headgear with an expanded inner bow in Class II correction. *Angle Orthod.* 70 (4): 317–325.

12 Stuani, M.B., Stuani, A.S., and Stuani, A.S. (2005). Modified Thurow appliance: a clinical alternative for correcting skeletal open bite. *Am. J. Orthod. Dentofac. Orthop.* 128 (1): 118–125.

13 You, Z., Fishman, L., Rosenblum, R., and Subtelny, D. (2001). Dentoalveolar changes related to mandibular forward growth in untreated Class II persons. *Am. J. Orthod. Dentofac. Orthop.* 120 (6): 598–607. quiz 676.

14 Pancherz, H. (1997). The effects, limitations, and long-term dentofacial adaptations to treatment with the Herbst appliance. *Semin. Orthod.* 3 (4): 232–243.

15 Le Cornu, M., Cevidanes, L.H.S., Zhu, H. et al. (2013). Three-dimensional treatment outcomes in Class II patients treated with the Herbst appliance: a pilot study. *Am. J. Orthod. Dentofac. Orthop.* 144 (6): 818–830.

16 Huang, G.J., English, J., Ferguson, D.J. et al. (2005). Ask Us - Functional appliances and long-term effects on mandibular growth. *Am. J. Orthod. Dentofac. Orthop.* 128 (3): 271–272.

17 Pancherz, H., Ruf, S., and Kohlhas, P. (1998). "Effective condylar growth" and chin position changes in Herbst treatment: a cephalometric roentgenographic long-term study. *Am. J. Orthod. Dentofac. Orthop.* 114 (4): 437–446.

18 Araujo, A.M., Buschang, P.H., and Melo, A.C.M. (2004). Adaptive condylar growth and mandibular remodeling changes with bionator therapy – an implant study. *Eur. J. Orthod.* 26 (5): 515–522.

19 Rogers, K., Campbell, P., Tadlock, L. et al. (2018). Treatment changes of hypo- and hyperdivergent Class II Herbst patients. *Angle Orthod.* 88 (1): 3–9.

20 Konik, M., Pancherz, H., and Hansen, K. (1997). The mechanism of Class II correction in late Herbst treatment. *Am. J. Orthod. Dentofac. Orthop.* 112 (1): 87–91.

21 Croft, R.S., Buschang, P.H., English, J.D., and Meyer, R. (1999). A cephalometric and tomographic evaluation of Herbst treatment in the mixed dentition. *Am. J. Orthod. Dentofac. Orthop.* 116 (4): 435–443.

22 Proffit, W.R. and Tulloch, J.F. (2002). Preadolescent Class II problems: treat now or wait? *Am. J. Orthod. Dentofac. Orthop.* 121 (6): 560–562.

23 Tulloch, J.F.C., Proffit, W.R., and Phillips, C. (2004). Outcomes in a 2-phase randomized clinical trial of early Class II treatment. *Am. J. Orthod. Dentofac. Orthop.* 125 (6): 657–667.

24 Ghafari, J., Shofer, F.S., Jacobsson-Hunt, U. et al. (1998). Headgear versus functional regulator in the early treatment of Class II, division 1 malocclusion: a randomized clinical trial. *Am. J. Orthod. Dentofac. Orthop.* 113 (1): 51–61.

25 Risinger, R.K. and Proffit, W.R. (1996). Continuous overnight observation of human premolar eruption. *Arch. Oral Biol.* 41 (8-9): 779–789.

26 Jakobsson, S.O. (1967). Cephalometric evaluation of treatment effect on Class II, Division 1 malocclusions. *Am. J. Orthod.* 53 (6): 446–457.

27 Tulloch, J.F., Phillips, C., Koch, G., and Proffit, W.R. (1997). The effect of early intervention on skeletal pattern in Class II malocclusion: a randomized clinical trial. *Am. J. Orthod. Dentofac. Orthop.* 111 (4): 391–400.

28 Wheeler, T.T., McGorray, S.P., Dolce, C. et al. (2002). Effectiveness of early treatment of Class II malocclusion. *Am. J. Orthod. Dentofac. Orthop.* 121 (1): 9–17.

29 Dolce, C., McGorray, S.P., Brazeau, L. et al. (2007). Timing of Class II treatment: skeletal changes comparing 1-phase and 2-phase treatment. *Am. J. Orthod. Dentofac. Orthop.* 132 (4): 481–489.

30 Almeida-Pedrin, R.R., Almeida, M.R., Almeida, R.R. et al. (2007). Treatment effects of headgear biteplane and bionator appliances. *Am. J. Orthod. Dentofac. Orthop.* 132 (2): 191–198.

31 Thurman, M.M., King, G.J., Ramsay, D.S. et al. (2011). The effect of an anterior biteplate on dental and skeletal Class II correction using headgears: a cephalometric study. *Orthod. Craniofac. Res.* 14 (4): 213–221.

32 Baccetti, T., Franchi, L., and Stahl, F. (2009). Comparison of 2 comprehensive Class II treatment protocols including the bonded Herbst and headgear appliances: a double-blind study of consecutively treated patients at puberty. *Am. J. Orthod. Dentofac. Orthop.* 135 (6): 698. e1–698.e10. discussion 698-9.

33 Southard, T.E., Marshall, S.D., Allareddy, V. et al. (2013). An evidence-based comparison of headgear and functional appliance therapy for the correction of Class II malocclusions. *Semin. Orthod.* 19 (3): 174–195.

34 Sloss, E.A.C., Southard, K.A., Qian, F. et al. (2008). Comparison of soft-tissue profiles after treatment with headgear or Herbst appliance. *Am. J. Orthod. Dentofac. Orthop.* 133 (4): 509–514.

35 Tsiouli, K., Topouzelis, N., Papadopoulos, M., and Gkantidis, N. (2017). Perceived facial changes of Class II division 1 patients with convex profiles after functional orthopedic treatment followed by fixed orthodontic appliances. *Am. J. Orthod. Dentofac. Orthop.* 152 (1): 80–91.

36 Demisch, A., Ingervall, B., and Thüer, U. (1992). Mandibular displacement in Angle Class II, division 2 malocclusion. *Am. J. Orthod. Dentofac. Orthop.* 102 (6): 509–518.

37 El-Dawlatly, M. and Mostafa, Y. (2018). Mandibular skeletal changes following orthodontic treatment of an adult case with Class II Division 2 malocclusion. *Acta Sci. Dent. Sci.* 2 (4): 41–45.

38 Keeling, S.D., Wheeler, T.T., King, G.J. et al. (1998). Anteroposterior skeletal and dental changes after early Class II treatment with bionators and headgear. *Am. J. Orthod. Dentofac. Orthop.* 113 (1): 40–50.

39 O'Brien, K. (2006). Is early treatment for Class II malocclusions effective? Results from a randomized controlled trial. *Am. J. Orthod. Dentofac. Orthop.* 129 (4 Suppl): S64–S65.

40 O'Brien, K., Wright, J., Conboy, F. et al. (2009). Early treatment for Class II div 1 malocclusion with the Twin-block appliance: a multi-center, randomized, controlled trial. *Am. J. Orthod. Dentofac. Orthop.* 135 (5): 573–579.

41 Mellion, Z.J., Behrents, R.G., and Johnston, L.E. (2013). The pattern of facial skeletal growth and its relationship to various common indexes of maturation. *Am. J. Orthod. Dentofac. Orthop.* 143 (6): 845–854.

42 Keski-Nisula, K., Keski-Nisula, L., and Varrela, J. (2020). Class II treatment in early mixed dentition with the eruption guidance appliance: effects and long-term stability. *Eur. J. Orthod.* 42 (2): 151–156.

43 O'Brien, K. (2019). Long term effects of eruption guidance look impressive? kevinobrienorthoblog.com/ eruption-guidance-therapy-look-impressive/ ().

44 Thiruvenkatachari, B., Harrison, J., Worthington, H., and O'Brien, K. (2015). Early orthodontic treatment for Class II malocclusion reduces the chance of incisal trauma: results of a Cochrane systematic review. *Am. J. Orthod. Dentofac. Orthop.* 148 (1): 47–59.

45 Thiruvenkatachari, B., Harrison, J.E., Worthington, H.V., and O'Brien, K.D. (2013). Orthodontic treatment for prominent upper front teeth (Class II malocclusion) in children. *Cochrane Database Syst. Rev.* 3: CD003452.

46 Koroluk, L.D., Tulloch, J.F.C., and Phillips, C. (2003). Incisor trauma and early treatment for Class II Division 1 malocclusion. *Am. J. Orthod. Dentofac. Orthop.* 123 (2): 117–125. discussion 125-6.

47 Nakasima, A., Ichinose, M., Nakata, S., and Takahama, Y. (1982). Hereditary factors in the craniofacial morphology of Angle's Class II and Class III malocclusions. *Am. J. Orthod.* 82 (2): 150–156.

48 Rabie, A.B. and Gu, Y. (1999). Orthodontics: management of pseudo Class III malocclusion in southern Chinese children. *Br. Dent. J.* 186 (4): 183–187.

49 Chung, C.H. and Dugoni, S.A. (2015). Appropriate timing for correction of malocclusions. In: *Mosby's Orthodontic Review*, 2e (eds. J.D. English, S. Akyalcin, T. Peltomäki and K. Litschel), 24–35. St. Louis: Elsevier.

50 Nagahara, K., Murata, S., Nakamura, S., and Tsuchiya, T. (2001). Prediction of the permanent dentition in deciduous anterior crossbite. *Angle Orthod.* 71 (5): 390–395.

51 Tweed, C.H. (1966). *Clinical Orthodontics*, vol. 2. C.V. Mosby: St. Louis.

52 Vasilakos, G., Koniaris, A., Wolf, M. et al. (2018). Early anterior crossbite correction through posterior bite opening: a 3D superimposition prospective cohort study. *Eur. J. Orthod.* 40 (4): 364–371.

53 Ngan, P., Hägg, U., Yiu, C. et al. (1996). Treatment response to maxillary expansion and protraction. *Eur. J. Orthod.* 18 (2): 151–168.

54 Ngan, P. (2005). Early timely treatment of Class III malocclusion. *Semin. Orthod.* 11 (3): 140–145.

55 Kim, J.H., Viana, M.A., Graber, T.M. et al. (1999). The effectiveness of protraction face mask therapy: a meta-analysis. *Am. J. Orthod. Dentofac. Orthop.* 115 (6): 675–685.

56 Jäger, A., Braumann, B., Kim, C., and Wahner, S. (2001). Skeletal and dental effects of maxillary protraction in patients with angle class III malocclusion: a meta-analysis. *J. Orofac. Orthop.* 62 (4): 275–284.

57 Wells, A.P., Sarver, D.M., and Proffit, W.R. (2006). Long-term efficacy of reverse pull headgear therapy. *Angle Orthod.* 76 (6): 915–922.

58 Vaughn, G.A., Mason, B., Moon, H.B., and Turley, P.K. (2005). The effects of maxillary protraction therapy with and without rapid palatal expansion: a prospective, randomized clinical trial. *Am. J. Orthod. Dentofac. Orthop.* 128 (3): 299–309.

59 Tortop, T., Keykubat, A., and Yuksel, S. (2007). Facemask therapy with and without expansion. *Am. J. Orthod. Dentofac. Orthop.* 132 (4): 467–474.

60 Baik, H.S. (1995). Clinical results of the maxillary protraction in Korean children. *Am. J. Orthod.* 108 (6): 583–592.

61 Liou, E.J.W. (2005). Effective maxillary orthopedic protraction for growing Class III patients: a clinical application simulates distraction osteogenesis. *Prog. Orthod.* 6 (2): 154–171.

62 Masucci, C., Franchi, L., Giuntini, V., and Defraia, E. (2014). Short-term effects of a modified Alt-RAMEC protocol for early treatment of Class III malocclusion: a controlled study. *Orthod. Craniofac. Res.* 17 (4): 259–269.

63 Liu, W., Zhou, Y., Wang, X. et al. (2015). Effect of maxillary protraction with alternating rapid palatal expansion and constriction vs. expansion alone in maxillary retrusive patients: a single-center, randomized controlled trial. *Am. J. Orthod. Dentofac. Orthop.* 148 (4): 641–651.

64 Wilmes, B., Ngan, P., EJW, L. et al. (2014). Early Class III facemask treatment with the hybrid hyrax and Alt-RAMEC protocol. *J. Clin. Orthod.* 48 (2): 84–93.

65 Sar, C., Arman-Özcirpici, A., Uçkan, S., and Yazici, A.C. (2011). Comparative evaluation of maxillary protraction with and without skeletal anchorage. *Am. J. Orthod. Dentofac. Orthop.* 139 (5): 636–649.

66 Cha, B.-K. and Ngan, P.W. (2011). Skeletal anchorage for orthopedic correction of growing Class III patients. *Semin. Orthod.* 17 (2): 124–137.

67 Major, M.P., Wong, J.K., Saltaji, H. et al. (2012). Skeletal anchored maxillary protraction for midface deficiency in children and early adolescence with Class III malocclusion: a systematic review and meta-analysis. *J. World Fed. Orthod.* 1 (2): e47–e54.

68 Woon, C. and Thiruvenkatachari, B. (2017). Early orthodontic treatment for Class III malocclusion: a systematic review and meta-analysis. *Am. J. Orthod. Dentofac. Orthop.* 151 (1): 28–52.

69 Mandall, N., Cousley, R., DiBiase, A. et al. (2016). Early class III protraction facemask treatment reduces the need for orthognathic surgery: a multi-centre, two-arm parallel randomized, controlled trial. *J. Orthod.* 43 (3): 164–175.

70 Macdonald, K.E., Kapust, A.J., and Turley, P.K. (1999). Cephalometric changes after the correction of Class III malocclusion with maxillary expansion/facemask therapy. *Am. J. Orthod. Dentofac. Orthop.* 116 (1): 13–24.

71 Turley, P.K. (2002). Managing the developing Class III malocclusion with palatal expansion and facemask therapy. *Am. J. Orthod. Dentofac. Orthop.* 122 (4): 349–352.

72 Deguchi, T., Kuroda, T., Minoshima, Y., and Graber, T.M. (2002). Craniofacial features of patients with Class III abnormalities: growth-related changes and effects of short-term and long-term chin cup therapy. *Am. J. Orthod. Dentofac. Orthop.* 121 (1): 84–92.

73 Wendell, P.D., Nanda, R., Sakamoto, T., and Nakamura, S. (1985). The effects of chin cup therapy on the mandible: a longitudinal study. *Am. J. Orthod.* 87 (4): 265–274.

74 Deguchi, T. and McNamara, J. (1999). Craniofacial adaptations induced by chin cup therapy in Class III patients. *Am. J. Orthod. Dentofac. Orthop.* 115 (2): 175–182.

75 Deguchi, T., Kuroda, T., Hunt, N.P., and Graber, T.M. (1999). Long-term application of chin cup force alters the morphology of the dolichofacial Class III mandible. *Am. J. Orthod. Dentofac. Orthop.* 116 (6): 610–615.

76 Mitani, H. (2002). Early application of chincap therapy to skeletal Class III malocclusion. *Am. J. Orthod. Dentofac. Orthop.* 121 (6): 584–585.

77 Barrett, A.A.F., Baccetti, T., and McNamara, J.A. Jr. (2010). Treatment effects of the light-force chin cup. *Am. J. Orthod. Dentofac. Orthop.* 138 (4): 468–476.

78 De Clerck, H., Cevidanes, L., and Baccetti, T. (2010). Dentofacial effects of bone-anchored maxillary protraction: a controlled study of consecutively treated

Class III patients. *Am. J. Orthod. Dentofac. Orthop.* 138 (5): 577–581.

79 Elnagar, M.H., Elshourbagy, E., Ghobashy, S. et al. (2016). Comparative evaluation of 2 skeletally anchored maxillary protraction protocols. *Am. J. Orthod. Dentofac. Orthop.* 150 (5): 751–762.

80 De Toffol, L., Pavoni, C., Baccetti, T. et al. (2008). Orthopedic treatment outcomes in Class III malocclusion. A systematic review. *Angle Orthod.* 78 (3): 561–573.

81 Wheeler, R.C. (1974). *Dental Anatomy, Physiology, and Occlusion*, 5e. Philadelphia: W.B. Saunders.

82 Angle, E.H. (1907). Malocclusion. In: *Treatment of Malocclusion of the Teeth: Angle's System*, 7e (ed. E.H. Angle), 41. Philadelphia: SS White.

83 Orsini, M.G., Huang, G.J., Kiyak, H.A. et al. (2006). Methods to evaluate profile preferences for the anteroposterior position of the mandible. *Am. J. Orthod. Dentofac. Orthop.* 130 (3): 283–291.

84 Gonzáles-Ulloa, M. and Stevens, E. (1968). The role of chin correction in profileplasty. *Plast. Reconstr. Surg.* 41 (5): 477–486.

85 Harrison, J.E., O'Brien, K.D., and Worthington, H.V. (2007). Orthodontic treatment for prominent upper front teeth in children. *Cochrane Database Syst. Rev.* 18 (3): CD003452. https://doi.org/10.1002/14651858. CD003452.pub2.

86 Rebellato, J., Lindauer, S.J., Rubenstein, L.K. et al. (1997). Lower arch perimeter preservation using the lingual arch. *Am. J. Orthod. Dentofac. Orthop.* 112 (4): 449–456.

87 Viglianisi, A. (2010). Effects of lingual arch used as space maintainer on mandibular arch dimension: a systematic review. *Am. J. Orthod. Dentofac. Orthop.* 138 (4): 382e1–382e4.

88 Naini, F.B. and Gill, D.S. (2018). Oral surgery: labial frenectomy: indications and practical implications. *Br Dent.* 225 (3): 199–200.

89 Mann, K.R., Marshall, S.D., Qian, F. et al. (2011). Effect of maxillary anteroposterior position on profile esthetics in headgear-treated patients. *Am. J. Orthod. Dentofac. Orthop.* 139 (2): 228–234.

90 Ng, J., Major, P.W., Heo, G., and Flores-Mir, C. (2005). True incisor intrusion attained during orthodontic treatment: a systematic review and meta-analysis. *Am. J. Orthod. Dentofac. Orthop.* 128 (2): 212–219.

91 Bernstein, R.L., Preston, C.B., and Lampasso, J. (2007). Leveling the curve of Spee with a continuous archwire technique: a long term cephalometric study. *Am. J. Orthod. Dentofac. Orthop.* 131 (3): 363–371.

92 Marshall, S., Dawson, D., Southard, K.A. et al. (2003). Transverse molar movements during growth. *Am. J. Orthod. Dentofac. Orthop.* 124 (6): 615–624.

93 Miner, R.M., Al Qabandi, S., Rigali, P.H., and Will, L.A. (2012). Cone-beam computed tomography transverse analysis. Part I: Normative data. *Am. J. Orthod. Dentofac. Orthop.* 142 (3): 300–307.

94 Lux, C.J., Conradt, C., Burden, D., and Komposch, G. (2003). Dental arch widths and mandibular-maxillary base widths in Class II malocclusions between early mixed and permanent dentitions. *Angle Orthod.* 73 (6): 674–685.

95 Hansen, K., Koutsonas, T.G., and Pancherz, H. (1997). Long-term effects of Herbst treatment on the mandibular incisor segment: a cephalometric and biometric investigation. *Am. J. Orthod. Dentofac. Orthop.* 112 (1): 92–103.

96 Tweed, C.H. (1954). The Frankfort mandibular incisor angle (FMIA) in orthodontic diagnosis, treatment planning and prognosis. *Angle Orthod.* 24 (3): 121–169.

97 Pirttiniemi, P., Kantomaa, T., and Lahtela, P. (1990). Relationship between craniofacial and condyle path asymmetry in unilateral corset patients. *Eur. J. Orthod.* 12 (4): 408–413.

98 Pinto, A.S., Buschang, P.H., Throckmorton, G.S., and Chen, P. (2001). Morphological and positional asymmetries of young children with functional unilateral posterior crossbite. *Am. J. Orthod. Dentofac. Orthop.* 120 (5): 513–520.

99 Kilic, N., Kiki, A., and Oktay, H. (2008). Condylar asymmetry in unilateral posterior crossbite patients. *Am. J. Orthod. Dentofac. Orthop.* 133 (3): 382–387.

100 Almeida, M.R., Henriques, J.F., Almeida, R.R. et al. (2004). Treatment effects produced by the Bionator appliance. Comparison with an untreated Class II sample. *Eur. J. Orthod.* 26 (1): 65–72.

101 Rodrigues de Almeida, M., Castanha Henriques, J.F., Rodrigues de Almeida, R., and Ursi, W. (2002). Treatment effects produced by Fränkel appliance in patients with class II, division 1 malocclusion. *Angle Orthod.* 72 (5): 418–425.

102 Andlin-Sobocki, A. (1993). Changes of facial gingival dimensions in children. A 2-year longitudinal study. *J. Clin. Periodontol.* 20 (3): 212–218.

103 Frodel, J.L., Sykes, J.M., and Jones, J.L. (2004). Evaluation and treatment of vertical microgenia. *Arch. Facial Plast. Surg.* 6 (2): 111–119.

104 Knott, V.B. and Meredith, H.V. (1966). Statistics on eruption of the permanent dentition from serial data for North American white children. *Angle Orthod.* 36 (1): 68–79.

105 Sugawara, J., Asano, T., Endo, N., and Mitani, H. (1990). Long-term effects of chincap therapy on skeletal profile in mandibular prognathism. *Am. J. Orthod. Dentofac. Orthop.* 98 (2): 127–133.

106 Björk, A. and Skieller, V. (1983). Normal and abnormal growth of the mandible. A synthesis of longitudinal cephalometric implant studies over a period of 25 years. *Eur. J. Orthod.* 5 (1): 1–46.

107 Koora, K., Muthu, M.S., and Rathna, P.V. (2007). Spontaneous closure of midline diastema following frenectomy. *J. Indian Soc. Pedod. Prev. Dent.* 25 (1): 23–26.

108 Björk, A. and Skieller, V. (1972). Facial development and tooth eruption: an implant study at the age of puberty. *Am. J. Orthod.* 62 (4): 339–383.

109 Steedle, J.R. and Proffit, W.R. (1985). The pattern and control of eruptive tooth movements. *Am. J. Orthod.* 87 (1): 56–66.

110 Buschang, P.H. and Jacob, H.B. (2014). Mandibular rotation revisited: what makes it so important? *Semin. Orthod.* 20 (4): 299–315.

111 Levander, E. and Malmgren, O. (1988). Evaluation of the risk of root resorption during orthodontic treatment: a study of upper incisors. *Eur. J. Orthod.* 10 (1): 30–38.

112 Sarikaya, S., Haydar, B., Ciğer, S., and Ariyürek, M. (2002). Changes in alveolar bone thickness due to retraction of anterior teeth. *Am. J. Orthod. Dentofac. Orthop.* 122 (1): 15–26.

113 Scolozzi, P. (2008). Distraction osteogenesis in the management of severe maxillary hypoplasia in cleft lip and palate patients. *J. Craniofac. Surg.* 19 (5): 1199–1214.

114 Epker, B.N., Stella, J.P., and Fisch, L.C. (1998). Transverse maxillomandibular discrepancies. In: *Dentofacial Deformities Integrated Orthodontic and Surgical Correction*, 2e (eds. B.N. Epker, J.P. Stella and L.C. Fisch). St Louis, MO: Mosby.

115 Profitt, W.R. and White, R.P. Jr. (2003). Combining surgery and orthodontics. In: *Contemporary Treatment of Dentofacial Deformity* (eds. W.R. Profitt, R.P. White Jr. and D.M. Sarver). St Louis, MO: Mosby.

116 DeLuke, D.M., Marchand, A., Robles, E.C., and Fox, P. (1997). Facial growth and the need for orthognathic surgery after cleft palate repair: literature review and report of 28 cases. *J. Oral Maxillofac. Surg.* 55 (7): 694–697. discussion 697-8.

117 Yun-Chia Ku, M., Lo, L.-J., Chen, M.-C., and Wen-Ching, K.E. (2018). Predicting need for orthognathic surgery in early permanent dentition patients with unilateral cleft lip and palate using receiver operating characteristic analysis. *Am. J. Orthod. Dentofac. Orthop.* 153 (3): 405–414.

118 Rosenstein, S., Kernahan, D., Dado, D. et al. (1991). Orthognathic surgery in cleft patients treated by early bone grafting. *Plast. Reconstr. Surg.* 87 (5): 835–892. discussion 840-2.

119 World Health Organization (2007). Human genomics in global health. Typical orofacial clefts – cumulative data by register. http://www.who.int/genomics/anomalies/cumulative_data/en/ (accessed 31 January 2021).

120 Parker, S.E., Mai, C.T., Canfield, M.A. et al. (2010). Updated national birth prevalence estimates for selected birth defects in the United States, 2004–2006. *Birth Defects Res. A Clin. Mol. Teratol.* 88 (12): 1008–1016.

121 Allori, A.C., Mulliken, J.B., Meara, J.G. et al. (2017). Classification of cleft lip/palate: then and now. *Cleft Palate Craniofac. J.* 54 (2): 175–188.

122 Vig, K.W. and Mercado, A.M. (2015). Overview of orthodontic care for children with cleft lip and palate, 1915–2015. *Am. J. Orthod. Dentofac. Orthop.* 148 (4): 543–556.

123 Ahmed, M.M., Brecht, L.E., Cutting, C.B., and Grayson, B.H. (2012). 2012 American board of pediatric dentistry college of diplomates annual meeting: the role of pediatric dentists in the presurgical treatment of infants with cleft lip/cleft palate utilizing nasoalveolar molding. *Pediatr. Dent.* 34 (7): e209–e214.

124 Grayson, B.H., Santiago, P.E., Brecht, L.E., and Cutting, C.B. (1999). Presurgical nasoalveolar molding in infants with cleft lip and palate. *Cleft Palate Craniofac. J.* 36 (6): 486–498.

125 Santiago, P.E., Schuster, L.A., and Levy-Bercowski, D. (2014). Management of the alveolar cleft. *Clin. Plast. Surg.* 41 (2): 219–232.

126 Attiguppe, P.R., Karuna, Y.M., Yavagal, C. et al. (2016). Presurgical nasoalveolar molding: a boon to facilitate the surgical repair in infants with cleft lip and palate. *Contemp. Clin. Dent.* 7 (4): 569–573.

127 Sasaki, H., Togashi, S., Karube, R. et al. (2012). Presurgical nasoalveolar molding orthopedic treatment improves the outcome of primary cheiloplasty of unilateral complete cleft lip and palate, as assessed by naris morphology and cleft gap. *J. Craniofac. Surg.* 23 (6): 1596–1601.

128 Grayson, B.H. and Maull, D. (2004). Nasoalveolar molding for infants born with clefts of the lip, alveolus, and palate. *Clin. Plast. Surg.* 31 (2): 149–158.

129 Latham, R.A., Kusy, R.P., and Georgiade, N.G. (1976). An extraorally activated expansion appliance for cleft palate infants. *Cleft Palate J.* 13 (3): 253–261.

130 Allareddy, V., Ross, E., Bruun, R. et al. (2015). Operative and immediate postoperative outcomes of using a Latham-type dentomaxillary appliance in patients with unilateral complete cleft lip and palate. *Cleft Palate Craniofac. J.* 52 (4): 405–410.

131 Bronkhorst, A., Allareddy, V., Allred, E. et al. (2015). Assessment of morbidity following insertion of fixed preoperative orthopedic appliance in infants with complete cleft lip and palate. *Oral Surg. Oral Med. Oral Pathol. Oral Radiol.* 119 (3): 278–284.

132 Prahl, C., Kuijpers-Jagtman, A.M., van't Hof, M.A., and Prahl-Andersen, B. (2001). A randomised prospective clinical trial into the effect of infant orthopaedics on maxillary arch dimensions in unilateral cleft lip and palate (Dutchcleft). *Eur. J. Oral Sci.* 109 (5): 297–305.

133 Bongaarts, C.A.M., van't Hof, M.A., Prahl-Andersen, B. et al. (2006). Infant orthopedics has no effect on maxillary arch dimensions in the deciduous dentition of children with complete unilateral cleft lip and palate (Dutchcleft). *Cleft Palate Craniofac. J.* 43 (6): 665–672.

134 Uzel, A. and Alparslan, Z.N. (2011). Long-term effects of presurgical infant orthopedics in patients with cleft lip and palate: a systematic review. *Cleft Palate Craniofac. J.* 48 (5): 587–595.

135 van der Heijden, P., Dijkstra, P.U., Stellingsma, C. et al. (2013). Limited evidence for the effect of presurgical nasoalveolar molding in unilateral cleft on nasal symmetry: a call for unified research. *Plast. Reconstr. Surg.* 131 (1): 62e–71e.

136 (1993). Parameters for the evaluation and treatment of patients with cleft lip/palate or other craniofacial anomalies. American cleft palate-craniofacial association. *Cleft Palate Craniofac. J.* 30 (Suppl 1): s1–s16. Revised edition, January 2018. http://journals. sagepub.com/doi/full/10.1177/1055665617739564 (accessed 15 March 2018).

137 Vander Woude, D.L. and Mulliken, J.B. (1997). Effect of lip adhesion on labial height in two-stage repair of unilateral complete cleft lip. *Plast. Reconstr. Surg.* 100 (3): 567–572. discussion 573-4.

138 Coots, B.K. (2012). Alveolar bone grafting: past, present, and new horizons. *Semin. Plast. Surg.* 26 (4): 178–183.

139 Eppley, B.L. (1996). Alveolar cleft bone grafting (Part I): Primary bone grafting. *J. Oral Maxillofac. Surg.* 54 (1): 74–82.

140 Ochs, M.W. (1996). Alveolar cleft bone grafting (Part II): secondary bone grafting. *J. Oral Maxillofac. Surg.* 54 (1): 83–88.

141 Rosenstein, S.W. (2003). Early bone grafting of alveolar cleft deformities. *J. Oral Maxillofac. Surg.* 61 (9): 1078–1081.

142 Kazemi, A., Stearns, J.W., and Fonseca, R.J. (2002). Secondary grafting in the alveolar cleft patient. *Oral Maxillofac. Surg. Clin. North Am.* 14 (4): 477–490.

5

Vertical Problems

Introduction

Problems in the vertical dimension are some of the most challenging problems that an orthodontist must deal with. This chapter provides a review of the etiology, diagnosis, and early treatment of vertical problems: dental deep bites, skeletal deep bites, dental open bites, skeletal open bites, and posterior open bites.

Q: What is overbite (OB), and what is the ideal OB magnitude?

A: Overbite is a measure of vertical maxillary incisor overlap of mandibular incisors, with the teeth in centric occlusion (CO) and the occlusal plane oriented to the horizontal. It is measured as the vertical distance from the mandibular incisor incisal edges to the maxillary incisor incisal edges projected on the coronal or sagittal plane or estimated as the percentage of vertical overlap of the clinical crown length of the mandibular central incisors. The ideal OB magnitude is 10–20% maxillary incisor coverage of mandibular incisors (Figures 5.1a and 5.1b).

When you examine a child with ideal OB but then have them open slightly, maxillary and mandibular permanent incisal edges should be approximately even and incisal edges should either be on the same level as the canine cusp tips or just slightly apical to the canine cusp tips (Figures 5.1c and 5.1d). The posterior occlusal plane should be relatively flat (Figures 5.1e and 5.1f) or the mandibular arch may have a 1–2 mm deep curve of Spee (Figure 5.1g) with the maxillary arch having a corresponding 1–2 mm compensating curve (Figure 5.1h) [1].

Figures 5.1i and 5.1j illustrates patients with an excessive overbite (80% and 100% OB, respectively). Traditionally, mandibular incisor palatal impingement is also defined as 100% overbite (Figures 5.1k–5.1m). Examples of inadequate overbite (anterior open bite) are shown in Figures 5.1n and 5.1o.

(a) 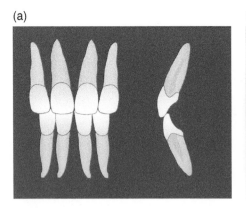 (b)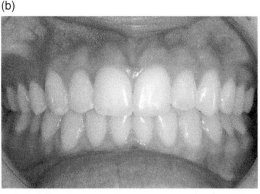

Figure 5.1 (a and b) Ideal overbite, or approximately 10–20% vertical maxillary incisor overlap of mandibular incisors; (c and d) incisal edges should either be on the same level as the canine cusp tips or just slightly apical to the canine cusp tips; (e and f) the posterior occlusal plane should be relatively flat, or (g) the mandibular arch may have a 1–2 mm deep curve of Spee with (h) the maxillary arch having a 1–2 mm compensating curve. Excessive overbites of approximately (i) 80% and (j) 100%. (k) Traditionally, mandibular incisor palatal impingement is also defined as 100% overbite (l, same patient open, m, patient closed). (n and o) Anterior open bites.

Practical Early Orthodontic Treatment: A Case-Based Review, First Edition. Thomas E. Southard, Steven D. Marshall, Laura L. Bonner, and Kyungsup Shin.
© 2023 John Wiley & Sons, Inc. Published 2023 by John Wiley & Sons, Inc.
Companion website: www.wiley.com/go/southard/practical

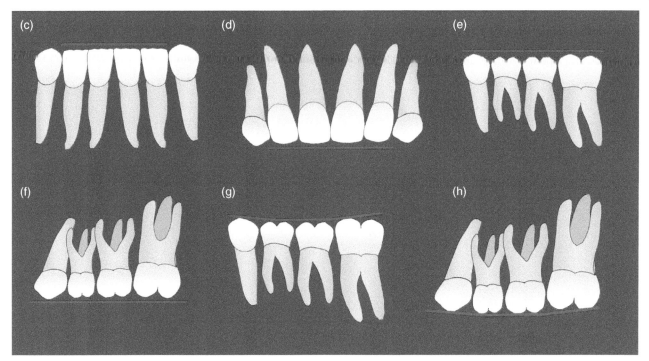

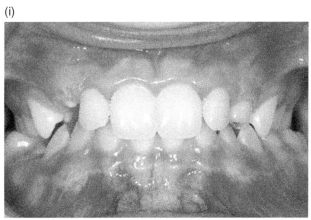

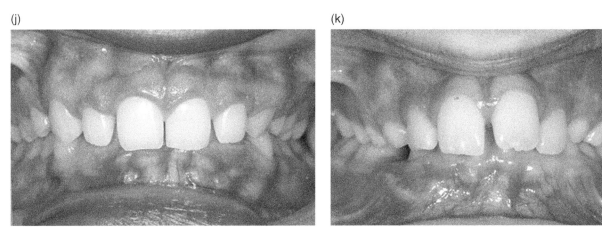

Figure 5.1 (Continued)

(l)
(m)
(n)
(o)

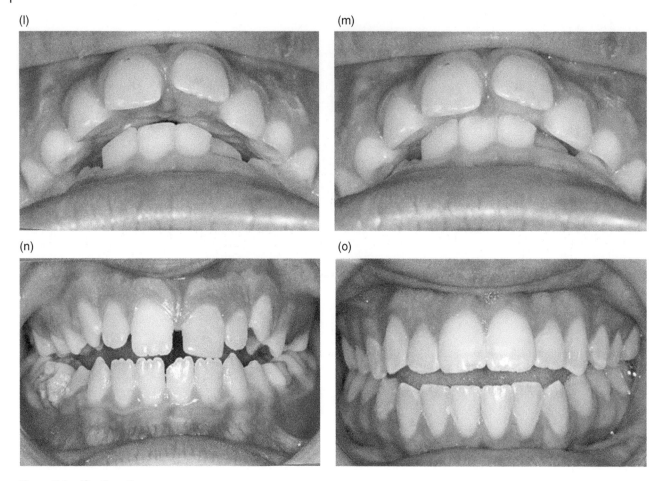

Figure 5.1 (Continued)

Q: How does ideal OB occur? How can a deep bite occur?

A: Teeth erupt between the tongue and cheeks, or between the tongue and lips, until opposed by occlusal or soft tissue forces great enough to halt their eruption. In a Class I patient, this eruption (Figure 5.2a, left) can result in contact with opposing incisors and ideal OB (Figure 5.2a, right). In a Class II patient (Figure 5.2b, left), mandibular incisors erupt until they occlude with the maxillary incisor cingulum or hard palate, maxillary incisors erupt until they occlude with mandibular incisors or are stopped by the mandibular lip, and excessive OB results (Figure 5.2b, right).

Q: Carson is a nine-year, nine-month-old boy (Figure 5.3) who presents to you with his parents' complaint, "Carson needs braces." Past medical history (PMH) and Past dental history (PDH) are within the range of normal (WRN). Centric relation (CR)=CO. Temporomandibular joint (TMJs), periodontal tissues, and mucogingival tissues are WRN. Can you list Carson's *primary* problems in each dimension (plus other primary problems)?

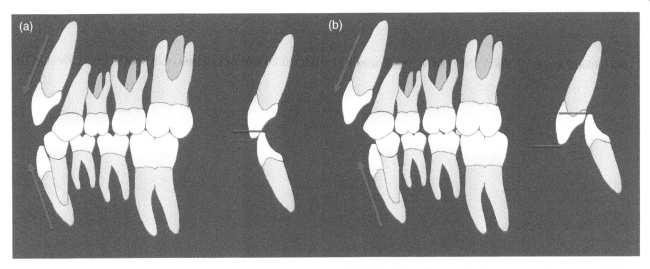

Figure 5.2 (a) Incisor eruption in a Class I patient can result in ideal OB. (b) In a Class II patient, incisor overeruption can result in a deep bite.

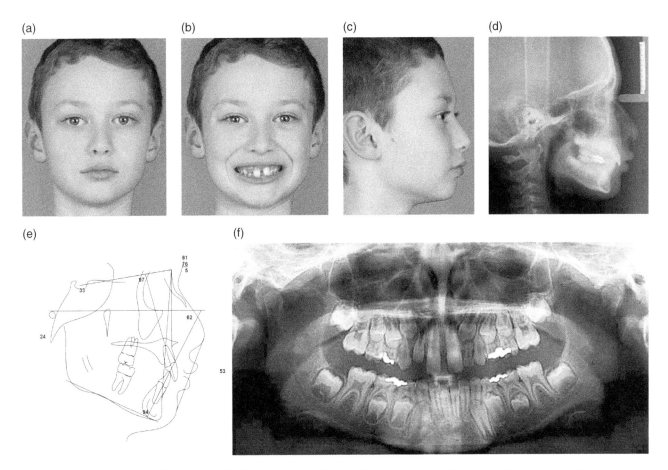

Figure 5.3 Initial records of Carson. (a–c) facial photographs; (d and e) lateral cephalometric radiograph and tracing; (f) panoramic image; (g–l) intraoral images; (m–q) model images.

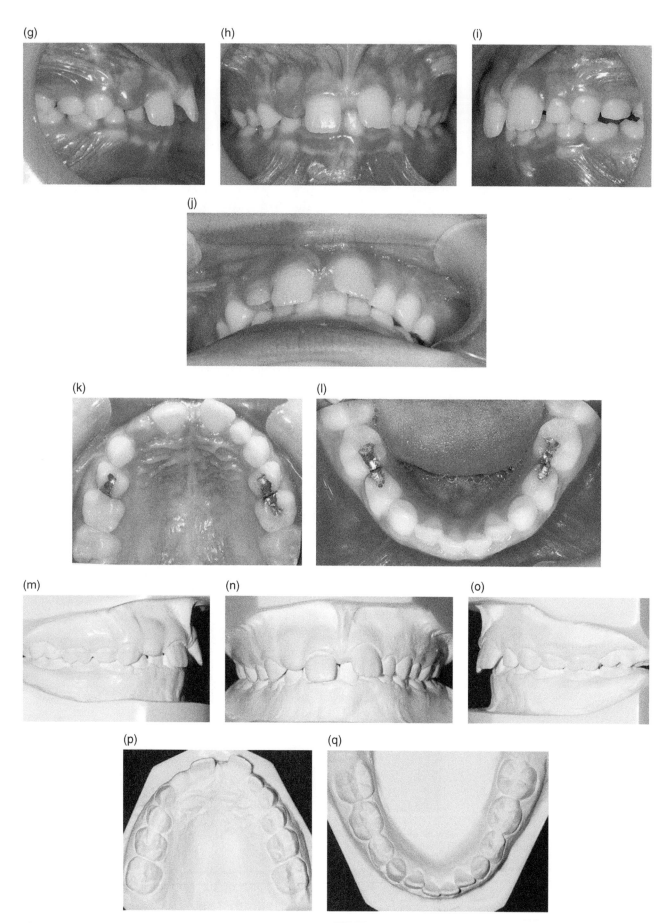

Figure 5.3 (Continued)

A:

Table 5.1 Primary problems list for Carson.

AP	Angle Class II division 2
	Iowa Classification: II(1 mm) I I II(2 mm)
	Mandibular skeletal anteroposterior deficiency
Vertical	LAFH WRN (LAFH/TAFH × 100% = 53%)
	OB 100% (palatal impingement by mandibular incisors)
Transverse	—
Other	Congenital absence of maxillary left permanent lateral incisor
	Upright maxillary incisors (U1 to SN = 97° measured to the right maxillary central incisor. However, the left maxillary central incisor is approximately 5° more proclined as seen in Figures 5.3m–5.3p)
	Mildly proclined mandibular incisors (FMIA = 62°)
	Thick maxillary midline frenum, with its inferior attachment confluent with the interproximal papilla between the maxillary central incisors (Figure 5.3h)
	~3 mm maxillary midline diastema
	2 mm mandibular anterior crowding

Q: What is the cause of Carson's deep bite (100% OB)?

A: By and large, his deep bite resulted from excessive mandibular anterior teeth eruption above the plane of his posterior teeth (Figures 5.4a and 5.4b) which is also seen in the sagittal plane as a deep curve of Spee (Figure 5.4c).

Q: Looking at Figure 5.5, did overeruption of Carson's *maxillary* incisors contribute to his deep bite?

A: Looking at Figure 5.5, Carson's maxillary central incisal edges are at approximately the same level as his maxillary posterior occlusal plane, with the right maxillary central incisor slightly below the occlusal plane

(a)

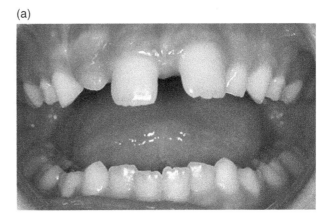

(b)

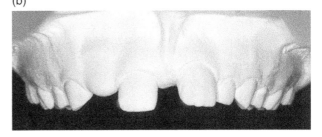

Figure 5.5 (a and b) View along Carson's maxillary occlusal plane.

(a)

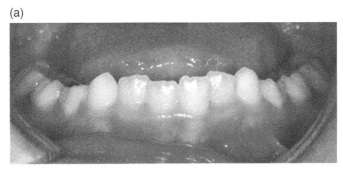

(b)   (c)

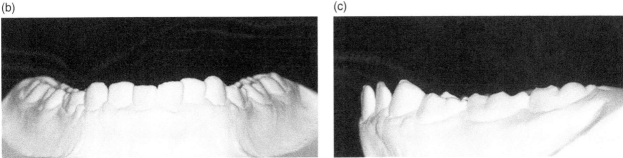

Figure 5.4 (a–c) Overeruption of mandibular anterior teeth has produced an excessively deep bite and deep curve of Spee.

(see also Figures 5.3m and 5.3o). That is, maxillary incisor overeruption has contributed a little to his deep bite.

Q: Does Carson have a *dental* deep bite, a *skeletal* deep bite, or a combination of both? Why?

A: Carson has a dental deep bite. His excessive OB resulted primarily from *mandibular incisor overeruption*.

His vertical skeletal measurements are within the range of normal:

- Soft tissue LAFH is WRN (LAFH approximately equal to midface height, Figure 5.6)
- Skeletal LAFH is WRN (Figure 5.3e, LAFH/total anterior face height (TAFH)$\times 100\%$ = 53%; normal = 55%, standard deviation = 2%) [2].
- Mandibular plane angle (MPA) is WRN (Franfort horizontal to mandibular plane angle (FMA) = 24°; SNMP = 33°)

Q: We classified Carson as a dental deep bite because he has normal vertical skeletal/soft tissue relationships and because his deep bite resulted from mandibular incisor overeruption. Can you describe the vertical soft tissue and skeletal features of a patient we would classify as a *skeletal* deep bite?

A: Yes – Sydney (Figure 5.7) is an example of a patient with a *skeletal* deep bite:

- Soft tissue LAFH *shorter* than midface height
- Short skeletal LAFH (LAFH/TAFH$\times 100\%$ = 52%, Figure 5.7b and c)
- Flat MPA (FMA = 18°; Sella – Nasion to mandibular plane angle (SN-MP) = 26°)
- MPA relatively parallel to FH and SN lines.

In fact, Sydney also exhibits a *dental* deep bite (Figures 5.7i–5.7p). Sydney exhibits a combination of dental deep bite *and* skeletal deep bite.

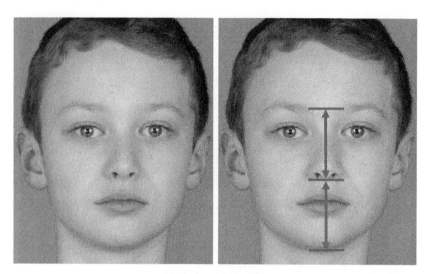

Figure 5.6 Carson's soft tissue LAFH is approximately equal to his soft tissue midface height.

(a)

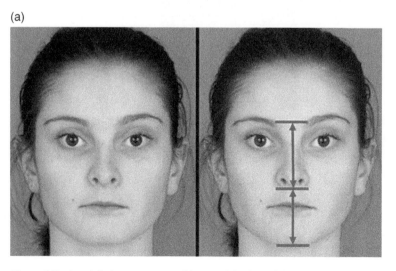

Figure 5.7 (a–p) Sydney presents with a combination of dental *and* skeletal deep bite.

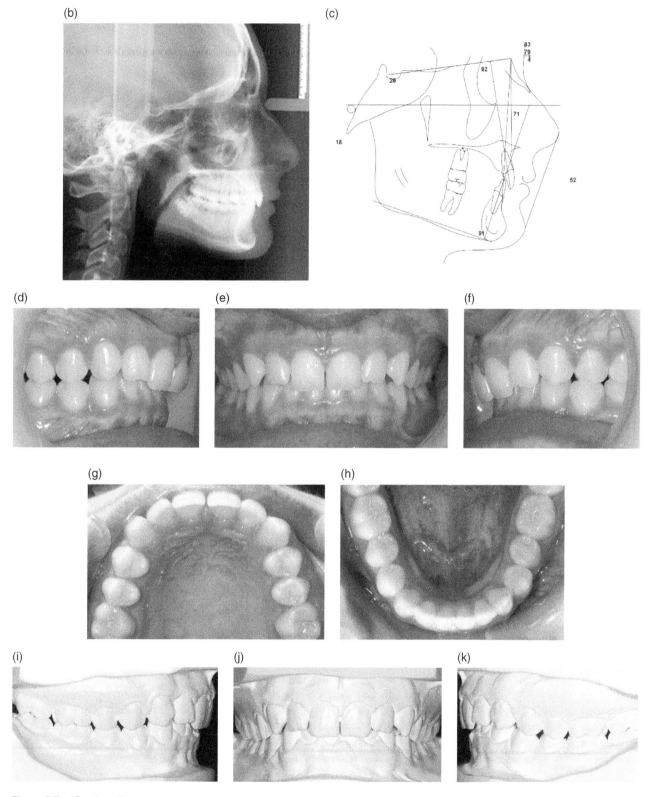

Figure 5.7 (Continued)

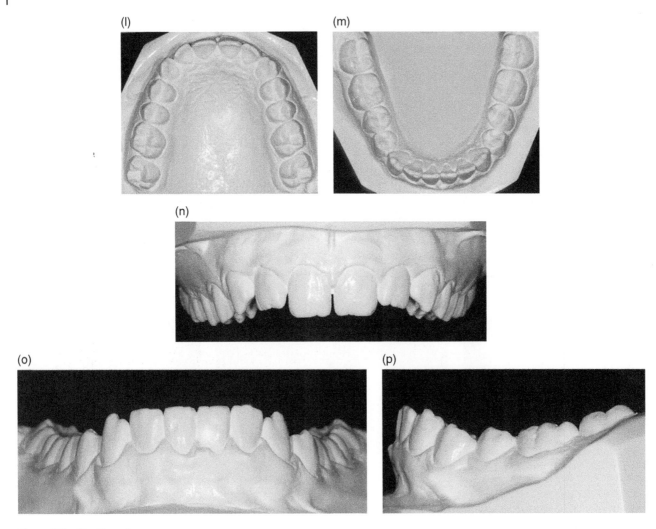

(l) (m)

(n)

(o) (p)

Figure 5.7 (Continued)

Q: What is the etiology of Sydney's *dental* deep bite?

A: Sydney's mandibular anterior teeth have overerupted (Figures 5.7o and 5.7p) resulting in a dental deep bite and deep curve of Spee. Her maxillary incisal edges are level with her maxillary posterior occlusal plane (Figure 5.7n) and have not contributed to her deep bite. In fact, her maxillary lateral incisors and canines are stepped *up* relative to the maxillary posterior occlusal plane.

Q: Contrast vertical facial growth of *dental* deep bite patients with vertical facial growth of *skeletal* deep bite patients. What is the etiology of skeletal deep bites?

A: Vertical growth of the lower anterior face depends upon several variables:
- Magnitude and direction of condylar growth
- Magnitude of maxillary corpus descent
- Maxillary and mandibular bony surface remodeling
- Maxillary molar eruption
- Mandibular molar eruption [3–10]

Contrasted to an individual with a dental deep bite (normal vertical facial growth, Figure 5.8a), an individual with a developing skeletal deep bite (Sydney, Figure 5.8b) generally exhibits *more vertical condylar growth, more forward rotation of the mandible (internal rotation), and a combination of maxillary descent and maxillary and mandibular molar eruption associated with the development of relatively greater posterior face height and relatively less anterior face height*. As the mandible rotates upward and forward in a skeletal deep bite patient, a deep bite results from the increased vertical overlap of maxillary and mandibular incisors.

(a)

(b)

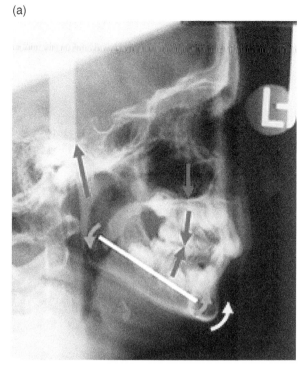
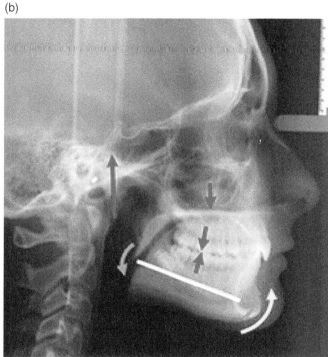

Figure 5.8   The growth pattern of a patient with a dental deep bite (a, normal vertical facial growth pattern) contrasts with the growth pattern of a patient with a skeletal deep bite (b) in terms of magnitude and direction of condylar growth, maxillary and mandibular bony surface remodeling (mandibular internal/true rotation), vertical descent of the maxillary corpus, and maxillary/mandibular molar eruption. In severe skeletal deep bite cases, there is marked forward mandibular rotation affecting the ratio of posterior face height (increased) to anterior face height (decreased). Vertical molar eruption (shown here as relatively decreased) may also be within the range of normal, compensating for the increase in posterior face height.

Q: If the etiology of *dental* deep bites is overeruption of anterior teeth, then how would you recommend treating them?

A: Treat dental deep bites by reversing their etiology – *intruding* maxillary and mandibular overerupted incisors (Figure 5.9a). Also, if incisors are upright, then the deep overbite can be reduced by *proclining* incisors (Figure 5.9b, left) which rotates them forward around their apices to open the bite (Figure 5.9b, right).

Finally, deep bites are opened by *erupting posterior teeth* (e.g. leveling the curve of Spee, Figure 5.9c). That is, using fixed orthodontic appliances, increasingly larger archwires are placed to erupt mandibular premolars, erupt permanent first molars, and upright mandibular second molars – tipping them distally which erupts them. The result is that the mandible is rotated down and back around the condyle which opens the bite (curved yellow arrow).

We would like to share a few thoughts about the maxillary incisal display, facial esthetics, and intruding (or extruding) maxillary incisors. At rest, maxillary incisal display varies with age and gender [11], but 3–4 mm is generally considered ideal in adolescents.

Maxillary incisal display decreases with age as philtrum length increases, and men generally have less incisal display than women [12, 13]. If a young girl's maxillary incisors are intruded to the point where there is no incisal display at rest, then she will have an aged/less feminine appearance.

Brynne (Figure 5.9d) exhibits excess maxillary incisal display (about 10 mm) when her teeth are separated, and her lips are relaxed (Figure 5.9e). Her maxillary central incisors are overerupted compared to her maxillary posterior occlusal plane (Figure 5.9f). Therefore, intrusion of Brynne's maxillary central incisors would be appropriate both to decrease her OB and decrease her maxillary incisal display at rest to 3–4 mm.

Jerin (Figure 5.9g) also exhibits excess maxillary incisal display at rest. However, Jerin's maxillary central incisors are *stepped up* relative to his maxillary posterior occlusal plane (Figure 5.9h). Leveling his maxillary arch will erupt his maxillary central incisors and increase (worsen) Jerin's incisal display. Therefore, we may wish to leave a compensating curve in Jerin's maxillary archwire during leveling/aligning so that his maxillary incisors do not erupt.

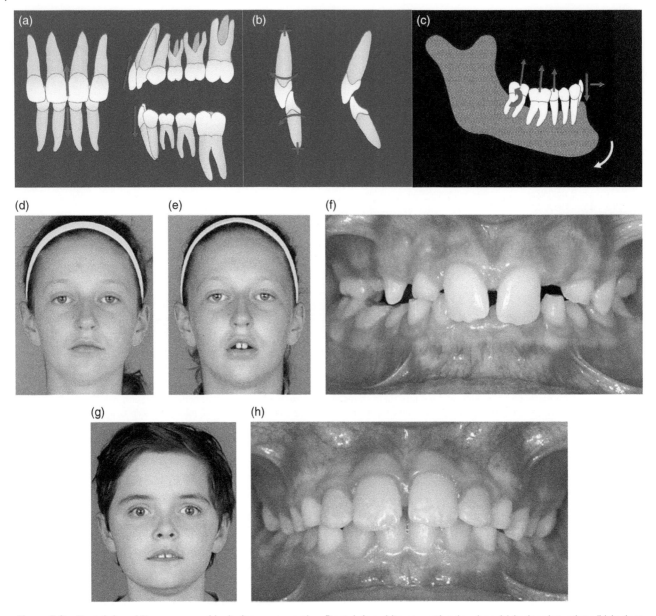

Figure 5.9 Dental deep bites are caused by incisor overeruption. Dental deep bite correction involves (a) incisor intrusion; (b) incisor proclination of upright incisors using their apices as the center of incisor rotation in the sagittal plane; or (c) eruption of posterior teeth which promotes downward and backward rotation of the mandible. In a child who presents with excessive maxillary incisor display at rest (d and e), intrusion of overerupted maxillary incisors (f) by leveling the arch may be beneficial both to reduce OB and to provide a more ideal incisal display. In a child who presents with excessive maxillary incisor display but has stepped-up maxillary incisors (g and h), care must be taken not to erupt maxillary incisors during arch leveling because this would increase (worsen) maxillary incisor display.

Our point is this – *you must consider maxillary incisal display, and future maxillary incisal display following lip growth, when deciding whether to intrude (or extrude) maxillary incisors during arch leveling/aligning.*

Q: The etiology of *skeletal* deep bites is upward and forward mandibular rotation resulting in increased vertical overlap of mandibular incisors by maxillary incisors. Skeletal deep bites often exhibit deficient vertical facial growth. How would you recommend treating skeletal deep bites?

A: There are three general ways to treat any skeletal discrepancy (anteroposterior, vertical, or transverse): orthopedics, masking (camouflage), and surgery.
  - *Orthopedics* (Figure 5.10) – enhancing downward maxillary corpus growth, increasing maxillary

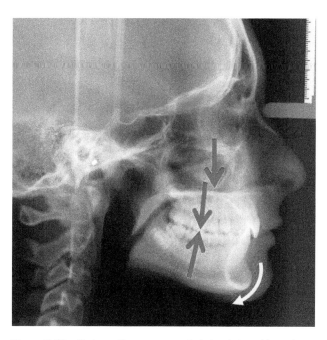

Figure 5.10 Orthopedic treatment of skeletal deep bites aims to increase maxillary corpus descent and/or molar eruption which results in downward/backward mandibular rotation (yellow arrow), bite opening, and increased LAFH.

molar eruption, and increasing mandibular molar eruption – lengthens the lower anterior face height, increases the MPA, opens the deep bite, eliminates lip redundancy, and reduces an overclosed facial appearance. The mandible rotates down and back (Figure 5.10, curved yellow line) – worsening a Class II molar relationship but improving a Class III molar relationship.

Specific appliances/techniques to achieve these movements include:

1) Cervical-pull headgears (CPHGs) during Class II correction. CPHGs rotate the anterior palatal plane downward/backward [14, 15] and erupt maxillary first permanent molars slightly (less than 1 mm on average) potentially increasing lower anterior face height and gingival display. The question of whether cervical traction causes a clinically significant change in vertical facial proportions remains equivocal [16].

2) Headgears with bite plates. Studies have reported headgear/bite plate treatment effects to range from a slight increase in MPA (1.3°) [17] to non-significant changes in the MPA and LAFH [18]. We consider these findings equivocal.

3) Straight-pull headgears (SPHGs). One study reported a slight increase in SN-MP angle (1°) [19]. We consider this finding equivocal.

4) Activators/bionators during Class II correction. The reported effects range from a slight vertical increase when measured at Menton [20] to non-significant changes in the MPA and LAFH [17, 18]. We consider these vertical effects equivocal.

5) The Frankel regulator (FR-II). One study reported a slight decrease in the SN-MP angle (decrease of 0.6°) [19]. We consider this result equivocal.

6) Herbst appliances, unfortunately, increase face height in *hyperdivergent* patients but not in hypodivergent patients [21].

7) Leveling the curve of Spee. Traditionally, leveling the curve of Spee was reported to occur primarily through eruption and uprighting of posterior teeth [22]. Mandibular premolars erupt because a flat archwire must be deflected down to engage premolar brackets in the presence of a curve of Spee. Mandibular molars tip distally/erupt because they are initially tipped mesially in the presence of a curve of Spee. Posterior tooth eruption during curve of Spee leveling rotates the mandible down and back – increasing vertical face height. In addition, mandibular incisors are intruded and proclined which opens the bite. Why do we consider curve of Spee leveling to be orthopedics? Because vertical alveolar process bone is grown during tooth eruption.

   A recent study considered the effect of MPA on curve of Spee leveling. The authors reported that while curve of Spee leveling occurs through eruption and uprighting of posterior teeth in *high-angle* patients, curve of Spee leveling occurs through buccal tooth movement plus mandibular incisor intrusion in *low-angle* patients [23].

8) Anterior bite plates disclude posterior teeth thereby eliminating occlusal forces. This assists curve of Spee leveling, erupting posterior teeth, and theoretically increasing LAFH.

9) Anterior bite plates used in conjunction with posterior vertical elastics can accelerate posterior tooth eruption (alveolar bone growth), potentially increasing vertical facial dimension.

● *Masking* (camouflage) – correcting the child's deep bite dentally without addressing the underlying vertical skeletal deficiency. *Masking is probably the way most skeletal deep bites are corrected in children and adults.* Specific skeletal deep bite masking techniques include:

1) Intruding maxillary and mandibular incisors with fixed appliances by increasing archwire size during curve of Spee leveling; bonding maxillary and mandibular incisors more incisal than

ideal – so that when archwires are inserted, the incisors are intruded; and placing artistic steps in the archwires to intrude incisors. Anterior teeth can also be intruded using aligners with temporary anchorage devices (TADs) for intrusion anchorage and buttons bonded directly to the clear aligners (elastics are worn from the buttons on the aligner to the TADs).

2) Proclining upright incisors during alignment which rotates the incisors forward about their apices to open the bite.

3) Leveling the curve of Spee by the eruption of mandibular premolars and distal tipping/eruption of mesial-tipped mandibular molars. Eruption of posterior teeth opens the bite and increases LAFH.

4) Masking could include prosthodontics (overlay prosthesis, implants, crowns, or bridges) in order to increase the vertical facial dimension and open the bite – within limits dictated by freeway space.

Masking is generally considered only in adult dentition patients and not during early treatment.

- *Surgery* – unlike orthopedics which attempts to open the bite via vertical facial growth; or masking which opens the bite dentally without addressing the short LAFH; surgery increases the vertical facial dimension by moving the maxilla downward (LeFort I maxillary downgraft osteotomy). Surgery is generally considered only in adult dentition patients.

Q: How can a child's mandibular growth (condylar growth direction, mandibular internal rotation) impact skeletal deep bite treatment?

A: Favorable mandibular growth (posterior-superior condylar growth, less forward rotation of the mandible) can make skeletal deep bite treatment more effective. Unfavorable mandibular growth (vertical condylar growth, more forward rotation of the mandible) can make skeletal deep treatment less effective.

Q: What two factors could persuade you to attempt, or dissuade you from attempting, orthopedic treatment of a skeletal deep bite patient?

A: As with all orthopedic treatment, the *magnitude* of the skeletal discrepancy and the potential *time* for remaining growth must be weighed. If the patient has a mild (borderline) skeletal deep bite and many years of anticipated growth, then you could attempt orthopedic treatment in the hope of correcting the problem. Of course, if the condition is mild, then you could treat successfully with masking in the permanent dentition.

If the patient has a very severe skeletal deep bite with little future anticipated growth, then it would be heroic to attempt orthopedic correction (and successful masking may not be possible). In this latter instance, if the short lower face height is a concern to the patient or parent, then surgery to increase the face height should be considered.

Q: We have touched on some important concepts regarding deep bites. A question remains. *Why* correct deep bites? Can you list five possible reasons?

A: Reasons for correcting (opening) excessively deep bites include:

1) Creating OJ in order to bond brackets on mandibular anterior teeth (Figure 5.11a).

2) Creating OJ to permit maxillary incisor retraction, or mandibular incisor proclination. In the presence of a deep bite (Figure 5.11b, left) the maxillary incisors contact the mandibular brackets during maxillary incisor retraction (maxillary space closure), or mandibular incisor proclination. The bite must be opened (Figure 5.11b, right) in order to create enough overjet to permit either of these tooth movements.

3) Creating space in order to permit restoration of teeth. Opening a deep bite creates OJ for restorative material in severely abraded incisors.

4) Eliminating pain and tissue trauma. In cases of excessively deep bites, mandibular incisors can bite into the palate (Figures 5.12a–5.12c) causing pain and tissue trauma. Likewise, upright maxillary incisors can injure soft tissue labial to mandibular incisors.

5) Eliminating lip trapping. "Trapping" of the mandibular lip is often seen in Class II patients with deep OB (Figure 5.13). The mandibular lip gets caught, or trapped, by the maxillary incisors creating a deep labiomental sulcus. Eliminating the deep bite and excess OJ can resolve lip trapping and open the labiomental sulcus.

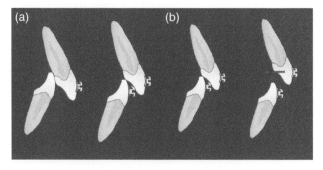

Figure 5.11 Opening a deep bite to create OJ (a) to bond mandibular anterior teeth and (b) to allow retraction of maxillary incisors or proclination of mandibular incisors.

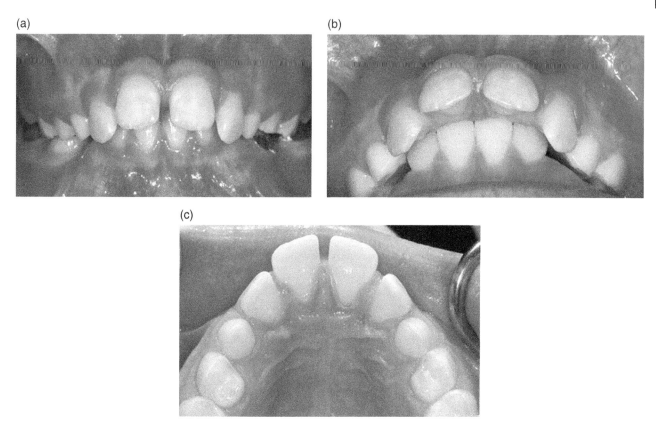

Figure 5.12 Deep bites can result in mandibular incisors biting into the palate. (a) Patient with a 100% OB as defined by palatal incisor impingement; (b) when viewed from below (note soft tissue incisor impingement); (c) indentations left by mandibular central incisors on palatal tissue lingual to maxillary central incisors (note incipient recession of palatal tissue lingual to the maxillary left central incisor).

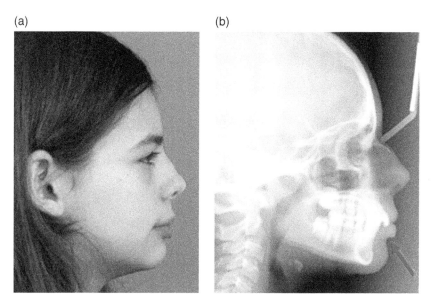

Figure 5.13 (a and b) Lip "trapping" by maxillary incisors with a resulting deep labiomental sulcus.

Q: Of the above reasons, which one clearly justifies *early* deep bite correction?

A: *Elimination of tissue trauma including pain when biting.* The other reasons justify deep bite reduction but can be dealt with later during comprehensive orthodontic treatment.

Q: Based upon the above, should you treat Carson's deep bite now (Figure 5.3, early mixed dentition) or recall? What questions should you ask him and his parents to determine the answer?

A: Ask Carson if he feels any pain from mandibular incisor impingement on his palate (Figure 5.3j). He denies any pain. Since there does not appear to be any tissue damage to the teeth, mandibular labial gingiva, or palatal soft tissue (Figures 5.3k and 5.4a), we feel that there is no need to correct his deep bite early. His deep bite can be addressed later during comprehensive treatment. However, tell Carson to inform his parents if he ever feels pain, and be sure to check for tissue damage during recall visits.

Q: Does *unlocking* the bite in Class II division 2 children by proclining upright maxillary incisors and reducing the deep bite *free the mandible* from the maxillary anterior teeth and thereby enhance mandibular growth?

A: The answer is unknown. We do know that when maxillary incisors are proclined in Class II division 2 patients, and the deep bite is corrected with an upper removable plate, the distance between mandibular retruded contact position and intercuspal position remains unchanged [24]. That is, the mandible does not immediately shift forward.

However, we are unaware of studies that have examined the effect of unlocking the bite on mandibular long-term growth. *Because no harm occurs from proclining upright maxillary incisors and reducing overbite in Class II division 2 children, we generally recommend unlocking the bite during Class II orthopedics in the hope that potential mandibular growth restriction is eliminated.*

Q: Assume that an early mixed dentition patient presents to you with a deep bite resulting from overeruption of mandibular incisors (dental deep bite). You are concerned that soft tissue damage may occur because the mandibular incisors bite into the palate. Can you suggest ways to correct (open) the deep bite?

A: Band or bond the mandibular first permanent molars and overerupted mandibular permanent incisors with fixed orthodontic appliances. Then, place a utility arch to intrude the mandibular incisors and erupt the mandibular first molars. Both effects will open the bite.

A utility arch, or intrusion arch, is a 2×4 appliance ("two-by-four" appliance). Two permanent first molars and four incisors have fixed orthodontic appliances placed with a tip-back bend (V-bend, intrusion bend, and anchor bend) placed in the archwire slightly mesial to the first molar brackets (Figure 5.14a). As the archwire is lifted incisally to engage the incisor brackets (Figure 5.14b), an intrusive force (F1) is placed on the incisors, an extrusive force (F2) is applied against the molars, a distal-tipping moment (M1) is applied against the molars, and the curve of Spee is leveled. The effectiveness of this technique to intrude overerupted incisors is illustrated in Figure 5.14c.

If maxillary incisors are overerupted, then a maxillary utility arch can be used in a similar fashion (Figure 5.14d). Figures 5.14e–5.14j illustrates OB reduction by maxillary incisor intrusion and proclination.

Deep bite reduction by posterior tooth eruption can be effective (anterior bite plate worn to disclude posterior teeth and allow them to erupt). Deep bite reduction by anterior bite plate wear *plus* vertical elastic wear is also an option (Figures 5.14k and 5.14l). However, we recommend this technique during comprehensive treatment in the permanent dentition and not during early treatment.

Q: Once you have opened the bite by intruding mandibular incisors, how can you *retain* them to prevent their re-eruption and contact with the palate?

A: Fabricate and place an LLHA (Figure 5.15) with the anterior portion of the arch laying on the incisor lingual surfaces. Or, after removing edgewise brackets, have the patient wear a clear mandibular vacuum-formed retainer.

Q: Can you think of a simple, but effective, way to prevent mandibular incisor impingement into palatal soft tissue – without braces?

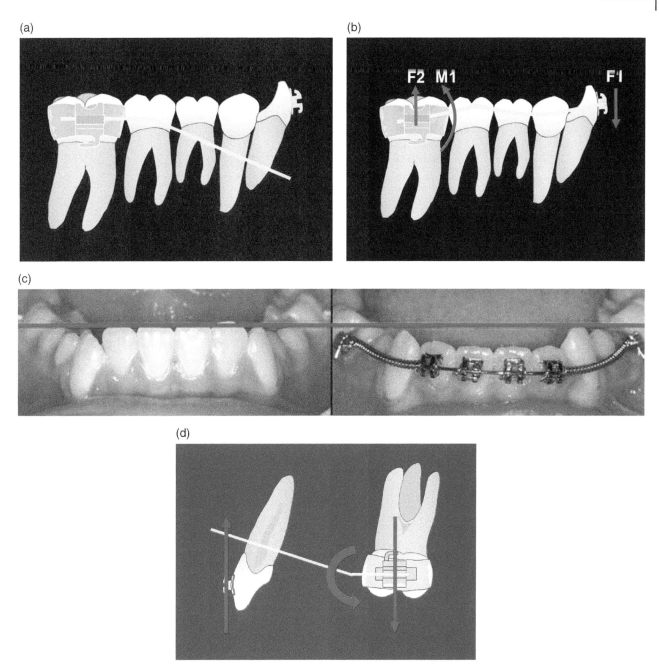

Figure 5.14 Techniques to reduce OB: (a) a "V bend" is placed just mesial to the first molar bracket in a utility arch. When the utility arch is engaged in the incisor brackets (b), an intrusive force is applied to overerupted mandibular incisors, an eruptive force is applied to the permanent first molars, and a distal tipping moment is applied to the molars. These forces and moment open a deep bite. The intrusive effect of a utility archwire on overerupted incisors is evident in (c). Note in this patient that the mandibular *primary* second molars were bonded with brackets instead of the permanent first molars – eliminating any eruptive/distal tipping effects on the permanent first molars; (d) a utility archwire (intrusion archwire) can likewise be designed to intrude overerupted maxillary incisors and erupt maxillary molars – thereby opening the bite; (e–j) reduction of OB via maxillary incisor intrusion (and proclination); vertical elastics (k and l) worn between the arches, in the presence of an anterior bite plate to disclude the posterior teeth, can be effective in erupting posterior teeth in order to open a deep bite. However, we limit our use of this technique to patients in the adult, not mixed, dentition.

(e)

(f)

(g)

(h)

(i)

(j)

(k)

(l)

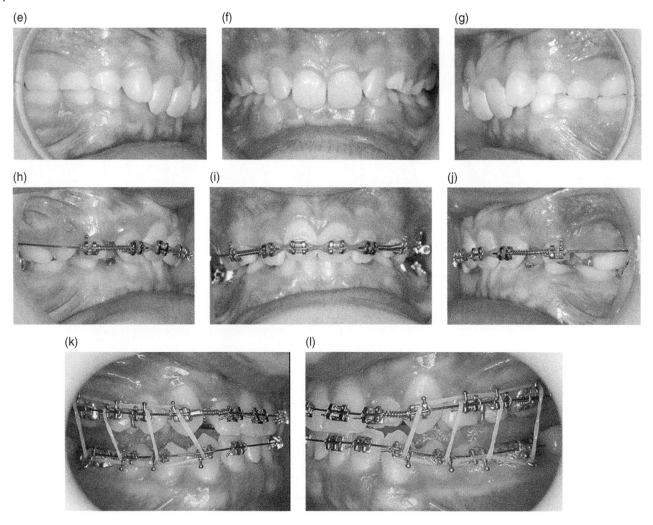

Figure 5.14   (Continued)

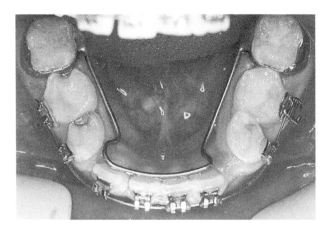

Figure 5.15   Following mandibular incisor intrusion, an LLHA can be placed to prevent the incisors from re-erupting.

A: Have the patient wear a clear, maxillary vacuum-formed retainer (Figure 5.16a) to prevent the mandibular incisal edges from impinging on palatal soft tissues. However, a drawback to full coverage of maxillary posterior teeth is that the retainer prevents differential eruption of posterior teeth. Such posterior teeth eruption normally aids opening the deep bite during growth.

A better design is to cover the *anterior teeth and palate only* with the retainer (Figure 5.16b). This modification permits posterior tooth eruption/OB reduction since the posterior teeth are left uncovered. Such a retainer is illustrated in a patient (Figure 5.16c) whose mandibular incisors were initially biting into her anterior palate. With the retainer in place, she was immediately relieved of pain when biting. After one month of

(a)

(b)

(c)

(d)

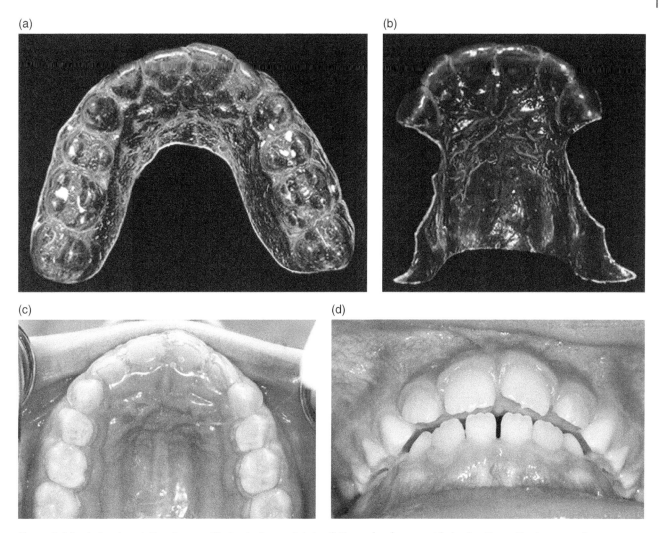

Figure 5.16 A simple solution to mandibular incisor palatal soft tissue impingement is having the patient wear a clear maxillary vacuum-formed retainer (a). However, occlusal coverage of all the teeth will tend to inhibit differential eruption of posterior teeth. A better solution is to *cover only the anterior teeth and palate* with the retainer (b). This modification protects the palatal tissue and permits posterior teeth to erupt, thereby decreasing the OB. (c) Successful use of a retainer covering only the anterior teeth and palate in a patient whose mandibular incisors were initially biting painfully into her anterior palate. The retainer permitted the posterior teeth to erupt slightly – thereby opening the bite and eliminating mandibular incisor palatal impingement (d).

retainer wear (Figure 5.16d), posterior teeth had erupted to the point where anterior teeth were no longer impinging on the palate, and she reported no pain when biting without the retainer. We have asked her to wear the retainer, full time, for three months and then nights only.

Q: Adam is a ten-year-old male (Figures 5.17a–5.17r) who presents to you for "correction of my bite." His PMH, PDH, and TMJ evaluation are WRN. His periodontal evaluation is WRN and CR=CO. List diagnostic findings and problems. What is your diagnosis?

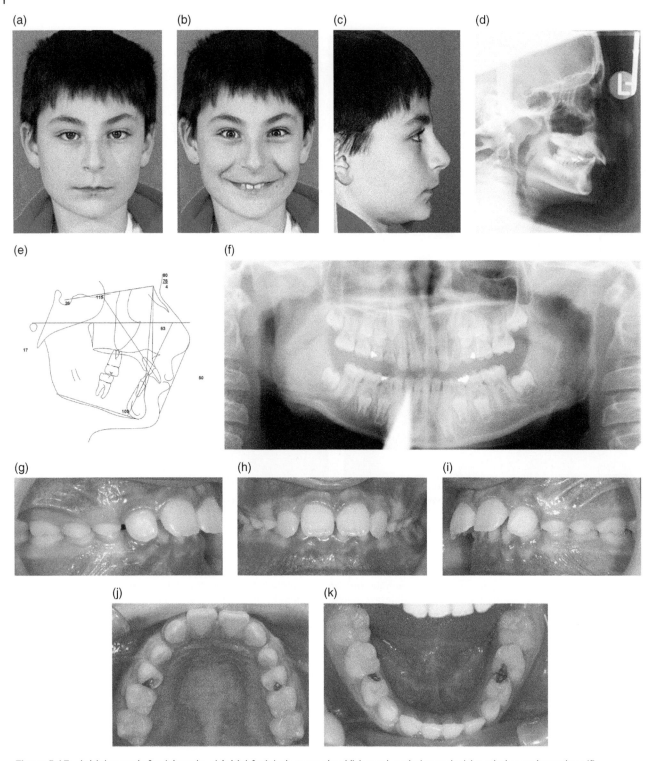

Figure 5.17 Initial records for Adam: (a–c) initial facial photographs; (d) lateral cephalograph; (e) cephalometric tracing; (f) pantomograph; (g–k) intraoral photographs; (l–p) models; (q) articulated models tipped up; (r) frontal view of separated models.

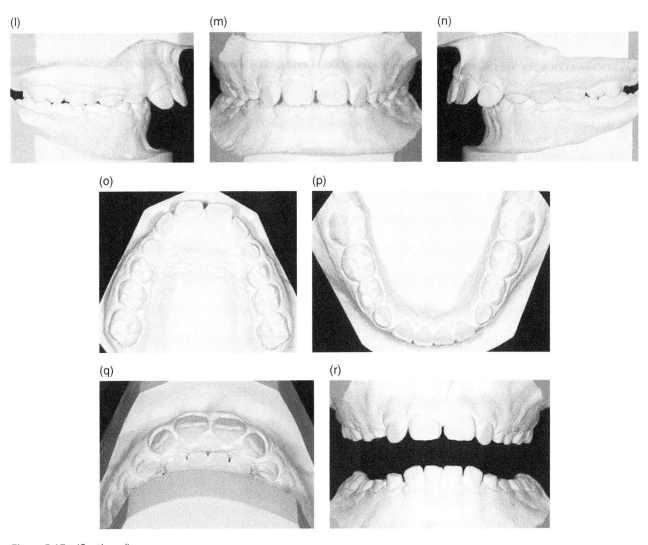

Figure 5.17 (Continued)

A:

Table 5.2 Diagnostic findings and problem list for Adam.

Full face and Profile	**Frontal View**
	Face is symmetric
	Short soft tissue LAFH (Subnasale – soft tissue Menton shorter than soft tissue Glabella – Subnasale)
	Lip competence
	Thin maxillary and mandibular lip
	UDML WRN
	Inadequate incisal display in a posed smile (maxillary central incisor gingival margins are positioned above border of maxillary lip)
	Profile View
	Convex profile
	Obtuse NLA
	Retrusive chin
	Deep labiomental sulcus

(Continued)

Table 5.2 (Continued)

Ceph Analysis	**Skeletal**
	Maxillary anteroposterior position WRN
	Mild mandibular skeletal deficiency (ANB = 4° with normal maxilla)
	Vertical skeletal deficiency (LAFH/TAFH × 100% = 50%; ideal = 55%)
	Flat mandibular plane angles (FMA = 17° and SNMP = 26°)
	Relatively parallel SN, FH, and MP lines
	Mandibular lip trapping
	Prominent soft tissue Pogonion
	Dental
	Proclined maxillary incisors (U1 to SN = 115°)
	Mildly proclined mandibular incisors (FMIA = 63°)
Radiographs	Early mixed dentition stage
	Enlarged adenoids (Figure 5.17d)
Intraoral Photos and Models	Angle Class II division 1
	Iowa Classification: II(6 mm) II(6 mm) II(6 mm) II(6 mm) (Note: Models illustrate the actual relationship, Adam postured his mandible forward in intraoral photographs)
	OJ: 10 mm (Figure 5.17q)
	OB: 100% (palatal impingement but Adam does not exhibit pain when his incisors impinge on his palate, and no damage to his palate is observed)
	3 mm COS (Figure 5.17r)
	Mandibular incisors stepped up relative to mandibular primary canines and posterior teeth
	Mild maxillary and mandibular anterior spacing
	Midlines are approximately coincident
Other	—
Diagnosis	Angle Class II division 1 malocclusion with 100% deep bite

Q: How should you manage Adam's enlarged adenoids?

A: You should discuss breathing history with every patient regardless of whether their adenoids are enlarged or not. *When in doubt, refer them out* – to the appropriate specialist when a breathing problem is identified or suspected. Under the direction of the physician, you may be asked to provide orthodontic procedures such as the maxillary expansion after a tonsillectomy and adenoidectomy. Adam and his parents deny any breathing problems.

Q: Is Adam's 100% OB (palatal impingement) a *dental* deep bite, a *skeletal* deep bite, or a combination of both?

A: Adam displays both dental deep bite and skeletal deep bite features. His *dental deep bite features* include:

- Mandibular incisors stepped up (overerupted, Figure 5.17r) relative to mandibular primary canines and mandibular posterior teeth (deep curve of Spee). His *skeletal deep bite features* include:
- Short soft tissue LAFH
- Short skeletal LAFH (LAFH/TAFH × 100% = 50%)
- Flat mandibular plane angles
- Mandibular plane relatively parallel to FH and SN.

Adam is a combination of dental and skeletal deep bites.

Q: What are Adam's primary problems in each dimension (plus other)?

A:

Table 5.3 Primary problems list for Adam.

AP	Angle Class II division 1
	Iowa Classification: II(6 mm) II(6 mm) II(6 mm) II(6 mm)
	Mandibular skeletal deficiency
Vertical	100% OB
	Skeletal and dental deep bite
Transverse	—
Other	—

Q: Considering Adam's primary problems, age, dental development and other features, should you begin early treatment now or should you wait? If you begin now, what early treatment would you recommend? If you wait, what treatment do you recommend when you begin?

A: We spoke to Adam's mother. Because Adam was in the early mixed dentition, he did not exhibit good statural growth velocity, and exhibited neither palatal soft tissue damage nor pain from his mandibular incisor impingement, we recommended waiting/monitoring until he either entered his late mixed dentition or showed good statural growth velocity.

When Adam entered his late mixed dentition stage of development, we placed him on a high-pull headgear (HPHG) to restrict his maxillary forward growth and distalize his maxillary permanent first molars – while his mandible grew forward. He also wore an anterior bite plate to disclude his posterior teeth. The anterior bite plate can be viewed as skeletal deep bite orthopedic treatment because the posterior teeth are encouraged to erupt – growing alveolar process bone vertically.

Note: By encouraging molar eruption with the anterior bite plate, we attempted to increase Adam's LAFH by rotating his mandible down and back. This rotation has an impact on the vertical and anteroposterior position of B-point and the mandibular first molars [25]. In skeletal deep bite patients (low FMA, hypodivergent), the effect is more vertical than anteroposterior

(i.e. B-point and the mandibular first molars move more downward than backward with a greater increase on LAFH and less worsening of Class II relationship). In contrast, backward mandibular rotation in skeletal open bite patients (high FMA, hyperdivergent) results in more backward than a downward movement of B-point and mandibular first molars and thus a greater worsening of Class II relationships. Given Adam's low FMA, we reasoned the effect of backward mandibular rotation on worsening his Class II relationship would be minimal, and likely would be overcome by differential forward growth of his mandible.

Adam was very compliant. He wore the bite plate full time and the headgear every night from about eight o'clock until the next morning – until his molars were corrected to Class I. The new Class I molar position was held with a light headgear force during sleep until all permanent teeth erupted (including his second molars). Early treatment ended at that time. Comprehensive treatment was begun, fixed appliances were placed, arches were leveled and aligned, finishing was successfully completed, and Adam was debanded (Figure 5.18).

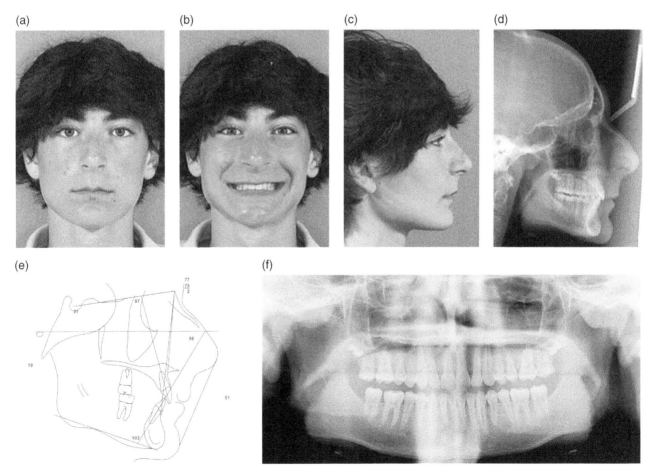

Figure 5.18 (a–k) Adam's deband records.

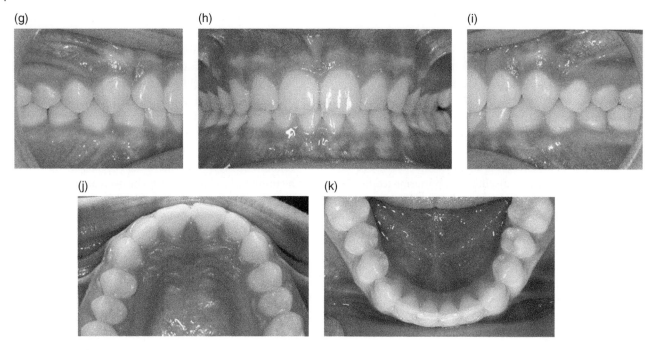

(g) (h) (i)

(j) (k)

Figure 5.18 (Continued)

Q: Adam presented with a combination of skeletal and dental deep bite but did *not* have tissue damage as a result of mandibular incisor impingement on his palate. But what if a mixed dentition patient presents to you with a combination of skeletal deep bite, dental deep bite, and *tissue damage* from mandibular incisor impingement? What treatment, if any, would you recommend?

A: Except for severe skeletal deep bites where the patient/parents express concerns with LAFH deficiency esthetics, skeletal deep bites are generally treated the same way as dental deep bites – *incisor intrusion; incisor proclination; and eruption of posterior teeth during curve of Spee leveling.* For skeletal deep bites, this is masking. It is treating the condition dentally and not addressing the underlying skeletal condition. Therefore, if a mixed dentition patient presents with a combination dental deep bite, *mild* skeletal deep bite, and palatal tissue pain/damage, we recommend that you treat him/her the same as a dental deep bite – by opening the deep bite to prevent incisor palatal impingement or by covering the anterior palatal with a vacuum-formed bite plate.

On the other hand, if a patient presents with a combination of dental deep bite and *severe* skeletal deep bite, then you should consider treating the dental deep bite early (to stop ongoing tissue damage and prevent future tissue damage). You should then consider treating the skeletal deep bite later, after growth completion, with orthognathic surgery (maxillary LeFort I downgraft). For example, the patient in Figure 5.19 presented with a severe skeletal deep bite (a very short LAFH), which was esthetically concerning. Definitive treatment was provided with maxillary downgraft surgery after growth cessation. Figures 5.19e–5.19g also illustrates this surgical procedure.

Q: Let's move to the other end of the vertical spectrum – anterior open bites. Elijah is a nine-year-old boy (Figure 5.20) who is in his permanent dentition. He presents to you with his parents' chief complaint, "Elijah has an open bite, and his teeth have come forward." PMH, PDH, and TMJs are WRN. CR=CO. The periodontal tissue covering his mandibular anterior teeth has a thin biotype. Can you list Elijah's *primary* problems in each dimension (plus other primary problems)?

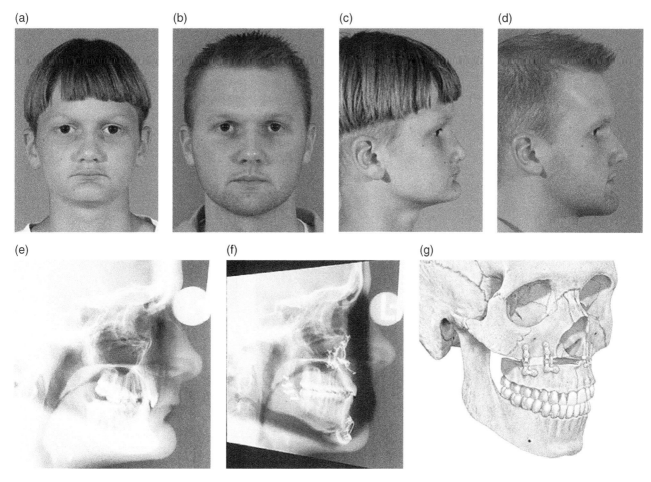

Figure 5.19 Downgraft osteotomy surgery to treat severe skeletal deep bites: ectodermal dysplasia patient presenting (a, c – initial photos) with a skeletal deep bite and dissatisfaction with short LAFH. Treatment included a maxillary LeFort I downgraft after growth cessation (b, d – final photos); (e and f) changes in a patient presenting with a skeletal deep bite and treated with maxillary downgraft osteotomy, mandibular advancement, and genioplasty downgraft; (g) drawing illustrating a maxillary downgraft osteotomy with osseous graft rigidly fixated between the bony segments.

A:

Table 5.4 Primary problem list for Elijah.

AP	Angle Class I
	Iowa Classification: I II(3 mm) II(3 mm) I
Vertical	LAFH WRN (soft tissue and skeletal tissue)
	Anterior open bite
Transverse	"Tight" posterior transverse relationship/ minimal posterior OJ
Other	Bimaxillary dental protrusion (U1 to SN angle = 112°; FMIA = 57°)
	~1 mm mandibular anterior crowding
	~2 mm maxillary anterior spacing

Q: What is the cause of Elijah's anterior open bite? What questions should you ask Elijah and his parents about his open bite?

A: His open bite is due to *inadequate maxillary incisor eruption.* Compare Elijah's maxillary incisor vertical positions to his maxillary posterior occlusal plane (Figure 5.21a). Note that his maxillary incisors are "stepped up." Inadequate eruption of his maxillary incisors is the cause of his open bite and exaggerated compensating curve (Figure 5.21b). His mandibular incisors are overerupted relative to his mandibular posterior teeth (Figure 5.22a) resulting in a deep curve of Spee (Figure 5.22b).

You should ask Elijah if he has any habits that prevent his maxillary teeth from erupting. Elijah says that, occasionally, he sucks on two digits.

Q: Is Elijah's anterior open bite a *dental* open bite, a *skeletal* open bite, or a combination of both? Why?

A: Elijah has a dental (functional) open bite. Why? His open bite resulted exclusively from the inadequate eruption of his maxillary incisors, and he is vertically normal. That is, his:

- Soft tissue LAFH is WRN (approximately the same height as his midface, Figure 5.23)

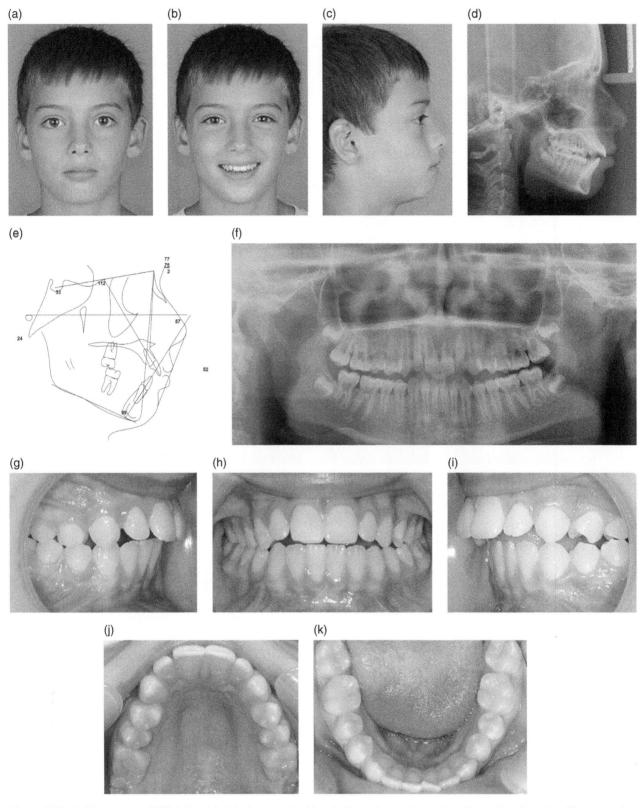

Figure 5.20 Initial records of Elijah. (a–c) facial photographs; (d and e) lateral cephalometric radiograph and tracing; (f) panoramic image; (g–k) intraoral images; (l–p) model images.

(l)   (m)   (n)

(o)   (p)

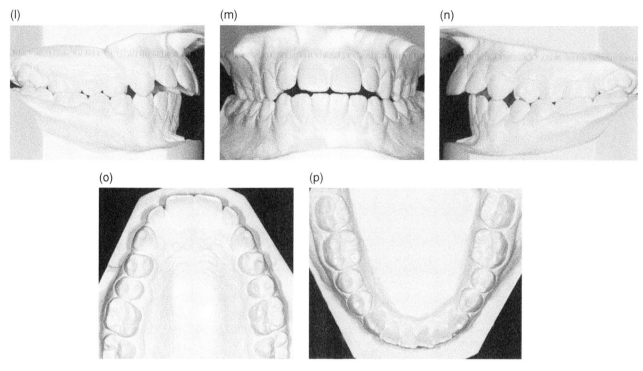

Figure 5.20   (Continued)

(a)   (b)

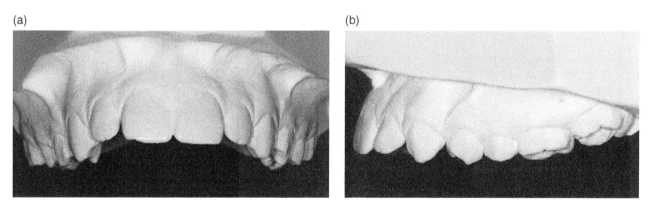

Figure 5.21   Inadequate maxillary incisor eruption (a) has resulted in Elijah's anterior open bite and exaggerated compensating curve (b).

(a)   (b)

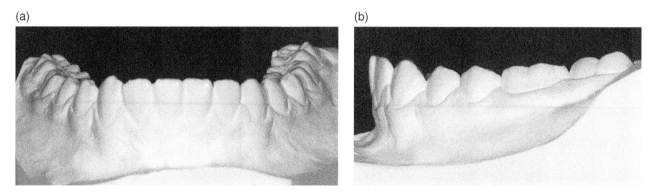

Figure 5.22   Excessive mandibular incisor eruption (a) has resulted in an exaggerated curve of Spee (b).

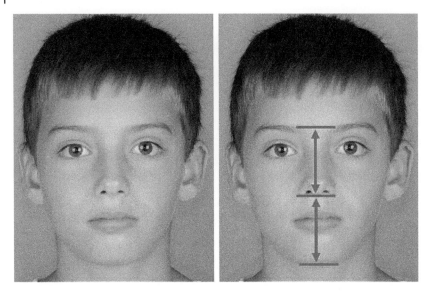

Figure 5.23 Elijah's soft tissue LAFH is approximately equal to his soft tissue midfacial height.

- Lips are competent
- Skeletal LAFH is mildly short (LAFH/TAFH × 100% = 52%, Figure 5.21e).

Q: Can you describe features of a *skeletal* open bite?

A: Let's use Jessa as an example (Figure 5.24) as she demonstrates many of the features of a skeletal open bite. Jessa exhibits:

- Soft tissue LAFH longer than midface height (Figure 5.24a)
- Relaxed interlabial gap (ILG) of 4–5 mm (as opposed to lip competence or an ILG ≤ 2 mm [26] which is considered normal). Note her mentalis strain to achieve lip competence (Figure 5.24b) even though she has a normal maxillary lip length

- Skeletal LAFH of 57% which is WRN but slightly long (Figure 5.24d, versus a normal LAFH/TAFH × 100% = 55%, standard deviation = 2%) [2]
- Steep MPA (FMA = 33°; SNMP = 46°)
- Short posterior ramus height
- Palatal plane tipped down in posterior (Figure 5.24c)
- Maxillary first permanent molar root apices erupted away from (down from) palatal plane.

Jessa also exhibits a *dental* open bite (Figures 5.24f, 5.24k, and 5.24o) due to inadequate maxillary incisor eruption. Therefore, Jessa exhibits a *combination* of skeletal and dental open bite.

(a)

(b)

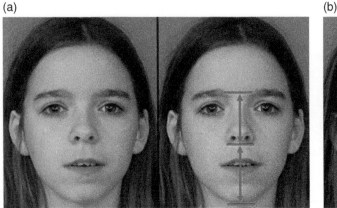
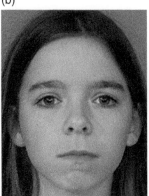

Figure 5.24 (a–r) Jessa, a child presenting with a combination dental open bite *and skeletal* open bite.

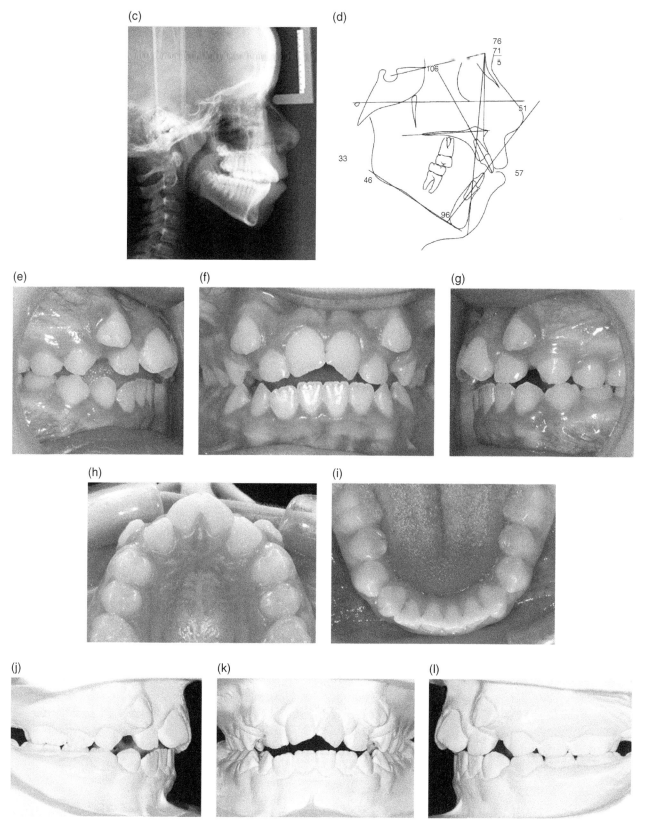

Figure 5.24 (Continued)

(m)

(n)

(o)

(p)

(q)

(r)

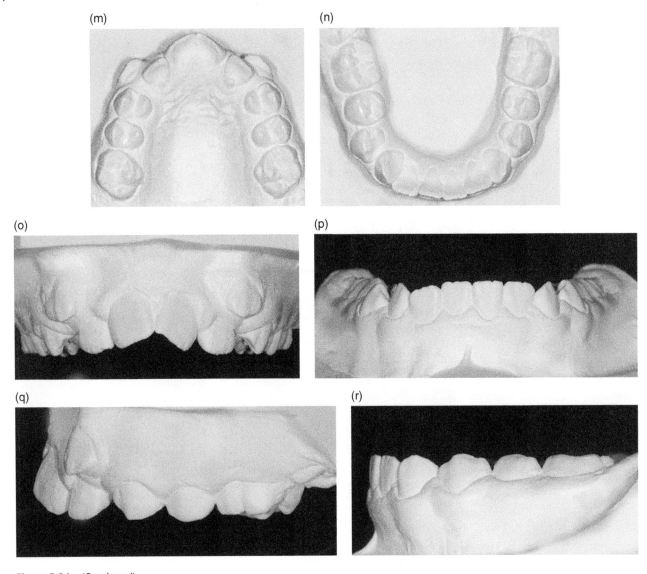

Figure 5.24 (Continued)

Q: Contrast the vertical facial growth found in dental open bite patients with the vertical facial growth found in *skeletal* open bite patients.

A: Vertical growth of the lower anterior face depends upon the following: magnitude and direction of condylar growth, maxillary and mandibular bony surface apposition and resorption, vertical descent of the maxillary corpus, maxillary molar eruption, and mandibular molar eruption [3–10, 27]. In contrast with an individual exhibiting a dental open bite (*normal* vertical facial growth, Figure 5.25a), a patient with a skeletal open bite exhibits:

- Posterior-superior condylar growth (Figure 5.25b, curved red arrow) as opposed to more vertical condylar growth

- A shorter posterior ramus height
- A more obtuse gonial angle
- A retrognathic mandible
- Less forward mandibular internal rotation or even backward internal rotation (curved blue arrows)
- A maxilla which may descend more than normal (palatal plane may rotate down posteriorly)
- Molars which often erupt more than normal (red arrows, maxillary molars most commonly)
- As the mandible rotates backward (yellow arrow), the MPA steepens, the anterior face height increases, and an anterior open bite may result – depending upon the influence of the tongue in preventing anterior tooth compensatory dental eruption.

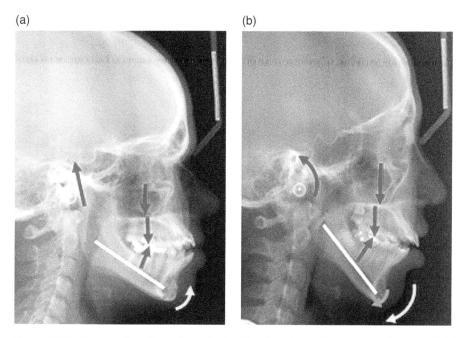

Figure 5.25 The growth pattern of a patient with a dental open bite (a, normal vertical facial growth) contrasts with that of a patient with a skeletal open bite (b) in terms of magnitude and direction of condylar growth, ramus height, maxillary and mandibular bony surface apposition/resorption (mandibular internal rotation, blue arrows), vertical descent of the maxillary corpus, and molar eruption.

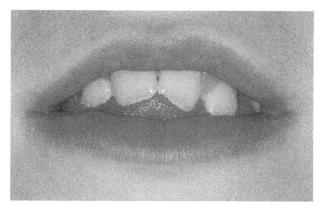

Figure 5.26 A close-up photo of Jessa while she was relaxed and distracted.

Q: We noted that Jessa (Figures 5.24a–5.24r) exhibits a combination of skeletal and dental open bite. Look at Figure 5.26, which was made while Jessa relaxed. Can you identify the probable etiology of Jessa's *dental* (functional) open bite?

A: Jessa's habit of posturing her tongue between her anterior teeth has reduced maxillary incisor eruption and caused her dental open bite.

Q: Jessa's ILG permitted easy visualization of her tongue-interposition habit. But how can you check for a tongue-interposition habit when the patient has lip competence?

A: Ask the patient to close their eyes. Talk to their parents or your staff for a minute. Then, ask the patient to open their eyes. As they open their eyes (they will be distracted), gently and quickly retract their lips. If they have a tongue-interposition habit, you should be able to see it.

Q: Why should we conclude that Jessa's dental open bite is due to a tongue-interposition habit (resting tongue habit) and not due to a tongue-*thrusting* habit when she swallows?

A: Remember this saying – *tongue thrust NO, tongue posture YES*. The fact is the cumulative time of daily tongue thrusting when swallowing is far too short and too intermittent to inhibit incisor eruption. Tongue *thrust* is merely an adaptation to seal an anterior open bite during swallowing. On the other hand, continuous tongue pressure exerted by an interposition resting habit is enough to prevent incisor eruption [28–30]. *Tongue thrust NO, tongue posture YES.*

Q: Jessa's open bite extended distally, but only to her first premolars (Figures 5.24f and 5.24k). Would you consider this unusual for a skeletal open bite?

A: Yes. Generally, *dental* anterior open bites (Figure 5.27a) extend no further distally than the primary first molars or first premolars. Why? Because dental open bites are caused by habits, and habits

(a)

(b)

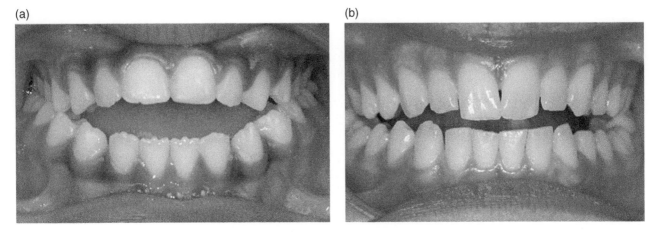

Figure 5.27 (a) Anterior *dental* open bites usually extend no further distally than the primary first molars or first premolars while (b) anterior *skeletal* open bites can extend to the first permanent molars or even second permanent molars.

(digit-sucking, tongue-interposition, and lip-biting) usually extend no further than the primary first molars or first premolars.

On the other hand, *skeletal* anterior open bites (Figure 5.27b) can extend distally to the permanent first molars of even permanent second molars. Why? Because skeletal open bites result from excess vertical growth and excess molar eruption which rotates the mandible down and back until only the molars contact during closure.

Q: In addition to tongue-interposition habits, can you suggest other common causes of anterior dental open bites?

A: Non-habit causes include the transition from primary to permanent dentition, ankylosis of teeth, and presence of blocked out/impacted teeth. Habit causes include resting tongue habits, thumb-sucking habits (Figure 5.28a), digit-sucking habits such as the habit Elijah is demonstrating (Figure 5.8b), and lip-biting habits (Figure 5.28c). Such habits impede tooth eruption and cause open bites.

(a)

(b)

(c)

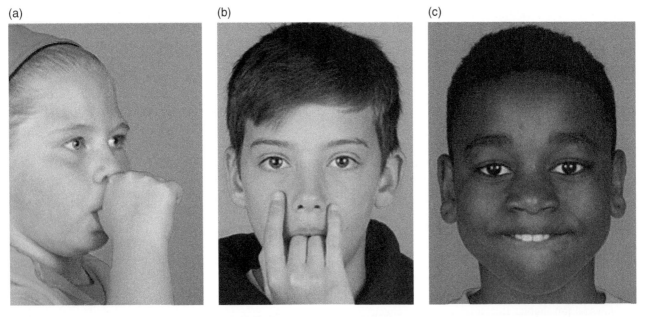

Figure 5.28 (a) thumb-sucking habits; (b) digit-sucking habits such as Elijah is demonstrating (see Figure 5.20); and (c) lip-biting habits can all cause dental (functional) anterior open bites.

(a)

(b)

(c)

(d)

(e)

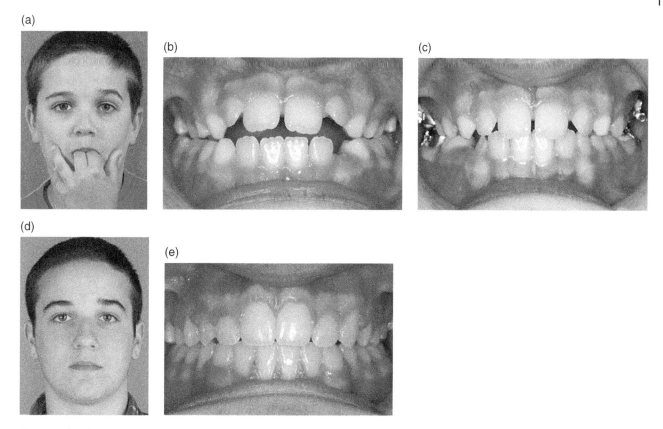

Figure 5.29 Closure of an anterior dental open bite which resulted from a digit-sucking habit. When the child presented with the habit and open bite (a and b), he was encouraged to end the habit. He stopped it, and the open bite closed spontaneously (c). Closure of his open bite was stable ten years later (d and e) because he ended the habit.

Q: Considering the etiology of anterior dental open bites, how would you recommend treating them?

A: Anterior dental open bites are treated by reversing their etiology – that is, by *eliminating the habit* so that the anterior teeth can continue erupting into occlusion (Figures 5.29a–5.29e).

First, talk to the patient. Using a mirror, show him/her the open bite and explain that the anterior teeth cannot come together if the habit persists.

If the habit is a thumb-sucking habit, digit-sucking habit, or lip-biting habit, and if the patient is interested in stopping the habit, ask him/her *when* the habit occurs. If it occurs when awake, ask them to try decreasing the habit over time. Tell them that even with occasional relapses, if they keep trying to end the habit, then they will eventually win over the habit. If the habit occurs when asleep, then this psychological approach may not work. However, ask them to try to stop the habit if they wake up to find they are doing it.

On the other hand, if they are not interested in stopping the habit, it may be better to wait until they mature to attempt stopping it. Our point is this, *win the patient over. To be successful, the patient must have a desire to quit.*

Q: Can you suggest non-compliance-based options for dealing with digit-sucking habits?

A: Various *thumb paints*, such as Mavala Stop (Figure 5.30a), can be used. Parents can also try having the child wear a sock over his/her hand when asleep. Various wearable *thumb guard* appliances are commercially available, and *thumb cribs* can be fabricated by a lab (Figures 5.30b and 5.30c). If the child requires maxillary skeletal expansion, then the rapid maxillary expansion (RME) appliance itself can act as a thumb deterrent.

None of these treatments is guaranteed to stop a digit-sucking habit in the face of a noncooperative child. To be successful, the patient must have a desire to quit the habit.

(a)

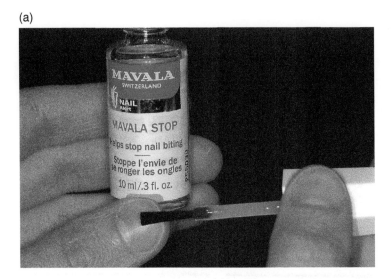

(b)   (c)

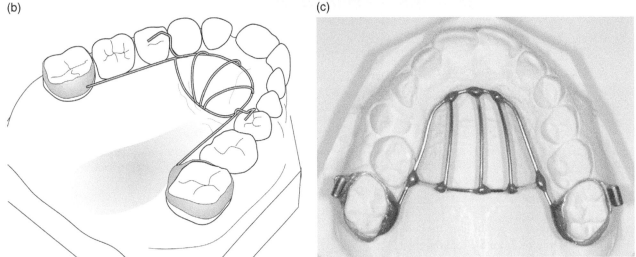

Figure 5.30 Thumb paints (a) and thumb cribs (b and c) can be used to deter digit-sucking habits.

Q: Are there potential problems associated with the use of thumb cribs?

A: We have received concerns from orthodontists that patients with intractable thumb-sucking habits may pull the maxillary posterior teeth forward with a thumb crib or RME. The potential for such an effect should be monitored. One of our colleagues (Dr. Mike Callan) abandoned the use of molar-borne thumb cribs altogether because of this effect. Instead, Mike bonds brackets to the lingual of maxillary incisors as a deterrent to thumb-sucking.

Q: A mixed dentition patient presents to you with an anterior dental open bite due to a tongue interposition (resting tongue) habit. How would you deal with the habit?

A: Start with the same approach you would use with a thumb-sucking/digit-sucking/lip-biting habit. That is, talk to the patient and explain that the habit is preventing the anterior teeth from erupting and coming together. Demonstrate this using a mirror.

If they are interested in stopping the habit, then ask them to avoid resting their tongue on the incisal edges of their anterior teeth. Have them demonstrate. When they swallow, ask them to touch the tip of their tongue to their anterior palate. If they are not interested in stopping the habit, then wait until they are more mature before attempting to stop it.

Q: Suggest at least two additional appliances or techniques that could remind patients to keep their tongues off their anterior teeth.

A: Appliances or techniques include:
- Short blunted spurs soldered to an LLHA (Figure 5.31a)

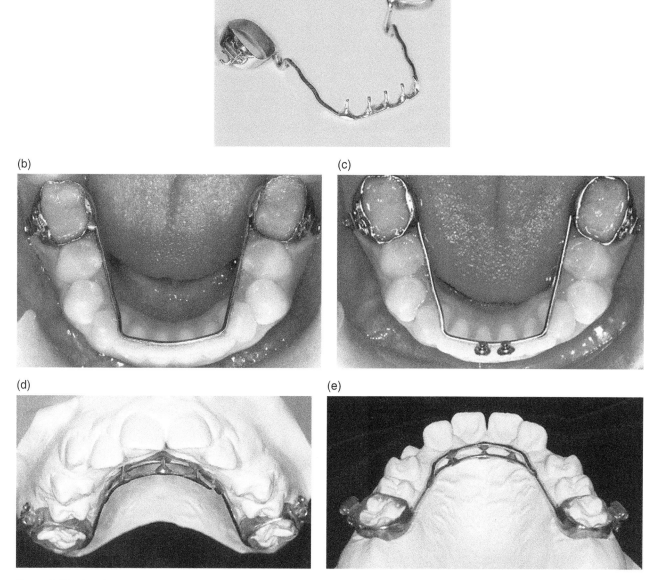

Figure 5.31 Appliances may be used to remind a child to stop anterior tongue-interposition habits (resting tongue habits). These include (a) a lingual arch with soldered anterior blunted reminders or "spurs;" (b–c) bondable buttons attached to the lingual of the mandibular incisors (easily placed even in the presence of an LLHA); and (d–e) a tongue crib designed to block the tongue.

- Blunted spurs embedded in the anterior acrylic of a mandibular Hawley retainer
- Buttons bonded to the lingual of the mandibular incisors (Figures 5.31b and 5.31c)
- Small amounts of composite cement bonded to the lingual of the mandibular incisors
- Maxillary clear (vacuum-formed) retainer with a hole placed in the anterior palate to attract the tongue tip

- Maxillary tongue crib designed to block the tongue (Figures 5.31d and 5.31e)
- Bluegrass palatal appliance
- Occasionally, the anterior resting tongue habit will cease (tongue will be retrained) if the open bite is closed with fixed orthodontic appliances
- Myofunctional therapy (combined with orthodontic treatment) has been reported in one study to be helpful in closing dental open bites [31]. However, this

study suffers from sample selection biases [32]. In our clinical experience, we have found that patients who are willing to perform daily myofunctional exercises are the most compliant. These patients would probably correct their resting tongue habits by themselves once the habit was explained to them.

Q: How would you deal with Elija's digit-sucking habit (Figure 5.28b) – especially since he has a "tight" posterior transverse relationship (minimal posterior OJ, Figures 5.20h and 5.20m). In other words, is there a way to improve his transverse relationship *and* deter his digit-sucking habit? Finally, how would you respond if Elijah's parents ask whether his open bite will close spontaneously?

A: Elijah sucks his fingers, but he says he is ready to quit. We spoke to him about ending the habit, and he agreed to let his parents put thumb paint on his fingers and a sock over his hand when he sleeps. In addition, an RME was placed to expand his maxilla (Figure 5.32) *and* deter his digit-sucking habit. A few weeks later, Elijah and his parents stated that his digit-sucking habit had ended.

With regards to the question of spontaneous open bite closure, tell Elijah's parents there is no guarantee. Worms et al. [33] reported that 80% of simple anterior open bites (open from canine to canine) corrected spontaneously in the mixed dentition. However, this was a cross-sectional study, so the results should be interpreted with caution.

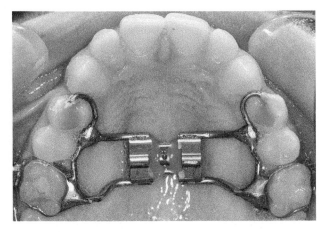

Figure 5.32 To address his anterior dental open bite (due to a digit-sucking habit), Elijah allowed his parents to apply thumb paint to his fingers and to place a sock over his hand when he slept. In addition, an RME was placed to expand his maxilla and deter his digit-sucking habit.

Q: We have discussed habit control – which alone can result in anterior dental open bite closure and without which open bite closure will relapse. However, can you list dental (functional) open bite *treatments*?

A: Dental open bite treatments include:
- *Erupting stepped-up maxillary anterior teeth and erupting stepped-down mandibular anterior teeth* during arch leveling using fixed orthodontic appliances. Vertical elastics (Figures 5.33a–5.33c) may aid in this eruption.

(a)

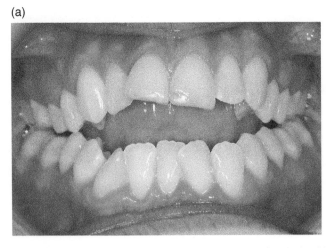

Figure 5.33 (a–c) Open bite closed by erupting anterior teeth with fixed orthodontic appliances and vertical elastics.

(b)

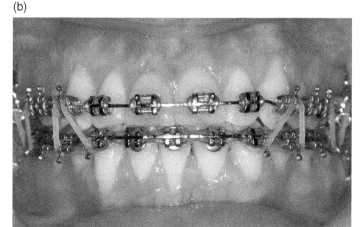

(c)

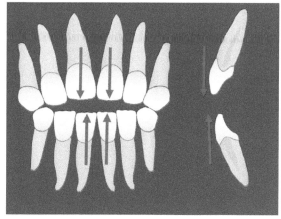

Figure 5.33   (Continued)

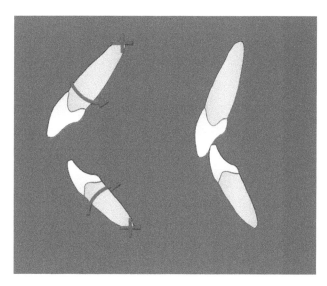

Figure 5.34   Proclined incisors with spacing can be retracted to increase vertical incisor overlap and close the open bite. As they retract, they rotate closed around their apices.

- *Adding curve of Spee to the mandibular archwire* which erupts mandibular incisors.
- *Retracting/uprighting proclined incisors* with spacing (Figure 5.34, left) to rotate them about their apices – thereby "erupting" them (Figure 5.34, right).

Q: When would you recommend *early* dental open bite correction?

A: We recommend early dental open bite correction, through habit control, *when the patient is interested in stopping the habit*. Otherwise, we recommend waiting to correct the open bite until the child matures.

Q: Does correction of childhood anterior open bites have a positive impact on quality of life?

A: Yes. Correction of anterior open bites has a positive impact on oral health-related quality of life and failure to correct it has a negative impact [34].

Q: Based upon the etiology of *skeletal* open bites (Figure 5.25b), how would you recommend treating them?

A: Skeletal open bites are skeletal discrepancies resulting from *excess* lower anterior face height during growth. There are three general ways to treat all skeletal discrepancies between the jaws (orthopedics, masking or camouflage, and surgery). Let's consider each.

Orthopedics (Figure 5.35a) – *closing the skeletal open bite by reducing molar eruption/intruding molars and reducing descent of the maxillary corpus*. The result is autorotation of the mandible upward and forward, open bite closure, and reduction in LAFH. Note that as the mandible rotates upward and forward – a Class II molar relationship will improve but a Class III molar relationship will worsen.

Two factors must be considered before attempting orthopedic treatment: the *magnitude* of the skeletal open bite and the *time* of growth remaining. In a cooperative child with a mild skeletal open bite and years of anticipated growth, you may be successful in closing the open bite with orthopedics. In a child with a severe skeletal open bite and little anticipated growth, your success is unlikely – *unless you intrude the maxillary and mandibular molars with TAD anchorage.*

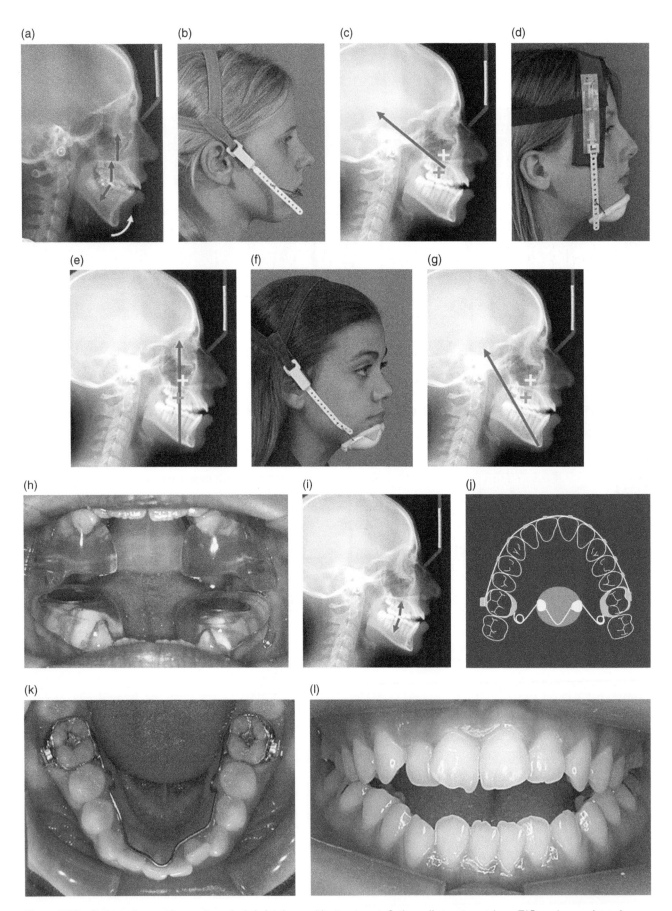

Figure 5.35 Orthopedic, masking, and surgical skeletal open bite treatment. Orthopedic treatment (a–n, TAD anchorage intrusion images graciously provided courtesy of Dr. Young-Chel Park, DDS, PhD) seeks to reduce maxillary corpus descent, intrude molars, or reduce molar eruption (relative intrusion). As a result, the mandible autorotates upward and forward, the LAFH decreases, and the open bite closes (a). Masking, or camouflage, consists of erupting anterior teeth (o, left) to close the open bite (o, right) without reducing the excessively long LAFH. Surgical treatment (p) consists of a LeFort I osteotomy with the removal of a wedge of the maxillary bone. As a result, the maxilla is impacted, and the mandible autorotates upward and forward closing the anterior open bite; (q and r) adult skeletal anterior open bite patient who underwent LeFort I impaction and genioplasty impaction osteotomies.

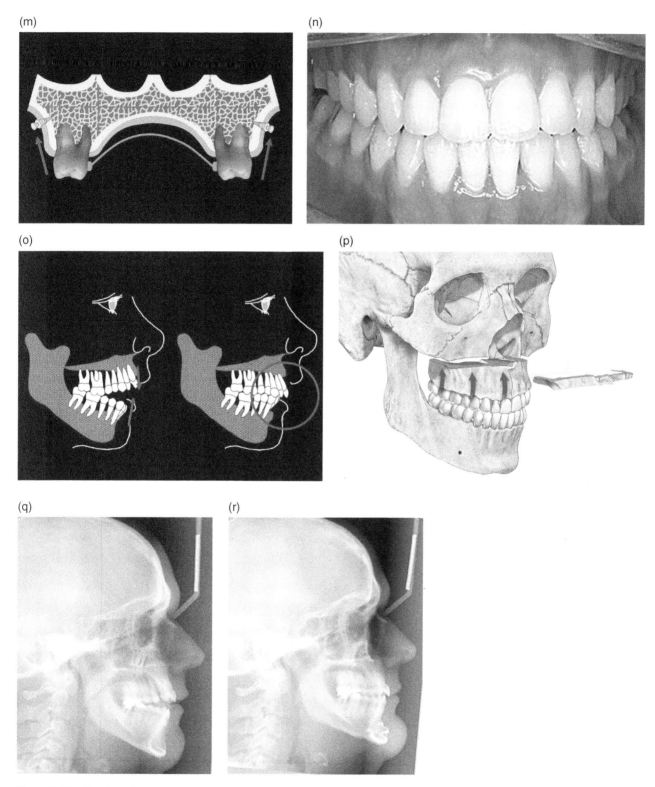

Figure 5.35 (Continued)

Specific orthopedic treatments to reduce molar eruption/intrude molars or reduce maxillary corpus descent include: [25]

- HPHG (Figures 5.35b and 5.35c) to reduce maxillary vertical descent and restrict maxillary molar eruption [14, 35].
- Vertical-pull chin cup (Figures 5.35d and 5.35e) to reduce maxillary vertical descent and reduce molar eruption [36, 37].
- High-pull chin cup (Figures 5.35f and 5.35g) to improve A point – Nasion – B Point angle (ANB) angle in Class III patients without increasing LAFH compared to controls [38, 39].
- Full occlusal coverage posterior bite plates with and without repelling magnets (Figures 5.35h and 5.35i) to stretch the masseteric sling and thereby create an intrusive force against the posterior teeth [40–43].
- Modified Herbst appliance (acrylic splints covering posterior teeth plus HPHG).
- Transpalatal arch with acrylic palatal button (Figure 5.35j) to transmit tongue pressure to the maxillary molars and reduce molar eruption [44].
- Lower lingual holding arch (Figure 5.35k) to reduce mandibular molar eruption by 1–2 mm compared to controls [45]. Reducing molar eruption is *relative molar intrusion* compared to controls.
- TADs used as molar intrusion anchors (Figures 5.35l and 5.35n, images courtesy of Dr. Young-Chel Park, DDS, PhD) [46–52]
- Chewing exercises to reduce the MPA [53, 54]
- Posterior buildups of light-cured orthodontic resin cement bonded on the occlusal surfaces of posterior teeth should provide the same masseteric sling stretch and intrusive force against posterior teeth as full coverage posterior bite plates. However, in a recent study, 2–3 mm-thick resin blocks bonded to palatal cusps of maxillary posterior teeth in seven to eleven-year-old children resulted in relative intrusion of maxillary molars but not counterclockwise (CCW) rotation of the mandible [55].

In our opinion, the skeletal open bite orthopedic treatment with the greatest chance of success and least need for patient cooperation is *TAD-supported maxillary and mandibular molar intrusion*. If attempted, we recommend that you intrude *both* maxillary and mandibular molars. Why? As molars in both arches intrude, the rate of open bite closure will be greater compared to molar intrusion in one arch only. Also, by intruding molars in both arches, you will avoid compensatory molar eruption in the non-intruded arch which occurs if only one arch is intruded.

Masking – closing the skeletal open bite by erupting anterior teeth but not by reducing the excess vertical facial growth (Figure 5.35o). Masking a skeletal open bite is equivalent to closing a dental open bite since eruption of anterior teeth occurs in both. Specific skeletal open bite masking techniques include:

- Anterior tooth eruption using fixed orthodontic appliances while wearing anterior vertical elastics. This treatment is inherently unstable for skeletal open bites greater than a few millimeters.

To increase post-treatment stability: (i) *overcorrect* – achieve an overbite > 20–40%; (ii) hold the correction for many months before debanding to give time for the soft and hard tissues to remodel; and (iii) *gradually* diminish vertical elastic wear and monitor relapse before debanding. In retention, have the patient wear clear, vacuum-formed, full occlusal coverage retainers with small composite blebs placed on the labial surfaces of the anterior teeth. The composite blebs will allow the retainer to "snap on" and hold the anterior teeth vertically. Have the patient wear the occlusal coverage retainers full-time in the hope that some posterior tooth intrusion will occur due to the thickness of the plastic and masseteric sling stretch.

- Bonding maxillary and mandibular incisors more gingivally in order to erupt the incisors more
- Placing archwire bends to increase anterior tooth eruption relative to posterior teeth
- Adding curve of Spee to the mandibular archwire to erupt incisors
- Retracting/uprighting proclined incisors with spacing to erupt incisal edges as they rotate about their apices
- Extracting second molars (if second molars are the only teeth in occlusion). The mandible will autorotate upward and forward closing the open bite until the first molars contact.
- Performing occlusal adjustment on posterior teeth. Since molars are about one-half the distance from the condyles to the incisors, removing 1 mm of enamel from molar occlusal contacts in both arches (2 mm total) will cause the mandible to autorotate upward and forward resulting in open bite closure up to 4 mm depending on the vertical and horizontal spatial relationships of the dentition to the condyles viewed in the sagittal plane [25].

We do not recommend masking in early skeletal open bite treatment. We will consider this option in some adult dentition patients.

Surgery – (Figures 5.35p and 5.35r) *closing the open bite by decreasing vertical face height.* Usually this includes performing a LeFort I osteotomy, removing a wedge of the maxillary bone, moving (impacting) the maxilla upward, and autorotating the mandible upward and forward, thereby closing the open bite. Surgery to close an anterior open bite is contraindicated until growth is complete. Why? The excessive vertical growth pattern will continue post-surgery if growth is not complete.

Q: You attend your study club where another orthodontist states, "The concept behind anterior open bite treatment is simple – *extrude anterior teeth* for dental open bites and *intrude posterior teeth* for skeletal open bites. It is simple." Is he correct?

A: Yes, your friend is basically correct. Let us review:

- Dental open bites are generally found in patients with normal vertical facial development and under-erupted anterior teeth due to a habit. No attempt is made to change the vertical facial dimension because it is normal. Elimination of the digit sucking, tongue interposition, of lip-biting habit may be enough to allow spontaneous *eruption of anterior teeth* and closure of the open bite. Or, the anterior teeth can be erupted using fixed orthodontic appliances and elastics (Figure 5.36, top right).
- Skeletal open bites result from excessive vertical facial development. Treatment consists of reducing the vertical dimension by *intruding posterior teeth* (Figure 5.36, bottom right). This can be accomplished by absolute posterior tooth intrusion (using TAD anchors), relative posterior tooth intrusion (e.g. using an LLHA to reduce mandibular molar eruption compared to controls), relative maxillary corpus intrusion (using an HPHG during growth), or absolute maxillary corpus intrusion (using a Lefort I impaction osteotomy). Of course, masking a skeletal open bite does not involve posterior tooth intrusion but consists of erupting anterior teeth.
- Finally, an anterior open bite can be a dental *and* skeletal open bite – resulting from a habit and from excess vertical facial growth. In such a case, orthodontic treatment consists of both anterior tooth eruption and posterior tooth intrusion.

Q: Rachael (Figure 5.37) is age nine years and four months and presents to you with the comment, "I want good teeth." Her PMH, TMJ evaluation, and periodontal evaluation are WRN. She fractured her maxillary right permanent central incisor at age eight years, and the tooth was restored with a composite veneer restoration. CR=CO. List diagnostic findings and problems. What is your diagnosis?

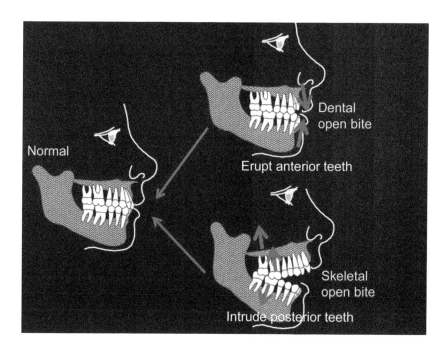

Figure 5.36 There are only two ways to close anterior open bites – either *erupt anterior teeth or intrude posterior teeth.* Anterior tooth eruption is the technique of choice in dental open bites where the facial skeleton is normal but a habit has prevented the anterior teeth from erupting. Posterior tooth intrusion is the technique of choice in skeletal open bites where the facial skeleton is vertically excessive.

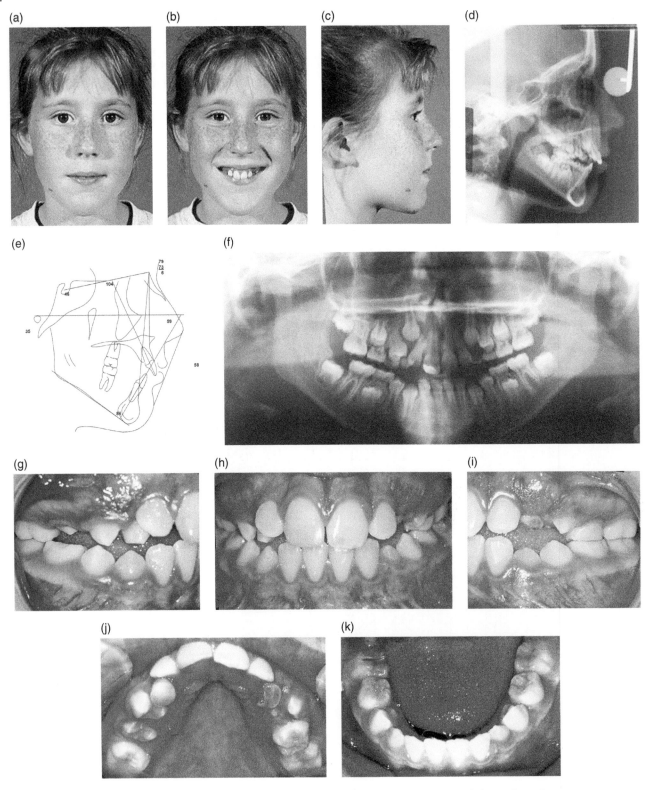

Figure 5.37 Initial records of Rachael. (a–c) facial photographs; (d) lateral cephalograph; (e) cephalometric tracing; (f) pantomograph; (g–k) intraoral photographs; (l–u) model photographs.

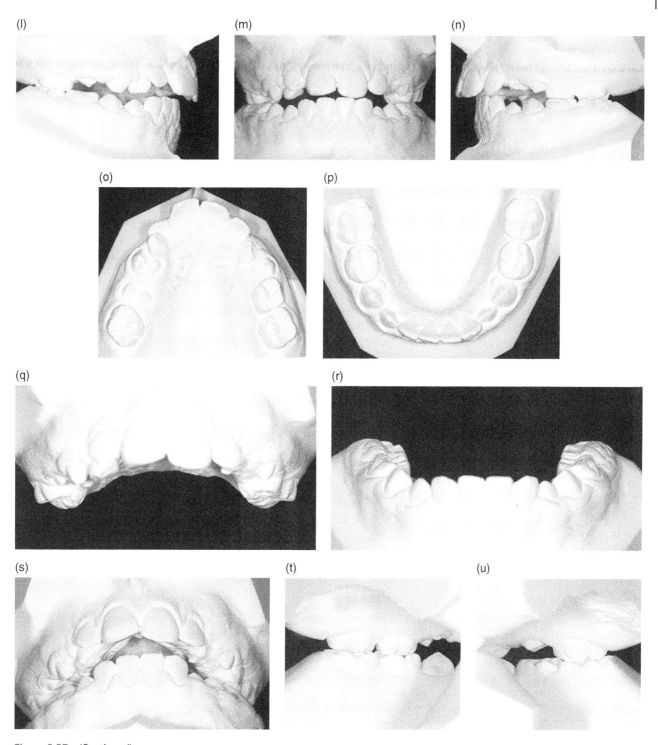

Figure 5.37 (Continued)

A:

Table 5.5 Diagnostic findings and problem list for Rachael.

Full face and Profile	**Frontal View**
	Chin appears deviated slightly to the right
	Mildly long LAFH (soft tissue Glabella-Subnasale < Subnasale-soft tissue Menton)
	Excess gingival display in a posed smile (maxillary lip border should be congruent with maxillary central incisor gingival sulci)
	UDML ~1–2 mm R
	Profile View
	Mildly convex profile
	Obtuse NLA
	ILG ~ 2 mm
	Retrusive chin
Ceph Analysis	**Skeletal**
	Maxilla anteroposterior position WRN (A-Point lies approximately on Nasion-perpendicular line)
	Mandibular deficiency (ANB = 6° with maxilla WRN)
	LLAFH (LAFH/TAFH × 100% = 58% which is one and one-half standard deviations longer than normal of 55%, sd = 2%)
	Steep cant of the palatal plane (PNS much lower than ANS due to excess vertical growth of posterior maxilla compared to anterior maxilla)
	Steep MPA (FMA = 35°; SNMP = 46°)
	Short posterior ramal height
	Vertical maxillary excess (VME)
	Dental
	Proclination of mandibular incisors (FMIA = 59°)
	Maxillary incisor angulation WRN (U1 to SN = 104°)
Radiographs	Late mixed dentition
	Incisal display at rest ~ 4 mm (Figure 5.37d)
Intraoral Photos and Models	Angle Class II division 1 malocclusion
	Iowa Classification: II (4–5 mm) II (4 mm) II (3–4 mm) II (3–4 mm)
	OJ: 7 mm (Figure 5.37s)
	Anterior open bite extending to right first permanent molar and left primary second molar
	Erupting premolars are not in occlusion
	Maxillary incisor edges are on the same level as maxillary posterior teeth (Figures 5.37l and 5.37n)
	Curve of Spee ~0 mm (Figures 5.37l and 5.37n)
	3.7 mm of maxillary anterior crowding
	Aligned mandibular anterior teeth with bilateral mandibular "E-space" present 38 mm maxillary permanent first molar intermolar width (mesiolingual cusp to mesiolingual cusp)
	40 mm mandibular intermolar width (central fossa to central fossa)
	Minimal permanent first molar OJ ("tight" transverse relationship, but no posterior crossbites)
	Maxillary first molars rotated mesially (Figure 5.37o)
	Thin mandibular anterior labial keratinized attachment (Figure 5.37h)
	Maxillary posterior buccal crown torque (Figure 5.37q, transverse compensations)
	Mandibular posterior lingual crown torque (Figure 5.37r, transverse compensations)
Other	—
Diagnosis	Class II Division 1 malocclusion secondary to mandibular skeletal deficiency with skeletal open bite (VME)

Q: We noted that Rachael's maxillary first permanent molars are mesially rotated. What direction should we look at the molars from? Why is this important?

A: We need to view the molar relationships from the lingual (Figures 5.37t and 5.37u). We note that both molar relationships remain Class II when viewed from the lingual.

This is important because mesially rotated molars appear more Class II when viewed from the buccal than from the lingual. If mesially rotated Class II molars are rotated distally around their palatal roots into proper alignment, then their buccal anteroposterior relationships will look improved – in some cases approaching Class I. But because Rachael's permanent molars still appear Class II when viewed from the lingual, we know that she will remain Class II even after her maxillary molars are rotated distally.

Q: What will be the effect of rotating Rachael's maxillary first permanent molars to the distal on her posterior *transverse* relationship?

A: Rotating her maxillary first permanent molars to the distal will swing the mesiobuccal cusps outward creating greater posterior OJ.

Q: Look at Rachael's posterior pharyngeal wall on her lateral cephalometric radiograph (Figure 5.37d). What do you observe?

A: Enlarged adenoids.

Q: Should you refer Rachael for adenoidectomy and tonsillectomy?

A: Not necessarily. Remember that lymphatic tissue size first increases, and then decreases, during the developmental years [56]. So, enlarged adenoids are not, by themselves, an indication for adenoidectomy.

Q: What are the current pediatric indications for tonsillectomy and adenoidectomy?

A: Indications include:
- Recurrent episodes of pharyngitis (7× strep sore throat in one year, or five each in two consecutive years, or three in three years with temps of 100.9°, white tonsil coverings, lymphadenopathy, and positive strep tests)
- Sleep apnea
- Severe difficulty with respiration [57].

Q: Does the fact that Rachael exhibits lip incompetence (ILG, Figures 5.37a and 5.37d) indicate that she is a mouth breather?

A: No. Lip incompetence does not necessarily indicate mouth breathing [58, 59]. Furthermore, Rachael has an ILG of only ~ 2 mm. An ILG of up to 2 mm may be considered normal [26].

Q: How would you decide if Rachael is a mouth breather and when would you refer her to an otolaryngologist for an airway evaluation?

A: First, try to *observe* if she breathes through her mouth. *Ask* Rachael and her parents whether she breathes through her nose or mouth. Ask her and her parents if she snores or has ever stopped breathing while asleep. If Rachael has difficulty breathing, is an obligatory mouth breather, snores, or presents with a history of sleep apnea, refer her for an airway evaluation. *Rachael is found to breathe nasally.*

Q: Mouth breathers may suffer from nasal obstruction. Can you name at least five causes of nasal obstruction?

A: Allergic rhinitis, adenoid hypertrophy, polyps, congenital nasal deformities, neoplasms, and recurrent upper respiratory infections. [60]

Q: Do otolaryngologists validate the use of conventional lateral cephalometric radiographs to assess possible airway obstruction?

A: No. [61, 62] The problem with using cephalometric radiographs to assess airway is that they are 2-D representations of a 3-D airway structure.

Q: Do we have evidence of a relationship between mouth breathing and facial morphology?

A: *We have evidence of an association between nasal obstruction and facial morphology, but the interaction is complex and the evidence for a direct cause-and-effect relationship remains weak.* Case studies have suggested that some children with nasal obstruction display a hyperdivergent pattern of facial growth with downward and backward mandibular rotation, and an increased lower face height [63, 64]. Children suffering from allergic rhinitis tend to have increased TAFH, increased lower anterior face height, and hyperdivergent MPA [60]. Long-faced adolescent subjects have significantly smaller components of nasal respiration [65].

On the other hand, some children with nasal obstruction do not display hyperdivergent facial patterns [66] and some children with morphologic characteristics associated with mouth breathing do not display significant nasal obstruction or mouth breathing [67]. In a sample [68] of 400 children, two to twelve years old (mean age six years) at an outpatient clinic for mouth breathers:
- Adenoid/tonsil obstruction was detected in 71.8%
- Allergic rhinitis alone was found in 18.7%

- Nonobstructive mouth breathing was diagnosed in 9.5%
- The prevalence of anterior open bites, Class II malocclusions, and posterior crossbites was higher in mouth-breathing children than in the general population. Posterior crossbite was detected in almost 30% of the children during primary and mixed dentitions and 48% in permanent dentition. During mixed and permanent dentitions, anterior open bite and Class II malocclusions were highly prevalent. However, more than 50% of the mouth-breathing children carried a normal inter-arch relationship in the sagittal, transverse and vertical planes. This finding is supported by findings of another study suggesting no differences in prevalence of malocclusion for children with obstructed nasal breathing compared to a normal population [68]. Furthermore, in a comparison of severely obstructed mouth-breathing and nasal-breathing children [69], mouth-breathing children had a hyperdivergent cephalometric pattern, but against all expectations, CCW mandibular rotation was the average observation. In a recent study of prepubertal severely obstructed mouth-breathing children and prepubertal nasal-breathing children, after adenoidectomy the mouth-breathing children showed greater maxillary transverse development [70]. As with children, adult subjects with obstructed nasal breathing tend to show mandibular plane hyperdivergence, but the correlation is too weak to support direct cause and effect [71].

Simply put, the data supporting a cause-and-effect relationship between nasal obstruction and altered craniofacial form is inconsistent. The exact connection between obstructed nasal breathing and craniofacial morphology remains to be elucidated.

Q: Is there *clear* evidence showing that correction of mouth breathing will result in normal vertical facial growth?

A: *No*. In a 2004 study [72], adenoidectomies were performed in a group of mouth-breathing children (nasal obstruction caused by enlarged adenoids) at age seven years which caused a change from mouth to nose breathing. This group was compared to an age- and sex-matched group of unoperated control subjects and re-examined at twelve years. Results indicated that adenoidectomy improved vertical facial growth and balance. On the other hand, the sum of upper and lower first molar height changes (amount of molar eruption) was 9.2 mm in the adenoidectomized group and 5.8 mm in the control group. This would indicate that corrected mouth breathers continued to grow more vertically. Other problems with this study have been reported [57]. *We do not have clear evidence that correction of nasal obstruction will transform a long face growth pattern into a normal face height growth pattern.*

Q: Are there other questions you should ask Rachael and her parents about her open bite? Is there anything else should you check for?

A: Additional questions you should ask or things you should check for include:
- You should show her parents the open bite and inquire how long she has had it. They respond that they have never noticed it before.
- Ask whether Rachael has any functional habits that could prevent her anterior teeth from erupting. None is noted, and Rachael denies any habits.
- Ask Rachael if she knows what could be preventing her front teeth from erupting into contact. Rachael has no idea.
- Check for permanent teeth that are erupting which could cause a temporary anterior open bite. Rachael's permanent maxillary canines and premolars are only partially erupted, which is consistent with her dental stage of development.
- Check for ankylosed teeth and blocked out teeth that are not fully erupted that could cause an open bite. There appears to be adequate space and no teeth appear to be ankylosed.
- Check for anterior tongue posturing. Ask Rachael to close her eyes. Talk to her parents for a minute. Then, to distract Rachael, ask her to open her eyes as you quickly and gently draw her lower lip forward and down. You find that her tongue is not anteriorly interposed between her front teeth.
- Confirm that she has not sustained jaw trauma and that her condyles appear normal (Figure 5.37f). She has not sustained jaw trauma, and her condyles appear normal.

Q: Can you list Rachael's skeletal and dental open bite features?

A: Her *skeletal* open bite features include:
- Mildly long soft tissue LAFH (soft tissue Glabella – Subnasale < Subnasale – soft tissue Menton, Figures 5.37a and 5.37c)
- ILG (even though her 2 mm ILG is considered WRN, an ILG in the presence of long soft tissue LAFH without a short upper lip suggests that her facial soft tissue growth has not kept pace with her excess vertical skeletal growth)

- Skeletal long lower anterior face height (LLAFH) (LAFH/TAFH×100% = 58% which is one and one-half standard deviations longer than normal)
- Steep cant of palatal plane (Posterior nasal spine (PNS) much lower than anterior nasal spine (ANS) due to excess vertical growth of posterior maxilla compared to anterior maxilla)
- Vertical maxillary excess (VME)
- Steep MPA (FMA = 35°; SNMP = 46°)
- Short posterior ramal height
- Anterior open bite extending to right permanent first molar and left primary second molar (however recall that she is transitioning into the permanent dentition) Her *dental* open bite features include:
- None. Rachael lacks habits which could be inhibiting tooth eruption and her maxillary and mandibular incisors are not intruded relative to their respective posterior occlusal planes (Figures 5.37l and 5.37m).

Q: Does Rachael have a dental open bite, a skeletal open bite, or a combination of both? What is the etiology of her open bite?

A: Rachael has a mild skeletal open bite resulting from an excessive vertical pattern of growth:
- Condyles growing more posterior-superiorly (Figure 5.37d)
- Reduced ramal height development
- Maxilla descending more in the posterior than normal (palatal plane tipped down posteriorly)
- Probable decreased forward mandibular internal rotation or even backward internal rotation.

As a result of this excess vertical growth pattern, her mandible rotated downward and backward, MPA steepened, lower anterior face height increased, and an anterior open bite occurred.

Q: What features constitute VME? Does Rachael exhibit these features?

A: VME features typically include:
- Long skeletal and soft tissue LAFH
- ILG (growth of facial soft tissue drape not keeping pace with vertical skeletal growth)
- Palatal plane tipped down in posterior (excessive maxillary posterior vertical growth)
- Maxillary first molar root apices erupted below the palatal plane (excessive molar eruption)
- Short ramal height
- Steep MPA
- Mandibular skeletal retrusion (due to mandible rotating down and back as a result of excessive maxillary vertical growth)

- Pronounced antegonial notching
- Anterior open bite (depending upon the amount of anterior tooth compensatory eruption).

Rachael exhibits many, but not all, of these features which is not unusual for any VME patient. In our opinion, Rachael exhibits VME.

Q: How will Rachael's skeletal open bite etiology affect her treatment?

A: Rachael lacks a dental open bite component. Her maxillary and mandibular incisor edges have erupted to the same plane as her posterior teeth, and she shows ~4 mm of incisal display at rest – which is normal (Figure 5.37d). For these reasons, you should avoid closing her open bite by erupting anterior teeth (masking). Why? You may increase her incisal display at rest, and possibly worsen her mildly excessive gingival display.

Instead, treatment of Rachael's open bite must focus on her excessive vertical facial growth. The treatment of choice for adolescent Class II skeletal open bite patients like Rachael is to:
- Reduce descent and forward growth of her maxillary corpus
- Reduce eruption or intrude maxillary and mandibular molars.

If the above can be accomplished, then the growing mandible can autorotate upward and forward, closing the open bite. This approach minimizes unwanted extrusion of her maxillary incisors to close her anterior open bite.

Rachael's vertical growth pattern may continue until she is finished growing. Even if Rachael cooperates with treatment, and even if you are successful in controlling her vertical growth during treatment, her growth pattern will not be normalized. So, you must either treat her until she is finished growing or gamble that she only has an inconsequential amount of growth remaining after you finish treatment.

We wish to emphasize one key point – Rachael has a relatively *mild* skeletal open bite. If she had a severe skeletal open bite, then it would be prudent to consider letting her finish growing before initiating treatment. At that time, you could consider treating her with orthognathic surgery. Of course, you could consider reducing her LLAFH at any time with TAD molar intrusion.

Finally, you should tell Rachael's parents that, depending upon growth and compliance, you may not be able to close her open bite or keep it closed. You should tell them that your goal is to correct the open bite completely, but you may only be able to improve it.

Q: What are the *primary* problems in each dimension you must stay focused on for Rachael?

A:

Table 5.6 Primary problems list for Rachael.

AP	Angle Class II division 1 malocclusion
	Iowa Classification: II (4–5 mm) II (4 mm) II (3–4 mm) II (3–4 mm)
	Mandibular skeletal deficiency
Vertical	Skeletal open bite
	VME
Transverse	Minimal first molar buccal OJ
	Transverse dental compensations
Other	—

Q: If you decide to treat Rachael's Class II relationship and skeletal open bite orthopedically, then when should treatment begin? Should you start now or wait?

A: Begin *now*, while Rachael is in the late mixed dentition and we can take advantage of growth [17, 19, 73–77]. Extensive, randomized prospective clinical trials examining skeletal open bite orthopedic treatment are lacking. However, if you are going to begin Class II treatment, then we recommend choosing biomechanics that will also correct/improve Rachael's vertical excess.

Q: What unknowns do you face?

A: The most significant unknown is Rachael's remaining jaw growth (magnitude and direction).

- How much will her maxilla descend or her maxillary posterior teeth erupt (rotating her mandible down and back – worsening her open bite and Class II relationship)?
- How much will her maxilla grow forward (worsening her Class II relationship)?
- How much will her mandibular posterior teeth erupt?
- How much will her mandible grow?
- Will the direction of her condylar growth help, or hurt, her mandibular forward growth?
- Will her mandible rotate forward internally or will it rotate backward?

The answers to these questions are unknown. Additional unknowns include her *cooperation, hygiene, and presence of an undetected CR-CO shift*. Rachael's unknowns are significant.

Q: What specific early treatment(s) do you recommend for Rachael?

A: We began by *reducing unknowns* (growth/compliance). A trans palatal arch (TPA) was placed and activated to rotate Rachael's maxillary first permanent molars into proper alignment at which time HPHG treatment began. An LLHA was placed to reduce eruption of mandibular first molars and prevent mandibular molars from drifting mesially – thereby forcing Class II correction via headgear. Rachael wore the headgear faithfully until her molar relationship was corrected to Class I. She continued wearing it at night while we monitored growth. Once all permanent teeth erupted, we re-evaluated progress and decided to proceed with non-extraction treatment. Rachael was placed in fixed orthodontic appliances (excluding her permanent second molars), her arches leveled and aligned, and the treatment finished.

Deband records are shown in Figures 5.38a–5.38l. She had an excellent result. Rachael's compliance with headgear wear was demonstrated by the fact that maxillary first permanent molar eruption halted (Figure 5.38f, top right). Her Class II correction was made via differential jaw growth – her maxilla grew down while her mandible grew forward (Figure 5.38f, left). B-Point came forward as much as it did because the maxillary first permanent molars did not erupt, and the mandibular first permanent molars erupted minimally (LLHA effect). B-Point would have come forward even more if the maxilla had not descended. Maxillary descent, and molar eruption, rotate the mandible (B-Point) down and back.

Although Rachael's maxilla descended, her anterior open bite closed because of mandibular forward growth, minimal mandibular first molar eruption, absence of maxillary first molar eruption, and ~2 mm maxillary incisor eruption (Figure 5.38f, top right). Overcorrection of her OB (final OB = 30%) was prudent in anticipation of future relapse. Her maxillary incisor extrusion was congruent with the vertical growth of her upper lip. Consequently, her mildly excessive gingival display was maintained (compare Figures 5.37b and 5.38b).

Q: Descent of the maxilla and molar eruption hinders skeletal open bite closure. How does *mandibular growth* impact skeletal open bite closure?

A: Favorable mandibular growth (more vertical condylar growth, more forward internal rotation) can aid skeletal open bite closure. Unfavorable mandibular growth (greater posterior-superior condylar growth, greater downward-backward internal rotation of the mandible) can impede skeletal open bite closure.

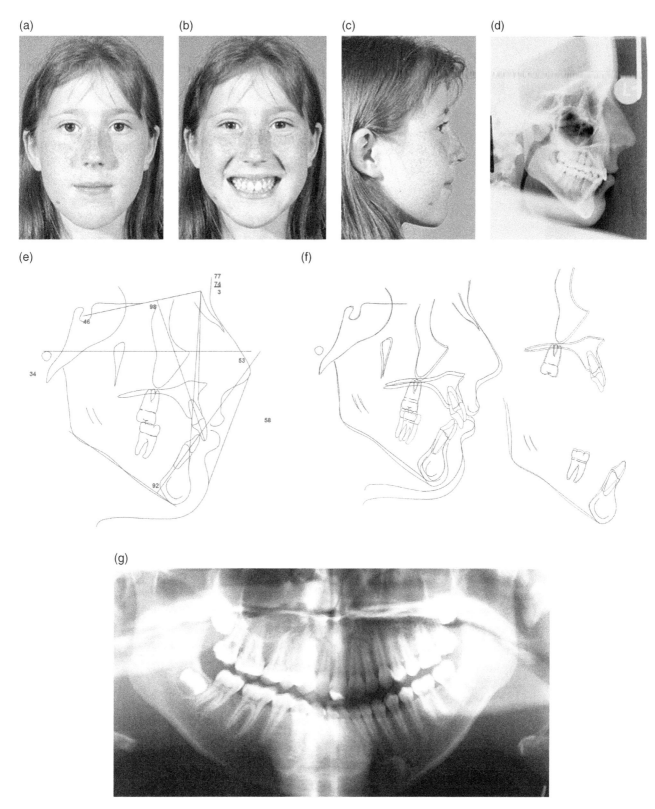

(a) (b) (c) (d)

(e) (f)

(g)

Figure 5.38   (a–l) Rachael's deband records.

(h)   (i)   (j)

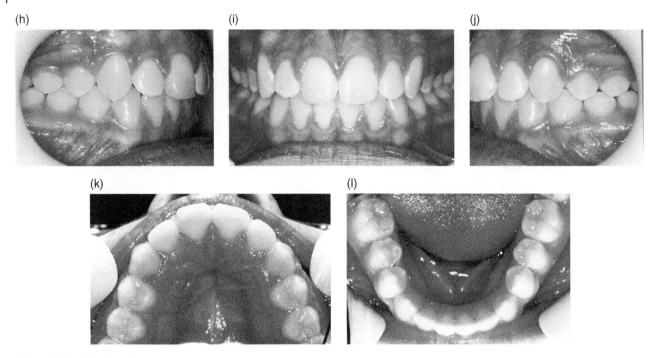

(k)   (l)

Figure 5.38 (Continued)

Q: Finally, can you list reasons for *early* dental or skeletal open bite treatment?

A: Reasons include the following:
- Providing the patient with the ability to incise food
- Improving smile esthetics in patients with minimal maxillary incisal display and significant esthetic concerns (dental open bites with stepped up maxillary incisors)
- Improving speech (we recommend consulting a speech therapist before treatment)

- Attempting to avoid future orthognathic surgery (mild-to-moderate skeletal open bites if orthopedics is employed).

Q: Anisa is a girl aged eight years and eleven months (Figure 5.39) who presents to you with her parents' concern, "Anisa has been referred by her general dentist for orthodontics." PMH and PDH are WRN. CR=CO. TMJs, periodontal tissues, and mucogingival tissues are WRN. Can you list Anisa's *primary* problems in each dimension (plus other)?

(a)   (b)   (c)   (d)

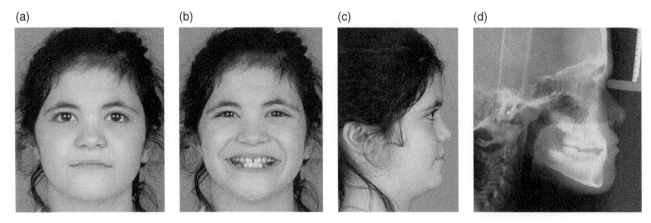

Figure 5.39 Initial records of Anisa. (a–c) facial photographs; (d and e) lateral cephalometric radiograph and tracing; (f) panoramic image; (g–k) intraoral images; (l–t) model images.

(e)

(f)

(g)

(h)

(i)

(j)

(k)

(l)

(m)

(n)

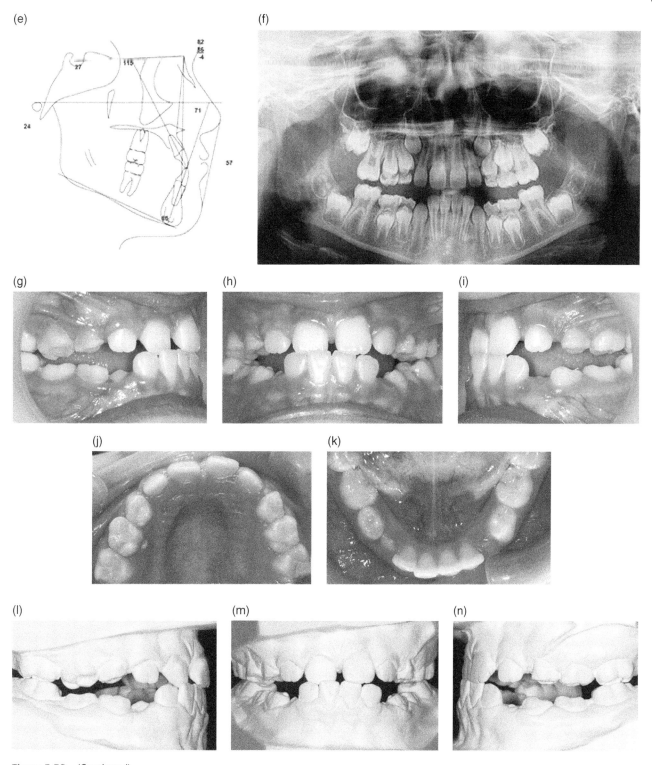

Figure 5.39 (Continued)

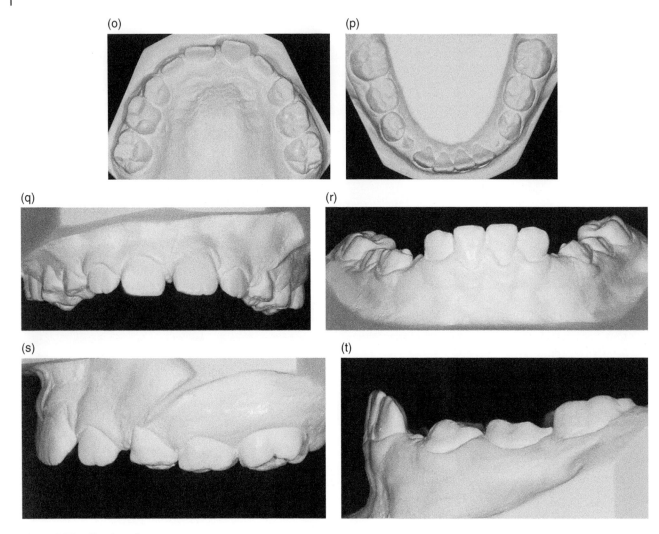

Figure 5.39 (Continued)

A:

Table 5.7 Primary problems list for Anisa.

AP	Angle Class II division 1 subdivision right
	Iowa Classification: II (2 mm) X X I
	Maxillary skeletal anteroposterior deficiency (A-Point lies behind Nasion-perpendicular line)
	Mandibular skeletal anteroposterior excess (See Appendix: since the Nasion-B Point line appears to be coincident with the Nasion-perpendicular line, the angle between both lines is 0° and the mandible is therefore excessive)
Vertical	Long soft tissue LAFH (soft tissue Glabella-Subnasale < Subnasale-soft tissue Menton)
	Skeletal LAFH WRN (LAFH/TAFH × 100% = 57%; versus ideal of 55%, sd = 2%)
	OB 10%
	Bilateral posterior open bite
Transverse	—
Other	Right central incisors are in crossbite
	Proclined maxillary incisors (U1- SN = 115°)
	Upright mandibular incisors (FMIA = 71°)
	Possible future impaction of maxillary permanent canines (lack of space)
	8 mm of maxillary arch crowding currently present (7 mm of anterior space but 15 mm of anticipated room needed for two maxillary permanent canines)

Q: Why does Anisa exhibit right Class II and left Class I permanent molars instead of *Class III* permanent molars? In other words, she is maxillary skeletal *deficient* and mandibular skeletal *excessive* (ANB = – 4°) with Class III dental compensations (upright mandibular incisors/proclined maxillary incisors) – so we would expect her to be Class III at her molars.

A: We speculate that premature loss of her maxillary primary canines resulted in the mesial drift of her maxillary posterior teeth, distal drift of her maxillary incisors, and spacing between her maxillary incisors. The maxillary molar mesial drift created the Class II molar relationship on her right and Class I on the left.

Q: With Anisa, we now begin discussion of our final vertical problem – *posterior open bites*. Anisa has a bilateral posterior open bite. A posterior open bite exists when some anterior teeth occlude with the opposing arch while some posterior teeth do not. Anisa's bite is open from her lateral incisors to her primary second molars. Why correct posterior open bites?

A: Reasons include:
- Increasing posterior occlusal chewing surface area
- Improving smile esthetics
- Reducing anterior tooth wear because of reduced posterior occlusal support.

Q: Can you list at least five causes of posterior open bites? Are any of these the cause of Anisa's posterior open bites?

A: Posterior open bite etiology includes the following:
- *Posterior tongue-interposition habit.* I asked Anisa to close her eyes for a minute while I spoke to her mother. Then, I distracted Anisa by asking her to open her eyes while I quickly, but gently, retracted her lips (Figure 5.40). I saw her tongue interposed between her posterior teeth and concluded that this resting tongue habit was possibly responsible for her posterior open bites.
- *Digit interposition habits.* Anisa and her parents denied any such habit.
- *Temporary posterior open bite occurring during the transition from late mixed to permanent dentition* – It is true that Anisa's erupting permanent mandibular canines, and potentially impacted maxillary permanent canines, are adding to her open bite. However, these are anterior locations which do not explain her primary molar open bites.
- *Ankylosis of teeth* – preventing their eruption into occlusion. Except for her potentially impacted maxillary canines, Anisa's permanent teeth appear to be erupting normally (Figure 5.39f). Furthermore, a step in the alveolar process bone crests between adjacent teeth is the clearest indication of an ankylosed primary molar (as adjacent teeth continue to erupt). Anisa does not exhibit such a step anywhere.
- Very *constricted dental arches* – where the tongue is forced to find space laterally in order to maintain a patent airway. Anisa does not appear to have severely constricted dental arches (Figures 5.39o and 5.39p).
- *Class III growth* resulting in an edge-to-edge incisor relationship – could potentially create a posterior open bite as the mandibular incisal edges occlude with the maxillary incisor edges. Such a Class III growth pattern (maxillary skeletal deficiency, mandibular skeletal excess) could be partially responsible for her posterior open bite, especially if her posterior tongue-interposition habit resulted from this growth pattern.
- *Lack of space* for complete tooth eruption (teeth blocked out). As we examine her records, we feel that this does partially explain the open bite at the canines (potentially impacted maxillary canines), but we do not feel that this is the cause of her posterior open bites.
- *Systemic factors* found in patients with certain syndromes, such as cleidocranial dysplasia, ectodermal dysplasia, Gardner syndrome, and Apert syndrome. Anisa's parents deny any such systemic factors.
- *Some treatments for sleep apnea* may create posterior open bites [78]. Anisa's parents deny any such problems.
- *Primary failure of eruption (PFE).* PFE refers to failure of a non-ankylosed tooth to erupt due to a disturbance of the eruption mechanism [79]. The following signs are characteristic of PFE: [79–83]
  1) Permanent first molars are always involved and present with no apparent barrier to eruption (100% for genetically confirmed PFE).

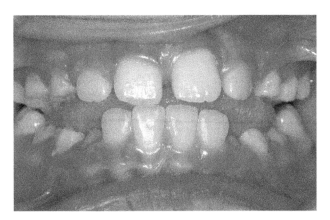

Figure 5.40 Anisa demonstrated a bilateral resting tongue habit.

2) Posterior teeth are more frequently affected.

3) *If a tooth in a more anterior position is affected, teeth more posterior are usually affected as well* (i.e. when premolars are affected, molars are also likely to be affected).

4) Both primary and permanent teeth can be affected.

5) The condition is often bilateral (50/50 for PFE patients versus – 80/20 unilateral/bilateral for ankylosis of molars only).

6) Teeth in both arches are often affected (91% of those with genetically confirmed PFE).

7) Affected teeth resorb the alveolar bone above the crown, may erupt into initial occlusion and then cease to erupt further, or may fail to erupt entirely.

8) Involved teeth may be displaced back and forth with manual pressure (indicating that they are not, initially, ankylosed). However, involved teeth tend to become ankylosed as soon as orthodontic eruptive forces are applied.

9) If a small area of ankylosis is broken by manipulating the ankylosed tooth, it might be possible to move the tooth for a short time, but re-ankylosis is inevitable.

10) Other concurrent skeletal problems (Class III malocclusion for 63% of genetically confirmed PFE patients) and dental anomalies (tooth agenesis, microdontia of maxillary lateral incisors, and anomalous root morphology) may be present.

11) There are two clinical phenotypes – Type 1 (all quadrants involved) and Type 2 (quadrants vary in severity). There is much variation seen and possible overlap with other genetic disorders of the eruption mechanism.

12) Possible treatment options for posterior open bites resulting from PFE include: restoring the involved teeth with buildups or crowns after vertical growth is complete; extraction of the involved teeth and replacement with bone grafts/implants; with first and second molar involvement, leaving the affected teeth in place and accepting a premolar occlusion; a segmental osteotomy or distraction osteogenesis to close the posterior open bite; a removable prosthetic (overlay) partial denture to provide posterior occlusion.

13) Finally, it is our clinical experience that cases involving permanent first molar ankylosis are frequently, and incorrectly, diagnosed as PFE. However, if a series of radiographs demonstrate continued permanent *second* molar eruption, then it is probably not a case of PFE.

Anisa's posterior open bite is probably *not* an example of PFE. Why? Her permanent first molars have erupted and are in occlusion (Figures 5.39g, 5.39i, 5.39l, 5.39n).

Q: To summarize, what is the probable cause of Anisa's posterior open bite?

A: Her *interposition tongue habit* is the probable cause. However, her Class III growth pattern could be playing a role and must be monitored.

Q: Can you contrast the treatment of *anterior* open bites with the treatment of *posterior* open bites?

A: Anterior open bites are treated by erupting anterior teeth (dental open bites and masking skeletal open bites) and by intruding posterior teeth (orthopedics or surgery for skeletal anterior open bites). In contrast, *posterior* open bites are treated *only* by erupting posterior teeth (Figure 5.41).

Q: Figures 5.41c and 5.41d illustrates crisscross elastics for posterior open bite closure (patient closed Figure 5.41c, patient open Figure 5.41d). Can you explain the advantage of crisscross elastics?

A: As shown, crisscross elastics consist of two crossbite elastics per side of the arch. One crossbite elastic is worn from the maxillary buccal to the mandibular lingual, and one crossbite elastic is worn from the maxillary lingual to the mandibular buccal. The advantage of using crisscross elastics is that the *horizontal* force components of the two elastics *cancel* each other – leaving only the vertical forces. This contrasts with vertical elastics worn from the maxillary buccal to the mandibular buccal – which tend to roll the teeth to the lingual.

Q: How difficult are posterior open bites to correct?

A: Clinical experience has taught us that posterior open bites can be one of the, if not *the*, most difficult orthodontic problems to correct (and to maintain once corrected).

Q: Treatment of a posterior open bite depends upon its specific etiology. How would you treat Anisa's posterior open bite? How would you treat her anterior crossbite?

A: You must address Anisa's posterior tongue-interposition habit (resting tongue habit) to correct, and maintain correction of, her posterior open bite. Otherwise, even if you close her posterior open bite, it may return.

Note: Before you attempt to close a posterior open bite due to a tongue-interposition habit, *confirm the absence of a breathing problem (snoring, sleep apnea, and partial/complete airway obstruction). It is imprudent*

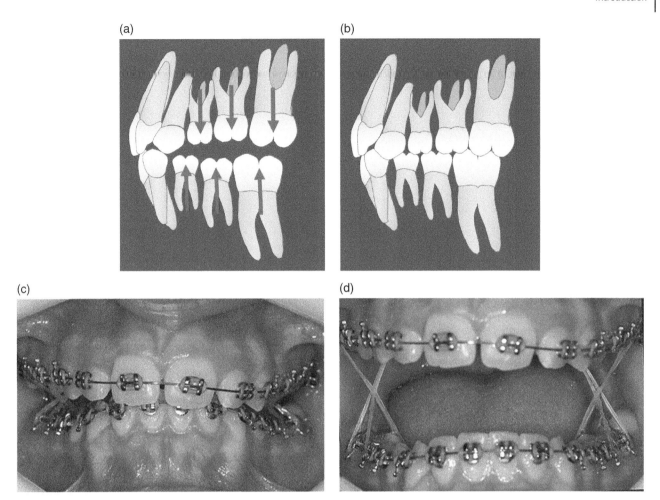

Figure 5.41 Posterior open bites are corrected by (a and b) erupting teeth:
- *Eliminate habits* that are preventing an eruption
- Fabricate and wear prostheses (e.g. crowns, implants or overlay dentures)
- Surgery such as segmental osteotomies
- (c and d) Erupt teeth with fixed orthodontic appliances and vertical elastics (crisscross elastics shown).

to reduce space for the tongue (forcing it back into the pharynx) if a breathing problem exists. If a breathing problem exists, first seek consultation with an otolaryngologist. Anisa did not have a breathing problem.

Contrasted with anterior dental open bites due to tongue-interposition habits, we have not had success correcting posterior tongue-interposition habits through patient discussions (psychological approach). Therefore, we decided to attempt training Anisa's tongue by fabricating an LLHA with bilateral soldered wire loops to block her tongue (Figures 5.42a–5.42d). Our hope was that if her resting tongue habit was eliminated and her posterior teeth erupted into occlusion, then the erupted teeth themselves would confine her tongue to the lingual.

Following placement of the LLHA with soldered loops, the posterior teeth began to erupt (Figures 5.42e–5.42j). Due to the 8 mm of maxillary crowding and the possibility of maxillary canine impaction, her maxillary first premolars were extracted. Correction of the anterior crossbite was achieved by asking her to bite on a soft suction tip at home as much as possible (Figures 5.42k and 5.42l). Her jaw growth was monitored, and at age ten years and eleven months, her maxilla and mandible appeared to have maintained a reasonable relationship (Figures 5.42m–5.42o). Also, by this time, her posterior open bite had closed (Figures 5.42p–5.42t). Was this open bite closure due to the action of the LLHA with soldered loops restricting lateral tongue interposition? Or, was this open bite closure due to normal permanent tooth eruption? We cannot be sure, but we are delighted with the open bite closure. Anisa will be followed for an eruption of her maxillary canines, but her early treatment was completed at this point.

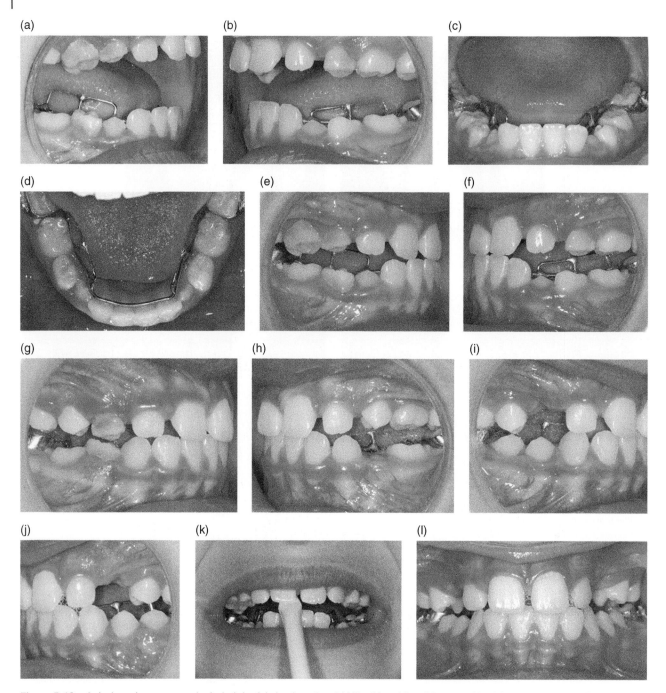

Figure 5.42 Anisa's early treatment included the fabrication of an LLHA with soldered loops to block her tongue (a–d). Over a period of seventeen months (e–j), her posterior open bite appeared to be closing as permanent teeth erupted (maxillary first premolars were extracted to permit eruption of maxillary canines). Her anterior crossbite was corrected by having Alisa bite on the end of a soft suction tip (k–l). By age ten years and eleven months (m–t), her maxillary and mandibular jaws appeared to be well related, and her posterior open bite had closed. She will be recalled in six months to follow her maxillary canine eruption.

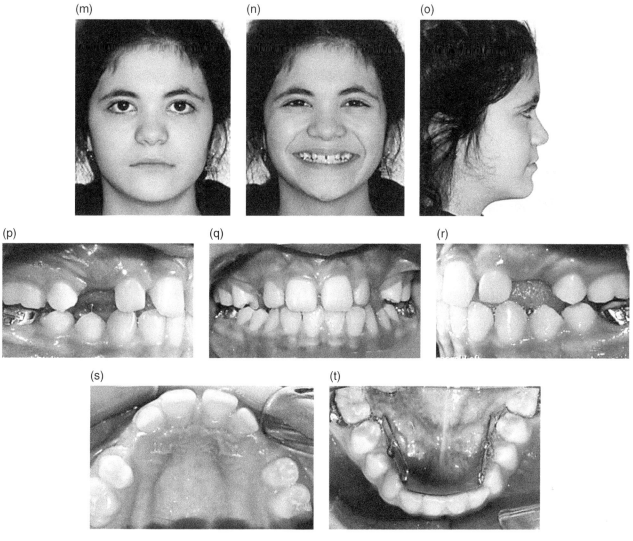

(m) (n) (o)

(p) (q) (r)

(s) (t)

Figure 5.42   (Continued)

Q: Other than the placing of an LLHA with bilateral soldered loops, can you suggest two additional appliances
or techniques to help correct a posterior interposition
tongue habit?

A: Possible appliances, or techniques, include:
- Wire loops embedded in a *removable* retainer to
block the tongue
- *Tooth positioner* wear to block the tongue
- Placement of fixed appliances with *vertical elastics*
worn between maxillary and mandibular posterior
teeth to block the tongue *and* erupt teeth
- *RME*, if you believe a constricted maxillary arch is
forcing the patient's tongue laterally.

Q: Digit habits creating posterior open bites can be dealt
with in the same way as digit habits causing anterior
open bites (e.g. thumb-sucking paints). Temporary

posterior open bites occurring as a result of the transition
from primary to permanent dentition are of little concern
unless a tongue-interposition habit develops. Posterior
open bites resulting from constricted dental arches
(tongue is forced laterally to maintain a patent airway)
are dealt with by skeletal/dental arch expansion. Posterior
open bites resulting from a Class III growth pattern are
dealt with by treating the Class III growth pattern.

But what about posterior open bites resulting from
ankylosed teeth or from PFE? Can you suggest treatment options for them?

A: Options include the following:
- If the posterior open bite is due to ankylosed primary
molars *with permanent successors* in a good position,
no treatment is needed. A normal occlusion should
eventually result, although a six-month delay can be
expected in the eruption of the premolar [84].

- For ankylosed primary molars *without permanent successors – generally extract the primary molars in young children*. Why? As adjacent permanent teeth erupt, the ankylosed primary molar is left behind, and a large vertical bony defect will develop. Later vertical bone grafting can be difficult in such situations. With the extraction of the ankylosed primary molar, an hourglass-shaped ridge will result as alveolar process bone resorbs and the ridge width decreases, *but* the ridge height will decrease by less than 2% [85] making later lateral bone grafting easier. In contrast, in older children with little future growth anticipated, a decision may be made to retain the ankylosed primary molar if the vertical bony defect is small, the tooth is cleansable, the tooth crown is in good shape, and the primary roots are well-formed.
- For ankylosed permanent posterior teeth in children, extraction must be considered. Why? A significant vertical defect will result as adjacent teeth continue to erupt.
- For mild posterior open bites resulting from permanent posterior tooth ankylosis/PFE in older children, restoring the involved tooth with a composite buildup or crown after vertical growth is complete is an option [86].
- For moderate posterior open bites resulting from permanent posterior tooth ankylosis/PFE in older children, extraction of the involved teeth and replacement with bone grafts/implants should be considered.

- In patients with first *and* second permanent molar ankylosis/PFE, consider leaving the affected teeth in place and accept a premolar occlusion.
- A segmental osteotomy [79, 87] or distraction osteogenesis [88] to close the posterior open bite may be entertained in severe posterior open bite cases due to ankylosis/PFE.
- Implant replacement with elongated crowns, or overlay removable partial dentures (RPD) can also be used to provide posterior occlusion [78].

Q: Closure of posterior open bites is performed to increase chewing surface area, improve smile esthetics, and reduce anterior tooth wear due to lack of posterior occlusal support. When do you recommend *early* posterior open bite treatment?

A: *We recommend early posterior open bite treatment through habit control if the open bite is due to a tongue-interposition habit or digit habit – if the patient is interested in stopping the habit.* Early treatment of posterior open bites due to other causes must be considered on a case-by-case basis addressing the etiology – as described earlier.

Q: Mark (Figure 5.43) is a boy aged ten years and two months who presents to you with the chief complaint, "I would like to have straight teeth and not have spaces between my teeth." PMH includes seasonal allergies and ADHD (Rx: Adderall), PDH WRN. TMJ and periodontal evaluations are WRN. CR=CO. List diagnostic findings and problems. What is your diagnosis?

(a)   (b)   (c)   (d)

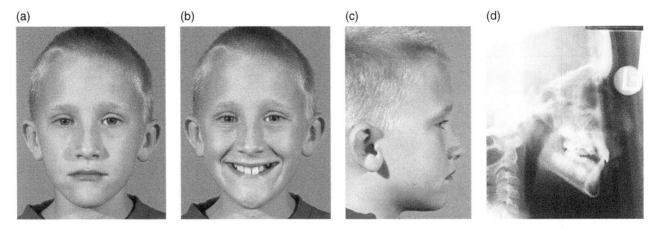

Figure 5.43 Initial records of Mark: (a–c) facial photographs; (d) lateral cephalograph; (e) cephalometric tracing; (f) pantomograph made before other records; (g–k) intraoral photographs; (l–p) model photographs.

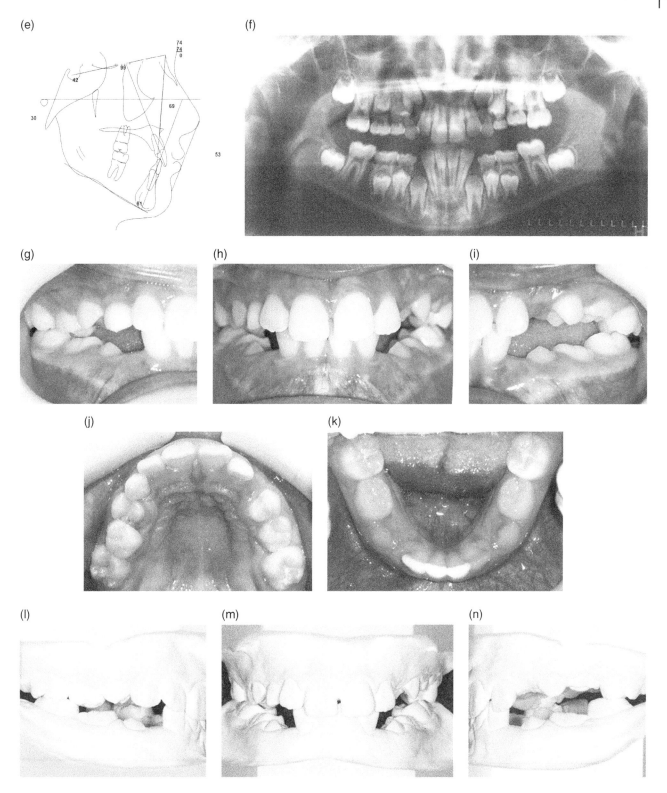

Figure 5.43 (Continued)

(o)

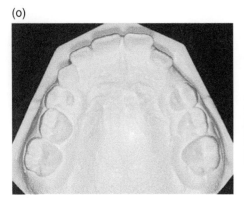

(p)

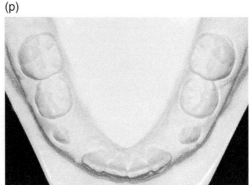

Figure 5.43 (Continued)

A:

Table 5.8 Diagnostic findings and problem list for Mark.

Full face and Profile	**Frontal View**
	Facial symmetry
	Soft tissue LAFH WRN (soft tissue Glabella – Subnasale = Subnasale – soft tissue Menton)
	Lip competence
	Adequate incisal display in a posed smile (maxillary incisors stepped down relative to the occlusal plane)
	UDML WRN
	Profile View
	Slightly convex profile
	NLA WRN
	Mildly retrusive chin
Ceph Analysis	**Skeletal**
	Maxilla retrusive (A-Point lies behind Nasion-perpendicular line)
	Mandible retrusive (ANB angle = 0° but maxilla is retrusive and angle between Nasion-B Point line and Nasion-perpendicular line = 4°)
	Maxillary molar root apices positioned *above* the palatal plane
	Steep MPA (FMA = 30°; SNMP = 42°)
	Skeletal LAFH WRN (LAFH/TAFH×100% = 53%; ideal is 55% with s.d. = 2%)
	Dental
	Maxillary incisor angulation appears WRN (U1 to SN = 99° but low Sella makes this angle smaller)
	Mandibular incisor angulation upright (FMIA = 69°)

Table 5.8 (Continued)

Radiographs	Mandibular primary second molar occlusal surfaces are stepped *below* mandibular permanent first molar occlusal surfaces, but their alveolar process crest heights appear even. In other words, a short primary second molar crown height created this occlusal step, but it was not created by primary second molar ankylosis.
	Maxillary left primary second molar alveolar crest height appears stepped up compared to the maxillary left permanent first molar crest height (possible ankylosed primary second molar)
Intraoral Photos and Models	Angle Class III subdivision left
	Iowa Classification: I X X III (1 mm)
	OJ: 1 mm
	OB: 50 %
	Maxillary incisors are stepped down relative to maxillary posterior teeth (Figure 5.43 m)
	Bilateral posterior open bite
	Late mixed dentition (panoramic image was made before models and photos)
	4 mm maxillary anterior crowding currently present (5 mm of total space, 1 mm maxillary right lateral incisor crowding, 7 mm width of right primary canine, and space needed for two 7.5 mm permanent canines)
	1.2 mm of maxillary "E-space" present per side 9 mm mandibular anterior crowding currently present (5 mm of total space, and 14 mm of space needed for two 7 mm permanent canines)
	2.9 mm of mandibular "E-space" present per side LDML 1.5 mm right of UDML
Other	—
Diagnosis	Angle Class III subdivision left malocclusion with bilateral posterior open bite

Q: Can you list *all* possible etiologies of Mark's bilateral posterior open bite (presented earlier in this section)? As you list them, suggest whether each could be contributing to his posterior open bite.

A: Possible posterior open bite etiologies include:

- *Interposition tongue habit*: Mark has a "football" shape to his posterior open bites, especially on his left which leads us to suspect that his tongue fits into it and is preventing the posterior teeth from erupting. You should have Mark relax while you talk to his parents, then ask Mark to open his eyes (to distract him) as you quickly/gently separate his lips and check for an interposition tongue habit. This was not done, but a tongue habit could be contributing to his open bite.
- *Digit interposition-sucking habits*: No inquiry was made regarding possible digit habits. This should have been done but was overlooked. A digit-sucking habit could be contributing to his open bite.
- *Temporary posterior open bite occurring while permanent teeth are erupting*: Transient eruption of posterior teeth could be playing a role in Mark's posterior open bite, especially in the first premolar area.
- *Ankylosis of teeth preventing their complete eruption into occlusion:* It looks like the maxillary left primary second molar could be ankylosed and partially contributing to the left posterior open bite.
- *Class III growth* with mandibular incisors "riding down" the maxillary incisor lingual surfaces, creating a posterior open bite: does not explain Mark's significant open bites.
- *Lack of space* for complete tooth eruption (teeth blocked out): Lack of space for the mandibular canines could be contributing to the open bites at those locations, but these are anterior areas.
- *Systemic factors*: Does not apply to Mark.
- *Primary failure of eruption (PFE)*: Since Mark's first permanent molars are in occlusion, this does not appear to be a case of PFE.
- *Treatments for sleep apnea*: Does not apply to Mark.

In summary, an interposition tongue habit, digit-sucking habit, transient eruption of first premolars, and ankylosis of maxillary left second primary molar are probable factors which could be contributing to Mark's posterior open bite. However, the precise posterior open bite etiology remains unknown. Finally, the open bite may be transient, closing with a normal eruption of the permanent canines and premolars.

Q: Let's focus on Mark's (possibly) ankylosed maxillary left *primary* second molar? What are your options for dealing with it?

A: Options include the following:

- Since the maxillary left permanent first molar does not appear to be erupting over the occlusal surface of the maxillary left primary second molar (Figures 5.43f and 5.43n), you could simply monitor the eruption of the maxillary left second premolar. Eruption of the second premolar may be delayed by six months in the case of an ankylosed primary second molar, but the bone level should be normal after the maxillary left second premolar erupts [89–91].
- If the maxillary left permanent first molar begins to erupt over the maxillary left primary second molar (potentially impacting the second premolar), then you may need to tip the maxillary left permanent first molar distally (space regaining) and maintain it there with a Nance holding arch.
- Another option is to extract the maxillary left primary second molar and place a Nance holding arch to maintain the anteroposterior position of the maxillary left permanent first molar. However, since the maxillary left second premolar root (Figure 5.43f) is < ½ developed, this extraction could actually slow its eruption as bone heals over it.

Q: What are Mark's primary problems in each dimension (plus other)?

A:

Table 5.9   Primary problems list for Mark.

AP	Angle Class III subdivision left Iowa Classification: I X X III (1 mm)
Vertical	Bilateral posterior open bite Anterior OB: 50%
Transverse	—
Other	9 mm mandibular anterior crowding

Q: What unknowns exist? What unknowns should you eliminate before you define Mark's final treatment plan or before you do something irreversible (e.g. extract permanent teeth)?

A: *The etiology of both posterior open bites is unknown.* Additional unknowns include Mark's growth (Class III growth due to deficient maxilla?), compliance, an undetected CR-CO shift, and future dentition development.

Q: What treatment, if any, do you recommend for Mark?

A: A decision was made to monitor his posterior open bite for one year. An LLHA was placed so that his mandibular "E-space" could provide room for his erupting mandibular permanent canines. Unfortunately, no attempt was made to check for tongue interposition or digit-sucking habits.

Mark was recalled one year later. At that time, it was noted that his maxillary left primary second molar was not erupting and a periapical radiograph was made (Figure 5.44). We noted that Mark's maxillary left second premolar was resorbing his maxillary left primary second molar roots, but that the maxillary left permanent first molar was *tipping mesially over the primary second molar* (potentially impacting the maxillary left second premolar).

Q: How would you deal with this situation (mesial tipping of the maxillary left first permanent molar over the primary second molar)?

A: The situation could be dealt with by *regaining the space* that was lost. Mark was placed on an asymmetric left headgear to upright/distalize his maxillary left first permanent molar and create space for the maxillary left second premolar to erupt.

Six months later, normal tooth eruption was judged to be occurring. The LLHA was removed, fixed orthodontic appliances were placed, arches were leveled and aligned, headgear discontinued, and a panoramic image was made (Figure 5.45). A posterior open bite was still noted on Mark's left side, and he was asked to wear left posterior vertical elastics to close it. The posterior open bite closed with elastic wear, and Mark was debanded (Figures 5.46a–5.46e).

Q: Let's compare the maxillary right and left second molars seen in Figures 5.43f and 5.45. What difference do you note?

A: Both second molars started at about the same level and developmental stage (Figure 5.43f). However, the

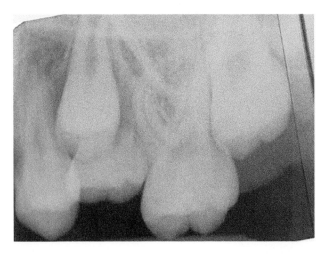

Figure 5.44 One year later, a periapical radiograph was made of Mark's maxillary left primary second molar and erupting permanent second premolar.

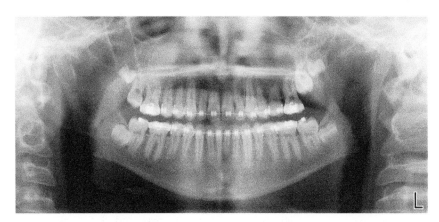

Figure 5.45 Mark's progress panoramic image following leveling and aligning of his dental arches.

(a)

(b)

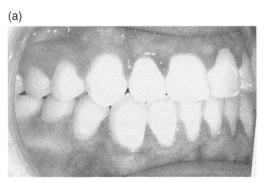

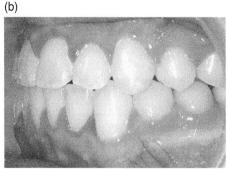

Figure 5.46 (a–e) Deband models of Mark.

(c)

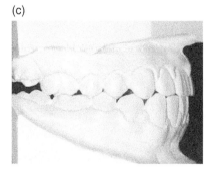

(d)

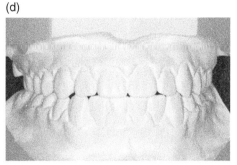

(e)

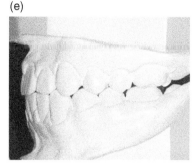

Figure 5.46   (Continued)

maxillary right second molar now appears to be erupting normally while the left is delayed (Figure 5.45).

Q: What could be happening to the maxillary left second molar? What could this be an example of?

A: The maxillary left second molar could be ankylosed or an example of PFE.

Q: What are your options for managing the unerupted maxillary left *permanent* second molar?

A: Options include the following:
- Since Mark exhibits good occlusal interdigitation, the simplest option is to monitor the eruption of the maxillary left second molar. Monitoring reduces your unknowns.
- If you think it is ankylosed, then you could surgically expose it, luxate it to break the bony union, and then attempt to erupt it immediately (before ankylosis recurs). Or, you could extract the ankylosed second molar and allow the maxillary left third molar to erupt and replace it.
- If you think this is an example of PFE, then you could consider:
    1) extracting the maxillary left permanent second molar and replacing it with a bone graft/implant (this option is heroic)
    2) leaving it unerupted and accepting a left first molar occlusion
    3) treating it with a segmental osteotomy or distraction osteogenesis to erupt it (heroic).

Q: Of the above options, how would you manage the unerupted maxillary left permanent second molar?

A: After discussions with Mark and his parents, a decision was made to continue monitoring the maxillary left second molar's eruption.

Q: Three years later, Mark presented for a retention check (Figure 5.47). What do you observe?

A: He has become Class III (2 mm) on the left side. His maxillary left second premolar is "stepped up" compared to his maxillary left first premolar and maxillary left permanent first molar (compare Figures 5.46b and 5.46e to 5.47a and 5.47d).

Q: How (why) did the "step-up" of the maxillary left second premolar occur?

A: Possible reasons include:
- Maxillary left second premolar became ankylosed
- An interposition tongue habit, or other habits, began or continued. This was never evaluated.

Q: Compare the maxillary left second molar vertical position in Figures 5.43f and 5.47a. What do you observe?

A: It appears that the maxillary left second molar has not erupted further.

Q: What treatment options would you consider *now* for the unerupted maxillary left second molar?

A: The options have not changed from three years ago. Please review them from the previous page.

Q: How would you proceed?

A: Mark was offered, and accepted, retreatment. His maxillary left second molar (considered to be ankylosed), and all third molars, were extracted. Both arches were placed in fixed orthodontic appliances, the arches were leveled/aligned, and vertical elastics were worn on the left side to close the open bite.

The left posterior open bite *worsened* (Figures 5.48a–5.48c), and a right-to-left cant of the maxillary arch developed in spite of the fact that Mark wore left vertical elastics. Why did this happen? How do you now recommend proceeding?

The maxillary left "stepped-up" second premolar was very likely ankylosed, and its inclusion in the arch has resulted in the intrusion of the other maxillary left

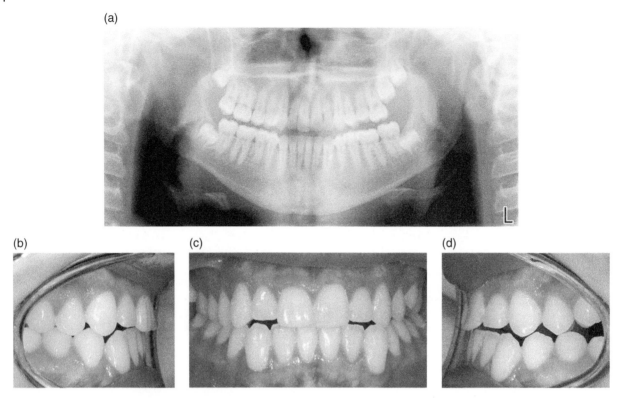

Figure 5.47 Recall records of Mark three years following deband. (a) Three year posttreatment pantomograph. (b–d) Three year posttreatment intraoral photographs.

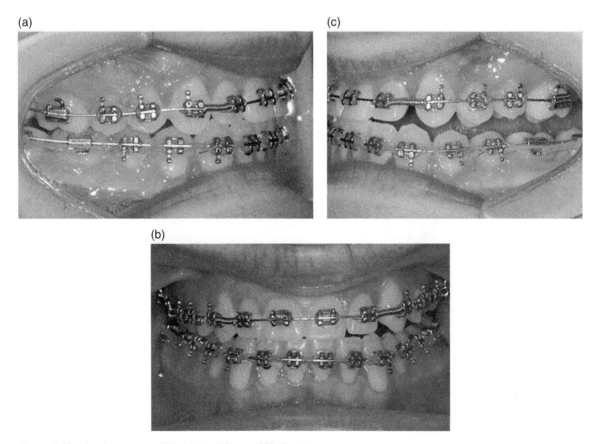

Figure 5.48 (a–c) Re-treatment progress photos of Mark.

posterior teeth and in the right-to-left cant. We removed the maxillary left second premolar bracket and continued with left vertical elastics to try to close the left posterior open bite. Mark was very compliant in wearing his vertical elastics, but the left posterior open bite did not close, and the Class III relationship did not improve.

We told Mark and his parents that late mandibular growth could be occurring, along with the possibility of a tongue-interposition habit, ankylosis of the maxillary left second premolar and first molar, and the possibility of PFE. Since Mark was complying with vertical elastic wear (elastics would block his tongue to the lingual), we did not believe that the cause of the open bite was a tongue-interposition habit. Further, we did not believe that the small amount of Class III growth could cause such a large open bite.

Q: What do you now consider the most likely cause of Mark's left posterior open bite?

A: The most likely cause of the left posterior open bite is *PFE*.

Q: How would you proceed?

A: A discussion was held with Mark and his parents. Genetic testing for PFE was recommended. A decision was made to correct his Class III relationship and close his left posterior open bite *only* to the first premolars (first premolar occlusion).

The maxillary archwire was sectioned distal to the left first premolar to free the arch from the ankylosed left second premolar and first molar. Mark was placed on Class III elastics on the right (elastics worn from the maxillary right first molar to the mandibular right canine), and on the left, he wore a Class III elastic from the maxillary left first premolar to the mandibular left canine. Anterior vertical elastics (triangle elastics) were worn bilaterally.

Within a few months, Mark's occlusion improved dramatically. He was debanded (Figure 5.49). We are not pleased with the excessive distal root tip of his maxillary left canine (Figure 5.49f), and we informed Mark and his parents of multiple teeth exhibiting root resorption.

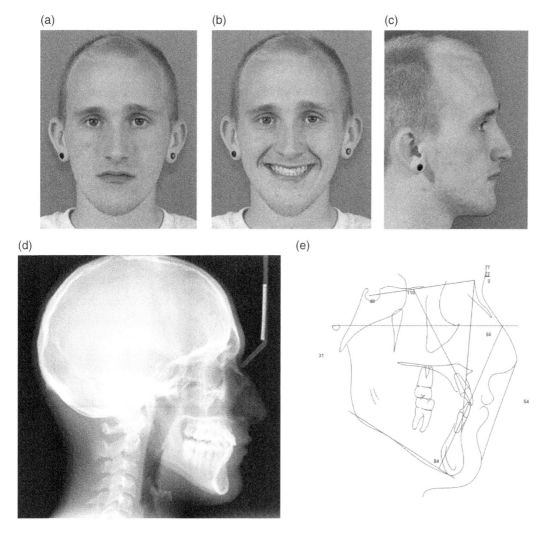

(a) (b) (c)

(d) (e)

Figure 5.49 (a–k) Re-treatment deband records of Mark.

(f)

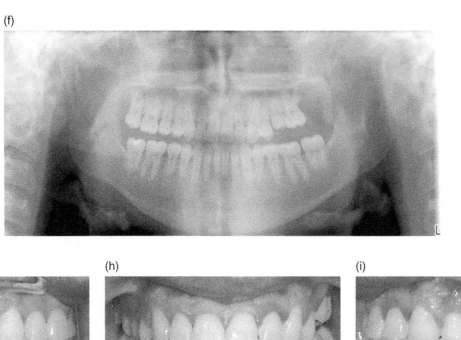

(g) (h) (i)

(j) (k)

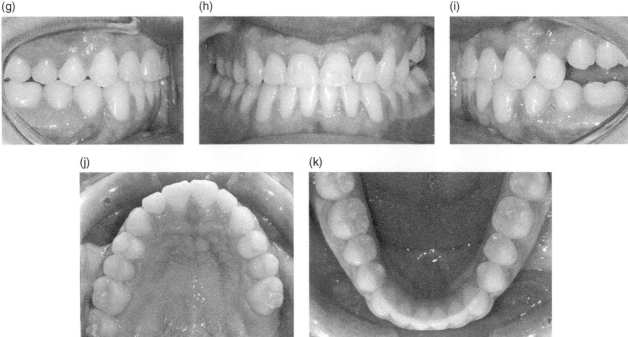

Figure 5.49 (Continued)

Q: Is Mark an example of a posterior open bite due to PFE?

A: *Mark is very likely an example of PFE.* The maxillary left second premolar and the first molar initially erupted but ankylosed during orthodontic treatment. The maxillary left second molar never erupted and was extracted.

Let's look at how PFE features relate to Mark:

- Permanent first molars are always involved: Mark's maxillary left permanent first molar was involved.
- Posterior teeth are more frequently affected: Mark's maxillary left second premolar, first molar, and second molar were affected.
- First and second molars are more frequently affected than premolars and canines: but premolars *can* be affected. Mark's maxillary left second premolar was affected.
- If a tooth in a further anterior position is affected, then more posterior teeth are usually affected as well: all teeth on Mark's maxillary left side distal to the maxillary left first premolar were affected.
- Both primary and permanent teeth can be affected: Mark's maxillary left primary second molar could have been affected.
- The condition is often bilateral: this was not true for Mark.
- Teeth in both arches are often affected: this was not true for Mark.

- Affected teeth resorb the alveolar bone above the crown and may erupt into initial occlusion and then cease to erupt further, or may fail to erupt entirely: Mark's maxillary left second premolar and first molar erupted into occlusion but ceased to erupt later with vertical elastic pull. The maxillary left second molar never erupted into occlusion.

- Involved teeth may be displaced back and forth with manual pressure (indicating that they are not initially ankylosed). However, involved teeth tend to become ankylosed as soon as orthodontic forces are applied. If an eruptive force is applied to the affected teeth, then the force will cause them to ankylose. Mobility of Mark's maxillary second premolar and first molar was never checked. However, even if these teeth were initially mobile, they became ankylosed when erupted forces were applied.

- In cases of PFE, if a small area of ankylosis is broken by manipulating the ankylosed tooth, then it might be possible to move the tooth for a short time. However, re-ankylosis is inevitable. It was wise to discontinue attempts to bring Mark's maxillary left second premolar and first molar into occlusion orthodontically. Freeing these teeth from the rest of the arch allowed his large left open bite to be closed from the first premolars forward.

- Other concurrent skeletal problems (Class III malocclusion for 63% of genetically confirmed PFE patients) and dental anomalies (tooth agenesis, microdontia of maxillary lateral incisors, anomalous root morphology) may be present. Mark exhibited Class III skeletal growth.

- There is much clinical variation seen for PFE owing to possible overlap with other genetic disorders of the eruption mechanism. Mark did not exhibit a "classic" sequence of PFE.

Q: What are your future options for Mark's ankylosed maxillary left second premolar and first molar?

A: Let's consider each possible option:

- Restoring the involved teeth with buildups or crowns after vertical growth is complete: would not be reasonable for Mark because of the large magnitude of the left open bite (Figure 5.49i)

- Extraction of the involved teeth and replacement with bone grafts/implants: would be reasonable, especially if Mark desired more chewing surface on his left side

- Leaving the affected teeth in place and accepting a first premolar occlusion: would be reasonable if Mark is satisfied with his current left occlusion

- Performing a segmental osteotomy or distraction osteogenesis to close the left posterior open bite: this is a possible (heroic) treatment

- Fabrication of a removable prosthetic (overlay) partial denture to provide greater left occlusion: this is a reasonable alternative, although not likely accepted by a young man.

- Of these options, Mark chose to maintain the left first premolar occlusion with a left posterior open bite. He was given Hawley retainers and will wear them at night.

Q: In summary, what are your "take-home pearls" regarding the etiology and early treatment of deep bites, anterior open bites, and posterior open bites?

A: "Take-home pearls" include the following:

- Dental deep bites result from mandibular and maxillary *incisor overeruption* usually in the presence of *normal* vertical facial growth.

- Skeletal deep bites result from a pattern of growth including: more vertical condylar growth, more forward rotation of the mandible (internal rotation), and a combination of maxillary descent and maxillary and mandibular molar eruption associated with the development of relatively more posterior face height and relatively less anterior face height. As the mandible rotates upward and forward, a deep bite results from increased vertical overlap of maxillary and mandibular incisors.

- Skeletal deep bites can present combined with dental deep bites.

- Dental deep bites are treated by: intruding overerupted maxillary and mandibular incisors; proclining anterior teeth (which is desirable if incisors are initially upright but undesirable if incisors are initially proclined); and by eruption of premolars/molars (elimination of a deep curve of Spee) which tends to increase the LAFH and rotate the mandible down and back (worsening a Class II relationship but improving a Class III relationship).

- Skeletal deep bites are treated with orthopedics (attempting to enhance downward maxillary growth plus increasing molar eruption), masking (intruding/proclining anterior teeth and erupting premolars/molars while leveling the curve of Spee), and surgery.

- In our opinion, *most deep bites (dental, skeletal, or a combination) are treated the same way – by intrusion/proclination of anterior teeth plus curve of Spee leveling*.

- Deep bites should be overcorrected to 10% OB in anticipation of post-treatment relapse.

- *We recommend early treatment of deep bites in the presence of palatal impingement with pain, soft tissue damage, or hard tissue damage.* Otherwise, we suggest treating the deep bite later as part of comprehensive orthodontics (adult dentition orthodontics).
- Dental (functional) anterior open bites feature inadequate incisor eruption usually as a result of a tongue-interposition habit (resting tongue habit), digit-sucking habit, or lip-biting habit. The hallmark of a pure dental anterior open bite is an anterior open bite in a patient who is otherwise normal in the vertical dimension.
- Skeletal anterior open bites result from a growth pattern including posterior-superior condylar growth, diminished ramus height growth, less forward mandibular internal rotation or even backward internal rotation, a maxilla which may descend more than normal (palatal plane may rotate down posteriorly), and molars which often erupt more than normal. As the mandible rotates downward and backward, the MPA steepens, the anterior face height increases, and an anterior open bite may result – depending upon the influence of the tongue/lips in preventing anterior tooth-compensatory dental eruption. When facial soft tissue growth does not keep pace with vertical skeletal growth, an ILG results.
- Skeletal open bites can present combined with dental open bites.
- Dental (functional) anterior open bites are corrected by eliminating the habit and erupting anterior teeth into occlusion.
- *We recommend early dental open bite treatment through habit control when the patient is interested in stopping the habit.* Otherwise, we generally wait until the child matures.
- Skeletal anterior open bites are treated with orthopedics, masking, or surgery. Orthopedic treatment of skeletal anterior open bites consists of restricting maxillary downward growth plus reducing/halting maxillary and mandibular molar eruption (or intruding molars). Masking treatment consists of erupting anterior teeth and ignoring the LLAFH. The intrusion of posterior teeth with TADs offers tremendous potential in correcting skeletal open bites without headgears, bite plates, or even surgery.
- *We recommend attempting early (orthopedic) treatment of skeletal open bites in mild-to-moderate cases only. We have found skeletal open bite cases to be very challenging* and successful in only the most cooperative children. Childhood TAD-supported intrusion of posterior teeth will likely change this in the future.

- When a patient presents with some skeletal open bite features, we recommend treating them as if they had all the skeletal open bite features. It is always better to prepare for the worst and hope for the best.
- When skeletal open bite orthopedics is attempted, discussions of future "fallback" options (contingency plans, including masking or surgery) should be discussed with the parents in the event that orthopedics fails. Orthopedics requires years of treatment and frequently leads to patient burnout.
- Anterior open bites should be overcorrected to 20–40% OB in anticipation of relapse, and the correction should be held for some time, before debanding. Monitor your patient in retention for as long as possible. We recommend retaining with clear aligners to take advantage of the posterior bite plate effect of the retainer material thickness to slow/halt residual posterior tooth eruption.
- Posterior open bites can result from a range of causes, including interposition tongue posture habits, digit-sucking habits, the transition from mixed-to-permanent dentition, ankylosis of teeth which prevents their eruption into occlusion, lack of space for complete tooth eruption (teeth blocked out), systemic factors found in patients with certain syndromes, PFE, and Class III growth resulting in edge-to-edge incisors. The hallmark of posterior open bites is anterior tooth contact in the absence of posterior occlusal contact at one or more teeth. The patient is otherwise normal in the vertical dimension.
- Treatment of posterior open bites consists of erupting posterior teeth until they are in occlusion. If a habit caused an open bite, then the habit must be eliminated. Orthodontic eruption of posterior teeth could include using fixed appliances with posterior vertical elastics or leveling a curve of Spee with archwires (to erupt premolars/molars). Other treatments include prosthodontics or surgery.
- Closure of posterior open bites, and retention of closed posterior open bites, can be one of the most difficult problems an orthodontist can face. Tell your patient that you may not be able to close, or to keep closed, a posterior open bite. Tell them to expect relapse and the possible need for retreatment. Retain your patient for life.
- *We recommend early posterior open bite treatment through habit control if the open bite is due to a tongue-interposition habit or digit habit – if the patient is interested in stopping the habit.* Early treatment of posterior open bites due to other causes must be considered on a case-by-case basis and addressing the etiology, as discussed earlier.

Case Lynnear

Q: Lynnear is a six-year-old girl (Figure 5.50), who presents for a consultation with her parent's chief complaint, "Our dentist says Lynnear's mouth is too small, and she bites the roof of her mouth." Her mother gives you her smartphone with a blurred picture showing what appears to be the incisive papilla of a maxillary palate. She says that the swelling resulted from Lynnear biting on the roof of her mouth. PMH and TMJ evaluations are WRN. CR=CO. *Compile your diagnostic findings and problem list.* State your *diagnosis.*

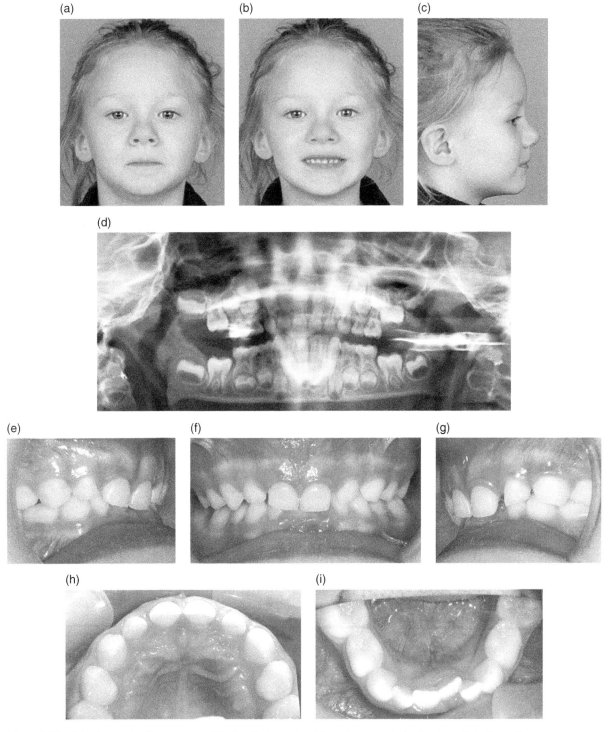

Figure 5.50   Initial records of Lynnear. (a–c) facial photographs; (d) pantomograph; (e–i) intraoral photographs.

A:

Table 5.10 Diagnostic findings and problem list for Lynnear.

Full face and Profile	***Frontal View*** Face is symmetric LAFH WRN (soft tissue Glabella – Subnasale = Subnasale – soft tissue Menton) Lip competence UDML to the right of facial midline by 1–2 mm Excess gingival display in posed smile ***Profile View*** Straight profile Upturned nasal tip Obtuse NLA Chin projection WRN Lip-chin-throat angle WRN Chin-throat length WRN
Radiographs	Early mixed dentition (mandibular permanent central incisors are erupted)
Intraoral Photos	Angle Class I Iowa Classification I I I I OJ 0 mm OB 100% (palatal impingement) Maxillary primary central incisors are overerupted Mandibular anterior labial keratinized attached gingivae WRN 4 mm of maxillary anterior spacing currently present 0.8 mm of maxillary arch crowding is anticipated following the eruption of all permanent teeth (if appropriate space maintenance is employed) 3 mm mandibular anterior crowding currently present 2.6 mm of mandibular arch crowding is anticipated following the eruption of all permanent teeth (if appropriate space maintenance is employed)
Other	—
Diagnosis	Class I malocclusion with 100% deep bite and mild mandibular anterior crowding

Q: Lynnear is six years old with an upturned nasal tip, adequate chin projection, and adequate chin-throat length. What changes do you anticipate in her nasal tip, chin projection, and chin-throat length as she grows and develops?

A: We anticipate that Lynnear's nasal tip angle will *decrease* with age [92] and both her chin projection and chin-throat length will *increase* with age [93].

Q: When you have Lynnear bring her teeth into occlusion, it appears that her mandibular central incisors *are* contacting her palatal gingiva. However, Lynnear states that the roof of her mouth *does not hurt* when she brings her teeth into occlusion. Looking closely at Figure 5.50h, do you see any soft tissue trauma? What do you tell Lynnear's mother?

A: The incisive papilla does not appear to be swollen. There is a slight tissue indentation along the anterior aspect of the incisive papilla. You confirm that this indentation is where the incisal edge of the mandibular right permanent central incisor makes contact in centric occlusion.

You should tell her mom that Lynnear's mandibular incisors appear to be occluding with the palate when she bites, but it is occurring at the same time all the other mandibular teeth are contacting their antagonists, so the tissue is being indented but not traumatized. The enlarged tissue she sees (the incisive papilla) is normal anatomy.

Q: Provide a detailed space analysis for Lynnear's maxillary and mandibular arches. How were the 0.8 mm of maxillary arch crowding and 2.6 mm of mandibular arch crowding calculated (if space maintenance is employed)?

A:

Average mesiodistal widths of permanent teeth (mm): [94]

Maxillary Central Incisor	8.5	Mandibular Central Incisor	5.0
Maxillary Lateral Incisor	6.5	Mandibular Lateral Incisor	5.5
Maxillary Canine	7.5	Mandibular Canine	7.0
Maxillary First Premolar	7.0	Mandibular First Premolar	7.0
Maxillary Second Premolar	7.0	Mandibular Second Premolar	7.0
Maxillary First Molar	10.0	Mandibular First Molar	11.0
Maxillary Second Molar	9.0	Mandibular Second Molar	10.5

Average mesiodistal widths of *primary* teeth (mm): [94]

Maxillary Central Incisor	6.5	Mandibular Central Incisor	4.2
Maxillary Lateral Incisor	5.1	Mandibular Lateral Incisor	4.1
Maxillary Canine	7.0	Mandibular Canine	5.0
Maxillary First Molar	7.3	Mandibular First Molar	7.7
Maxillary Second Molar	8.2	Mandibular Second Molar	9.9

MAXILLARY ARCH (permanent incisors are unerupted)

+4 mm of maxillary anterior spacing currently present (Figure 5.30h)

+5.1 mm primary maxillary right lateral incisor width

−6.5 mm permanent maxillary right lateral incisor width anticipated

+6.5 mm primary maxillary right central incisor width

−8.5 mm permanent maxillary right central incisor width anticipated

+6.5 mm primary maxillary left central incisor width

−8.5 mm permanent maxillary left central incisor width anticipated

+5.1 mm primary maxillary left lateral incisor width

−6.5 mm permanent maxillary left lateral incisor width anticipated

+2 mm of anticipated leeway space (1 mm/side)

Balance = +4 mm +5.1 mm −6.5 mm +6.5 mm −8.5 mm +6.5 mm −8.5 mm +5.1 mm −6.5 mm +2 mm = −0.8 mm

MANDIBULAR ARCH (permanent lateral incisors are unerupted)

−3 mm of anterior crowding is currently present

+4.1 mm primary mandibular left lateral incisor width

−5.5 mm permanent mandibular left lateral incisor width anticipated

+4.1 mm primary mandibular right lateral incisor width

−5.5 mm permanent mandibular right lateral incisor width anticipated

+3.2 mm of anticipated leeway space (1.6 mm per side)

Balance = −3 mm +4.1 mm −5.5 mm +4.1 mm −5.5 mm +3.6 mm = −2.6 mm

That is, *0.8 mm of maxillary arch crowding and 2.6 mm of mandibular arch crowding is anticipated following the eruption of all permanent teeth (if proper space maintenance is employed).*

Q: What would you say are Lynnear's *primary* problems that you must stay focused on?

A:

Table 5.11   Primary problem list for Lynnear.

AP	—
Vertical	100% deep bite (palatal impingement of mandibular incisors)
	Overeruption of maxillary primary central incisors
Transverse	—
Other	—

Q: Discuss Lynnear in the context of three principles, which should be applied to every early treatment patient.

A:

1) The goal of early treatment is to correct developing problems – get the patient *back to normal for their stage of development* (including preventing complications such as resorption of adjacent tooth roots, reducing later treatment complexity, or reducing/eliminating unknowns). Improving Lynnear's deep bite by intruding maxillary incisors would put her back on track for her stage of development. Intruding her mandibular incisors would prevent palatal pain/tissue trauma when biting.

2) Early treatment should address *very specific problems with a clearly defined end point*, usually begun and ended within six to nine months (not protracted over many years except for some orthopedic problems). Placing limited fixed orthodontic appliances in the maxillary and mandibular arches in order to level the arches, intrude incisors, and correct her deep bite addresses a focused problem which could be corrected in less than nine months.

3) Always ask: Is it necessary that I treat the patient early? *What harm will come if I choose to do nothing now?* Currently, there is no tissue damage from mandibular incisor palatal impingement, and Lynnear denies having pain when she bites. If her mandibular incisor palatal impingement is not corrected, then we cannot guarantee the absence of future palatal tissue damage or pain. We could ask Lynnear to tell her mother if she ever does have pain when biting, but for now, no harm will come from monitoring only.

Q: Is Lynnear's mouth *too small*?

A: No. Lynnear does not exhibit *microstomia* (reduction in oral aperture size affecting appearance, function, or quality of life). Furthermore, with timely space maintenance, we anticipate that Lynnear will have only 0.8 mm of crowding in her maxillary arch and 2.6 mm of crowding in the mandibular arch. Of course, the final crowding values will depend upon the actual size of her erupted permanent teeth. Lynnear does not have a small mouth.

Q: What treatment options would you consider for Lynnear?

A: Options include the following:
   • *Recall* (no treatment, monitor only) – is a viable option especially since Lynnear denies having pain when

biting and since her palatal tissue appears normal. You should speak to her mother and ask her mother to report to you any future palatal pain on biting. If it does not occur, then recall Lynnear in one year.

- *Wearing a clear vacuum-formed maxillary retainer* – is a viable option and would eliminate mandibular incisor impingement on the palatal soft tissue. If the retainer covers *only the maxillary anterior teeth and palate* (not the maxillary posterior teeth), then the maxillary posterior teeth will erupt – opening the bite. Note: Lynnear will be exfoliating primary anterior teeth soon, so you should anticipate making a series of these retainers over the next year to fit her permanent teeth.

- *Improve her deep bite using fixed orthodontic appliances to intrude her maxillary and mandibular incisors* – is not recommended for a number of reasons. Intruding primary incisors may have an undesirable effect on the position of the developing permanent incisor crowns, or cause premature exfoliation of the primary incisors due to the intrusion forces accelerating their root resorption. Moreover, the vertical incisor overbite of her permanent maxillary incisors cannot be predictably influenced by this approach nor can retention of this improvement. Simply put, it is best to address deep incisor overbite by modifying anteroposterior and vertical positions of *permanent* incisors after they erupt.

Finally, Lynnear's palatal impingement is due, in part, to overeruption of mandibular permanent central incisors. If we chose to intrude these now, then we must maintain our appliances until we can include the mandibular permanent lateral incisors to influence their vertical position. This creates a need for an extended treatment time and is not aligned with our principle of focused early treatment of short duration.

- *Space maintenance* – placing an LLHA and/or Nance holding arch is not recommended at this time. Why? It will be years before Lynnear begins to exfoliate her primary canines and primary first molars.

Q: What treatment do you recommend at this consultation?

A: Discussions were held with Lynnear and her mom. Since Lynnear is not in pain and her palatal tissues appear normal, a decision was made to recall her in one year. Mom promised to notify us if Lynnear complains of pain upon biting.

Case Sydney

Q: Sydney (Figure 5.51) is ten years old and presents for a consultation with her parents' chief complaint, "Sydney's teeth hit the roof of her mouth, and she says it hurts." PMH and TMJ evaluations are WRN. CR=CO. *Compile your diagnostic findings and problem list*. State your *diagnosis*.

(a) (b) (c)

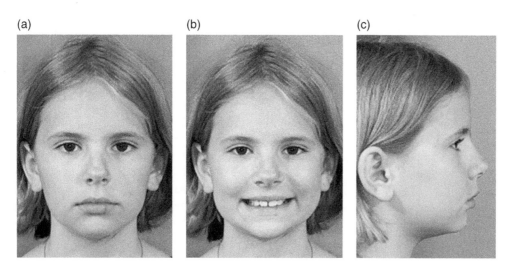

Figure 5.51 Initial records of Sydney: (a–c) facial photographs; (d) pantomograph; (e–j) intraoral photographs.

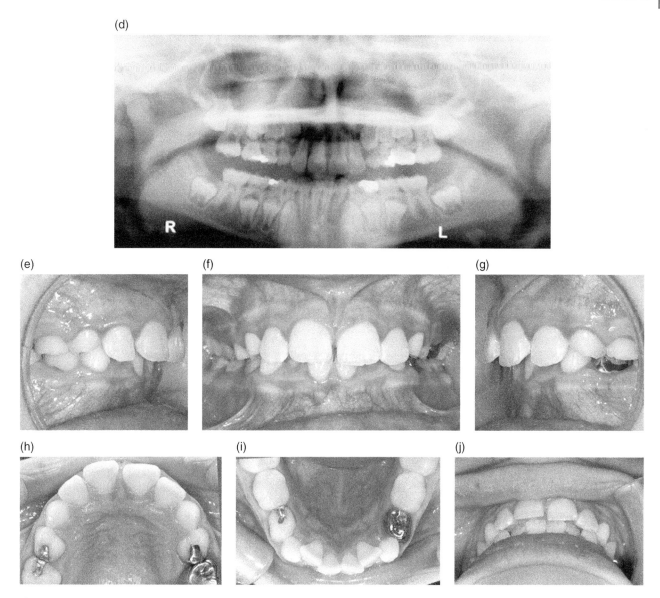

(d)

(e) (f) (g)

(h) (i) (j)

Figure 5.51   (Continued)

A:

Table 5.12   Diagnostic findings and problem list for Sydney.

Full face and Profile	***Frontal View*** Face is symmetric LAFH WRN (soft tissue Glabella – Subnasale = Subnasale – soft tissue Menton) Lip competence UDML WRN Incisal display inadequate in posed smile (gingival margin should be congruent with maxillary lip border) Large buccal corridors ***Profile View*** Convex profile Upturned nasal tip

Table 5.12 (Continued)

	Obtuse NLA
	Chin projection inadequate (chin positioned behind zero-meridian line)
	Obtuse lip-chin-throat angle
Radiographs	Early mixed dentition
Intraoral Photos	Angle Class I
	Iowa Classification I I I I
	Maxillary midline diastema
	Thick maxillary midline labial frenum
	OJ 2–3 mm
	OB 100% (mandibular incisors occluding with palate)
	Maxillary incisors are stepped down relative to posterior teeth
	Mandibular incisors are stepped up relative to occlusal plane of mandibular posterior teeth (Figure 5.51d)
	LDML and UDML are coincident
	Only a minimal band of keratinized attached tissue exists labial to the mandibular central incisors
	1.5 mm of maxillary anterior spacing currently present
	3.5 mm of maxillary arch spacing is anticipated following the eruption of all permanent teeth (if appropriate space maintenance is employed)
	4 mm mandibular anterior crowding currently present
	0.8 mm of mandibular arch crowding is anticipated following the eruption of all permanent teeth (if appropriate space maintenance is employed)
	—
Diagnosis	Class I malocclusion in the early mixed dentition
	Deep (100%) incisor overbite
	Moderate mandibular permanent incisor crowding with adequate leeway space anticipated

Q: Looking closely at Figure 5.51h, do you see evidence of soft tissue trauma resulting from mandibular incisor impingement?

A: It is difficult to tell. The tissue on either side of the incisive papilla appears erythematous. When we pressed down lightly on these areas, Sydney said it felt sore. But there does not appear to be any overt soft tissue damage.

Q: Provide a detailed space analysis for Sydney's maxillary and mandibular arches. How were the 3.5 mm of maxillary arch spacing and 0.8 mm of mandibular arch crowding calculated (if space maintenance is employed)?

A:

Average mesiodistal widths of permanent teeth (mm): [94]

Maxillary Central Incisor	8.5	Mandibular Central Incisor	5.0
Maxillary Lateral Incisor	6.5	Mandibular Lateral Incisor	5.5
Maxillary Canine	7.5	Mandibular Canine	7.0
Maxillary First Premolar	7.0	Mandibular First Premolar	7.0
Maxillary Second Premolar	7.0	Mandibular Second Premolar	7.0
Maxillary First Molar	10.0	Mandibular First Molar	11.0
Maxillary Second Molar	9.0	Mandibular Second Molar	10.5

Average mesiodistal widths of *primary* teeth (mm): [94]

Maxillary Central Incisor	6.5	Mandibular Central Incisor	4.2
Maxillary Lateral Incisor	5.1	Mandibular Lateral Incisor	4.1
Maxillary Canine	7.0	Mandibular Canine	5.0
Maxillary First Molar	7.3	Mandibular First Molar	7.7
Maxillary Second Molar	8.2	Mandibular Second Molar	9.9

MAXILLARY ARCH

+1.5 mm of maxillary anterior spacing currently present (Figure 5.51h)
+2 mm of anticipated leeway space (1 mm/side)
Balance = +1.5 mm + 2 mm = +3.5 mm

MANDIBULAR ARCH

−4 mm of anterior crowding is currently present (Figure 5.51i)
+3.2 mm of anticipated leeway space (1.6 mm per side)
Balance = −4 mm +3.2 mm = −0.8 mm

That is, *3.5 mm of maxillary arch spacing and 0.8 mm of mandibular arch crowding is anticipated following the eruption of all permanent teeth (if proper space maintenance is employed).*

Q: What would you say are Sydney's *primary* problems that you must stay focused on?

A:

Table 5.13 Primary problem list for Sydney.

AP	—
Vertical	100% deep bite (palatal impingement)
	Overeruption of maxillary and mandibular incisors
Transverse	—
Other	Moderate mandibular permanent incisor crowding

Q: Discuss Sydney in the context of three principles, which should be applied to every early treatment patient.

A:

1) The goal of early treatment is to correct developing problems – get the patient *back to normal for their stage of development* (including preventing complications such as resorption of adjacent tooth roots, reducing later treatment complexity, or reducing/eliminating unknowns). Correcting Sydney's deep bite by intruding her maxillary and mandibular permanent incisors would put her back on track for her stage of development and eliminate palatal pain when biting. Mandibular space maintenance would improve her moderate (4 mm) crowding via leeway space.

2) Early treatment should address *very specific problems with a clearly defined end point*, usually begun and ended within six to nine months (not protracted over many years except for some orthopedic problems). Sydney's deep bite with mandibular incisor palatal impingement could be corrected with fixed orthodontic appliances (2×4 appliances) in six to nine months by intruding her incisors plus erupting her permanent first molars.

3) Always ask: Is it necessary that I treat the patient early? *What harm will come if I choose to do nothing now?* Sydney's palatal irritation will continue, or worsen, if her deep bite is not corrected.

Q: We noted that Sydney has large buccal corridors (Figure 5.51b, dark spaces between posterior teeth and cheeks). Should we consider the maxillary expansion to reduce these dark spaces?

A: *Large* buccal corridors in the permanent dentition are considered unesthetic by laypersons, and large buccal corridors should be noted in your problem list. If large buccal corridors exist because a maxilla is constricted and the patient is in posterior crossbite, then you should consider expanding the maxilla in order to correct the crossbite and reduce the buccal corridors. If large buccal corridors exist because a maxilla is constricted and the patient has significant posterior [95] dental compensations (labial maxillary molar torque, lingual mandibular molar torque), then you should consider expanding the maxilla to make posterior OJ in order to eliminate compensations and reduce the buccal corridors.

We consider Sydney's maxilla to be mildly constricted, but she is not in crossbite and does not exhibit significant transverse dental compensations. We decided *not* to address her buccal corridors at this time but to re-evaluate them once her permanent posterior teeth had erupted.

Q: We note Sydney has a thick maxillary midline labial frenum. How do we classify the inferior attachment point of this frenum?

A: The most common attachment point is at the mucogingival junction, termed *mucosal* attachment. The attachment below the mucogingival junction into the keratinized attached gingivae is termed *gingival* attachment. The attachment to the interdental papilla is termed *papillary* attachment. Finally, the attachment that penetrates the interdental papilla and inserts into the premaxillary alveolar crest or the incisive papilla is termed *papillary penetrating* [96].

Q: How would you classify Sydney's maxillary midline labial frenum?

A: Looking at Figure 5.51f, Sydney's frenum attachment is *papillary*. Looking at Figure 5.51h, it may also be *papillary penetrating*. One accepted clinical test for the presence of papillary penetrating attachment is the blanching test. This is accomplished by pulling the upper lip to stretch the frenum and simultaneously inspecting whether or not the incisive papilla is blanching [97]. This was not done for Sydney.

Q: Does Sydney's maxillary midline frenum require treatment now?

A: No. It requires monitoring during growth. The maxillary midline frenum is a dynamic structure, and can change in size, shape, and position during growth. With the eruption and vertical drift of the maxillary incisors, and the associated growth and vertical drift of the maxillary alveolar process, the maxillary midline frenum generally displays a more superior insertion point with time [98].

Q: Will Sydney's maxillary midline frenum impede the closure of her maxillary midline diastema as she transitions to the adolescent dentition?

A: Possibly. One histologic study suggests that when a frenum attachment is papillary penetrating, the fibers of the frenum disrupt the transseptal fiber arrangement at the midline which impedes normal diastema closure by the transseptal fiber system [99].

If we do not provide early treatment for Sydney, then we will monitor her frenum and be able to observe any effect on diastema closure. If the diastema does not close as she develops her adolescent dentition (especially permanent canine eruption), then we will close it during comprehensive orthodontic treatment. We will monitor during treatment and retention for evidence of tissue bunching in the area of the midline papilla, or a tendency for relapse of the diastema. If either of these issues arises, then we may refer to Sydney for a frenectomy. Our recommendation is to consider frenectomy as an option *after* orthodontic treatment, not before [100]. Also, if the midline diastema does not close spontaneously during the permanent canine eruption, and must be closed with orthodontics, then we recommend retaining its closure with a fixed lingual retainer.

Q: What treatment options would you consider for Sydney?
A: Options include the following:
- *Recall* (no early treatment, monitor) – is reasonable if Sydney feels that the irritation/pain from mandibular incisor palatal impingement is mild and occasional. You could show mom and Sydney (with a mouth mirror) what the palatal tissue looks like and ask them to keep an eye on it. Tell them that you will correct the deep bite during comprehensive orthodontic treatment after permanent canines and premolars erupt. However, if Sydney states that the pain is moderate and occurs every time she bites, then corrective early treatment *now* would be recommended.
- *Wearing a clear vacuum-formed maxillary retainer* – is a viable option and would immediately reduce/eliminate mandibular incisor impingement on the palatal soft tissue. If the retainer covered only the maxillary anterior teeth and palate, then the posterior teeth would be slightly separated and with full-time wear, the posterior teeth would erupt and open the bite.

- *Opening her bite with fixed appliances* – is a viable option if her biting irritation/pain was frequent/moderate or if her incisor palatal impingement was causing tissue damage. If her bite was opened with fixed appliances, then she would need to wear retainers at night to prevent the deep bite from recurring.
- *Space maintenance* – placing an LLHA is recommended to reduce her moderate mandibular anterior crowding using leeway space (mandibular permanent canine and premolar root development is ≥ half complete and these teeth are erupting). However, if a mandibular 2×4 appliance is used to intrude Sydney's incisors, then the LLHA should be fabricated/placed after the incisors are intruded.

Q: Based upon these options, what treatment do you recommend for Sydney at this consultation?
A: Sydney's situation differs from that of Lynnear (our previous patient). Sydney is older, all her permanent incisors have erupted, and her permanent canines and premolars should erupt within ~one year.

We discussed options with Sydney and her mom. Sydney feels that the irritation/pain from mandibular incisor palatal impingement is mild and occasional. We gave Sydney a clear maxillary vacuum-formed retainer (covering anterior teeth and palate only) which she will wear occasionally when her palate is irritated. We will correct her deep bite/incisor palatal impingement later using fixed appliances during comprehensive orthodontic treatment. This will be performed as soon as all her permanent canines and premolars erupt. We also recommended placement of an LLHA now.

Case Ned

Q: Ned is an eleven-year-old boy (Figure 5.52) who presents to you with his parent's chief complaint, "Ned needs orthodontics. He bites the roof of his mouth, and it hurts." His PMH, PDH, periodontal evaluation, and TMJ evaluation are WRN. He exhibits a right 1–2 mm CR-CO shift. Compile your diagnostic findings and problem list. Also state your diagnosis.

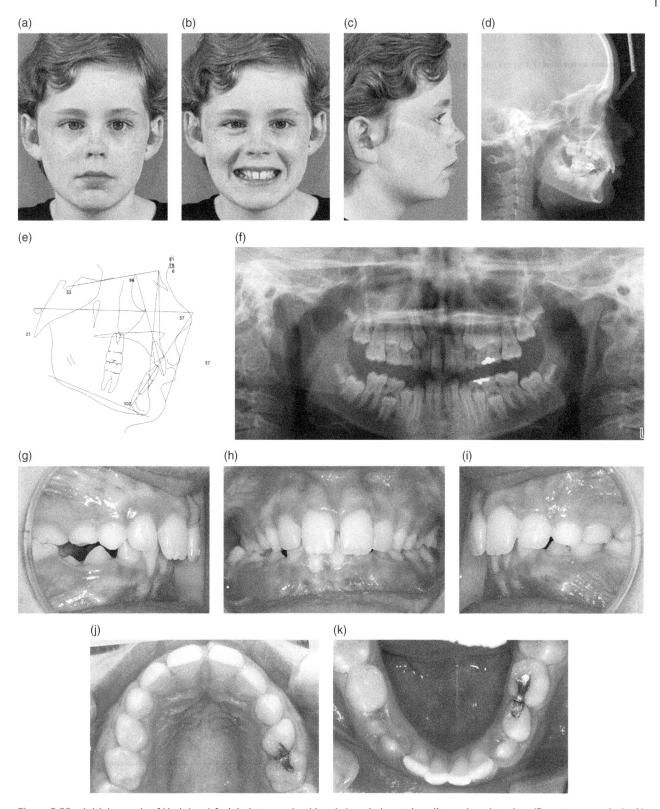

Figure 5.52 Initial records of Ned: (a–c) facial photographs; (d and e) cephalometric radiograph and tracing; (f) pantomograph; (g–k) intraoral photographs; (l–w) models.

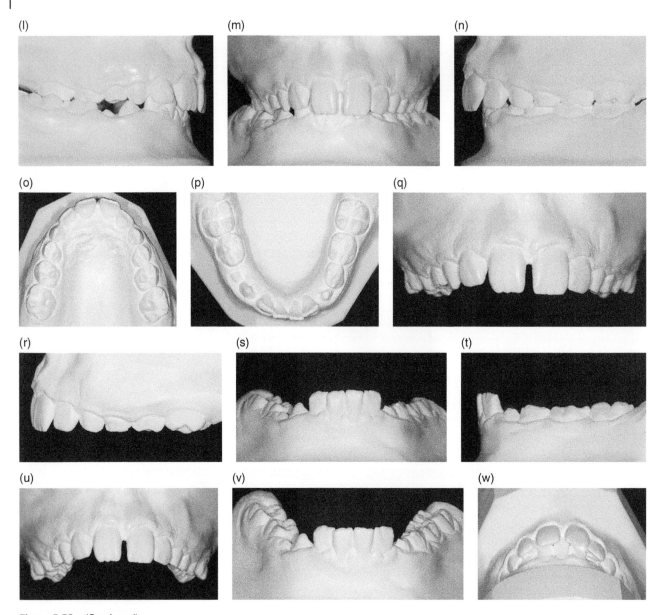

Figure 5.52 (Continued)

A:

Table 5.14 Diagnostic findings and problem list for Ned.

Full face and Profile	***Frontal View***
	Mild chin deviation to right in CO (Figure 5.52a)
	Medial strabismus of the right eye
	Long soft tissue LAFH (soft tissue Glabella – Subnasale < Subnasale – soft tissue Menton)
	Lip competence
	UDML left ~2 mm of facial midline
	Gingival display in posed smile slightly excessive (maxillary central incisor gingival margins slightly below the maxillary lip border)
	Large buccal corridors

Table 5.14 (Continued)

	Profile View
	Convex profile
	Upturned nose
	Obtuse NLA
	Protrusive lower lip
	Deep labiomental sulcus
	Mildly retrusive chin
	Obtuse lip-chin-throat angle
Ceph Analysis	***Skeletal***
	Maxillary anteroposterior position WRN (A-Point slightly ahead of Nasion-perpendicular line, but maxillary incisors are upright)
	Mandible is deficient anteroposteriorly (ANB angle = 6° with normal maxilla)
	Skeletal LAFH WRN (ANS-Menton/Nasion-Menton × 100% = 57%; normal = 55% with s.d. = 2%)
	Mandibular plane WRN (FMA = 21°; SNMP = 32°)
	Effective bony Pogonion (Pogonion ahead of line through N-B)
	Dental
	Upright maxillary incisors (U1 to SN = 96°). However, Sella is low (FH-SN = 11° instead of 7°) which makes U1-SN less. Proclined mandibular incisors (FMIA = 57°)
Radiographs	Late mixed dentition
Intraoral Photos and Models	Angle Class II division 2 malocclusion
	Iowa Classification: II (6 mm) II (6 mm) II (2 mm) II (3 mm)
	OJ ~ 3–4 mm
	OB 100% (palatal impingement)
	1.5 mm maxillary central diastema
	3.5 mm maxillary arch spacing anticipated following the eruption of all permanent teeth (if proper space maintenance is employed)
	1.0 mm of mandibular incisor crowding is currently present
	5.5 mm of mandibular arch spacing is anticipated following the eruption of all permanent teeth (if proper space maintenance is employed)
	Maxillary arch asymmetry – right side slightly ahead
	Right posterior lingual crossbite
	LDML to right of UDML by ~ 2–3 mm
	Stepped up mandibular incisors (Figures 5.52s–5.52t)
	Stepped down maxillary central incisors
	Posterior transverse compensations (Figures 5.52q and 5.52s, maxillary first permanent molar buccal crown torque, mandibular first permanent molar lingual crown torque)
Other	None
Diagnosis	Class II malocclusion with right posterior lingual crossbite and 100% OB

Q: Why would Ned's upright maxillary incisors lead us to conclude that his maxillary anteroposterior position was WRN?

A: As we noted, A-Point is slightly ahead of Nasion-perpendicular line (maxilla slightly ahead of normal). However, Ned's maxillary incisors are upright which makes A-point positioned forward. In other words, the root apices of the maxillary central incisors are positioned forward relative to the maxillary central incisor crowns (maxillary central incisor labial root torque/lingual crown torque; see Figure 5.52d).

Let's assume the equal forward movement of Nasion and A-point during Ned's continuing growth. If we improve maxillary incisor inclination, then the root apices will move posteriorly relative to the crowns, A-point will follow the root apices, and A-point will be more in line with Nasion-perpendicular.

In other words, Ned's upright maxillary incisors are the reason A-point lies slightly ahead of Nasion-perpendicular (Figure 5.52d). His maxillary anteroposterior position is WRN.

Q: Ned has a protrusive lower lip and deep labiomental sulcus. Can you identify two factors contributing to these features?

A: His lower lip is "trapped" or pushed down and forward by his maxillary incisors (Figure 5.52d) because he is Class II (secondary-to-mandibular deficiency) with a deep bite. This lip trapping creates a deep labiomental sulcus and protruded lower lip. His proclined mandibular incisors add to the lower lip protrusion.

Q: How would you classify Ned's maxillary midline frenum?

A: Ned has a *papillary attachment* of his maxillary frenum (Figures 5.52h and 5.52j). We cannot confirm that it penetrates the papilla, as pulling the lip to check for incisive papilla blanching was not done [96].

Q: Do Ned's maxillary midline frenum and diastema need treatment now?

A: No. We will monitor his frenum during growth and treatment. If during retention after comprehensive treatment, there is evidence of tissue bunching in the area of the midline papilla or incisive papilla, or a tendency for relapse of the diastema, then we may refer Ned for a frenectomy [99, 100].

We will monitor the closure of his midline diastema during the maxillary permanent canine eruption. If the midline diastema must be closed orthodontically during comprehensive treatment, then we will place a maxillary fixed lingual retainer to maintain its closure.

Q: Provide a detailed space analysis for Ned's maxillary and mandibular arches. In other words, how were the anticipated 3.5 mm maxillary arch spacing and 5.5 mm mandibular arch spacing calculated *(if proper space maintenance is employed)*?

A:

Average mesiodistal widths of permanent teeth (mm): [94]

Maxillary Central Incisor	8.5	Mandibular Central Incisor	5.0
Maxillary Lateral Incisor	6.5	Mandibular Lateral Incisor	5.5
Maxillary Canine	7.5	Mandibular Canine	7.0
Maxillary First Premolar	7.0	Mandibular First Premolar	7.0
Maxillary Second Premolar	7.0	Mandibular Second Premolar	7.0
Maxillary First Molar	10.0	Mandibular First Molar	11.0
Maxillary Second Molar	9.0	Mandibular Second Molar	10.5

Average mesiodistal widths of *primary* teeth (mm): [94]

Maxillary Central Incisor	6.5	Mandibular Central Incisor	4.2
Maxillary Lateral Incisor	5.1	Mandibular Lateral Incisor	4.1
Maxillary Canine	7.0	Mandibular Canine	5.0
Maxillary First Molar	7.3	Mandibular First Molar	7.7
Maxillary Second Molar	8.2	Mandibular Second Molar	9.9

MAXILLARY ARCH
+1.5 mm maxillary diastema (Figure 5.52j)
+2 mm of anticipated leeway space (1 mm/side)
Balance = +1.5 mm +2 mm = +3.5 mm

MANDIBULAR ARCH (permanent canines and right first premolar appear to have adequate room to erupt; leeway space cannot be used because primary canines and primary right first molar have exfoliated).
−1.0 mm incisor crowding (Figure 5.52k)
+2.9 mm left mandibular "E space" (difference in mesiodistal widths between mandibular left primary second molar and mandibular left second premolar, or 9.9 mm – 7.0 mm = 2.9 mm).
+7.7 mm mesiodistal width of the left primary first molar
−7.0 mm anticipated mesiodistal width of the left first premolar
+2.9 mm right mandibular "E space"
Balance = −1.0 mm +2.9 mm +7.7 mm −7.0 mm +2.9 mm = +5.5 mm

That is, *3.5 mm of maxillary arch spacing and 5.5 mm of mandibular arch spacing is anticipated following the eruption of all permanent teeth (if proper space maintenance is employed).*

Q: What are Ned's *primary* problems in each dimension, plus other problems?

A:

Table 5.15 Primary problems list for Ned.

AP	Angle Class II division 2 malocclusion
	Iowa Classification: II (6 mm) II (6 mm) II (2 mm) II (3 mm)
	Mandibular anteroposterior skeletal deficiency
Vertical	OB 100% (palatal impingement with pain)
Transverse	Right posterior lingual crossbite with a right lateral CR-CO shift of 1–2 mm
Other	Maxillary arch asymmetry – right slightly ahead

Q: Discuss Ned in the context of three principles applied to every early treatment patient.

A:

1) The goal of early treatment is to correct developing problems – get the patient *back to normal for their stage of development* (including preventing complications such as resorption of adjacent tooth roots, reducing later treatment complexity, or reducing/eliminating unknowns). Correcting Ned's Class II relationship, reducing his deep bite to alleviate mandibular incisor palatal impingement, correcting his right posterior crossbite and lateral CR-CO shift, and eliminating his maxillary arch asymmetry would get Ned back on a normal track for his stage of development.

2) Early treatment should address *very specific problems with a clearly defined end point*, usually within six to nine months (except in the case of some orthopedic problems). Orthopedic correction of his Class II relationship is a very specific problem but will take longer than nine months depending upon growth. Correction of his right posterior crossbite and lateral shift are focused problems, which could be addressed with RME in less than nine months. His deep bite could be corrected by leveling arches with fixed orthodontic appliances in less than six to nine months. Finally, his maxillary arch asymmetry will take longer than nine months to correct because his permanent canines and incisors have not erupted.

3) Always ask: Is it necessary that I treat the patient now? *What harm will come if I choose to do nothing now?* If we do not begin Class II orthopedic treatment now, then useful jaw growth could be missed. Correction of the right posterior cross could be postponed for a year, but the longer Ned is left with the lateral CR-CO shift, the greater the chance that he will develop a mandibular asymmetry. If we do not correct his deep bite now, then he will continue to be in pain when his mandibular incisors bite into his palate, and we run the risk of palatal tissue damage. Finally, correction of the maxillary asymmetry is not necessary now because his permanent canines and incisors have not erupted.

Q: Should you extract permanent teeth (i.e. institute serial extractions) to create space for uprighting Ned's proclined mandibular incisors?

A: Incisor proclination may, or may not, justify extraction of permanent teeth. Extraction of mandibular permanent teeth depends upon a number of factors including the degree of incisor proclination, the amount of mandibular arch crowding, and the patient's desire for less or more lip fullness/lip protrusion.

As far as serial extraction is concerned, remember that the ideal serial extraction patient is in the *early* mixed dentition stage of development and is *normal in every way except severe anterior crowding (≥ 9 mm per arch)*. Ned is entering the late mixed dentition stage of dental development. Let's examine the factors that would qualify/disqualify him for serial extraction:

- *Class I first molars*. Ned is Class II at the molars.
- *Vertically normal-to-slightly long soft tissue and skeletal LAFH, with minimal OB or possibly a mild open bite, but* not *a deep bite*. Ned has a long soft tissue LAFH, a normal skeletal LAFH, but a 100% deep bite.
- *Normal incisor angulation or proclined incisors, but* not *upright incisors*. Ned has proclined mandibular incisors but upright maxillary incisors.
- *Normal posterior transverse relationship (normal intermolar arch widths with good posterior interdigitation; absence of posterior crossbites; and absence of significant transverse compensations)*. Ned has a right posterior crossbite.
- *Severe (≥ 9 mm) anterior crowding*: Ned currently has a maxillary midline diastema and only 1.0 mm of mandibular incisor crowding.

Based upon the above features, Ned is *not* a good candidate for serial extraction.

Q: Ned has a significant Class II skeletal discrepancy (mandibular deficiency). There are three general ways to treat any skeletal discrepancy. Can you offer specific Class II treatments for each?

A: Anteroposterior, vertical, and transverse skeletal discrepancies can be treated with orthopedics, masking (camouflage), or surgery.

Class II orthopedics for Ned (restrict maxillary growth while permitting the mandible to continue growing forward or accelerate mandibular growth). Options include:

- Headgears: High-pull, straight-pull, and cervical-pull headgears restrict maxillary corpus forward growth, allow the mandible to continue growing forward, and move maxillary molars to the distal – all of which could correct Ned's Class II relationship. An HPHG is the best choice for Ned because it may reduce descent of his maxillary corpus and maxillary first permanent molars which aids Class II correction by mandibular forward rotation [14, 35, 101]. A disadvantage of CPHGs is that they tend to rotate the anterior palatal plane down and back which will increase (worsen) Ned's maxillary incisor display.

A further disadvantage of CPHGs is that they extrude maxillary first molars slightly (< 1 mm) [14, 15, 101], which would tend to rotate his mandible down and back – worsening his Class II relationship. SPHGs are a combination of high-pull and cervical-pull headgears and produce an effect somewhere between that of a high pull and a cervical pull.

- Class II functional appliances: The Herbst appliance is a typical Class II functional appliance. In growing individuals, it restricts maxillary forward growth, retracts maxillary posterior teeth, uprights maxillary incisors, moves mandibular posterior teeth to the mesial, proclines mandibular incisors, accelerates condylar growth, and displaces the glenoid fossae anteriorly [102, 103].

Class II functional appliances *accelerate* mandibular growth in growing individuals but *do not enhance* mandibular horizontal growth beyond that found in control subjects [104]. In fact, the *direction* of condylar growth from functional appliances (posterior superiorly) may not correct the mandibular skeletal deficiency or improve chin projection [105, 106], and *hyperdivergent* patients experience a deleterious backward mandibular rotation and increases in face height with Herbst treatment [21].

The ideal Class II functional appliance patient has a short LAFH, flat MPA, proclined maxillary incisors (since they will be upright), and upright mandibular incisors (since they will procline). Since Ned has upright maxillary incisors (U1 to SN = 96°) and proclined mandibular incisors (FMIA = 57°), he is *not* an ideal candidate for a Class II functional appliance.

Masking or camouflage (achieving an ideal occlusion *dentally* without correcting the underlying skeletal discrepancy). We generally recommend masking during comprehensive treatment in adult dentition when:

- Class II orthopedic treatment outcome was unsatisfactory
- Growth is complete or nearly complete (i.e. *avoid doing anything irreversible such as extracting permanent teeth until unknowns such as growth are eliminated*)
- Obtaining Class I canines dentally is reasonable and will not result in unacceptable dental compensations or unfavorable esthetics.
- *First Principle of Masking – the smaller the skeletal discrepancy, the more normal the patient looks, and the smaller the dental compensation – the more successful masking (camouflage) will be; the larger the* *skeletal discrepancy, the less normal the patient looks, and the larger the dental compensations – the less successful masking (camouflage) will be.*

Class II masking options include:

- Extraction of maxillary first premolars to permit retraction of maxillary anterior teeth (achieving a Class I canine relationship but leaving molars Class II). This is an example of intra-arch mechanics.
- Using TADs as anchors to distalize the entire maxillary arch. For example, a pendulum appliance can be used to distalize maxillary posterior teeth if supported by a TAD attached to the palatal acrylic button. Also, TADs could be placed into the right and left infrazygomatic crests and used as anchors to retract the entire maxillary arch (non-extraction). These are examples of intra-arch mechanics.
- The use of Class II correctors such as Class II elastics or Class II springs. These are examples of inter-arch mechanics.

Surgery (mandibular advancement) is generally considered only during comprehensive treatment in adult dentition. However, if an orthopedic outcome is unfavorable, and if masking is deemed inappropriate, and then surgery may be Ned's best option. Ned and his parents should be informed of this at his case presentation.

Q: If you chose to treat Ned's Class II skeletal discrepancy with orthopedics – *when* should you begin? Also, is it reasonable to attempt orthopedics considering the *magnitude* of his discrepancy?

A: Now is the appropriate time to attempt Class II orthopedic treatment for Ned. Prospective clinical trials consistently report no advantage in treating Class II relationships in the *early* mixed dentition (except for a possible decrease in incisal trauma as a result of excess overjet) [17, 19, 73–77], and we subscribe to this guideline unless the patient shows good statural growth, in which case, we will begin Class II treatment in the early mixed dentition. Ned is in the late mixed dentition, and now is the time to attempt Class II orthopedics.

Looking at Ned's lateral cephalometric tracing (Figure 5.52e), we see that his anteroposterior skeletal discrepancy is moderate with an ANB angle of 6° which is slightly inflated due to the influence of his upright maxillary incisors on the position of A-Point. Being age eleven years, he is ~one and a half years from reaching the average age for the onset of pubertal growth acceleration for boys [107], and we will not miss the acceleration of growth if we begin orthopedics now. If Ned is cooperative, then we have a chance to fully correct his Class II relationship. Even if he does not fully correct with orthopedics, he may be able to improve to the point where we can acceptably mask (camouflage) his Class II discrepancy.

Q: Would you classify Ned's deep bite as a skeletal deep bite, a dental deep bite, or a combination?

A: Ned has a *dental* deep bite. Why? He has a *long* soft tissue LAFH and a normal skeletal LAFH. He does not have a short LAFH which would be seen in a skeletal deep bite. Ned's deep bite resulted from overeruption of his mandibular incisors (Figures 5.52s and 5.52t) and a slight overeruption of his maxillary incisors.

Q: What would be the ideal way to correct Ned's dental deep bite?

A: Apply orthodontic forces to provide relative intrusion of his overerupted incisors.

Q: What does *relative* intrusion mean?

A: During childhood and adolescence (~ages six to sixteen years), erupted permanent teeth continue to drift vertically. On average, mandibular molars and incisors drift vertically ~2 mm/year during this period [108]. If orthodontic force is applied to impede vertical drift of overerupted mandibular incisors, then the mandibular molars will continue to erupt relatively to the mandibular incisors. That is, the mandibular incisors are *relatively* intruded.

Such force application has the potential to improve deep overbites while maintaining the spatial orientation of the mandibular incisors to the mandibular body (i.e. the mandibular incisor angulation in the sagittal plane).

Q: Are there other approaches to achieve relative intrusion of mandibular incisors?

A: Yes. Tipping mandibular incisors forward (proclining mandibular incisors) rotates their incisal edges downward relative to the occlusal plane – thus, opening the bite. If mandibular incisors begin with an upright inclination (i.e. FMIA > 65°), this may be a useful approach to open a deep bite because it will result in improved FMIA. However, if the mandibular incisors are initially proclined (i.e. FMIA < 62°), then the benefit of bite opening will be offset by worsening of mandibular incisor proclination.

Q: Is there a compelling reason to correct Ned's dental deep bite now?

A: Yes. Ned demonstrates an OB of 100% (palatal impingement), he bites into the roof of his mouth, and he says it hurts when he bites. There is no palatal tissue damage yet, but it could develop in the future.

Q: Given his stage of dental development, what options can you suggest to open Ned's dental deep bite?

A: Since his deep bite is primarily a result of excessive mandibular incisor eruption, correction of his deep bite would ideally occur via mandibular incisor relative intrusion. Options include:

- Using mandibular fixed appliances to apply an intrusion force against the mandibular incisors. Mandibular incisors are typically intruded during the curve of Spee leveling with fixed orthodontic appliances by incisor proclination, which reduces the vertical height of their incisal edges relative to the posterior occlusal plane. In Ned's case, his mandibular incisors are initially proclined (FMIA = 57°, see Figure 5.52e), and additional incisor proclination to level the mandibular dental arch *would not be prudent*.

- Curve of Spee leveling with fixed appliances to erupt and upright posterior teeth [22]. Mandibular premolars erupt when a flat archwire is deflected apically to engage premolar brackets. Mandibular molars tip distally/erupt because they are initially tipped mesially in a curve of Spee, and archwires act to upright them. However, erupting posterior teeth will rotate Ned's mandibular plane down and back – potentially worsening his Class II relationship and increasing FMIA.

- Using a maxillary removable appliance with an anterior bite plane. The use of this appliance discludes the posterior teeth while the mandibular incisors maintain occlusal contact with the bite plate. Posterior teeth will erupt and thereby achieve relative intrusion of mandibular incisors without a significant change in their sagittal inclination. The use of a bite plate would also eliminate mandibular incisor palatal impingement. However, the relative incisor intrusion gained by this approach may take longer than nine months, and the mandibular plane may steepen as posterior teeth erupt.

- Relative mandibular incisor intrusion, without a reactive eruption of posterior teeth, by inserting mandibular anterior TAD anchors to limit vertical drift of the mandibular incisors during growth. This is an excellent way of achieving relative mandibular incisor intrusion while minimizing a change in the inclination of these teeth. However, given Ned's stage of permanent tooth development, this is not a short term treatment. It is best accomplished when the mandibular posterior permanent teeth are undergoing vertical drift after their eruption (i.e. the adolescent dentition stage). Ned is at least two years from reaching this stage of dentition development.

- Gain improvement of Ned's dental deep bite as a result of treatments used to address anteroposterior and transverse problems. For instance, RME often opens the bite as posterior teeth slide along cuspal inclines in the opposing arch. Although the improvement may not achieve complete bite opening, it may alleviate the pain from mandibular incisor palatal impingement. Complete mandibular arch leveling can then be accomplished later during comprehensive treatment.

Given that the above options are not short-term, we felt it might be best to consider the effect of treatment for anteroposterior and transverse problems on his palatal impingement before deciding on how to manage Ned's dental deep bite.

Q: Ned has a right posterior lingual crossbite (Figures 5.52l and 5.52m) with a 1–2 mm right CR-CO shift. He also has mandibular permanent first molar lingual crown torque (Figure 5.52v) and maxillary permanent first molar buccal crown torque (Figure 5.52u). How will these transverse dental compensations affect the correction of Ned's crossbite?

A: The transverse compensations (mandibular permanent first molar lingual crown torque and maxillary first permanent molar buccal crown torque) increase the magnitude of the transverse correction needed. That is, when we finish treatment, we want upright posterior teeth. As we upright his permanent first molars, the mandibular crowns will move *buccally*, and the maxillary crowns will move *lingually*, worsening the right crossbite and decreasing his left posterior overjet.

Q: Does Ned have a dental, or skeletal, posterior crossbite? Why?

A: It is skeletal. If you remove posterior compensations (upright posterior teeth transversely), then his crossbite will worsen. This reflects a discrepancy between his maxillary transverse skeleton and mandibular transverse skeleton. If uprighting posterior teeth improved his crossbite, then this would indicate an absence of transverse skeletal discrepancy and his crossbite would be dental. Ned has a *skeletal* crossbite.

Q: One orthodontic treatment objective is upright posterior teeth (as viewed transversely). What will be the effect on the *vertical* position of Ned's permanent first

molars if we upright them (i.e. decrease the existing mandibular permanent molar lingual crown torque and decrease the existing maxillary permanent molar buccal crown torque)? How will this affect his dental deep bite?

A: Uprighting mandibular molars, by tipping them buccally, will cause the cusps to move upward and buccally along an arc described by the radius bisecting the cusp tips and the molar center of rotation viewed in the coronal plane. The effect will be to "open the bite" by extrusion of the mandibular molars relative to the mandibular incisors. Uprighting maxillary molars, by tipping them lingually, will cause the crowns to move down and lingually.

The effect of uprighting Ned's molars will therefore be a tendency to open his dental deep bite. That is, achieving this transverse objective will help improve his vertical problem.

Q: There are three general ways to treat a skeletal discrepancy. Can you list specific treatments for Ned's transverse skeletal discrepancy using each way?

A: Skeletal (apical base) discrepancies can be treated using orthopedics, masking (camouflage), or surgery.

Orthopedics (widening his maxilla by separating the midpalatal suture). Options include using a/an:

- RME appliance – expansion can be performed rapidly (0.25 mm or 0.5 mm per day) or slowly (0.25 mm or 0.5 mm) per week.
- Quad-helix appliance – can generate enough force to separate the midpalatal suture only if Ned's facial skeletal resistance is low. Otherwise, only dental movements will occur.

Masking (correcting the posterior crossbite by increasing dental compensations – adding maxillary posterior *buccal* crown torque and mandibular posterior *lingual* crown torque). Masking would not be our first choice since RME (orthopedics) – should be successful at Ned's age, requires only minimal patient compliance, and can create enough posterior overjet to permit uprighting of permanent first molars and elimination of the lateral shift. Masking to correct posterior crossbites is generally considered an option in adult dentition during comprehensive treatment.

Surgery – such as a surgically assisted RME (SARME) is not recommended for the same reason that masking (camouflage) is not recommended. That is, RME (orthopedics) should be successful. Surgery is generally considered an option in adult dentition.

Q: It is important to *reduce unknowns* – especially before proceeding with irreversible treatment options (e.g.

extraction of permanent teeth). What are Ned's unknowns?

A: Future jaw growth magnitude and direction, patient compliance, an undetected (worse) CR-CO shift, and the ability to achieve a midpalatal suture separation with RME.

Q: What are your *long-term* (comprehensive) treatment goals for Ned?

A: Improve his profile and smile – decreasing profile convexity, increasing chin projection, reducing buccal corridors, positioning canines (and maxillary molars if he is treated non-extraction) into Class I relationships, correcting his right posterior crossbite, correcting the CR-CO shift, and obtaining minimal overbite and overjet.

Q: Should you start early treatment now or recall? If you start treatment, what options would you consider?

A: Treatment options include the following:

- *Recall* (no treatment, monitor only) – re-evaluate in one year. We do *not* recommend this option. Now is the perfect time to begin Class II orthopedic treatment. If we wait a year, then we may miss out on favorable jaw growth. Now is also the perfect time to correct Ned's right posterior crossbite. If we delay RME for years, then his facial skeletal resistance will increase making it harder to achieve midpalatal suture separation and harder to maximize transverse skeletal expansion. Further, not correcting his right lateral CR-CO shift may result in asymmetric mandibular growth. Finally, if we do not address Ned's dental deep bite, then his pain upon biting will continue and palatal tissue damage may occur.
- *Space maintenance* – placement of an LLHA and possibly a Nance holding arch. Ned has 1.0 mm of mandibular incisor crowding. If we place an LLHA, then we anticipate 5.5 mm of mandibular space following the eruption of all permanent teeth. This space could be used to upright Ned's proclined mandibular incisors. If we choose RME to address his transverse problem, then we would recommend LLHA placement after mandibular permanent molars were uprighted.

Placement of a Nance holding arch would prevent maxillary first permanent molar mesial drift, and subsequent worsening of his Class II relationship, during the transition to permanent dentition. However, this would be unnecessary if we used an HPHG or Herbst appliance to retract the maxillary molars distally.

- *Class II orthopedics (headgear or functional appliance wear)* – would help correct Ned's Class II skeletal/molar relationship if he has favorable growth and is compliant. Functional appliance wear would increase his mandibular incisor proclination.
- *Wearing a clear, vacuum-formed maxillary retainer* – would immediately eliminate palatal pain from mandibular incisor palatal impingement. If only the maxillary incisors and palate were covered by the retainer, then the posterior teeth would erupt – opening the bite. We look upon such clear retainer wear as a temporary deep bite solution for Ned.
- *Transverse orthopedics (RME or quad-helix posterior crossbite correction) including CR-CO shift elimination* – is recommended. If the posterior crossbite is corrected, and adequate posterior OJ created, then Ned's permanent molars can be uprighted. This treatment may also produce a beneficial opening of his dental deep bite.
- *Dental deep bite correction with fixed orthodontic appliances* – to intrude Ned's mandibular incisors, erupt mandibular posterior teeth, open his bite, and eliminate his mandibular incisor palatal impingement. This treatment is not recommended yet – at least not until we evaluate the effect of RME on Ned's deep bite.
- *Space regaining* – is unnecessary. There does not appear to be loss of space following exfoliation of primary teeth (Figures 5.52j and 5.52k).
- *Extraction of maxillary and mandibular primary canines* – is not recommend. All of Ned's teeth, including his permanent canines, appear to be erupting normally.
- *Serial extraction* – for the reasons discussed earlier, Ned is *not* a good candidate for serial extraction.

Q: What are the drawbacks of placing an LLHA in a Class II mixed-dentition patient?

A: If an LLHA is placed, then *mandibular first permanent molar mesial drift is significantly reduced*, spontaneous improvement in the Class II molar relationship will not occur through mesial molar drift, and Class II molar correction must occur by some other means (e.g. headgear wear, functional appliance treatment).

Also, if mandibular first permanent molars move *slightly* to the mesial with an LLHA in place, then they will push the mandibular incisors forward through the lingual arch bar (proclining the incisors) [109, 110]. Since skeletal Class II patients usually exhibit proclined mandibular incisors (dental compensations for the underlying deficient mandible), this additional proclination is undesirable.

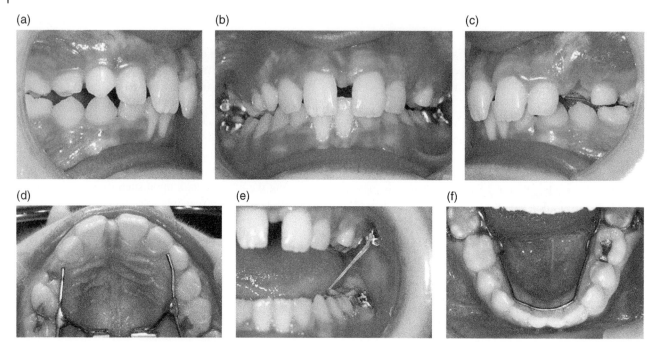

(a) (b) (c)

(d) (e) (f)

Figure 5.53 (a–f) Progress records of Ned.

Q: What is your recommended treatment? How would you proceed?

A: We elected to *reduce unknowns*. At his case presentation appointment, Ned's CR-CO shift and Class II molar relationship were confirmed. An RME appliance was fabricated with arms extending mesial from the first permanent molar bands to incorporate maxillary primary teeth as anchorage (Figures 5.53a–5.53d). However, these arms were not bonded to the primary teeth. If we were to retreat Ned today, then we would etch the lingual surfaces of the primary teeth and bond them directly to the RME appliance wires. This would rigidly incorporate the primary teeth as anchors.

During RME, Ned's left posterior overjet became excessive before the right posterior crossbite was corrected. To prevent Ned from going into left buccal crossbite, he was placed on left crossbite elastics to upright the mandibular left first permanent molar and reduce overjet (Figure 5.53e). An LLHA was placed (Figure 5.53f) after the right crossbite was corrected.

Ned wore an HPHG each night. Our plan was to overcorrect Ned to Class III at the permanent first molars by 1–2 mm and then to slowly taper off headgear wear as we monitored his corrected molar relationship and his remaining permanent teeth erupted. Once all premolars and permanent canines erupted, the LLHA was removed.

Q: Compare Figures 5.52h and 5.53b. What happened to Ned's mandibular incisor palatal impingement during RME?

A: Ned's deep bite opened, and his mandibular incisor palatal impingement was corrected. Bite opening during RME usually occurs as maxillary posterior teeth cusp inclines ride up mandibular posterior teeth cusp inclines (mandible forced down and back slightly). Additionally, we uprighted his mandibular left first molar buccally, increasing the vertical height of this tooth's occlusal surface.

Q: Records were made one year later (Figure 5.54). What changes do you note?

A: Changes include:
- Chin deviation eliminated
- Maxillary midline diastema closed
- Buccal corridors reduced
- Labiomental sulcus has opened (compare Figures 5.52c and 5.54c)
- Mandibular lip procumbency (lip trapping) has reduced
- All permanent teeth have erupted
- Right posterior crossbite has been corrected
- Anteroposterior relationship has corrected to Class I (note maxillary first premolars are Class I, maxillary left canine is Class I, maxillary right canine is Class II by 1–2 mm but with 2 mm space distal to it)

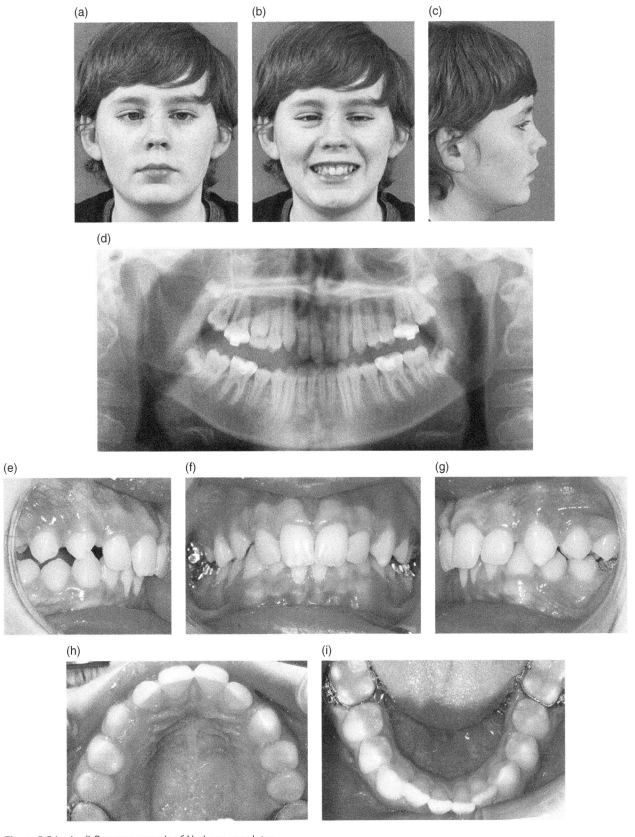

Figure 5.54 (a–i) Progress records of Ned one year later.

- OB 60% but without palatal impingement
- 1 mm of mandibular anterior crowding is present
- 5 mm of maxillary spacing is present
- Thin attached keratinized tissue labial to mandibular central incisors.

Q: You can see that the RME appliance was removed (Figure 5.54h). Should it have been left in place for retention?

A: Yes and no. For expansion stability, we typically leave RME appliances in place for as long as nine to twelve months post-expansion. However, because Ned was compliant with headgear, we removed the RME appliance after his crossbite was corrected and maintained the maxillary expansion by expanding the headgear inner bow.

Q: Was it prudent to remove the LLHA once all permanent canines and premolars erupted?

A: No. Look at Figure 5.53f. See how nearly aligned the mandibular incisors are? And, we still anticipated "E-space" at that time (2.9 mm per side = 9.9 mm width of mandibular primary second molar minus 7 mm width of mandibular second premolar).

   If we had left the LLHA in place, then we would have ended with mandibular arch *spacing* instead of mandibular arch crowding (Figure 5.54i). Further, Ned would have been forced to correct his Class II relationship entirely by headgear wear (potentially improving his profile more) and not with the assistance of mandibular first permanent molar mesial drift.

Q: We anticipated 3.5 mm of maxillary spacing if a Nance holding arch had initially been placed. A Nance holding arch was never placed, but we ended up with about 5 mm of maxillary spacing. How can this be?

A: RME created maxillary dental arch space.

Q: With the eruption of all permanent teeth except third molars, early treatment was finished. What comprehensive treatment would you now recommend?

A: A discussion of treatment progress was held with Ned and his parents. A decision was made to continue with non-extraction treatment. Maxillary and mandibular arches were bonded with fixed orthodontic appliances, arches were leveled and aligned, and maxillary spaces were closed. Ned continued to wear his headgear while his maxillary anterior teeth were retracted and we were sure that his Class II correction was maintained.

Q: Should you be concerned with aligning Ned's crowded mandibular anterior teeth in the presence of the thin mandibular anterior labial periodontal biotype?

A: Yes, we were concerned that labial gingival recession could occur if the crowded mandibular anterior teeth were aligned by incisor proclination. This concern was explained to Ned's parents. However, the amount of mandibular anterior crowding was minimal, and Ned had some attached keratinized tissue, so we felt that the risk of gingival recession would be minimal during arch leveling and aligning.

Q: Treatment was completed. His deband records (fifteen years old) are shown in Figure 5.55. What changes do you note?

A: Changes include:
- A significant improvement in Ned's facial appearance compared to the initial presentation
- Broad smile with reduced buccal corridors and wider maxilla
- Maxillary midline diastema closed
- Maxillary midline 1–2 mm to the left of the facial midline
- Maxillary midline coincident with the mandibular dental midline
- Smile arc, formed by maxillary anterior teeth edges, reasonably congruent with the lower lip
- Right posterior crossbite corrected
- Nasal tip has descended on profile
- Naso labial angle (NLA) has decreased
- Profile convexity has diminished as chin projection has improved
- Deep labiomental sulcus has opened
- ANB angle decreased from 6° to 1°
- Mandibular plane angle has flattened (FMA decreased from 21 to 20°; SNMP angle decreased from 32 to 30°)
- Mandibular incisors have uprighted relative to the face (FMIA increased from 57 to 60°) and relative to the mandible (IMPA decreased from 102 to 100°)
- Maxillary incisors proclined (U1 to SN increased from 96 to 110°)
- Initial to deband lateral cephalometric superimposition (Figure 5.55f) demonstrates significant mandibular growth with B-point growing down and forward, maxillary descent with A-point growing vertically, maxillary and mandibular molar eruption with mesial movement, maxillary and mandibular incisor eruption, and maxillary incisor proclination.
- Blunting (mild resorption) of maxillary incisor and second premolar root tips (Figure 5.55 g)
- Well-seated Class I occlusion
- OB decreased to 20%
- When viewed from the occlusal, maxillary lateral incisors have greater labial crown torque compared to maxillary central incisors

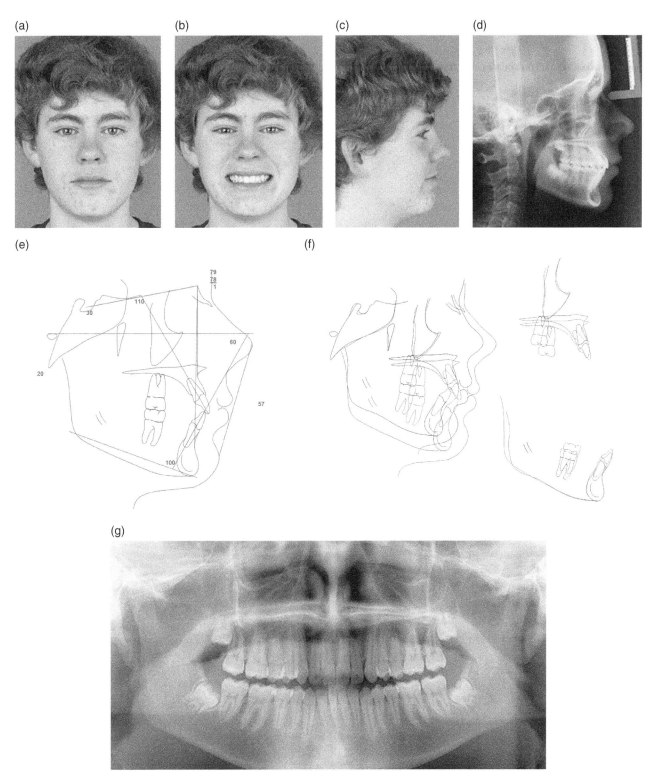

Figure 5.55 (a–l) Deband records of Ned.

(h)　　　　(i)　　　　(j)

(k)　　　　(l)

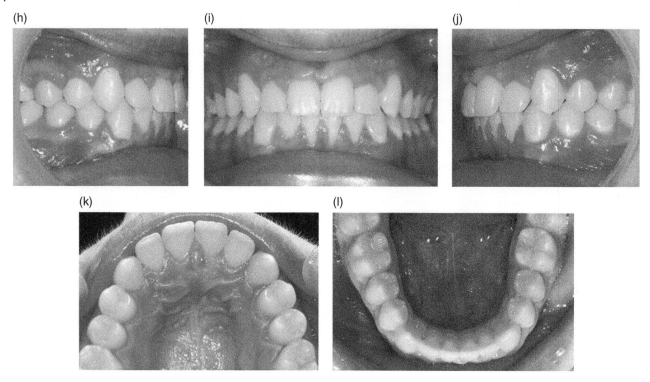

Figure 5.55 (Continued)

- Significant gingival hyperplasia and generalized decalcification due to poor hygiene, but the mandibular gingival recession has not occurred
- Medial strabismus of the right eye has been corrected
- Dental arch asymmetries, if present, are minimal

Q: Why did Ned's labiomental sulcus open?

A: Because his lip trapping was eliminated – by correcting his Class II relationship and by correcting his deep bite (compare Figures 5.52d and 5.55d).

Q: Can you describe the effect of Ned's HPHG wear?

A: Headgear wear resulted in *differential jaw growth*. Ned's maxilla grew minimally forward while his mandible continued to grow forward, resulting in improved profile, skeletal, and dental relationships (compare forward movement of PNS, ANS, and Pogonion in overall superimposition, Figure 5.55f).

Q: Ned's facial convexity decreased. But, could it have been improved even more? How?

A: Yes, it could have been improved more. If his maxillary and the mandibular molar eruption was reduced, then his mandible would have rotated CCW more – improving his B-Point and chin projection. The molar eruption can be halted/reduced with the use of TAD anchors, increased HPHG wear for maxillary molars, longer use of an LLHA, occlusal bite plates, and possibly chewing exercises. Also, if we had left the LLHA in place longer, then Class I molar correction would have been achieved with additional headgear wear/differential jaw growth (and not mandibular molar mesial drift) and improved chin projection.

Q: Why did his maxillary incisor angulation increase from 96° to 110°?

A: We were surprised by this increase in maxillary incisor angulation. With RME, and subsequent maxillary midline diastema closure, we expected to see maxillary incisor *uprighting*.

But, let's take a closer look. When we examine the maxillary superimposition (Figure 5.55f, top right), we see that the maxillary incisors tipped within the maxilla. This tipping could be a compensatory response to the significant differential between maxillary and mandibular forward growth. Then, look at the overall facial superimposition (Figure 5.55f, left). See how the maxillary palatal plane rotated CCW during growth. This maxillary rotation added to the increased inclination of the incisors.

Q: How was Ned's deep bite corrected?

A: Ned's deep bite was corrected by (Figure 5.55f):

- Maxillary and mandibular molar eruption
- Maxillary incisor proclination

Note that we did not procline Ned's mandibular incisors. His dental deep bite was improved by the *relative* intrusion of the mandibular incisors (compared to mandibular molars) without changing their inclination.

Q: Ned initially presented with a maxillary midline diastema. Midline diastemas will often reopen after they are closed orthodontically – even with good removable retainer wear. Should we have bonded a fixed maxillary lingual retainer between Ned's maxillary central incisors to prevent the diastema from reopening?

A: Not necessarily. In most cases, mixed dentition diastemas will close spontaneously as the permanent canines erupt [111]. Ned's diastema closed spontaneously, even after RME (Figures 5.54a–5.54i). In the deband photos, it is difficult to classify his diastema attachment (Figure 5.55i). It may still have a papillary attachment. We did not test for incisive papilla blanching when the upper lip is gently pulled forward [96]. However, we should inform Ned and his parents that the diastema could open and ask them to inform us if it does. If it does, then we will place a maxillary lingual fixed retainer between the central incisors.

Q: Ned had some cephalometric characteristics of a bimaxillary protrusive pattern at deband (Figure 5.55e). Specifically, he shows increases in maxillary and mandibular incisor angulations. However, he is very close to normal for three other parameters used to classify bimaxillary protrusion. His inter-incisal angle is just below the normal range (120° compared to normal of 130° $\pm$ 8°), his maxillary and mandibular incisors are positioned slightly forward (0.5 to 1 mm) of the A-point to Pogonion line compared to averages, and his lips lie behind the E-plane [112]. Should Ned have been treated with four first premolar extractions (or four second premolar extractions) instead of non-extraction?

A: The concept is that extraction of four premolars provides space to retract (distalize) canines, retract incisors, and upright incisors as they are retracted. Ned's bimaxillary incisor proclination could have been eliminated with premolar extractions, and an excellent outcome may have resulted. Or, depending upon the biomechanics employed, extraction of premolars could have resulted in incisor over-retraction. Had Ned's non-extraction treatment resulted in a markedly decreased inter-incisal angle, protrusive incisors well in front of the A-Point to Pogonion line, and lip protrusion well in front of the E-plane, four premolar extraction treatment would have been impactful in reducing these parameters to within the normal range. However, Ned's growth and non-extraction treatment resulted in maintaining these parameters within the normal range.

The burden on the orthodontist is to make the optimal treatment decision for the patient at every appointment based upon the best science, his/her best clinical judgment, and the patient's desires. We feel that we did this for Ned. Initially, he was Class II and extraction of four premolars would have been imprudent. Why? Without guaranteed good growth and compliance, we may never have been able to correct his Class II relationship if mandibular canines had been retracted through extraction spaces the same amount as maxillary canines. So, it was initially wise not to extract premolars but to reduce unknowns instead (RME, headgear, LLHA).

At the time of progress records (Figure 5.54), Ned's facial esthetics were improving, and he had only minimal mandibular anterior crowding. So, proceeding non-extraction was reasonable. Ned's final esthetics (Figure 5.55) were much improved compared to his initial esthetics. Maxillary incisors were proclined, but we would not wish to reduce his maxillary lip support by retracting maxillary incisors. Non-extraction treatment resulted in a pleasing profile, good maxillary lip support, an esthetic smile, an excellent occlusion, and healthy tissue. Ned and his parents were delighted with his treatment outcome.

We have friends who would demand that Ned be treated with premolar extractions, if only to satisfy ideal cephalometric incisor angulation norms. We use cephalometric measurements in making extraction decisions, but cephalometric norms should not dictate treatment decisions.

We have friends who would demand that Ned be treated with premolar extractions to guarantee treatment stability. However, only lifelong retention guarantees lifelong alignment stability. If we were to treat Ned again, then we would treat him non-extraction again – but with even greater emphasis on oral hygiene and with leaving the LLHA in place until fixed orthodontic appliances were bonded in the mandibular arch.

Q: Was early treatment justified for Ned?

A: Yes – his deep bite, palatal impingement with pain, posterior crossbite, and Class II relationship were corrected with early treatment, and his facial esthetics were improved.

Q: What retention protocol would you recommend for Ned?

A: He was placed in removable Hawley retainers and asked to wear them at night, for life. Lifelong retention is the only guarantee that alignment of teeth can be maintained. The maxillary Hawley retainer included an anterior bite plate to disclude his posterior teeth slightly when he wears it. This feature will help prevent his OB from deepening long-term.

Q: What "take-home" messages can you draw from Ned's treatment?

A: "Take-home" messages include the following:

- Ned was an eleven-year-old boy who presented as he was entering the late mixed dentition stage of dental development. He had a Class II molar relationship secondary to mandibular skeletal deficiency, a right posterior lingual crossbite with right CR-CO lateral shift, a dental deep bite, and mandibular incisor palatal impingement causing pain. He was successfully treated early with RME, headgear, and LLHA. Comprehensive treatment in adult dentition included fixed orthodontic appliances to level/align arches, close spaces, and finish. All treatment goals were achieved.

- Decisions to treat anteroposterior, vertical, or transverse skeletal discrepancies orthopedically, with masking (camouflage), or surgically depend upon two factors: *the age of the patient and the magnitude of the underlying skeletal discrepancy* (in addition to patient desires). Ned's two dimensions with skeletal discrepancies (anteroposterior and transverse) were treated with orthopedics successfully.

- *Reduce unknowns before committing to irreversible treatments.*

- HPHG was a good Class II orthopedic appliance choice, and Ned was very compliant in wearing it. If Ned had not been cooperative, then a fixed functional appliance (Herbst appliance) would have been a reasonable alternative but additional mandibular incisor proclination would have been anticipated.

- If you attempt headgear treatment, then set a fixed trial period (three to four months) to judge patient compliance with it (reducing unknowns). If compliance is not forthcoming, switch to another treatment approach.

- Large buccal corridors alone may not justify RME. However, large buccal corridors combined with a right posterior lingual crossbite justified RME in this case.

- The longer we have practiced, the longer we are leaving our RME appliances in post-expansion (for stability).

- Post-maxillary expansion, if a child is wearing and compliant with headgear, then the RME appliance can be removed (after three to four months) and the maxillary expansion maintained by expanding the headgear inner facebow.

- Ned's soft tissue LAFH was long, his skeletal LAFH was WRN, but his mandibular incisors were overerupted – leading to his *dental deep bite*. His deep bite was corrected through molar eruption and maxillary incisor proclination. OB reduction did not occur through *absolute* mandibular incisor intrusion during arch (curve of Spee) leveling. OB reduction did occur through the *relative* intrusion of the mandibular incisors (compared to mandibular molars)

- The compelling reason for *early* deep bite treatment is tissue damage or pain as a result of mandibular incisor palatal impingement. Otherwise, deep bite treatment may be postponed until comprehensive treatment in adult dentition.

- Ned's OB was reduced to 20%. Further OB reduction, say to 10%, would have been even better. Why? No matter how you retain deep bite corrections, you should expect an increase in OB post-treatment.

- *Principle: overcorrect deep bites to a shallow OB, overcorrect open bites to a deep bite.*

- As a rule, leave LLHAs in place until you are ready to bond the mandibular arch with fixed appliances.

Case Anna

Q: Anna is a seven-year-old girl in the early mixed dentition who presents to you for a consultation (Figure 5.56). Her pediatric dentist is concerned with her anterior open bite. PMH and TMJ evaluations are WRN. Using only facial and intraoral frontal views (no lateral cephalometric radiograph, right or left intraoral photos, or models), what features classify her open bite as a *dental* open bite (open bite due to a habit, vertical skeletal growth normal)? What features classify her open bite as a *skeletal* open bite (open bite due to excessive vertical growth)? Do you feel that she is one or the other, or a combination of both?

A: Anna's *dental* open bite features include the following:

- Soft tissue LAFH WRN (soft tissue Glabella – Subnasale approximately equal to Subnasale – soft tissue Menton)

- Lip competence (absence of ILG)

- Maxillary incisors are stepped up (apically) relative to the corresponding posterior teeth (Figure 5.56d).

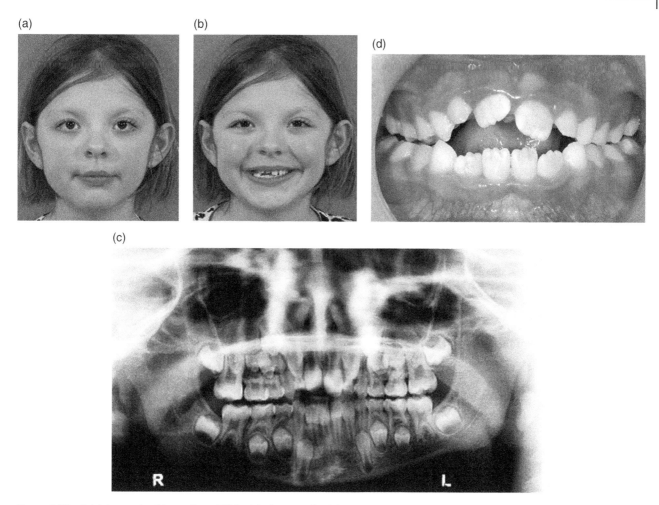

Figure 5.56 Initial records of Anna: (a and b) facial photographs; (c) pantomograph; (d) intraoral frontal photograph.

- Anterior open bite is football-shaped and extends only to the right and left canines.

  Her *skeletal* open bite features include:

- None, as seen in these views.

  Anna has a dental open bite.

Q: Why do *dental* anterior open bites typically extend no further posteriorly than the primary first molars or first premolars? Why do *skeletal* anterior open bites often extend to the permanent molars?

A: Dental (functional) open bites are caused by habits (lip-biting, resting tongue interposition, and digit-sucking), which prevent anterior teeth from erupting. Because these habits usually extend from canine to canine, dental open bites usually extend from canine to canine.

Skeletal open bites can be the result of excessive vertical (maxillary) skeletal growth, or more commonly, the result of excessive vertical maxillary dentoalveolar growth. Either of these characteristics, alone or in concert, are associated with a backward, or less-than-average forward mandibular rotation during growth – which rotates the mandible down and back around the condyles. An excessive eruption of mandibular posterior teeth is also associated with backward mandibular rotation and skeletal open bites [27]. The presence of one or more of these characteristics, and mandibular down and back rotation, can result in an anterior open bite extending to the first, or even second, permanent molars.

It is important to remember that skeletal anterior open bite is a subcategory of the *hyperdivergent* phenotype. Excessive vertical maxillary skeletal growth, excessive maxillary and mandibular posterior dentoalveolar growth, backward mandibular growth rotation, short mandibular ramus, large gonial angle, and excessive LAFH can be associated with hyperdivergent individuals with *and without* anterior open bite (Figure 5.57) [27].

(a)

(b)

(c)

(d)

(e)

(f)

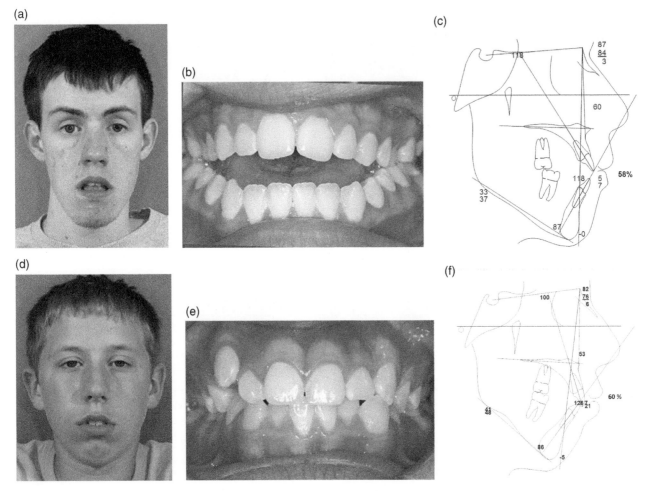

Figure 5.57 Hyperdivergent individuals. (a–c) Owen is hyperdivergent with a skeletal open bite. (d–f) Mitchell is hyperdivergent without an open bite.

Q: What questions should you ask Anna and her parents about her open bite? What else should you check for?

A:

- Ask them how long Anna has had her open bite. They do not recall her having an open bite until their dentist pointed it out.
- Ask Anna if she has ever had a thumb-sucking (digit) habit or lip-biting habit. Her parents state that Anna sucked her thumb but stopped the habit a long time ago.
- Check for an anterior interposition tongue habit. Ask Anna to close her eyes while you talk to her parents. Then, ask her to open her eyes (to distract her) while you gently and quickly retract her lips to see if her tongue is resting between her anterior teeth. Anna does not have an anterior tongue interposition habit.
- Check to see if the open bite could be due to TMJ degeneration. Ask if Anna suffered jaw trauma or

has a history of generalized musculoskeletal problems. Her parents deny a history of trauma, generalized musculoskeletal problems, TMJ pain, or TMJ dysfunction. Examine the condyles on Anna's panoramic image (Figure 5.56c). Her condyles appear well corticated, and no condylar degeneration is noted. Without additional signs or symptoms of TMJ degeneration, Anna's open bite is probably *not* due to condylar degeneration and additional imaging is unwarranted.

- Check for incisor ankylosis that could be preventing incisor eruption. Her incisors exhibit normal mobility.
- Check for crowding which could be blocking out incisors and preventing incisor eruption. Crowding is not evident.
- Check for a *temporary* anterior open bite due to normal tooth eruption. You contact Anna's pediatric

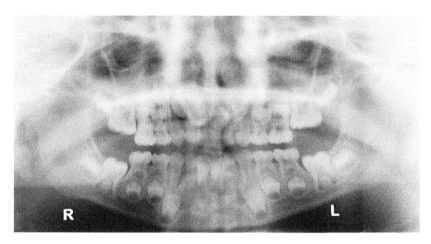

Figure 5.58 Previous panoramic image of Anna in the primary dentition. Note that the primary maxillary and mandibular incisors appear to have erupted to the same approximate level as the primary posterior teeth. That is, Anna does not appear to have had an anterior open bite in the primary dentition.

dentist and request a previous panoramic image (Figure 5.58). What do you see? It appears that Anna's primary maxillary and mandibular incisors were erupted to the level of her primary posterior teeth. In other words, it does not appear that Anna had an anterior open bite until her primary incisors exfoliated.

Q: What is the average eruption age of maxillary permanent incisors?

A: Examine the permanent tooth eruption timing values below [113]. On average, maxillary central incisors erupt between seven and eight years of age and maxillary lateral incisors erupt between eight and nine years of age.

	Maxillary	Mandibular
Central incisor	7–8	6–7
Lateral incisor	8–9	7–8
Canine	11–12	9–10
First premolar	10–11	10–12
Second premolar	10–12	11–12
First molar	6–7	6–7
Second molar	12–13	11–13

Q: Based upon answers to the above questions and observations, what is the most likely cause of Anna's open bite?

A: Her open bite is probably temporary and occurring during the transition from primary to permanent dentitions.

Q: In addition to her anterior open bite, Anna also exhibits a unilateral right posterior lingual crossbite

(Figure 5.56d). What did we fail to check for that could affect this crossbite?

A: We failed to check for a CR-CO shift. *Always check for a CR-CO shift in every patient at every appointment.* As seen in Figure 5.59, Anna has a unilateral right posterior lingual crossbite in CO (Figure 5.59a), but shifts to a *bilateral* transverse discrepancy in CR (Figure 5.59b). Note in Figure 5.56a that Anna exhibits a slight chin deviation to the right in CO.

Q: Which crossbite is generally easier to treat – a unilateral crossbite or a bilateral crossbite?

A: A *bilateral* maxillary transverse deficiency, such as Anna demonstrates in Figure 5.58b, is generally easier to treat. Why? RME can correct this problem readily by applying *bilateral* expansion forces – which are easier to create than unilateral expansion forces. Further, the bilateral correction needed on each side in CR is smaller than the unilateral correction that would have been needed on her right side in CO.

Q: What can result if Anna's shift into a unilateral right crossbite is not corrected?

A: A *mandibular asymmetry* may result [114–116].

Q: If Anna develops a mandibular asymmetry due to her lateral shift, what happens if we correct the crossbite and shift early enough with RME?

A: If her unilateral crossbite and shift are treated in the early mixed dentition, then *the mandibular asymmetry can be eliminated* [115–119]. Of course, this assumes that the mandibular asymmetry is developing as a result of the shift and not as a result of inherent asymmetric mandibular growth. If asymmetric mandibular

(a)

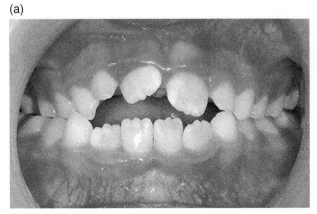

(b)

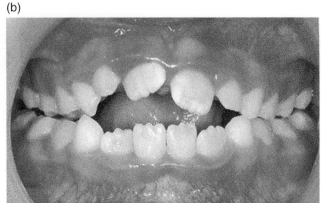

Figure 5.59 Frontal intraoral photographs of Anna in CO (a) and CR (b).

(condylar) growth is causing the mandibular asymmetry, then it must be treated orthopedically (e.g. with unilateral Class III elastics supported by TADs) or surgically.

Q: *When* should we treat Anna's crossbite?

A: *Now* is an ideal time to correct her posterior crossbite. Why? There was no urgency to treat her crossbite in the primary dentition, and treatment relapse in the primary dentition could require later re-treatment. Further, Anna is years away from puberty, so the chance of maximizing skeletal expansion is excellent now, her first permanent molars have erupted and will provide excellent RME appliance anchorage, and Anna's cooperation should be good at this age.

Q: Focusing *only* on her anterior open bite and unilateral right posterior crossbite, discuss Anna in the context of three principles, which should be applied to every early treatment patient.

A:

1) The goal of early treatment is to correct developing problems – get the patient *back to normal for their stage of development* (including preventing complications such as resorption of adjacent tooth roots, reducing later treatment complexity, or reducing/eliminating unknowns). Correcting her anterior open bite, CR-CO shift, and unilateral posterior crossbite would put Anna back on track.

2) Early treatment should address *very specific problems with a clearly defined end point*, usually begun and ended within six to nine months (not protracted over many years except for some orthopedic problems).
   - Correction of her anterior open bite has a clear end point, and it may self-correct in a few months if it is

due to the normal transition from primary to permanent dentition. However, if it is due to an undetected habit, then it will not correct until Anna eliminates the habit.
   - Correction of the posterior crossbite has a clear end point. Because the crossbite is a *bilateral* transverse problem in CR (Figure 5.59b, maxillary transverse deficiency), RME should correct the problem quickly.

3) Always ask: Is it necessary that I treat the patient early? *What harm will come if I choose to do nothing now?* No harm will come from monitoring Anna's open bite. In fact, it may close spontaneously.

   If we do not correct her lateral shift into crossbite, then she may develop a mandibular asymmetry. However, she is only 7 years old, so minimal harm should result if we wait one year to treat it.

Q: If we focus *only* on her anterior open bite, CR-CO shift, and right posterior crossbite, then what treatment options will you consider? Would you start treatment now or recall?

A: Treatment options include the following:
   - *Recall* (no treatment now, monitor only) – re-evaluate in one year. We *do* recommend monitoring her open bite since it will most likely close as her maxillary incisors erupt (assuming the absence of a habit). We *do not* recommend monitoring her unilateral posterior crossbite since it will not self-correct and asymmetric mandibular growth may result.
   - *Fixed orthodontic appliances* – to level her maxillary arch, force maxillary incisor eruption, and close Anna's anterior open bite. We do not recommend this option without giving her maxillary incisors time to erupt naturally.

- *RME (or possibly quad-helix maxillary skeletal expansion)* – is recommended. If posterior overjet is increased with maxillary skeletal expansion, then Anna's maxillary transverse deficiency can be corrected, her right crossbite and CR-CO shift eliminated, and possible future asymmetric mandibular growth prevented (if due to the CR-CO shift).
- *Thumb habit, or tongue-interposition habit, correction* – are not recommended yet because Anna and her parents deny such habits and because the open bite is probably due to the normal transition from primary to permanent dentition.

Q: What is your recommended treatment for Anna? How would you proceed?

A: We decided to monitor Anna's anterior open bite under the assumption that it could close spontaneously. We employed RME, and Anna's lateral shift and transverse posterior discrepancy corrected. Four months later (Figure 5.60a), our orthodontic resident removed the RME appliance, and a TPA was fabricated to maintain the maxillary expansion. Unfortunately, Anna never returned for placement of the TPA (the RME appliance should have been re-cemented until the TPA was delivered). Later, we received the photo of Anna in Figure 5.60b from another orthodontist.

Q: Contrasting Figure 5.59b with Figures 5.60a and 5.60b, what do you observe?

A: The anterior open bite continued to close with the eruption of the maxillary permanent central incisors. The maxillary primary lateral incisors exfoliated and the maxillary permanent lateral incisors continued to erupt. There was an inadequate expansion of the maxillary arch during RME, and the maxillary right first premolar is erupting nearly in crossbite.

Q: What is the ideal amount of RME?

A: When the mandibular first permanent molars are upright, the ideal amount of RME is to expand until the maxillary first permanent molar lingual cusps are end-to-end with the mandibular first permanent molar buccal cusps. This amount of expansion is *overexpansion* and permits uprighting buccally tipped maxillary permanent first molars. Also, overexpansion is important in anticipation of some post-expansion collapse (relapse).

When the mandibular first permanent molars are not upright, but tipped lingually instead, the mandibular first permanent molars should be uprighted before or during RME. Uprighting mandibular first permanent molars is performed using either a Schwarz appliance, an expanded LLHA, or crossbite elastics worn from the buccal of the RME appliance to buttons bonded on the lingual of the mandibular molars.

Q: We assumed that Anna's open bite resulted from normal maxillary incisor eruption during the transition from primary to permanent dentition. What if it was actually due to a habit – could RME have helped?

A: Yes. If her open bite had been due to a thumb habit, then placement of a palatal expander may have discouraged the habit. If her open bite had been due to an anterior tongue-interposition habit, then expanding the maxilla may have created more room for the tongue and lessened the need for the tongue to posture forward (to maintain a patent airway).

Q: Can you suggest "take-home pearls" regarding Anna?

A: "Take-home pearls" include the following:
- Dental (functional) open bites result from inadequate tooth eruption, *not* from excessive vertical facial growth. The hallmark of a *dental* open bite is an open bite in a patient who is vertically normal.

(a)

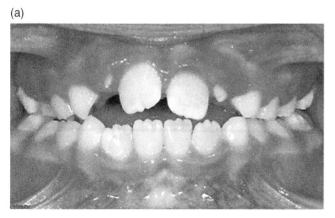

(b)

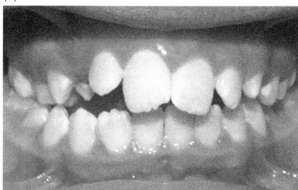

Figure 5.60 Progress photos of Anna. (a) Four months post-RME after removal of the expansion appliance (TPA was never delivered). (b) A photograph sent to us later.

- Dental anterior open bites usually result from tongue-interposition habits (resting tongue habits), digit-sucking habits, or lip-biting habits. However, other causes include ankylosed teeth, blocked out (impacted) teeth, or incompletely erupted teeth during the transition from primary to permanent dentitions.
- Dental (functional) open bites correct by eliminating any habit and allowing the teeth to erupt naturally or by erupting the teeth with orthodontics. In Anna's case, during the transition from primary to permanent dentitions, monitoring was prudent.
- We recommend *early* dental open bite closure via habit control when the patient is interested in stopping the habit. Otherwise, we wait until the child matures.
- A mandibular asymmetry may result if a lateral CR-CO shift into a posterior crossbite is not corrected during growth.
- If a unilateral posterior crossbite and lateral shift are treated in a timely manner (early mixed dentition), then a mandibular asymmetry developing from the lateral shift can be largely eliminated. If a unilateral posterior crossbite has resulted from asymmetric mandibular growth, then the asymmetric mandibular growth must be dealt with.
- You must retain RME in order to prevent relapse. In addition to holding the maxillary expansion for three or more months post-RME with the appliance in place, *we strongly recommend overexpansion followed by placement of a TPA for twelve or more months post-RME.* The longer we practice, the longer we retain the maxillary expansions.

Case Emily

Q: Emily is six years and ten months old (Figure 5.61), and she presents to you for a consultation. Her parents' chief complaint is, "We are concerned because Emily cannot bite off food." Her PMH, PDH, periodontal evaluation, and TMJ evaluation are WRN. Do you need any additional records in order to decide whether to perform early treatment, or recall, Emily?

A: No additional records are required. A decision to treat, or recall, Emily can be made using the above records.

Q: Compile your diagnostic findings and problem list for Emily using the above records. Also, state your diagnosis.

A:

Table 5.16 Diagnostic findings and problem list for Emily.

Full face and Profile	*Frontal View*
	Face is symmetric
	Soft tissue LAFH WRN (soft tissue Glabella – Subnasale approximately equal to Subnasale – soft tissue Menton)
	Lip competence
	UDML WRN (based upon mesial of left central incisor)
	Gingival display in posed smile is inadequate (maxillary central incisor gingival margins are apical to border of maxillary lip)
	Profile View
	Convex profile
	Chin projection retrusive
	Tipped-up nose
	Obtuse NLA
	Obtuse lip-chin-throat angle
Radiographs	Early mixed dentition
	Developing maxillary second premolar crowns are not observed (the left maxillary second premolar crown could be partially overlapping the left first premolar crown)
Intraoral Photos and Models	Angle Class II subdivision left
	Iowa Classification: I I II (2 mm) II (2 mm)
	OJ ~ 3 mm
	Anterior open bite
	Maxillary midline diastema with low maxillary labial frenum
	Maxillary labial frenum has a papillary penetrating attachment
	0.6 mm maxillary anterior space is currently present (8.5 mm of space with a right primary lateral incisor of 5.1 mm width but two unerupted maxillary permanent lateral incisors of 6.5 mm width each)
	2.6 mm of maxillary space is anticipated following the eruption of all permanent teeth (if appropriate space maintenance is employed)
	2.5 mm mandibular anterior space is currently present
	5.7 mm of mandibular space is anticipated following the eruption of all permanent teeth (if appropriate space maintenance is employed)
	Maxillary arch asymmetric with left side 2 mm ahead
	Mandibular arch symmetric
	Maxillary central incisors stepped up relative to maxillary posterior teeth (Figure 5.61f)
	Left posterior lingual crossbite
	Mandibular dental midline left of maxillary dental midline
	Poor hygiene
Other	None
Diagnosis	Class II subdivision left malocclusion with left posterior lingual crossbite

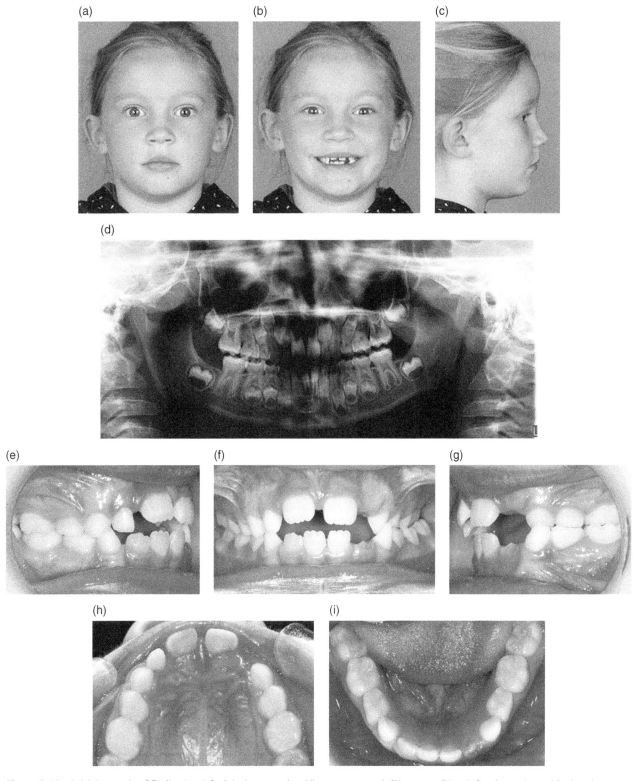

Figure 5.61 Initial records of Emily: (a–c) facial photographs; (d) pantomograph [Note: maxillary left primary lateral incisor has exfoliated subsequent to this image]; (e–i) intraoral photographs.

Q: What did we fail to check for?

A: We failed to check for the presence of a CR-CO shift. When we finally did this, we found CR=CO. Emily did *not* have a shift.

Q: What is the average age for maxillary and mandibular permanent incisor eruption?

A:

Mandibular central incisors: six to seven years
Mandibular lateral incisors: seven to eight years
Maxillary central incisors: seven to eight years
Maxillary lateral incisors: eight to nine years [113].

Q: How do these eruption times relate to Emily's anterior open bite?

A: Emily is almost seven years old. So, the eruption of her maxillary and mandibular permanent incisors appears to be on track. In other words, her anterior open bite could be a result of the normal transition from primary to permanent dentition.

Q: We noted the possible absence of maxillary second premolar crown calcification. The average age for *completion* of maxillary second premolar crown calcification is six to seven years. Should we assume that Emily is an example of maxillary second premolar agenesis? What recommendation would you make regarding them?

A: Her maxillary second premolars could be missing. However, their development could simply be delayed.

Q: How would you recommend dealing with the possible missing maxillary second premolars?

A: For now, we would recommend monitoring their development for at least another year.

Q: Provide a detailed space analysis for Emily's maxillary and mandibular arches. In other words, how were the 2.6 mm of maxillary space and 5.7 mm of mandibular space calculated (if appropriate space maintenance is employed).

A:

Average mesiodistal widths of permanent teeth (mm): [94]

Maxillary Central Incisor	8.5	Mandibular Central Incisor	5.0
Maxillary Lateral Incisor	6.5	Mandibular Lateral Incisor	5.5
Maxillary Canine	7.5	Mandibular Canine	7.0
Maxillary First Premolar	7.0	Mandibular First Premolar	7.0
Maxillary Second Premolar	7.0	Mandibular Second Premolar	7.0
Maxillary First Molar	10.0	Mandibular First Molar	11.0
Maxillary Second Molar	9.0	Mandibular Second Molar	10.5

Average mesiodistal widths of *primary* teeth (mm): [94]

Maxillary Central Incisor	6.5	Mandibular Central Incisor	4.2
Maxillary Lateral Incisor	5.1	Mandibular Lateral Incisor	4.1
Maxillary Canine	7.0	Mandibular Canine	5.0
Maxillary First Molar	7.3	Mandibular First Molar	7.7
Maxillary Second Molar	8.2	Mandibular Second Molar	9.9

MAXILLARY ARCH
+8.5 mm of anterior space is present (Figure 5.61h)
+5.1 mm maxillary right primary lateral incisor mesiodistal width
−6.5 mm required for maxillary right permanent lateral incisor
−6.5 mm required for maxillary left permanent lateral incisor
+2 mm of anticipated leeway space (1 mm/side)
Balance = +8.5 mm + 5.1 mm −6.5 mm −6.5 mm +2 mm = + 2.6 mm

MANDIBULAR ARCH
+2.5 mm anterior space currently present (Figure 5.61i)
+3.2 mm of anticipated leeway space (1.6 mm/side)
Balance = +2.5 mm +3.2 mm= +5.7 mm

That is, *2.6 mm of maxillary space and 5.7 mm of mandibular space are anticipated following the eruption of all permanent teeth (if appropriate space maintenance is employed).*

Q: What are Emily's *primary* problems in each dimension, plus other problems?

A:

Table 5.17 Primary problems list for Emily.

AP	Class II subdivision left
	Iowa Classification: I I II (2 mm) II (2 mm)
Vertical	Anterior open bite
Transverse	Left posterior lingual crossbite
Other	Possible agenesis of maxillary second premolars
	Papillary penetrating maxillary labial frenum attachment

Q: What features indicate Emily's open bite is a *dental (functional)* open bite? A skeletal open bite? Is her open bite a combination of both?

A. Emily's dental open bite features include the following:

- Soft tissue LAFH WRN (soft tissue Glabella – Subnasale approximately equal to Subnasale – soft tissue Menton)
- Lip competence (absence of an ILG, Figure 5.61a) indicating that her soft tissue vertical growth has kept pace with her skeletal vertical growth
- Maxillary incisors stepped apically relative to the corresponding posterior teeth (Figure 5.61f) indicating that incisor under-eruption is the cause of her open bite
- Anterior open bite football-shaped and restricted to the incisors – indicating that her open bite is limited to the area of a possible habit.

Her *skeletal* open bite features include:

- None.
  Emily has a dental open bite.

Q: To help determine the etiology of Emily's open bite, what questions should you ask and what should you check for?

A: Questions you should ask and things you should check for include the following:

- Ask how long her open bite has been present. Emily and her parents cannot recall.
- Contact her dentist, ask for any previous panoramic images, and try to determine if her *primary* incisors were stepped apically compared to her posterior teeth (i.e. whether the open bite was present in her primary dentition). No previous panoramic images are available.
- Ask Emily if she has ever had a thumb-sucking habit (digit habit) or lip-biting habit. Emily states that she sucks her thumb – mostly at night (Figure 5.62).
- Check for an anterior tongue-interposition habit. Do this by asking Emily to close her eyes while you talk to her parents. Ask her to open her eyes (distracting her) while you gently/quickly retract her lips – noting if her tongue is resting between her anterior teeth. She does not exhibit an anterior tongue interposition habit.
- Inquire as to whether Emily has suffered jaw trauma (resulting in condylar degeneration, upward and backward movements of her condyles, and an anterior open bite). Her parents and Emily deny any history of trauma, generalized musculoskeletal problems, TMJ pain, or TMJ dysfunction. Further,

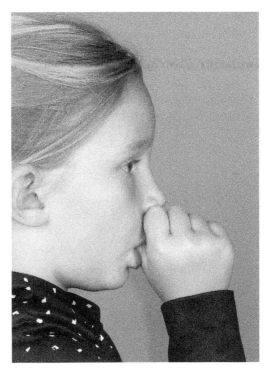

Figure 5.62 Emily demonstrates her thumb habit.

there does not appear to be any degeneration of her condyles, radiographically (Figure 5.61d). Her condyles appear well corticated.

- Check incisor mobility. Her incisors exhibit normal mobility, so dental ankylosis is not the cause of her open bite.
- Check for anterior tooth crowding which could be blocking out incisors and preventing eruption. Crowding is not the cause of her open bite.
- Check for a *temporary* anterior open bite due to normal tooth eruption. Since Emily is undergoing the transition from primary to permanent incisor dentition, this could be a contributing factor to her open bite.

Q: Based upon the above, what is the most likely cause of Emily's anterior open bite?

A: The open bite is probably due to her thumb habit, but the fact that she is in transition from primary to permanent incisor dentition cannot be discounted.

Q: Emily exhibits a maxillary midline diastema with low labial frenum. Should this diastema be closed with early treatment?

A: No. In most cases, mixed dentition diastemas close spontaneously as the permanent canines erupt [111]. Also, the vertical position of the frenum attachment tends to improve (migrates superiorly relative to the papilla) with growth and development [100]. Therefore, we recommend monitoring the diastema for now.

If the diastema persists, then it can be closed orthodontically in the permanent dentition. If you must close the diastema orthodontically, then we recommend the placement of a bonded fixed lingual retainer between the central incisors to maintain closure.

Q: Emily has a left lingual crossbite. Will this crossbite *create* asymmetric mandibular growth?

A: No. Since CR=CO (no lateral shift) the right mandibular condyle is seated in the right glenoid fossa. That is, the right condyle is not distracted out of the right glenoid fossa by a left lateral shift – which would accelerate right mandibular growth like a Class II functional appliance. Therefore, the left crossbite should not cause asymmetric mandibular growth.

Q: Could her left crossbite be a sign of *asymmetric mandibular growth*?

A: Yes. If the right side of a patient's mandible grows forward more than their left, their right buccal occlusion will become more Class III than their left, their mandibular midline will shift to the left, their chin will deviate to the left, and they will develop a left posterior lingual crossbite.

Of these features, Emily is Class I on the right but Class II on the left (i.e. more Class III on the right), her mandibular midline is to the left of her maxillary midline, and she is in the left posterior lingual crossbite. However, a chin asymmetry is not observed (Figure 5.61a), and a maxillary dental arch asymmetry exists which explains the left Class II relationship. Even so, *mandibular asymmetric growth cannot be ruled out and must be monitored*.

Q: Is it easier to treat a patient who presents with a lateral CR-CO shift into a unilateral posterior crossbite (*functional unilateral crossbite*), or is it easier to treat a patient with a unilateral posterior crossbite without a CR-CO shift (*true unilateral crossbite*)?

A: It is easier to treat a patient with a lateral CR-CO shift into a unilateral posterior crossbite. Why? When the lateral shift is eliminated, the transverse discrepancy becomes bilateral *but smaller on the crossbite side*. Also, bilateral arch forces (expansion, constriction) to correct a crossbite are easier to generate than unilateral forces. Further, if the unilateral crossbite is due to asymmetric mandibular growth (no CR-CO shift), then the same growth pattern will continue during adolescence and cause crossbite correction relapse.

Q: *When* should Emily's left posterior crossbite be corrected?

A: We recommend correcting Emily's left posterior crossbite any time now but before puberty. Why?

- Emily is in the early mixed dentition. Her maxillary permanent first molars are erupted and will provide excellent anchorage for an RME appliance.
- The most marked RME skeletal effects occur *before/during* the pubertal growth spurt, and expansion after the pubertal growth spurt is primarily dentoalveolar (not orthopedic/skeletal) [120–126]. Do not wait until after puberty to attempt RME.
- Cooperation should be ideal at Emily's age. Cooperation may decline later.
- Emily does not present with a lateral CR-CO shift into the posterior crossbite. If she did, then we would recommend correcting the lateral shift and crossbite *immediately* – to prevent the shift from causing asymmetric mandibular growth.
- Although posterior crossbites can be treated in the *primary* dentition [127–129], there is generally no urgency to treat them that early. Of course, if a patient in the primary dentition has a posterior crossbite due to a lateral shift of a simple occlusal interference, then we would recommend treating it in the primary dentition with minor occlusal adjustment.

Q: How do you decide whether to treat Emily's left Class II relationship orthopedically?

A: We lack a cephalometric radiograph to determine whether an anteroposterior skeletal discrepancy exists. However, Emily exhibits a convex profile, so mandibular skeletal deficiency (and/or ineffective bony Pogonion) is likely.

The magnitude of her left Class II relationship is small (2 mm), and we may choose to treat it with masking (e.g. Class II elastics) during comprehensive treatment in adult dentition. Furthermore, Emily's mandible may be growing asymmetrically, and we recommend caution when considering Class II treatment because she may require Class III orthopedics (e.g. TAD-supported Class III elastics) on her right.

To summarize, considering her mild unilateral Class II relationship, her age, her dental developmental stage, and the fact that her mandible may be growing asymmetrically, we do not feel that Emily is a good candidate for early left Class II orthopedic correction. We recommend monitoring growth for now.

Q: Discuss Emily in the context of three principles applied to every early treatment patient.

A:

1) The goal of early treatment is to correct developing problems – get the patient *back to normal for their stage of development* (including preventing complications such as resorption of adjacent tooth roots, reducing later treatment complexity, or reducing/eliminating unknowns). Correcting her anterior open bite, left posterior crossbite, left Class II relationship, possible asymmetric mandibular growth, and possible maxillary second premolar agenesis would put Emily back on track.

2) Early treatment should address *very specific problems with a clearly defined end point*, usually begun and ended within six to nine months (not protracted over years except for some orthopedic problems).
   - Assuming that her anterior open bite is due to a thumb habit, open bite closure has a clear end point *only* if she stops her habit. If her open bite is due to the normal transition from primary to permanent dentition, then closure has a clear end point and is virtually guaranteed.
   - Correction of her left posterior crossbite can be readily performed and has a clear end point (using RME) if the underlying cause is not asymmetric mandibular growth. If the crossbite has resulted from asymmetric mandibular growth, then we will be dealing with it until growth is complete.
   - Correction of her left Class II relationship has a clear end point but we recommend addressing it during comprehensive treatment in the permanent dentition. We recommend monitoring her growth for now.
   - Determination of second premolar agenesis could take longer than six to nine months.

3) Always ask: Is it necessary that I treat the patient early? *What harm could come from doing nothing now?*
   - No harm will come if we choose to monitor Emily's open bite. Her anterior teeth will simply not erupt if the open bite is due to a thumb-sucking habit. They will erupt if due to a normal transition to permanent dentition.
   - Since a CR-CO lateral shift is lacking, we anticipate no harm from monitoring her left posterior crossbite. The crossbite can be readily addressed any time before puberty with RME if it is not due to asymmetric mandibular growth.
   - No harm will come from postponing Class II treatment, monitoring growth for a year, or monitoring second premolar development for a year.

Q: Should you begin early treatment now, or recall Emily? If you begin now, what treatment options would you consider?

A: Treatment options include the following:
   - *Recall* (no treatment now, monitor only) – re-evaluate in one year. This is a good option. Why? Emily may end her thumb habit, incisors may erupt, and her open bite may close spontaneously. Or, the open bite will close if it is due to the transition to permanent dentition. Also, since a lateral CR-CO shift is absent, there is no pressing needed to correct her left crossbite. Finally, when she returns in one year, we can better evaluate her growth pattern and maxillary second premolar development.
   - *Attempt to discourage her thumb habit through discussion and encouragement* – is recommended if Emily is interested in trying to stop the habit. Even if she attempts and fails, with time, she will succeed if she is determined. We recommend giving her a chance to end the habit on her own before resorting to thumb paint or a thumb crib.
   - *Forced maxillary incisor eruption using fixed orthodontic appliances* – to close Emily's anterior open bite is *not* recommended without giving Emily an opportunity to end the habit first. Why? If she does not end her habit, then the open bite will return after a forced eruption.
   - *Maxillary skeletal expansion* with RME or possibly a quad-helix – will eventually be recommended to correct her left posterior crossbite. However:
     1) Since a lateral CR-CO shift is absent, we do not see a compelling reason to perform RME yet.
     2) Before we correct the crossbite, we recommend monitoring Emily's growth to determine whether asymmetric growth is the cause of the crossbite.
     3) With the maxillary expansion, we must be careful not to *overexpand her right* maxillary dentition into a buccal crossbite.
   Note: When a palatal expansion appliance is used, it will act as a thumb-sucking habit deterrent.
   - *Space maintenance* – placement of an LLHA is not *recommended* at this time. Emily currently has 2.5 mm of mandibular anterior space, her permanent canines and premolar roots are < ½ developed, and their eruption is not imminent.
   - *Extraction of maxillary right primary lateral incisor* – to encourage eruption of the right permanent lateral incisor is not recommended because Emily is less than seven years old and the average age for maxillary permanent lateral incisor eruption is eight and nine years [113]. That is, maxillary permanent lateral incisor eruption is on track.
   - *Left Class II (2 mm) correction* using orthopedics or Class II elastics (masking) – is not recommended at this time. As previously stated, we recommend

caution when considering Class II treatment because Emily may require asymmetric Class III orthopedics (e.g. TAD-supported Class III elastics) on her right, later. We recommend monitoring growth for now.

Q: Based upon the above options, what is your recommended treatment for Emily? How would you proceed?

A: We held a thoughtful discussion with Emily, encouraging her to stop sucking her thumb. She was enthusiastic about ending the habit, and we asked her parents to encourage her. She was recalled nine months later at which time her parents stated that she was no longer sucking her thumb. We decided to recall her one year later.

Q: Emily presented for another recall/consultation appointment (Figure 5.63). She was now 8 years and 8 months old. Records were made and a *left lateral 2 mm shift* from CR to CO was detected. An intraoral photograph was not taken in CR to illustrate the shift, but if you look closely at Figure 5.63b, you can see that Emily's maxillary and mandibular midlines appear coincident when her teeth are separated. Identify diagnostic findings and problems that differ from her initial records list (Table 5.16) made two years earlier.

A: Initial (six years and ten months of age) to recall (eight years and eight months of age): Diagnostic findings and problem list differences for Emily include the following:
- Moderate buccal corridors (Figure 5.63b)
- Maxillary skeletal position WRN (Figure 5.63e)
- Mandibular anteroposterior skeletal position WRN (ANB = 3° with a normal maxilla)
- Skeletal LAFH WRN (LAFH/TAFH × 100% = 53%)
- Flat MPA (FMA = 20°, SN-MP = 28°)
- Proclined maxillary incisors (U1 to SN angle = 112°)
- Proclined mandibular incisors (FMIA = 55°)
- Entering late mixed dentition stage of development (Figure 5.63f, mandibular right permanent canine eruption imminent)
- Maxillary second premolar crowns are developing (Figure 5.63f)
- Maxillary left second premolar erupting ectopically (rotated by 90°)
- Maxillary lateral incisors are erupting and on track for age
- Anterior central incisor open bite has closed (OB 10%)
- Mandibular midline is to the left of the maxillary midline by 2 mm but a 2 mm left lateral CR-CO shift is present.
- Maxillary labial frenum has migrated superiorly, relative to the papilla, and the midline diastema is reduced.

Q: How does detection of a 2 mm left lateral CR-CO shift influence your decision to begin early treatment?

A: Detection of this shift compels us to begin treatment. Why? If Emily's lateral shift into crossbite *is not* corrected, then a mandibular asymmetry may develop [114–116]. However, if her shift *is* corrected, then an asymmetry developing from it can be eliminated [115–119]. It is unfortunate that we did not identify this shift earlier.

Q: How does the lateral shift affect Emily's *anteroposterior* relationship?

A: As Emily shifts to the left (Figure 5.64a, red arrow) from CR to CO:
- Her left condyle rotates in the glenoid fossa (Figure 5.64b)
- Her right condyle and right dentition *translate anteriorly* (Figure 5.64b and c, yellow arrows).

Therefore, the left CR-CO shift has little effect on her left anteroposterior relationship but results in her *right* anteroposterior relationship appearing more Class III than it really is in CR.

Q: I am confused. If her right condyle and right dentition are translated forward during the left lateral CR-CO shift, then why isn't Emily Class III on the right?

A: It is true that Emily should be more Class III on the right *relative* to the left in CO – and she is. In other words, Emily is Class I on the right but Class II on the left.

Q: How will this finding of a 2 mm left lateral shift impact Emily's treatment?

A: The most important impact is that *asymmetric mandibular growth is now unlikely*. This is wonderful news. Once the lateral shift is eliminated, we anticipate that Emily will be slightly Class II in CR on the left *and on the right*.

Treating a mild bilateral Class II is far easier than treating asymmetric mandibular jaw growth. Furthermore, the finding of a left lateral shift means that in CR, Emily has a milder left posterior lingual crossbite and can be treated with bilateral RME force.

Q: Would you recommend extraction of Emily's maxillary left primary second molar in order to increase the chance that her ectopically erupting maxillary left second premolar will erupt (Figure 5.63f)?

A: No, at least not yet. Why? Although the maxillary second premolar crowns appear to be fully calcified, their roots are only beginning to form. If we extract the maxillary left primary second molar before the root of the

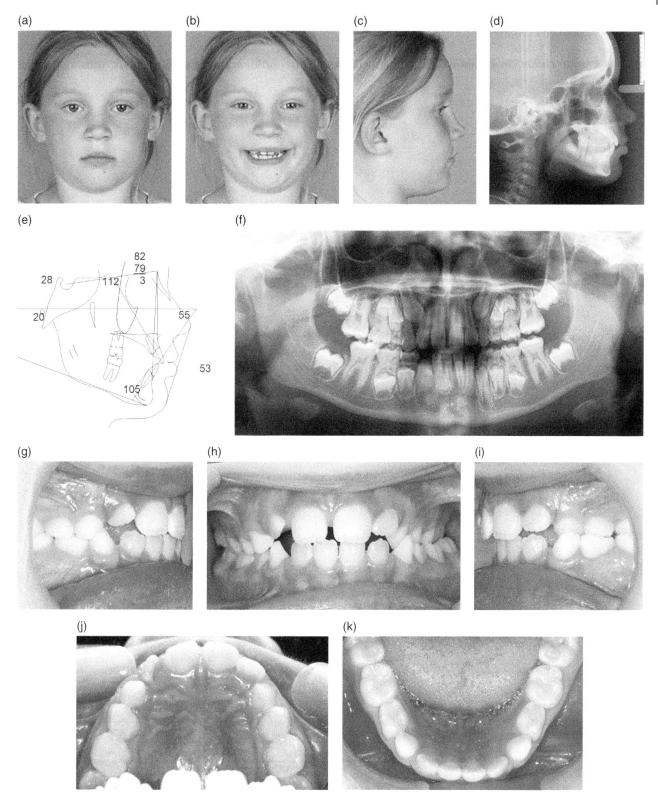

Figure 5.63 Recall records of Emily [Note: Emily has a *2 mm left CR-CO shift and intraoral photographs are made in CO*].

(a)

(b)

(c)

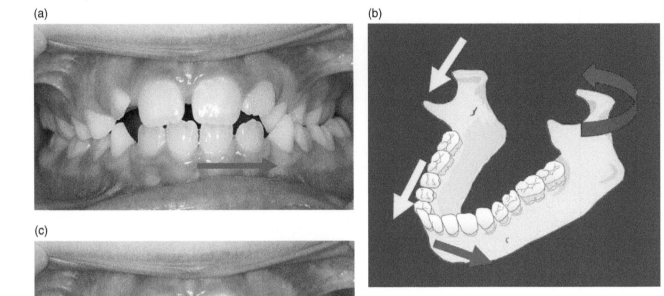

Figure 5.64 Emily's left lateral shift from CR to CO moves her mandibular midline to the left (a, red arrow), places her in a left lingual crossbite, rotates her mandible around her left condyle (b), *translates her mandibular right condyle anteriorly* (b), and translates her mandibular right condyle and dentition forward (b and c, yellow arrows).

maxillary left second premolar is half formed, then we will delay the second premolar eruption as the bone heals over it.

However, if the maxillary left second premolar ectopic eruption continues, then we may consider extracting the maxillary left primary second molar in the future. If we decide to extract the maxillary left primary second molar, then we will want to prevent mesial drift of the maxillary left permanent first molar with either headgear wear or placement of a Nance holding arch.

Q: Should an LLHA be delivered to Emily?

A: We do not feel that space maintenance (an LLHA) is necessary. Why? Emily currently has 2.5 mm mandibular anterior space, and leeway space is not needed to eliminate anterior crowding.

Also, she has a reasonable profile and is skeletally normal (Figures 5.63c and 5.63e). As her mandibular primary molars exfoliate without an LLHA, the mandibular permanent first molars will drift forward from bilateral "end-on" Class II (in CR) toward Class I, and the proclined mandibular incisors will upright. Orthopedic Class II treatment will probably be unnecessary.

Q: What unknowns do you face with Emily?

A: Emily's bilateral first permanent molar relationship once the left CR-CO shift has been eliminated. We anticipate that she will be bilaterally ("end-on") Class II, but until the shift is eliminated, we cannot be sure. Other unknowns include future jaw growth magnitude and direction, patient compliance with treatment, whether her midpalatal suture will separate if we employ RME, and whether her maxillary left second premolar will continue to erupt ectopically.

Q: Would you recommend recalling Emily in another year or would you recommend proceeding with early treatment now? If you recommend proceeding, then what early treatment would you suggest?

A: We recommend RME now to eliminate Emily's left lateral shift and crossbite, reduce the size of her buccal corridors, and determine her true permanent first molar anteroposterior relationships. If she is bilateral Class II, then we will consider either Class II orthopedics or monitoring her molar relationships during the transition to permanent dentition.

We will explain to Emily's parents that eventual extraction of her maxillary left primary second molar, and possible surgical exposure of her ectopically erupting maxillary left second premolar, may be necessary. A Nance holding arch may also be considered for maxillary space maintenance. Following the eruption of all permanent teeth, records will be made and the need for comprehensive orthodontic treatment determined and discussed.

Q: Can you suggest "take-home" pearls regarding Emily's consultations?

A: "Take-home pearls" include the following:

- Emily presented at six years and ten months of age. She was an Angle Class II subdivision left with an anterior dental open bite, unilateral left posterior lingual crossbite, and possible agenesis of maxillary second premolars. A CR-CO shift was not detected. Her open bite was discussed with her, and she was encouraged to stop sucking her thumb. She successfully stopped her habit, and her central incisor open bite closed. At her eight-year, eight-month recall/consultation appointment, a 2 mm left lateral CR-CO shift was discovered.
- Emily's maxillary central incisors were stepped up relative to her maxillary posterior teeth (Figure 5.61f), but her facial proportions were WRN and she exhibited lip competence. The hallmark of a dental (functional) anterior open bite is an open bite in a patient who is *vertically normal*. Emily was normal.
- Emily's dental (functional) open bite was due to a thumb-sucking habit. Other causes of dental anterior open bites include tongue-interposition habits (resting tongue habits), lip-biting habits, ankylosed

teeth, blocked out (crowded) teeth, or incompletely erupted teeth during the transition from primary to permanent dentition.

- Her anterior open bite self-corrected by habit elimination which allowed her maxillary central incisors to erupt. We recommend early dental anterior open bite treatment through habit control *when the patient is interested in stopping the habit*. Otherwise, we generally wait until the child matures.
- When in doubt, it is prudent to monitor the development of missing teeth before concluding agenesis. Remember this when you see a similar patient in practice.
- We cannot overstate the importance of checking for the presence of a CR-CO shift at every appointment (*check for a shift the first time and every time you see a patient*). If you do not know where your starting point is, then you cannot determine the treatment course to take you to your destination.
- We checked for a CR-CO shift when Emily was six years and ten months of age, but we failed to detect one. It was fortunate that we discovered the 2 mm left lateral CR-CO shift when she returned to our clinic at eight years and eight months of age. If we had not detected this lateral shift, then Emily could have developed a mandibular asymmetry.
- Elimination of the left lateral shift with RME should move Emily's mandibular right dentition posteriorly, from a Class I into a slight Class II molar relationship. This should make Emily Class II, bilaterally. Also, elimination of the left shift converts her unilateral left lingual crossbite into a *bilateral* transverse discrepancy (constricted maxilla). Bilateral maxillary transverse deficiencies are generally easier to treat than true unilateral crossbites.

Case Gabby

Q: Gabby is a ten-year-old girl (Figure 5.65) who presents to you with her parent's chief complaint, "Gabby cannot bite off food. Her front teeth do not touch." Her PMH, PDH, periodontal evaluation, and TMJ evaluation are WRN. CR=CO. Compile your diagnostic findings and problem list for Gabby. Also state your diagnosis.

A:

Table 5.18 Diagnostic findings and problem list for Gabby.

Full face and Profile	***Frontal View***
	Face is symmetric
	Soft tissue LAFH WRN (soft tissue Glabella – Subnasale approximately equal to Subnasale – soft tissue Menton)
	Lip competence
	UDML WRN
	Midlines are coincident
	Inadequate incisal display
	Inadequate gingival display in posed smile (maxillary central incisor gingival margins not coincident with border of maxillary lip)
	Large buccal corridors
	Smile is asymmetric (facial musculature elevates left oral commissure higher than right commissure)
	Profile View
	Convex profile
	Nasal tip up
	Protrusive maxillary lip
	Obtuse NLA (angle appears normal at Subnasale but increases toward the nasal tip)
	Deficient chin projection
	Obtuse lip-chin-throat angle
Ceph Analysis	***Skeletal***
	Protrusive maxillary position (A-Point ahead of Nasion-perpendicular line)
	Mandibular deficient *relative* to maxilla (ANB angle = 5°)
	Skeletal LAFH WRN (ANS-Menton/Nasion-Menton × 100% = 56%; normal skeletal LAFH=55%, sd = 2%)
	MPA WRN (FMA = 25°; SNMP = 38°)
	Effective bony Pogonion (Pogonion lies on Nasion-B Point line)
	Dental
	Maxillary incisor angulation appears WRN (U1 to SN = 102°), but Sella is low (SN to FH = 13°). Adjusting for SN to FH being +6° more than average, maxillary incisors are mildly proclined (adjusted U1 to SN = 102° + 6° = 108°)
	Mandibular incisors mildly proclined (FMIA = 60°; ideal FMIA = 65°)
Radiographs	Late mixed dentition stage of development
Intraoral Photos and Models	Angle Class II division 1
	Iowa Classification: II(3 mm) II(3 mm) II(3 mm) II(2 mm)
	OJ ~3 mm
	Anterior open bite
	0.5 mm of maxillary incisor crowding is currently present
	0.9 mm of maxillary arch spacing is anticipated following the eruption of all permanent teeth (if proper space maintenance is employed)
	2.0 mm of mandibular incisor crowding is currently present
	4.3 mm of mandibular arch spacing is anticipated following the eruption of all permanent teeth (if proper space maintenance is employed)
	Symmetric maxillary dental arch
	Asymmetric mandibular dental arch – left molar slightly ahead of right
	Small maxillary lateral incisors
	Mildly tapered maxillary dental arch (Figures 5.65j and 5.65o)
	Transverse compensations – maxillary first permanent molar buccal crown torque (Figure 5.65q) and mandibular first permanent molar lingual crown torque (Figure 5.65r)
	Maxillary incisors stepped up relative to maxillary posterior teeth
Other	None
Diagnosis	Class II malocclusion with anterior open bite

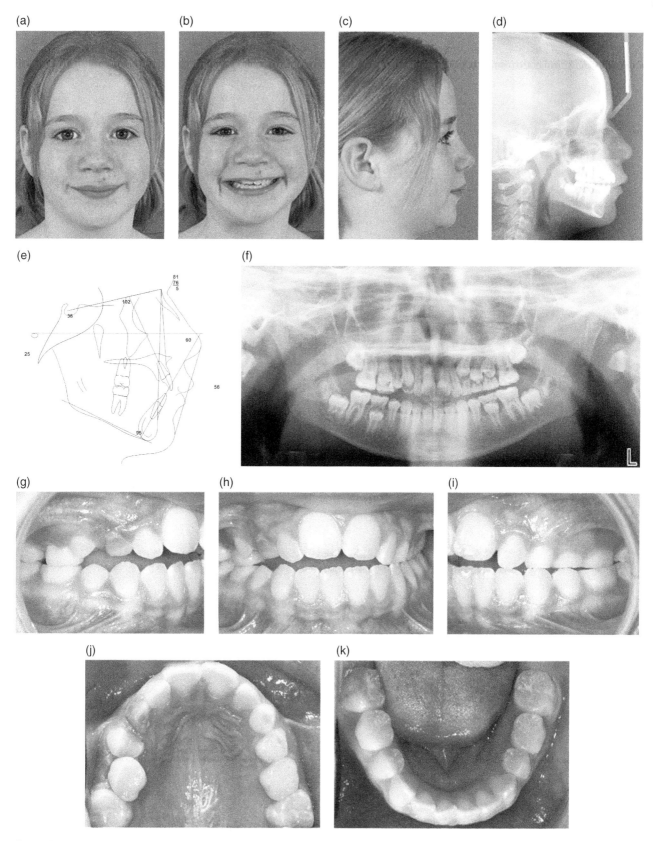

Figure 5.65 Initial records of Gabby: (a–c) facial photographs; (d and e) lateral cephalometric radiograph and tracing; (f) pantomograph; (g–k) intraoral photographs; (l–t) models.

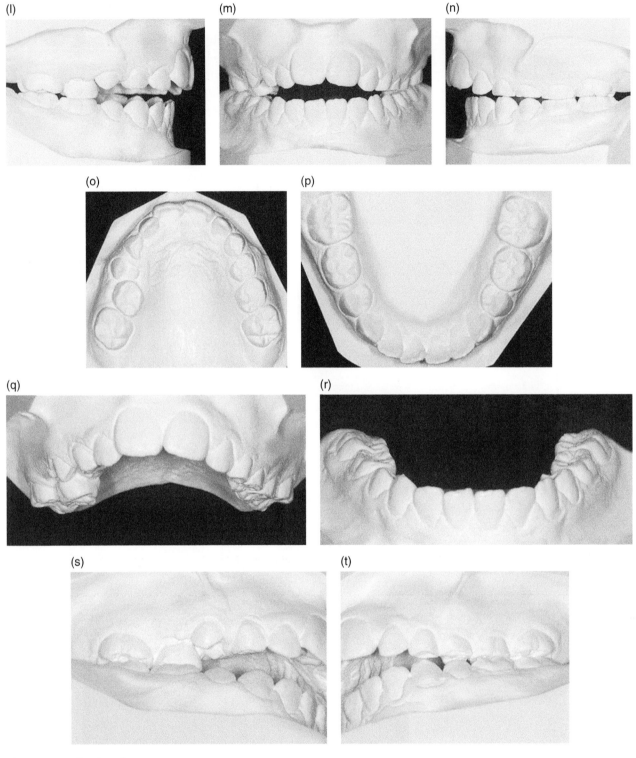

(l) (m) (n)

(o) (p)

(q) (r)

(s) (t)

Figure 5.65   (Continued)

Q: We noted that Gabby exhibits *inadequate incisal display*. But how can we make this observation without a photograph of Gabby with her lips relaxed and held slightly apart?

A: You can make this observation from the lateral cephalometric radiograph (Figure 5.65d) taken with relaxed lips. Observe that Gabby's maxillary incisal edges are *stepped above* her maxillary lip border – instead of being stepped below the border by 2–4 mm (ideal adolescent incisal display). Therefore, Gabby has an inadequate incisal display.

Note: If a patient is over-closed with redundant lips, then you cannot use this technique. You would first need to have the patient open to where their lips were relaxed and just touching before you make the cephalometric radiograph. Why? As the over-closed patient opens, the redundant maxillary lip will descend and reduce the incisal display.

Q: Gabby's anteroposterior jaw descriptions are presented in Table 5.18. Can you discuss Gabby's jaw positions, and chin position, in more detail?

A: Let's start with her maxilla. It is skeletally protrusive because A-Point is ahead of an imaginary line drawn from Nasion vertically downward, perpendicular to Frankfort Horizontal (Figure 5.66a, Nasion-perpendicular line in red). While it is true that SNA = 81° which is WRN, Sella appears low which leads to a smaller SNA. If Sella was higher (normally positioned), then SNA would be greater and indicate a protrusive maxilla. *Gabby's maxilla is skeletally protrusive.*

Next, let's consider Gabby's mandible. Since Gabby's maxilla is skeletally protrusive, we cannot use her ANB angle to judge her mandibular skeletal position (see Appendix). Instead, we relate her mandible to Nasion-perpendicular by measuring the angle formed between Nasion-perpendicular and the Nasion-B Point line. The angle is ~2° (Figure 5.66a) which indicates that her *mandible is skeletally normal.*

Finally, we can judge Gabby's chin position using her profile photograph (Figure 5.66b) and the zero-meridian line – a vertical line drawn perpendicular to clinical Frankfort horizontal, passing through Nasion.

A normally positioned chin should lie on this line or just short of it [130, 131]. Since Gabby's soft tissue Pogonion lies on the zero-meridian line, her chin position is judged to be normal.

Because Frankfort horizontal varies considerably from true horizontal established when a patient is postured in natural head position [132], many consider the zero-degree meridian to be a true vertical line present in a cephalometric radiograph or lateral photograph taken with the patient in physiological *natural head position*. A perpendicular to this line establishes true horizontal for the patient [133].

Q: What points can be drawn from the above two questions?

A: There are no cephalometric analyses, which describe bone, teeth, and soft tissue relationships perfectly in every patient. Gabby's low Sella vertical position had a dramatic impact on her SNA and SNB angles. In patients with high or low Sella, you must take care when using SNA and SNB angles to assess maxillary and mandibular anteroposterior positions. The ANB angle is a more reliable measurement of anteroposterior skeletal discrepancies *between* jaws.

Cephalometric measurements should *corroborate* clinical findings/features. If your clinical findings differ from your cephalometric findings, ask why they differ. Your clinical impression usually trumps your cephalometric impression if they differ. We treat patients – not cephalograms. Radiographs are tools that work for us. We do not work for radiographs.

Q: In terms of Gabby's MPA, how can her FMA be average (FMA = 25°; average FMA = 25°), while her SN-MP angle is *greater* than average (SN-MP = 38°; average SN-MP = 32°)?

Figure 5.66 Evaluating Gabby's (a) maxillary and mandibular anteroposterior position (Nasion-perpendicular line drawn in red); (b) chin position using the zero-meridian line.

(a)

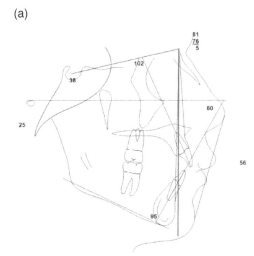

(b)

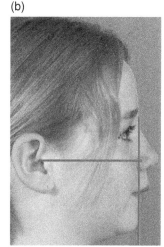

A: Although FMA and SN-MP generally differ by about 7°, because Gabby's Sella is low (Figure 5.65e), SN is steeper than normal, SN-MP is greater than average, while FMA remains average.

Q: Provide a detailed space analysis for Gabby's maxillary and mandibular arches. In other words, how were the anticipated 0.9 mm maxillary arch spacing and 4.3 mm mandibular arch spacing calculated *(if proper space maintenance is employed)*?

A:

Average mesiodistal widths of permanent teeth (mm): [94]

Maxillary Central Incisor	8.5	Mandibular Central Incisor	5.0
Maxillary Lateral Incisor	6.5	Mandibular Lateral Incisor	5.5
Maxillary Canine	7.5	Mandibular Canine	7.0
Maxillary First Premolar	7.0	Mandibular First Premolar	7.0
Maxillary Second Premolar	7.0	Mandibular Second Premolar	7.0
Maxillary First Molar	10.0	Mandibular First Molar	11.0
Maxillary Second Molar	9.0	Mandibular Second Molar	10.5

Average mesiodistal widths of *primary* teeth (mm): [94]

Maxillary Central Incisor	6.5	Mandibular Central Incisor	4.2
Maxillary Lateral Incisor	5.1	Mandibular Lateral Incisor	4.1
Maxillary Canine	7.0	Mandibular Canine	5.0
Maxillary First Molar	7.3	Mandibular First Molar	7.7
Maxillary Second Molar	8.2	Mandibular Second Molar	9.9

MAXILLARY ARCH (right leeway space cannot be used since maxillary right first premolar has erupted)
+7.3 mm space held by the maxillary right primary second molar (lingually positioned)
−7 mm of space required for the maxillary right second premolar
+7.6 mm maxillary right canine space available
−7.5 mm of space required for the maxillary right permanent canine
−1 mm crowding (maxillary right permanent central incisor-lateral incisor, Figure 5.65j)
+0.5 mm space, maxillary left permanent central incisor-lateral incisor

+1 mm of anticipated leeway space maxillary left side
Balance = +7.3 mm −7.0 mm +7.6 mm −7.5 mm −1.0 mm +0.5 mm +1.0 mm = +0.9 mm

MANDIBULAR ARCH (we cannot use leeway space since the permanent canines and first premolars have erupted)
+ 2.9 mm left "E space" (9.9 mm width of primary second molar minus 7 mm anticipated width of the second premolar)
−2.0 mm of incisor crowding (Figure 5.65k)
+0.5 mm of space between mandibular right primary second molar and first premolar
+2.9 mm right "E space"
Balance = +2.9 mm −2.0 mm +0.5 mm +2.9 mm = +4.3 mm

That is, *0.9 mm of maxillary arch spacing and 4.3 mm of mandibular arch spacing is anticipated following the eruption of all permanent teeth (if proper space maintenance is employed).*

Q: What are Gabby's *primary* problems in each dimension, plus other problems?

A:

Table 5.19   Primary problems list for Gabby.

AP	Angle Class II division 1
	Iowa Classification: II(3 mm) II(3 mm) II(3 mm) II(2 mm)
	Mandible is skeletally normal – but retrusive *relative* to her protrusive maxilla (ANB angle = 5°)
Vertical	Anterior open bite
Transverse	Mildly tapered maxillary dental arch with transverse (posterior) dental compensations
Other	—

Q: Discuss Gabby in the context of three principles applied to every early treatment patient.

A:

1) The goal of early treatment is to correct developing problems – get the patient *back to normal for their stage of development* (including preventing complications such as resorption of adjacent tooth roots, reducing later treatment complexity, or reducing/eliminating unknowns). Correcting Gabby's Class II relationship, anterior open bite, and transverse dental compensations (uprighting permanent first molars) would get her back on track.

2) Early treatment should address *very specific problems with a clearly defined end point*, usually within six to nine months (except for some orthopedic treatments). Gabby's Class II relationship is a specific problem, but its correction could take longer than nine months depending upon growth and cooperation. Correction of her open bite is a specific problem which could be corrected quickly by maxillary incisor eruption – *if any underlying habit is eliminated*. Transverse dental compensations are a specific problem, which could be corrected by first increasing posterior overjet with RME and then uprighting first permanent molars with crossbite elastics.

3) Always ask: Is it necessary that I treat the patient now? *What harm may come if I chose to do nothing now?* If we wait a year to begin Class II orthopedic treatment, then we may miss useful jaw growth. Not correcting Gabby's anterior open bite would result in the continued inability to incise food. Correction of her posterior dental compensations could be postponed without harm. However, if we decide to treat Gabby with RME, and if we wait until postpuberty to attempt RME, then achieving a midpalatal sutural separation will become increasingly difficult as the facial bones and sutures mature.

Q: What features would lead you to classify Gabby as a dental open bite? Skeletal open bite?

A: Gabby's *dental* open bite features include the following:
- Soft tissue LAFH WRN
- Skeletal LAFH WRN
- Lip competence (absence of ILG)
- Mandibular plane WRN (FMA = 25°, SNMP is excessive because Sella has a low position)
- Maxillary first permanent molar root apices located above the palatal plane (Figure 5.65d). That is, excessive molar eruption, resulting in maxillary first permanent molar root apices below the palatal plane, has *not* occurred
- Maxillary incisors are stepped up relative to the maxillary posterior teeth (Figures 5.65g and 5.65i).
- Anterior open bite has a "football shape" and extends only to the right first premolars.

Her s*keletal* open bite features include the following:

- Palatal plane tipped down in posterior by 3°. This is a small deviation from normal and not significant in Gabby's case. Larger CCW rotations of the palatal plane may be associated with greater hyperdivergence and skeletal open bite.

Q: Anterior *dental* open bites usually extend no further distally than the primary first molars or first premolars while anterior *skeletal* open bites often extend to the permanent first molars or permanent second molars. Why?

A: Dental (functional) open bites are usually due to habits preventing teeth from erupting. The effects of lip-biting, resting tongue posture, and digit-sucking habits are limited to areas where those habits take place – from the anterior to the primary first molars or first premolars. Skeletal open bites are associated with a hyperdivergent growth pattern and masticatory muscle weakness that increases the LAFH, MPA, gonial angle, and rotates the mandible down and back (clockwise) – often leaving occlusion only on the first or second permanent molars.

Q: We've stated that Gabby's PMH is normal. What important breathing-related questions should be included in your medical history evaluation, not only for open bite patients, but for all prospective orthodontic patients?

A: Questions regarding snoring, sleep habits, nasal congestion, and difficulty breathing. Answers to these questions are important to establish whether referral for obstructive sleep apnea (airway) evaluation is necessary. Gabby's parents deny any breathing issues, and she does not need a referral for airway evaluation.

Q: What questions should you ask Gabby and her parents about her open bite? What else should you check for?

A: Ask or check for the following:
- How long has she had her open bite? Gabby and her parents respond that she has always had her open bite.
- Does she have a lip-biting or digit-sucking habit that could prevent her anterior teeth from erupting? Yes, Gabby and her parents state that she sucks her thumb when she sleeps.
- Ask Gabby to close her eyes while you talk to her parents. Then, ask Gabby to open her eyes (to distract her) while you gently/quickly separate her lips to see if she exhibits an anterior tongue-interposition habit (resting tongue habit). You do not observe a resting tongue habit.
- Inquire whether Gabby suffered jaw trauma or has a history of generalized musculoskeletal problems. Her parents deny a history of trauma, generalized musculoskeletal problems, TMJ pain, or dysfunction. Examine the condyles on her panoramic image (Figure 5.65f). Note no overt condylar head roughness or degeneration. With a history of always having had her open bite, and without additional signs or symptoms of TMJ degeneration, Gabby's open bite is probably *not* due to condylar degeneration and additional imaging is unwarranted.

- Check for a temporary open bite due to erupting permanent teeth, ankylosed teeth that are not fully erupted, or teeth that are not completely erupted due to lack of space. None of these is the probable cause of her open bite.

Q: Does Gabby have a dental (functional) open bite, a skeletal open bite, or a combination of both?

A: Gabby has a dental open bite. Although she exhibits a mild increase of one feature of a skeletal open bite, she presents with a predominance of dental open bite features. She has a *dental* open bite.

Q: It is not unusual for anterior open bite patients to present with features of both a dental open bite *and* a skeletal open bite. An open bite can be a combination of both types. Gabby's anterior open bite exhibits a predominance of dental open bite features, and we will treat her as a dental (functional) open bite. But, does that mean we should ignore her skeletal open bite feature?

A: Absolutely not. Although we will treat her as a dental open bite, we should continually monitor Gabby's growth for signs of developing hyperdivergence and skeletal open bite (lengthening LAFH, developing ILG, and open bite extending further distally). If you perceive that a skeletal open bite is developing, and if its magnitude is mild enough to consider treating it orthopedically, then we recommend treating it aggressively by attempting to decrease maxillary corpus descent and by inhibiting molar eruption.

In an analogous fashion, over your career, you may begin treating Class I patients who have some Class III features (for instance, Class I molars with a straight profile, but an ANB angle of −1°). Many of these patients will maintain their Class I molar relationship throughout treatment. But some will begin growing into a Class III molar relationship. It is incumbent upon you to stay alert to these changes. When you see Class III growth beginning, you must decide if your treatment plan should change to address it.

Our point is this: *You must continually monitor your adolescent patient's growth. You must examine each patient's primary problems in each dimension at every appointment. When you see unexpected changes, you must regroup, re-evaluate, and deal with those changes.*

Q: What is the etiology of Gabby's dental open bite?

A: Incompletely erupted maxillary incisors resulting from a thumb-sucking habit.

Q: Is habit *duration* or force *magnitude* more important in inhibiting tooth eruption?

A: Habit duration [134–137]. Research reveals that even light continuous force against erupting rodent incisors will inhibit their eruption.

Q: What is your recommendation for dealing with the thumb habit?

A: First, talk to Gabby. Using a mirror, show her the anterior open bite and explain that it will not close (her anterior teeth will not erupt) until the thumb habit ends.

Q: Gabby states that she understands. She wants to stop, but she sucks her thumb when sleeping. What do you recommend now?

A: Since she sucks her thumb when sleeping, the psychological approach (encouraging her to win over the habit) will probably not work – although you should encourage her to stop if she wakes to find herself sucking her thumb. The good news is that Gabby wants to stop. *To be successful, the patient must have a desire to quit the habit causing the open bite.*

Options now include:
- Applying thumb paint, such as Mavala Stop, before she goes to bed
- Wearing a sock over her hand when she sleeps
- Wearing any of the commercially available thumb guard appliances
- Fabricating and cementing a palatal thumb crib
- Using an RME appliance as a thumb-sucking deterrent, if you decide that Gabby could benefit from RME

Q: Gabby has a significant Class II discrepancy (mandibular skeletal deficiency relative to her maxilla, ANB angle = 5°). There are three general ways to deal with any skeletal discrepancy. Can you list specific treatments for Gabby based on each of these three?

A: Skeletal discrepancies can be treated using orthopedics, masking (camouflage), or surgery.

Orthopedics (restrict maxillary growth while the mandible continues growing forward or accelerate mandibular growth). Specific options include:
- Headgears: High-pull, straight-pull, and cervical-pull headgears restrict maxillary corpus forward growth, allow the mandible to continue growing forward, and move maxillary molars to the distal – all of which could correct Gabby's Class II relationship. Since she has a protrusive maxilla, headgear wear (restriction of forward maxillary growth) should be ideal.

HPHG wear could offer a further benefit of reducing maxillary corpus descent and maxillary first permanent molar descent – both effects improving anteroposterior correction by mandibular forward CCW rotation [14, 35, 101]. CPHG wear would extrude maxillary first molars slightly (< 1 mm) [14, 15, 101], which would tend to rotate her mandible down and back – worsening her Class II relationship. SPHGs (a combination of HPHG and CPHG) will produce an effect somewhere between that of a high pull and a cervical pull.

- Class II functional appliances: We prefer Herbst appliances when we use Class II functional appliances because patient compliance is greatly reduced. Herbst appliances restrict maxillary forward growth, retract (distalize) maxillary posterior teeth, upright maxillary incisors, move mandibular posterior teeth to the mesial, procline mandibular incisors, accelerate condylar growth, and displace the glenoid fossae anteriorly [102, 103].

The ideal Class II functional appliance patient has a short LAFH, flat MPA, and upright mandibular incisors (since they will be proclined). Gabby has neither a short LAFH nor flat MPA. The fact that Class II functional appliances procline mandibular incisors makes their use less than ideal for Gabby since her mandibular incisors are already mildly proclined (FMIA = 60°; ideal FMIA = 65°).

When Class II functional appliances were introduced into the United States, some orthodontists made claims that these appliances could grow mandibles more than would have occurred naturally. Research over the past decades has revealed that Class II functional appliances accelerate mandibular growth in growing individuals but do not enhance mandibular horizontal growth beyond that found in control subjects [104]. The advantage of this accelerated growth is that you have a better idea of the Class II improvement sooner. The disadvantage of this accelerated growth is that the *direction* of condylar growth (posterior superiorly) may not correct the mandibular skeletal deficiency or improve chin projection [105, 106]. In fact, *hyperdivergent* patients experience a deleterious backward mandibular rotation and increases in face height with Herbst treatment [21].

Masking or camouflage (achieving an ideal Class I occlusion *dentally* without correcting the underlying skeletal discrepancy). We generally recommend masking later, during comprehensive treatment in adult dentition if:

- Class II orthopedic outcome is unsatisfactory
- Growth is complete or nearly complete (i.e. *avoid doing anything irreversible such as extracting permanent teeth until unknowns such as growth are eliminated*)

- Achieving Class I canines dentally is reasonable and will not result in unacceptable dental compensations or unfavorable esthetics.
- *First Principle of Masking – the smaller the skeletal discrepancy, the more normal the patient looks,* and *the smaller the dental compensations, the more successful masking (camouflage) will be; the larger the skeletal discrepancy, the less normal the patient looks, and the larger the dental compensations, the less successful masking (camouflage) will be.*

Masking options for Gabby include intra-arch (single arch) and inter-arch mechanics:

- Extraction of maxillary first premolars to create space and permit retraction of maxillary anterior teeth (achieving a Class I canine relationship but leaving molars Class II). This is an example of intra-arch mechanics.
- Extraction of maxillary first premolars and mandibular second premolars will create space – in the maxillary arch to retract maxillary canines and incisors, in the mandibular arch to protract permanent first molars into a Class I relationship, and in the mandibular arch to retract/upright proclined incisors. Such treatment will result in Class I canines and molars. This is an example of intra-arch mechanics in both arches.
- Using TADs as anchors to distalize the entire maxillary arch. This is an example of intra-arch mechanics.
- Class II elastics, Class II springs, or other Class II correctors to move maxillary teeth distally and mandibular teeth mesially. These are examples of inter-arch mechanics.

Surgery (mandibular advancement) would not be considered for Gabby. Even if Class II orthopedics is unsuccessful, we would probably treat Gabby with masking and not surgery. Why? Her convex profile (Figure 5.65c) is not severe. At most, we might consider a chin advancement (genioplasty advancement) if Gabby requested a stronger chin as an adult.

Q: Considering the *magnitude* of Gabby's Class II discrepancy, is it reasonable to attempt orthopedics?

A: Yes. Radiographically, she exhibits only a moderate skeletal discrepancy (ANB angle = 5°, Figure 5.65e), and, clinically, she exhibits only a 2–3 mm Class II molar relationship. Lastly, she is only ten years old and has significant growth remaining. She is about one year from the female average age for the peak of pubertal acceleration [107]. If Gabby is cooperative, then we should be able to achieve full orthopedic correction to

Class I. Even if we do not achieve full correction, a fall-back masking option is reasonable.

Q: Gabby is ten years old and in her *late* mixed dentition stage of dental development. Now is the ideal time to attempt Class II orthopedic treatment [17, 19, 73–77]. But what if Gabby were ten years old and still in the *early mixed* dentition – would you initiate Class II orthopedic treatment?

A: If Gabby were demonstrating *good statural growth*, then we would consider beginning Class II orthopedic treatment in the early mixed dentition.

Q: Does Gabby have a *transverse* skeletal discrepancy?

A: Yes, although she does not exhibit a posterior crossbite. Let's examine the facts. She has:
- Large buccal corridors (Figure 5.65b)
- Minimal OJ in the canine/premolar/primary molar areas (Figures 5.65h and 5.65m)
- A mildly tapered maxillary arch (Figures 5.65j and 5.65o)
- Transverse posterior compensations – maxillary first permanent molar buccal crown torque (Figure 5.65q) and mandibular first permanent molar lingual crown torque (Figure 5.65r)

Ideally, we will upright, in the transverse dimension, Gabby's first permanent molars. As we do, her maxillary first permanent molar crowns will tend to move *lingually*, and her mandibular first permanent molar crowns will tend to move *buccally* – reducing her posterior overjet or even putting her into posterior lingual crossbite. If uprighting permanent molars creates or worsens a posterior crossbite, then a transverse skeletal discrepancy generally exists. Gabby has a transverse skeletal discrepancy – a mildly *narrow* (anteriorly tapered) maxillary arch.

Q: Would you treat Gabby's transverse skeletal discrepancy with orthopedics, masking (camouflage), or surgery?

A: We recommend using orthopedics, but let's discuss all three options:

Orthopedics (widening the maxilla by separating the midpalatal suture). Gabby is at a perfect age for RME since the *most marked RME skeletal effect occurs before/during the pubertal growth spurt*, and expansion after the pubertal growth spurt is mainly dentoalveolar (not orthopedic/skeletal) [120–126]. Even if Gabby was in her mid- to late-teens, we would still *attempt* (TAD-supported) RME before choosing either masking or surgery.

RME (0.25 mm or 0.5 mm screw expansion per day) results in both maxillary skeletal and dental expansion. As the maxillary dental arch is widened, enough posterior overjet could be created to permit uprighting first permanent molars (removing transverse dental compensations) and coordinating dental arches. Also, Gabby's maxillary arch is mildly tapered toward the anterior (Figure 5.65j). RME will result in more skeletal widening in the anterior than in the posterior [138, 139], which is perfect for broadening the taper.

Depending upon Gabby's facial skeletal maturity and skeletal resistance, a quad-helix appliance might exert enough force to separate her midpalatal suture. However, we prefer RME which virtually guarantees a midpalatal sutural separation at Gabby's age.

Masking or camouflage (creating posterior overjet by increasing maxillary first permanent molar buccal crown torque, increasing mandibular first permanent molar lingual crown torque, but not by addressing the underlying transverse skeletal discrepancy). For Gabby, masking would include *leaving or increasing* the transverse dental compensations of her permanent first molars. At her age and maturity level, we do not recommend masking. We generally consider transverse masking in the permanent dentition.

Surgery (SARME – surgically assisted RME; MPMO – multiple piece maxillary osteotomy expansion) could achieve the desired increase in maxillary width. However, we do not recommend surgery at Gabby's age or for the magnitude of her mild transverse skeletal discrepancy.

Q: If Class II orthopedics results in Gabby's mandible growing forward relative to her maxilla, how will this growth affect her transverse relationship? How would this relative movement affect your decision to treat, or not to treat, with RME?

A: If her mandible grows forward more than her maxilla, then a wider part of her mandibular dental arch is brought forward into a narrower part of the maxillary dental arch – tending to worsen Gabby's transverse relationship. This potential worsening of her transverse relationship is another reason to treat her with RME.

Q: Gabby has proclined mandibular incisors. Would you consider extracting mandibular first premolars in order to create space to retract and upright these teeth?

A: No. Her mandibular incisors are only *mildly* proclined (FMIA = 60°; ideal FMIA = 65°). Extractions performed solely to address such mild proclination are unwarranted. Furthermore, she currently has only 2.0 mm of mandibular incisor crowding, and 4.3 mm of mandibular arch *spacing* is anticipated following the eruption of all permanent teeth If proper space maintenance is employed. This 4.3 mm of mandibular space could be used to retract/upright her incisors. For these reasons, we do not feel that she is a candidate for mandibular premolar extractions.

Let's examine this question from another perspective. If Gabby was in the early mixed dentition, then would she be a suitable serial extraction candidate? Does she exhibit features of an ideal serial extraction candidate? These features include:

- *Class I first permanent molars.* Gabby is molar Class II. If we extract first premolars without first correcting her to Class I, then achieving a final Class I relationship would be challenging. Gabby does not meet this criterion.
- *Vertically normal to slightly long soft tissue and skeletal LAFH, with minimal OB or possibly a mild open bite, but* not *a deep bite.* Gabby meets these criteria.
- *Normal incisor angulation or proclined incisors, but* not *upright incisors.* She meets this criterion.
- *Normal posterior transverse relationship (normal intermolar arch widths with good posterior interdigitation; absence of posterior crossbites; and absence of significant transverse compensations).* Gabby has minimal OJ in the canine/premolar/primary molar areas and significant permanent molar transverse compensations. She does not meet this criterion.
- *Severe (≥ 9 mm) anterior crowding:* Gabby currently has only mild anterior crowding in both arches. Furthermore, she has anticipated spacing in both arches if proper space maintenance is employed.

Based upon the above features, Gabby would *not* be a good candidate for serial extractions if she was in the early mixed dentition.

Q: Before you commit to a final treatment plan, especially to a plan which includes irreversible treatment (e.g. permanent tooth extractions), you should reduce/eliminate what?

A: *Reduce or eliminate unknowns.* Gabby's unknowns include future jaw growth magnitude and direction, cooperation with treatment (including thumb-sucking habit elimination), the presence of an undetected CR-CO shift, and our ability to achieve a midpalatal suture separation during maxillary skeletal widening.

Q: What are your *long-term* treatment goals (comprehensive treatment goals) for Gabby?

A: Improved maxillary incisor display, decreased buccal corridors, anterior open bite closure, positioning canines (and molars if she is treated non-extraction) into a Class I relationship, uprighting posterior teeth, increasing posterior OJ, achieving minimal anterior OJ, and obtaining 20–30% OB.

Q: Should you start early treatment or recall? If you start early treatment, what treatment options would you consider?

A: Treatment options include the following:

- *Recall* (no treatment now, monitor only) – re-evaluate in one year. We do *not* recommend this option. Since Gabby is in the late mixed dentition, now is the perfect time to begin Class II orthopedic treatment. If we wait, we may miss out on favorable jaw growth. Because she is prepubertal, now is also the perfect time to treat her transverse skeletal discrepancy (maxillary transverse deficiency). If we delay RME for years, then her facial skeletal resistance will increase – making it harder to achieve midpalatal suture separation and maximization of skeletal widening. Finally, if we do not address her anterior open bite (thumb habit), then she will be unable to incise food.
- *Headgear or functional appliance* – Class II orthopedic correction – would help correct Gabby's Class II molar relationship if she has favorable growth and is compliant. Functional appliance wear would increase proclination of her mandibular incisors.
- *Thumb habit correction* – could correct her anterior open bite as incisors erupt.
- *Fixed orthodontic appliances and forced incisor eruption* – to close Gabby's anterior open bite. We do not recommend this treatment without first attempting to correct her thumb-sucking habit. Even if we can close Gabby's open bite with fixed appliances, without habit cessation, the open bite could return.
- *RME* – is strongly recommended. If posterior overjet is increased through maxillary skeletal expansion, then Gabby's posterior teeth can be uprighted. Further, an RME appliance could deter Gabby's thumb-sucking.
- *Space maintenance* – placement of an LLHA, and possibly a Nance holding arch. Gabby currently has 2 mm of mandibular incisor crowding. But if we place an LLHA, then we will anticipate 4.3 mm of mandibular arch spacing following the eruption of all permanent teeth. This space could be used to upright Gabby's mildly proclined mandibular incisors. Also, the LLHA could be expanded to upright

her lingually inclined mandibular permanent first molars. Placement of a Nance holding arch would prevent maxillary first permanent molar mesial drift and worsening of her Class II molar relationship. It would also convert 0.5 mm of maxillary anterior crowding into 0.9 mm of maxillary anterior spacing. However, placement of a Nance holding arch would not be recommended until after RME and Class II correction with headgear or functional appliance.

- *Extraction of maxillary left primary canine* (to prevent impaction of maxillary left permanent canine) – is not recommend. Why? The left permanent canine appears to be erupting normally (Figure 5.65f).
- *Extraction of maxillary left primary fist molar and primary canine* – would accelerate eruption of maxillary left first premolar since its root length > ½ developed. This could be a reasonable option if we plan RME and desire using the first premolars as anchorage.
- *Extraction of permanent teeth/serial extraction* – is not reasonable for the reasons we discussed earlier.

Q: Placement of an LLHA will reduce mandibular first permanent molar mesial drift which will occur when Gabby's mandibular primary second molars exfoliate. How will LLHA placement affect Class II molar correction?

A: Since mandibular first permanent molar mesial drift is reduced with an LLHA, correction of Gabby's Class II molar relationship by other means (e.g. headgear wear or functional appliance treatment) is increased.

Q: What is your recommended treatment? How would you proceed?

A: Thumb-sucking habit cessation was reinforced. Gabby's maxillary left primary first molar and primary canine were extracted in order to accelerate the first premolar eruption. An LLHA was fabricated, expanded to upright mandibular first permanent molars, and delivered.

After the maxillary left first premolar erupted, an RME appliance was fabricated and inserted. The RME appliance included banded maxillary first premolars and maxillary first permanent molars as anchorage. The maxillary expansion proceeded, a midpalatal sutural separation was noted (a large maxillary midline diastema formed), and expansion continued until maxillary first permanent molar lingual cusps were edge-to-edge with mandibular first permanent molar buccal cusps. The RME appliance was left in place for stability, and e.g. headgear treatment was initiated.

Gabby stated that with the presence of her RME appliance, her thumb-sucking habit had stopped completely. Compliant headgear wear resulted in the first permanent molar overcorrection to Class III (1 mm) bilaterally. Headgear force and time of wear were decreased slowly while the anteroposterior relationship was monitored.

Once her maxillary incisors had erupted, her anteroposterior correction achieved, and her transverse relationship improved, early treatment was complete. After all other permanent teeth erupted (excluding wisdom teeth), comprehensive treatment began. The LLHA and RME appliance were removed, fixed orthodontic appliances were placed, arches were leveled and aligned, and all spaces closed. Gabby continued wearing headgear, and the maxillary expansion was maintained with the expanded headgear inner bow. Her open bite and vertical facial growth were monitored, and will continue to be monitored, until she has completed growth.

Q: Records following deband are shown in Figure 5.67. What changes do you note?

A: Changes include:

- Gabby has an excellent esthetic, and functional, result. She has an attractive posed smile with increased maxillary incisal display (although her maxillary lip border is not ideal – laying incisal to her maxillary gingival margins).
- The left buccal corridor is not observed but the right buccal corridor is reduced (compare Figures 5.65b and 5.67b).
- Midlines are coincident but to the left of her facial midline by 1–2 mm.
- Facial convexity has diminished slightly (compare Figures 5.65c and 5.67c).
- NLA appears unchanged, but the nasal tip has descended with growth and maxillary lip prominence has diminished.
- The maxillary protrusion has decreased (compare Figures 5.65e and 5.67e).
- ANB angle has decreased from 5° to 2°.
- Skeletal LAFH has decreased from 56 to 54%.
- FMA is unchanged.
- IMPA has decreased from 95° to 91°.
- FMIA has increased from 60° to 65°.
- The anterior open bite has been eliminated.
- Maxilla (Figure 5.67f) has grown downward with A-point moving relatively back.
- Upper lip has been retracted.
- Mandible has grown downward and slightly forward.
- Incisors have erupted.
- Maxillary molars erupted and moved slightly to the mesial.

- Mandibular molars have erupted slightly and moved to the mesial slightly.
- All permanent teeth (excluding wisdom teeth) have erupted.

- Bilateral Class I occlusion achieved.
- OB of 10% now present (Figure 5.67i).
- Dental arches are well aligned, except rotation of mandibular central incisors present.

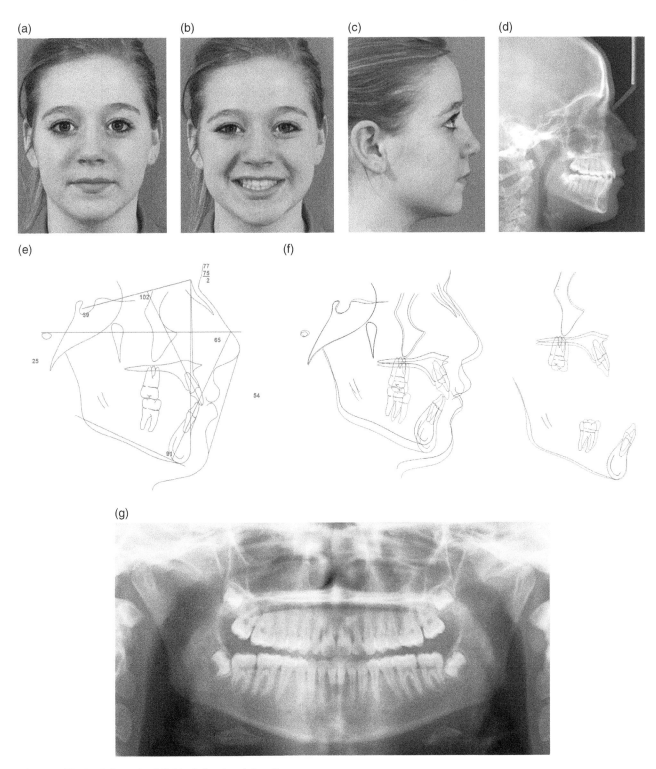

Figure 5.67 (a–l) Records of Gabby following debanding.

(h)　　　　　　　　　　　(i)　　　　　　　　　　　(j)

(k)　　　　　　　　　　　(l)

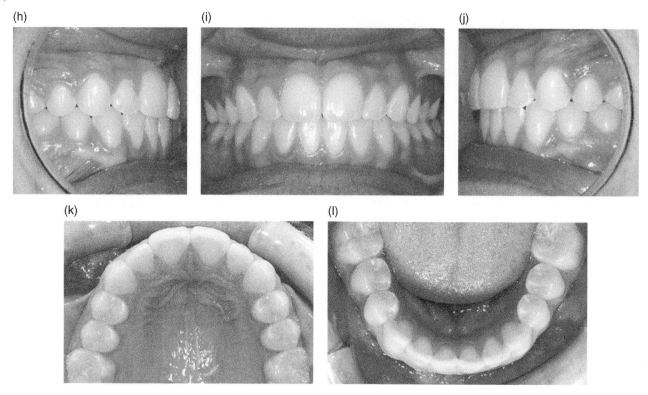

Figure 5.67　(Continued)

Q: How was her Class II molar relationship corrected?

A: Through a combination of mandibular forward growth and mandibular first permanent molar mesial movement. The combination of these two effects was enough to correct the original Class II molar relationship and to overcome mesial movement of the maxillary first permanent molars, molar eruption, and downward growth of the maxilla.

Q: How was her facial convexity diminished (Figure 5.67f, left)?

A: By mandibular forward growth and maxillary lip retraction. Mandibular forward growth brought soft tissue Pogonion slightly forward.

Q: If Gabby had not cooperated with headgear, what fallback options would you have suggested to correct her Class II relationship?

A: Alternative treatment options we would have considered include:

1) *Herbst appliance treatment* (orthopedics). The advantage of Herbst appliance treatment is that it is a *cemented* Class II corrector. The need for patient compliance is greatly reduced compared to headgear wear. A distinct disadvantage is that it would procline Gabby's mandibular incisors.

2) *Extraction of either maxillary first or second premolars* and space closure (masking the underlying skeletal discrepancy).

3) *Extraction of maxillary first premolars plus mandibular second premolars* (masking).

4) *Infrazygomatic, palatal, or maxillary buccal TADs (masking)* to retract the entire maxillary dental arch into a Class I relationship.

5) *Class II elastics, Forsus, or other Class II correctors* (masking).

Q: Is the amount of deband overbite adequate (10%, Figure 5.67i)?

A: Not ideally. Since Gabby began with an anterior open bite, we should have overcorrected her to 20–40% overbite – anticipating future relapse (rebound).

Q: Does the above question lead you to a principle for orthodontic treatment?

A: Yes. *Overcorrect, hold, monitor.* In many (most?) instances, do not just correct – *overcorrect*. For example, in cases of deep overbite, you should *overcorrect* to a shallow overbite. Then, you should *hold* this overcorrection for as long as reasonable during treatment. Then, you should *monitor* the patient post-treatment – knowing that the patient will tend to relapse to a deeper bite over time.

As another example, if your patient is wearing headgear to achieve Class I molars, overcorrect slightly to Class III (1–2 mm). Then, hold this overcorrection as you slowly decrease headgear wear and monitor to see if the patient rebounds (relapses) to a Class I molar relationship. *Overcorrect, hold, monitor.*

Q: What factors will determine whether Gabby's open bite returns?

A: The most important factor is whether her thumb-sucking habit has ended. If the habit has not ended, then the open bite will likely return. Another factor is whether soft tissue stretch (periodontal ligament, transeptal fiber, etc.) which occurred during maxillary arch leveling is stable. If not, the open bite could return.

Q: Gabby stated that with the help of her RME appliance, her thumb habit ended. This led to incisor eruption and closure of her open bite. However, even with habit cessation, fixed appliances are sometimes used to close anterior open bites. Can you describe the biomechanics of dental anterior open bite closure using fixed orthodontic appliances?

A: The easiest way to close an anterior open bite with fixed appliances is to have the patient wear vertical elastics between the maxillary and mandibular anterior teeth. Anterior teeth will erupt, and the open bite will close. However, deflected archwires themselves, without elastics, tend to close an anterior open bite by erupting stepped up maxillary incisors and stepped down mandibular incisors.

Let's first review the simple biomechanics involved in opening dental *deep* bites using a 2×4 appliance (Figures 5.68a–5.68c). When archwires with tip-back bends ("V bends," anchor bends) are inserted into permanent first molar bracket slots, the anterior of the archwires sit apical to the overerupted incisors (Figure 5.68b). When the wires are next inserted in the incisor brackets (Figure 5.68c), the incisors are intruded (opening the bite), the molars are erupted (opening the bite), and the molars are tipped distally (uprighting mesially tipped molars and opening the bite).

In fact, tip-back wire bends may not be required for these same forces and moments to be produced. All that is required is for the anterior of the archwires to lay apical to the incisor brackets before being engaged.

Next, let's apply the same logic to closing dental *open bites*. As shown in Figures 5.69a–5.69c, when plain archwires (no bends) are inserted into permanent first molar bracket slots, the anterior of the wires sit incisal to the incisor brackets (Figure 5.69b). When the wires are inserted into the incisor brackets (Figure 5.69c), the incisors are extruded (closing the bite), the molars *tend* to be intruded (tending to close the bite), and the molars are tipped mesially (increasing the curve of Spee and tending to close the bite).

Q: Why did we wait to include maxillary first premolars in Gabby's RME appliance instead of proceeding with only maxillary permanent first molar anchorage?

A: *Midpalatal suture expansion is 2.5 greater when using a 4-banded RME appliance* compared to a 2-banded RME appliance [140]. Since we wanted to maximize maxillary skeletal expansion, we included the first premolars.

Q: What if Gabby's maxillary first premolars were not going to erupt for years? Would you have to wait for them to erupt before RME?

A: No, you would not have to wait. If a patient has years before puberty (low facial skeletal resistance to RME), then you can attempt RME using only the maxillary

(a)

(b)

(c)

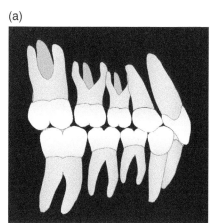 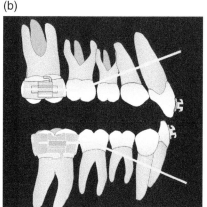 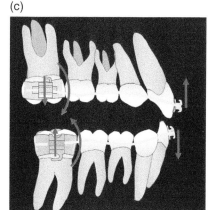

Figure 5.68   (a–c) Archwire biomechanics during deep bite opening.

(a) (b) (c)

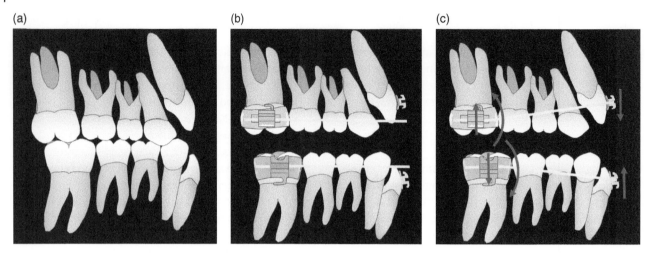

Figure 5.69 (a–c) Archwire biomechanics during open bite closure.

first permanent molars as anchorage. Or, to gain additional anchorage, you can extend lingual soldered metal arms from the maxillary first permanent molar bands forward and bond those metal arms to the maxillary first and/or second primary molars.

Q: Gabby's mandibular incisors erupted during treatment (Figure 5.67f). What additional mandibular incisor change occurred? Can you explain why this change took place?

A: Gabby's mandibular incisors *uprighted* (FMIA increased by 5°, IMPA decreased by 4°). This uprighting movement was likely due to "E-space" closure following removal of the LLHA.

Q: Was early treatment warranted?

A: Let's answer this question in the context of three principles applied to every early treatment patient:

1) The goal of early treatment is to correct developing problems – get the patient *back to normal for their stage of development*. Gabby's anteroposterior skeletal discrepancy was corrected via HPHG wear, her anterior open bite was closed via thumb-sucking habit cessation (incisor eruption), and her maxillary transverse deficiency was corrected via RME. She was put back on track before her remaining permanent teeth erupted and before braces were placed.

2) Early treatment should address *very specific problems with a clearly defined end point*, usually within six to nine months. Gabby's Class II discrepancy was a specific problem, but its correction required over a year. This is not unusual for orthopedic treatment. Her habit cessation/dental open bite correction was

a specific problem that was treated during RME and took less than six months.

3) Always ask: Is it necessary that I treat the patient now? *What harm will come if I choose to do nothing?* By starting at age ten, we were able to capitalize on mandibular forward growth to achieve an ideal Class I relationship. We may have missed out on this growth if we had waited. By starting RME treatment, we maximized skeletal expansion and the RME was an aid in habit cessation.

Based upon the above, early treatment (treatment before the eruption of all permanent teeth) was justified.

Q: What retention protocol would you recommend for Gabby?

A: Gabby was placed in removable Hawley retainers and asked to wear them at night, for life. Lifelong retention is the only guarantee that alignment of teeth can be maintained. A mandibular fixed canine-to-canine retainer could also have been used instead of a mandibular Hawley retainer.

If we treated Gabby today, we would place small labial maxillary incisor bumps of composite resin at deband so that a clear (vacuum-formed) retainer would "snap" over the bumps and hold the erupted maxillary incisors in place.

Q: Can you suggest "take-home pearls" from Gabby's treatment?

A: "Take-home pearls" include the following:
- Gabby was ten years old when she presented in the late mixed dentition with a Class II (2–3 mm) molar relationship, protrusive maxilla, dental (functional)

anterior open bite due to a thumb-sucking habit, and maxillary transverse skeletal deficiency. The Class II relationship was corrected orthopedically using an HPHG which improved her skeletal relationship and profile. Her dental open bite was corrected via incisor eruption because Gabby was motivated to stop her thumb-sucking habit. RME corrected her maxillary transverse skeletal deficiency and acted as a thumb-sucking habit deterrent.

- It is not unusual for anterior open bite patients to present with features of both skeletal open bites and dental open bites. In fact, anterior open bites can be *combinations* of skeletal open bites (excess vertical facial growth) and dental open bites (functional habits). Even though Gabby exhibited a predominance of dental open bite features, it was wise to monitor her growth for progression to a skeletal open bite (lengthening LAFH, steepening MPA, ILG development, anterior open bite extending further distally). If we had observed her developing into a skeletal open bite, then we would have initiated aggressive orthopedics by attempting to decrease maxillary corpus descent and/or by inhibiting/intruding molar eruption. Also, we would have evaluated her for condylar degenerative changes (e.g. idiopathic condylar resorption).
- *You must monitor your patient's growth and primary problems in each dimension at every appointment.* When you see unexpected changes, you must regroup, re-evaluate, and deal with those changes. If you become complacent, it is time to leave the practice of dentistry.
- Functional habits must be eliminated in order to achieve, and maintain, dental open bite closure. Functional habits may sometimes be corrected by forcing dental open bite closure first with fixed orthodontic appliances and anterior vertical elastics, but never depend on this. *Correct your patient's habit first before open bite closure using fixed appliances.*
- For you to be successful in closing a dental open bite, the patient must have a *desire to end the habit*.
- Cephalometric measurements should *corroborate* your clinical findings. If your clinical findings differ from your cephalometric findings, ask yourself why they differ. Clinical impressions generally trump cephalometric findings when they differ.
- If the magnitude of the (anteroposterior, vertical) skeletal discrepancy is mild and the time of remaining growth is long, then attempting orthopedics is usually a good option.

- If the magnitude of the skeletal discrepancy is moderate and the time of remaining growth is long, then orthopedics may be attempted with the understanding that masking or surgery may be required.
- If the magnitude of the skeletal discrepancy is severe and the time of remaining growth is long, then orthopedics may be attempted with the hope that the discrepancy can be reduced to a point where masking can be successful (surgery avoided). However, the patient must be informed that surgery may be the best ideal option.
- Principle of Masking – *the smaller the skeletal discrepancy between the jaws, the more normal the patient looks, and the smaller the dental compensations, the more successful masking (camouflage) will be; the greater the skeletal discrepancy, the less normal the patient looks, and the larger the dental compensations, the less successful masking (camouflage) will be.*
- Reduce *or eliminate unknowns before committing to irreversible, or final, treatment.* Gabby's unknowns of future jaw growth magnitude and direction, compliance with treatment, elimination of thumb-sucking habit, and ability to achieve a midpalatal suture separation with RME were all eliminated – before comprehensive treatment.
- Overcorrect, *hold, monitor.* Whether using headgears, functional appliances, RPHGs, archwires to close open bites, archwires to open deep bites, or Class II elastics – do not just correct and release. If you correct and release, then your correction may relapse and the original problem resurface. Instead, overcorrect, hold the overcorrection, and slowly reduce appliances wear over time to monitor your correction.
- We failed to overcorrect Gabby's open bite. We should have overcorrected her to a deep bite of 20–40%. We are monitoring her for relapse, and so far, she is stable.

Case Carter

Q: Carter is eleven years and ten months of age (Figure 5.70) and presents with his parents for a consultation. Their chief complaint is, "We do not like his open bite." His mother states that Carter acts immaturely for his age. His PMH, PDH, periodontal evaluation, and TMJ evaluation are WRN. CR=CO. Compile your diagnostic findings and problem list for Carter. Also, state your diagnosis.

A:

Table 5.20 Diagnostic findings and problem list for Carter.

Full face and Profile	***Frontal View***
	Face is symmetric
	Long soft tissue LAFH (soft tissue Glabella – Subnasale < Subnasale – soft tissue Menton)
	Mentalis muscle strain to achieve lip closure (note the 18 mm interlabial gap when Carter relaxed during lateral cephalometric radiograph exposure, Figure 5.70d)
	UDML 1 mm left of facial midline
	Anterior open bite
	Excessive incisal display when relaxed (Figure 5.70d, ideal adolescent incisal display 2–4 mm)
	Maxillary lip border coincident with maxillary central incisor gingival margin in posed smile
	Large buccal corridors
	Profile View
	Convex profile
	Deficient chin projection
	Obtuse lip-chin-throat angle
Ceph Analysis	***Skeletal***
	Maxillary anteroposterior position WRN (A-Point lies on Nasion-perpendicular line)
	Mandibular anteroposterior position deficient (ANB angle = 6°)
	Long skeletal LAFH (ANS-Menton/Nasion-Menton × 100% = 58%; normal skeletal LAFH=55%, sd = 2%)
	Steep MPA (FMA = 29°; SNMP = 37°)
	Effective bony Pogonion (bony Pogonion lies ahead of Nasion-B Point line)
	Dental
	Maxillary incisors proclined (U1 to SN = 116°)
	Mandibular incisors proclined (FMIA = 55°; ideal FMIA = 65°)
Radiographs	Late mixed dentition stage of development
Intraoral Photos and Models	Angle Class II division 1
	Iowa Classification: II(4 mm) II (6 mm) II (6 mm) II(3 mm)
	OJ ~ 4 mm
	Anterior open bite
	Maxillary incisors stepped up relative to maxillary posterior teeth
	Mandibular midline to right of maxillary midline by ~2 mm
	0.2 mm maxillary anterior spacing currently present (+7.6 mm space for maxillary right and left permanent canines each, −7.5 mm width of maxillary right and left permanent canines)
	4.9 mm maxillary spacing is anticipated following the eruption of all permanent teeth (if proper space maintenance is employed)
	0.0 mm mandibular anterior crowding currently present
	6.8 mm of mandibular spacing is anticipated following the eruption of all permanent teeth (if proper space maintenance is employed)
	Maxillary dental arch is asymmetric – right permanent first molar ahead of left
	Mandibular dental arch is symmetric
	Left posterior complete buccal crossbite (scissor bite, Figures 5.70i and 5.70n)
	Maxillary first permanent molar buccal crown torque (Figure 5.70q)
	Mandibular first permanent molar lingual crown torque (Figure 5.70r)
	Poor hygiene
Other	None
Diagnosis	Class II malocclusion with anterior open bite

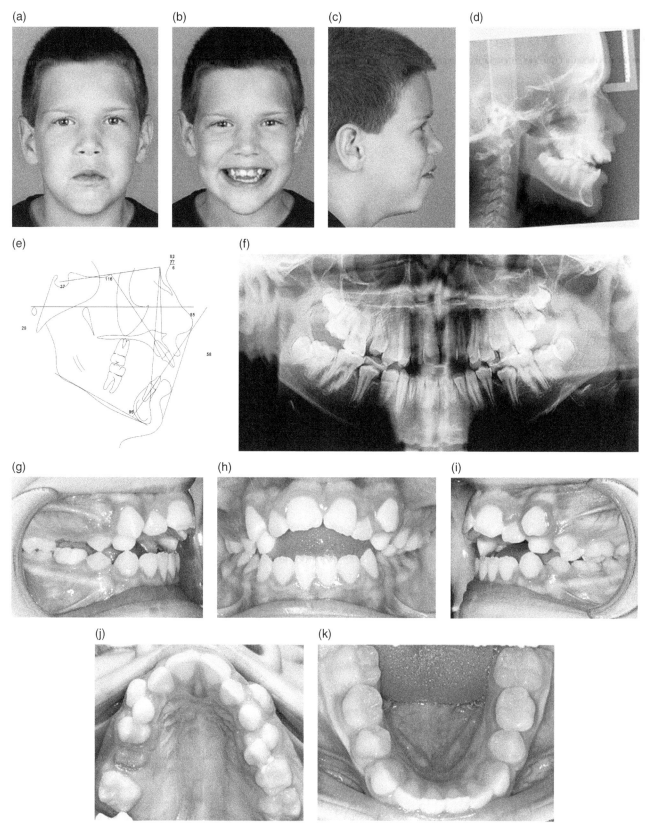

Figure 5.70 Initial records of Carter: (a–c) facial photographs; (d and e) lateral cephalometric radiograph and tracing; (f) pantomograph; (g–k) intraoral photographs; (l–r) intraoral scans.

(l)   (m)   (n)

(o)   (p)

(q)   (r)

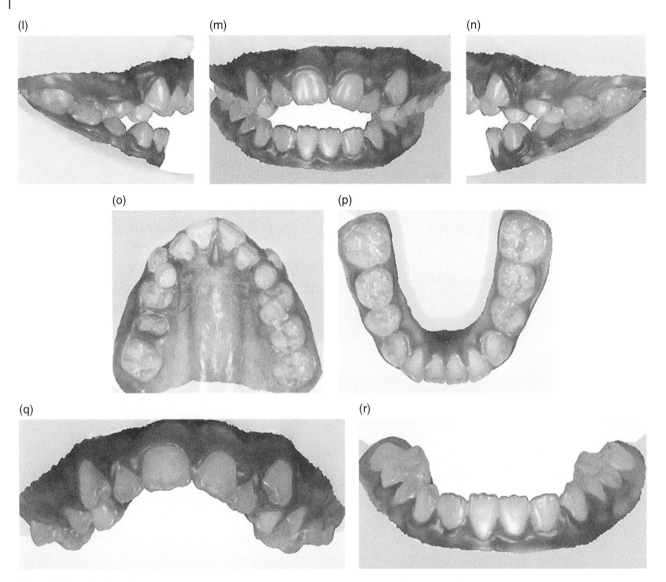

Figure 5.70 (Continued)

Q: A vertically normal patient should present with lip competence or at most a 1–2 mm ILG [26]. Carter presents with a very large ILG (18 mm). How do lip growth and lower anterior face skeletal growth combine to produce either lip competence or lip incompetence (an ILG)? Why does Carter have such a large ILG?

A: During normal facial growth, soft tissue length keeps pace with lower anterior skeletal length. The result is lip competence.

  With excessive facial lower anterior skeletal growth, the maxillary corpus descends more than normal and/or molars erupt more than normal – rotating the mandible down and back and lengthening the lower face excessively. Facial soft tissue growth (including lip length) cannot keep pace with lower anterior skeletal growth, and an ILG results.

  The normal range of maxillary lip length for adolescent girls is 17–23 mm and for adolescent boys 22–26 mm [141]. Carter's maxillary lip length is only 15 mm (Figure 5.70d) – much shorter than average. Combine his very short maxillary lip length with his long skeletal LAFH, and Carter ended up with an 18 mm ILG.

Q: What features would lead you to classify Carter as a dental open bite? A skeletal open bite?

A: Carter's *dental* open bite features include:
  • Maxillary incisors stepped up relative to maxillary posterior teeth
  • Anterior open bite extends only to the canines
  • Maxillary first molar root apices are located above the palatal plane (Figure 5.70d). Excessive molar

eruption, resulting in maxillary first permanent molar root apices *below* the palatal plane, has not occurred

His *skeletal* open bite features include:
- Long soft tissue LAFH (soft tissue Glabella – Subnasale < Subnasale – soft tissue Menton)
- Long skeletal LAFH (ANS-Menton/Nasion-Menton × 100% = 58%; normal skeletal LAFH = 55%, sd = 2%)
- Mentalis muscle strain to achieve lip competence (18 mm ILG when relaxed, Figure 5.70d)
- Short posterior face height
- Steep MPA (FMA = 29°, SNMP = 37°).

Q: What questions should you ask Carter and his parents regarding the etiology of his open bite? What should you check for?

A: Ask or check for the following:
- How long has Carter had his open bite? Carter's mother says he has always had it.
- Whether Carter has any habits which would inhibit his teeth from erupting? Carter's mother states that he sucks his thumb. She says that they tried tying socks over his hands to deter him from sucking his thumb, but he pulled the socks off. She says she has never seen Carter biting his lip.
- Ask Carter to close his eyes while you talk to his mother. Then, ask Carter to open his eyes (to distract him) while you gently/quickly retract his lips to see if he exhibits an anterior (resting) tongue-interposition habit. Carter has an anterior resting tongue habit (see Figures 5.70b and 5.70h).
- Check his mandibular condylar heads on the panoramic image for signs of degeneration. His left condyle has a smooth surface, but we are unable to examine his right condylar head due to anatomic overlap with the base of his skull. Carter and his mother deny any history of trauma, generalized musculoskeletal problems, TMJ pain, or TMJ dysfunction. Lacking such history, we conclude that Carter's open bite is probably not due to condylar degeneration, and we do not pursue additional joint imaging.
- Check for a temporary open bite due to erupting permanent teeth, ankylosed teeth that are not fully erupted, and teeth that are not completely erupted due to lack of space. Carter's central incisors are mobile (not ankylosed), and none of these causes appears to be the likely etiology of his anterior open bite.
- Although evidence demonstrating a relationship between mouth breathing and facial morphology is not of the highest level [60, 63–65, 68–70], you need to ask questions related to Carter's airway and breathing. Pediatric sleep questionnaires are useful in evaluating children for referral to investigate obstructive sleep apnea [142]. The American Association of Orthodontists has published a White Paper on this topic, including guidance on history taking for patients with suspected breathing difficulties [143].

Observe Carter to see if he is a mouth breather. Ask Carter and his mother whether he breathes through his nose or mouth, if he snores, or if he has ever stopped breathing while asleep. Does Carter have tonsil or adenoid conditions, nasal congestion, or sinus problems? Does he have difficulty sleeping or suffer from daytime fatigue? Based upon answers to these questions, seek a physician referral. *Carter does not appear to have any breathing difficulties.*

Q: Does Carter have a dental (functional) open bite, a skeletal open bite, or a combination of both? What is the etiology of his open bite?

A: Carter has a combination of skeletal and dental open bites. His skeletal open bite pattern (hyperdivergence) is illustrated by his excessively long soft tissue and skeletal LAFH which resulted from a combination of excessive vertical maxillary growth, deficient vertical ramus, condylar growth magnitude and direction, and excessive posterior maxillary and/or mandibular vertical dentoalveolar growth. His dental open bite is illustrated by his stepped-up maxillary incisors, by the open bite extending only to his canines, and by his reported thumb habit and observed tongue posture habit.

Q: Provide a detailed space analysis for Carter's maxillary and mandibular arches. In other words, how were the anticipated 4.9 mm maxillary spacing and 6.8 mm mandibular spacing calculated *(if proper space maintenance is employed)*?

A:

Average mesiodistal widths of permanent teeth (mm): [94]

Maxillary Central Incisor	8.5	Mandibular Central Incisor	5.0
Maxillary Lateral Incisor	6.5	Mandibular Lateral Incisor	5.5
Maxillary Canine	7.5	Mandibular Canine	7.0
Maxillary First Premolar	7.0	Mandibular First Premolar	7.0
Maxillary Second Premolar	7.0	Mandibular Second Premolar	7.0
Maxillary First Molar	10.0	Mandibular First Molar	11.0
Maxillary Second Molar	9.0	Mandibular Second Molar	10.5

Average mesiodistal widths of *primary* teeth (mm): [94]

Maxillary Central Incisor	6.5	Mandibular Central Incisor	4.2
Maxillary Lateral Incisor	5.1	Mandibular Lateral Incisor	4.1
Maxillary Canine	7.0	Mandibular Canine	5.0
Maxillary First Molar	7.3	Mandibular First Molar	7.7
Maxillary Second Molar	8.2	Mandibular Second Molar	9.9

MAXILLARY ARCH (Figure 5.70j, leeway space cannot be used because premolars are erupting)

+8.5 mm space for maxillary right second premolar

−7.0 mm width of the right second premolar

+7.6 mm space for maxillary right permanent canine

−7.5 mm width of maxillary right permanent canine

+7.6 mm space for maxillary left permanent canine

−7.5 mm width of maxillary left permanent canine

+2.0 mm space distal to left first premolar

+8.2 mm maxillary left primary second molar width

−7.0 mm anticipated width of maxillary left second premolar

Balance = +8.5 mm −7.0 mm +7.6 mm −7.5 mm +7.6 mm −7.5 mm + 2.0 mm + 8.2 mm −7.0 mm = +4.9 mm

MANDIBULAR ARCH (leeway space cannot be used because permanent canines and first premolars have erupted)

+0.0 mm anterior crowding (Figure 5.70k)

+9.9 mm left primary second molar width

−7.0 mm anticipated width of the mandibular left second premolar

+1.0 mm space between right permanent canine and first premolar

+9.9 mm right primary second molar width

−7.0 mm anticipated width of the mandibular right second premolar

Balance = +0.0 mm +9.9 mm −7.0 mm + 1.0 mm +9.9 mm −7.0 mm = +6.8 mm

That is, *4.9 mm maxillary arch spacing and 6.8 mm mandibular arch spacing are anticipated following the eruption of all permanent teeth (if proper space maintenance is employed).*

Q: What are Carter's *primary* problems in each dimension, plus other problems?

A:

Table 5.21   Primary problems list for Carter.

AP	Angle Class II division 1 malocclusion secondary to mandibular skeletal anteroposterior deficiency
	Iowa Classification: II(4 mm) II (6 mm) II (6 mm) II(3 mm)
Vertical	Skeletal anterior open bite pattern (hyperdivergence) and dental anterior open bite
Transverse	Left posterior complete buccal crossbite (scissor bite)
	Transverse (posterior) dental compensations in both arches
Other	—

Q: Discuss Carter in the context of three principles applied to every early treatment patient.

A:

1) The goal of early treatment is to correct developing problems – get the patient *back to normal for their stage of development* (including preventing complications such as resorption of adjacent tooth roots, reducing later treatment complexity, or reducing/eliminating unknowns). Carter has severe skeletal discrepancies in all three facial dimensions. Correcting his Class II dental relationship to Class I, improving his profile from convex to straight, correcting his dental open bite, correcting his skeletal open bite, correcting his unilateral left posterior crossbite, and eliminating his posterior transverse compensations would get Carter back on a normal track.

2) Early treatment should address *very specific problems with a clearly defined end point*, usually within six to nine months (except for some orthopedic problems). Of Carter's three facial dimensions, only his left posterior scissor bite could be corrected in less than a year. The magnitude of his anteroposterior and vertical skeletal discrepancies is so large that orthopedic correction with a clearly defined end point is uncertain. A clear end point for correction of his dental open bite cannot be guaranteed unless Carter stops his thumb-sucking and tongue-interposition habits.

3) Always ask: Is it necessary that I treat the patient now? *What harm will come if I chose to do nothing now?* At eleven years and ten months, Carter is at the average age for the onset of pubertal acceleration in boys (11.9–12.0 years), and he likely has ~three years of significant facial growth remaining [107]. Waiting a year to begin Class II orthopedic treatment could result in missing important jaw growth. Waiting a year to begin skeletal open bite

orthopedics could result in a worsening of his open bite. There is no harm in monitoring Carter's dental open bite other than his inability to incise food.

Since Carter does not have a CR-CO shift, asymmetric mandibular growth is not a concern if we chose to monitor his left crossbite for one year. However, if his transverse correction requires RME in order to eliminate compensations, then we will want to use it before Carter reaches puberty because the most marked RME skeletal effects occur before/during the pubertal growth spurt [120–126].

Q: There are only two general ways to close anterior open bites. What are they? Specifically, how would they relate to Carter's treatment?

A: Anterior open bites are closed either by *erupting anterior teeth or intruding posterior teeth*. We generally close anterior dental open bites by erupting (unerupted) anterior teeth – since the anterior vertical skeletal dimension is normal. We generally close anterior skeletal open bites by intruding posterior teeth (and possibly decreasing descent of the maxillary corpus). This reduces the anterior vertical facial skeletal dimension.

Carter has a combination of dental and skeletal anterior open bites. We would therefore close his open bite through a combination of anterior tooth eruption (specifically, eruption of his under-erupted maxillary incisors) and posterior tooth intrusion/reduction in maxillary corpus descent (Figure 5.71).

Q: What is *relative*, as opposed to absolute, intrusion of posterior teeth?

A: If molars are intruded in an adult, that is *absolute intrusion*. But if early treatment reduces the amount molars would normally erupt, then this is *relative* intrusion. For example, LLHAs reduce mandibular first permanent molar eruption by 1–2 mm over a one to two-year period – compared to controls [45]. This is relative intrusion.

Q: What is your recommendation for early dental open bite treatment, in general? What is your recommendation for Carter's dental open bite treatment, in particular?

A: In general, *we recommend early treatment of dental open bites by habit control when the child is interested in stopping*. Otherwise, we generally wait until the child matures.

Using a mirror, demonstrate to Carter how his thumb habit and tongue posture habit are preventing his maxillary teeth from erupting. Carter says he

(a)

(b)

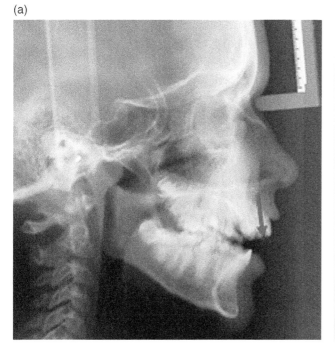
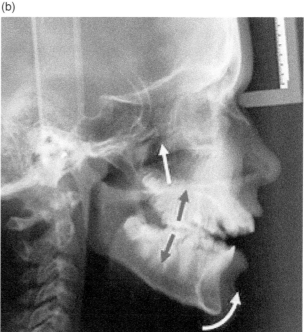

Figure 5.71 Since Carter's anterior open bite is a combination of dental and skeletal open bites, treatment should include a combination of maxillary incisor eruption (a) to close his dental open bite plus posterior tooth intrusion/reduction of maxillary corpus descent (b) to address his skeletal open bite (autorotating his mandible upward/forward and reducing his excessive LAFH, curved yellow line).

understands and wants to stop these habits. However, previous attempts failed to stop the thumb habit (tying socks to his hands). Other approaches can be attempted:

- Applying thumb paint (e.g. Mavala Stop) to his thumbs before he goes to bed
- Wearing a commercially available thumb guard appliance
- Fabricating and cementing a palatal thumb crib
- Using an RME appliance to deter his habit if an expansion appliance is indicated.

In terms of the tongue-interposition habit, ask Carter to avoid resting his tongue on the incisal edges of his anterior teeth. Have him demonstrate. When he swallows, ask him to touch the tip of his tongue to his anterior palate. Other appliances or techniques can remind him to keep his tongue off his anterior teeth:

- Short blunted spurs soldered to an LLHA or embedded in a retainer
- Buttons or composite bonded to the lingual of the mandibular incisors
- Maxillary clear (vacuum-formed) retainer with a hole placed in the anterior palate to attract the tongue tip
- Maxillary tongue crib designed to block the tongue
- Sometimes, the anterior resting tongue habit will cease (tongue will be retrained) if the open bite is closed with fixed orthodontic appliances
- Myofunctional therapy. However, we are not enthusiastic about this approach. In our experience, the patients who respond to myofunctional therapy would probably correct their resting tongue habits by themselves once the habit was explained to them.

To be successful long term, Carter must demonstrate a desire to quit his habits. If Carter does not wish to stop, then it will be better to wait until he matures to address the habits.

Q: What about Carter's skeletal open bite pattern? Can you suggest treatment guidelines to follow in dealing with it?

A: Guidelines include the following:

- Successful early (orthopedic) treatment of skeletal open bites is very difficult and should be attempted in only the *most cooperative patients*. If Carter is not cooperative, then do not attempt orthopedic treatment. Discontinue treatment if he becomes uncooperative – and wait until he has finished growing to treat his skeletal open bite with masking (erupting anterior teeth if facial esthetics will permit) or with orthognathic surgery.

- The more severe the skeletal open bite, the less successful your orthopedic treatment will be to correct it.
- The older the patient, the less likely you will be to correct the skeletal open bite with orthopedics.
- Successful orthopedic correction must be monitored until the patient has completed growth. Orthopedic treatment does not normalize growth. The same pattern of excessive vertical facial growth will continue once orthopedic treatment ends.
- Always have a fallback plan (contingency plan) to deal with unsuccessful orthopedic treatment. Your plan may include masking or jaw surgery. Discuss these with the patient and parents.

Q: How can Carter's skeletal open bite be treated? Suggest specific orthopedic treatments and possible masking/surgery treatments if orthopedics fails.

A: *Orthopedics* (treatment to reduce downward descent of the growing maxilla and/or reduce molar eruption). The advantage of treating Carter's skeletal open bite with orthopedics is that he is also Class II skeletally. Treatment to reduce descent of his maxillary corpus and reduce molar eruption will tend to rotate his mandible upward and forward – reducing his excess vertical dimension *and* reducing his distocclusion/retrusive profile. Specific orthopedic treatments include:

- High-pull headgear (HPHG)
- Vertical-pull chin cup
- Full posterior occlusal coverage bite plates (with and without repelling magnets)
- Transpalatal arch with acrylic button
- Lower lingual holding arch
- Temporary anchorage devices (TADs) used as molar intrusion anchors
- Chewing exercises
- Modified Herbst appliance (acrylic splints covering posterior teeth plus HPHG).

The skeletal open bite orthopedic treatment with the greatest chance of success and least need for patient cooperation is *TAD-supported maxillary and mandibular molar intrusion* – intrusion of *both* maxillary and mandibular molars. Why? As molars in both arches intrude, the rate of open bite closure will be greater compared to molar intrusion in one arch only. Further, intrusion of molars in both arches avoids compensatory molar eruption in the non-intruded arch which occurs if only one arch is intruded.

Masking or camouflage – (treatment to achieve open bite closure via anterior tooth eruption without reducing the underlying excess vertical skeletal dimension). Masking treatments include:

- Vertical elastics to erupt anterior teeth
- Bonding incisor brackets gingivally (bonding for an open bite) to erupt anterior teeth
- Steps placed in archwires to erupt anterior teeth
- Curve of Spee placement in mandibular archwire to erupt mandibular anterior teeth.

At his present age and considering the significant magnitude of Carter's vertical skeletal excess, we would strongly advise against masking at this time. We would consider masking only during later comprehensive orthodontic treatment. Also, the stability of Carter's open bite closure with masking would be questionable.

Surgery (maxillary impaction osteotomy) could correct Carter's skeletal open bite. Although presurgical orthodontics (preparing Carter's arches to coordinate at surgery) can be performed at any time once all permanent teeth erupt, the *surgical procedure itself should not be performed until Carter's growth is complete* in order to reduce postsurgical relapse due to postsurgical vertical growth.

Q: Do you consider Carter's open bite mild, moderate, or severe? Are you concerned with his mother's comment that Carter is emotionally immature? How do these two factors influence your decision to treat early (or not to treat) and how do they influence your estimation of probable treatment success?

A: In our opinion, Carter's dental and skeletal open bites are moderate to severe. Two early treatment principles we adhere to are described in the Foundations section: (i) generally avoid early treatment cases that require correction of *severe* skeletal discrepancies; and (ii) generally avoid cases if the patient is *severely* challenged (poor cooperation).

Both factors weigh against orthopedic success for Carter and should be sensitively discussed with his parents. You should tell them that you may not be able to close his open bite or keep it closed. Success will depend upon growth and treatment compliance. If you decide to attempt orthopedic treatment, then tell his parents that your goal is to correct the open bite but improvement may be all that you can achieve.

Q: How can Carter's moderate Class II skeletal discrepancy be addressed? Suggest specific orthopedic treatments – and masking/surgery treatments if orthopedics fails.

A: *Orthopedics* (restrict his maxillary growth while permitting his mandible to continue growing – or accelerate mandibular growth). Two points must be emphasized: (i) Carter has a *hyperdivergent* growth pattern (skeletal LAFH = 58%, FMA = 29°). Anything you can do to reduce Carter's maxillary descent and molar eruption will help minimize clockwise (CW) rotation of the mandible downward and backward – helping to close Carter's open bite and improving his anteroposterior relationship; (ii) Carter has proclined incisors. Treatment should seek to upright, not procline, his incisors.

Orthopedic options include:

- HPHG – would reduce forward growth (and may reduce descent) of the maxillary corpus, distalize maxillary molars, reduce descent of the maxillary first molars [14, 35], and allow the mandible to grow forward. This is an ideal option for Carter if he will wear it.
- CPHG – would reduce maxillary forward growth and distalize maxillary molars. However, it would not restrict descent of the maxillary corpus, could result in slight CW rotation of Carter's palatal plane, and could result in slight (< 1 mm) extrusion of his maxillary first molars compared to controls [14, 15, 35]. CPHG would not be an ideal treatment for Carter.
- SPHG – would produce an effect somewhere between that of high-pull and cervical-pull headgears and would not be an ideal treatment.
- Herbst appliance (or other Class II functional appliance) – would not be ideal due to Carter's hyperdivergent skeletal features and proclined mandibular incisors. Recall that the ideal Class II functional appliance patient is growing with a *short* lower anterior face height (*hypodivergent*), deep bite, and *upright* mandibular incisors.

Herbst appliance treatment effects include inhibition of maxillary growth (a tendency for restraint of maxillary growth occurs with all Class II functional appliances), distal movement of maxillary teeth, acceleration of mandibular growth, and mesial movement of mandibular teeth (mandibular incisor proclination) [102, 105, 144]. However, the *direction* of condylar growth from Class II functional appliance wear may not correct the mandibular skeletal deficiency or improve chin projection, and a significant part of the Class II correction is dental movement – not skeletal change [21, 106]. Specifically, hyperdivergent patients like Carter undergo a deleterious *backward mandibular rotation and increases in face height* with Herbst appliances [21].

- Any orthopedic treatment that tends to rotate the mandible CCW (up and forward) will improve Carter's Class II relationship. These treatments include *vertical-pull* chin cup wear, TADs to intrude molars, chewing exercises, bite plates to stretch the masseteric sling, TPAs with acrylic buttons, and LLHAs.

Masking or camouflage (achieving a Class I canine relationship without addressing the underlying Class II skeletal discrepancy). We would consider masking in the permanent dentition to get his teeth together if Carter did not respond to orthopedics – but only if his skeletal discrepancy improved to the point where his appearance was relatively normal and where masking would not produce unacceptable dental compensations. *Class II masking will probably be compromised treatment*. Options include the following:

- Extraction of maxillary first premolars to permit retraction of maxillary anterior teeth (achieving Class I canines but leaving molars Class II)
- Placing maxillary buccal, palatal, or infrazygomatic crest TADs as anchors for distalizing the entire maxillary arch.
- Use of Class II elastics (Forsus™ appliance or other inter-arch Class II correctors) would *not* be ideal because the lower incisors would procline further [145–147]. Also, the mandible will tend to rotate down and back with Class II elastic wear as mandibular molars erupt.
- Aligning permanent teeth only (not correcting canines to Class I).

Surgery (mandibular advancement) could be considered in conjunction with a maxillary impaction osteotomy, but not until Carter completed growth.

Q: *When* should Carter's skeletal Class II and skeletal open bite treatment begin?

A: If you decide to attempt orthopedics, then begin *now* while Carter is in the late mixed dentition and is near or at the inception of pubertal growth acceleration. Prospective clinical trials consistently report no advantage in treating Class II relationships in the *early* mixed dentition (except for a possible decrease in incisal trauma as a result of excess overjet) [17, 19, 73–77]. But Carter is in the late mixed dentition, and if we wait longer, then we may miss some favorable growth for orthopedic change.

We wish to reinforce three points:

- Dental age may not coincide with skeletal age. Although we generally wait to begin Class II treatment until the late mixed dentition, we will begin Class II treatment in the *early mixed dentition when a patient exhibits good growth velocity*.

- Prospective clinical trials of skeletal open bite orthopedic treatment are lacking. Therefore, a recommendation to begin Carter's skeletal open bite treatment now is based upon our clinical judgment.
- If you begin early orthopedic treatment now to address Carter's Class II relationship, then you should choose biomechanics that simultaneously reduces his vertical excess.

Q: How would you recommend correcting Carter's crossbite?

A: Before we recommend treatment, let's first review the transverse problems Carter is presenting with:

- Unilateral left complete buccal crossbite (scissor bite)
- CR=CO
- Maxillary first permanent molars have buccal crown torque (Figure 5.70q)
- Mandibular first permanent molars have lingual crown torque (Figure 5.70r)

We would like to expand Carter's maxillary arch in order to create an overjet on his right side, then use that overjet to upright his buccally inclined maxillary right first molar toward the lingual and upright his lingually inclined mandibular right first molar toward the buccal. However, the maxillary expansion would worsen his left scissor bite. Therefore, the maxillary expansion is not a good idea.

Similarly, we would like to expand his mandibular arch with a Schwarz appliance in order to improve the left scissor bite. However, expanding the mandibular left with a Schwarz appliance would also expand the mandibular right and put his right side into lingual crossbite.

Therefore, instead of *bilateral* maxillary or mandibular expansion, we recommended unilateral treatment – placing Carter on crossbite elastics from the buccal of his banded maxillary left first molar to the lingual of his banded mandibular left first molar. This reciprocal force would improve/correct the left scissor bite and upright the left molars. We will deal with the right molar crown torques later, during comprehensive treatment.

Q: Hypothetically speaking, if we do not correct Carter's left crossbite but his skeletal Class II orthopedics succeeds – how will this affect Carter's transverse relationship?

A: With mandibular forward growth relative to maxillary forward growth, a broader portion of Carter's mandibular arch will move into a narrower portion of his maxillary arch. This movement would improve his left buccal crossbite but worsen his right side – tending toward the right lingual crossbite.

Q: What unknowns do you face in treating Carter?

A: Growth magnitude and direction, cooperation, and presence of an undetected CR-CO shift.

Q: After considering all the above, would you recommend treatment for Carter at this consultation appointment, or recall? If you recommend treatment, then how would you proceed?

A: We recommended *reducing unknowns (growth/compliance)*, and then re-evaluating. A discussion was held with Carter and his parents about compliance. Considering the magnitude of his skeletal Class II and skeletal open bite relationships, coupled with his emotional immaturity, we were not optimistic about achieving correction with orthopedics. We were not even sure that we could gain enough improvement to successfully mask/camouflage him later. However, Carter and his parents implored us to attempt orthopedics. We agreed, with the understanding that orthognathic surgery would likely be needed to achieve an ideal result.

All four permanent first molars were banded, and Carter was placed on a HPHG (250 gm per side, twelve hours per night) for a six-month trial period. He was asked to wear crossbite elastics from the buccal of his maxillary left first molar to the lingual of his mandibular left first molar to correct his crossbite. If he could correct the left crossbite, then an LLHA would be placed to reduce the eruption of mandibular first permanent molars. Carter agreed to use thumb paint to help control his thumb-sucking habit. No treatment was initiated at this time to address his resting tongue habit.

At his headgear-fitting appointment, Carter cried and jumped out of the chair. After repeated attempts, we became exasperated and discussed the situation with his mother. We decided not to attempt headgear, to emphasize the thumb-sucking habit control for three months, and then to reattempt headgear wear. Three months later, a headgear was successfully fitted and delivered.

During the following four months, we received mixed reports from Carter and his mother regarding his thumb habit, elastic wear, and headgear wear. When questioned, Carter began to cry and stated that he could not fall asleep without sucking his thumb. At the end of four months, I asked Carter how much he was wearing his headgear. He said fewer than half the nights.

Q: How would you proceed?

A: I spoke to his mother and advised that we discontinue treatment for now. She agreed. We recommended against using a thumb crib appliance for habit control because Carter admitted to having no interest in quitting his habit.

We decided to let him mature before attempting habit control again. We removed his first molar bands and began monitoring his growth. When he completes growth and quits his thumb habit, we intend to proceed with orthognathic surgery or possibly TAD molar intrusion.

Q: Can you suggest "take-home pearls" regarding Carter's treatment?

A: "Take-home pearls" include the following:
- Carter was eleven years and ten months of age in the late mixed dentition when he presented for a consultation with his parent's chief complaint, "We do not like his open bite." He was Angle Class II division 1 secondary to mandibular skeletal anteroposterior deficiency with an open bite and left posterior complete buccal crossbite.
- Carter's anterior open bite was severe (10 mm) – a combination of dental open bite resulting from a thumb-sucking habit/resting tongue habit and skeletal open bite resulting from excessive vertical facial growth.
- Dental (functional) anterior open bites are corrected by eliminating the habit and erupting anterior teeth into occlusion.
- *We* recommend *early dental open bite treatment through habit control when the patient is interested in stopping the habit.* Otherwise, we wait until the child matures. Even thumb paints and thumb cribs will fail unless a patient is internally motivated to quit. Carter was not motivated to quit.
- Skeletal anterior open bites are treated with orthopedics, masking, or surgery. Early orthopedic treatment of skeletal open bites consists of restricting downward maxillary corpus growth plus reducing maxillary/mandibular molar eruption.
- *We* recommend *attempting early (orthopedic) treatment of skeletal open bites in mild-to-moderate cases only. Skeletal anterior open bites are very challenging* and successfully treated in only the most cooperative children. The purpose of including Carter in this textbook was to reinforce this point.
- Be wary of treating early *severe skeletal discrepancy cases.* There are exceptions to this guideline. We will recommend early treatment of severe skeletal

discrepancy cases in some Class III patients, maxillary transverse deficiency patients, when there is a clear psychosocial (cosmetic) benefit, or when early treatment will dramatically simplify future treatment. If you attempt early orthopedic treatment in severe cases, do not aim for ideal correction. Instead, aim for improvement.

- Be circumspect of treating early cases *when the patient is severely mentally/physically disabled*. We love and are empathetic with all our children. But orthodontics is a heavily compliance-based specialty.
- Although we were reluctant to begin early treatment on Carter due to the severity of his open bite, Class II relationship, and emotional immaturity, we attempted treatment because he and his parents were very supportive and enthusiastic. You can never be sure of a patient's response to treatment until you try it. If we had obtained some orthopedic skeletal improvement, then we might have been able to treat Carter later with masking or at least reduce the magnitude of surgical correction.
- Attempting headgear treatment was reasonable. An HPHG would restrict maxillary forward growth while allowing the mandible to continue growing. HPHG treatment could prevent maxillary first molar eruption and possibly reduce maxillary corpus descent. These effects would help Carter's Class II and excess vertical skeletal relationships. An LLHA would reduce mandibular first permanent molar eruption by 1–2 mm which would also aid vertical *and* anteroposterior improvement.
- Principle: *Always reduce unknowns before committing to a final (especially irreversible) treatment plan.* In Carter's case, we started with a six-month headgear/crossbite/thumb habit treatment period. He failed. We succeeded by knowing that we at least attempted orthopedics and by determining how Carter will need to be treated later.
- Any time you attempt orthopedic treatment, you must have a *fallback* (contingency) plan. To achieve an ideal result, the fallback plan for Carter is a maxillary LeFort I impaction osteotomy (or TAD-supported molar intrusion) coupled with a mandibular advancement osteotomy.
- A fundamental precept of practical early orthodontic treatment is periodic, and frequent, patient reassessment. If you are unsure whether treatment is proceeding in the desired direction, then make records of the patient and re-evaluate.

Case Tricia

Q: Tricia is seven years and seven months of age (Figure 5.72). She presents to you with her parent's chief complaint, "Tricia has an open bite." PMH includes tonsillectomy, adenoidectomy, and placement of tympanostomy tubes. PDH includes a thumb-sucking habit until age five years and maxillary primary incisor avulsion at age six. Periodontal and TMJ evaluations are WRN. CR=CO. Compile your diagnostic findings and problem list for Tricia. Also state your diagnosis.

A:

Table 5.22 Diagnostic findings and problem list for Tricia.

Full face and Profile	*Frontal View*
	Face is symmetric
	Long soft tissue LAFH (soft tissue Glabella – Subnasale < Subnasale – soft tissue Menton)
	Possible mentalis strain
	Lip competence
	UDML WRN
	Large buccal corridors
	Inadequate gingival display in posed smile (maxillary central incisor gingival margins are above maxillary lip border)
	Profile View
	Convex profile
	NLA WRN
	Chin projection inadequate
	Obtuse lip-chin-throat angle
Ceph Analysis	*Skeletal*
	Maxillary anteroposterior position WRN (A-Point lies approximately on Nasion-perpendicular line)
	Mandibular anteroposterior position mildly deficient (ANB angle = 4° with a normal maxillary anteroposterior position)
	Long skeletal LAFH (LAFH/TAFH × 100% = 60%; normal = 55%, sd = 2%)
	Palatal plane cant (PNS much lower than ANS due to excess vertical growth of posterior maxilla)
	Steep MPA (FMA = 30°; SNMP = 37°)
	Effective bony Pogonion (Pogonion lies on extended Nasion-B Point line)
	Short posterior face height
	Dental
	Proclined maxillary incisors (U1 to SN = 113°)
	Proclined mandibular incisors (FMIA = 60°)

Table 5.22 (Continued)

Radiographs	Early mixed dentition
Intraoral Photos and Models	Angle Class II division 1
	Iowa Classification: II(3) II(2) II(2) II(2)
	OJ ~ 7 mm
	Anterior open bite
	Maxillary incisors are stepped up relative to the maxillary posterior teeth
	1 mm of maxillary anterior spacing is currently present (Figure 5.72j)
	3.0 mm of maxillary arch spacing is anticipated following the eruption of all permanent teeth (if proper space maintenance is employed)
	1 mm of mandibular incisor crowding is currently present (Figure 5.72k)
	2.2 mm of mandibular arch spacing is anticipated following the eruption of all permanent teeth (if proper space maintenance is employed)
	UDML and LDML are coincident
	Maxillary and mandibular dental arches are symmetric
	"Hour-glass" shape to maxillary arch (Figure 5.72o)
	Minimal posterior OJ of primary canines, primary first molars, and primary second molars (Figure 5.72h)
	Maxillary first permanent molars are rotated to the mesial (Figure 5.72o)
	Maxillary permanent first molar buccal crown torque (transverse compensations, Figure 5.75a)
	Mandibular permanent first molar lingual crown torque (transverse compensations, Figure 5.75b)
Other	None
Diagnosis	Class II division 1 open bite malocclusion

Q: Tricia's maxillary first permanent molars are rotated to the mesial. How does this fact affect her Class II relationship?

A: When maxillary first permanent molars are rotated to the mesial, their molar relationship appears more Class II when viewed from the buccal than they really are. That is, when fixed orthodontic appliances are placed and the maxillary first permanent molars are rotated distally into normal alignment, then the crowns will appear more Class I.

Tricia's scans should have been viewed from the lingual to ascertain whether the maxillary first permanent molar lingual cusps were seated in the mandibular first permanent molar central fossa (Class I) or are still

Class II. This was not done. However, we can assume that her molars will become more Class I when they are aligned.

Q: We noted the possibility of mentalis strain in the frontal view, but there was no mention of an ILG in the clinical notes (once Tricia relaxed her lips). Besides facial photographs, what other images might reveal Tricia exhibiting an ILG?

A: Patients with mentalis strain sometimes relax when they move from the photography room to the radiography suite. If you suspect mentalis strain in photographs, look for an ILG on the cephalometric radiograph. In Figure 5.72d, we do not see an ILG. Tricia probably does not have an ILG.

Q: In profile, Tricia's chin projection was inadequate. What *soft tissue* reference do you use to judge soft tissue chin projection (soft tissue Pogonion projection)? What *skeletal* reference do you use to judge skeletal chin projection (bony Pogonion projection)?

A: The *zero-meridian line* is used to judge soft tissue chin projection. The zero-meridian line is a vertical line drawn perpendicular to the Frankfort horizontal line and passing through soft tissue Nasion. A normally positioned chin should lie on this line or just short of it [130, 131]. Note in Figure 5.73, Tricia's chin (soft tissue Pogonion) lies behind zero meridian. Therefore, her chin projection is deemed *inadequate*.

An effective *bony* Pogonion is one positioned at, or anterior, to a line extended from Nasion through B-Point. An ineffective bony Pogonion is one that lies behind a line extended from Nasion through B-Point. Therefore, as shown in Figure 5.72e, Tricia possesses an *effective* bony Pogonion.

Q: Tricia had a tonsillectomy and adenoidectomy at an earlier age. However, look at the posterior pharyngeal wall on her lateral cephalometric radiograph (Figure 5.72d). What do you observe?

A: She appears to have mildly enlarged adenoids.

Q: Is regrowth of adenoidal tissue following adenoidectomy possible?

A: Yes. Using transnasal fibroscopy, a recent study reported some adenoidal tissue regrowth in approximately 19% of patients, more often occurring in children under 5 years old [148]. However, the authors concluded that nasal obstruction after adenoidectomy is not due to adenoidal tissue regrowth but rather is of rhinogenic origin.

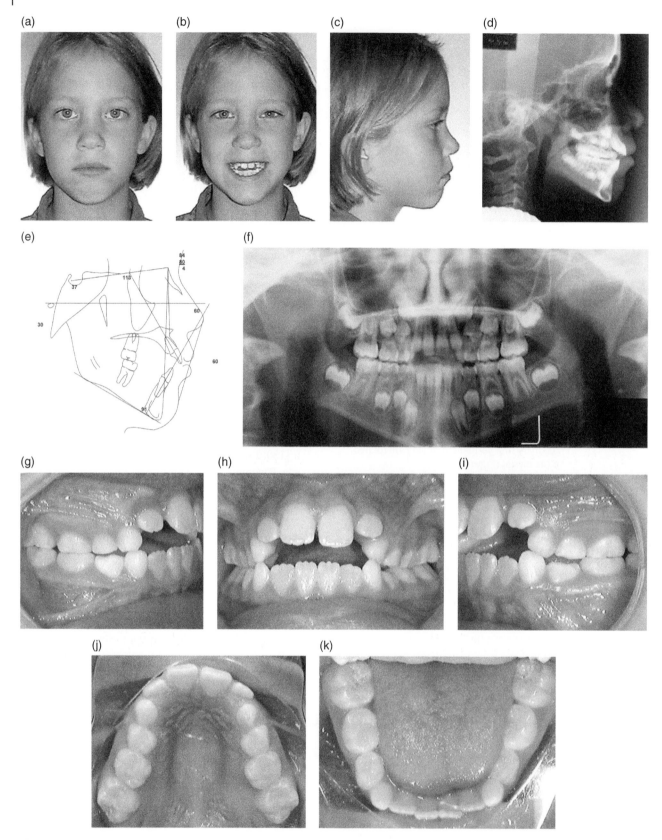

Figure 5.72 Initial records of Tricia: (a–c) facial photographs; (d) cephalometric radiograph; (e) cephalometric tracing; (f) pantomograph; (g–k) intraoral photographs; (l–q) intraoral scans.

(l) (m) (n)

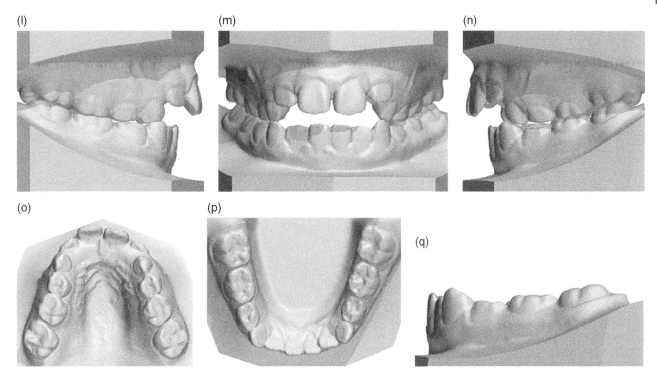

(o) (p) (q)

Figure 5.72 (Continued)

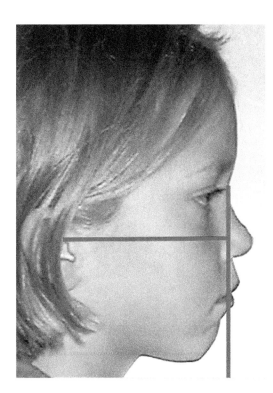

Figure 5.73 Zero-meridian line is drawn perpendicular to FH at soft tissue Nasion. The chin should lie on or just short of zero-meridian line to be considered effective. As illustrated, Tricia's chin lies behind zero meridian and is therefore inadequate/ineffective.

Q: Should you refer Tricia for a second adenoidectomy based solely upon her mildly enlarged adenoids in Figure 5.72d?

A: No. Remember that lymphatic tissue size first increases, and then decreases, during the developmental years [56]. So, enlarged adenoids are not, by themselves, an indication for adenoidectomy. Further, based upon the Lesinskas and Drigotas study [148], if Tricia was found to be mouth breathing, the obstruction is probably not due to the adenoids but is of rhinogenic origin.

If she was mouth breathing, snoring, or showing other signs of breathing difficulty (e.g. sleep apnea), then we would refer Tricia to an otolaryngologist for an airway evaluation.

Q: What are "adenoidal facies"?

A: Adenoidal facies [149], or *long-face syndrome*, are terms traditionally used to describe patients who exhibit an LLAFH, narrow face, ILG, narrow alar base, constricted maxillary arch (posterior crossbite), anterior open bite, high palatal vault, and frequent self-reported mouth breathing.

Q: Why has adenoidal facies been thought to result from nasal obstruction and mouth breathing?

A: The traditional view is that if the posterior teeth are held apart because of mouth breathing, then they will continue erupting and the face will lengthen. Consequently, an anterior open bite will result, an ILG will result, and the stretched cheeks will prevent the maxilla from growing wider.

Q: The traditional view links mouth breathing to adenoidal facies, but what does the current scientific evidence show?

A: *We have evidence of an association between nasal obstruction and facial morphology, but the interaction is complex and the evidence for a direct cause-and-effect relationship remains weak.*

Let's look at some of the research. Case studies have suggested that some children with nasal obstruction display a hyperdivergent pattern of facial growth with downward and backward mandibular rotation, and an increased lower face height [63, 64]. Children suffering from allergic rhinitis tend to have increased TAFH, increased lower anterior face height, and hyperdivergent MPA [60]. Long-faced adolescent subjects have significantly smaller components of nasal respiration [65].

On the other hand, some children with nasal obstruction do not display hyperdivergent facial patterns [66], and some children with morphologic characteristics associated with mouth breathing do not display significant nasal obstruction or mouth breathing [67]. In a sample [68] of 400 children aged two to twelve years (mean age 6 years) at an outpatient clinic for mouth breathers, the prevalence of anterior open bites, Class II malocclusions, and posterior crossbites was higher in mouth-breathing children than in the general population. However, more than 50% of the mouth-breathing children carried a normal inter-arch relationship in the sagittal, transverse, and vertical planes. This finding is supported by findings from another study suggesting no differences in the prevalence of malocclusion for children with obstructed nasal breathing compared to a normal population [67]. Furthermore, in a comparison of severely obstructed mouth-breathing and nasal-breathing children [69], mouth-breathing children had a hyperdivergent cephalometric pattern, but against all expectations, CCW mandibular rotation was the average observation. In a recent study of prepubertal severely obstructed mouth-breathing children and prepubertal nasal-breathing children, after adenoidectomy, the mouth-breathing children showed greater maxillary transverse development [70]. As with children, adult subjects with obstructed nasal breathing tend to show mandibular

plane hyperdivergence, but the correlation is too weak to support direct cause and effect [71].

Q: Does Tricia exhibit any features of adenoidal facies?

A: Yes, some. She exhibits an LLAFH, constricted maxillary arch, anterior open bite, and high palatal vault. She does not exhibit a narrow face, an ILG, a narrow alar base, or mouth breathing. Tricia should *not* be considered a traditional adenoidal face.

Q: Tricia exhibits lip *competence* which we associate with nasal breathing. However, she also exhibits an LLAFH, constricted maxillary arch, and anterior open bite – features often associated with mouth breathing. What questions should you ask Tricia and her parents to determine whether Tricia is a mouth breather or has trouble breathing? When would you refer her to an otolaryngologist for an airway evaluation?

A: First, try to observe whether Tricia breathes through her mouth. *Ask* her if she normally breathes through her nose or her mouth. Ask her parents the same question. Ask Tricia and her parents if she snores or has ever stopped breathing while asleep. If she has difficulty breathing, snores, is an obligatory mouth breather, or has a history of sleep apnea, refer her for an airway evaluation. If her parents are unsure of answers to these questions, ask them to pay close attention to Tricia and let you know what they observe. Alternatively, you may consider asking the parents to fill out a pediatric sleep questionnaire. Pediatric sleep questionnaires are useful in evaluating children for referral to investigate obstructive sleep apnea [142]. The American Association of Orthodontists has published a White Paper on this topic, including guidance on history taking and referral for patients with suspected breathing difficulties [143].

Tricia is found to breathe nasally and normally. She lacks any history of mouth breathing, snoring, sleep apnea, or other breathing difficulties.

Q: Discuss Tricia in the context of three principles applied to every early treatment patient.

A:

1) The goal of early treatment is to correct developing problems – get the patient *back to normal for their stage of development* (including preventing complications, reducing later treatment complexity, and/or reducing unknowns). The key to getting Tricia back on track is to correct her:
   - Open bite
   - Excess vertical maxillary corpus growth and maxillary dentoalveolar growth

- Hyperdivergence by promoting forward mandibular rotation
- Class II dental and skeletal relationships
- Transverse molar compensations (upright her molars)
- Minimal posterior transverse OJ.

2) Early treatment should address *very specific problems with a clearly defined end point*, usually within six to nine months (except for some orthopedic problems). Tricia's excess vertical growth and Class II dental/skeletal relationships have clearly defined end points, but orthopedics to address these problems will take longer than six to nine months. If the open bite has a dental (habit) component, then the time for correction will also depend upon habit cessation. Increasing posterior OJ and elimination of posterior compensations could be quickly accomplished with RME and mandibular molar uprighting.

3) Always ask: Is it necessary that I treat the patient now? *What harm will come if I choose to do nothing now?* If we do not treat Tricia now, then she will not be able to incise her food. Even though she is in the early mixed dentition, if she demonstrates good statural growth velocity and we wait, then we may miss an opportunity to modify growth in order to improve her skeletal problems. In terms of her transverse relationship, we see no harm in placing her on recall – as long as we treat her transverse problem before she reaches her peak of pubertal growth acceleration.

Q: Are there questions you should ask Tricia and her parents about her open bite? Is there anything else should you check for?

A: Do the following:
- Show her parents the open bite and ask how long she has had it. They respond that she has had the open bite for as long as they can remember.
- Tricia stopped sucking her thumb at age five, but ask if she has any other current habits (e.g. lip biting) that could prevent her anterior teeth from erupting? Tricia and her parents deny any habits.
- Ask Tricia if she has any idea what could be preventing her maxillary front teeth from erupting. She says she has no idea.
- Check whether the open bite is temporary due to the transition from primary to permanent dentition. In this case, we will consider the maxillary incisors since the maxillary incisors are stepped up relative to her posterior teeth (Figures 5.72h and 5.72m). Because Tricia is seven and a half years old, and because the normal age for maxillary incisor eruption ranges from seven to nine years [113], it is possible that her open bite could be due to the transition from primary to permanent dentition.

- Check for ankylosed maxillary incisors and blocked out incisors that are not fully erupted. No incisors appear to be ankylosed (all have normal mobility), and there appears to be adequate space for them to erupt.
- Check for anterior tongue posturing. Ask Tricia to close her eyes. Talk to her parents for a minute. Then, to distract Tricia, ask her to open her eyes as you quickly and gently draw her lower lip forward and down. You find that her tongue is anteriorly interposed between her incisors. *She does have a tongue-interposition habit.*
- Confirm that Tricia has not sustained jaw trauma and that her condyles appear normal (Figure 5.72f). Her parents state that Tricia has not sustained jaw trauma, and her condyles are difficult to see on her initial panoramic image. However, Tricia does not complain of any TMD symptoms and degenerative joint signs (e.g. crepitus) are absent. Based upon these findings, no additional joint imaging was requested.

Q: Can you list Tricia's skeletal open bite features? Dental open bite features?

A: Her *skeletal* open bite features include the following:
- Long soft tissue LAFH (soft tissue Glabella – Subnasale < Subnasale – soft tissue Menton)
- Long skeletal LAFH (ANS-Menton/Nasion-Menton × 100% = 60%; normal = 55%, sd = 2%)
- Palatal plane cant (PNS much lower than ANS due to excess vertical growth of posterior maxilla compared to anterior maxilla)
- Steep MPA (FMA = 30°; SNMP = 37°)
- Lack of posterior face height development

Typical skeletal open bite features that are missing in Tricia include:
- ILG (soft tissue growth appears to have kept pace with vertical skeletal growth, although she does show signs of mild mentalis muscle strain to achieve lip closure, Figure 5.72a)
- Maxillary first molar root apices have not erupted below the palatal plane (excess molar eruption is absent).

It is not unusual for skeletal open bites to lack some skeletal open bite features.

Her *dental* open bite features include the following:
- Active anterior tongue-interposition habit
- Anterior open bite extends only from canine to canine (where the interposed tongue rests)
- Maxillary incisors are stepped up relative to the maxillary posterior teeth. That is, her open bite is due to either the transition from primary to permanent dentition or to the interposed tongue habit.

Q: Does Tricia have an anterior *dental* open bite, *skeletal* open bite, or a combination of both? What is the etiology of her open bite?

A: Tricia has a combination of dental open bite *and* skeletal open bite. The etiology of her dental open bite probably includes:
- Transition from the primary to permanent maxillary dentition
- Anterior tongue-interposition habit.

Her skeletal open bite features resulted from a pattern of hyperdivergent growth including (Figure 5.74):
- Condyles growing posterior-superiorly

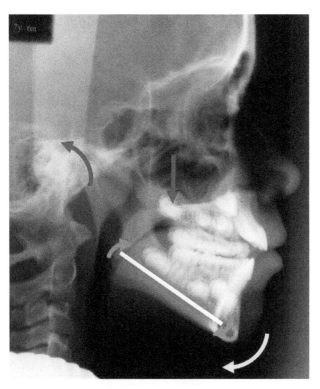

Figure 5.74 Tricia's hyperdivergent growth pattern resulting in many features of a skeletal open bite.

- Lack of posterior face height development
- Less forward mandibular internal rotation or even backward internal rotation (blue arrows)
- Vertical maxillary excess growth (VME, palatal plane rotated down posteriorly).

As a result of hyperdivergent growth, Tricia's mandible rotated downward and backward (yellow arrow), the MPA steepened, and the lower anterior face height increased. However, contrasted with many skeletal open bite patients, her maxillary molars are not overerupted (maxillary first permanent molar root apices are at the palatal plane – *not erupted below it*).

Q: Should you treat Tricia as a dental open bite or as a skeletal open bite?

A: You should treat her as both. Clearly, you must correct her tongue-interposition habit in order to achieve, and maintain, anterior open bite closure. However, you should also treat her as a skeletal open bite.

Q: Tricia has minimal posterior overjet at her primary canines and primary molars. What else should you examine in the *transverse* dimension beyond the presence of posterior overjet or posterior crossbite?

A: Look at her separated models from the front to check the torques of her posterior teeth (Figure 5.75). Note the *labial crown torque of her maxillary first molars and lingual crown torque of her mandibular first molars*. These teeth inclinations are dental compensations for an underlying narrow maxillary bony base (relative to the mandibular bony base).

Q: Will you want posterior crown torques (transverse dental compensations) to remain?

A: No, ideally you will want to upright these posterior teeth. However, uprighting her maxillary first permanent molars will tend to bring the crowns lingually,

(a)

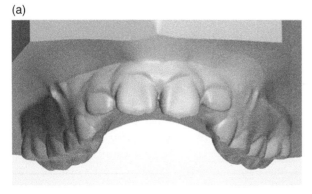
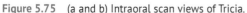

(b)

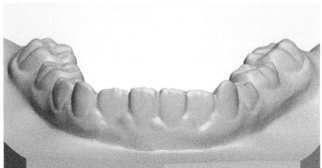

Figure 5.75 (a and b) Intraoral scan views of Tricia.

while uprighting her mandibular molars will tend to bring the crowns buccally. These movements could produce a posterior lingual crossbite.

It will be prudent to first expand the maxilla with RME so that you create enough buccal overjet to permit uprighting the posterior teeth without creating a posterior crossbite.

Q: Provide a detailed space analysis for Tricia's maxillary and mandibular arches. In other words, how were the anticipated 3.0 mm maxillary arch spacing and 2.2 mm mandibular arch spacing calculated *(if proper space maintenance is employed)?*

A:

Average mesiodistal widths of permanent teeth (mm): [94]

Maxillary Central Incisor	8.5	Mandibular Central Incisor	5.0
Maxillary Lateral Incisor	6.5	Mandibular Lateral Incisor	5.5
Maxillary Canine	7.5	Mandibular Canine	7.0
Maxillary First Premolar	7.0	Mandibular First Premolar	7.0
Maxillary Second Premolar	7.0	Mandibular Second Premolar	7.0
Maxillary First Molar	10.0	Mandibular First Molar	11.0
Maxillary Second Molar	9.0	Mandibular Second Molar	10.5

Average mesiodistal widths of *primary* teeth (mm): [94]

Maxillary Central Incisor	6.5	Mandibular Central Incisor	4.2
Maxillary Lateral Incisor	5.1	Mandibular Lateral Incisor	4.1
Maxillary Canine	7.0	Mandibular Canine	5.0
Maxillary First Molar	7.3	Mandibular First Molar	7.7
Maxillary Second Molar	8.2	Mandibular Second Molar	9.9

MAXILLARY ARCH

+1.0 mm of maxillary anterior spacing is currently present (Figure 5.72j)

+2.0 mm of anticipated leeway space (1 mm/side)

Balance = +1 mm +2 mm = +3 mm

MANDIBULAR ARCH

−1.0 mm of incisor crowding is currently present (Figure 5.72k)

+3.2 mm of anticipated leeway space (1.6 mm/side)

Balance = −1 mm +3.2 mm = +2.2 mm

That is, *3.0 mm of maxillary arch spacing and 2.2 mm of mandibular arch spacing is anticipated following the eruption of all permanent teeth (if proper space maintenance is employed).*

Q: What are Tricia's *primary* problems in each dimension, plus other problems?

A:

Table 5.23   Primary problems list for Tricia.

AP	Angle Class II division 1
	Iowa Classification: II(3) II(2) II(2) II(2)
	Mild mandibular anteroposterior deficiency
Vertical	Long soft tissue and skeletal LAFH (hyperdivergent growth pattern, VME)
	Anterior dental and skeletal open bite
Transverse	Minimal posterior OJ of primary canines and primary molars
	Transverse compensations
Other	—

Q: What are your options for dealing with Tricia's 1 mm of mandibular incisor crowding?

A: Options include the following:

- *Monitoring* – since her mandibular permanent canine roots are only half developed, and since the roots of her premolars are < half developed, monitoring would be a reasonable option.

- *Space maintenance* – since over 2 mm of mandibular spacing is anticipated following the eruption of all permanent teeth (if proper space maintenance is employed), placement of an LLHA is reasonable – at a future date. This space could be used during comprehensive treatment to upright mandibular incisors slightly. The advantage of placing an LLHA now is that you will not forget to place it later. The disadvantage of placing it now is that the banding cement could wash out over a period of years.

- *Incisor alignment with fixed appliances* – is not recommended at this time for only 1 mm of mandibular anterior crowding. Further, aligning proclined mandibular incisors would only procline them further.

- *Serial extraction* – would not be recommended. Exhibiting only mild crowding, Tricia is not an ideal candidate for serial extraction.

- *Interproximal reduction (IPR)* – is not recommended at this time. Incisor IPR could eliminate the 1 mm of crowding, but we would first recommend space maintenance to deal with it.

Q: How does Tricia's open bite etiology affect treatment?

A: Because Tricia's maxillary incisors are stepped up relative to her maxillary posterior teeth (*dental* open bite), and because she exhibits inadequate maxillary incisor display in both relaxed lip position (Figure 5.72d) and during posed smile (Figure 5.72b), it will be crucial to eliminate her anterior tongue-interposition habit so the maxillary incisors can erupt spontaneously. If the habit is corrected and the incisors do not erupt spontaneously, then they can be erupted with orthodontics. If the habit is not corrected, then we may never be able to close her open bite or maintain closure.

Tricia's *skeletal* anterior open bite features have resulted from excessive vertical facial growth. The treatment of choice for adolescent Class II patients with skeletal open bite features like Tricia is to:
- Reduce descent of her maxillary corpus
- Reduce/halt the maxillary molar eruption
- Reduce/halt the mandibular molar eruption.

If the above can be done, then the growing mandible can autorotate upward and forward, helping to close the open bite, reduce skeletal open bite features, *and* improve the Class II relationship/chin position. Also, the more condylar growth and more forward internal rotation of the mandible Tricia has, the more her mandible will autorotate upward and forward. The less condylar growth and less forward internal rotation of the mandible Tricia has, the less her mandible will autorotate upward and forward.

One key point – Tricia's excess vertical facial growth pattern will probably continue until growth is complete. Even if Tricia cooperates with orthopedics, and even if you are successful in controlling her vertical growth during treatment, her growth pattern will not be normalized after treatment. So, you must either treat her until she is finished growing or gamble that she will not grow out of treatment after you finish.

Another key point – Tricia has relatively mild skeletal open bite features. If she had severe skeletal open bite features, then it could be prudent to let her finish growing before initiating treatment – and plan on treating her with orthognathic surgery.

Finally, you should tell Tricia's parents that you may not be able to close her open bite or keep it closed. It will all depend upon her habit correction, her future growth, and her compliance with treatment. You should tell her parents that your goal is to correct the open bite completely, but you may only be able to reduce it.

Q: How would you address Tricia's dental open bite?

A: First and foremost, we always recommend discussing habit control with patients. If Tricia does not wish to end her anterior tongue-interposition habit, then the habit may win in the end – even if we force open bite closure with fixed orthodontic appliances and vertical elastics. If she does not wish to end the habit, then it is probably better to wait until she matures to address it.

If Tricia wants to end her tongue-interposition habit, then ask her to keep her tongue back behind her incisors (not interposed over them). Various "reminders" can be placed to help her remember to keep her tongue back:
- Short soldered spurs attached to an LLHA or maxillary U-arch
- Buttons bonded to the lingual surfaces of mandibular incisors
- Small blebs of composite bonded to the lingual surfaces of mandibular incisors
- "Blue Grass" appliance across the palate which acts to attract the tongue tip to it
- Hole through the anterior palate of a clear vacuum-formed retainer to attract the tongue to it.

It is possible that Tricia keeps her tongue forward to maintain a patent airway. Tricia does not have a breathing problem now but ask her parents to monitor her and report any changes to you.

Q: How would you address Tricia's skeletal open bite (hyperdivergent growth pattern, vertical skeletal excess) with orthopedics, masking, or surgery? Suggest specific options for each.

A: *Orthopedics – closing the skeletal open bite by reducing molar eruption/intruding molars and reducing descent of the maxillary corpus.* If we reduce/prevent molar eruption, then condylar growth will tend to rotate the mandible forward – improving her Class II molar relationship, improving chin projection, and reducing ANB angle. The same is true if we reduce her downward maxillary growth. Specific orthopedic treatments to reduce maxillary corpus descent or prevent molar eruption include:
- HPHG wear which may restrict vertical and anterior maxillary growth and restrict eruption of the maxillary molars [14, 35].
- Vertical-pull high-pull wear to inhibit dentoalveolar growth (inhibit posterior tooth eruption) [36, 37, 150].
- Temporary anchorage devices (TADs, attached to a transpalatal arch in the maxilla or an LLHA in the mandible) to halt eruption of the maxillary and mandibular first molars or intrude molars [46–49]. Care must be taken to ensure that the TADs do not damage developing tooth buds.

- Exercising (chewing gum) to reduce her MPA compared to controls [53, 54, 151].
- Posterior bite plates to stretch the masseteric sling and cause an intrusive force against the posterior teeth, or active vertical correctors (posterior repelling magnets) to reduce molar eruption [40–43, 152].
- Tongue pressure from a TPA with an acrylic button several millimeters off the palate to reduce increases in lower face height [44].
- LLHAs to reduce eruption of mandibular molars by 1–2 mm compared to controls [45].
- Modified Herbst appliance (Herbst appliance combined with acrylic splints and HPHG wear) that have been reported to control the vertical dimension in hyperdivergent adolescents (reducing Go-Gn-SN angle −1° compared to a reduction of −0.3° in control group, Bolton standards) [153].

Masking (camouflage) – closing the skeletal open bite by erupting anterior teeth but not by reducing the excess vertical facial growth. Options include:

- Leveling her maxillary arch with archwires to erupt her stepped up maxillary incisors. This could be performed with or without vertical elastics.
- Premolar extractions and space closure to retract her proclined anterior teeth. This will deepen her bite as incisors upright/rotate around their apices.
- Bonding incisors gingivally (bonding for open bite) to extrude anterior teeth relative to posterior teeth during leveling.
- Placing steps in archwires to erupt incisors.
- Adding a curve of Spee to her mandibular archwire to erupt mandibular incisors.
- Aggressive posterior occlusal adjustment (enameloplasty) to close the anterior open bite.

We would recommend masking as a fallback (contingency) option in the permanent dentition only if Tricia's vertical excess did not worsen and if her orthopedic outcome was unsatisfactory.

Surgery (maxillary impaction osteotomy) – could correct Tricia's skeletal open bite features (reduce her LLAFH, palatal cant, and steep MPA). However, she is too young to consider surgery. Why? If she has surgery before growth is complete, then she will continue to grow vertically, postsurgically, and your treatment will relapse.

In summary, we recommend treating Tricia as a dental open bite *and* skeletal open bite. We are willing to attempt orthopedics because she is a *mild* skeletal open bite. However, we must inform Tricia and her parents that depending upon growth and cooperation, surgery may be required to provide an ideal result. Correction

of her tongue-interposition habit is necessary for orthopedic, masking, or surgical treatment to be stable.

Q: Would you describe Tricia's Class II relationship as mild, moderate, or severe?

A: Her Class II relationship is mild. Dentally, she is Class II by 3 mm and 2 mm at her right and left permanent first molars, respectfully. However, her maxillary molars are rotated to the mesial, and the molar relationships will improve when they are aligned. Skeletally, her maxilla is in a normal position and her mandible is only slightly deficient (ANB angle is 4° which is 1° greater than a normal 2–3°).

Q: If Tricia's mandible is only slightly deficient, then why does her profile appear convex?

A: Her profile is convex through a combination of her mandible being slightly deficient plus bony Pogonion laying on a line extending from Nasion through B-Point. That is, Pogonion is effective by definition – but just barely so and not effective enough to compensate for the slightly deficient mandibular position.

Q: How could you improve Tricia's convex profile?

A: Tricia's convex profile resulted from inadequate mandibular forward growth relative to her maxillary forward growth and VME which rotated her mandible down and back. Her convex profile could be improved by reversing these growth patterns with orthopedics or surgery.

Q: Let's consider Class II orthopedics (restriction of maxillary growth while permitting the mandible to continue growing forward – or, acceleration of mandibular forward growth). *We would like Tricia's Class II orthopedics to complement her vertical orthopedics.* So, let's examine the vertical orthopedics list we considered earlier and see if any of these options would also be effective as Class II orthopedic treatments.

A: Options include:

- HPHG wear – would be ideal for Tricia because its force vector tends to restrict maxillary forward growth, maxillary downward growth, and maxillary molar eruption. Also, it would retract maxillary molars distally. All these effects could benefit Tricia – assuming, of course, that she was also placed in an LLHA to reduce mandibular molar eruption (mandibular molar compensatory eruption) [14, 35, 45].
- Vertical-pull chin cup wear – would be ideal because it inhibits/reduces maxillary *and* mandibular posterior tooth eruption [36, 37, 150]. Therefore, condylar growth would be translated into more forward

mandibular growth than if the molar eruption was not inhibited.

- Temporary anchorage devices (TADs, attached to a transpalatal arch in the maxilla or an LLHA in the mandible) – would be ideal if used to halt molar eruption/intrude molars in both arches and retract maxillary molars [46–49]. Condylar growth would translate into more forward mandibular growth than if molars were allowed to erupt unimpeded. Care must be taken to ensure that the TADs do not damage developing tooth buds.
- Exercising (chewing gum) – would help by reducing Tricia's MPA (compared to controls) [53, 54, 151], thereby rotating her mandibular forward into a more Class I relationship.
- Posterior bite plates (stretching the masseteric sling and causing an intrusive force against the posterior teeth), active vertical correctors (posterior repelling magnets), tongue pressure from a TPA with an acrylic button several millimeters off the palate, or an LLHA – would be helpful by reducing molar eruption and reducing increases in lower face height [40–45, 152]. Condylar growth would be translated into forward mandibular growth and toward Class I.
- Modified Herbst appliance (Herbst appliance combined with acrylic splints and HPHG wear) [153] – may be helpful by controlling the vertical dimension in hyperdivergent adolescents like Tricia. Once again, condylar growth would then be translated into forward mandibular growth.

If you attempt orthopedics now, then you must inform Tricia and her parents that, depending upon growth and cooperation, masking or surgery are fallback options that may be required later.

Q: Would you consider masking or surgical treatment to address Tricia's mild Class II skeletal relationship? What specific options would you consider?

A:

Masking (camouflage) – treatment to correct her Class II molar relationship dentally without addressing her underlying skeletal Class II relationship. Options include:
- *Intra-arch* mechanics to retract maxillary teeth to the distal (headgear, TAD anchorage to retract maxillary teeth, extraction of maxillary premolars to create space to retract anterior teeth).
- *Inter-arch* mechanics to retract maxillary teeth to the distal while simultaneously advancing mandibular teeth to the mesial (Herbst or other Class II functional appliances, Class II elastics, or Class II

correctors such as Jasper Jumpers, Forsus, etc.). Inter-arch mechanics would be less ideal than maxillary intra-arch mechanics because Class II inter-arch mechanics would procline Tricia's mandibular anterior teeth. Class II elastics would also erupt mandibular molars – worsening Tricia's excess LAFH.

We strongly recommend attempting orthopedics first. We also recommend rotating Tricia's maxillary first permanent molars into proper alignment first in order to more accurately assess her Class II relationship. Masking is a contingency option considered in the permanent dentition if Tricia's orthopedic response is unsatisfactory and if she remains Class II following maxillary molar alignment.

Surgery (mandibular advancement osteotomy, maxillary impaction osteotomy) could correct Tricia's Class II skeletal relationship. However, that is a significant amount of surgery to treat a mild Class II problem. An advancement/impaction genioplasty alone could benefit her profile and reduce her vertical dimension. We do not recommend orthognathic surgery yet because Tricia is too young.

Q: How would you deal with Tricia's posterior transverse relationship?

A: As is true with so many orthodontic problems, the answer depends upon the transverse problem's *magnitude*. The magnitude of Tricia's transverse problem is mild. Look at the facts:
- An overt posterior crossbite is absent.
- Although her primary canines and primary molars exhibit minimal posterior OJ (Figures 5.72h and 5.72m), her mesially rotated maxillary first permanent molars have adequate OJ at their distal. Further, if we rotate her maxillary first permanent molars distally to a correct alignment (rotate them around their lingual roots), then their mesiobuccal cusps will rotate to the buccal – providing the molars with adequate OJ along their entire buccal surfaces.
- The permanent first molar transverse compensations (maxillary molar buccal crown torque and mandibular molar lingual crown torque) are moderate, not severe. Uprighting the permanent first molars may, or may not, place them in posterior lingual crossbite.
- Tricia is only seven and a half years old. We have years before she reaches puberty and plenty of time to expand her maxilla with RME.

Based upon these facts, one could suggest dealing with Tricia's transverse relationship now, using RME to expand her maxilla and an expanded LLHA (or Schwarz appliance) to upright her mandibular molars. Or, one could suggest dealing with Tricia's transverse relationship later after all permanent teeth erupt to better judge her transverse and treat with RME or perhaps archwires.

Q: What unknowns do you face?

A: By far, the most significant unknown is Tricia's future jaw growth (magnitude and direction). We do not know how much her maxilla will descend or how much her posterior teeth will erupt (rotating her mandible down and back, worsening her open bite, and worsening her Class II relationship). We do not know how much her maxilla will grow forward (worsening her Class II relationship). We do not know how much her condyles will grow and in what direction. We do not know if her mandible will undergo forward or backward internal rotation.

Additional unknowns include her cooperation, interest in ending her tongue-interposition habit), hygiene, and presence of an undetected CR-CO shift. Tricia's unknowns are significant.

Q: Should you guarantee to Tricia's parents that you will be able to close her open bite and maintain open bite closure?

A: No. Tricia's open bite closure will depend upon variables out of your control (e.g. growth and cooperation). Unless she can end her anterior tongue-interposition habit, you have little chance of closing her open bite – or keeping it closed. Inform Tricia and her parents that you will do your best to care for her and that, with reasonable growth and cooperation, you have a good chance of correcting her open bite. But, never guarantee outcomes.

Q: *When* should you begin Tricia's Class II and open bite treatment?

A: If Tricia is interested and willing, then habit control to address her anterior tongue interposition should begin immediately.

As far as her Class II relationship is concerned, prospective clinical trials consistently report no advantage in treating Class II relationships in the *early* mixed dentition (except for a possible decrease in incisal trauma as a result of excess overjet) [17, 19, 73–77]. However, since dental age may not coincide with skeletal age, we recommend beginning Class II treatment in the early mixed dentition *if the patient has good statural growth velocity*. Tricia's parents monitor her growth and tell us that she is *not growing*.

We lack extensive, prospective clinical trials examining early orthopedic skeletal open bite treatment. However, since we hope to address her Class II

relationship and excess vertical growth simultaneously, we recommend *delaying those orthopedic treatments until Tricia reaches the late mixed dentition stage of development or demonstrates good statural growth velocity*.

Q: Based upon these discussions, would you recommend early treatment for Tricia or recall her? If you recommend early treatment, what treatment would you recommend?

A: We recommend:

- Interposition tongue habit control (discussions/encouragement plus placement of small composite reminder "blebs" on mandibular incisor lingual surfaces)
- RME followed by conversion of the RME appliance into a TPA to maintain the expansion. An expanded LLHA would upright the lingually inclined mandibular molars.
- Monitoring growth and development until Tricia reaches the late mixed dentition or until she demonstrates good statural growth velocity. Then, we would begin Class II orthopedics which simultaneously addresses her excess vertical growth (HPHG, vertical-pull chin cup, TAD molar intrusion, exercises (e.g. chewing gum daily), LLHA, or posterior bite plate.
- Once all permanent teeth erupt, early treatment would be finished. At this time, orthodontic records would be made, growth and patient compliance assessed, and a comprehensive treatment plan established.

Tricia was treated by Dr. Bradley L. Pearson. He held conversations with Tricia and her parents and proceeded as follows:

- Maxillary molars were banded, and a constricted 0.032 stainless steel wire lingual U-arch (removable) was placed to eliminate maxillary transverse compensations (eliminate buccal crown torque). Once the maxillary molars were upright, a bonded RME appliance was placed, and the maxilla was expanded.
- The RME appliance was removed, and a soldered maxillary U-arch (with spurs to help control the anterior tongue habit) was placed to maintain the transverse correction.
- A Schwarz appliance was used to upright/expand the mandibular dental arch. Spurs were placed in the anterior portion of the Schwarz appliance to remind Tricia to control her anterior tongue-interposition habit.
- Growth was monitored.
- Tricia began wearing a vertical-pull chin cup which she wore until growth was complete.
- All permanent teeth erupted (*early treatment was finished* at this time).

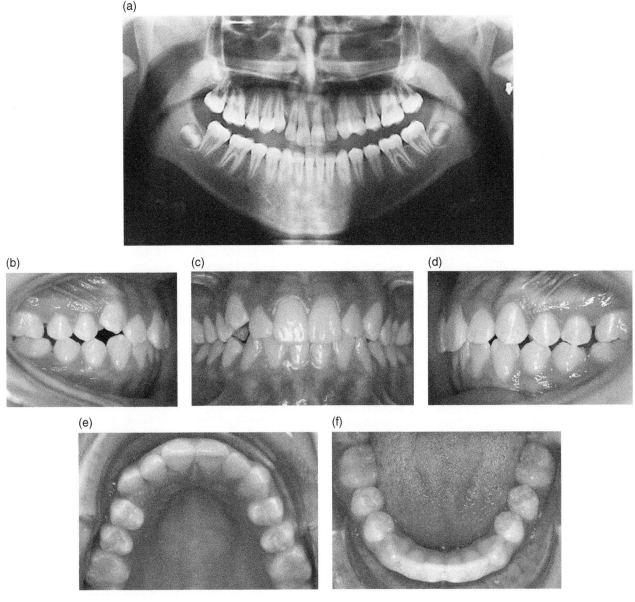

Figure 5.76 (a–f) Progress records of Tricia.

The maxillary U-arch was removed, and progress records were made (Figure 5.76) along with a decision to proceed with non-extraction comprehensive treatment. Tricia was bonded with fixed 0.022-inch edgewise appliances which included lingual arches to maintain the maxillary arch expansion. Spurs were soldered to the mandibular lingual arch to help control the tongue habit. Arches were leveled and aligned, spaces were closed, arches were finished, Class II elastics were worn for two months, and Tricia was debanded.

Q: Deband records are shown in Figure 5.77. The cephalometric radiograph was taken six months post-deband. What changes occurred during treatment?

A: Changes include the following:
- Closure of her open bite *during early treatment* (Figure 5.76c) to an OB of 20%
- Reduction in skeletal LAFH from 60% (Figure 5.72e) to 57% (Figure 5.77e)
- Significant facial growth (Figure 5.77f) over seven years. Her maxilla grew downward. Her mandible grew downward and slightly forward relative to the maxilla – resulting in a decrease of ANB angle from 4° to 0° and greater chin prominence. Her maxillary molars, mandibular molars, and incisors erupted. Her maxillary molars moved mesially, and her U1 to SN angle decreased by 9°.
- She has a beautiful smile, straight profile, coincident midlines, aligned dental arches, a Class II (2 mm)

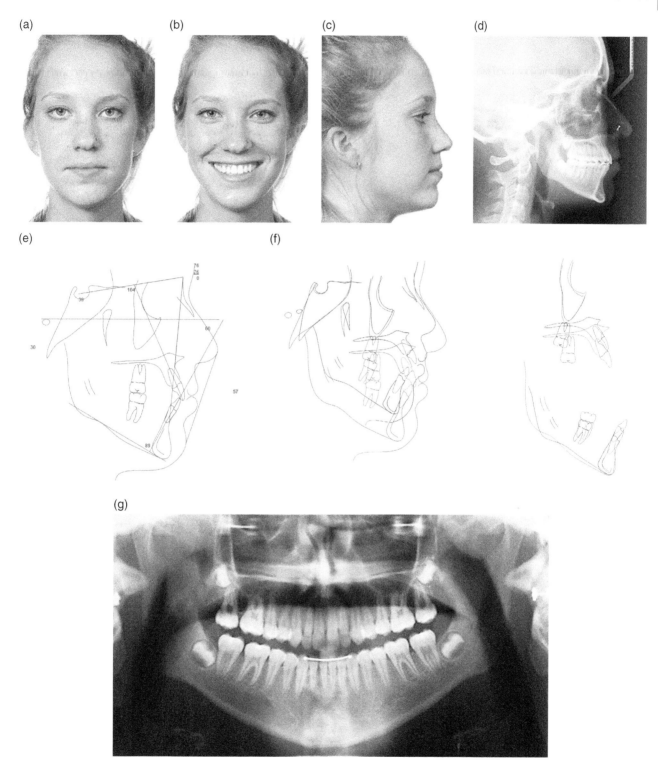

Figure 5.77 (a–l) Post-treatment records of Tricia.

(h)   (i)   (j)

(k)   (l)

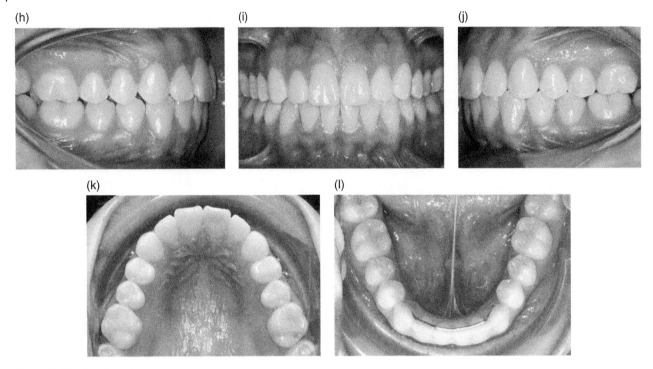

Figure 5.77 (Continued)

right molar and canine relationship, and a Class I left molar and canine relationship. No mentalis muscle strain is noticeable.

- Development/eruption of her wisdom teeth will be monitored.

Q: How was Tricia's open bite closed (Figures 5.72h, 5.76c, and 5.77f)?

A: Her open bite closed primarily via *incisor eruption*. Tricia was motivated and cooperative in eliminating her anterior tongue-interposition habit. Habit reminders (tongue spurs) probably helped. We wish to emphasize that her open bite closed during *early* treatment, before fixed orthodontic appliances were placed.

We will never know whether vertical-pull chin cup wear prevented Tricia from developing a severe skeletal open bite. What we do know is that her skeletal LAFH decreased by 3% during treatment. Finally, mandibular growth (Figure 5.77f, lower right) was more than adequate to keep pace with combined downward maxillary growth, maxillary molar eruption, and mandibular molar eruption. Without this mandibular growth, the mandible would have rotated CW significantly (down and back).

Q: What is the advantage of vertical-pull chin cup wear versus HPHG wear in Tricia's case, specifically?

A: Vertical-pull chin cups apply an intrusive force against maxillary molars, mandibular molars, and maxillary corpus. Vertical facial growth (skeletal LAFH) reduced and, with accompanying mandibular condylar growth, the chin came forward – improving Tricia's profile and Class II relationship.

HPHGs apply an intrusive force only against the maxillary molars and maxillary corpus. If maxillary molars erupt less than normal (relative intrusion), then mandibular molars may erupt more than normal (*compensatory eruption*) – leaving little vertical skeletal improvement and reducing forward chin movement. If an HPHG is worn, then its effect can improve, and mandibular molar compensatory eruption can be reduced, with an LLHA.

Finally, HPHGs apply a distal force to the maxillary molars and maxilla – potentially improving the Class II relationship. Vertical-pull chin cups do not.

Q: What was the advantage of using a *bonded* RME for Tricia instead of a conventional Hyrax RME appliance.

A: Due to their bite block effect (stretching of the masseteric sling), bonded RME appliances cause less initial vertical opening than banded RMEs. Studies have reported an average of 0.8 mm maxillary first molar intrusion and a reduction of 0.5 mm downward movement of PNS [154, 155] with bonded RME appliances compared to banded RME appliances.

Q: What retention protocol would you recommend for Tricia?

A: Tricia was placed in a maxillary removable Hawley retainer and a fixed mandibular canine-to-canine retainer (Figure 5.77l). We would recommend retaining Tricia with occlusal coverage clear vacuum-formed retainers – to be worn full time for at least a year. Why? The plastic occlusal coverage acts as a bite plate to reduce/halt molar eruption.

Q: Can you suggest "take-home pearls" regarding Tricia's treatment?

A: "Take-home pearls" include the following:
- Tricia was seven and a half years old when she presented with a dental open bite and skeletal open bite. Her dental open bite features included the presence of an anterior tongue-interposition habit, an anterior open bite extending to primary canines only, and the fact that her maxillary incisors were stepped up relative to the maxillary posterior teeth.

  Her skeletal open bite features included long soft tissue and skeletal LAFHs, posterior downward cant of the palatal plane, steep MPA, and lack of posterior face height development. Skeletal open bite features that were missing included lack of an ILG (mentalis strain to achieve lip competence?) and the fact that her maxillary first molar root apices were in the palatal plane.

- Tricia's dental open bite probably started with a thumb-sucking habit and then continued with an anterior tongue-interposition habit. Her skeletal open bite features were most likely due to a traditional skeletal open bite (hyperdivergent) growth pattern –
  a) More posterior-superior condylar growth as opposed to superior or superior-anterior condylar growth
  b) Shorter posterior ramus height development
  c) Less forward mandibular internal rotation or even backward internal rotation
  d) Maxilla which descends more than normal (palatal plane rotated down posteriorly)
  e) Molars which often erupt more than normal
  f) As the mandible rotates backward, the MPA steepens, the anterior face height increases, and an anterior open bite may result – depending upon the influence of the tongue in preventing anterior teeth compensatory dental eruption

- Her tongue anterior interposition habit was successfully treated by asking her to discontinue the habit and by placing reminders (spurs) to help her remember to stop. We have found that putting a hole in the anterior palate of a maxillary retainer also works well to correct these habits. Why? The retainer modification attracts the tongue.

- If a patient does not wish to end a habit causing an anterior dental open bite, then the habit will win in the end. Even if you force closure of the open bite with fixed orthodontic appliances and vertical elastics, the habit may win in the end and the open bite return. If the child does not wish to end the habit, then it is best to postpone open bite closure until she/he matures.

- Tricia presented with many features of a skeletal open bite. When a patient presents with many skeletal open bite features, it is wise to treat them as if they had *all* the skeletal open bite features. This was how Tricia was successfully treated.

- Skeletal open bites can be challenging to treat orthopedically. Because the vertical maxillary growth/molar eruption that causes the open bite is not normalized with orthopedic treatment, this growth must be addressed (in active treatment and in retention) until growth is complete.

- We will *attempt* orthopedic treatment in children with mild-to-moderate skeletal open bites, but correction is successful in only the most cooperative patients. Orthopedic correction of severe skeletal open bites can be heroic.

- In treating skeletal open bites, you must have a fallback plan (contingency plan) including masking/orthognathic surgery and inform parents of this plan if orthopedics is not successful.

- Orthopedic treatment of skeletal open bites aims at reducing maxillary corpus descent and reducing maxillary/mandibular molar eruption. A vertical-pull chin cup was successfully used for Tricia and helped reduce her skeletal LAFH. She had significant maxillary corpus descent and molar eruption but probably less than she would have had without the vertical-pull chin cup.

- Tricia is a perfect example of the need to *reduce unknowns* before making irreversible treatment decisions. Tricia's tongue habit correction, vertical-pull chin cup wear compliance, and treatment response were determined *before* the final decision made to treat her without extracting teeth or without surgery.

- Patient compliance does not last forever. Trying to decide when to begin orthopedics in order to maximize change (while avoiding patient "burnout") is challenging. Tricia was exceptionally compliant. Part of an orthodontist's job is being a cheerleader.

- Overcorrection of OB should be a goal for open bite cases.

Case Nora

Q: Nora is nine years and three months old (Figure 5.78). She is referred to you for correction of her anterior crossbite. PMH and TMJ evaluations are WRN. She exhibits a 1 mm anterior shift from CR into CO. When she closes into CR, her mandibular incisors contact edge-to-edge with her maxillary lateral incisors. She then shifts forward slightly into CO. Do you need any additional records to decide whether to begin early treatment or to recall her?

A: No additional records are necessary. However, a cephalometric radiograph and tracing were made (Figure 5.79).

Q: Using the above records, *compile your diagnostic findings and problem list*. State your *diagnosis*.

A:

Table 5.24   Diagnostic findings and problem list for Nora.

Full face and Profile	***Frontal View***
	Face is symmetric
	LAFH WRN (soft tissue Glabella – Subnasale = Subnasale – soft tissue Menton)
	Lip competence
	UDML WRN
	Incisal display during posed smile is inadequate (maxillary central incisor gingival margins are apical to maxillary lip border)
	Profile View
	Mildly convex profile
	Upturned nasal tip
	Obtuse NLA
	Chin projection WRN
	Lip-chin-throat angle WRN
	Chin-throat length WRN
Radiographs	Early mixed dentition
Ceph Analysis	***Skeletal***
	Mildly deficient maxillary anteroposterior position (A-Point lies behind Nasion-perpendicular line)
	Mandibular anteroposterior position WRN (ANB angle = 1° with maxillary anteroposterior position slightly deficient)
	Skeletal LAFH WRN (ANS-Menton/Nasion-Menton × 100% = 55%)
	Mandibular plane WRN (FMA = 23°; SNMP = 36°)
	Effective bony Pogonion (Pogonion lies anterior to a line drawn extending from Nasion to B-Point)
	Dental
	Maxillary incisor inclination WRN (U1 to SN = 99°, but Sella is low)
	Mandibular incisor inclination WRN (FMIA = 65°)

Table 5.24   (Continued)

Intraoral Photos	Angle Class I
	Iowa Classification: I I I I
	OJ 0 mm
	OB 60%
	LDML 1 mm to left of UDML
	Periodontal biotype WRN
	0.5 mm of maxillary anterior crowding currently present
	1.5 mm of maxillary arch spacing is anticipated following the eruption of all permanent teeth (if appropriate space maintenance is employed)
	0 mm mandibular anterior crowding currently present
	3.2 mm of mandibular arch spacing is anticipated following the eruption of all permanent teeth (if appropriate space maintenance is employed)
	Bilateral anterior crossbite of maxillary lateral incisors
	Bilateral posterior open bite of primary molars
	Dental arches are symmetric
	Significant posterior transverse compensations (Figure 5.78o, maxillary first permanent molar buccal crown torque; Figure 5.78p, mandibular first permanent molar lingual crown torque)
	Mandibular first permanent molars appear to be tipping over the mandibular primary second molars
Other	—
Diagnosis	Class I malocclusion with bilateral anterior crossbite and bilateral posterior open bite

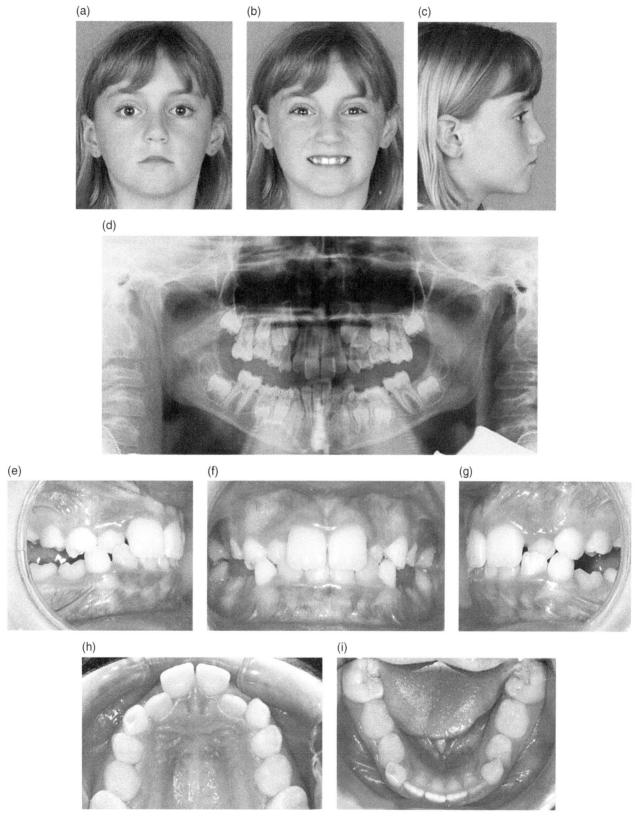

Figure 5.78 Initial records of Nora. (a–c) facial photographs; (d) pantomograph; (e–i) intraoral photographs; (j–r) model photographs.

(j)

(k)

(l)

(m)

(n)

(o)

(p)

(q)

(r)

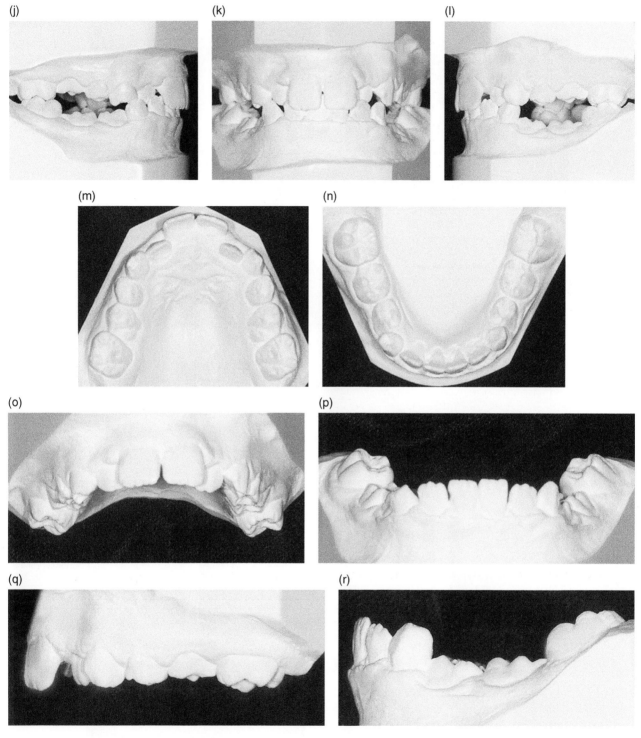

Figure 5.78 (Continued)

Q: The normal range of U1 to SN angles = 101–104°, but Nora's U1 to SN = 99° (suggesting upright maxillary central incisors). So, why did we conclude that her maxillary incisal angulation was *normal*?

A: It was because the long axis of her maxillary incisors (Figure 5.79b) *appear* to have a normal angulation. In fact, U1 to SN measures less than normal because Sella is low – not because maxillary incisors are upright. This

(a)   (b)

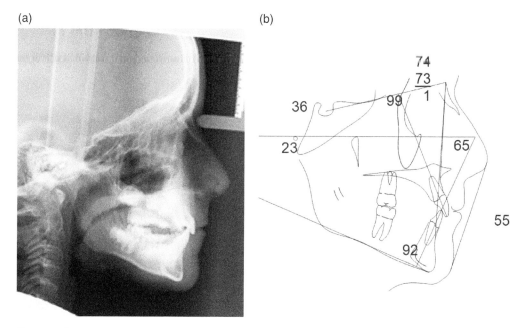

Figure 5.79   Initial records of Nora. Cephalometric radiograph (a) and tracing (b).

is evidenced by the fact that the normal angular difference between SN and FH is 7°, but Nora's difference between these lines is 13° (Sella is low). Adding 6° to the measured 99° gives an approximation closer to normal.

Our point is that you should *look* at the incisors on the cephalometric tracing and ask – how do they appear. Do they look upright? Do they look proclined? To us, Nora's maxillary incisors appear to have a normal inclination.

First principle of cephalometric analysis – use cephalometric measurements to corroborate what you see. If the measurements do not reflect what you see, then try to determine why they do not.

Q: Provide a detailed space analysis for Nora's maxillary and mandibular arches. How were the 1.5 mm of maxillary arch spacing and 3.2 mm of mandibular arch spacing calculated (if space maintenance is employed)?

A:

Average mesiodistal widths of permanent teeth (mm): [94]

Maxillary Central Incisor	8.5	Mandibular Central Incisor	5.0
Maxillary Lateral Incisor	6.5	Mandibular Lateral Incisor	5.5
Maxillary Canine	7.5	Mandibular Canine	7.0
Maxillary First Premolar	7.0	Mandibular First Premolar	7.0
Maxillary Second Premolar	7.0	Mandibular Second Premolar	7.0
Maxillary First Molar	10.0	Mandibular First Molar	11.0
Maxillary Second Molar	9.0	Mandibular Second Molar	10.5

Average mesiodistal widths of *primary* teeth (mm): [94]

Maxillary Central Incisor	6.5	Mandibular Central Incisor	4.2
Maxillary Lateral Incisor	5.1	Mandibular Lateral Incisor	4.1
Maxillary Canine	7.0	Mandibular Canine	5.0
Maxillary First Molar	7.3	Mandibular First Molar	7.7
Maxillary Second Molar	8.2	Mandibular Second Molar	9.9

MAXILLARY ARCH

−1.0 mm crowding right lateral incisor–central incisor contact (Figure 5.78h)

+0.5 mm spacing midline diastema

+2 mm of anticipated leeway space (1 mm/side)

Balance = −1.0 mm +0.5 mm +2.0 mm = +1.5 mm

MANDIBULAR ARCH

0 mm of anterior crowding is currently present

+3.2 mm of an anticipated leeway space (1.6 mm/side)

Balance = +3.2 mm

That is, *1.5 mm maxillary arch spacing and 3.2 mm mandibular arch spacing is anticipated following the eruption of all permanent teeth (if proper space maintenance is employed).*

Q: What are Nora's *primary* problems that you must stay focused on?
A:

Table 5.25   Primary problems list for Nora.

AP	Bilateral anterior crossbite of permanent lateral incisors
Vertical	Deep bite of 60% Bilateral posterior open bite
Transverse	Significant posterior transverse compensations without posterior crossbites
Other	

Q: In terms of Nora's anterior crossbite (maxillary lateral incisors), what should you check for?
A: Incisor trauma.

Q: When she opens (Figure 5.80), what do you see?
A: Attrition on the mesial one-half of the facial surfaces of her maxillary lateral incisor crowns. Note the left lateral incisor has significant facial surface attrition along the mesial one-half of the incisal edge.

Q: Do you recommend treating Nora's anterior crossbite early (now)?
A: Yes. When Nora closes into CR, her mandibular incisors contact edge-to-edge with her maxillary lateral incisors. She then shifts forward slightly into CO. Elimination of her anterior crossbite will eliminate this shift and eliminate additional lateral incisal wear.

Q: Let's discuss this 1 mm CR-CO shift into anterior crossbite further. Could this forward shift (forward jaw posturing) act like a Class II functional appliance?

A: Yes, at least theoretically. That is, a forward shift distracts the mandibular condylar head out of the glenoid fossa and could result in accelerated mandibular growth, maxillary forward growth restriction, uprighting of maxillary incisors, and proclination of mandibular incisors. However, considering the magnitude of Nora's forward shift (1 mm), these effects may be undetectable.

Q: Nora presents with bilateral posterior open bites. These are *posterior* open bites because her anterior teeth occlude but her primary molars do not. What should you check for during your examination?
A: Check for a posterior tongue-interposition habit (resting tongue habit). A clue that this is relevant is visible in Figure 5.78f where her tongue is observed posteriorly. Ask Nora to relax while you gently retract her right cheek and then her left cheek.

Q: As you retract her cheeks, what do you observe (Figure 5.81)?
A: We observe bilateral posterior tongue (resting) interposition habits.

Q: Is pressure from her tongue-interposition habit inhibiting tooth eruption and causing her bilateral posterior open bite?
A: Possibly, but there may be other causes as well.

Q: Can you exhaustively list other possible causes?
A: Other possible causes of her posterior open bites include:
- Ankylosis of primary molars
- Digit-sucking habit
- Temporary transition to permanent dentition
- Rapid Class III growth
- Inadequate space for tooth eruption
- Systemic factors
- Sleep apnea treatments
- Primary failure of eruption

(a)

(b)

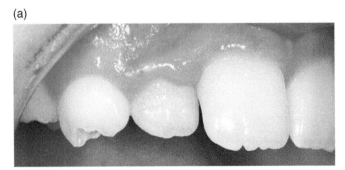
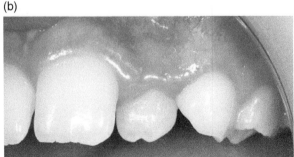

Figure 5.80   Nora's maxillary right (a) and left (b) anterior teeth.

(a)   (b)

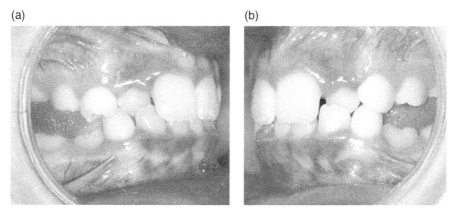

Figure 5.81   (a and b) Nora with her cheeks retracted.

Q: Can you eliminate any of the above possible causes using Nora's records and questions to her and her parents?

A: Let's consider each possible cause:

- Ankylosis of primary molars – preventing their eruption into occlusion. To judge the presence of primary molar ankylosis, compare alveolar bone crest levels between suspected primary teeth and adjacent erupting teeth. In the presence of ankyloses, the adjacent erupting teeth leave the bone level of the ankylosed teeth behind – and an alveolar bone crest step is seen.

  Looking at Nora's panoramic image (Figure 5.78d), a step between the alveolar crest of her primary second molars and permanent first molars is not obvious. To explore this possibility further, periapical radiographs (or a CBCT) would need to be made. This was not done. However, Nora's bilateral posterior open bites are so large that one would expect to see a distinct bone step if ankylosis was the cause.

- Digit-sucking habit – Nora denies any such habit.

- Temporary posterior open bite occurring from the time of normal primary molar exfoliation until premolar eruption into occlusion. Since Nora is still in the early mixed dentition stage of development, this cannot be the cause.

- Rapid Class III growth resulting in an edge-to-edge incisor relationship and posterior open bite – is not a potential cause since Nora is Class I.

- Lack of space for complete tooth eruption (teeth blocked out) – is not a potential cause since Nora appears to have adequate room for tooth eruption.

- Systemic factors found in patients with certain syndromes, such as cleidocranial dysplasia, ectodermal dysplasia, Gardner syndrome, and Apert syndrome – is not a potential cause since Nora's parents deny any such conditions.

- Treatments for sleep apnea [78] – Nora's parents deny any history of sleep apnea treatment.

- Primary failure of eruption (PFE) – is not a likely cause. Why? Because:

  1) *Permanent first molars are always involved* with PFE and present with no apparent barrier to eruption. Nora does not exhibit this sign. Her permanent first molars occlude.

  2) *If a tooth in a more anterior position is affected, then teeth more posteriorly positioned are usually affected as well.* Nora does not exhibit this sign since her permanent first molars occlude [79–83].

Q: Below is a list of other possible signs/facts of PFE [79–83]. Which are true and which are false?

1) Posterior teeth are more frequently affected
2) Only permanent teeth are affected
3) PFE is often bilateral
4) Teeth in both arches are often affected
5) Affected teeth resorb the alveolar bone above the crown, may erupt into initial occlusion and then cease to erupt further, or may fail to erupt entirely
6) Involved teeth may be displaced back and forth with manual pressure (indicating that they are not initially ankylosed)
7) If a small area of ankylosis is broken by manipulating the ankylosed tooth, it might be possible to move the tooth for a short time, but re-ankylosis is inevitable
8) Other concurrent skeletal problems and dental anomalies are never present.

A:

1) True
2) False
3) True
4) True

5) True
6) True
7) True
8) False

Q: Based upon the above, what is the probable cause of Nora's bilateral posterior open bite?

A: The most likely cause is a tongue-interposition habit (resting tongue habit).

Q: How will you deal with this tongue-interposition habit?

A: First, verify that Nora does not have a breathing problem (partial/complete airway obstruction, snoring, or sleep apnea). *Do nothing that will reduce space for her tongue if she has a breathing problem.* Nora's parents deny that she has a breathing problem – awake or asleep. Options for dealing with the resting tongue habit include the following:

- Psychological approach – discuss with Nora the need to retrain her tongue not to rest between her posterior teeth. Unlike anterior open bites due to tongue-interposition habits, we have not had success using this approach for the treatment of posterior open bites. Why? We suspect because the tongue must lay somewhere. Trying to train someone to retract the sides of their tongue medially would be very challenging.
- LLHA with posterior *bilateral* soldered wire loops to block the tongue
- Bilateral loops to block the tongue incorporated into a removable appliance
- Full-time tooth positioner wear to block the tongue
- Placing fixed orthodontic appliances in order to wear posterior vertical elastics between maxillary and mandibular arches to block the tongue. Crisscross elastics (paired crossbite elastics – maxillary buccal to mandibular lingual plus maxillary lingual to mandibular buccal) achieve the desired tongue blocking and tooth eruption effects while avoiding any horizontal side effects.
- RME to make space for her tongue, if you believe Nora has a constricted maxillary arch forcing her tongue laterally.

Q: Nora has a 60% overbite (deep bite). Would you classify her deep bite as being a skeletal deep bite, a dental deep bite, or a combination of both? Why?

A: Nora has a *dental* deep bite. Why? Her soft tissue LAFH is normal (soft tissue Glabella – Subnasale = Subnasale – soft tissue Menton), and her skeletal LAFH is normal (ANS-Menton/Nasion-Menton × 100% = 55%). In other words, Nora's vertical growth is normal.

Her 60% overbite has resulted primarily from mandibular incisor overeruption (Figures 5.78p and 5.78r), and possibly a small amount of maxillary incisor overeruption (Figure 5.78q). Nora has a dental deep bite.

Q: What would be the ideal way to reduce Nora's dental deep bite?

A: The ideal way would be to intrude her overerupted incisors. Proclining her incisors would also open the bite by rotating their crowns forward around their root apices. Lastly, erupting her premolars (and molars) during the curve of Spee leveling would open her bite by rotating her mandible down and back.

Q: A member of your study club suggests that Nora undergo RME, but another member questions this suggestion because Nora's first permanent molars are not in crossbite (Figures 5.78j–5.78l). Can you think of any reasons why you should consider RME?

A: We can think of two reasons. First, Nora demonstrates significant posterior transverse compensations (Figures 5.78o and 5.78p – maxillary first permanent molar *buccal* crown torque and mandibular first permanent molar *lingual* crown torque). If we upright these molars, then she will likely develop a bilateral posterior lingual crossbite. This fact illustrates that she has a maxillary transverse deficiency. Performing RME would widen her maxilla, increase her posterior overjet, and permit us to upright her permanent first molars.

Second, if a posterior resting tongue habit is the cause of her posterior open bite, then widening her maxilla and moving her mandibular molar crown to the buccal to upright them would make room for her tongue – possibly eliminating the need for the tongue to rest between the teeth and allowing her primary molars to erupt.

Q: Discuss Nora in the context of three principles applied to every early treatment patient.

A:

1) The goal of early treatment is to correct developing problems – get the patient *back to normal for their stage of development* (including preventing complications such as resorption of adjacent tooth roots, reducing later treatment complexity, or reducing/eliminating unknowns). Eliminating her anterior crossbites, anterior deep bite, bilateral posterior open bites, and posterior transverse compensations (uprighting her first permanent molars) would get Nora back on track for her stage of development.

2) Early treatment should address *very specific problems with a clearly defined end point*, usually begun and ended within six to nine months (not protracted over many years except for some orthopedic problems).

  - Eliminating her anterior crossbites can be accomplished in six to nine months. Maxillary lateral incisor crossbites will sometimes self-correct with RME. That is, the bite is opened as occlusal planes of maxillary posterior teeth cusps ride up opposing mandibular occlusal planes with expansion – permitting the lateral incisors to pass over the mandibular lateral incisors and primary canines.

  Or, Nora's bite could be opened using a posterior bite plate and the maxillary lateral incisors moved anteriorly with a removable appliance or fixed orthodontic appliances. However, care must be taken not to drive the maxillary lateral incisor roots into the erupting permanent canine crowns (causing resorption of the maxillary lateral incisor roots).

  - Opening Nora's deep bite could be readily accomplished by leveling her mandibular arch with fixed orthodontic appliances (intruding/proclining mandibular incisors, erupting mandibular permanent first molars). Or, her deep bite may open spontaneously with RME as maxillary posterior teeth cusp occlusal planes ride up opposing mandibular posterior occlusal planes.

  - Her bilateral posterior open bites will be difficult (impossible?) to correct if caused by a resting tongue habit unless the habit stops. Methods to attempt habit correction include an LLHA (or removable appliance) with bilateral posterior loops to block the tongue, full-time positioner wear to block the tongue, or posterior vertical elastics worn between fixed appliances in both arches to block the tongue. If RME is employed, then the resting tongue habit may resolve spontaneously because the room is made for the tongue. Finally, the open bites may close spontaneously during permanent tooth eruption which will take years.

  - Elimination of posterior transverse compensations (uprighting first permanent molars) can be readily achieved following RME with increased posterior overjet. Mandibular molars can be uprighted using crossbite elastics connected from the lingual of the mandibular molars to the RME appliance. Maxillary molars can be uprighted later during comprehensive orthodontic treatment.

3) Always ask: Is it necessary that I treat the patient early? *What harm can come if I choose to do nothing now?* If we do nothing, then continued maxillary lateral incisor attrition will occur as she closes and shifts from CR into CO. No harm is anticipated from her deep bite (no palatal impingement/soft tissue damage), posterior open bites, or transverse compensations if she is recalled.

Q: Should you start treatment now or recall Nora? If you start treatment, what treatment options would you consider?

A: Treatment options include the following:

  - *Recall* (no treatment now, monitor only) – re-evaluate in one year. We would anticipate continued attrition to Nora's maxillary lateral incisors and do not recommend this option.

  - *Space maintenance* – placement of an LLHA and Nance holding arch would be beneficial:
    1) to provide an anticipated 1.5 mm of maxillary arch spacing and 3.2 mm of mandibular arch spacing following the eruption of all permanent canines and premolars.
    2) to prevent further tipping of permanent first molars over primary second molars.

  However, we would recommend placement of an LLHA only *after* RME and uprighting of mandibular first permanent molars (with a Schwarz appliance or with elastics) or after RME with an expanded LLHA used to upright mandibular first permanent molars.

  - *LLHA with bilateral tongue-blocking soldered loops* – would provide mandibular space maintenance *and* prevent the tongue from inhibiting posterior tooth eruption.

  - Removable *appliance with posterior tongue-blocking loops or tooth positioner wear* – could provide mandibular space maintenance *and* block the tongue from inhibiting posterior tooth eruption. Of course, the tooth positioner would need to be fabricated with the posterior open bites closed and room for permanent canines and premolars to erupt.

  - *RME* – is recommended and would:
    1) create room for the tongue (possibly achieving spontaneous closure of the posterior open bites if they are due to a resting tongue habit)
    2) increase posterior overjet to permit uprighting of permanent molars (removal of posterior transverse compensations)
    3) possibly correct the anterior lateral incisor crossbite spontaneously.

  - Anterior crossbite correction with fixed, or removable, appliances – is recommended especially since there appears to be adequate room to advance the maxillary lateral incisor crowns (Figure 5.78h).

However, as the lateral incisor crowns are advanced, care must be taken not to drive the roots of the maxillary lateral incisors reciprocally into the erupting permanent canine crowns (resulting in lateral incisor root resorption).

- *Extraction of other primary teeth (e.g. primary canines)* – is not recommended. Why? All permanent teeth appear to be erupting normally.

Q: What early treatment, if any, do you recommend?

A: We decided to proceed with RME (Figure 5.82) to provide posterior overjet and increase tongue space in the hope of eliminating her interposition resting tongue habit. Concurrently, Nora began wearing bilateral crossbite elastics from the buccal of her maxillary first molar bands to the lingual of her mandibular first molar bands in order to upright her mandibular first molars.

Once the maxillary diastema created by RME closed, we planned to place fixed orthodontic appliances in the maxilla and advance the maxillary lateral incisors out of crossbite. However, as seen in Figure 5.82, her lateral incisor crossbites corrected spontaneously with RME.

Q: Take a close look at Figure 5.82. Can you make four observations regarding treatment progress from these images?

A: Observations include the following:

- Significant posterior overjet has been created with RME (Figure 5.82b). Note opening of the RME appliance expansion screw (Figure 5.82d). Also note that the screw has been tied off with a steel ligature to prevent it from reversing.
- Soldered metal arms, extending to the mesial from the RME appliance, were bonded to the maxillary primary second molars (Figure 5.82d) to increase anchorage. The bonding to the right primary second molar is intact. The bonding to the left primary second molar has separated. The left arm appears to have "ridden up" the lingual of the maxillary left primary canine.
- Excess expansion on Nora's left side has resulted in a complete buccal crossbite of her left permanent first molars (Figure 5.82b)
- Spontaneous correction of the maxillary permanent lateral incisor crossbites has occurred with RME.
- Overbite has been reduced to 40% with RME as the transverse movement of maxillary posterior teeth has resulted in their cusp occlusal inclines "riding up" mandibular posterior cusp inclines – forcing the jaws apart.
- The tongue no longer appears to be resting (interproximally) on either side.

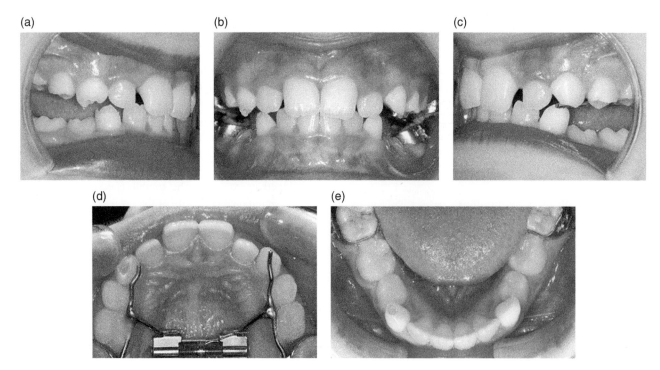

Figure 5.82   (a–e) Progress records of Nora following RME and during mandibular first permanent molar uprighting.

(a)

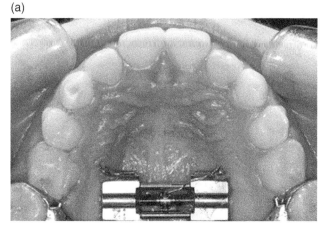

(b)

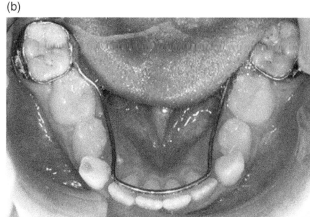

Figure 5.83　(a) Conversion of the RME appliance into a TPA, and (b) delivery of the LLHA.

Q: How would you proceed?

A: Nora was asked to continue wearing her posterior cross-bite elastics in order to upright her mandibular first permanent molars and correct her left buccal crossbite.

Q: The RME appliance was converted into a TPA by removing the mesial arms (Figure 5.83a), and an LLHA was placed (Figure 5.83b). Do you see a potential problem with the LLHA?

A: The mandibular right permanent canine cusp tip is erupting to the *lingual* of the LLHA. Unless the LLHA is redesigned, the canine could continue to erupt this way.

Q: Nora was recalled five months later (Figure 5.84). What do you observe? How would you proceed?

A: Observations include the following:
- No closure of right and left posterior open bites.
- Creating tongue space (RME plus mandibular first permanent molar uprighting) did not eliminate the tongue resting habit (Figures 5.84b and 5.84e).
- We neglected to solder tongue-blocking loops to her LLHA.
- Her mandibular permanent canines are erupting lingual to the LLHA (Figure 5.84g).

A decision was made to remake the LLHA with wires lingual to the mandibular canines so that they can erupt. Wire loops were soldered to block her tongue (Figure 5.85). Nora was recalled in three months. At that time, she stated that she could not tolerate the loops. A new LLHA (without loops and with metal arms lingual to the mandibular permanent canines) was fabricated and placed.

Q: She returned eight months later, and a panoramic image was made (Figure 5.86). What do you observe? How would you recommend proceeding?

A: Compared to Figure 5.78d, a step now clearly exists between the alveolar bone crest of the mandibular primary second molars and permanent first molars – indicating ankylosis of the primary second molars. Furthermore, the mesial roots of the mandibular primary second molars do not appear to be resorbing readily. We decided to extract all four primary second molars and monitor permanent tooth eruption. After the second premolars erupted, the RME and LLHA were removed.

Q: Records were made when Nora reached thirteen years of age (Figure 5.87). What changes do you observe? How would you recommend proceeding?

A: Changes include the following:
- All permanent teeth have erupted – early treatment is complete, and Nora can begin comprehensive orthodontic treatment if desired.
- Her bilateral posterior open bite has closed significantly.
- Nora has excellent facial esthetics and a mildly convex profile.
- Iowa Classification: I II(2 mm) II(3 mm) II(2 mm)
- 40–50% OB
- Good dental alignment

We recommended non-extraction comprehensive orthodontic treatment. Both arches will be bonded with fixed orthodontic appliances, arches leveled and aligned, and anterior OB reduced to create OJ. Note: *You must have OJ in order to correct a Class II relationship* – otherwise anterior teeth will be moved into crossbite.

Her 2 mm molar Class II relationship will be corrected using Class II elastics. We recommend Class II elastics since her mandibular incisors have a normal inclination (FMIA = 65°), they are aligned, and they

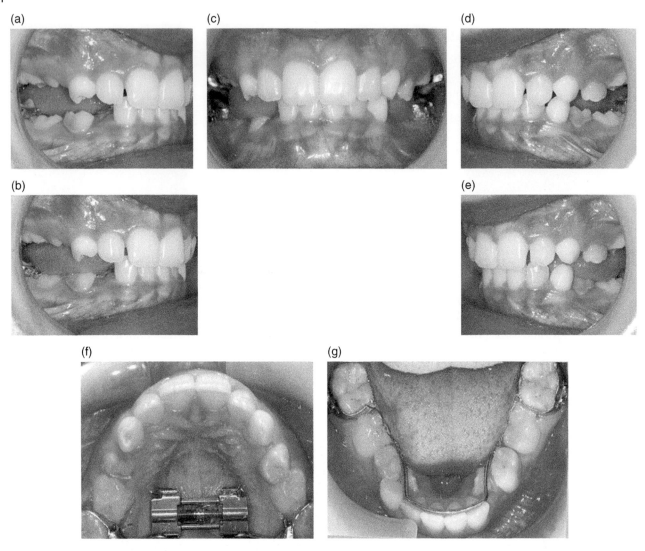

Figure 5.84 Progress records five months later; (a) tongue retracted showing posterior open bite; (b) tongue when resting; (c) frontal view with tongue resting; (d) tongue retracted showing posterior open bite; (e) tongue when resting; (f and g) occlusal views.

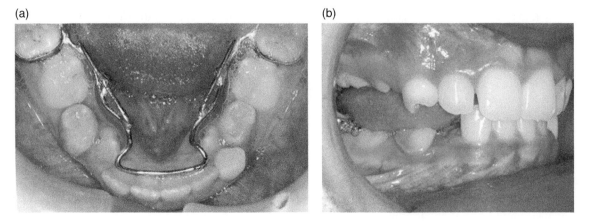

Figure 5.85 LLHA with soldered wire loops to block Nora's tongue.

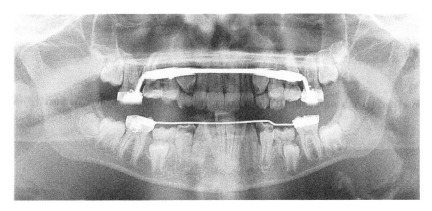

Figure 5.86   Progress panoramic image made at eleven years of age.

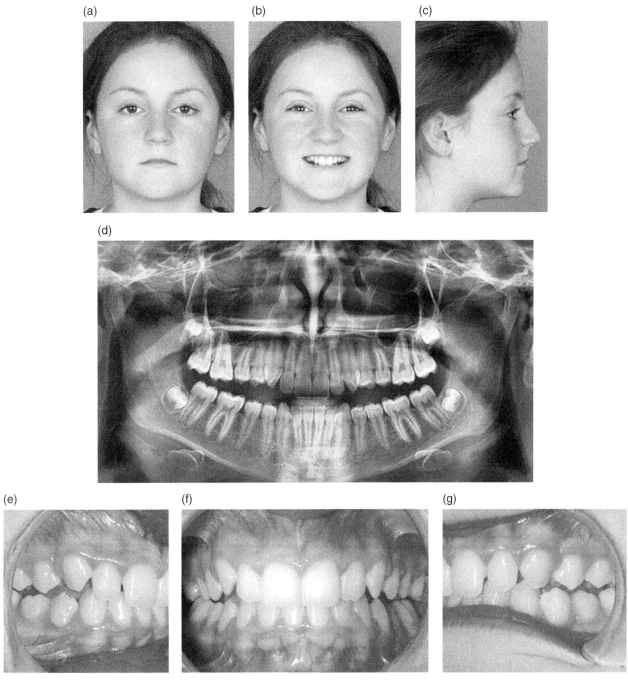

Figure 5.87   (a–n) Progress records of Nora made at age thirteen years.

(h) (i)

(j) (k) (l)

(m) (n)

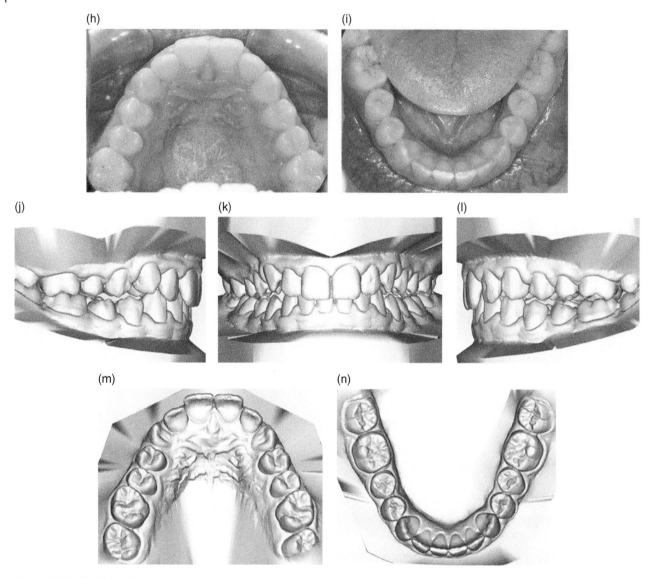

Figure 5.87 (Continued)

have a good labial periodontal biotype. We will use *crisscross vertical* posterior elastics to block the tongue and help close the remaining posterior open bite. At deband, we will ask Nora to wear a tooth positioner as a retainer in order to block the tongue habit.

Q: Can you identify "take-home pearls" for Nora?
A: "Take-home pearls" include the following:
   - Nora was nine years old in the early mixed dentition when she presented for correction of an anterior crossbite. She exhibited a Class I molar relationship, anterior dental deep bite, anterior lateral incisor crossbites, and bilateral posterior open bites.

Nora underwent RME to provide posterior overjet, permit posterior teeth uprighting, and increase tongue space. She wore bilateral crossbite elastics in order to upright her mandibular first molars and make additional room for her tongue. An LLHA was placed once her mandibular molars were upright. Our plan was to correct the anterior crossbite following RME, but her lateral incisor crossbites corrected spontaneously with RME.
   - What was the cause of Nora's bilateral posterior open bites? Initially, we observed a tongue-interposition habit and assumed that the tongue was preventing the primary molars from erupting. However, RME (making room for the tongue) did not result in habit cessation or in open bite closure (Figures 5.84b

and 5.84e). A later panoramic image (Figure 5.86) revealed a clear step between the alveolar bone crests of the mandibular primary second molars and permanent first molars – indicating ankylosis of primary second molars. This ankylosis was not observed initially (Figure 5.78d).

Because the posterior open bites are closing (Figures 5.87e and 5.87g) following primary second molar extraction and permanent tooth eruption, we believe that primary molar ankylosis was the major cause of her open bite development. However, the interposition tongue habit could still be playing a role.

Q: Are the following statements true or false?

1) Posterior open bites are easy problems to correct and maintain.
2) RME used to create space for Nora's tongue, eliminate her resting tongue habit, permit eruption of her posterior teeth, and eliminate her bilateral posterior open bite was a failure.
3) Early treatment was warranted for Nora.
4) Cephalometric measurements should determine your treatment plan.

A:

1) False. Depending upon the etiology, posterior open bites can be one of the most difficult problems to correct and to maintain correction of. If the etiology is ankylosed primary molars and erupting premolars are present, then the posterior open bite may self-correct once the ankylosed primary molars are exfoliated and the premolars erupt. If the etiology is a resting tongue habit, then the open bite can only be closed if the habit is corrected. If the etiology is PFE, then the posterior open bite may never be corrected. Depending upon the etiology, inform your patient that you may not be able to close the posterior open bite or to keep it closed. Tell them to expect relapse and the possible need for retreatment.
2) False. Although it is true that creating additional space for her tongue did not result in *immediate* posterior open bite closure, RME:
   - Spontaneously improved her anterior deep bite
   - Spontaneously corrected her anterior crossbites
   - Provided posterior overjet to permit uprighting of permanent first molars (elimination of transverse dental compensations)
   - May have helped improve her bilateral posterior open bite *long term*, by age thirteen years.
3) True. Correction of her anterior crossbite alone was justification for early treatment in order to prevent further maxillary lateral incisor attrition.

4) False. Information gleaned from cephalometric radiographs, or any imaging modality, should be considered together with clinical observations, your clinical experience, the best scientific evidence, and the patient's desires to determine your treatment plan. *Use cephalometric measurements to corroborate what you see clinically. If cephalometric measurements do not reflect what you see clinically, then try to determine why they do not.*

Case Mara

Q: Mara is nine years and five months old (Figure 5.88). She was referred to you for a consultation by her pediatric dentist. Her PMH includes a heart murmur, but her pediatric cardiologist states that prophylaxis is no longer necessary. PDH, periodontal/mucogingival evaluation, and TMJ evaluation are WRN. She exhibits a minimal (< 1 mm) right lateral shift from CR to CO. You contact her pediatric dentist who states that he is concerned with her right crossbite and her left posterior open bite. Compile your diagnostic findings and problem list for Mara. Also state your diagnosis.

A:

Table 5.26 Diagnostic findings and problem list for Mara.

Full face and Profile	*Frontal View*
	Face is symmetric
	Short soft tissue LAFH (Subnasal to soft tissue Menton < Glabella to Subnasal)
	Lip competence
	UDML ~2 mm to right of facial midline (Figure 5.88b)
	Gingival display in posed smile inadequate (maxillary central incisor gingival margins are significantly apical to border of maxillary lip)
	Significant left buccal corridor
	Profile View
	Relatively straight profile
	Chin projection WRN (soft tissue Pogonion at zero-meridian line)
	Obtuse NLA
	Mildly deep labiomental sulcus
	Lip-chin-throat angle WRN
Radiographs	Late mixed dentition (mandibular left permanent canine has erupted)

(Continued)

Table 5.26 (Continued)

Intraoral Photos and Models	Angle Class I Iowa Classification: I I I I OJ ~ 0 mm OB 30% 1.0 mm of maxillary anterior crowding is currently present 1.0 mm of maxillary arch spacing is anticipated following the eruption of all permanent teeth (if proper space maintenance is employed) 1.0 mm of mandibular incisor crowding is currently present 4.2 mm of mandibular arch spacing is anticipated following the eruption of all permanent teeth (if proper space maintenance is employed) Mesiobuccal cusp of maxillary right permanent first molar is in lingual crossbite (Figure 5.88o) Right primary canines are in crossbite Transverse dental compensations (buccal crown torque) of maxillary first permanent molars and (lingual crown torque) of mandibular left first permanent molar Mandibular midline to right of maxillary midline by 1–2 mm Maxillary and mandibular dental arches are symmetric (Figures 5.88m and 5.88n) Resting tongue habit left side (Figure 5.88g) Bilateral posterior open bites (Figures 5.88j and 5.88l)
Other	Maxillary left primary second molar is ankylosed Poor hygiene
Diagnosis	Class I malocclusion with right posterior crossbite and bilateral posterior open bites

Q: We noted that Mara's maxillary left primary second molar is ankylosed. What is the best way to diagnose primary tooth ankylosis?

A: *Radiographically* – ankylosis is definitively diagnosed when a *step in the alveolar bone crest height* is observed between the primary molar and adjacent teeth. Why? A step in bone height indicates that the ankylosed primary tooth has stopped erupting compared to the adjacent teeth.

Look at Mara's maxillary left primary second molar (Figure 5.88d). The maxillary left permanent first molar alveolar bone crest height is *coronal* to the maxillary left primary second molar bone crest height. The maxillary left permanent first molar has continued to erupt while the (ankylosed) maxillary left primary second molar stopped erupting.

Other techniques to determine ankylose, such as tapping the suspect tooth with an intraoral mirror handle in order to detect a difference in sound pitch compared to adjacent teeth, or checking for the mobility of the suspect tooth (an ankylosed tooth is fused to the bone and cannot move), may be of value. But the *best* way to confirm ankylosis of a primary molar is to look for a difference in alveolar bone crest height between the suspect tooth and adjacent teeth.

Q: Do Mara's other three primary second molars appear ankylosed?

A: Her maxillary and mandibular right primary second molars do not appear ankylosed. That is, they appear to have alveolar bone crest heights *level* with their adjacent permanent first molar bone crest heights.

On the other hand, the mandibular left primary second molar has a bone crest level which appears stepped down on the distal compared to the mandibular left permanent first molar bone crest level. Therefore, the mandibular left primary second molar could be ankylosed and should be monitored.

Q: Can primary second molar ankylosis be diagnosed simply by noting a clinical *occlusal step* between the permanent first molar and primary second molar?

A: No. Primary second molar crowns are generally shorter, coronal-apically, than permanent first molar crowns. So, a clinical step between the two can be normal and not indicate ankylosis.

Look at Figure 5.88q. Both Mara's right and left sides exhibit occlusal steps between permanent first molars and primary second molars. But her right mandibular primary second molar is *not* ankylosed (Figure 5.88d).

Q: Should Mara's ankylosed maxillary left primary second molar be extracted? What will happen if it is left in place?

A: Her ankylosed maxillary left primary second molar should *not* be extracted – at least for now. In the presence of a permanent successor in a normal position, the ankylosed tooth should be left in place and eruption of the second premolar monitored [84, 91, 156]. Exfoliation of the ankylosed primary second molar may be delayed approximately six months, but the eventual alveolar bone height of the erupted second premolar will be normal.

However, this is assuming that her maxillary left second premolar continues to resorb her primary second molar. If we find that resorption of the maxillary left primary second molar does not progress, then we would recommend extracting it.

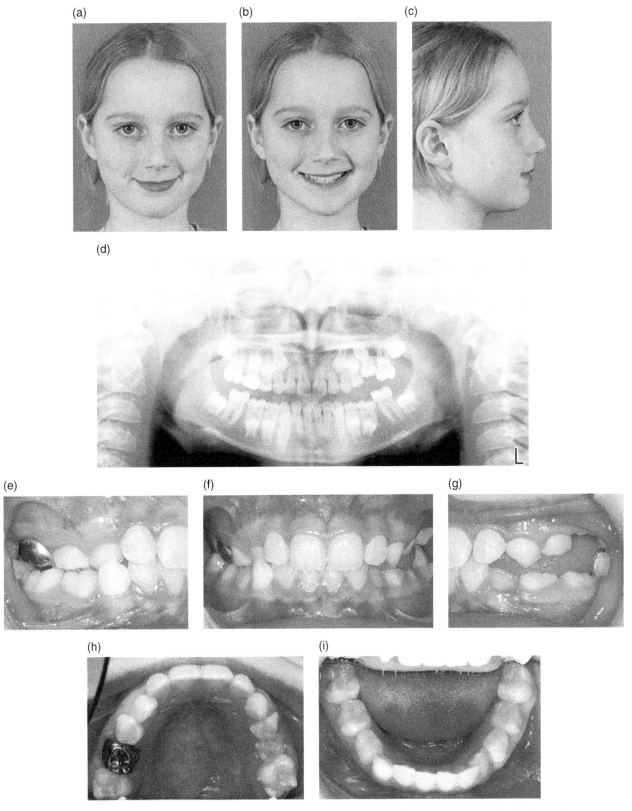

Figure 5.88 Initial records of Mara: (a–c) facial photographs; (d) pantomograph; (e–i) intraoral photographs; (j–s) models.

(j)　　　　　　　　(k)　　　　　　　　(l)

(m)　　　　　　　　(n)　　　　　　　　(o)

(p)　　　　　　　　　　　　(q)

(r)　　　　　　　　　　　　(s)

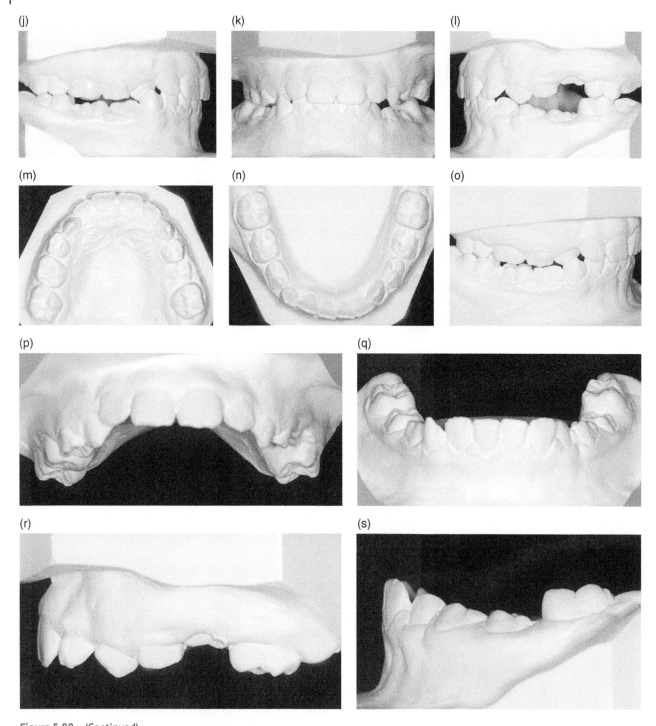

Figure 5.88　(Continued)

Q: What can happen to permanent first molars in the presence of an ankylosed primary second molar?

A: As the permanent first molar continues to erupt relative to the ankylosed primary second molar, the first molar may tip mesially (over the ankylosed primary second molar) and the unerupted second premolar can become impacted (Figure 5.89).

Q: What simple treatment can prevent permanent first molar mesial tip over ankylosed second primary molars?

A: Placement of a Nance holding arch in the maxilla, or an LLHA in the mandible, can prevent first molar mesial tipping. If significant first molar mesial tipping has already occurred, then the permanent first molar

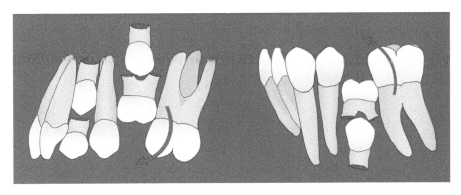

Figure 5.89 Eruption and mesial tipping of maxillary (left) and mandibular (right) permanent first molars relative to ankylosed primary second molars. As the permanent first molars erupt over the ankylosed primary second molars, space for the unerupted second premolars is lost, and the second premolar may become impacted.

should first be uprighted and tipped distally (space regaining), using either a removable appliance or fixed orthodontic appliances. After it is upright, the Nance holding arch or LLHA can be placed.

Q: Mara exhibits bilateral, *posterior* open bites. What features lead us to this observation?

A: Her anterior teeth occlude while her primary molars do not (Figures 5.88j and 5.88l).

Q: Can you exhaustively list the possible cause(s) of her posterior open bites?

A: Possible causes include the following:

- *Interposition (resting) tongue habit* – the pressure from which could prevent tooth eruption. Mara appears to exhibit a resting tongue habit on her left side (Figures 5.88f and 5.88g).
- *Digit-sucking habit* – Mara denies any such habit.
- *Temporary posterior open bite occurring after normal exfoliation of primary molars but before permanent teeth have time to erupt into occlusion* – is not the cause of her posterior open bites except for the left mandibular permanent canine which is partially erupted (Figure 5.88g).
- *Ankylosis of teeth* – preventing their eruption into occlusion. The ankylosed maxillary left primary second molar and (possibly) ankylosed mandibular left primary second molar appear to be contributing to Mara's left posterior open bite.
- *Very constricted dental arches* forcing a resting tongue habit – because the tongue must find space laterally to maintain a patent airway. This is not a likely cause of Mara's posterior open bite. Even though Mara has a right posterior crossbite and transverse dental compensations, her arches do not appear severely constricted (Figures 5.88h, 5.88i, 5.88m, and 5.88n).

- *Rapid Class III growth* resulting in an edge-to-edge incisor relationship – is not a potential cause since Mara is Class I.
- *Lack of space* for complete tooth eruption (teeth blocked out) – is not a potential cause since Mara appears to have adequate room for tooth eruption.
- *Systemic factors* found in patients with certain syndromes, such as cleidocranial dysplasia, ectodermal dysplasia, Gardner syndrome, and Apert syndrome – is not a potential cause since Mara's parents deny any such problems.
- *Some treatments for sleep apnea* [78] – Mara's parents deny any history of sleep apnea treatment.
- *Primary failure of eruption (PFE)*. Let's review the signs of PFE [79–83] and see whether Mara exhibits these signs:
  1) *Permanent first molars are always involved* and present with no apparent barrier to eruption. Mara does not exhibit this sign.
  2) Posterior teeth are more frequently affected. Mara exhibits this sign.
  3) *If a tooth in a more anterior position is affected, then teeth more posterior are usually affected as well* (i.e. when premolars are affected then molars are also likely to be affected). Mara does not exhibit this sign since her first permanent molars have erupted into occlusion.
  4) Both primary and permanent teeth can be affected. Mara may exhibit this sign.
  5) The condition is often bilateral (50/50 for PFE patients versus – 80/20 unilateral/bilateral for ankylosis of molars only). Mara may exhibit this sign.
  6) Teeth in both arches are often affected (91% of those with genetically confirmed PFE). Mara may exhibit this sign (maxillary and mandibular primary second molars could be affected).

7) Affected teeth resorb the alveolar bone above the crown, may erupt into initial occlusion and then cease to erupt further, or may fail to erupt entirely. Mara may exhibit this sign.

8) Involved teeth may be displaced back and forth with manual pressure (indicating that they are not, initially, ankylosed). However, involved teeth tend to become ankylosed as soon as orthodontic eruptive forces are applied. It is unknown whether Mara exhibits this sign.

9) If a small area of ankylosis is broken by manipulating the ankylosed tooth, it might be possible to move the tooth for a short time, but re-ankylosis is inevitable. It is unknown whether Mara exhibits this sign.

10) Other concurrent skeletal problems (Class III malocclusion for 63% of genetically confirmed PFE patients) and dental anomalies (tooth agenesis, microdontia of maxillary lateral incisors, anomalous root morphology) may be present. Mara does not exhibit any of these signs.

Considering these ten signs of PFE together, we concluded that Mara was *not* an example of PFE.

Q: Based upon the above, what is the cause of Mara's *left* posterior open bite.

A: The most likely cause of Mara's left posterior open bite is ankylosis of her left primary second molar(s) and a resting tongue habit.

Q: What is the cause of Mara's right (smaller) posterior open bite?

A: Possible resting tongue habit, possible (undetected) primary molar ankylosis.

Q: This is confusing. How could the posterior open bite result from two different causes?

A: Look at Figure 5.88g. The cause of the more distal portion of the open bite (primary second molar ankylosis as viewed on the panoramic image) is obvious. The more mesial portion of the open bite, the open bite existing between the left primary first molars, is more difficult to explain. However, the tongue does appear to be resting between the teeth, so we feel that this interposition tongue habit is contributing to the open bite.

Q: If Mara's posterior open bite is partially caused by an interposition (resting) tongue habit, then how will you deal with the habit?

A: First, *before closing a posterior open bite due to a resting tongue habit, confirm that a breathing problem (partial/complete airway obstruction, snoring, or sleep apnea) is not present.* Why? *If you force the tongue lingually, then obstruction of the airway could worsen.* If a breathing problem exists, seek consultation with an otolaryngologist. Mara's parents state that she does not have a breathing problem.

We have not had success correcting *posterior* tongue-interposition habits through patient education. Instead, options to correct (block) a resting posterior tongue habit include:

- LLHA with *bilateral* soldered posterior wire loops
- Bilateral posterior loops to block the tongue incorporated into a removable retainer
- Nearly full-time wear with a tooth positioner
- Placing fixed orthodontic appliances and wearing posterior vertical elastics (crisscross elastics) between maxillary and mandibular arches
- RME, if you believe a constricted maxillary arch is forcing Mara's tongue laterally.

Inform Mara and her parents of the difficulty in correcting, and in maintaining the correction of, posterior open bites.

Q: Provide a detailed space analysis for Mara's maxillary and mandibular arches. In other words, how were the anticipated 1.0 mm maxillary anterior spacing and 4.2 mm mandibular arch spacing calculated (*if proper space maintenance is employed*)?

A:

Average mesiodistal widths of permanent teeth (mm): [94]

Maxillary Central Incisor	8.5	Mandibular Central Incisor	5.0
Maxillary Lateral Incisor	6.5	Mandibular Lateral Incisor	5.5
Maxillary Canine	7.5	Mandibular Canine	7.0
Maxillary First Premolar	7.0	Mandibular First Premolar	7.0
Maxillary Second Premolar	7.0	Mandibular Second Premolar	7.0
Maxillary First Molar	10.0	Mandibular First Molar	11.0
Maxillary Second Molar	9.0	Mandibular Second Molar	10.5

Average mesiodistal widths of *primary* teeth (mm): [94]

Maxillary Central Incisor	6.5	Mandibular Central Incisor	4.2
Maxillary Lateral Incisor	5.1	Mandibular Lateral Incisor	4.1
Maxillary Canine	7.0	Mandibular Canine	5.0
Maxillary First Molar	7.3	Mandibular First Molar	7.7
Maxillary Second Molar	8.2	Mandibular Second Molar	9.9

MAXILLARY ARCH

−1.0 mm anterior crowding currently present (Figures 5.88h and 5.88m)

+2.0 mm of anticipated leeway space (1 mm/side)

Balance = −1.0 mm +2.0 mm = +1.0 mm

MANDIBULAR ARCH (left leeway space cannot be used because the mandibular left permanent canine has already erupted)

+9.9 mm space held by the mandibular left primary second molar (Figures 5.88i and 5.88n)

−7.0 mm space required by the mandibular left second premolar

+7.7 mm space held by the mandibular left primary first molar

−7.0 mm space required by the mandibular left first premolar

−1.0 mm of incisor crowding currently present

+1.6 mm mandibular right side leeway space

Balance = +9.9 mm −7.0 mm +7.7 mm −7.0 mm −1.0 mm +1.6 mm = +4.2 mm

That is, *1 mm of maxillary arch spacing and 4.2 mm of mandibular arch spacing is anticipated following the eruption of all permanent teeth (if proper space maintenance is employed).*

Q: Is Mara's 30% OB a skeletal deep bite, a dental deep bite, or a combination of both?

A: Mara's 30% may be a combination of both, but it is principally a dental deep bite. Why? Mara's soft tissue LAFH is only mildly short. She looks normal (not overclosed). On the other hand, her mandibular incisors are overerupted (Figures 5.88q and 5.88s) – leading to a dental deep bite.

Q: Is Mara's right crossbite a dental crossbite or a skeletal crossbite?

A: It is a skeletal crossbite. Why? First, let's review her transverse features:

- Significant left buccal corridor (Figure 5.88b)
- Minimal right lateral CR-CO shift
- Mesiobuccal cusp of maxillary right permanent first molar is in lingual crossbite (Figure 5.88o)
- Right primary canines are in crossbite
- Transverse dental compensations (buccal crown torque) of maxillary first permanent molars (Figure 5.88p)
- Transverse dental compensation (lingual crown torque) of mandibular left first permanent molar (Figure 5.88q)

Next, let's perform a mind experiment. Imagine uprighting Mara's maxillary first permanent molars, uprighting her mandibular left first permanent molar, and eliminating her small right CR-CO shift. As you do this, her:

- Maxillary first permanent molar crowns will tend to move lingually
- Mandibular left first permanent molar crown will tend to move labially
- Right first permanent molar crossbite worsens
- Left first permanent molar overjet decreases.

In other words, as we upright permanent molars (and remove the CR-CO shift), the transverse problem worsens. Even though her maxillary arch does not appear constricted (Figure 5.88m), a mild transverse skeletal discrepancy exists. *Relative to her mandibular arch the maxillary arch is constricted.* Mara has a skeletal posterior crossbite.

Q: Based upon the above, can you state our principle for differentiating between a skeletal and dental posterior crossbite?

A: *If uprighting permanent molars (removing transverse compensations) creates, or worsens, a posterior crossbite, then a transverse skeletal discrepancy exists (skeletal crossbite exists).* If uprighting permanent molars improves a crossbite, then a dental crossbite probably exists.

Q: What are Mara's *primary* problems in each dimension, plus other problems?

A:

Table 5.27 Primary problems list for Mara.

AP	—
Vertical	Bilateral posterior open bites
	30% overbite
Transverse	Crossbite of right permanent first molars and right primary canines
	Transverse posterior dental compensations
Other	Ankylosed maxillary left primary second molar
	Possible anklyosis of mandibular left primary second molar
	Poor hygiene

Q: Why would poor hygiene be listed as a primary problem?

A: Years of treatment are frequently required to provide an excellent orthodontic outcome, and patients must practice superb oral hygiene during this time. Poor hygiene can result in gingival hyperplasia, enamel decalcification, and caries – forcing premature removal of braces. Poor oral hygiene should always be considered a primary problem.

Q: Discuss Mara in the context of three principles applied to every early treatment patient.

A:

1) The goal of early treatment is to correct developing problems – get the patient *back to normal for their stage of development*. This can include preventing complications, reducing later treatment complexity, or reducing/eliminating unknowns. Eliminating Mara's deep bite, posterior open bites, ankylosed molar(s), crossbite, and small CR-CO shift would get her back on track.

2) Early treatment should address *very specific problems with a clearly defined endpoint*, usually within six to nine months except for some orthopedic treatment.

   - Opening Mara's deep bite could be readily accomplished by leveling her mandibular arch with a 2×4 fixed orthodontic appliance (intruding/proclining mandibular incisors, erupting mandibular permanent first molars).
   - The posterior open bites may self-correct following exfoliation of her ankylosed primary molar(s) and eruption of her premolars, but this will take longer than nine months. An uncorrected interposition tongue habit may prevent her bilateral open bite from ever closing, or the habit may take a very long time to correct.
   - Her right posterior crossbite and small CR-CO shift can be readily corrected with RME which will create posterior overjet to permit uprighting of permanent first molars.

3) Always ask: Is it necessary that I treat the patient now? *What harm will come if I choose to do nothing now?* It is not necessary to treat Mara now. Correction of her 30% OB can be delayed without harm until Mara undergoes later comprehensive orthodontic treatment. She has permanent first molar occlusion for chewing – so, postponed treatment of her posterior open bites can be delayed without harm. However, without space maintenance, her permanent first molar(s) could erupt and tip to the mesial over the ankylosed left primary second molar(s) and potentially impact the left second premolar(s). Correction of her right posterior crossbite, and transverse dental compensations, could be postponed for a year without harm. However, if we wait until puberty or postpuberty to attempt RME, then achieving a midpalatal sutural separation (maxillary skeletal expansion) will become increasingly difficult as the facial bones mature and skeletal resistance increases.

Q: Should you start early treatment or recall Mara? If you start treatment, what treatment options would you consider?

A: Your treatment options include the following:

- *Recall* (no treatment, monitor only) – re-evaluate in one year. The potential harm would be eruption and mesial drift of Mara's left permanent first molar(s) over her ankylosed primary second molar(s). If such drift occurred, then her left second premolar(s) could become impacted. We do not anticipate a problem in postponing RME for one year nor in delaying OB reduction.
- *RME* – would permit correction of Mara's right crossbite, eliminate the CR-CO shift, and create posterior overjet to allow uprighting permanent first molars.
- *Space maintenance* – placement of an LLHA and Nance holding arch would be beneficial for two reasons – it would prevent mesial drift of permanent first molars over ankylosed primary second molars and it would alleviate crowding via leeway space. However, we would not recommend placing space maintainers until RME was complete and the mandibular left first permanent molar was upright.
- *LLHA with bilateral posterior loops* – would provide space maintenance *and* prevent the tongue from interfering with tooth eruption. Again, we would wait until after RME to do this.
- *Opening the 30% overbite with a mandibular 2×4 fixed appliance* – is not recommended. No tissue damage or pain is resulting from this overbite which can be dealt with during comprehensive treatment.
- *Left ankylosed primary second molar extraction(s)* – is not recommend. Why? The roots of the second premolars are < half developed, so extraction of the primary second molars would slow premolar eruption as tissue healed over them. Also, eruption of second premolars is delayed by six months if ankylosed primary second molars are left in place – but normal eruption will eventually occur [84, 91, 156].
- *Extraction of other primary teeth* (e.g. *primary canines*) – is not recommended at this time. Why? Except for the left ankylosed primary second molar(s), Mara's tooth eruption appears normal.

  However, if Mara's mandibular right primary canine does not demonstrate significant mobility or exfoliate by recall, then it will be extracted. Why? Its root does not appear to be resorbing (Figure 5.88d). Also, if the mandibular right permanent canine erupts into crossbite with the maxillary right primary canine, then the maxillary right primary canine will be extracted.
- *Emphasis on improved oral hygiene* – is recommended and necessary.

Q: Based upon the above options, what is your recommended treatment? How would you proceed?

A: Oral hygiene was emphasized. Mara and her parents were informed that depending upon their etiology, posterior open bites can be difficult to close and to maintain closed. We decided to recall Mara in nine months and monitor tooth eruption.

Q: Mara returned eight months later. Clinical examination revealed that her mandibular right permanent canine was erupting lingual to the (nonmobile) mandibular right primary canine. Is there a clue on the initial panoramic radiograph that suggested this? How would you proceed?

A: Looking at Figure 5.88d, the mandibular right permanent canine image is significantly larger in mesiodistal dimension than the mandibular left permanent canine. This difference can be the result of the right canine being displaced to the lingual, causing its image to be enlarged in a panoramic radiograph. Remember, the x-ray source for a panoramic radiograph is behind the patient, so teeth displaced to the lingual (or palatal) often show image enlargement. At the time this radiograph was taken, palpation of the area may have confirmed a lingually displaced canine. This was not done.

Q: How would you deal with the lingually displaced mandibular right permanent canine?

A: The mandibular right primary canine was extracted. Four months later, Mara returned. A decision was made to extract her maxillary left primary canine (nonmobile compared to the maxillary right primary canine).

Q: A panoramic image was made at age eleven years and one month (Figure 5.90). What do you note? Can you suggest how you would now proceed?

A: Compared to her initial presentation at nine years of age (Figure 5.88d), all mandibular primary teeth exfoliated, mandibular right canine and first premolars erupted, and mandibular second premolars are erupting. The intraoral assessment suggested that adequate arch space existed for both mandibular second premolars to erupt.

The maxillary left primary canine had exfoliated, maxillary left premolar roots appeared to be half complete, and the maxillary right primary first molar exfoliated. The maxillary left permanent first molar was erupting to the mesial over the ankylosed maxillary left primary second molar. A decision was made to extract the maxillary left primary first molar in order to accelerate eruption of the maxillary left first premolar. We hoped that the maxillary second premolars would continue to erupt on their own.

Q: Mara was recalled at age twelve years and one month. Another panoramic radiograph was made (Figure 5.91). What do you note?

A: All permanent teeth erupted except for wisdom teeth and the maxillary left second premolar. Further resorption of the maxillary left second primary molar was minimally evident.

Q: How would you proceed?

A: A decision was made to extract the maxillary left primary second molar. A series of clear retainers were provided to prevent further mesial drift of Mara's maxillary left permanent molars, but the family dog kept eating them, and they were never worn.

Q: Three months later, progress records shown in Figure 5.92 were made. *Mara is now in her adult dentition and ready for comprehensive treatment.* A CR-CO shift could no longer be detected. Compile your

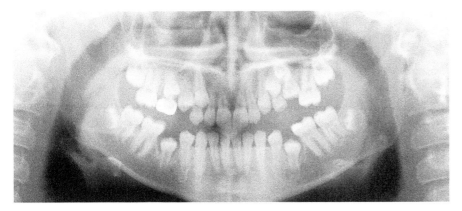

Figure 5.90 Progress panoramic image made at age eleven years and one month.

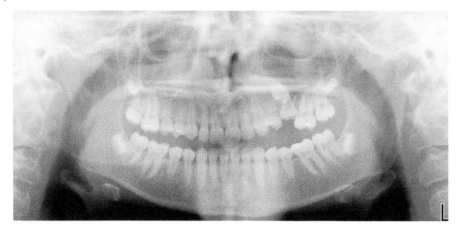

Figure 5.91 Progress panoramic image made at age twelve years and one month.

cephalometric findings. What changes do you note from the facial photographs, intraoral photographs, and model photographs?

A:

Table 5.28 Cephalometric findings for Mara.

Ceph Analysis	*Skeletal*
	Maxillary anteroposterior position slightly deficient (A-Point lies slightly behind a line drawn vertically from Nasion and perpendibular to Frankfort Horizontal)
	Mandibular anteroposterior position WRN
	Skeletal LAFH is WRN but tending toward short (ANS-Menton/Nasion-Menton × 100% = 53%; normal is 55% with 2% sd)
	Flat MPA (FMA = 20°; SNMP = 29°)
	Effective bony Pogonion (Pogonion lies ahead of extended Nasion-B Point line)
	Dental
	Upright maxillary incisors (U1 to SN = 90°)
	Mandibular incisor proclination WRN (FMIA = 64°; ideal FMIA = 65°)

Changes include the following:
- Mara has a straight profile
- More maxillary incisal display is observed in a posed smile (Figure 5.92b compared to 5.88b), but maxillary central incisor gingival margins are still apical to the maxillary lip border
- Right permanent canines are not in crossbite
- Right permanent first molar crossbite is still present (Figure 5.92p)
- Posterior transverse compensations are still present (Figures 5.92q and 5.92r) and now include buccal crown torque of maxillary permanent second molars

and lingual crown torque of the mandibular second molars
- Right premolars have erupted into occlusion (right posterior open bite is corrected)
- Midlines are nearly coincident (Figures 5.92g and 5.92l)
- Left permanent canines have erupted nearly into occlusion (Figure 5.92l)
- Left posterior open bite is still present
- Maxillary left permanent first molar has tipped/drifted mesially into a Class II relationship (2 mm) with the mandibular left permanent first molar
- Maxillary left first premolar has drifted distally
- Inadequate room exists for the erupting maxillary left second premolar – it is impacted (Figures 5.92i and 5.92n)
- Mandibular incisors are aligned (Figures 5.92j and 5.92o)
- Oral hygiene is still poor (Figures 5.92f–5.92h)

Q: What is your diagnosis?

A: Angle Class II division 2 subdivision left malocclusion, Iowa Classification: I I I II(2 mm), with left posterior open bite, impacted maxillary left second premolar, and right posterior lingual crossbite.

Q: We judged Mara's maxilla to be slightly deficient anteroposteriorly because A-Point is distal to where it should be ideally (A-Point should lie on a line drawn vertically down from Nasion and perpendicular to FH). What do you anticipate will happen to A-point during comprehensive orthodontic treatment?

A: We anticipate that A-point will move further to the distal as Mara's maxillary incisors are torqued to a proper inclination (and their apices move posteriorly). At that time, her maxilla will be judged to be even more deficient.

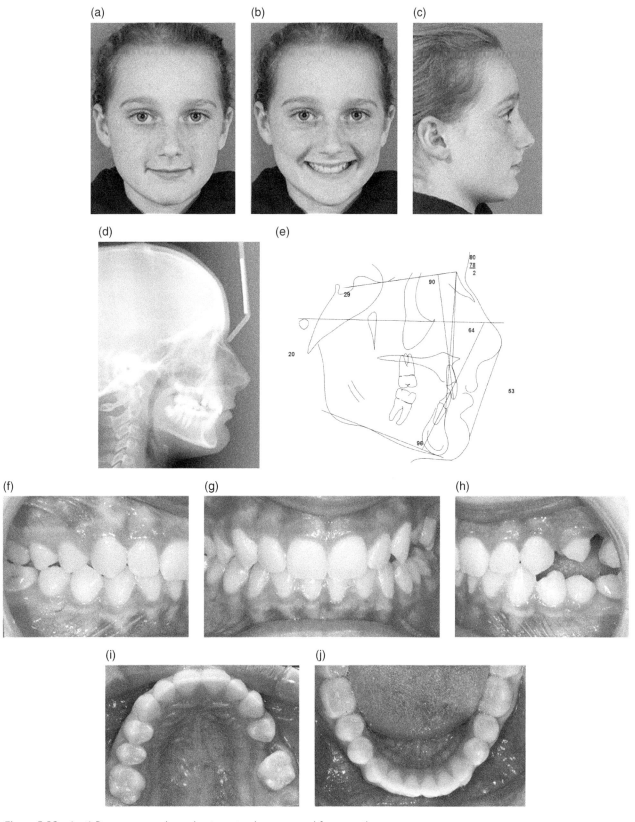

Figure 5.92 (a–t) Progress records made at age twelve years and four months.

(k)

(l)

(m)

(n)

(o)

(p)

(q)

(r)

(s)

(t)

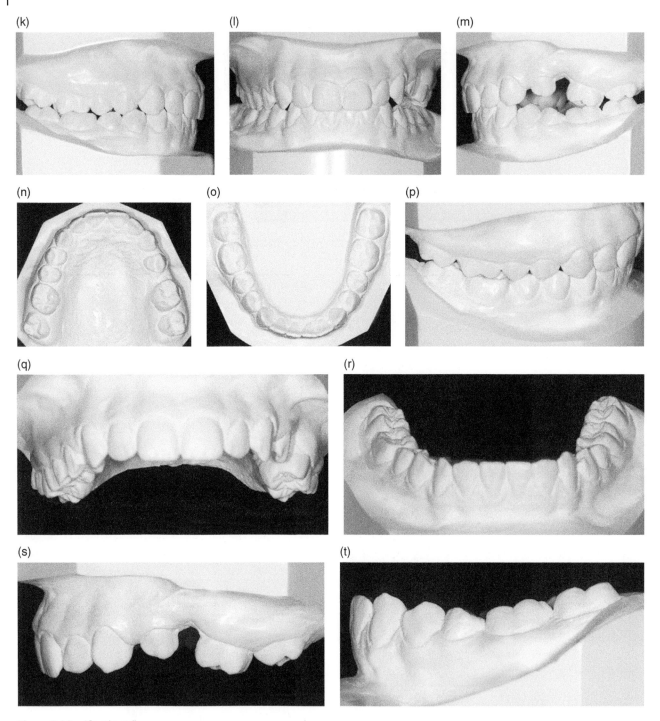

Figure 5.92 (Continued)

Q: Initially, a small *right* posterior open bite existed (Figures 5.88e and 5.88j) which has now closed following premolar eruption (Figure 5.88k). Does the fact that the right posterior open bite closed spontaneously provide you with any insight regarding its etiology?

A: Perhaps, but we cannot be sure. A potential resting tongue habit (interposition habit) was never addressed. So, either the habit never existed or the habit self-corrected on the right side. An alternate explanation, that the right primary molars were ankylosed at a later age will never be validated. We cannot be sure why the right posterior open bite closed spontaneously.

Q: Can you list two options for dealing with the impacted maxillary left second premolar?

A: Options include the following:

- *Extract it surgically* – then place fixed orthodontic appliances and attempt to protract the maxillary left molars forward to close the space. We do not recommend this option. Why? There is no indication that the maxillary left second premolar is ankylosed. It may erupt spontaneously if we create room for it. Further, the root of the maxillary left permanent first molar is tipped to the distal and will need to be moved to the mesial 10 mm in order to close the space – a movement that may result in maxillary left molar root resorption.

- *Open space for it (space regaining)*, using:
  1) A removable appliance with springs or screws trapped between the maxillary left first premolar and first permanent molar. The appliance should be designed to reciprocally push the maxillary left first permanent molar distally and the maxillary left first premolar mesially.
  2) Fixed appliances with archwires to level the maxillary arch – which will cause the distally tipped maxillary left first premolar to upright to the mesial and the mesially tipped maxillary left permanent first molar to upright to the distal (opening space between them).
  3) Fixed appliances with archwires and a compressed spring trapped between the maxillary left permanent first molar and maxillary left first premolar to reciprocally push them apart.
  4) Fixed appliances with a Class II corrector on the left (Forsus™, Class II elastics plus jig, etc.) to drive the maxillary left permanent first molar distally.
  5) Fixed appliances with TADs used as anchors on the maxillary left – to distalize the maxillary left permanent first molar.
  6) A headgear to move the maxillary left permanent first molar to the distal.

Q: You discuss the above options with members of your study group. One doctor says, "Headgear, why would you consider using headgear on this patient who has a *deficient* maxilla! You will ruin her profile." What is your response to his statement?

A: This is a question that we asked ourselves years ago. In answer, we conducted a study and found that in Class II growing patients with protrusive, normally positioned, or *retrusive maxillae* headgear treatment used in con-

junction with fixed orthodontic appliances is effective in *improving* facial profile esthetics. In fact, we found that the greater the initial ANB angle, the greater the profile esthetic improvement with treatment [157]. So, using a headgear on Mara to regain space for the maxillary left second premolar remains a viable alternative.

Q: Can you list options for dealing with Mara's right posterior crossbite?

A: Options include:

- *Leave it uncorrected* – we do not recommend this option. If Mara was an adult, then leaving the right crossbite could be considered and discussed – especially if a surgical procedure was required to correct it. However, she is a child, and we would want the crossbite corrected if she was our daughter.

- *Increase transverse dental compensations* (masking the skeletal discrepancy) by torquing the maxillary right first molar buccally and/or the mandibular right first molar lingually. This could be accomplished using:
  1) A maxillary removable appliance with springs or screws to push the permanent first molar buccally;
  2) An LLHA with the right molar band torqued lingually, or with the LLHA constricted (recall that constricting the LLHA will have a *bilateral* effect tending to also move the left molar lingually);
  3) Fixed orthodontic appliances with right crossbite elastics worn from the lingual of the maxillary right first permanent molar to the buccal of the mandibular right permanent first molar.
  4) An expanded TPA to move the maxillary right permanent first molar labially (recall that expanding a TPA will have a bilateral effect tending to also move the maxillary left first permanent molar labially);
  5) An expanded inner bow of a headgear frame to move the maxillary right permanent first molar labially (recall that expanding the inner bow of a headgear will have a bilateral effect tending to also move the maxillary left first permanent molar labially). This option could be considered if Mara was asked to wear a headgear for Class II correction.

Since Mara is in permanent dentition, and since the magnitude of her transverse discrepancy is not large, masking could be a viable option.

- *RME* – is a viable option. We spoke to Mara and her parents who stated that she had not reached puberty. So, we should be able to achieve midpalatal suture separation with RME. Maxillary skeletal expansion would not only allow correction of Mara's right permanent first molar lingual crossbite but would create posterior overjet for uprighting molars.

Q: How do you recommend proceeding?

A: Hygiene instructions were reinforced. These included asking Mara to stop drinking carbonated sodas. She was placed on an asymmetric (left) CPHG to distalize/upright her maxillary left permanent first molar. The inner bow of the headgear frame was expanded.

A progress panoramic radiograph was made at age thirteen years and four months (Figure 5.93a). Her maxillary left second premolar was erupting but lacked room to erupt completely (Figure 5.93b). The maxillary left permanent first molar still appeared to be tipped mesially.

Q: How do you recommend proceeding?

A: Fixed orthodontic appliances were placed in both arches. We planned to have Mara wear left crisscross elastics (buccal maxillary to lingual mandibular elastic plus buccal mandibular to lingual maxillary elastic) to block her tongue if the left open bite persisted. A compressed spring was inserted between the maxillary left permanent first molar and the first premolar in order to tip the maxillary left first permanent molar distally, tip the maxillary left first premolar mesially, and make space for the erupting maxillary left second premolar.

Mara continued to wear her asymmetric (left) CPHG. The maxillary left second premolar erupted and was bonded. Both arches were leveled and aligned with increasingly stiffer archwires, remaining spaces were closed, and detailing bends were placed in the archwires to finish her treatment.

Q: Can you explain how a left *asymmetric* headgear works to distalize Mara's maxillary left first permanent molar?

A: Look at Figure 5.94a. Note that the left side of the facebow outer bow has been bent away from the left cheek. The red arrows (Figure 5.94b) represent the force vectors resulting from the springs in the plastic force modules. These force vectors combine to create a resultant force (yellow vector, Figure 5.94c). Since this resultant force is closer to the maxillary left permanent first molar than the right molar (Figure 5.94d), the left first molar absorbs more of the force and should be retracted more than the right.

(a)

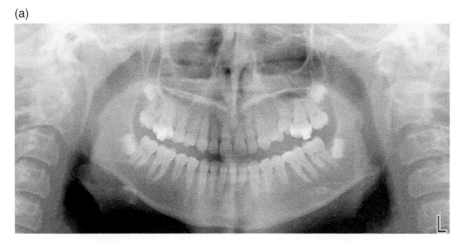

(b)

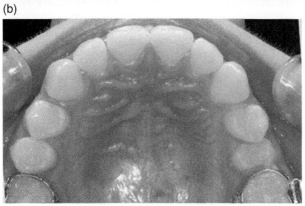

Figure 5.93 (a and b) Progress records of Mara at age thirteen years and four months during maxillary left *space regaining* and left Class II molar correction using an asymmetric left CPHG.

(a)

(b)

(c)

(d)

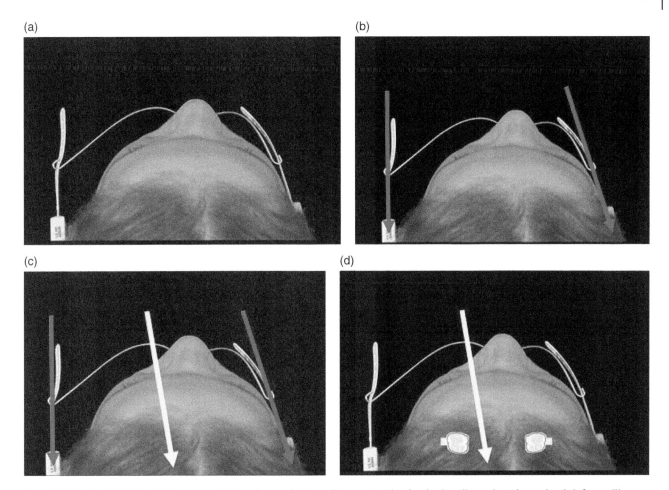

Figure 5.94 (a–d) Effect of left asymmetric headgear, which applies a retraction load primarily against the patient's left maxillary first molar.

Q: Mara was debanded at age fourteen years and nine months (Figure 5.95). The cephalometric superimposition (Figure 5.95f) illustrates changes from age twelve years and four months to deband (Figures 5.92e–5.95e). What changes do you note?

A: Changes include the following:
- Mara has grown into a beautiful young lady with an esthetic smile and nice occlusion.
- Noticeable buccal corridors are present in a posed smile (Figure 5.95b), and the border of her maxillary lip is not ideally positioned relative to her central incisor gingiva (ideally, the maxillary lip border and maxillary central incisor gingival margins are congruent).
- Her profile has not changed dramatically and is still straight. Her NLA is obtuse, and she has a moderately deep labiomental sulcus.
- Her maxilla is WRN (Figure 5.95e), but her ANB angle has decreased from 2° to −1°. Her skeletal LAFH increased to 54% and her MPA increased slightly as her mandible rotated down and back.

- Significant facial growth occurred (Figure 5.95f) during the two and a half years of headgear and fixed appliance treatment. Mara's nose, lips, and chin grew downward and forward. Her maxilla descended but (A-Point) did not grow forward (headgear effect). Her mandible underwent condylar/ramus growth (bottom right, mandibular superimposition), and B-Point descended and grew forward. Her maxillary molars erupted and tipped distally, her mandibular molars erupted, her maxillary incisors proclined, and her mandibular incisors erupted and proclined.
- Mara's mandibular left canine and mandibular first premolar roots (Figure 5.95g) are not parallel. The mandibular left first premolar is stepped up and has excessive lingual root torque.
- She exhibits bilateral Class I canines and molars, an upper dental midline (UDML) slightly to the right of the LDML, minimal overbite, incisal embrasures, and minimal overjet. A slight space is present between her maxillary left central incisor and lateral incisor (Figure 5.95k). Maxillary and mandibular

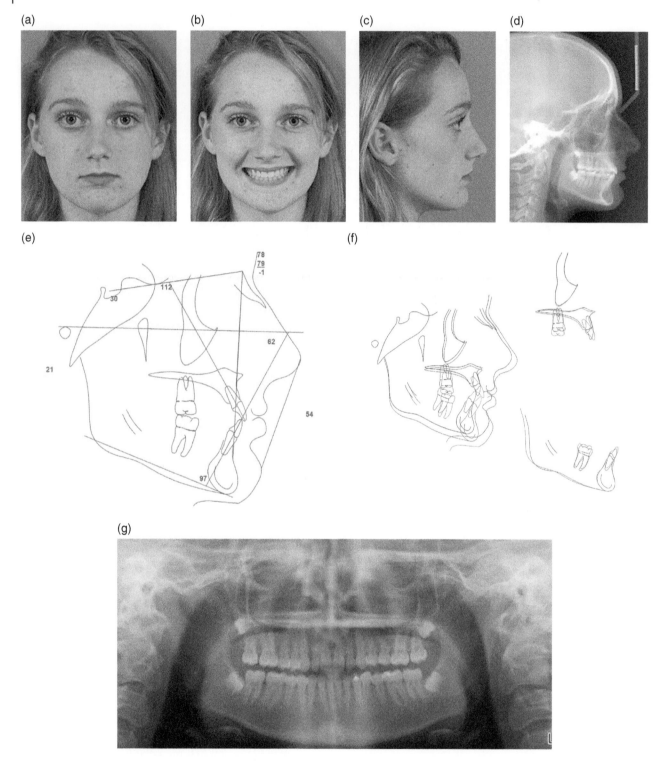

Figure 5.95 (a–u) Deband records of Mara. (f) lateral cephalometric superimposition between age twelve years and four months and fourteen years and nine months.

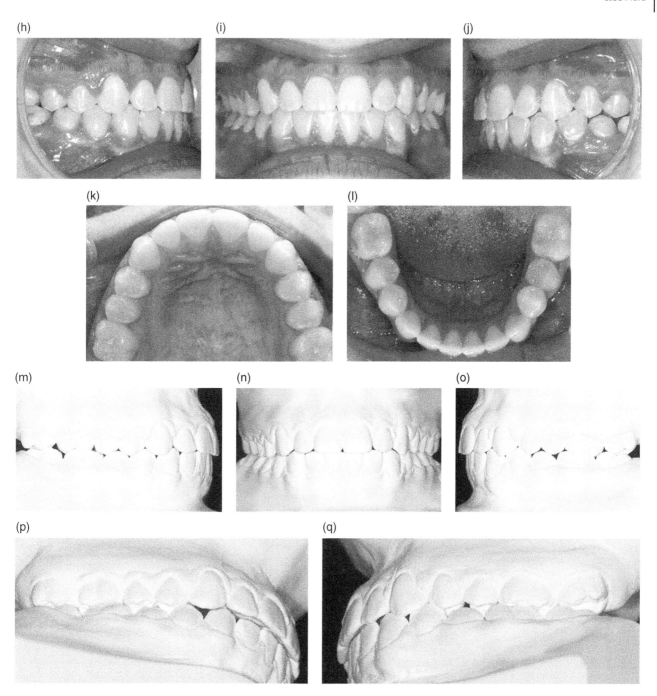

Figure 5.95 (Continued)

(r)   (s)

(t)   (u)

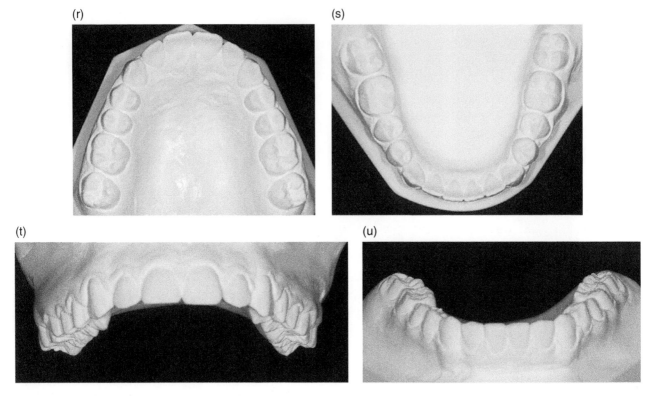

Figure 5.95 (Continued)

permanent first molar band space is noted (Figures 5.95r and 5.95s).

- Her right posterior crossbite has been corrected (Figure 5.95p).
- Neither the maxillary left second premolar nor the mandibular left second premolar is fully seated (Figure 5.95j, a mild left posterior open bite still exists).
- Maxillary second molar labial crown torque, and mandibular second molar lingual crown torque, is noted (Figure 5.95t and u).

Q: What were the skeletal and dental effects of Mara's CPHG wear (Figure 5.95f)?

A: The most dramatic skeletal effect was differential jaw growth. A-Point was restricted horizontally while B-Point (mandible) came downward and forward. Unexpectedly, the maxilla grew vertically in a parallel fashion without anterior palatal plane tipping normally seen from CPHG wear [14, 15, 101]. Maxillary molars erupted, but distal maxillary molar tipping resulted not only from CPHG wear but also from the compressed spring action.

Q: We observed that neither the maxillary left second premolar nor the mandibular left second premolar erupted completely (are not seated fully). However, could it be that *only* the maxillary left second premolar is not fully erupted?

A: No, neither left second premolar is fully erupted. Look at Figure 5.95j. If only the maxillary left second premolar was not fully erupted, then the mandibular left second premolar would be in contact with the maxillary left first premolar. Because both maxillary and mandibular left second premolars are not fully erupted, neither is making occlusal contact on the mesial or distal.

Q: Why are the left second premolars not in occlusion?

A: The most likely cause was poor orthodontic bracket vertical positioning. Errors in vertical positioning are the most common errors in orthodontic bracket placement. The left second premolar brackets were probably bonded too occlusally, resulting in less than full eruption during arch leveling. Also, the mandibular left first premolar was probably bonded too apically, resulting in overeruption of that tooth.

Q: What should have been done to finish Mara with both left second premolars seated in occlusion?

A: It is disappointing to find that she was debanded with a left posterior open bite present. Before debanding, either:

- Both left second premolars should have been re-bonded with *brackets positioned more apically* and the arches re-leveled or,
- Second-order bends (step-up bends) should have been placed in both maxillary and mandibular archwires to erupt both left second premolars into occlusion.

Q: Should Mara have been treated with RME?

A: Yes. Although her right crossbite was corrected without RME, this treatment outcome was less than ideal – second molar transverse compensations are still present (maxillary molar buccal crown torque and mandibular molar lingual crown torque, Figures 5.95t and 5.95u). With RME:

- Greater posterior overjet could have been created to allow molar uprighting,
- Mandibular molars could have been uprighted by wearing crossbite elastics between the buccal of the RME appliance and lingual mandibular molar buttons or by mandibular dental expansion with a Swartz mandibular expansion appliance,
- Buccal corridors could have been reduced.

Q: Should an LLHA and Nance holding arch have been placed in Mara? If yes, then when would you have placed them?

A: If we could treat Mara again, then we would place an LLHA and Nance holding arch immediately after RME and after her mandibular first permanent molars were uprighted. Placement of a Nance holding arch would have prevented mesial drift of the maxillary left permanent first molar over the ankylosed primary second molar. An LLHA with bilateral, tongue-blocking, loops may have stopped the tongue from preventing posterior tooth eruption (assuming there was a resting tongue habit).

Q: Mara ended treatment with proclined maxillary and mandibular incisors. How could her incisor proclination have been reduced, *without extracting permanent teeth*?

A: RME would have widened the maxillary arch and created a midline diastema. Closure of this midline diastema would collapse the maxillary anterior dental arch slightly and upright the maxillary incisors (reducing incisor proclination, Figure 5.96a). Placement of an LLHA (space maintenance) would have given us an estimated 4.2 mm of mandibular space following premolar eruption. Closure of this space would collapse the mandibular arch slightly and upright the mandibular incisors (Figure 5.96b).

Q: What do you predict will happen to Mara's left second premolars? Will they erupt into occlusion or not?

A: There is never a guarantee of any outcome. However, Mara returned to our clinic eight years later (Figure 5.97), she had failed to wear her retainers as prescribed, and we noted that the left premolars were fully seated. Her occlusion looked good which is surprising considering her poor retention compliance. We can only assume that her tongue-interposition habit was corrected.

Q: Was early treatment warranted?

A: *Early* treatment consisted of mandibular right primary canine extraction (to aid eruption/alignment of the mandibular right permanent canine), maxillary left primary canine extraction (to aid the eruption of her

(a)

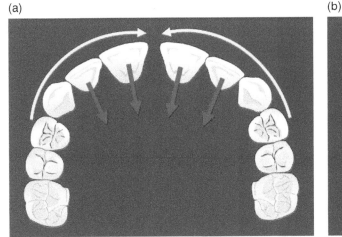

(b)

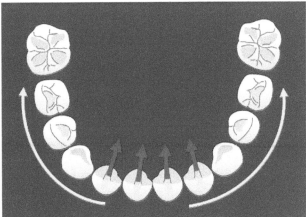

Figure 5.96 Maxillary midline diastema closure following RME (a, yellow arrows) and mandibular space closure after removal of an LLHA (b, yellow arrows) can upright incisors (red arrows).

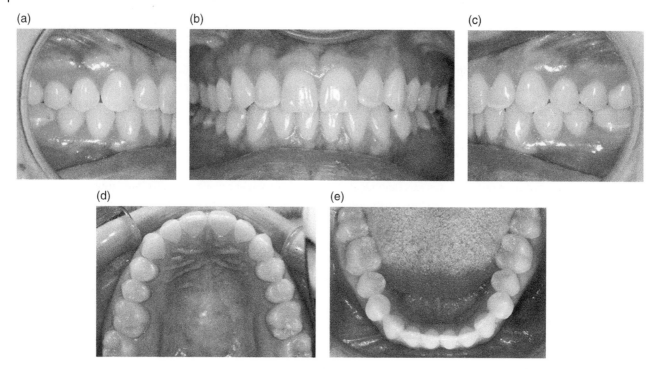

Figure 5.97   (a–e) Intraoral photos of Mara eight years later.

maxillary left permanent canine), maxillary left primary first molar extraction (to aid the eruption of her maxillary left first premolar), and extraction of the maxillary left second primary molar.

Extraction of teeth is a surgical procedure and never to be taken lightly, but this early treatment was limited and warranted. Additional early treatment (RME followed by placement of a Nance holding arch and placement of an LLHA with loops) would have been beneficial but was not performed.

Q: Can you suggest "take-home pearls" regarding Mara's treatment?

A: "Take-home pearls" include the following:
- Mara was nine years old when she presented with a right posterior crossbite and bilateral posterior open bites. She exhibited a Class I molar relationship, ankylosed maxillary left primary second molar, and mandibular left primary second molar that was probably ankylosed. Early treatment consisted of the primary teeth extractions to aid in permanent tooth eruption and alignment.

As Mara's maxillary left first permanent molar erupted, it tipped mesially over the ankylosed primary second molar into a Class II relationship, impacting the maxillary left second premolar. Comprehensive orthodontic treatment consisted of left asymmetric CPHG

wear to upright/distalize her maxillary left permanent first molar (space regaining) followed by bonding with fixed orthodontic appliances and leveling/aligning arches. A compressed open coil spring helped distalize her maxillary left first permanent molar and create space for the impacted premolar.
- Closure of posterior open bites, and maintenance of closure of posterior open bites, can be one of the most difficult problems encountered by an orthodontist. Inform your patient that you may not be able to close it, or keep it closed. Tell them to expect relapse and the possible need for retreatment in the future.
- Mara's left posterior open bite resulted from ankylosis of her maxillary left primary second molar (and probable ankylosis of her mandibular left primary second molar), a resting tongue habit, and possibly ankylosed right primary molars. Other causes of posterior open bites include digit-sucking habits, incomplete permanent tooth eruption during the transition from primary to permanent dentitions, lack of space for complete tooth eruption (teeth blocked out), PFE, and Class III growth resulting in an edge-to-edge incisor relationship.
- Treatment of posterior open bites consists of dealing with the etiology and erupting posterior teeth into occlusion.

If a tongue habit caused the open bite, then the habit may be eliminated using a tooth positioner or LLHA with soldered loops. In the permanent dentition, you can use fixed orthodontic appliances to level the arch and posterior vertical elastics (e.g. crisscross elastics) to block a tongue habit and erupt teeth.

For ankylosed primary molars with permanent successors, the open bite may close spontaneously with (delayed) premolar eruption. For ankylosed primary molars lacking permanent successors, or for ankylosed permanent teeth, treatment options include extraction, surgery (segmental maxillary downgraft osteotomy), and prosthodontics (buildups, crowns, implant replacement with elongated crowns, or overlay RPDs).

- Mara's mild right posterior open bite corrected spontaneously during premolar eruption. Her larger left posterior open bite corrected through a combination of:
  1) Space regaining/creation for the maxillary left second premolar
  2) Premolar eruption
  3) Posterior tooth eruption during arch leveling with fixed appliances.

Because the maxillary and mandibular left second premolar brackets were bonded too occlusally, and the mandibular left first premolar was bonded too apically, a mild left posterior open bite still existed at deband.

- Treatment for her tongue interposition habit (resting tongue habit) was never instituted, and we were fortunate that her left posterior open bite finally closed. Did we correct the tongue-interposition habit during comprehensive treatment via arch leveling (blocking her tongue)? We will never know. Our fallback plan was to have Mara wear crisscross (vertical) elastics during comprehensive treatment to aid in the open bite closure.

- Small posterior open bites (like the open bite Mara exhibited on her right side), occasionally develop during the transition from primary molars to premolar occlusion (Figure 5.98). We have discussed this phenomenon amongst ourselves, other orthodontists, and pediatric dentists. We speculate that these small posterior open bites result from continued eruption of the permanent first molars as the primary molar roots undergo resorption (interruption of their eruption mechanism); intrinsically faster permanent first molar eruption than primary molar eruption; transient resting tongue habits; or late primary molar ankylosis. As occurred with Mara, these small posterior open bites usually resolve as the premolars erupt.

- Mara exhibited a transverse *skeletal* discrepancy (relatively narrow maxilla compared to her mandible). If uprighting permanent molars creates, or worsens, a posterior crossbite (worsens a transverse relationship), then a transverse *skeletal* discrepancy generally exists. If uprighting permanent molars improves a crossbite, then a *dental* crossbite generally exists (i.e. the skeletal bases relate well).

- Mara's retention compliance has been poor. Only lifelong (nightly) retainer wear, or fixed retention, can assure continued ideal arch alignment.

- Mara had a nice outcome. However, we should have placed an LLHA and Nance holding arch immediately after RME and after her mandibular first permanent molars were uprighted. Placement of a Nance holding arch would have prevented mesial drift of the maxillary left permanent first molar over the ankylosed primary second molar. An LLHA with bilateral, tongue-blocking, loops may have stopped the tongue from inhibiting posterior tooth eruption.

(a)

(b)

(c)

(d)

(e)

(f)

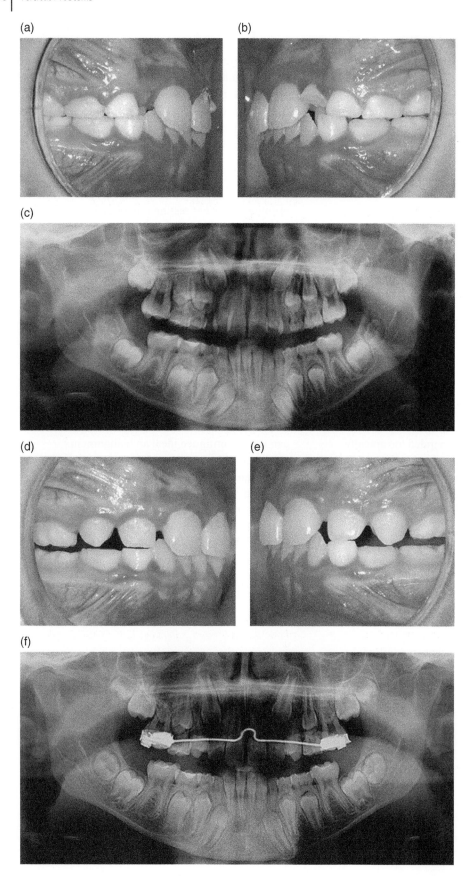

Figure 5.98 Spontaneous development of small posterior open bites during the transition from primary molars to premolar occlusion: (a–c) initial images with primary molars in occlusion; (d–f) one and a half years later.

References

1 Marshall, S.D., Caspersen, M., Hardinger, R.R. et al. (2008 Sep). Development of the curve of Spee. *Am. J. Orthod. Dentofac. Orthop.* 134 (3): 344–352.

2 Wylie, W.L. and Johnson, E.L. (1952 Jul). Rapid evaluation of facial dysplasia in the vertical plane. *Angle Orthod.* 22 (3): 165–182.

3 Schudy, F.F. (1965 Jan). The rotation of the mandible resulting from growth: its implications in orthodontic treatment. *Angle Orthod.* 35 (1): 36–50.

4 Schudy, F.F. (1968 Jan). The control of vertical overbite in clinical orthodontics. *Angle Orthod.* 38 (1): 19–39.

5 Björk, A. and Skieller, V. (1972 Oct). Facial development and tooth eruption. An implant study at the age of puberty. *Am. J. Orthod.* 62 (4): 339–383.

6 Nemeth, R.B. and Isaacson, R.J. (1974 Jun). Vertical anterior relapse. *Am. J. Orthod.* 65 (6): 565–585.

7 Björk, A. and Skieller, V. (1983 Feb). Normal and abnormal growth of the mandible. A synthesis of longitudinal cephalometric implant studies over a period of 25 years. *Eur. J. Orthod.* 5 (1): 1–46.

8 Björk, A. and Skieller, V. (1984 Dec). Contrasting mandibular growth and facial development in the long face syndrome, juvenile rheumatoid arthritis and mandibulofacial dysostosis. *J. Craniofac. Genet. Dev. Biol.* Suppl.1: 127–138.

9 Proffit, W.R. (2007). Later stages of development. In: *Contemporary Orthodontics*, 4e (ed. W.R. Proffit, H.W. Fields and D.M. Sarver), 107–129. St. Louis: Mosby.

10 Buschang, P.H. and Jacob, H.B. (2014 Dec). Mandibular rotation revisited: what makes it so important? *Semin. Orthod.* 20 (4): 299–315.

11 Vig, R.G. and Brundo, G.C. (1978 May). The kinetics of anterior tooth display. *J. Prosthet. Dent.* 39 (5): 502–504.

12 Zankl, A., Eberle, L., Molinari, L., and Schinzel, A. (2002 Sep 1). Growth charts for nose length, nasal protrusion, and philtrum length from birth to 97 years. *Am. J. Med. Genet.* 111 (4): 388–391.

13 Fundalej, P. (2008 Feb). Long-term changes of the upper lip position relative to the incisal edge. *Am. J. Orthod. Dentofac. Orthop.* 133 (2): 204–209.

14 Baumrind, S., Korn, E.L., Isaacson, R.J. et al. (1983 Nov). Quantitative analysis of the orthodontic and orthopedic effects of maxillary traction. *Am. J. Orthod.* 84 (5): 384–398.

15 Kirjavainen, M., Kirjavainen, T., Hurmerinta, K., and Haavikko, K. (2000 Aug). Orthopedic cervical headgear with an expanded inner bow in class II correction. *Angle Orthod.* 70 (4): 317–325.

16 Southard, T.E., Marshall, S.D., Allareddy, V. et al. (2013 Sep). An evidence-based comparison of headgear and functional appliance therapy for the correction of Class II malocclusions. *Semin. Orthod.* 19 (3): 174–195.

17 Dolce, C., McGorray, S.P., Brazeau, L. et al. (2007 Oct). Timing of Class II treatment: skeletal changes comparing 1-phase and 2- phase treatment. *Am. J. Orthod. Dentofac. Orthop.* 132 (4): 481–489.

18 Almeida-Pedrin, R.R., Almeida, M.R., Almeida, R.R. et al. (2007 Aug). Treatment effects of headgear biteplane and bionator appliances. *Am. J. Orthod. Dentofac. Orthop.* 132 (2): 191–198.

19 Ghafari, J., Shofer, F.S., Jacobsson-Hunt, U. et al. (1998 Jan). Headgear versus function regulator in the early treatment of Class II, division 1 malocclusion: a randomized clinical trial. *Am. J. Orthod. Dentofac. Orthop.* 113 (1): 51–61.

20 Jakobsson, S.O. (1967 Jun). Cephalometric evaluation of treatment effect on Class II, Division 1 malocclusions. *Am. J. Orthod.* 53 (6): 446–457.

21 Rogers, K., Campbell, P.M., Tadlock, L. et al. (2018 Jan). Treatment changes of hypo- and hyperdivergent Class II Herbst patients. *Angle Orthod.* 88 (1): 3–9.

22 Bernstein, R.L., Preston, C.B., and Lampasso, J. (2007 Mar). Leveling the curve of Spee with a continuous archwire technique: a long term cephalometric study. *Am. J. Orthod. Dentofac. Orthop.* 131 (3): 363–371.

23 Rozzi, M., Mucedero, M., Pezzuto, C., and Cozza, P. (2017 Apr). Leveling the curve of Spee in continuous archwire appliances in different vertical skeletal patterns: a retrospective study. *Am. J. Orthod. Dentofac. Orthop.* 151 (4): 758–766.

24 Demisch, A., Ingervall, U., and Thüer, U. (1992 Dec). Mandibular displacement in Angle Class II, division 2 malocclusion. *Am. J. Orthod. Dentofac. Orthop.* 102 (6): 509–518.

25 Southard, T.E., Bonner, L.L., and Marshall, S.D. (2015). *Orthodontics in the Vertical Dimension: A Case-Based Review*, 197. Hoboken, NJ: Wiley Blackwell.

26 Fridrich, K.L. and Casko, J.S. (1997). Genioplasty strategies for anterior facial vertical dysplasias. *Int. J. Adult Orthod. Orthognath. Surg.* 12 (1): 35–41.

27 Buschang, P.H., Jacob, H., and Carrillo, R. (2013 Dec). The morphologic characteristics, growth, and etiology of the hyperdivergent phenotype. *Semin. Orthod.* 19 (4): 212–226.

28 Davidovich, Z. and Shanfield, J.L. (1975 Sep). Cyclic AMP levels in alveolar bone of orthodontically-treated cats. *Arch. Oral Biol.* 20 (9): 567–574.

29 Davidovich, Z., Montgomery, P.C., Eckerdal, O., and Gustafson, G.T. (1976 Mar). Demonstration of AMP in bone cells by immuno-histochemical methods. *Calcif. Tissue Res.* 19 (4): 305–315.

30 Proffit, W.R. and Mason, R.M. (1975 Feb). Myofunctional therapy for tongue-thrusting: background and recommendations. *J. Am. Dent. Assoc.* 90 (2): 403–411.

31 Smithpeter, J. and Covell, D. Jr. (2010 May). Relapse of anterior open bites treated with orthodontic appliances with and without orofacial myofunctional therapy. *Am. J. Orthod. Dentofac. Orthop.* 137 (5): 605–614.

32 Turpin, D.L. (2010 Jan). Editor's choice. *Am. J. Orthod. Dentofac. Orthop.* 137 (1): 11A.

33 Worms, F.W., Meskin, L.H., and Isaacson, R.J. (1971 Jun). Open-bite. *Am. J. Orthod.* 59 (6): 589–595.

34 Pithon, M.M., Magno, M.B., da Silva Coqueiro, R. et al. (2019 Sep). Oral health-related quality of life of children before, during, and after anterior open bite correction: a single-blinded randomized controlled trial. *Am. J. Orthod. Dentofac. Orthop.* 156 (3): 303–311.

35 Firouz, M., Zernik, J., and Nanda, R. (1992 Sep). Dental and orthopedic effects of high-pull headgear in treatment of Class II, Division 1 malocclusion. *Am. J. Orthod. Dentofac. Orthop.* 102 (3): 197–205.

36 Pearson, L.E. (1978 Apr). Vertical control in treatment of patients having backward-rotational growth tendencies. *Angle Orthod.* 48 (2): 132–140.

37 Pearson, L.E. (1986 Jul). Vertical control in fully-banded orthodontic treatment. *Angle Orthod.* 56 (3): 205–224.

38 Wendell, P.D., Nanda, R., Sakamoto, T., and Nakamura, S. (1985 Apr). The effects of chin cup therapy on the mandible: a longitudinal study. *Am. J. Orthod.* 87 (4): 265–274.

39 Deguchi, T. and McNamara, J. (1999 Feb). Craniofacial adaptations induced by chincup therapy in Class III patients. *Am. J. Orthod. Dentofac. Orthop.* 115 (2): 175–182.

40 Dellinger, E.L. (1986 May). A clinical assessment of the Active Vertical Corrector – a nonsurgical alternative for skeletal open bite treatment. *Am. J. Orthod.* 89 (5): 428–436.

41 Barbre, R.E. and Sinclair, P.M. (1991 Summer). A cephalometric evaluation of anterior openbite correction with the magnetic active vertical corrector. *Angle Orthod.* 61 (2): 93–102.

42 Kiliaridis, S., Egermark, I., and Thilander, B. (1990 Nov). Anterior open bite treatment with magnets. *Eur. J. Orthod.* 12 (4): 447–457.

43 Kuster, R. and Ingervall, B. (1992 Dec). The effect of treatment of skeletal open bite with two types of bite-blocks. *Eur. J. Orthod.* 14 (6): 489–499.

44 DeBerardinis, M., Stretesky, T., Sinha, P., and Nanda, R.S. (2000 Jun). Evaluation of the vertical holding appliance in treatment of high-angle patients. *Am. J. Orthod. Dentofac. Orthop.* 117 (6): 700–705.

45 Villalobos, F.J., Sinha, P.K., and Nanda, R.S. (2000 Oct). Longitudinal assessment of vertical and sagittal control in the mandibular arch by the mandibular fixed lingual arch. *Am. J. Orthod. Dentofac. Orthop.* 118 (4): 366–370.

46 Umemori, M., Sugawara, J., Mitani, H. et al. (1999 Feb). Skeletal anchorage system for open-bite correction. *Am. J. Orthod. Dentofac. Orthop.* 115 (2): 166–174.

47 Sherwood, K.H., Burch, J.G., and Thompson, W.J. (2002 Dec). Closing anterior open bites by intruding molars with titanium miniplate anchorage. *Am. J. Orthod. Dentofac. Orthop.* 122 (6): 593–600.

48 Kuroda, S., Katayama, A., and Takano-Yamamoto, T. (2004 Aug). Severe anterior open-bite case treated using titanium screw anchorage. *Angle Orthod.* 74 (4): 558–567.

49 Kuroda, S., Sakai, Y., Tamamura, N. et al. (2007 Nov). Treatment of severe anterior open bite with skeletal anchorage in adults: comparison with orthognathic surgery outcomes. *Am. J. Orthod. Dentofac. Orthop.* 132 (5): 599–605.

50 Southard, T.E., Franciscus, R.G., Fridrich, K.L. et al. (2006 Aug). Restricting facial bone growth with skeletal fixation: a preliminary study. *Am. J. Orthod. Dentofac. Orthop.* 130 (2): 218–223.

51 Lee, H. and Park, Y. (2008 Feb). Treatment and posttreatment changes following intrusion of maxillary posterior teeth with miniscrew implants for open bite correction. *Korean J Orthod.* 38 (1): 31–40.

52 Sugawara, J., Baik, U.B., Umemori, M. et al. (2002). Treatment and posttreatment dentoalveolar changes following intrusion of mandibular molars with application of a skeletal anchorage system (SAS) for open bite correction. *Int. J. Adult Orthodon. Orthognath. Surg.* 17 (4): 243–253.

53 Ingervall, B. and Bitsanis, E. (1987 Feb). A pilot study of the effect of masticatory muscle training on facial growth in long-face children. *Eur. J. Orthod.* 9 (1): 15–23.

54 English, J.D. (2002 Jun). Early treatment of skeletal open bite malocclusions. *Am. J. Orthod. Dentofac. Orthop.* 121 (6): 563–565.

55 Aliaga-Del Castillo, A., Vilanova, L., Miranda, F. et al. (2021 Jan). Dentoskeletal changes in open bite treatment using spurs and posterior build-ups: a randomized clinical trial. *Am. J. Orthod. Dentofac. Orthop.* 159 (1): 10–20.

56 Tanner, J.M. (1962). *Growth at Adolescence*, 2e. Oxford: Blackwell Scientific Publications.

57 Bluestone, C. (1992 Jan). Current indications for tonsillectomy and adenoidectomy. *Ann. Otol. Rhinol. Laryngol.* 155 (Suppl): 58–64.

58 Gwynne-Evans, E. (1958 Apr). Discussion on the mouth-breather. *Proc. R. Soc. Med.* 51 (4): 279–282.

59 Hartgerink, D.V. and Vig, P.S. (1989 Spring). Lower anterior face height and lip incompetence do not predict nasal airway obstruction. *Angle Orthod.* 59 (1): 17–23.

60 Trask, G.M., Shapiro, G.G., and Shapiro, P.A. (1987). The effects of perennial allergic rhinitis on dental and skeletal development; a of sibling pairs. *Am. J. Orthod. Dentofacial Orthop.* 92 (4): 286–293.

61 Vig, P.S. and Hall, D.J. (1980 Feb). The inadequacy of cephalometric radiographs for airway assessment. *Am. J. Orthod.* 77 (2): 230–233.

62 Schwab, R.J. (1998 Mar). Upper airway imaging. *Clin. Chest Med.* 19 (1): 33–54.

63 Linder-Aronson, S. (1979 Apr). Respiratory function in relation to facial morphology and the dentition. *Br. J. Orthod.* 6 (2): 59–71.

64 McNamara, J.A. (1981 Oct). Influence of respiratory pattern on craniofacial growth. *Angle Orthod.* 51 (4): 269–300.

65 Fields, H.W., Warren, D.W., Black, K., and Phillips, C.L. (1991 Feb). Relationship between vertical dentofacial morphology and respiration in adolescents. *Am. J. Orthod. Dentofac. Orthop.* 99 (2): 147–154.

66 Katyal, V., Pamula, Y., Martin, A.J. et al. (2013 Jan). Craniofacial and upper airway morphology in pediatric sleep-disordered breathing: systematic review and meta-analysis. *Am. J. Orthod. Dentofac. Orthop.* 143 (1): 20–30.

67 Pliska, B.T., Lee, J., and Chadha, N.K. (2017). Prevalence of malocclusion in children with sleep-disordered breathing. *J. Dent. Sleep Med.* 4 (2): 41–44.

68 Souki, B.Q., Pimenta, G.B., Souki, M.Q. et al. (2009 May). Prevalence of malocclusion among mouth breathing children: do expectations meet reality? *Int. J. Pediatr. Otorhinolaryngol.* 73 (5): 767–773.

69 Franco, L.P., Souki, B.Q., Pereira, T.B. et al. (2013 Sep). Is the growth pattern in mouth breathers comparable with the counterclockwise mandibular rotation of nasal breathers? *Am. J. Orthod. Dentofac. Orthop.* 144 (3): 341–348.

70 Petraccone Caixeta, A.C., Andrade, I. Jr., Bahia Junqueira Pereira, T. et al. (2014 Apr). Dental arch dimensional changes after adenotonsillectomy in prepubertal children. *Am. J. Orthod. Dentofac. Orthop.* 145 (4): 461–468.

71 Miles, P.G., Vig, P.S., Weyant, R.J. et al. (1996 Feb). Craniofacial structure and obstructive sleep apnea syndrome – a qualitative analysis and meta-analysis of the literature. *Am. J. Orthod. Dentofac. Orthop.* 109 (2): 163–172.

72 Mahony, D., Karsten, A., and Linder-Aronson, S. (2004 Nov). Effects of adenoidectomy and changed mode of breathing on incisor and molar dentoalveolar heights and anterior face heights. *Aust Orthod J.* 20 (2): 93–98.

73 Proffit, W.R. and Tulloch, J.F. (2002 Jun). Preadolescent Class II problems: treat now or wait? *Am. J. Orthod. Dentofac. Orthop.* 121 (6): 560–562.

74 Tulloch, J.F., Proffit, W.R., and Phillips, C. (2004 Jun). Outcomes in a 2-phase randomized clinical trial of early Class II treatment. *Am. J. Orthod. Dentofac. Orthop.* 125 (6): 657–667.

75 Keeling, S.D., Wheeler, T.T., King, G.J. et al. (1998 Jan). Anteroposterior skeletal and dental changes after early Class II treatment with bionators and headgear. *Am. J. Orthod. Dentofac. Orthop.* 113 (1): 40–50.

76 O'Brien, K. (2006 Apr). Is early treatment for Class II malocclusions effective? Results of a randomized controlled trial. *Am. J. Orthod. Dentofac. Orthop.* 129 (4 Suppl): S64–S65.

77 O'Brien, K., Wright, J., Conboy, F. et al. (2009 May). Early treatment for Class II Division 1 malocclusion with the Twin-block appliance: a multi-center, randomized, controlled trial. *Am. J. Orthod. Dentofac. Orthop.* 135 (5): 573–579.

78 Perez, C.V., de Leeuw, R., Okeson, J.P. et al. (2013 Mar). The incidence and prevalence of temporomandibular disorders and posterior open bite in patients receiving mandibular advancement device therapy for obstructive sleep apnea. *Sleep Breath.* 17 (1): 323–332.

79 Proffit, W.R. and Vig, K.W. (1981 Aug). Primary failure of eruption: a possible cause of posterior open-bite. *Am. J. Orthod.* 80 (2): 173–190.

80 Stellzig-Eisenhauer, A., Decker, E., Meyer-Marcotty, P. et al. (2010 Jan). Primary failure of eruption (PFE) – clinical and molecular genetics analysis. *J. Orofac. Orthop.* 71 (1): 6–16.

81 Ahmad, S., Bister, D., and Cobourne, M.T. (2006 Dec). The clinical features and aetiological basis of primary eruption failure. *Eur. J. Orthod.* 28 (6): 535–540.

82 Rhoads, S.G., Hendricks, H.M., and Frazier-Bowers, S.A. (2013 Aug). Establishing the diagnostic criteria for eruption disorders based on genetic and clinical data. *Am. J. Orthod. Dentofac. Orthop.* 144 (2): 194–202.

83 Frazier-Bowers, S.A., Koehler, K.E., Ackerman, J.L., and Proffit, W.R. (2007 May). Primary failure of eruption: further characterization of a rare eruption disorder. *Am. J. Orthod. Dentofac. Orthop.* 131 (5): 578. e1–578.e11.

84 Kurol, J. (2006 Apr). Impacted and ankylosed teeth: why, when, and how to intervene. *Am. J. Orthod. Dentofac. Orthop.* 129 (4 Suppl): S86–S90.

85 Ostler, M.S. and Kokich, V.G. (1994 Feb). Alveolar ridge changes in patients congenitally missing mandibular second premolars. *J. Prosthet. Dent.* 71 (2): 144–149.

86 Yatani, H., Watanabe, E.K., Kaneshima, T. et al. (1998 Nov). Etched-porcelain resin bonded onlay technique for posterior teeth. *J. Esthet. Dent.* 10 (6): 325–332.

87 Piattelli, A. and Eleuterio, A. (1991 Sep). Primary failure of eruption. *Acta Stomatol. Belg.* 88 (3): 127–130.

88 Kater, W.M., Kawa, D., Schäfer, D., and Toll, D. (2004 Sep). Treatment of posterior open bite using distraction osteogenesis. *J Clin Orthod.* 38 (9): 501–504. quiz 487-8.

89 Kurol, J. (2002 Jun). Early treatment of tooth-eruption disturbances. *Am. J. Orthod. Dentofac. Orthop.* 121 (6): 588–591.

90 Kurol, J. and Koch, G. (1985 Jan). The effect of extraction of infraoccluded deciduous molars: a longitudinal study. *Am. J. Orthod.* 87 (1): 46–55.

91 Kurol, J. and Thilander, B. (1984 Nov). Infraocclusion of primary molars and the effect on occlusal development, a longitudinal study. *Eur. J. Orthod.* 6 (4): 277–293.

92 Sforza, C., Grandi, G., De Menezes, M. et al. (2011 Jan 30). Age- and sex-related changes in the normal human external nose. *Forensic Sci. Int.* 204 (1-3): 205. e1–205.e9.

93 Bergman, R.T., Waschak, J., Borzabadi-Farahani, A., and Murphy, N.C. (2014). Longitudinal study of cephalometric soft tissue profile traits between the ages of 6 and 18 years. *Angle Orthod.* 84 (1): 48–55.

94 Wheeler, R.C. (1974). *Dental Anatomy, Physiology, and Occlusion*, 5ᵗe. Philadelphia: W.B. Saunders.

95 Moore, T., Southard, K.A., Casko, J.S. et al. (2005 Feb). Buccal corridors and smile esthetics. *Am. J. Orthod. Dentofac. Orthop.* 127 (2): 208–213. quiz 261.

96 Mirko, P., Miroslav, S., and Lubor, M. (1974 Dec). Significance of the labial frenum attachment in periodontal disease in man. Part 1. Classification and epidemiology of the labial frenum attachment. *J. Periodontol.* 45 (12): 891–894.

97 Suter, V.G., Heinzmann, A.E., Grossen, J. et al. (2014 Jan). Does the maxillary diastema close after frenectomy? *Quintessence Int.* 45 (1): 57–66.

98 Díaz-Pizán, M.E., Lagravère, M.O., and Villena, R. (2006 Jan-Apr). Midline diastema and frenum morphology in the primary dentition. *J. Dent. Child (Chic).* 73 (1): 11–14.

99 Ferguson, M.W. and Rix, C. (1983 Apr 9). Pathogenesis of abnormal midline spacing of human central incisors. A histological study of the involvement of the labial frenum. *Br. Dent. J.* 154 (7): 212–218.

100 Delli, K., Livas, C., Sculean, A. et al. (2013 Feb). Facts and myths regarding the maxillary midline frenum and its treatment: a systematic review of the literature. *Quintessence Int.* 44 (2): 177–187.

101 Elder, J.R. and Tuenge, R.H. (1974 Dec). Cephalometric and histologic changes produced by extraoral high-pull traction to the maxilla in Macaca mulatta. *Am. J. Orthod.* 66 (6): 599–617.

102 Pancherz, H. (1997 Dec). The effects, limitations, and long-term dentofacial adaptations to treatment with the Herbst appliance. *Semin. Orthod.* 3 (4): 232–243.

103 Le Cornu, M., Cevidanes, L.H.S., Zhu, H. et al. (2013 Dec). Three-dimensional treatment outcomes in Class II patients treated with the Herbst appliance: a pilot study. *Am. J. Orthod. Dentofac. Orthop.* 144 (6): 818–830.

104 Huang, G.J. (2005 Sep 1). Ask Us – functional appliances and long-term effects on mandibular growth. *Am. J. Orthod. Dentofac. Orthop.* 128 (3): 271–272.

105 Pancherz, H., Ruf, S., and Kohlhas, P. (1998 Oct). "Effective condylar growth" and chin position changes in Herbst treatment: a cephalometric roentgenographic long-term study. *Am. J. Orthod. Dentofac. Orthop.* 114 (4): 437–446.

106 Araujo, A.M., Buschang, P.H., and Melo, A.C.M. (2004 Oct). Adaptive condylar growth and mandibular remodeling changes with bionator therapy – an implant study. *Eur. J. Orthod.* 26 (5): 515–522.

107 Mellion, Z.J., Behrents, R.G., and Johnston, L.E. Jr. (2013 Jun). The pattern of facial skeletal growth and its relationship to various common indexes of maturation. *Am. J. Orthod. Dentofac. Orthop.* 143 (6): 845–854.

108 Buschang, P.H., Roldan, S.I., and Tadlock, L.P. (2017 Dec). Guidelines for assessing the growth and development of orthodontic patients. *Semin. Orthod.* 23 (4): 321–335.

109 Rebellato, J., Lindauer, S., Rubenstein, L.K. et al. (1997 Oct). Lower arch perimeter preservation using the lingual arch. *Am. J. Orthod. Dentofac. Orthop.* 112 (4): 449–456.

110 Viglianisi, A. (2010 Oct). Effects of lingual arch used as space maintainer on mandibular arch dimension: a systematic review. *Am. J. Orthod. Dentofac. Orthop.* 138 (4): 382–383.

111 Huang, W.J. and Creath, C.J. (1995 May-June). The midline diastema: a review of its etiology and treatment. *Pediatr. Dent.* 17 (3): 171–179.

112 Bills, D.A., Handelman, C.S., and BeGole, E.A. (2005 May). Bimaxillary dentoalveolar protrusion: traits and orthodontic correction. *Angle Orthod.* 75 (3): 333–339.

113 ADA Division of Communications. For the dental patient (2006 Jan). Tooth eruption: the permanent teeth. *J. Am. Dent. Assoc.* 137 (1): 127.

114 O'Byrn, B.L., Sadowsky, C., Schneider, B., and BeGole, E.A. (1995 Apr.). An evaluation of mandibular asymmetry in adults with unilateral posterior crossbite. *Am. J. Orthod. Dentofac. Orthop.* 107 (4): 394–400.

115 Pinto, A.S., Buschang, P.H., Throckmorton, G.S., and Chen, P. (2001 Nov). Morphological and positional asymmetries of young children with functional unilateral posterior crossbite. *Am. J. Orthod. Dentofac. Orthop.* 120 (5): 513–520.

116 Pirttiniemi, P., Kantomaa, T., and Lahtela, P. (1990 Nov). Relationship between craniofacial and condyle path asymmetry in unilateral cross-bite patients. *Eur. J. Orthod.* 12 (4): 408–413.

117 Myers, D.R., Barenie, J.T., Bell, R.A., and Williamson, E.H. (1980 Sep). Condylar position in children with functional posterior crossbites: before and after crossbite correction. *Pediatr. Dent.* 2 (3): 190–194.

118 Yoshikane, T., Pullinger, A., Turley, P. (1987). Characteristics of functional posterior crossbites in the deciduous and mixed dentitions. Thesis. Los Angeles (CA): University of California, School of Dentistry.

119 Hesse, K.L., Artun, J., Joondeph, D.R., and Kennedy, D.B. (1997 Apr). Changes in condylar position and occlusion associated with maxillary expansion for correction of functional unilateral posterior crossbite. *Am. J. Orthod. Dentofac. Orthop.* 111 (4): 410–418.

120 Krebs, A. (1964 Dec). Midpalatal expansion studies by the implant method over a seven-year period. *Rep. Congr. Eur. Orthod. Soc.* 40: 131–142.

121 Krebs, A. (1959). Expansion of the midpalatal suture, studied by means of metallic implants. *Acta Odontol. Scand.* 17 (4): 491–501.

122 Hicks, E.P. (1978 Feb). Slow maxillary expansion. A clinical study of the skeletal versus dental response to low-magnitude force. *Am. J. Orthod.* 73 (2): 121–141.

123 Wertz, R. and Dreskin, M. (1977 Apr). Midpalatal suture opening: a normative study. *Am. J. Orthod.* 71 (4): 367–381.

124 Baccetti, T., Franchi, L., Cameron, C.G., and McNamara, J.A. Jr. (2001 Oct). Treatment timing for rapid maxillary expansion. *Angle Orthod.* 71 (5): 343–350.

125 Betts, N.J., Vanarsdall, R.L., Barber, H.D. et al. (1995 Jan). Diagnosis and treatment of transverse maxillary deficiency. *Int. J. Adult Orthodon. Orthognath. Surg.* 10 (2): 75–96.

126 Shetty, V., Caridad, J.M., Caputo, A.A., and Chaconas, S.J. (1994 Jul). Biomechanical rationale for surgical-orthodontic expansion in the adult maxilla. *J. Oral Maxillofac. Surg.* 52 (7): 742–749. discussion 750-1.

127 Schröder, U. and Schröder, L. (1984 Feb). Early treatment of unilateral posterior crossbite in children with bilaterally contracted maxillae. *Eur. J. Orthod.* 1: 65–69.

128 Kantomaa, T. (1986). Correction of unilateral crossbite in the deciduous dentition. *Eur. J. Dermatol.* 8 (2): 80–83.

129 Thilander, B., Wahlund, S., and Lennartsson, B. (1984 Feb). The effect of early interceptive treatment in children with posterior crossbite. *Eur. J. Orthod.* 6 (1): 25–34.

130 González-Ulloa, M. (1962 Feb). Quantitative principles in cosmetic surgery of the face (profileplasty). *Plast. Reconstr. Surg. Transplant. Bull.* 29 (2): 187–198.

131 González-Ulloa, M. and Stevens, E. (1968 May). The role of chin correction in profileplasty. *Plast. Reconstr. Surg.* 41 (5): 477–486.

132 Naini, F.B. (2013 Sep-Oct). The Frankfort plane and head positioning in facial aesthetic analysis – the perpetuation of a myth. *JAMA Facial Plast. Surg.* 15 (5): 333–334.

133 Naini, F.B. (2011). *Facial Aesthetics: Concepts and Clinical Diagnosis.* Wiley-Blackwell: Oxford, England.

134 Proffit, W.R. (1986 Jan). On the aetiology of malocclusion. The Northcroft lecture, 1985, presented to the British Society for the Study of Orthodontics, Oxford, April 18, 1985. *Br. J. Orthod.* 13 (1): 1–11.

135 Burn-Murdoch, R.A. (1981). The effect of applied forces on the eruption of rat maxillary incisors. *Arch. Oral Biol.* 26 (11): 939–943.

136 Steedle, J.R., Proffit, W.R., and Fields, H.W. (1983). The effects of continuous axially-directed intrusive loads on the erupting rabbit mandibular incisor. *Arch. Oral Biol.* 28 (12): 1149–1153.

137 Proffit, W.R. and Sellers, K.T. (1986 Feb). The effect of intermittent forces on eruption of the rabbit incisor. *J. Dent. Res.* 65 (2): 118–122.

138 Wertz, R.A. (1970 Jul). Skeletal and dental changes accompanying rapid and midpalatal suture opening. *Am. J. Orthod.* 58 (1): 41–65.

139 Garrett, B.J., Caruso, J.M., Rungcharassaeng, K. et al. (2008 Jul). Skeletal effects to the maxilla after rapid maxillary expansion assessed with cone-beam computed tomography. *Am. J. Orthod. Dentofac. Orthop.* 134 (1): 8–9.

140 Davidovitch, M., Eistathiou, S., Sarne, O., and Vardimon, A.D. (2005 Apr). Skeletal and dental response to rapid maxillary expansion with 2- versus 4-band appliances. *Am. J. Orthod. Dentofac. Orthop.* 127 (4): 483–492.

141 Burstone, C.J. (1967 Apr). Lip posture and its significance in treatment planning. *Am. J. Orthod.* 53 (4): 262–284.

142 Rohra, A.K. Jr., Demko, C.A., Hans, M.G. et al. (2018 Jul). Sleep disordered breathing in children seeking orthodontic care. *Am. J. Orthod. Dentofac. Orthop.* 154 (1): 65–71.

143 Behrents, R.G., Shelgikar, A.V., Conley, R.S. et al. (2019 Jul). Obstructive sleep apnea and orthodontics: an American Association of Orthodontists white paper. *Am. J. Orthod. Dentofac. Orthop.* 156 (1): 13–28.

144 Pancherz, H. (1985 Jan). The Herbst appliance – its biological effects and clinical use. *Am. J. Orthod.* 87 (1): 1–20.

145 Franchi, L., Alvetro, L., Giuntini, V. et al. (2011 Jul). Effectiveness of comprehensive fixed appliance

treatment used with the Forsus Fatigue Resistant Device in Class II patients. *Angle Orthod.* 81 (4): 678–683.

146 Heinig, N. and Göz, G. (2001 Nov). Clinical application and effects of the Forsus spring. A study of a new Herbst hybrid. *J. Orofac. Orthop.* 62 (6): 436–450.

147 Janson, G., Sathler, R., Fernandes, T.M. et al. (2013 Mar). Correction of Class II malocclusion with Class II elastics: a systematic review. *Am. J. Orthod. Dentofac. Orthop.* 143 (3): 383–392.

148 Lesinskas, E. and Drigotas, M. (2009 Apr). The incidence of adenoidal regrowth after adenoidectomy and its effect on persistent nasal symptoms. *Eur. Arch. Otorhinolaryngol.* 266 (4): 469–473.

149 Schendel, S.A., Eisenfeld, J., Bell, W.H. et al. (1976 Oct). The long-face syndrome: vertical maxillary excess. *Am. J. Orthod.* 70 (4): 398–408.

150 Kingsley, N.W. (1881). Die anomalien der zahnstellung und die defekte des gaumens. [The anomalies of the tooth alignment and the defects of the palate.] Leipzig: A. Felix.

151 Parks, L.R., Buschang, P.H., Alexander, R.A. et al. (2007 May). Masticatory exercises as an adjunctive treatment for hyperdivergent patients. *Angle Orthod.* 77 (3): 457–462.

152 Gurton, A.U., Akin, E., and Karacay, S. (2004 Aug). Initial intrusion of the molars in the treatment of anterior open bite malocclusions in growing patients. *Angle Orthod.* 74 (4): 454–464.

153 Schiavoni, R., Grenga, V., and Macri, V. (1992 Nov). Treatment of Class II high angle malocclusions with the Herbst appliance: a cephalometric investigation. *Am. J. Orthod. Dentofac. Orthop.* 102 (5): 393–409.

154 Wendling, L.K., McNamara, J.A. Jr., and Franchi, L. (2005 Jan). Baccetti T. A prospective study of the short-term treatment effects of the acrylic-splint rapid maxillary expander combined with the lower Schwarz appliance. *Angle Orthod.* 75 (1): 7–14.

155 Sarver, D.M. and Johnston, M.W. (1989 Jun). Skeletal changes in vertical and anterior displacement of the maxilla with bonded rapid palatal expansion appliances. *Am. J. Orthod. Dentofac. Orthop.* 95 (6): 462–466.

156 Kurol, J. and Olson, L. (1991 Oct). Ankylosis of primary molars: a future periodontal threat to the first permanent molars? *Eur. J. Orthod.* 13 (5): 404–409.

157 Mann, K.R., Marshall, S.D., Qian, F. et al. (2011 Feb). Effect of maxillary anteroposterior position on profile esthetics in headgear-treated patients. *Am. J. Orthod. Dentofac. Orthop.* 139 (2): 228–234.

6

Transverse Problems

Introduction

Posterior crossbite correction is the most common reason for early transverse treatment. This chapter provides a summary of the etiology, diagnosis, and treatment of transverse problems ranging from one-tooth dental crossbites in the primary dentition to bilateral skeletal crossbites in the permanent (adolescent) dentition.

Q: Can you describe the ideal permanent first molar transverse relationship? Can you describe common first molar transverse malocclusions (assume an absence of centric relation [CR]-centric occlusion [CO] shifts during closure)?

A: In the ideal permanent first molar transverse relationship (Figure 6.1a), maxillary first molar mesiolingual cusps are seated in the mandibular first molar central fossae, mandibular first molar distobuccal cusps are seated in the central fossae of the maxillary first molars, maxillary and mandibular first molar buccal and lingual cusps (Figure 6.1b) are oriented along a straight horizontal line, and posterior teeth are in a normal buccolingual inclination. Normal first molar transverse inclinations vary with age in individuals with normal occlusion, ranging from ~10 to ~4° of buccal inclination for maxillary molars (buccal crown torque decreases with age during growth) and from ~10 to ~3° of lingual inclination for mandibular molars (lingual crown torque decreases with age during growth) [1]. Large samples have confirmed individuals with normal transverse occlusion show mild maxillary molar buccal crown torque and mild mandibular molar lingual crown torque with the ideal cusp-fossae relationships noted above [2].

Variation in molar transverse occlusion can produce transverse malocclusion including:

- Excess maxillary buccal crown torque or excess mandibular lingual crown torque (Figure 6.1c, molars on left of illustration)
- Excess maxillary lingual crown torque or excess mandibular buccal crown torque (Figure 6.1d, molars on left of illustration)
- Inadequate posterior overjet (Figure 6.1e, bilateral)
- Lingual crossbite (Figure 6.1f, molars on right of illustration)
- Complete lingual crossbite (Figure 6.1g, molars on right of illustration)
- Excess posterior overjet (Figure 6.1h, bilateral)
- Complete buccal crossbite or scissors bite (Figure 6.1i, molars on the right of illustration)

Notes: Posterior crossbites can present as unilateral or bilateral malocclusions of the primary, mixed, or permanent dentitions. Canine involvement is often seen and considered part of a posterior crossbite even though canines are not posterior teeth.

Nomenclature is based on the position of the *maxillary* teeth. Posterior *lingual* crossbite, the most common posterior crossbite, exists when the buccal cusps of the maxillary teeth are lingual to the buccal cusps of the mandibular teeth. Posterior *buccal* crossbite occurs when the lingual cusps of the maxillary teeth are buccal to the opposing buccal cusps of the mandibular teeth.

Q: The terms *buccal crown torque* and *lingual crown torque* were used in the previous question. This is confusing. Isn't torque a physics concept, like force is a physics concept? In other words, force is an interaction that causes linear motion, and torque is an interaction that causes rotation. What does torque have to do with tooth position?

A: Good question. In physics, torque is indeed a tendency to cause rotation of a body. In fact, the term "torque" is often used interchangeably with other terms

Practical Early Orthodontic Treatment: A Case-Based Review, First Edition. Thomas E. Southard, Steven D. Marshall, Laura L. Bonner, and Kyungsup Shin.
© 2023 John Wiley & Sons, Inc. Published 2023 by John Wiley & Sons, Inc.
Companion website: www.wiley.com/go/southard/practical

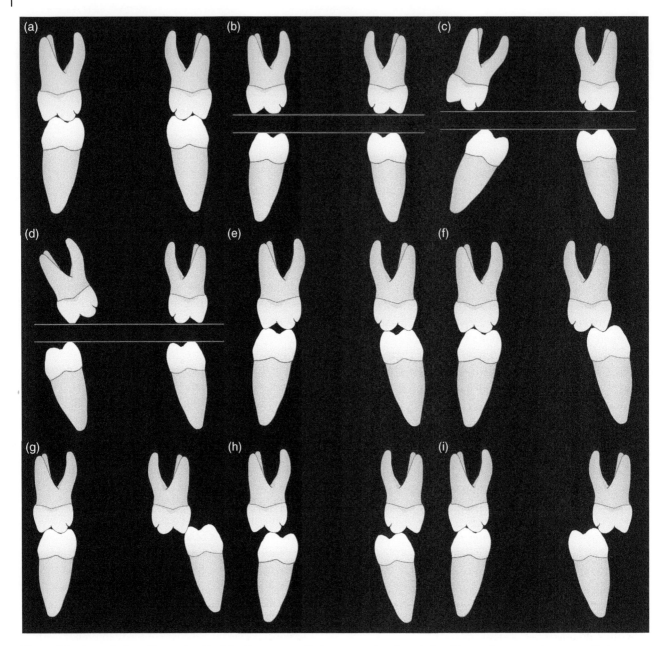

Figure 6.1 Frontal views illustrating ideal (a–b) transverse first permanent molar relationships and common transverse first permanent molar malocclusions (c–i).

(e.g. moment or couple) to describe a tendency to cause rotation of a body. Likewise, in orthodontics, torque is a tendency to cause rotation of a tooth or jaw.

Now, by convention, many orthodontists will also use the term torque to describe the *position* of a tooth, buccolingually. For instance, they will state that a maxillary molar has excess buccal crown torque or a mandibular molar has excess lingual crown torque (Figure 6.1c).

Q: In Figures 6.1a–6.1i, we assumed the absence of a lateral CR-CO shift. But, what if that was not the case?

What if a lateral CR-CO shift was present? How could Figures 6.1e–6.1f be related if a lateral CR-CO shift was present? How could Figures 6.1h–6.1i be related if a lateral CR-CO shift was present?

A: Let's start with Figure 6.1e, which illustrates inadequate posterior overjet. The bite is relatively unstable here because a cusp-to-fossa occlusion is absent. Instead, a cusp-to-cusp occlusion is present. In such cases, it is not unusual for the patient to close from CR to CO with a lateral shift into a more stable cusp-to-fossa relationship (Figure 6.1f).

Figure 6.1h illustrates excessive posterior overjet. Once again, the bite is relatively unstable because a cusp-to-fossa occlusion is absent. In such cases, it is not unusual for the patient to close from CR to CO with a lateral shift into a stable cusp-to-fossa relationship (Figure 6.1i).

Q: What is the incidence of posterior crossbites in the primary or early mixed dentition stage of development?

A: Studies report an incidence of posterior crossbites that range from 7–23% and a greater prevalence of unilateral crossbites with lateral CR-CO shift (functional unilateral crossbite) [3–7].

Q: How do transverse dental relationships develop?

A: Transverse (buccolingual) dental relationships develop in the same way, and for the same reasons, that incisor labiolingual dental relationships develop. Teeth tend to erupt along their long axes throughout life until sufficient occlusal, or soft tissue, forces prevent a further eruption. Their buccolingual inclination is governed by the soft tissue envelope (tongue-cheeks-lips), which directs them to erupt into occlusion with teeth from the opposing jaw. In the presence of an anteroposteriorly deficient maxilla, the tongue will tend to tip the maxillary incisors forward, and the mandibular lip will tend to tip the mandibular incisors lingually (anteroposterior dental compensations for an underlying skeletal discrepancy between the jaws). In this way, the incisors can erupt into normal occlusion.

In a similar fashion, in the presence of a transversely deficient maxilla, the tongue will tend to tip the maxillary molars buccally, and the cheeks will tend to tip the mandibular molars lingually. These are transverse dental compensations for an underlying transverse skeletal discrepancy between the jaws. In this way, the molars erupt into normal occlusion.

Q: A seven-year-old girl presents to you with a posterior crossbite. Her parents ask, "Will our daughter's crossbite correct spontaneously?" How do you respond?

A: Her posterior crossbite will *probably not* correct spontaneously. However, a range of spontaneous crossbite corrections (17–45%) [3, 4, 7, 8] has been reported. So, spontaneous correction is *possible*, just not probable. *One option is to monitor her crossbite for three to six months to see whether it corrects spontaneously before treating.*

Q: Is it easier to treat a patient who presents with a lateral CR-CO shift into a unilateral posterior crossbite (functional unilateral crossbite), or is it easier to treat a patient with a unilateral posterior crossbite without a CR-CO shift (a true unilateral crossbite)?

A: It is easier to treat a patient with a lateral CR-CO shift into a unilateral posterior crossbite. Why? When the lateral shift is eliminated, the transverse discrepancy becomes bilateral *but smaller on the crossbite side.* Also, bilateral arch forces to correct the bilateral discrepancy (expansion, constriction) are easier to generate than unilateral forces.

Q: What fact of diagnosis does this concept underscore?

A: It underscores the importance of checking for CR-CO shifts at every appointment. If a patient presents with a unilateral crossbite in CO, but shifts into a bilateral (smaller) transverse discrepancy in CR, then your transverse correction will generally be easier.

Q: What may result if a unilateral crossbite resulting from a lateral CR-CO shift (functional crossbite) is not corrected during growth?

A: A *mandibular growth asymmetry* may result. This fact stresses the importance of early correction of lateral shifts into crossbites.

The fact that most unilateral crossbites do not spontaneously correct and that functional shifts are rarely detected in adults with unilateral crossbites suggests that adaptive remodeling of the temporomandibular joint occurs and that children with unilateral crossbites and functional shifts develop asymmetries of the mandible [9–11].

Q: A child presents to you with a developing mandibular asymmetry due to a lateral shift into crossbite. What does the literature tell us about the asymmetry if the crossbite is corrected early enough with maxillary expansion?

A: *If the crossbite and functional shift are treated in a timely manner (early mixed dentition), then the asymmetry can be largely eliminated* [10–14].

Q: Anneke is a seven-year-old girl who presents to you in the early mixed dentition (Figure 6.2) with the parents' chief complaint, "Anneke has a crossbite." Past medical history (PMH) includes asthma. Past dental history (PDH) is within the range of normal (WRN), CR = CO, and upper dental midline (UDML) WRN. Temporomandibular joints (TMJs), periodontal tissues, and mucogingival tissues are WRN. Can you list her *primary* problems in each dimension (plus others)?

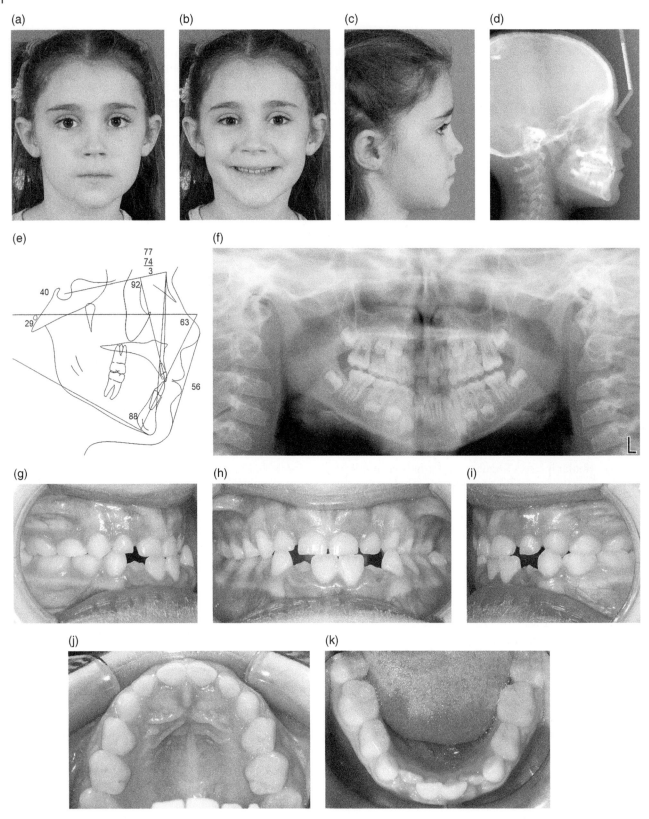

Figure 6.2 Initial records of Anneke. (a–c) facial photographs, (d–e) lateral cephalometric radiograph and tracing, (f) panoramic image, (g–k) intraoral images, (l–s) model images.

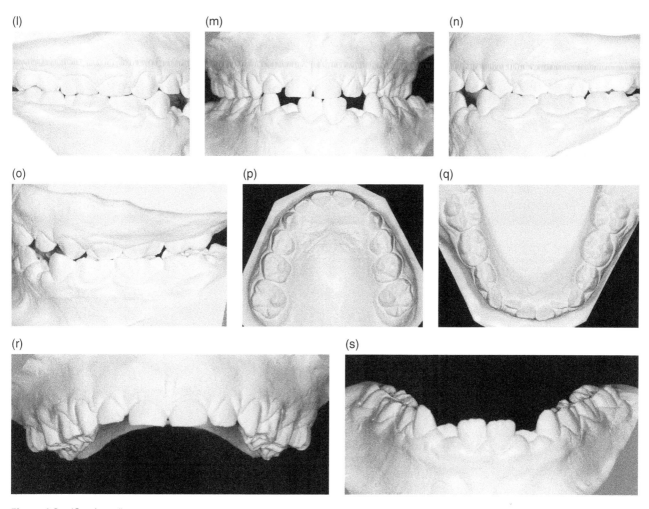

Figure 6.2 (Continued)

A:

Table 6.1 Primary problems list for Anneke.

AP	–
Vertical	OB 0%
Transverse	Left lingual crossbite
	Maxillary first permanent molar buccal crown torque (Figure 6.2r)
	Mandibular right first permanent molar lingual crown torque (Figure 6.2s)
	Maxillary first permanent molar interlingual cusp distance = 34.9 mm
	Mandibular first permanent molar intercentral fossa distance = 40.9 mm
Other	Mildly proclined mandibular incisors (FMIA = 63°)
	Edge-to-edge relationship of maxillary left primary central incisor and mandibular left permanent central incisor
	2–3 mm maxillary anterior spacing
	Mild (3–4 mm) mandibular incisor crowding

Q: Can you more fully describe Anneke's left crossbite?

A: It is a unilateral left lingual crossbite of her permanent first molars, primary canines, and primary molars (without CR-CO shift).

Q: We will return to Anneke later. For now, can you list at least four etiologic factors that cause transverse discrepancies?

A: Etiologic factors include: [4, 15–24]

- Ectopic tooth eruption. Figure 6.3a illustrates a developing (left to right) buccal crossbite resulting from an ectopic first permanent molar eruption.
- Soft tissue imbalance (e.g. resulting from prolonged digit sucking). Figure 6.3b shows the posterior crossbite (and anterior open bite) resulting from three decades of heavy thumb sucking. However, one study reported no difference in sucking habits of patients with or without spontaneous correction of a posterior crossbite [3].

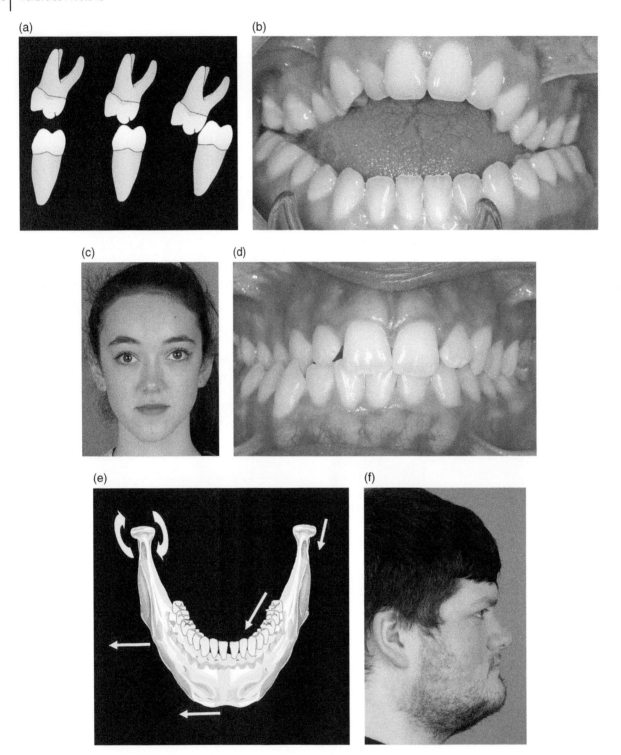

Figure 6.3 Factors causing transverse problems: (a) ectopic eruption of posterior teeth; (b) prolonged digit sucking; (c–e) asymmetric mandibular jaw growth; (f–h) deficient maxillary/excessive mandibular anteroposterior growth resulting in lingual crossbite with relative transverse discrepancy; (i–k) deficient maxillary transverse growth associated with a palatal cleft.

- A large tongue carried low in the mouth can cause excessive mandibular transverse dental widening resulting in a lingual posterior crossbite [25].
- Prolonged retention of primary teeth.

- Asymmetric mandibular growth (Figures 6.3c–6.3e) – note the right chin deviation and right posterior *unilateral* crossbite that has resulted from asymmetric mandibular growth.

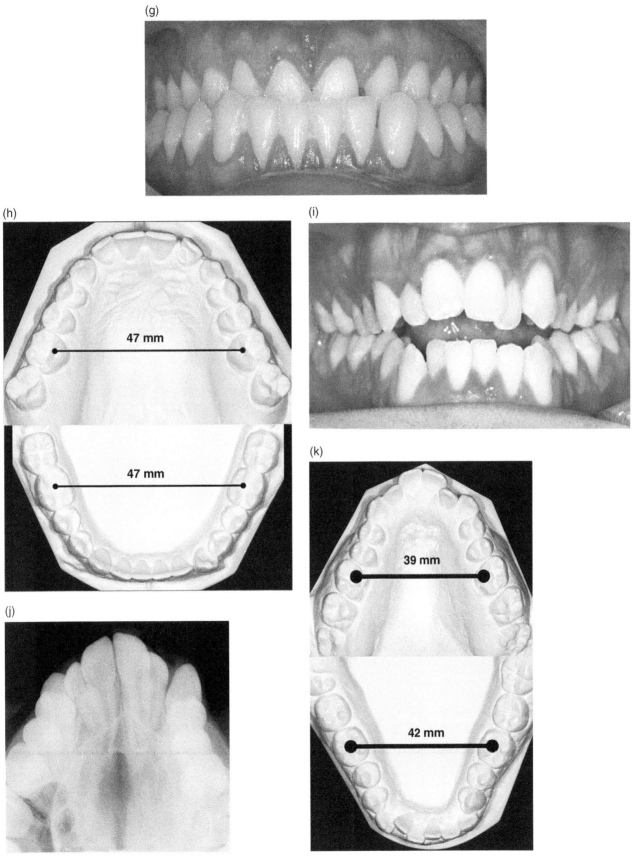

Figure 6.3 (Continued)

- A lateral CR-CO shift without an underlying skeletal problem.
- Excess or deficient anteroposterior growth of the maxilla or mandible. Figures 6.3f–6.3h illustrate a 19-year-old male with lingual crossbite of the entire dentition due to maxillary anteroposterior deficiency/mandibular anteroposterior excess.
- Some TMD issues. Temporomandibular joint dysfunction has been associated with skeletal asymmetries and crossbite occlusion.
- Excess or deficient maxillary or mandibular transverse growth. Figures 6.3i–6.3k illustrate a left posterior crossbite developed in a cleft lip and palate patient due to deficient maxillary transverse growth.

Q: A unilateral posterior crossbite often results from one of the two etiologies. What are they?

A: Either a lateral CR-CO shift into crossbite or asymmetric mandibular growth.

Q: Which of these two etiologies is the more difficult to treat?

A: A unilateral posterior crossbite resulting from asymmetric mandibular growth (Figure 6.3c–e) is more difficult to treat. Why? *Correcting the crossbite early does not normalize growth.* As asymmetric mandibular growth continues into adolescence, the unilateral crossbite is likely to return. This fact underscores the importance of determining whether a unilateral posterior crossbite is due to asymmetric mandibular growth or a CR-CO lateral shift.

Q: Can you discuss six factors that should be considered when formulating a diagnosis and treatment plan for patients with transverse discrepancies?

A: The following factors must be considered:
- *Magnitude of transverse discrepancy:* This is the single most important factor in your transverse treatment planning decision and will influence your decision to treat the child with orthopedics, masking/camouflage (adult dentition), or surgery (adult dentition).

As illustrated in Figures 6.4a–6.4c, the magnitude of a transverse discrepancy is not simply the linear difference between maxillary first molar intermolar width (lingual cusp to lingual cusp) and mandibular first molar intermolar width (central fossa to central fossa). This linear difference would reflect the magnitude of the discrepancy only if the molars displayed normal buccolingual inclinations (i.e. were initially *upright*).

Instead, transverse dental compensations (usually maxillary posterior buccal crown torque and mandibular posterior lingual crown torque) must be considered when determining the magnitude of the transverse discrepancy. Buccally tipped maxillary molar crowns will tend to move lingually as they are uprighted (unless a transpalatal arch is used to apply torque to upright their roots while maintaining the intermolar distance). Likewise, lingually tipped mandibular molar crowns will tend to move buccally as they are uprighted (unless a lower lingual holding arch is used to apply lingual root torque while maintaining the intermolar distance). Removal of these compensations by uprighting the molars can dramatically increase the transverse occlusal discrepancy magnitude and worsen a skeletal crossbite relationship.

Also, changes in the sagittal relationships between the jaws affect transverse relationships. If you move

(a)

(b)

(c)

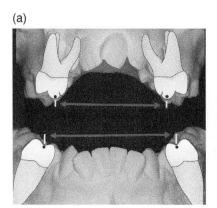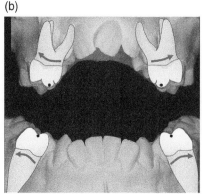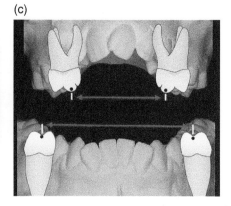

Figure 6.4 (a) The magnitude of a transverse discrepancy is not simply the linear difference between maxillary first molar intermolar width (lingual cusp to lingual cusp) and mandibular first molar intermolar width (central fossa to central fossa); (b) Instead, the magnitude of the transverse discrepancy must consider compensations, which will be removed by uprighting posterior teeth; (c) Uprighting posterior teeth usually increases the transverse discrepancy magnitude and can worsen, or create, a posterior crossbite.

the maxilla or mandible relative to each other via orthopedics or surgery, you must anticipate how these movements will affect the resulting posterior transverse relationships (e.g. see absolute vs. relative transverse discrepancy below).

- *Facial symmetry or asymmetry:* The *first* thing to do when compiling a problem list in the transverse dimension is to examine the patient's face in the frontal view. Unlike problems in either the anteroposterior or vertical dimensions, problems in the transverse dimension are frequently camouflaged by the overlying soft tissue. However, asymmetries can usually be spotted during a clinical examination. The use of a cone beam computed tomography (CBCT) scan can also be of value in assessing skeletal asymmetries and transverse skeletal discrepancies between the maxilla and mandible.

  We do *not* recommend using a 2-D posteroanterior cephalometric radiographs to determine transverse skeletal discrepancies between the maxilla and mandible because the alveolar process bone of the jaws, the bone that houses the roots of the teeth and is the bone of interest in diagnosing transverse skeletal discrepancies, is obscured in posteroanterior cephalometric films.

- *Presence of a lateral CR-CO shift:* You should always *check for a CR-CO shift in every patient at every appointment.* If you note an asymmetry, especially a deviation of the chin in the presence of a unilateral crossbite, try to establish whether the asymmetry is a result of the lateral shift or a developing mandibular growth asymmetry. In addition, check for lateral deviation upon opening.

  Have the patient tip his chin upward and touch his tongue to the back of their palate while he opens and closes slowly until his teeth just touch, to help seat the condyles in the glenoid fossa. Then, ask the patient to close into maximal intercuspation to check for a CR-CO shift. If there is any doubt about the presence or absence of a functional shift, you can place the patient on a flat-plane bite plate for a week or two to disarticulate the occlusion and deprogram. However, compliance with a removable appliance is never certain. We prefer to deprogram using either a fixed expansion appliance (in the presence of a constricted maxilla while attempting orthopedics), or by leveling/aligning with fixed orthodontic appliances.

  Principle of CR-CO shifts and treatment planning: if you detect a sizable CR-CO shift, inform the patient that you cannot establish your final treatment plan until the shift has been eliminated. It is only when

the shift is eliminated that you can observe the true relationship between the jaws and formulate a rational treatment plan.

- *Whether the transverse discrepancy is relative or absolute:* Haas [26] introduced the terms relative and absolute transverse discrepancy. A *relative* transverse discrepancy exists when the posterior teeth do not coordinate in centric relation but do coordinate when the canines of the models are placed in Class I occlusion. For instance, Figure 6.5a shows the models of an adult patient with a severe Class II malocclusion in CR. Note the significant transverse discrepancy. The patient was treatment planned for mandibular advancement surgery. Figure 6.5b shows the same models advanced to a Class I canine relationship. Note that the transverse discrepancy has disappeared. This patient had a *relative* transverse discrepancy.

  On the other hand, an *absolute* discrepancy exists when the posterior teeth do not coordinate even when the canines are placed into a Class I relationship. For instance, Figure 6.5c shows the models of a patient with a severe Class III malocclusion in a centric relationship. Note the significant transverse discrepancy. The patient was treatment planned for a mandibular setback osteotomy. Figure 6.5d shows the same models set back to Class I canines. Note that the transverse discrepancy is still present. In fact, the transverse discrepancy will be even worse when the mandibular molars are uprighted (Figure 6.5e, note mandibular molar lingual crown torque). This patient has an *absolute* transverse discrepancy.

- *How future anteroposterior growth/treatment will affect the transverse discrepancy:* Forward growth of the mandible relative to the maxilla brings a wider part of the mandibular arch forward relative to the maxillary arch. This relative mandibular arch forward movement can improve a posterior buccal crossbite but worsen a posterior lingual crossbite.

  For example, if the patient shown in Figure 6.5a was still growing, then orthopedically restricting the maxilla with headgear (while allowing the mandible to grow forward) could result in improvement/elimination of the transverse discrepancy (Figure 6.5b).

- *Magnitude of buccal corridors:* When a patient smiles, the buccal corridors are spaces existing between the lateral surfaces of the posterior teeth and the inner commissures of the lips or cheeks. Usually, a patient with a constricted maxilla and narrow maxillary arch will have large buccal corridors. Conversely, a patient with a wide maxilla, and a broad maxillary arch, will have small buccal corridors. Moore and colleagues

(a)

(b)

(c)

(d)

(e)

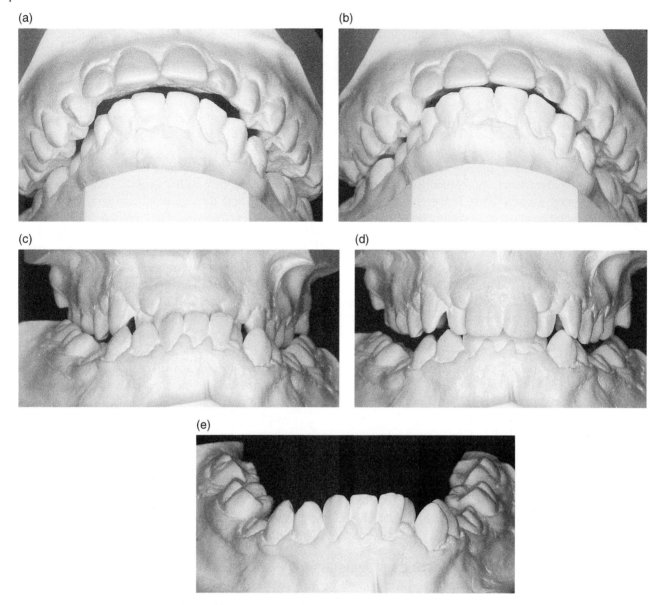

Figure 6.5 Transverse discrepancies: (a–b) patient with *relative* transverse discrepancy, (c–e) patient with absolute transverse discrepancy.

studied the effect of buccal corridor size on smile esthetics [27] and found that *large* buccal corridors are considered unaesthetic (compare Figures 6.6a and 6.6b). When examining a patient, we recommend recording the presence of large buccal corridors during a posed smile and sensitively discussing them with the patient.

- *Whether the posterior crossbite (transverse discrepancy) is dental or skeletal:* This factor will be considered in detail in the following series of questions.

Q: Assume that a patient presents to you with a unilateral right lingual posterior crossbite of only one to two

teeth (Figure 6.7). Further, assume that she is Class I without a functional shift. Is her crossbite a dental, or skeletal, crossbite? In other words, can dental crossbites be differentiated from skeletal crossbites by simply counting the number of teeth in crossbite? [28]

A: No – we cannot conclude that it is a dental crossbite because only one to two posterior teeth are in crossbite. Nor can we conclude that it is a skeletal crossbite if more than a few teeth are in crossbite.

Q: *Why* are we not able to differentiate skeletal from dental crossbites simply by counting the number of teeth in crossbite?

(a) (b)

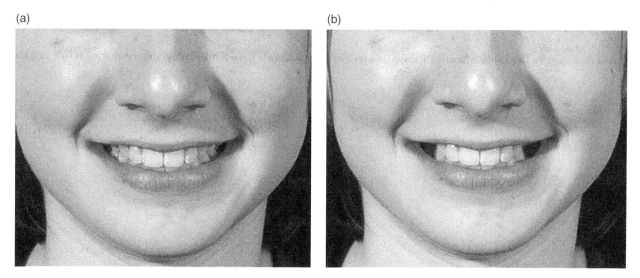

Figure 6.6   Effect of buccal corridors on smile esthetics. (a) Broad smiles, with small buccal corridors, are preferred by laypersons; (b) Very narrow smiles, usually resulting from maxillary transverse skeletal deficiency, combined with *large* buccal corridors are considered less attractive.

(a) (b)

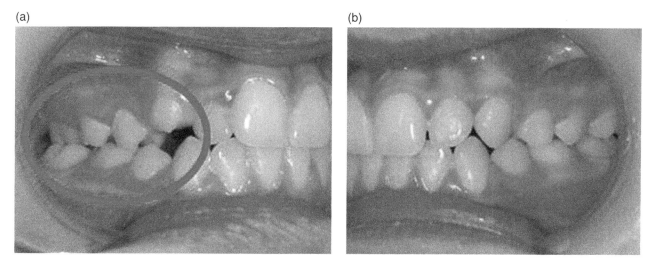

Figure 6.7   (a–b) Patient presenting with only mandibular right permanent first molars in crossbite. Posterior dental and skeletal crossbites cannot be differentiated simply by counting the number of teeth in crossbite.

A: Differentiation between dental and skeletal crossbites is not that simple. As recently reported [29], there is a large variation in transverse skeletal widths (and transverse dental compensations) in the *absence* of crossbites ranging from:

- Small maxillary skeletal widths compared to large mandibular skeletal widths (Figure 6.8a), to
- Comparable maxillary and mandibular skeletal widths (Figure 6.8b), to
- Large maxillary skeletal widths compared to small mandibular skeletal widths (Figure 6.8c).

In other words, a large transverse skeletal discrepancy can exist between the jaws in the absence of a crossbite, in the presence of only a few teeth in crossbite, or in the presence of a large number of teeth in crossbite. *Counting teeth to determine the presence or absence of a transverse skeletal discrepancy is ill-advised.* You must take into account the presence and magnitude of dental compensations in order to determine whether a transverse skeletal discrepancy exists.

Q: So, if we cannot simply count the number of posterior teeth in crossbite to determine whether it is dental or skeletal, then how do we differentiate between a dental and skeletal crossbite?

A: By visualizing what happens when we *upright the molars* (i.e. estimate the true intermolar width that

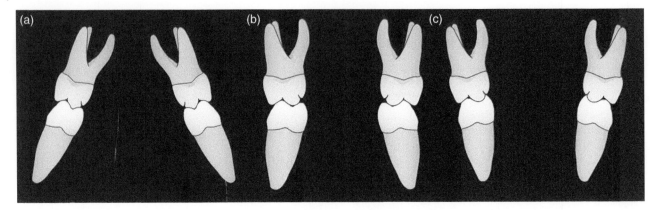

Figure 6.8 Variation in transverse skeletal widths in the *absence* of crossbites: (a) small maxillary skeletal width compared to a large mandibular skeletal width (note maxillary buccal crown torque and mandibular lingual crown torque), (b) comparable maxillary and mandibular skeletal widths (relatively upright molars), (c) large maxillary skeletal width compared to a small mandibular skeletal width (note maxillary lingual crown torque and mandibular buccal crown torque).

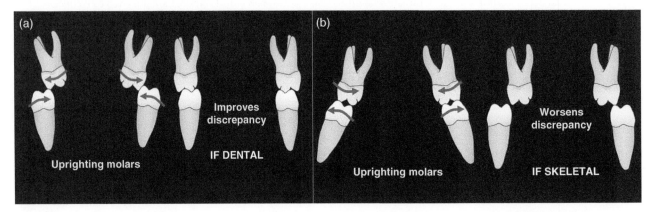

Figure 6.9 Determining whether a posterior crossbite is dental or skeletal: (a) uprighting molars will improve a *dental* crossbite because the maxillary and mandibular skeletal bases relate well, (b) uprighting molars (removing transverse compensations) will worsen a *skeletal* crossbite because the maxillary and mandibular bases do not relate well.

results from eliminating transverse compensations in each arch). For instance, since maxillary and mandibular skeletal bases relate well in a *dental* crossbite, uprighting molars should improve (eliminate) a dental crossbite (Figure 6.9a). On the other hand, since maxillary and mandibular skeletal bases do not relate well in a *skeletal* crossbite, uprighting molars should worsen a skeletal crossbite (Figure 6.9b).

Q: Let's apply the above concept to Anneke (Figure 6.2). Is Anneke's left lingual crossbite a dental crossbite or a skeletal crossbite?

A: It is a skeletal crossbite. If we upright Anneke's buccally inclined maxillary first molars (Figure 6.2r), then their crowns will tend to move lingually, worsen her left crossbite, and minimize her right posterior overjet. If we upright her lingually inclined mandibular right first permanent molar (Figure 6.2s), then its crown will tend

to move buccally – reducing her right posterior overjet. Since her transverse relationships worsen as the molars are uprighted, we conclude that her crossbite is *skeletal* (her skeletal bases do not relate well in the transverse).

Q: List goals of transverse treatment.

A: Goals of transverse treatment include:
- Correcting posterior crossbites and lateral CR-CO shifts
- Uprighting posterior teeth
- Creating a stable and coordinated posterior occlusion
- Reducing large buccal corridors
- Maintaining a healthy periodontium
- Increasing chewing efficiency (for example, in patients with scissor bites)

Q: Isn't cheek biting elimination a goal of transverse treatment?

A: Possibly, if the cause of cheek biting is the transverse discrepancy. In many patients, suggesting that they simply slow down when they chew can reduce/eliminate cheek biting.

Q: *When* should posterior crossbites be corrected? Should you correct posterior crossbites in the primary dentition or wait until the mixed dentition?

A: If *limited* occlusal interferences are causing a lateral shift into posterior crossbite, then perform occlusal adjustment as early as possible, even in the primary dentition (Figures 6.10a–6.10d). Why? Limited occlusal adjustment can be performed with minimal time, compliance, and cost to the patient. However, high failure rates have been reported with occlusal adjustments [3, 7, 30, 31].

If extensive occlusal interferences are causing a lateral shift into crossbite, or if an underlying transverse skeletal discrepancy is causing crossbite, then you should not use occlusal adjustment. Instead, we recommend *waiting until the permanent first molars erupt (early mixed dentition)* to begin treatment. Why? Although maxillary expansion plates, composite buildups, and Porter W appliances can be used to treat posterior crossbites in the primary dentition [3, 32, 33], there is generally no urgency to treat posterior crossbites that early. Further, the permanent first molars provide excellent anchorage for maxillary expansion, cooperation should be better if the patient is a little older, and treatment relapse in the primary dentition may require later re-treatment. *We recommend waiting until the early mixed dentition to treat posterior crossbites with maxillary expansion* [34].

Figures 6.10e–6.10j illustrate a seven-year-old girl in the early mixed dentition with a Class I right posterior lingual crossbite of all primary teeth and right first permanent molars. CR = CO. When would you recommend treatment of her crossbite?

Because a lateral shift is absent and she is facially symmetric, we see two options. You can wait to perform rapid maxillary expansion (RME) when she is a little older, say eight years of age, without harm. Or, you can proceed with RME now. We recommend speaking to the parents, assessing her maturity level, and using that information to decide which option to pursue.

Q: A child presents to you with a posterior crossbite. Can you list options for dealing with it?

A: There is no single treatment approach for every patient. Options include:
- No treatment – leave the crossbite
- Dental crossbite – upright the involved teeth, thus improving/correcting the crossbite

- Skeletal crossbite – the same three general options are available for dealing with transverse skeletal discrepancies as for dealing with anteroposterior or vertical skeletal discrepancies:
  - Orthopedics (attempting maxillary skeletal expansion)
  - Masking (camouflage, increasing transverse dental compensations without addressing the underlying skeletal discrepancy)
  - Orthognathic surgery

The challenge is deciding which option is the *best* option. You must consider all of the factors discussed earlier in coming to your decision: presence of a developing skeletal asymmetry, presence of a CR-CO shift, magnitude of the transverse discrepancy, whether the crossbite is of dental or skeletal origin, whether the transverse discrepancy is relative or absolute, how orthopedic or surgical correction in the anteroposterior direction will affect the transverse, the presence and magnitude of dental compensations (torques), which jaw is at fault, the presence of large buccal corridors, the patient's age, the condition of the periodontal tissues, and the patient's desires.

Q: Which jaw should be treated to correct a skeletal transverse discrepancy in a child?

A: If a child presents with a constricted maxilla, the obvious choice is to orthopedically expand the maxilla. If a child presents with an excessively wide mandible, a reasonable choice may still be to expand the maxilla. Surgery would be an option for treating an excessively broad maxilla (removing a wedge of bone to constrict the maxilla), or an excessively narrow mandible (midline osteotomy, with symphyseal distraction or graft).

Q: Let's spend some time discussing options for treating posterior crossbites in more detail. When is the option of *leaving the child in crossbite* (no transverse treatment) reasonable?

A: In contrast to adults, we generally do not consider this option in children. In children, we will almost always correct crossbites. Of course, this depends upon the transverse discrepancy magnitude, whether the crossbite is absolute or relative, current anteroposterior relationships, future growth potential, plans for future surgery, and periodontal biotype. Occasionally, we will finish a child's treatment with a permanent second molar left in crossbite, if the remaining occlusion has excellent interdigitation (no CR-CO shift), if correcting the crossbite would require placing too much second molar compensations, if the patient is not cheek biting

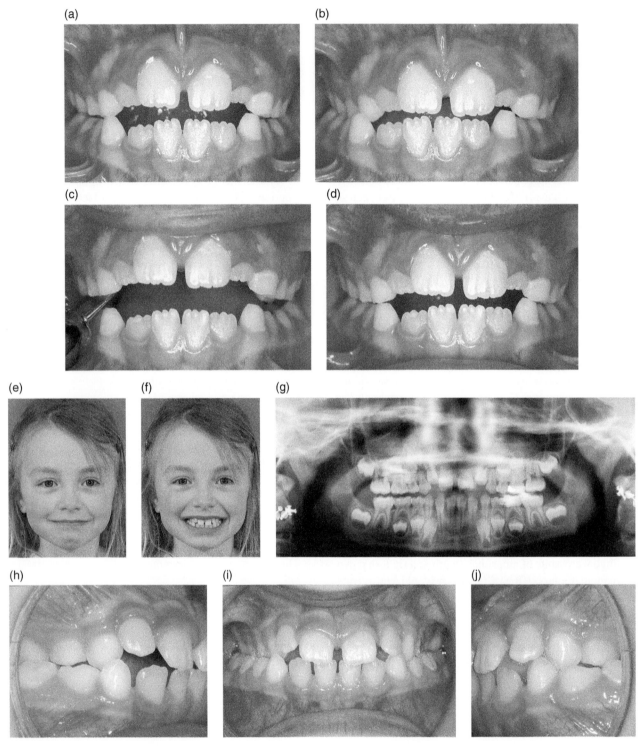

Figure 6.10 *When* to correct posterior crossbites. If limited occlusal interferences are causing a shift from CR (a) into a unilateral crossbite in CO (b), then consider occlusal adjustment (c) to correct the crossbite (d) – *even in the primary dentition*. However, we generally recommend waiting until the permanent first molars erupt as anchorage before beginning maxillary expansion to correct crossbites. (e–j) A seven-year-old girl with facial symmetry and a Class I right lingual crossbite of her permanent first molars. CR = CO. Because a lateral shift is absent, you could choose to treat her now with maxillary expansion, or wait a year without harm.

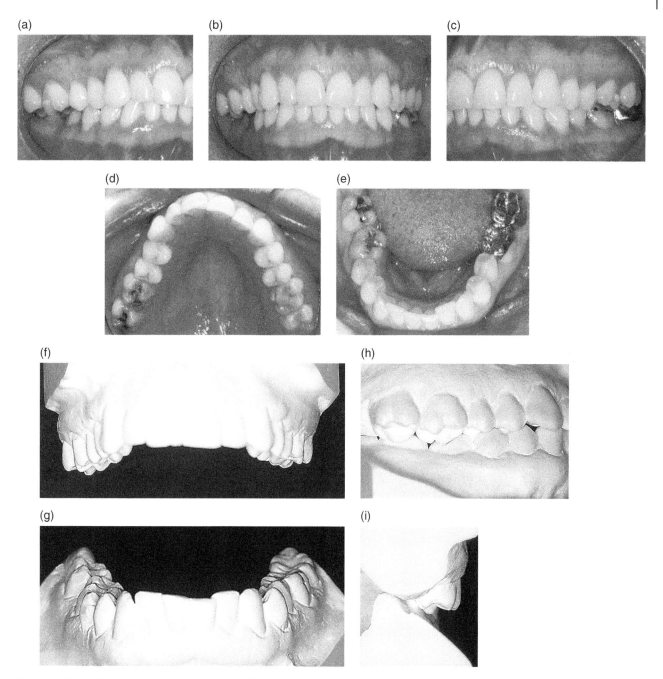

Figure 6.11 (a–i) Class I patient with a unilateral right buccal posterior crossbite and CR = CO.

with the second molars, and if the parents are in agreement with our decision.

In rare medical instances, we will elect to leave a child in crossbite. For example, we recently left a child in crossbite who suffered from chronic recurrent multifocal osteomyelitis. We were concerned with microhemorrhaging (surgical insult), which would occur as the midpalatal suture separated. Our pediatric rheumatologist concurred with our decision. Ideally, in situations where we leave a child in posterior crossbite, we

would at least finish treatment with canines in proper occlusion and with canine rise disclusion.

Q: Figure 6.11 illustrates a female patient with a right posterior buccal crossbite of her first and second molars. She is Class I and CR = CO. Does she have a skeletal or dental posterior crossbite?

A: Her unilateral posterior crossbite is a *dental* crossbite. Why? Clearly, her mandibular right molars have erupted with significant lingual crown torque (Figures 6.10e and

6.10g), while her maxillary right second molar exhibits mild buccal crown torque (Figure 6.10f). Since uprighting these teeth will improve or correct her crossbite, we conclude that she has a *dental* crossbite.

Q: In general terms, how would you correct her dental crossbite?

A: Since uprighting posterior teeth improves a dental crossbite (skeletal bases relate well in dental crossbites), you would move her right maxillary second molar crowns lingually and her mandibular right molar crowns buccally (Figure 6.12).

Q: What problems do you anticipate when uprighting her right molars?

A: The major problem is the magnitude of right molar *overbite*. In other words, her right molars have erupted so far past each other (Figures 6.11h–6.11i) that her vertical dimension may be opened significantly as the right molars upright and are brought into occlusion. These molars may become the only teeth in contact, and she may not be able to tolerate such an increase in vertical dimension. She may require significant occlusal adjustment (enameloplasty) to reduce this increased vertical dimension. Depending upon the amount the right molars must be cut down, she may even require molar endodontics and crowns. She must be informed of these possibilities.

Q: How would you proceed?

A: We placed fixed orthodontic appliances, and asked her to wear crossbite elastics from right mandibular molar lingual buttons to right maxillary molar buccal brackets. Surprisingly, no other treatment was necessary, not even an anterior biteplate to allow her right molars to pass across each other. She required no enameloplasty. Her deband photographs are shown in Figure 6.13.

Q: Let's discuss the treatment of *skeletal* crossbites, beginning with *orthopedic* treatment. What does transverse orthopedic treatment consist of?

A: Correcting dental arch width discrepancies by disarticulating the midpalatal suture with force and spreading the hemi-maxillae apart.

Q: Upon application of a transverse maxillary force (Figure 6.14a), what movements occur in the maxillary anchor teeth and in the maxilla?

A: The answer depends upon the *magnitude of the force and the maturity of the facial skeleton* [35–38]. If the force is too light to overcome the facial skeletal resistance, only buccal tipping/buccal translation of the maxillary posterior teeth will result. If the force is heavy enough to overcome the skeletal resistance, buccal tipping/buccal translation of the maxillary teeth will still occur, together with midpalatal suture disarticulation/separation (Figure 6.14b). This sutural separation may be asymmetric, depending upon the rigidity of the bony structures.

If the facial skeleton is fully mature, the skeletal resistance may be so large it will prevent midpalatal suture separation regardless of how great the force. In this instance, the alveolar process may fracture if a heavy enough force is applied.

Q: Assume that you wish to orthopedically expand a maxillary arch in an eight-year-old child. You are considering three appliances (Figure 6.15) to achieve expansion: a split plate, a quad-helix (Porter arch/W-appliance), or a Hyrax expansion screw appliance. Which should you use?

A: Let's first consider the effects of each appliance:
- Split plate – results in an increased rate of growth (widening) of the midpalatal suture when the screw is opened 0.5 mm/week [39]. The split plate acts as a bite plate to deprogram any shift.

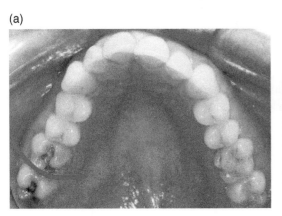

(a)

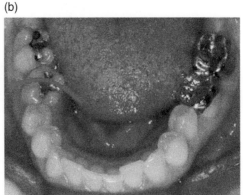

(b)

Figure 6.12 (a–b) To correct her right dental crossbite, upright her molars by moving her maxillary right second molar crown lingually and her mandibular right molar crowns buccally.

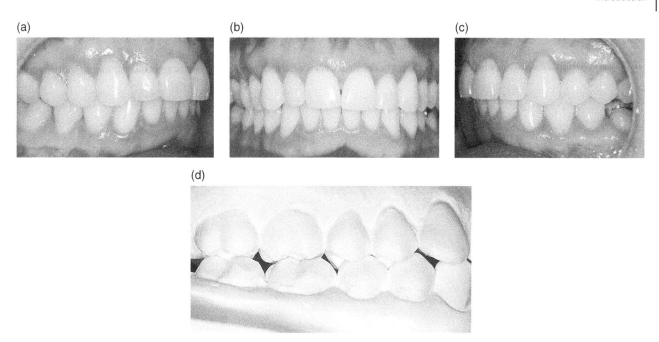

(a) (b) (c)

(d)

Figure 6.13 (a–d) Deband records of patient with the right dental crossbite. Note the large mandibular buccal wear facets in Figure 6.13d.

Figure 6.14 Depending upon the magnitude of applied transverse force (a) and the facial skeletal resistance, maxillary posterior teeth can tip/translate buccally, and the midpalatal suture can separate (b).

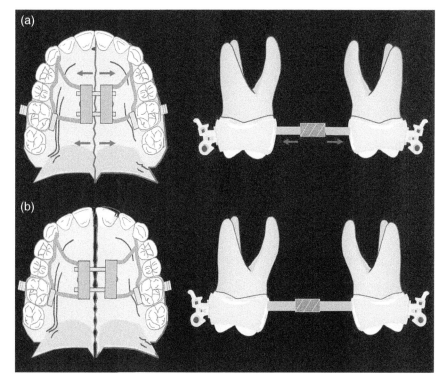

- Quad-helix – can achieve true midpalatal sutural separation if the facial skeletal resistance is low enough [40, 41].
- Hyrax expansion screw appliance – virtually guarantees true midpalatal sutural separation with skeletal expansion at this age.

Additionally:

- Tipping/buccal translation of maxillary anchor teeth will occur with each of these appliances.
- The quad-helix has significantly fewer failures, is more cost-effective, and has a shorter treatment time than an expansion plate [42, 43]. Early treatment

(a)

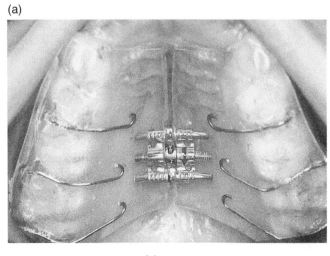

(b)

(c)

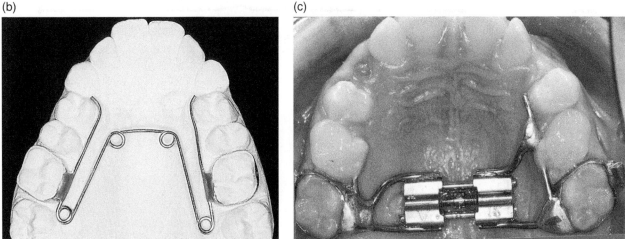

Figure 6.15 Appliance options for maxillary expansion: (a) split plate; (b) quad helix; (c) Hyrax expansion screw appliance.

with the quad-helix appliance is effective in increasing intermolar, palatal, and alveolar widths with the teeth moving through the alveolus, leading to substantial decreases in buccal bone thickness and increases in lingual bone thickness [44].

- No scientific evidence exists to show which treatment modality – expansion plate, quad-helix, Hyrax expansion screw appliance, or enameloplasty – is the most effective in crossbite correction [30].

In summary, which appliance should we use? Well, each of the above appliances may be effective in widening, or at least increasing growth of, the midpalatal suture in an eight-year-old child. However, of the three appliances, *we recommend using the Hyrax expansion screw appliance.* Why? With a Hyrax expansion screw appliance, patient compliance is minimal and skeletal expansion is virtually guaranteed before puberty.

Q: If the midpalatal suture disarticulates during RME, how do the hemi-maxillae separate? In other words, what pattern do you see with this separation? How do the maxillary teeth separate?

A: Skeletal expansion during RME is greatest in the anterior (Figure 6.16a), creating a "V" expansion of the suture [45, 46]. On the other hand, transverse movement of the maxillary first molars is approximately twice that of the maxillary canines, leading to a "reverse V" expansion of the dental arch.

Maxillary anchor teeth tip buccally [45–47]. Viewed in the frontal plane (Figures 6.16b–6.16d), a pyramidal opening occurs during RME with the fulcrum at the frontomaxillary suture [26, 48–50]. The RME creates a significant increase in nasal width, and the intermaxillary and maxillary frontal nasal sutures are the sutures primarily affected [51].

Q: When we apply a force during RME, the facial bones resist this force. What is the site of this facial skeletal resistance? Is the midpalatal suture the major site of facial skeletal resistance to RME force?

(a)

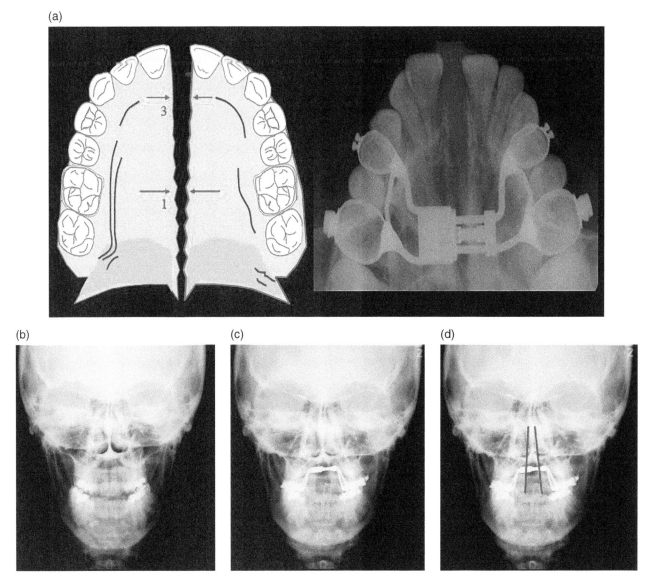

Figure 6.16 Movements of the hemi-maxillae during tooth-borne RME: (a) occlusal view; (b–d) frontal view.

A: No, the midpalatal suture is not the major site of skeletal resistance to RME. If the midpalatal suture (Figure 6.17a) was the major site of skeletal resistance to RME, then once the suture separated, the skeletal resistance would decrease dramatically. However, Isaacson and Ingram [52] reported no significant change in the RME force during the time the midpalatal suture opened.

Instead, it has been suggested that the zygomatic buttress (Figure 6.17b) is the *major* site of skeletal resistance to RME [53]. Other resistance sites include the palatal soft tissue, pterygomaxillary articulation, pterygoid plates (sphenoid bone), pyramidal processes (palatine bone), and pyriform aperture.

Q: What problem do we face in attempting RME in post-pubertal adolescents?

A: The problem we face is the increasing skeletal resistance to maxillary expansion that occurs with age. *The most marked RME skeletal effect occurs before/during the pubertal growth spurt*, and expansion after the pubertal growth spurt is mainly dentoalveolar (not orthopedic/skeletal) [18, 35, 50, 54–57]. In older adolescents, facial maturation may be too advanced and offer too much skeletal resistance to permit separation of the midpalatal suture.

In older adolescents, you may consider *attempting* RME at the rate of 0.25 mm per day, or 0.25 mm every other day, and monitor whether the midpalatal suture

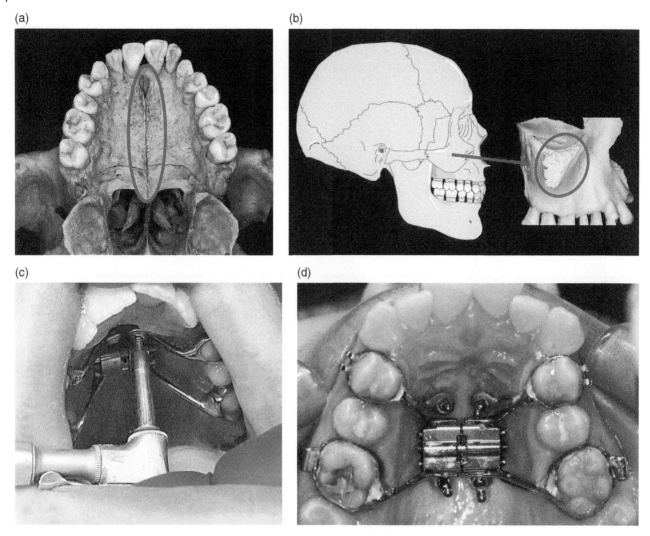

Figure 6.17 Possible sites of skeletal resistance to RME: (a) midpalatal suture, (b) zygomatic buttress – considered the *major* site of skeletal resistance, (c–d) mini-screws, inserted into palatal bone as part of the RME appliance, provide additional anchorage for overcoming skeletal resistance.

separates. On occasion, we have been able to achieve a midpalatal suture separation in women in their late teens or early twenties. The youngest person we were unable to achieve a midpalatal sutural separation in was a twelve-year-old girl.

Are there nonsurgical techniques to help overcome skeletal resistance to RME in postpubertal adolescents and young adults? Yes, in addition to including both maxillary first premolars and first permanent molars as anchors, temporary anchorage devices (TADs) (mini-screws) can be inserted into the palatal bone and attached to the Hyrax appliance (Figures 6.17c–6.17d). TAD-supported RME may help overcome skeletal resistance to RME, protect anchor teeth, and reduce buccal tipping of the posterior dentoalveolar segment [58–60].

Q: Can you offer age guidelines of when to use TAD-supported RME?

A: At the University of Iowa, we use *TAD-supported RME in children older than fifteen years* (especially in large-framed individuals).

Q: If you attempt RME in a child, how do you know whether the midpalatal suture has separated?

A: The most obvious sign of midpalatal suture separation is the development of a maxillary midline diastema (Figures 6.18a–6.18b) or radiographic evidence of midpalatal sutural separation (Figure 6.18d).

Q: If you attempt RME, how do you know when the midpalatal suture is *not* separating and you are getting only dental tipping/translation?

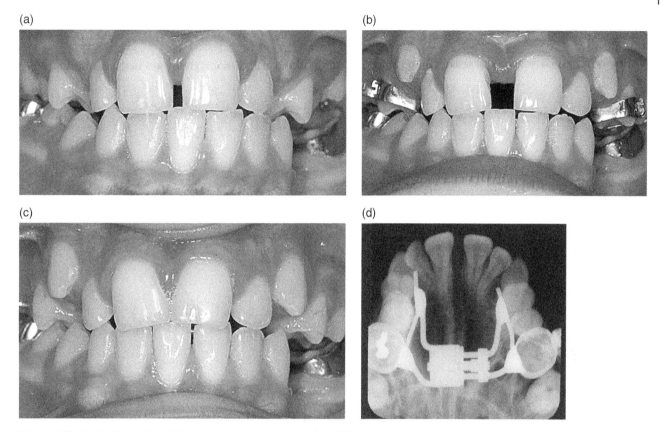

Figure 6.18 Indications of a midpalatal suture separation during RME. (a–b) development/increase of maxillary midline diastema. This diastema usually closes later (c). Radiographic widening of midpalatal suture separation (d).

A: Signs include:
- Absence of a midline diastema or absence of unequivocal radiographic midpalatal suture separation.
- Increasing impingement of the RME appliance's metal arms on the palatal alveolar process soft tissue (indicating lateral dental movement and absence of maxillary bony expansion).
- Patient sensation of expansion pressure from the screw for more than five or ten minutes after expansion screw activation.
- Patient complains of pain.

Q: When attempting RME, you must have a "fallback" plan if the midpalatal suture fails to separate (dental expansion only). Can you discuss such contingency plans?

A: Here is what we recommend:
- If the dental expansion already achieved is large compared to what you need to correct the crossbite, and if the maxillary posterior buccal periodontium is robust (thick biotype, thick buccal bone, thick keratinized attached tissue), and if you believe you can correct the crossbite by increasing posterior compensations further (masking), then your fallback plan may be continuing dental expansion slowly at the rate of 0.25 mm or 0.5 mm *per week*.
- If the dental expansion already achieved is small compared to what you need to correct the crossbite, or if the posterior buccal periodontium is of a thin biotype, then your fallback plan may be switching to a TAD-supported RME, surgical intervention (SARME), or leaving the crossbite.

Q: Is there a difference in outcome between rapid maxillary expansion (0.25–0.5 mm expansion per day) and slow maxillary expansion (0.25–0.5 mm or slower expansion per week)? Can you give a recommendation about which to use?

A: Since the 1800s, a debate has raged between those advocating rapid maxillary expansion and those claiming a slower process is less traumatic and more stable [61, 62]. The literature is mixed regarding this question:
- Hicks [35] compared his slow expansion patients to a subset of Krebs' [54] rapid expansion patients. Rapid expansion produced a greater maxillary skeletal width increase (45%) compared to slow expansion (28%). In a more recent study, RME skeletal

width increase ranged from 38 (first molar) to 55% (first premolar) [46].

- More molar bodily displacement and bone loss have been reported with slow maxillary expansion along with more molar inclination with rapid maxillary expansion [63].
- Approximately, one millimeter expansion per week is the maximum rate tissues of the midpalatal suture can adapt to so that tearing and hemorrhaging are minimized [35].
- In a systematic review [64], studies on slow maxillary expansion failed to achieve a higher level of scientific evidence, and the authors could not make strong conclusions regarding dental or skeletal changes with slow maxillary expansion.

  Recommendation – we use RME almost exclusively. However, because the skeletal and dental expansion components of RME long-term are approximately 50–50 (about the same as when done more slowly – 1 mm per week), some authors consider slow expansion to be equally effective and less traumatic than RME [25].

Q: In anticipation of transverse relapse and to permit post-expansion maxillary molar uprighting, overexpansion during RME is necessary [35, 45]. How much overexpansion do you recommend?

A: Haas recommended 50% overexpansion [65]. Assuming that any mandibular compensations have been removed (upright mandibular molars), we recommend *overexpanding until the maxillary first permanent molar lingual cusps contact the mandibular molar buccal cusps* (Figure 6.19).

Q: As the maxilla is widened during RME, how can lingually torqued mandibular posterior teeth crowns be uprighted so as to maintain arch coordination?

A: Lingually inclined mandibular posterior teeth can be uprighted by wearing crossbite elastics from the maxillary expansion appliance to mandibular molar lingual buttons (Figure 6.20a), by inserting an expanded lower lingual holding arch (LLHA), or by using a Schwarz expansion appliance (Figure 6.20b).

Q: What is the effect of RME on maxillary and mandibular anteroposterior or vertical positions?

A: The following effects have been reported during RME:
- Downward displacement of the maxilla [50, 66, 67]
- Forward displacement of the maxilla in some studies, but not all [50, 66–69]
- Downward and backward mandibular displacement (Figures 6.21a–6.21e) [50, 66–68].

- However, *long-term (> three to six years), RME has little effect on either vertical or anteroposterior facial dimensions, even in hyperdivergent patients* [70–72].

Q: Is long-term retention recommended following RME? Why?

A: Yes, long-term retention is recommended following RME. Let's look at some facts:
- There is only second-level evidence that maxillary expansion obtained with fixed appliances is stable long-term, and there is only weak indirect evidence of long-term stability using removable maxillary expansion appliances [73].
- The transversely displaced hemi-maxillae require a lengthy period of rigid stabilization in order to allow sutural readjustment and dissipation of accumulated residual forces at the contiguous articulations of the maxilla [74].
- Intermolar and intercanine relapse following RME has been shown to continue for up to *five years* post-RME [54].
- A meta-analysis reports that following a mean expansion of 6, 4.9 mm was maintained while wearing retainers, and only 2.4 mm was maintained long-term, post-retention (which the authors stated was no greater than normal growth) [75].
- *Based upon the above, we recommend lifelong retention for all RME patients.*

Q: Can you suggest a retention protocol post-RME?

A: Post-activation retention periods of three to six months, while the expansion appliance is still cemented in place, are normally recommended to allow reorganization and stabilization of rapidly expanded maxillary sutures [76]. However, *the longer we are in practice, the longer we keep the expansion appliance cemented in place*. If the patient will tolerate the appliance, then we will leave it cemented in place for nine to twelve months post-expansion. Removable retention following expansion seems less effective [35, 40, 54, 77].

In order to permit bracket bonding, leveling, and aligning of dental arches during the fixed retention period, we will convert the expansion appliance into a trans palatal arch (TPA) by cutting off the metal arms to the first premolars (Figures 6.22a–6.22b). The fact that the appliance jackscrew sits some millimeters away from the palate during this nine- to twelve-month retention period may reduce eruption of the maxillary first molars via tongue pressure. This may be desirable in patients with excess vertical

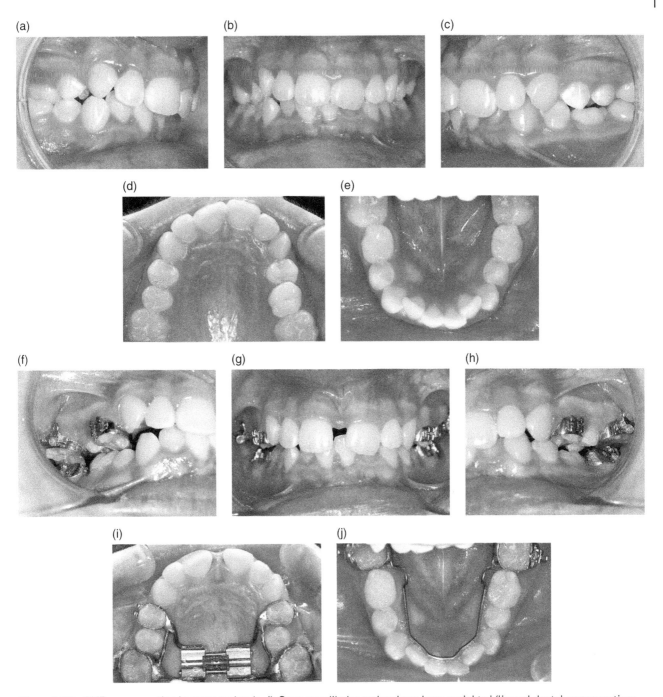

Figure 6.19 RME overcorrection/overexpansion (a–j). Once mandibular molars have been uprighted (lingual dental compensations removed), overexpand during RME until the maxillary molar lingual cusps contact the mandibular molar buccal cusps (f and h).

development but undesirable in patients with inadequate vertical development.

If the RME appliance must be removed, then another option to maintain the expansion is to insert a slightly expanded 0.032-inch stainless steel overlay wire (Figure 6.22c) into the 0.045-inch headgear tubes. Or, if the patient is wearing a headgear, simply expand the inner bow of the headgear.

Assuming the above protocol is followed post-RME, the transverse correction should be relatively stable once you have leveled and aligned the maxillary arch to stainless steel archwires of 0.018×0.025 inches or greater. However, you must continue to monitor the transverse dimension (in CR) at each visit during active treatment. Following deband, the patient should be placed in a well-fitting maxillary Hawley retainer to be worn at night for life.

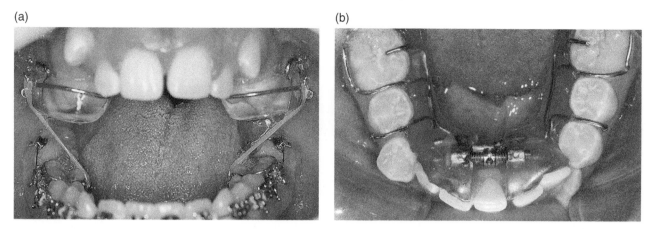

Figure 6.20 Uprighting lingually inclined mandibular posterior teeth during RME using (a) crossbite elastics to buttons on the lingual of the mandibular molars, (b) a Schwarz expansion appliance.

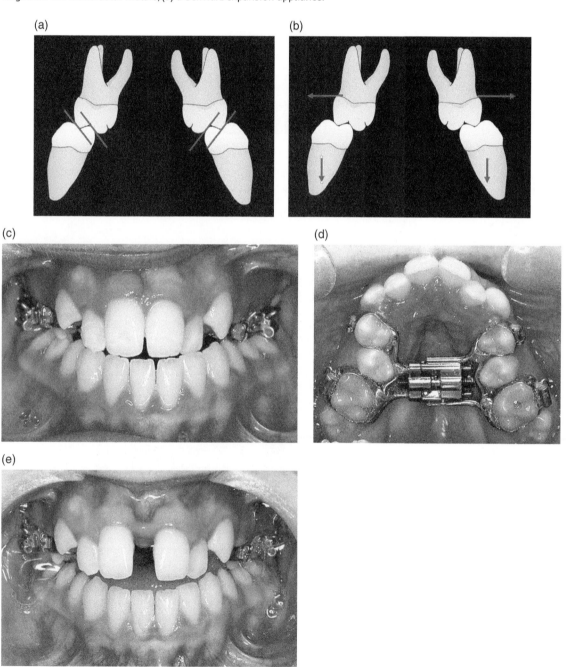

Figure 6.21 Short-term effect of RME on the vertical dimension. The presence of cuspal inclines (a) results in downward (and backward) mandibular movement (b). As the maxillary molars move buccally, bite opening results (c–e). Important note: *RME has little long-term effect on either vertical or anteroposterior facial dimensions.*

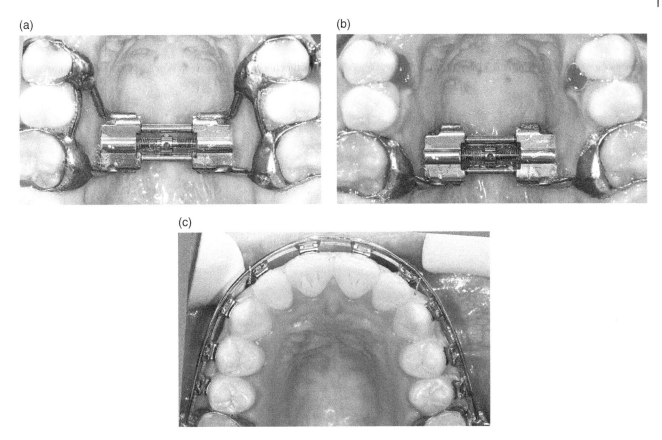

Figure 6.22 Post-RME fixed retention: (a–b) conversion of a Hyrax four-banded expansion appliance into a TPA, (c) placement of an expanded 0.032-inch stainless steel overlay wire through the molar band headgear tubes.

Q: Which expander provides greater *skeletal* expansion, a two-banded maxillary RME appliance (maxillary first permanent molars banded for anchorage) or a four-banded RME appliance (maxillary first molars and premolars banded for anchorage)?

A: *Sutural expansion is 2.5 times greater with four bands* [78, 79]. When maxillary premolars have erupted, we recommend RME using a 4-banded appliance. When maxillary premolars have not yet erupted, we recommend banding maxillary permanent first molars and bonding maxillary primary molars to metal arms extending forward from the maxillary permanent first molars.

Q: Can the maxilla be orthopedically expanded using only *primary* teeth for anchorage?

A: Yes, in young children, the facial skeletal resistance to expansion may be so small that the midpalatal suture will open using (nonmobile) maxillary primary second molars as anchor units (Figure 6.23). Using primary teeth exclusively for anchorage has been suggested as a way to avoid undesirable side effects of RME on maxillary permanent molars (e.g. root resorption) [80].

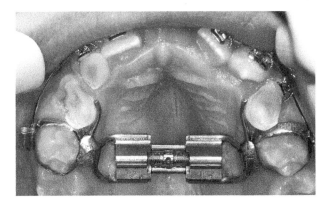

Figure 6.23 RME in a six-year-old child using banded maxillary primary second molars as anchor teeth.

Q: What do you do if the patient/parent *overexpands* the maxillary arch with the RME appliance (turns the screw too many times)?

A: First, attempt to turn the screw backward. We have had mixed results attempting this. Or, remove the expansion appliance and allow the expansion to relapse. If only the anchor teeth are overexpanded, you could remove the expansion appliance and place a Hawley retainer with the plastic selectively trimmed away lingual to the anchor teeth to permit relapse.

Q: You receive a maxillary expansion appliance back from the lab. The appliance fits very nicely on the model from which it was fabricated, so you know the laboratory did a good job. You try to seat the appliance in the patient's mouth but discover that it will not seat on the patient's left side due to the path of draw (Figure 6.24). What do you do?

A: Because maxillary molars erupt with buccal crown torque, problems with seating banded maxillary appliances are not unusual (due to their divergent path of draw). In this particular case, you could try:

- Opening the expansion screw slightly to see if that helps seat the appliance.
- Section one, or both, premolar bands from the appliance but leave the metal arms lingual to the premolars intact. Then, roughen the surface of the metal arms and bond them to the premolars (and maxillary left primary second molar if it is nonmobile) to provide anchorage in addition to the permanent first molars.
- Using larger bands for all anchor teeth (providing additional "play" during appliance seating) and having the appliance remade.
- Use a *bonded* expansion appliance instead of a banded appliance.

Q: What is the effect of RME on the periodontium?

A: *Study results appear mixed.* Of twenty eight children undergoing 4.6 mm of maxillary molar expansion [81], few children exhibited marked periodontal breakdown and minimal difference was found compared to a control group. However, in a group of eight girls, RME induced bony dehiscences on the buccal aspect of

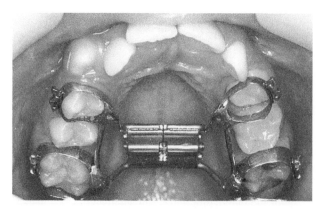

Figure 6.24 Expansion appliance which cannot seat completely.

anchor teeth, especially in children with thinner buccal plates, when measured by CT three months post-expansion [82]. Finally, Timms and Moss found histological evidence of buccal bone deposition two years post-expansion [83], and the possible long-term recovery of buccal bone remains to be investigated.

Q: Based on these mixed study results, do you have any recommendations regarding the condition of maxillary buccal periodontium before RME?

A: *Before performing maxillary expansion, confirm that the child has a thick buccal periodontal biotype (thick buccal bone, thick keratinized attached tissue) and not a thin buccal biotype (thin buccal bone, thin keratinized attached tissue).*

Figures 6.25a–6.25f illustrate a patient who presented with a thick maxillary buccal periodontal biotype, a bilateral posterior lingual crossbite, and underwent successful slow maxillary expansion. The maxillary buccal tissues were healthy before, and after, buccal expansion. On the other hand, Figures 6.25g–6.25h illustrate a patient with thin maxillary buccal bone plus gingival recession over the buccal of the maxillary left molar. Nonsurgical maxillary expansion in this patient would be ill-advised.

Even if you begin RME with a thick buccal periodontal biotype, you should visually monitor, and palpate, the buccal periodontium during expansion. *If you begin to feel the first molar roots, then you should consider discontinuing expansion.*

Q: Does RME cause root resorption?

A: Yes. Anchor premolars have been found to resorb with RME while non-anchor premolars have been shown not to resorb [84]. Further, the longer a tooth is held overcorrected, the greater the resorption. Two years after RME evidence of root resorption and repair are still present [83].

In our clinical experience the potential for significant root resorption from RME is small. However, *the risk of root resorption from any orthodontic treatment must be discussed with the patient before treatment begins.*

Q: The Haas maxillary expander (Figure 6.26) is similar to the Hyrax expander but includes acrylic pads seated against palatal alveolar process shelves. Has the Haas expander been shown to provide more orthopedic correction than a Hyrax expander?

A: No. *Hyrax and Haas expanders produce similar orthopedic effects* [85, 86]. The claims of treatment superiority with the Haas expander have not been substantiated.

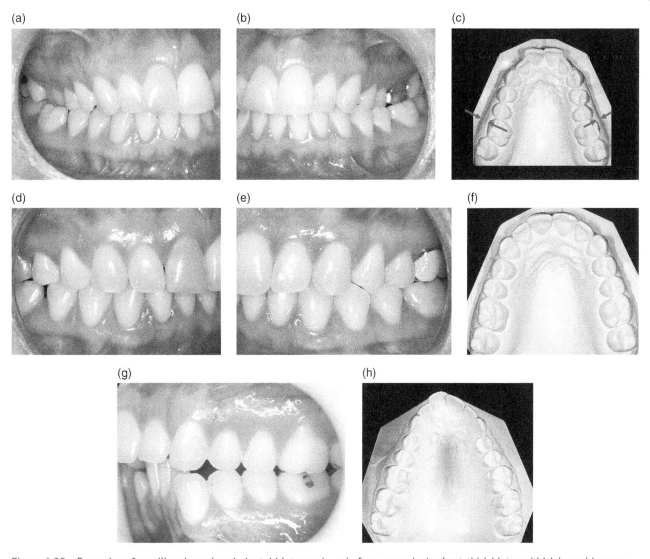

(a) (b) (c)

(d) (e) (f)

(g) (h)

Figure 6.25 Examples of maxillary buccal periodontal biotypes: (a–c, before expansion) robust, thick biotype (thick buccal bone as shown by red arrows, thick keratinized attached tissue) is favorable before buccal tooth movement/expansion, (d–f, after expansion); thin biotype (g–h, thin buccal bone with recession already present on the maxillary left first molar) is unfavorable for nonsurgical expansion.

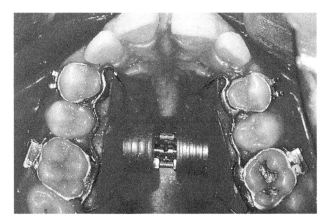

Figure 6.26 Haas maxillary expander.

Q: A child presents with a true unilateral crossbite (CR = CO, no lateral shift). Can you list the skeletal and dental differences between unilateral crossbites, bilateral crossbites, and control subjects?

A: Miner et al. [29] reported that the:
- Skeletal discrepancy in the bilateral crossbite group was due to a *narrow maxilla* and wider mandible [29].
- Molar inclination was not different between the control and bilateral crossbite groups.
- Skeletal discrepancy in the unilateral crossbite group was due to a *wider mandible*.
- Molar inclination on the crossbite side of the unilateral crossbite group was not significantly different from that of the control group.

- Dental compensations on the non-crossbite side of the unilateral crossbite group resulted in a normal transverse dental relationship on that side.

Q: A child presents with a *true unilateral lingual posterior (dental) crossbite which has not resulted from asymmetric mandibular growth.* CR = CO. How do you recommend treating it?

A: Figures 6.27a–6.27e illustrate models of a patient with a true unilateral right lingual posterior crossbite. Note the maxillary arch asymmetry (Figure 6.27d, maxillary right hour-glass shape) which is often found in these patients. On the right crossbite side, the mandibular teeth have normal buccolingual inclination (no transverse dental compensations), while on the non-crossbite side, the mandibular molars are torqued lingually (dental compensations).

First, confirm the absence of a lateral CR-CO shift. Although various acrylic appliances have been proposed for unilateral crossbite correction (Figures 6.27f–6.27h), we recommend RME using a conventional Hyrax expander (Figures 6.27i–6.27k). When using a Hyrax expander, the non-crossbite side of the maxillary arch will quickly become overexpanded. If the patient has lingual crown torque (transverse dental compensation) on the non-crossbite side of the arch, *place the patient on a crossbite elastic to upright the lingually torqued, non-crossbite side mandibular first molar – thus, moving it buccally, uprighting it, reducing the non-crossbite side overjet* (Figures 6.27l–6.27m), and allowing continued bilateral maxillary expansion (overexpansion). Figure 6.27n shows the resulting transverse relationship at the end of maxillary expansion with even left and right side posterior overexpansion.

Q: What are the advantages of bonded maxillary expanders compared to banded maxillary expanders?

A: Bonded maxillary expanders [87] (Figures 6.28a–6.28b):
- Act as bite plates to eliminate lateral CR-CO shifts
- Offer the potential of intruding (or at least reducing the eruption of) posterior teeth due to stretching of the masseteric sling by this bite plate effect
- Eliminate the need to place separators and fit bands
- Open the bite so that anterior teeth can be tipped forward out of crossbite.

Q: Does the biteplate effect of bonded RME appliances result in less vertical growth?

A: Yes, slightly. Studies report an average 0.8 mm maxillary first molar intrusion [88] and 0.5–1.5 mm reduction in downward movement of PNS [89, 90] with bonded RME appliances compared to banded RME appliances. Surprisingly, no significant difference in buccal tipping of posterior teeth has been demonstrated between bonded, and banded, RME [90].

Q: How does adolescent maxillary expansion compare when using tooth-borne versus bone-borne appliances?

A: *Results of studies appear mixed.* One study showed similar outcomes with both appliances [91], including: midpalatal suture separation; greater dental crown expansion than apical/skeletal expansion; no difference in molar apical expansion; and no difference in molar tipping. However, another study [92] reported that tooth-borne maxillary Hyrax expansion in adolescents produced more dental expansion, buccal rolling, and a greater increase in nasal width than did bone-borne expansion. Both expanders produced basal bone expansion at the level of the hard palate.

Q: What is the limit for maxillary arch expansion?

A: There are really two answers. First, a linear millimetric limit of maxillary arch expansion has never been established. At a Midwest Angle meeting, Dr. Andrew Haas (inventor of the Haas expander) once told me that 20 mm was the greatest maxillary expansion he had ever performed. We cannot recall ever expanding a maxilla more than this.

Second, another way of answering this question is to state that the *limit for maxillary arch expansion is the mandibular arch width.* The mandibular arch is the template for treatment. Ideal coordination and interdigitation with the mandibular arch are both the goals, and limits, for maxillary arch expansion at the time of deband.

Q: As a follow-up to the previous question's answer, what is the limit for mandibular arch expansion?

A: *The limit for mandibular arch expansion is the point where the mandibular posterior teeth are upright.* If the mandibular posterior teeth initially present with lingual crown torque, then it is reasonable to expand the mandibular posterior arch (assuming a thick buccal periodontal biotype) by moving the molar crowns buccally to the point where they are upright. The only way to achieve more mandibular expansion than this is to perform a symphyseal osteotomy and widen the mandible with a symphyseal bone graft or bony distraction.

Q: Can you estimate the amount of maxillary arch perimeter increase for every 1 mm of maxillary arch width increase at the first premolars during RME?

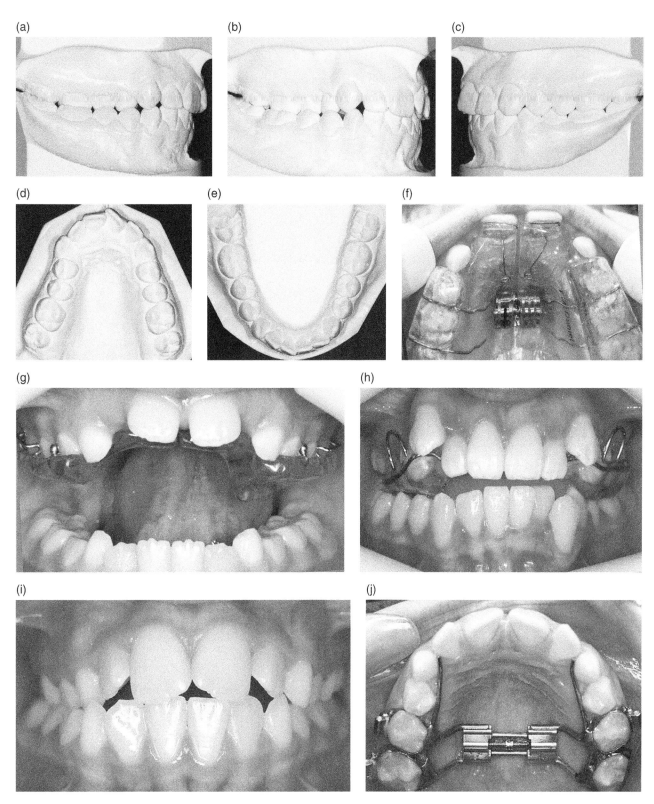

Figure 6.27 Orthopedic treatment of true unilateral crossbites: (a–e) models of a patient presenting with a true unilateral right posterior lingual crossbite (CR = CO). Note the right maxillary arch asymmetry (d), (f–g) Nord removable expander being used in a patient with a true unilateral right lingual crossbite. The right side of the appliance has a flat occlusal plastic biteplate so the maxillary teeth are free to move buccally. The left side of the appliance has an occlusal index intended to gain additional anchorage from the left mandibular arch so the maxillary teeth are prevented from moving buccally, (h) another bonded maxillary expander with the same right flat occlusal plastic biteplate and left occlusal index, (i–n) correction of a true unilateral right lingual posterior crossbite using a Hyrax appliance. Hyrax expansion results in overexpansion of the non-crossbite, left side (l). If the mandibular teeth on the non-crossbite side exhibit lingual crown torque (transverse dental compensations), they can be uprighted and moved buccally by having the patient wear an elastic from the lingual of the mandibular left molar to the buccal of the expansion appliance (l–m). The results in even left and right posterior overexpansion at the end of RME (n).

(k)

(l)

(m)

(n)

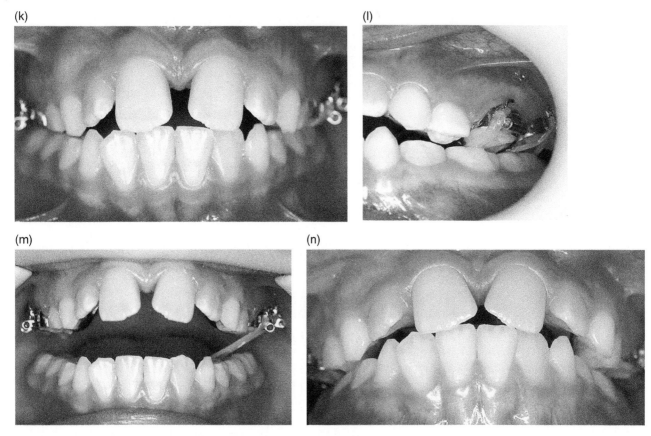

Figure 6.27 (Continued)

(a)

(b)

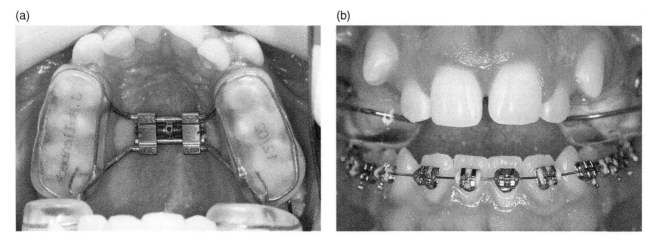

Figure 6.28 (a–b) Bonded RME appliance.

A: It has been estimated that for every 1 mm of maxillary arch width increase at the first premolars during RME, the maxillary arch perimeter increases by 0.7 mm [47].

Q: Should arch expansion be used to increase arch length (arch perimeter) in the absence of a crossbite?

A: Yes and no. *Maxillary and mandibular expansion increases arch perimeter, but the mandibular arch limits the amount of maxillary expansion that can be achieved. Expansion of both arches (at deband) beyond the point where the mandibular molar crowns are upright and excellent occlusal interdigitation achieved, is inherently unstable and not recommended.*

As previously stated, we reported that maxillary molars erupt with buccal crown torque and upright with age while mandibular molars erupt with lingual crown torque and upright with age [1]. Because this is an inherent part of normal human facial growth, uprighting lingually inclined mandibular molars to a more upright position is a reasonable orthodontic treatment (assuming the other goals of transverse treatment presented earlier can be achieved).

Expansion resulting from mandibular molar uprighting will create an additional arch perimeter. In cases with lingually inclined mandibular molars, the molar roots are lateral to the crowns and moving the crowns to a position directly over the roots can be appropriate. However, if the mandibular posterior teeth are already upright, then arch expansion that results in labial crown torque is ill-advised.

We again wish to emphasize that it is the intermolar width of upright mandibular molars that ultimately determines the limit of potential maxillary expansion. Unless the mandible is widened (surgically, e.g. symphyseal distraction), the mandibular basal bone width is fixed.

Finally, arch expansion (arch development) increases cheek pressure against the teeth, so instability can be a significant problem. As Little [93] has noted, arch development (widening arches) in the mixed dentition without lifetime retention yields unstable results.

Q: What is a non-extraction alternative to mandibular expansion to gain arch space?

A: *Place an LLHA in the mixed dentition to preserve leeway space.* Gianelly noted that 68% of patients with crowding will have adequate space for alignment if a lower lingual holding arch is used to preserve leeway space, and another 19% will have adequate space with only marginal crowding (up to 1 mm per side) [94]. Further, for mixed dentition cases with favorable leeway space, treatment results using a lower lingual holding arch appear stable [93]. Of course, interproximal enamel reduction (IPR, slenderizing) is another way to gain arch space.

Q: Do *mandibular* arch intercanine and intermolar widths spontaneously increase with RME (Figure 6.29)?

A: *Results of studies investigating the effect of RME on mandibular intercanine and intermolar widths are mixed.* The concept behind this question is intuitively appealing because as the maxilla is expanded, the cheeks are pushed buccally by the maxillary teeth. So, the tongue should push the mandibular canines and posterior teeth buccally, increasing intercanine and intermolar widths. However, mandibular intermolar width increases with RME have been found to range from 0 to over 3 mm and mandibular intercanine width increases

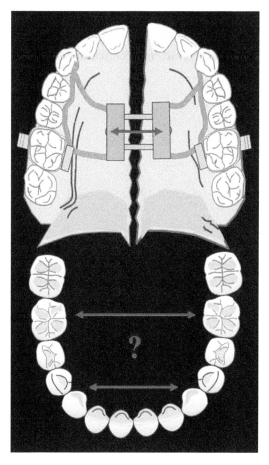

Figure 6.29 Effects of RME on the mandibular arch.

have been found to range from 0 to less than 1 mm [26, 47, 50, 69, 95–101]. We speculate that spontaneous mandibular effects relate to the magnitude of the maxillary expansion.

Q: Is mandibular arch expansion stable when used in conjunction with RME?

A: *Reports suggesting stability are mixed* [65, 97, 102–104]. Further study is necessary. We do not recommend that patients be told RME will improve mandibular arch expansion stability.

Q: Assume that you are seating an RME appliance and the maxillary left first premolar band splits (Figure 6.30a). What can you do?

A: Instead of remaking the expansion appliance, simply remove the split premolar band, prepare the lingual surfaces of the premolars for bonding, roughen the appliance steel arms next to the maxillary left premolars to better hold the bonding material, and bond the lingual of the premolars to the appliance arms (Figure 6.30b).

(a)

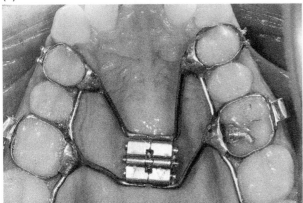

(b)

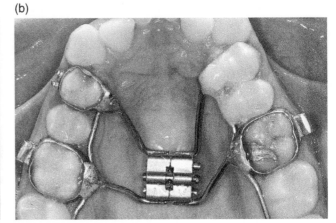

Figure 6.30 If the maxillary left first premolar band splits during RME placement (a), simply remove the band and bond the expansion appliance steel arms to the maxillary left premolars (b).

Q: In addition to expanding the maxillary bones, why else did RME gain popularity?

A: A belief that it could improve nasal breathing [105].

Q: What is the effect of RME on the nasal cross-sectional area? On upper airway volume?

A: RME increases nasal width, nasal cross-sectional area, [54, 55, 65, 106–111], and seems to be associated with an increase in the nasal cavity volume both in the short, and long, term [112]. However, changes in nasal volume are small [113].

Q: Should RME be used to treat obstructive sleep apnea in children?

A: We are fortunate that the American Association of Orthodontists provided the specialty with a White Paper discussing this topic [114]. We recommend following these guidelines:

- The definitive diagnosis of obstructive sleep apnea is appropriately made by a physician. If the patient is found to have OSA, the physician should decide on an appropriate course of action for the treatment of OSA.
- The orthodontist may choose to work in a collaborative way with the physician, providing orthodontic treatment when necessary and when it does not interfere with ongoing medical treatment.
- The primary objective of the RME appliance should be to improve the occlusion and address the underlying skeletal discrepancy.
- Secondary effects of this treatment may result in the reduction of nasal airway resistance and an increase in the volume of the nasopharynx and nasal cavity.
- An OSA patient might be referred for expansion who does not have a transverse discrepancy. The treatment

alternatives should be considered on a case-by-case basis by the medical and dental practitioners involved. In such situations, it is appropriate to prioritize the treatments to serve the best interests of the patient.

Q: Does prophylactic RME prevent the future development of obstructive sleep apnea?

A: There is no indication in the literature that prophylactic maxillary expansion prevents the future development of OSA [114].

Q: Has RME been suggested as a possible treatment for other medical problems?

A: Yes, *RME has been suggested as a treatment for nocturnal enuresis (NE, bed wetting)* [115–118]. NE is thought to result from an insufficient arousal response, insufficient vasopressin (ADH) production, increased intraabdominal pressure (pressure from respiratory efforts against an obstructed airway), and decreased oxygen saturation (resulting in myoclonus). Conventional NE treatments include ADH substitution and addressing any airway obstruction [119, 120].

Q: Can RME change the soft-tissue profile?

A: Yes, during RME use, but not post-retention [121].

Q: Some have suggested that in the absence of a posterior crossbite, RME be used to correct a Class II relationship. Is this notion true?

A: *Since Class II functional appliances, which actively posture the mandible forward, do not enhance mandibular forward growth in the long term, it is doubtful that RME enhances mandibular growth.* Any Class II improvement with RME in adolescence is probably due to unlocking of the occlusion. Since there is greater normal forward growth of the mandible during adolescence compared to the maxilla, unlocking the occlusion may allow the mandibular posterior teeth to move forward with mandible growth (improving the Class II relationship), instead of being held back by the maxillary teeth. Let's discuss this in more detail.

Short-term functional appliance studies by Stöckli and Willert [122], McNamara [123], and Woodside and coworkers [124] clearly demonstrate that if an appliance postures the mandible forward, then remodeling changes in the temporomandibular joint occur that tend to bring the mandible forward. In a magnetic resonance imaging study, Ruf and Pancherz demonstrated the same effect [125]. Thus, in the short term, Class II functional appliances have been shown to remodel the joint (accelerate growth).

However, acceleration in the short-term does not translate into enhanced growth, long term. DeVincenzo reported significant, short-term increases in mandibular length when children wore the twin-block appliance [126]. However, compared with controls, this significant increase gradually diminished with time. By the fourth year after treatment with the twin-block appliance, DeVincenzo reported no significant difference in mandibular length compared with controls. Wieslander, in a study of the headgear-Herbst treatment followed by activator appliance treatment, reported that the mandibular protrusive effect of these appliances decreased to insignificance years after treatment [127]. Wieslander stated that the long-term skeletal effect did not come from enhanced mandibular growth but rather from maxillary restriction with the Herbst appliance and activator. Pancherz [128] reported no long-term influence of Herbst treatment on mandibular growth. In other words, *in the short term, Class II functional appliances enhance (accelerate) mandibular growth; but in the long term, controls catch up.*

If in the long term, hyperpropulsive functional appliances do not enhance mandibular growth compared with controls, then how can one possibly anticipate improvement in Class II relationships through RME? There may be a simple explanation. Research has shown that during adolescence, the mandible usually grows forward more than the maxilla [129–131]. For this reason, orthodontists should typically see a spontaneous improvement in Class II patients during growth without any treatment at all. However, in fact, we do not see it. Most orthodontists would agree that Class II malocclusions are not self-correcting, and studies have demonstrated that minimal change occurs in a Class II relationship in growing patients [132, 133]. Reasons for this phenomenon need further evaluation.

You et al. [134] compared mandibular growth in a sample of untreated Class II malocclusion children to a sample of norms. Their findings confirmed earlier studies that forward growth of the mandible during adolescence exceeded that of the maxilla (by over 4 mm). However, they also reported that the effect of forward growth of the mandible, which could potentially bring the lower dentition forward, vanished because of *intercuspal locking.* In other words, without treatment, as the mandible outgrew the maxilla, intercuspal locking caused the mandibular teeth to drag the maxillary teeth mesially, the maxillary teeth to drag the mandibular teeth posteriorly, and the Class II relationship to be left intact. Lager [135] recommended the elimination of intercuspal locking in a growing Class II patient with a biteplate to allow forward movement of the mandibular dentition (improvement in the anteroposterior relationship) with mandibular growth.

In summary, *Class II improvement with RME in adolescence is probably due to unlocking of the occlusion and the greater normal forward growth of the mandible compared with the maxilla.*

Q: We have discussed the orthopedic treatment of skeletal crossbites. Let's next discuss *masking (camouflage)* as a means to treat skeletal crossbites. What is masking in the transverse dimension?

A: Masking is the correction of skeletal crossbites with dental movement – without treating the underlying skeletal discrepancy. Masking usually involves placing (or increasing) posterior transverse compensations, often in combination with transverse bodily tooth movement. We introduce masking here, but masking is generally reserved for treatment in adult dentition during comprehensive orthodontics.

For example, masking is illustrated in Figure 6.31 as a way to correct a bilateral lingual crossbite caused by a skeletally narrow maxilla. The maxillary first molars are tipped buccally (Figure 6.31a, buccal crown torque) while the mandibular molars are tipped lingually (Figure 6.31b, lingual crown torque). These torquing movements correct the lingual crossbite (Figure 6.31c) without addressing the underlying narrow maxilla. Masking could also consist of translating maxillary first molars buccally and/or translating mandibular first molars lingually. The point is that masking consists of dental, not skeletal, movements to improve the occlusion.

Q: Can you list five options for masking skeletal crossbites?

A: Options include the following:
- TPAs or LLHAs to *bilaterally* expand, or constrict, arches (Figure 6.32) by translating teeth through

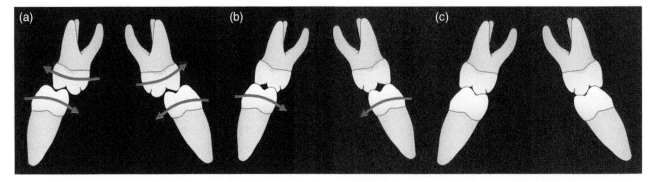

Figure 6.31 (a–c) Masking (camouflage) to correct a bilateral lingual skeletal crossbite caused by a narrow maxilla. *Masking consists of dental movements to improve the transverse occlusion* while orthopedics and surgery consist of skeletal change to improve the occlusion.

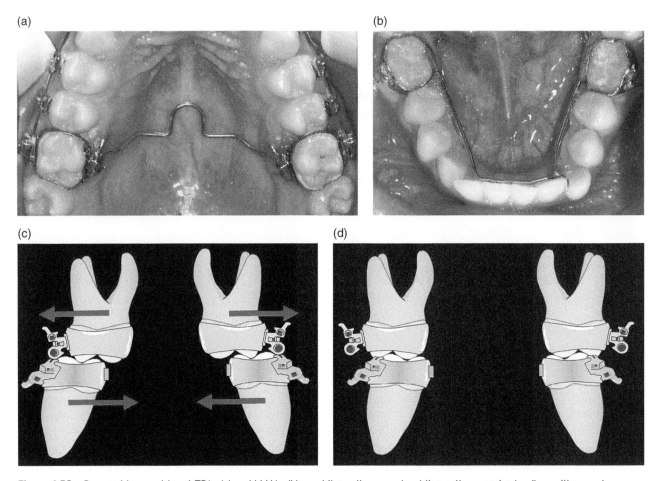

Figure 6.32 Removable or soldered, TPAs (a) and LLHAs (b) can *bilaterally* expand or bilaterally constrict (c–d) maxillary and mandibular molars.

bone. We italicized the word *bilaterally* for a reason. In correcting unilateral crossbites, orthodontic residents will frequently suggest using a TPA or LLHA but forget that the expansive/constrictive forces are exerted *bilaterally*.

- Note: If the skeletal resistance is low enough in a child, the bilateral expansive force of a TPA may be large enough to create midpalatal sutural separation (skeletal expansion).

- TPAs or LLHAs to increase molar compensations (buccal or lingual crown torques, Figures 6.31a–6.31c) bilaterally, or unilaterally.
- Bilateral maxillary dental expansion using a Hyrax appliance (RME appliance) if skeletal resistance prevents the midpalatal suture from opening.
- Crossbite elastics (Figure 6.33) to either place compensations or remove compensations. Crossbite elastics can be used unilaterally, or bilaterally. If the

crossbite involves permanent first molars *and* primary molars, then elastics should also include the primary molars. Why? Failure to correct the primary tooth crossbite will result in a high probability of the permanent premolars erupting into crossbite [7].

- Bilateral expansion (or constriction) using expanded (or constricted) archwires or overlay wires (Figures 6.34a–6.34c).

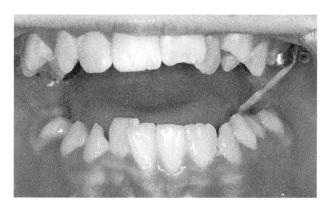

Figure 6.33 Crossbite elastic.

(a)

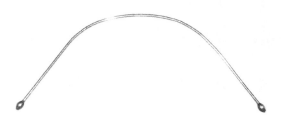

- Bilateral expansion using a maxillary split plate (Figure 6.15a) or mandibular Schwarz expansion appliance (Figures 6.35a–6.35b). Expansion with the Schwarz appliance is primarily dentoalveolar [136].

Removable expansion plates may be designed for correction of true unilateral crossbites involving one or two teeth. However, because removable plates exert equal but opposite bilateral forces when activated, an increasingly bilateral effect will result as more teeth are involved.

Q: With each of the previous masking options, can you state whether the teeth will be translated laterally, torqued (tipped) laterally, or undergo a combination of translation and torquing?

A: The exact movement will depend upon the force and moment applied at the *center of resistance (CR) of the tooth*.

For example, in Figure 6.36a, a lingual force is applied to the maxillary first molar crown, and a buccal force is applied to the mandibular first molar crown.

(b) (c)

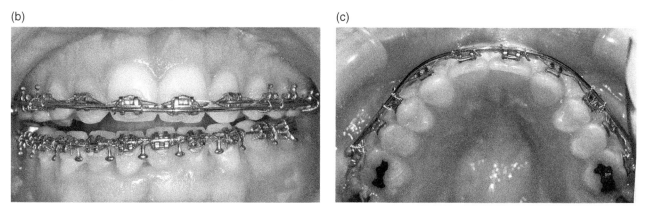

Figure 6.34 Expanded maxillary 0.032-inch stainless steel overlay wire (a) with tips covered in silver solder to reduce irritation, (b–c) expanded overlay wire secured with steel ligatures to maxillary brackets *over* the base maxillary archwire, which is ligated into the bracket slots.

(a)

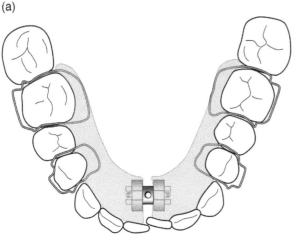

(b)

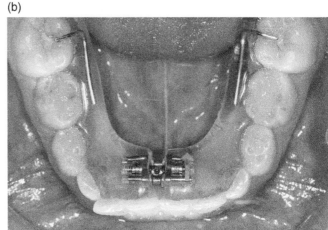

Figure 6.35 (a–b) Schwarz expanders.

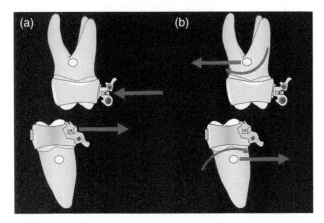

Figure 6.36 Application of forces to the molar crowns (a) equals the same force plus a moment (b) at CR (yellow dots).

For the maxillary molar, the lingual force equates to (Figure 6.36b) a lingual force plus a CW moment at CR (yellow dot), which results in maxillary molar lingual translation *and* lingual crown tip. For the mandibular molar, the buccal force equates to a buccal force plus CW moment at CR which results in mandibular molar buccal translation and buccal crown tip.

If a maxillary appliance, such as a TPA, can apply this force to the molar crown and *concurrently apply a CCW moment*, then this CCW moment can cancel the CW moment at CR, leaving only a pure lingual force acting at CR and resulting in pure lingual maxillary molar translation. A TPA is capable of adding a CCW moment, but a removable split plate or crossbite elastic is not.

Likewise, if a mandibular appliance, such as an LLHA, can apply this force to the molar crown and concurrently apply a CCW moment, then the CCW moment could cancel the CW moment at CR, leaving

only a pure buccal force acting at CR and resulting in pure buccal translation. An LLHA is capable of adding this CCW moment, but a Schwarz appliance or crossbite elastic is not.

Q: Do you have a recommendation regarding masking and the periodontium?

A: We suggest the same recommendation that we made earlier (Figure 6.25) – *before performing maxillary or mandibular buccal expansion, confirm that the patient has a thick buccal periodontal biotype (thick buccal bone, thick keratinized attached tissue) and not a thin buccal biotype (thin buccal bone, thin keratinized attached tissue).* If you fail to follow this principle, you may end up with bony dehiscences, fenestrations, or gingival recession.

Q: Do you have any recommendations regarding masking limits?

A: Yes, a *3–5 mm correction is a reasonable transverse correction to attempt with masking.* We recommend avoiding masking with a thin buccal periodontal biotype.

The literature does not offer limits on the amount of buccolingual tip (torque) which can be placed in molars, since a large variation in transverse dental compensations exists in the absence of crossbites [29]. There does not appear to be a scientific reason to prevent us from increasing posterior teeth compensations, even in children. However, molars normally upright with age [1]; upright molars are a standard required by the American Board of Orthodontics, and masking transverse discrepancies is a compromise treatment.

We may offer masking as a compromise crossbite treatment option for adults, but *in children, we recommend crossbite correction with orthopedics whenever*

(a)

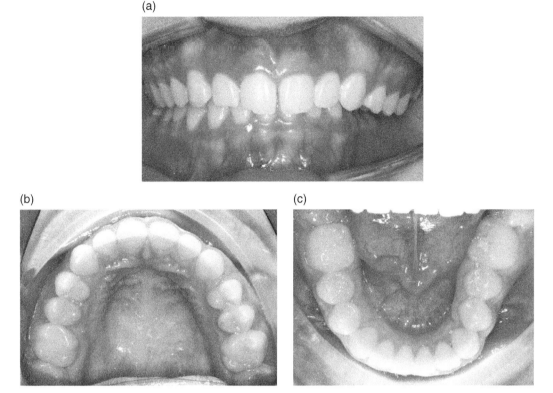

(b) (c)

Figure 6.37 (a–c) Patient with left scissor bite (photographs courtesy of Dr. Mike Callan).

possible in order to increase posterior overjet, permit elimination of transverse dental compensations, and finish with upright molars.

Q: Would you like to think outside the box? An older adolescent presents to you with a left scissor bite (left complete buccal crossbite), Class I relationship, and CR = CO (Figure 6.37a–c). Can you suggest *masking* options for correcting this scissor bite?

A: Options include:
- *Aligning the mandibular arch with a broad arch form.* Because the mandibular arch has an hourglass shape on the patient's left side, and because the mandibular left first molar appears to be torqued/tipped lingually, the mandibular left premolars and molars should move buccally with a broad arch form. This buccal movement will improve/correct the left crossbite and upright the lingually torqued mandibular molar.
- *Left crossbite elastics*, worn between fixed orthodontic appliances on both arches, from the maxillary left buccal to the mandibular left lingual.
- As a novel alternative, two *TADs* were placed in the palate (Figure 6.38) as TPA anchors to allow unilateral lingual translation of the maxillary left posterior teeth.

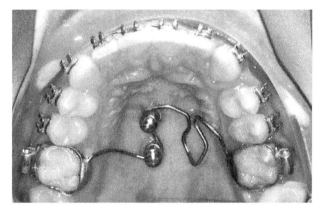

Figure 6.38 Palatal TADs used as anchors to move maxillary left posterior teeth lingually (note the lingual movement of the maxillary left first molar relative to the unbanded maxillary left second molar) (photographs courtesy of Dr. Michael Callan).

Q: Having covered orthopedic and masking treatment of skeletal crossbites, let's now turn our attention to *surgical* treatment of skeletal crossbites. Maxillary and mandibular surgeries are more appropriate for adult treatment – when growth is complete; when the maxillary facial bones offer too much skeletal resistance to attempt RME; and when the magnitude of the transverse correction needed, or the condition of the periodontium, prohibit masking. Orthognathic surgeries are

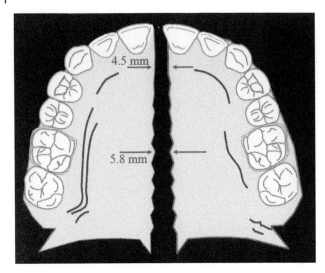

Figure 6.39 Maxillary expansion with SARME can produce significant *anterior* widening.

generally not considered in children unless growth is very nearly complete. We would like to review/introduce a few concepts of transverse surgeries for general background information.

Let's consider maxillary transverse surgeries first. Can you suggest guidelines for considering surgically assisted rapid maxillary expansion (SARME) versus multiple piece maxillary osteotomy (MPMO)?

A: Recommended guidelines include the following:

- SARME is chosen for *maxillary expansions of 10 mm or more* because the tissue is being grown with a SARME (histogenesis). The *limit of expansion with MPMO is 8–10 mm* due to soft tissue stretch, depending on the height of the palate.
- SARME is chosen when *only transverse widening is needed*. MPMO is chosen when the maxilla must also be moved in other directions (impaction, downgraft, advancement, setback). Why? MPMO requires downfracturing the maxilla which is necessary only if other maxillary movements are required.
- SARME is chosen (Figure 6.39) if significant maxillary *intercanine widening is desired* [137, 138] (e.g. patients with significant tapering of the maxillary arch). Incidentally, more posterior widening has been reported to occur with SARME than anterior widening.
- SARME is chosen in cases of a low palatal vault (where palatal soft tissue is quickly stretched during transverse expansion surgery). MPMO can be considered in cases of high palatal vault where palatal soft tissue stretch will be less restrictive.

- MPMO is chosen in patients with *significant anterior occlusal steps* – where the maxillary arch must be surgically treated in two planes. Research indicates that orthodontic leveling an anterior step up to 2 mm is stable post-treatment [139], but research is lacking regarding the stability of orthodontic leveling of anterior occlusal steps greater than 2 mm. Certainly, an anterior step of 6 mm or more would warrant maxillary surgery in two planes.
- MPMO is chosen in cases of maxillary transverse skeletal excess – where a wedge of maxillary bone is removed in order to narrow the maxilla.
- SARME exhibits minimal relapse and overcorrection is generally unnecessary. On the other hand, MPMO can be unstable. Surgical expansion with an MPMO should include overexpansion by 20%; a fixed occlusal splint placed at the time of surgery to hold the transverse correction for six weeks postsurgically; and the use of a palatal splint, TPA, or heavy overlay wire to hold the transverse correction for as long as possible after the occlusal splint is removed [18, 137, 140, 141].
- MPMO – the orthodontist should remove transverse compensations (upright posterior teeth) *before* surgery.
- MPMO – *the more pieces, the more the problems*. Keep the number of bony cuts to a minimum (ensuring an adequate blood supply).

Q: In terms of the surgery itself, what is the *principal* difference between SARME and an MPMO?

A: *Downfracture of the maxilla*. Both surgeries include a horizontal osteotomy of the lateral maxillary wall, separation of the lateral nasal wall, nasal septum disarticulation, and palatal osteotomy. But, the maxilla is downfractured in MPMO and not downfractured with SARME.

Q: Describe the difference between a two-piece and a three-piece MPMO.

A: In a traditional two-piece MPMO (Figures 6.40a–6.40b), a bony cut is made para-sagittally, and the maxilla is widened by opening (rotating) the two hemi-maxillae around the central incisors. Therefore, the intercanine width increases, but it increases less than the intermolar width increases. Two-piece MPMOs can also be designed with osteotomy cuts made, not para-sagittally, but instead involving only one posterior segment.

In a three-piece MPMO (Figures 6.40c–6.40d), the intercanine width is left unchanged because osteotomy cuts are made distal to the canines. Only the posterior maxilla is widened. Depending upon the surgical goals, three-piece MPMOs can also be designed with

(a)

(b)

(c)

(d)

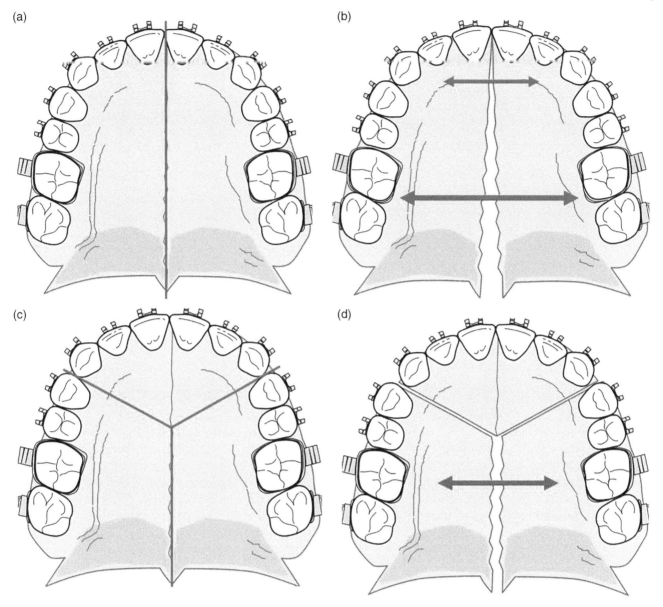

Figure 6.40 A two-piece (a–b) and three-piece (c–d) MPMO.

osteotomy cuts distal to one or both premolars – or without widening the posterior at all and only surgically leveling a significant anterior occlusal step.

Q: As an example of the decision-making involved in a transverse surgical case, Figures 6.41a–6.41b illustrate a patient's initial mandibular model advanced to its anticipated, postsurgical position following mandibular first premolar extractions, mandibular canine retraction, and mandibular advancement surgery. This is the same patient shown in Figures 6.25g–6.25h. In planning this patient's treatment with the mandibular model advanced, what do you note in terms of the resulting transverse relationship following the advancement?

A: The initial models, with mandibular model advanced to its anticipated postsurgical position, exhibit a bilateral crossbite, especially noticable in the anterior. The interach width of the patient's maxillary arch is inadequate by approximately 3–4 mm on each side (6–8 mm total), *especially in the canine area*. Looking at the initial maxillary model (Figure 6.41c), the reason for this intercanine discrepancy is patently clear – an anteriorly tapered maxillary arch.

Q: Although the previous question deals with an adult occlusion, let's continue with this exercise. What are your options for managing this anticipated post-advancement bilateral crossbite? Why would, or why would you not, choose each option?

(a)   (b)   (c)

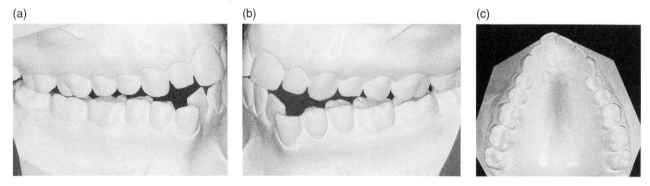

Figure 6.41 (a–c) Relationship of patient's initial models with mandibular model advanced to the anticipted, postsurgical, position (a–b). Initial maxillary model demonstrating a tapered maxillary anterior arch.

A: Options include the following:
- No treatment – leave the patient in crossbite. This option is unacceptable. If the patient is willing to undergo major surgery to improve appearance/bite, then not addressing the anticipated crossbite would be inexcusable.
- *Attempting* RME (orthopedics) – is *not recommended* due to the gingival recession buccal to the patient's maxillary left first molar (Figure 6.25g). Even if this site was grafted, the risk of further recession during RME is significant.
- Masking (camouflage; increasing buccal crown torque of the maxillary canines and maxillary posterior teeth, plus increasing lingual crown torque of the mandibular posterior teeth, plus translating the maxillary canines and posterior teeth buccally) – is *not recommended* due to the magnitude of his anticipated transverse discrepancy, the presence of maxillary buccal gingival recession, and the fact that our goal is an ideal outcome.
- SARME – would guarantee enough posterior overjet to correct the crossbite and upright posterior teeth without taxing the maxillary buccal gingiva. Another advantage of SARME is that it would provide significant *anterior* expansion, which the patient's anteriorly tapered maxilla needs. A drawback of SARME is that the patient will need to go through two major surgeries – first the SARME and then the mandibular advancement. Some patients refuse a second surgical procedure.
- MPMO – is not recommended. Why? The amount of maxillary intercanine widening we could achieve with a two-piece MPMO is inadequate. With a three-piece MPMO, the maxillary intercanine width would be left unchanged.

Q: Can you describe at least four mandibular surgeries that are used in treating skeletal posterior crossbites?

A: Possible surgeries include:
- Mandibular bilateral sagittal split osteotomy (BSSO) advancements can improve/correct posterior *buccal* crossbites by advancing a wider part of the mandibular arch into a narrower part of the maxillary arch (Figures 6.42a–6.42c). In a similar fashion, a mandibular BSSO setback can improve/correct a posterior *lingual* crossbite by moving a narrower part of the mandibular arch into a wider part of the maxillary arch.
- Mandibular bilateral sagittal split osteotomies can be used to advance, or set back, one side of an asymmetric mandible and improve/correct transverse relationships. Figure 6.42d and f illustrate a Class III subdivision left the patient with excessive left mandibular growth and resulting right posterior crossbite. A mandibular bilateral sagittal split setback osteotomy corrected her left Class III relationship and her right posterior crossbite (Figures 6.42e and 6.42g).
- To reduce the mandibular intermolar width, a mandibular midline osteotomy combined with "rolling the two hemi-mandibles lingually" (Figure 6.42h) has been proposed [142, 143].
- The mandible can be constricted by extracting a mandibular central incisor, performing a mandibular midline osteotomy, removing bone at the extraction site, and fixating the two hemi-mandibles in contact at the symphysis.
- The mandible can be widened by performing a mandibular midline osteotomy, separating the two hemi-mandibles at the midline, bridging the symphyseal defect with a bone graft, then fixating the two hemi-mandibles and bone graft.
- The mandible can be widened by symphyseal distraction [144–146] using either a tooth-borne, or bone-borne, distraction device. A mid-symphyseal bony cut is made, a four- to five-day latency period

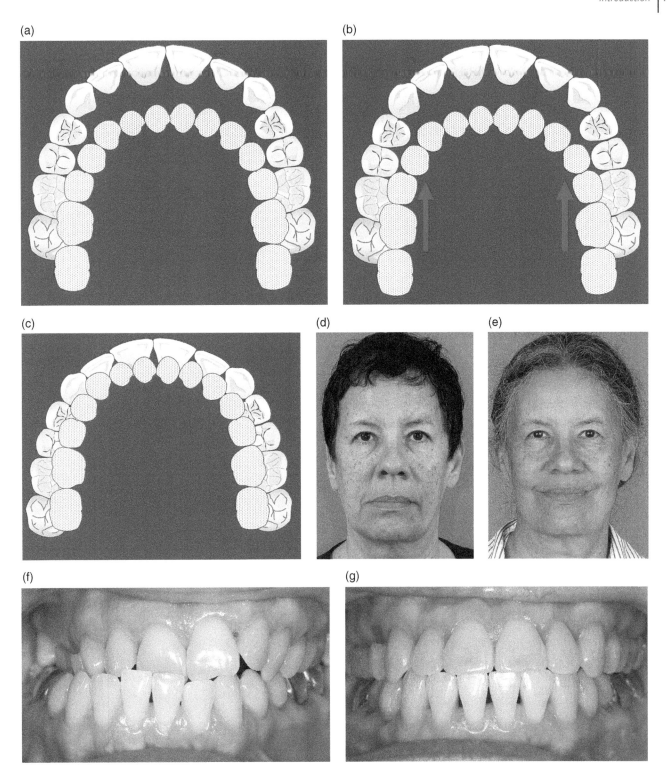

Figure 6.42 Mandibular surgeries used in correcting posterior crossbites: (a–c) a BSSO advancement will generally improve the transverse relationship in cases of buccal crossbite, (d, f) patient with right posterior crossbite and deviation of the chin to the right caused by excessive left condylar growth successfully treated (e, g) with an asymmetric BSSO setback, (h) midline osteotomy and "rolling lingually" of hemi-mandibles to reduce mandibular inter-canine and intermolar widths, (i–l) symphyseal distraction to widen mandibular inter-canine *and* intermolar widths.

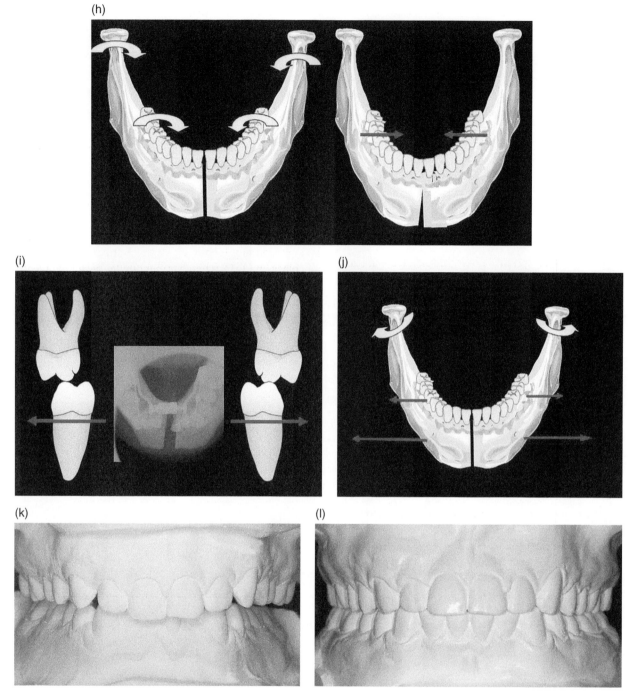

Figure 6.42 (Continued)

is allowed, and then activation of 0.75 mm per day (midline opening) is followed until the desired mandibular expansion is achieved (Figure 6.42i). Overexpansion is not performed, and the expansion device is left in place for a minimum of three months for stability. Prior studies have shown that osseous expansion achieved by mandibular symphyseal distraction osteogenesis is stable in the long term [147, 148]. During distraction osteogenesis, there is a progressive bone generation and expansion of the soft tissue envelope, which contributes to long-term stability.

We wish to emphasize that when widening the mandible using this technique or a midline osteotomy with bone graft, *widening of the entire mandibular arch takes place*, not just the intercanine width (Figure 6.42j). As an example, the patient whose models are shown in Figure 6.42k required mandibular expansion from the canines to the second molars. Symphyseal distraction was appropriate and resulted in the correction of his entire transverse relationship (Figure 6.42l).

Q: Now that we have reviewed the salient points regarding transverse discrepancies, let's return to Anneke (Figures 6.2a–6.2s). What are your options for dealing with Anneke's *unilateral left lingual posterior crossbite* (CR = CO)? Why would you choose, or not choose, each option?

A: Options include:

- No treatment – leaving her in the left posterior crossbite. This option is not recommended – at least not long term. However, since she is only seven years old, is in the early mixed dentition, and lacks a lateral CR-CO shift, there would be no harm in waiting one year to treat the posterior crossbite.
- RME (orthopedics) – is the recommended treatment. Her facial skeleton should offer little resistance to RME at age seven years, and her maxillary permanent first molars are available for anchorage.

If, during RME, she begins to overexpand on her right side before her left crossbite is corrected, then we will ask her to wear right crossbite elastics from lingual buttons on her mandibular right posterior teeth to the right buccal of her RME. These crossbite elastics will move her mandibular right posterior teeth buccally, upright her mandibular right permanent first molar, reduce her right posterior overjet, and allow us to continue RME.

- Masking (camouflage, increasing transverse compensations) – translating her maxillary left posterior teeth buccally, translating her mandibular left posterior teeth lingually, torquing her maxillary left posterior teeth crowns buccally, and/or torquing her mandibular left posterior teeth crowns lingually.

This option is not recommended. Masking may be a viable alternative in an adult dentition when an attempt at orthopedic correction failed and if the periodontium is robust. But placing compensations in a child (when ideal orthopedic treatment is possible) is a compromise and unacceptable.

- Surgery (SARME or MPMO) – would guarantee the skeletal correction of her unilateral posterior crossbite. However, surgery at Anneke's age to address a mild-to-moderate skeletal crossbite is ill-advised, especially since ideal orthopedic treatment is possible.

Q: Do you recommend early treatment to address Anneke's unilateral left posterior crossbite? If yes, what treatment do you recommend?

A: We decided to proceed with treatment. A Hyrax expansion appliance was fabricated and placed. RME proceeded. The Hyrax appliance was left in place for six months post-expansion, at which time it was removed (Figure 6.43). Thankfully, the left crossbite was corrected before the right (non-crossbite) side expanded into a buccal crossbite (Figure 6.43e).

Q: How do you recommend proceeding now?

A: Anneke was given a clear maxillary retainer to wear at night. She was scheduled for recall appointments every three months to monitor tooth eruption. We planned to place an LLHA when her mandibular permanent teeth were closer to eruption to utilize leeway space (note moderate mandibular anterior crowding). She kept her recall appointments for some time, but then failed recall appointments for two years.

Q: Anneke returned to our clinic when she was twelve years old at which time progress records were made (Figure 6.44). She had not worn her maxillary clear retainer. Can you identify her primary problems now?

A:

Table 6.2 Primary problems list for Anneke at age twelve years.

AP	Maxillary anteroposterior deficiency (A-Point lies behind Na-Perpendicular Line)
	Angle Class III subdivision right with a straight profile
	Maxillary right primary canine Class III (1–2 mm)
	Maxillary left primary canine Class I
Vertical	Soft tissue and skeletal LAFH WRN
	Steep MPA (FMA = 34°, SNMP = 44°)
	OB 10%
Transverse	–
Other	Maxillary incisors appear upright (U1 to SN = 98°), but Sella is low (FH – SN = 10° instead of an average 7°), (so adjusted U1 to SN = 101°)
	Slightly proclined mandibular incisors (FMIA = 61°)
	Maxillary permanent canine crowns overlap lateral incisor roots on panoramic radiograph (Figure 6.44f)
	Mild (1–2 mm) maxillary anterior crowding
	Moderate (4–5 mm) mandibular incisor crowding

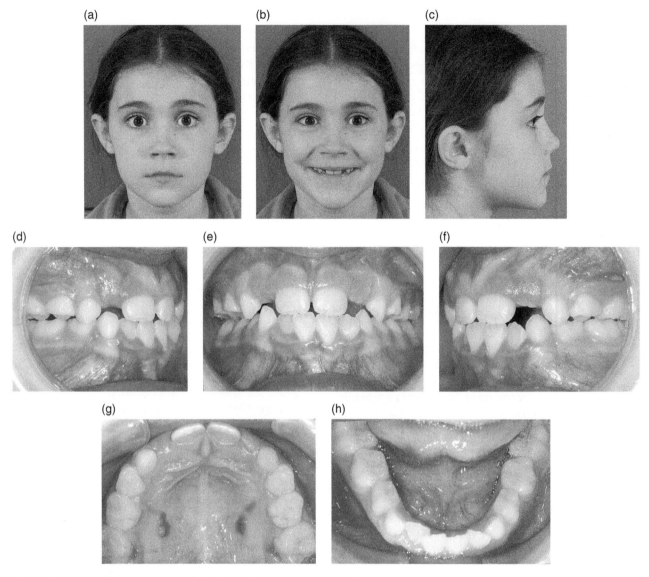

Figure 6.43 (a–h) Progress records of Anneke made when the maxillary Hyrax expander was removed (note palatal irritation from the expander, g).

Q: In Figure 6.44h, we see that Anneke's left posterior crossbite did not relapse in spite of poor retainer wear. We also see that her permanent central incisors are not edge-to-edge. We are delighted by these observations. However, a number of other observations are worrisome. What are they?

A: We are concerned by the fact that her maxillary right primary canine is Class III by 1–2 mm and her lower dental midline (LDML) is left of her UDML. These facts lead to the following questions:

- Is her mandible growing asymmetrically (more right mandibular growth than left)?
- If her mandible is growing asymmetrically, then was this asymmetric growth the underlying cause of

her left posterior crossbite when she was seven years old?

- If her mandible is growing asymmetrically, then will this growth result in a return of the left posterior crossbite?

Also concerning is the fact that Anneke never returned for an LLHA. If an LLHA had been placed, then the mandibular leeway space would have permitted spontaneous alignment of her mandibular anterior teeth as the mandibular primary canines and molars exfoliated. Instead, moderate mandibular anterior crowding exists, and the right "E-space" seen in Figure 6.44k may result in mesial drifting of the mandibular right first molar into a Class III relationship.

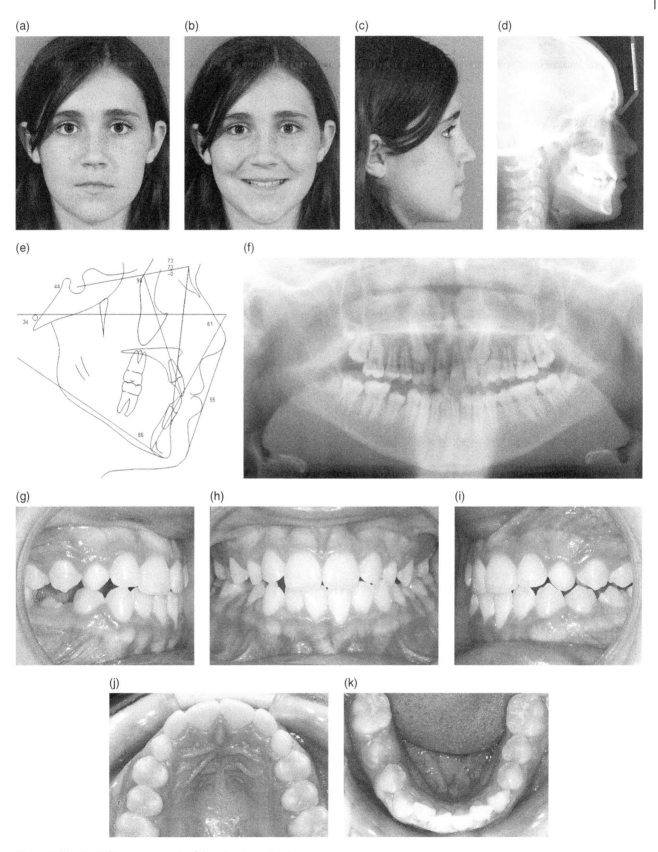

Figure 6.44 (a–k) Progress records of Anneke at age twelve years.

Also concerning is the radiographic overlap of the maxillary permanent canine crowns over the permanent lateral incisor roots (Figure 6.44f). However, both canine crowns overlap only the distal one-half of the lateral incisor roots. If we ensure space for their eruption, then the canines should erupt normally.

Q: In terms of Anneke's potential mandibular asymmetric growth, how does her age benefit us?

A: On average, females reach peak facial growth velocity at 10.9–12.3 years [149–151]. Therefore, if Anneke's mandible is growing asymmetrically, it is better that she is nearing the end of growth than if she was very young and had many more years of asymmetric growth left. Fortunately, even if mandibular asymmetric growth is occurring, it is small enough that a chin deviation is not noticeable (Figure 6.44a–b).

Q: We are nearly into the permanent dentition. How would you recommend proceeding?

A: We decided to monitor Anneke's growth. If her right Class III relationship worsened, we would consider unilateral Class III orthopedics (right Class III elastics worn between maxillary and mandibular TADs). If her asymmetric growth did not worsen, we would treat her with right Class III elastics during comprehensive orthodontic treatment.

Anneke's maxillary primary canines were extracted, fixed orthodontic appliances were placed in the maxillary arch, and spaces were opened for the maxillary permanent canines (Figure 6.45). The maxillary canines did not erupt for nine months. We surgically exposed them and erupted them into the arch. At this point, early treatment was complete.

Mandibular fixed appliances were placed, the arches were leveled and aligned, and Class III elastics were worn on her right side until a Class II(1 mm) overcorrected canine relationship was achieved – then, elastic wear was tapered off. Her treatment was finished.

Q: Deband records of Anneke are shown in Figure 6.46. Growth was complete. What changes do you note?

A: Changes include the following:
- Anneke completed treatment with a beautiful smile and occlusion.
- UDML is coincident with facial midline and LDML.
- Her lower lip appears slightly more protrusive (compare Figures 6.45c and 6.46c).
- Maxillary permanent canines were successfully erupted and positioned.
- Class I occlusion, bilaterally.
- Maxillary left first premolar is not fully erupted/seated.

Q: Do you have any "take-home pearls" regarding Anneke's treatment or other points made in this transverse introduction?

A: A number of important points can be made:
- When treating posterior crossbites in children, force yourself to reflect on the etiology. In addition to a small maxillary width, Anneke's left posterior crossbite could have been due to excessive right mandibular condylar growth. We were fortunate that Anneke's apparent asymmetric mandibular growth was limited and did not require correction via orthopedics (unilateral Class III elastic wear to TADs), extraction of permanent teeth (masking), or surgical treatment. But this may not be the case in the next patient we treat.
- Etiologic factors that cause transverse discrepancies include ectopic tooth eruption, soft tissue imbalance, prolonged retention of primary teeth,

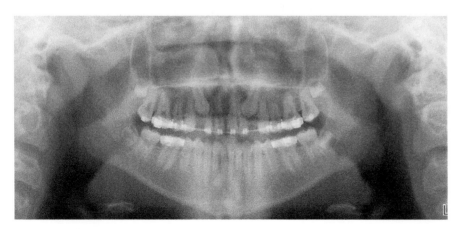

Figure 6.45 Progress panoramic image of Anneke at age thirteen years.

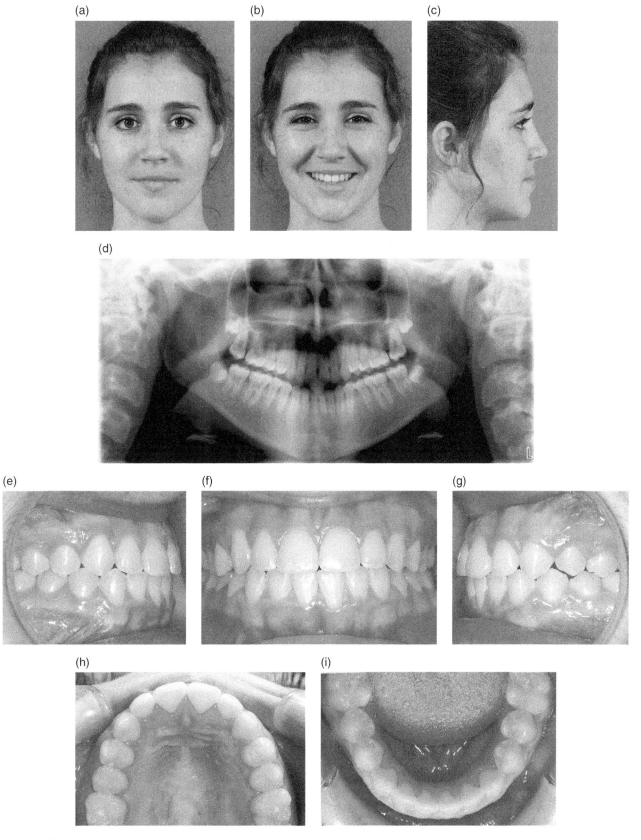

Figure 6.46 (a–i) Deband records of Anneke.

asymmetric mandibular growth, a lateral CR-CO shift, excess or deficient anteroposterior growth of the maxilla or mandible, some TMD issues, and excess or deficient maxillary or mandibular transverse growth.

- A unilateral posterior crossbite often results from either a lateral CR-CO shift or asymmetric mandibular growth. A unilateral posterior crossbite resulting from asymmetric mandibular is more difficult to treat.

- If a child presents with a developing mandibular asymmetry *due* to a lateral shift into crossbite, then the asymmetry can be largely eliminated if the crossbite and functional shift are treated in a timely manner (early mixed dentition).

- A number of factors should be considered when formulating a diagnosis and treatment plan for patients with transverse discrepancies, including magnitude of transverse discrepancy, facial symmetry or asymmetry, presence of a CR-CO shift, whether the transverse discrepancy is relative or absolute, how future anteroposterior growth/treatment will affect the transverse discrepancy, magnitude of buccal corridors, and whether the posterior crossbite (transverse discrepancy) is dental or skeletal.

- We differentiate between a dental and skeletal crossbite, not by counting teeth in crossbite, but by visualizing what happens when we *upright the molars* (eliminate transverse skeletal compensations). Since maxillary and mandibular skeletal bases relate well in a *dental* crossbite, uprighting molars should improve (eliminate) a dental crossbite. Since maxillary and mandibular skeletal bases do not relate well in a *skeletal* crossbite, uprighting molars should worsen a skeletal crossbite.

- Dental crossbites are corrected by uprighting the teeth in crossbite.

- Skeletal crossbites are treated via orthopedics (maxillary expansion), masking (correction of skeletal crossbites with dental movement – without treating the underlying skeletal discrepancy), and surgery. Masking and surgery are best reserved for treatment in adult dentition during comprehensive orthodontics.

- Before maxillary orthopedic expansion is begun, or before maxillary/mandibular dental expansion is begun, confirm the existence of a thick buccal periodontal biotype.

- We recommend waiting until the early mixed dentition to treat skeletal posterior crossbites with maxillary expansion.

- The most marked RME skeletal effect occurs before/during the pubertal growth spurt.

- The limit for maxillary arch expansion is the mandibular arch width, and the limit for mandibular arch expansion is the point where the mandibular posterior teeth are upright.

- Ideally, Anneke's left posterior crossbite would have been a *bilateral* crossbite with a functional CR-CO shift to the left. Why? If it was bilateral, then RME could have proceeded with even correction on the right *and* left sides. Instead, she had a true unilateral left lingual crossbite. True unilateral crossbites can be challenging because overexpansion with an RME appliance on the non-crossbite side frequently occurs before correction is achieved on the crossbite side. We were fortunate with Anneke. RME resulted in only mild overcorrection on her non-crossbite (right side, Figure 6.43e) by the time we had corrected her crossbite (left) side.

- If we could treat Anneke again, then we would have placed her on right crossbite elastics (buccal of the RME appliance to a bonded lingual button on the mandibular right permanent molar) to upright the mandibular right molar, reduce right posterior overjet, and permit additional overcorrection of her left side.

- The longer we practice orthodontics, the longer we maintain the RME appliance cemented in place post-expansion for retention (or convert it into a TPA for retention).

- Anneke disappeared for years. This was unacceptable. A hallmark of successful early orthodontic treatment is periodic, and frequent patient recall, monitoring, and plan revision.

- There is no indication in the literature that prophylactic maxillary expansion prevents the future development of obstructive sleep apnea.

- We thought that Anneke's maxillary permanent canines would erupt after we made space for them with RME. We were wrong. Her maxillary permanent canines were not ankylosed, but did not erupt on their own, even after we made space for them. *Spontaneous eruption of an unerupted tooth is never guaranteed.*

Case Jasmin

Q: Jasmin is five years old (Figure 6.47). She presents to you with her parents' chief complaint "Jasmin has a crossbite." Her PMH, PDH, periodontal evaluation,

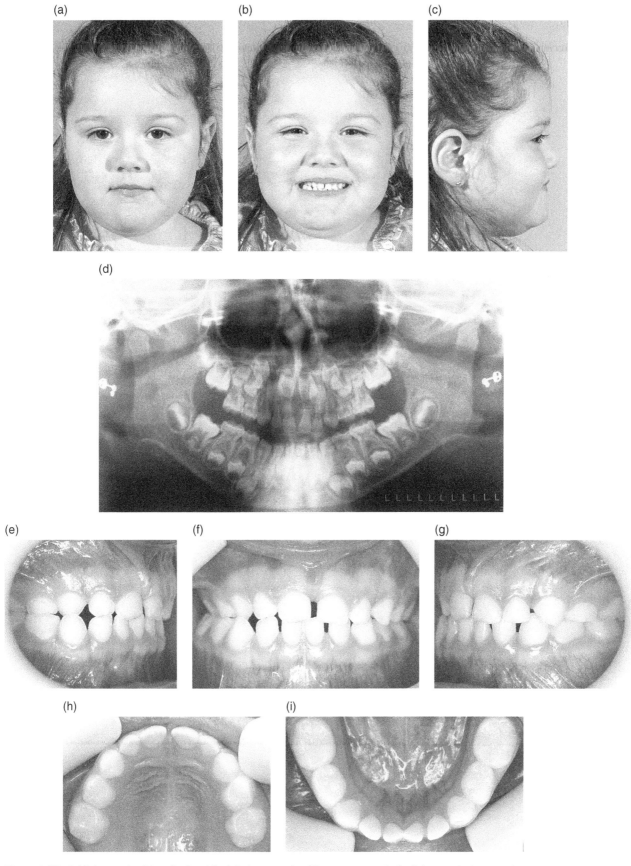

Figure 6.47 Initial records of Jasmin: (a–c) facial photographs; (d) pantomograph; (e–i) intraoral photographs.

and TMJ evaluations are WRN. Do you need any additional records in order to decide whether to recall Jasmin or to perform the early treatment?

A: No additional records are needed.

Q: Compile your diagnostic findings and problem list for Jasmin. Also, state your diagnosis.

A:

Table 6.3 Diagnostic findings and problem list for Jasmin.

Full face and profile	***FRONTAL VIEW***
	Face is turned slightly right in frontal view, but she appears symmetric.
	Soft tissue LAFH WRN (soft tissue Glabella-Subnasale approximately equal to
	Subnasale – soft tissue Menton)
	Lip competence
	UDML WRN
	PROFILE VIEW
	Straight profile
	Prominent chin projection
	Obtuse NLA
	Lip-chin-throat angle WRN
Radiographs	Primary dentition
Intraoral photos	Class II primary molar relationship right, Class I primary molar relationship left
	Iowa classification (primary dentition): II(2 mm) II(2 mm) I I
	Right posterior lingual crossbite
	OJ ~0 mm
	OB 10%
	LDML to right of UDML by ~2 mm
	Maxillary right posterior is slightly ahead of left posterior (Figure 6.47h)
	Mandibular dental arch is symmetric
	2 mm maxillary midline diastema with low labial frenum
	2 mm mandibular primary anterior spacing
Other	None
Diagnosis	Class II subdivision right primary molar relationship with right posterior lingual crossbite

Q: Should you be concerned with Jasmin's maxillary and mandibular incisor spacing?

A: No, we are concerned with eventual permanent incisor *crowding*. Let's do the math using the following data:

Average mesiodistal widths of permanent teeth (mm): [152]

Maxillary central incisor	8.5	Mandibular central incisor	5.0
Maxillary lateral incisor	6.5	Mandibular lateral incisor	5.5
Maxillary canine	7.5	Mandibular canine	7.0
Maxillary first premolar	7.0	Mandibular first premolar	7.0
Maxillary second premolar	7.0	Mandibular second premolar	7.0
Maxillary first molar	10.0	Mandibular first molar	11.0
Maxillary second molar	9.0	Mandibular second molar	10.5

Average mesiodistal widths of *primary* teeth (mm): [152]

Maxillary central incisor	6.5	Mandibular central incisor	4.2
Maxillary lateral incisor	5.1	Mandibular lateral incisor	4.1
Maxillary canine	7.0	Mandibular canine	5.0
Maxillary first molar	7.3	Mandibular first molar	7.7
Maxillary second molar	8.2	Mandibular second molar	9.9

Primary maxillary
incisors = 5.1 mm + 6.5 mm + 6.5 mm + 5.1 mm = 23.2 mm

Permanent maxillary
incisors = 6.5 mm + 8.5 mm + 8.5 mm + 6.5 mm = 30.0 mm

Difference −6.8 mm

Primary mandibular incisors = 4.1 mm + 4.2 mm + 4.2 mm + 4.1 mm = 16.6 mm

Primary mandibular incisors =
4.1 mm + 4.2 mm + 4.2 mm + 4.1 mm = 16.6 mm

Difference −4.4 mm

That is, an anticipated maxillary permanent incisor *space deficit* of −4.8 mm exists (−6.8 mm + 2 mm current spacing). An anticipated mandibular permanent incisor *space deficit* of −2.4 mm exists (−4.4 mm + 2 mm current spacing).

Q: What did we fail to check for during our examination?

A: We failed to check for a CR-CO shift (Figures 6.48a–6.48b). You must *check for a CR-CO shift in every patient – every time you examine them. If you do not know where you are starting from, then you cannot know what direction to take in order to reach your goal.* Jasmin demonstrates a 2 mm right lateral shift as she closes from CR into CO.

Q: How does this right lateral shift affect Jasmin's anteroposterior, vertical, and transverse findings?

A: As Jasmin shifts her occlusion from CR into CO, her mandible shifts to the right as it rotates around her right condyle. Her left condyle is distracted forward making Jasmin appear more Class III on the left in CO than she really is. In other words, in CR, Jasmin is probably slightly Class II bilaterally, and in CO, she shifts forward on the left into a Class I primary molar relationship.

(a)

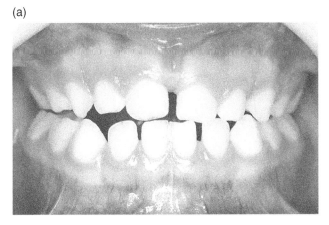

(b)

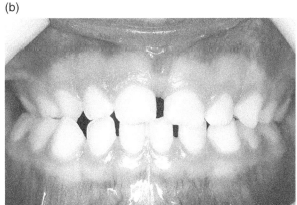

Figure 6.48 Initial intraoral frontal photos of Jasmin in (a) CR and (b) CO.

In CR (Figure 6.48a), Jasmin occludes cusp-to-cusp in the posterior (versus cusp-to-fossa), and her bite opens slightly into an open bite at the maxillary right incisors.

Finally, in CR, Jasmin has a mild bilateral posterior overjet deficit but not a crossbite. That is, in CR, the right posterior lingual crossbite has disappeared.

Q: A bilateral posterior overjet deficit will be much easier to treat than a true unilateral lingual crossbite. Why?

A: Two reasons:

- Equal but opposite expansion forces can be used to eliminate a bilateral posterior overjet deficit. Equal but opposite forces are generally easier to generate than unilateral forces.
- The magnitude of her right transverse problem has been reduced by one half compared to the magnitude if it was a true unilateral right posterior crossbite.

Q: What are Jasmin's *primary* problems in each dimension, plus other problems?

A:

Table 6.4 Primary problem list for Jasmin.

AP	Angle Class II primary molar relationship in CR
	Iowa classification in CO (primary dentition):
	II(2 mm) II (2 mm) I I
Vertical	Mild anterior open bite in CR
Transverse	Posterior overjet deficit bilaterally in CR
	Unilateral right posterior lingual crossbite in CO
Other	2 mm right lateral shift from CR into CO

Q: Discuss Jasmin in the context of three principles applied to every early treatment patient.

A:

1) The goal of early treatment is to correct developing problems – get the patient *back to normal for their stage of development* (including preventing complications such as resorption of adjacent tooth roots, reducing later treatment complexity, or reducing/eliminating unknowns). Correcting Jasmin's right posterior lingual crossbite, right CR-CO shift, and mild Class II relationship would bring her back to normal for her stage of development.

2) Early treatment should address *very specific problems with a clearly defined end point,* usually within six to nine months. Correcting her right crossbite and lateral shift are focused problems which could be treated in six to nine months. At five years old, it is simply too early to consider treatment of her mild Class II relationship.

3) Always ask: Is it necessary that I treat the patient now? *What harm will come if I choose to do nothing now?* It is not necessary to treat Jasmin now, at least not if we plan to recall her in one year. If we do not treat her now, then her CR-CO shift into right posterior lingual crossbite will remain.

Q: What harm may result if we chose to *never* treat Jasmin's CR-CO shift into the right posterior crossbite?

A: A mandibular growth asymmetry may result [9–11].

Q: Assume that Jasmin's mandible begins to grow asymmetrically as a result of her uncorrected right CR-CO shift. How would this asymmetric growth be affected if her crossbite and shift were corrected early enough with maxillary expansion?

A: If her crossbite and functional shift were corrected early enough (early mixed dentition), then the developing asymmetry could be largely eliminated [10–14].

Q: But what if Jasmin's right posterior lingual crossbite resulted from *excessive left mandibular growth*. Would correction of her right crossbite with RME prevent future asymmetric mandibular growth?

A: No. Correction of her right crossbite would be only temporary. The right crossbite would return as excessive left mandibular growth continued. This fact underscores the importance of determining whether a unilateral posterior crossbite is the result of a CR-CO shift or true asymmetric mandibular growth.

Q: How would you treat excessive unilateral mandibular growth?

A: Either with orthopedics (e.g. TAD-supported Class III elastics) in a growing child, masking (e.g. premolar extractions to achieve Class I permanent canines) in an adult, or surgery (e.g. asymmetric mandibular setback osteotomy) in an adult.

Q: What unknowns do you face in treating Jasmin?

A: Unknowns include future jaw growth magnitude and direction, an undetected (worse) CR-CO shift, and patient compliance.

Q: Should you start early treatment now or recall Jasmin? If you start treatment, what treatment options would you consider?

A: Treatment options include the following:

- *Recall* (no treatment, monitor only) – *is a recommended option*. No harm is anticipated in waiting for one year. Her right lateral CR-CO shift and right posterior lingual crossbite will remain, but her maxillary first permanent molars should erupt by then for use as maxillary expander anchorage. Further, she would likely be more compliant at six years old than at five years old.
- *Occlusal adjustment to remove interferences causing the CR-CO shift* – is not recommended. Why? Look at Figure 6.48a. There are multiple teeth causing the lateral shift and eliminating occlusal interferences would require flattening many/all posterior teeth occlusal surfaces. Even then, the maxillary dental arch would still be narrow compared to the mandibular dental arch.
- *Maxillary expansion with a split plate removable appliance* – could provide enough bilateral posterior overjet to eliminate the shift, eliminate the right crossbite, and seat the posterior occlusion in a cusp-fossa relationship. The advantage of a split plate is that it would act as a flat plane biteplate to permit unimpeded expansion. The disadvantage of the split

plate is that it will require Jasmin's compliance wearing it.

We would ask Jasmin's mother to open the split plate expansion screw at a rate of 0.25 to 0.50 mm per week. Opening faster than this would result in the split plate "riding up" the lingual surfaces of the maxillary posterior teeth. At five years old we will expect an increased rate of growth (widening) of the midpalatal suture with a split plate [39].

- *Maxillary expansion with a quad-helix appliance or RME* – could provide bilateral posterior overjet to eliminate the shift, eliminate the crossbite, and seat the posterior occlusion in a cusp-fossa relationship. These appliances could incorporate maxillary second primary molar bands. Since they are cemented in place, they would reduce the need for Jasmin's cooperation. Furthermore, midpalatal sutural separation (skeletal expansion) should occur because the facial skeletal resistance to expansion is minimal at five years of age [40, 41].
- *LLHA for space maintenance* – *is unnecessary*. Jasmin has many years of development before mandibular primary canines and molars approach exfoliation.
- *Extraction of primary canines or other primary teeth* – *is unnecessary*. We see no need to extract these teeth, and Jasmin's permanent teeth appear to be erupting uneventfully.
- *Closure of maxillary diastema* – *is unnecessary*. A future maxillary anterior space *deficit* is predicted, and the maxillary midline diastema may close spontaneously as the maxillary incisors and canines erupt.
- *Class II correction* – *is unnecessary*. Jasmin is only five years old, the Class II relationship is very mild, and science does not support Class II correction this early. Furthermore, we would recommend correcting her right lateral CR-CO shift first to reduce unknowns and to determine her true anteroposterior relationship in CR.

Q: What is your recommended treatment? How would you proceed?

A: We decided to expand her maxillary arch with a split plate (Figures 6.49a–6.49e) whose screw was opened at a rate of 0.5 mm per week until bilateral transverse overjet (OJ) overcorrection was achieved. She wore the expanded split plate as a full-time retainer until the maxillary first molars erupted (Figures 6.49f–6.49l, Jasmin in CR). She was occluding only on her permanent first molars.

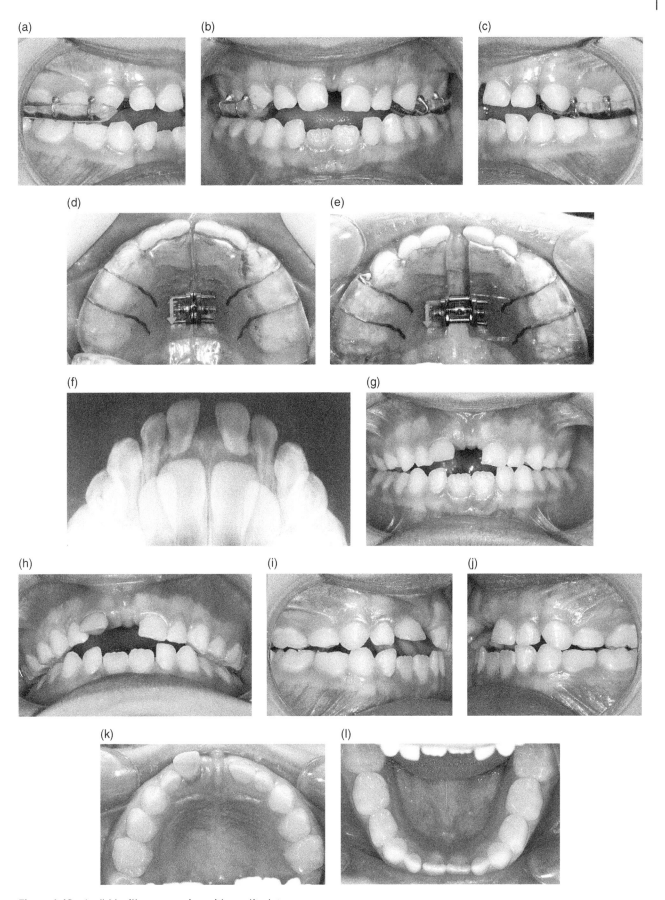

Figure 6.49   (a–l) Maxillary expansion with a split plate.

Q: Increased width of Jasmin's maxillary diastema, and overcorrection of her posterior overjet, are both apparent in Figure 6.49h. Was this maxillary expansion skeletal, or dental, expansion?

A: We suspect that her maxillary expansion was a combination of skeletal (midpalatal suture widening), and dental, expansion but we cannot state this with certainty. Skieller [39] reported that maxillary split plate expansion increased the rate of growth (widening) of the midpalatal suture. This may have occurred, but Jasmin's midpalatal suture (Figure 6.49f) does not appear particularly wide, especially in comparison to her diastema.

Q: Jasmin's right lateral CR-CO shift was eliminated with split plate expansion. How do you deal with her anterior open bite and excessive posterior overjet (Figure 6.49h)?

A: Unless she develops a habit of interposing her tongue between her teeth, the open bite should close as her permanent teeth erupt into occlusion. Jasmin was asked to stop wearing the split plate and to begin chewing gum to help settle her occlusion. A few months after the primary posterior teeth erupted into occlusion (Figures 6.50a–6.50e), she was given a vacuum-formed maxillary clear retainer to wear until her permanent teeth erupted. The retainer plastic covering the maxillary incisors was cut away to permit maxillary incisor eruption. Figures 6.50f–6.50j illustrate Jasmin's occlusion following incisor eruption. Placement of an LLHA was planned when the permanent mandibular canines and premolars were closer to eruption.

Q: Jasmin returned to our clinic in the late mixed dentition when she was ten years old (Figure 6.51). An LLHA had never been delivered, and she had lost her maxillary clear retainer years earlier. CR = CO. What are her primary problems?

A:

Table 6.5 Primary problem list for Jasmin.

AP	Angle Class II division 1
	Iowa classification: II (3 mm) x II (2 mm) II (2 mm)
	Maxillary anteroposterior position WRN (A-Point lies on Nasion-Perpendicular Line)
	Mandibular anteroposterior position WRN (ANB angle = 2° with normal maxillary position)
Vertical	OB 20%
	Skeletal LAFH WRN (LAFH/TAFH x 100% = 56%)
	MPA WRN (FMA = 22°; SN-MP = 32°)
Transverse	–
Other	Proclined mandibular incisors (FMIA = 55°)
	Unerupted maxillary second premolars

Q: Thankfully, Jasmin's transverse correction has held, she is normal vertically, and her maxillary and mandibular skeletal anteroposterior positions are normal. But *dentally*, her posterior teeth exhibit a 2–3 mm Class II relationship. In other words, she does not exhibit an anteroposterior skeletal discrepancy (apical base discrepancy), but she does exhibit a mild-to-moderate Class II molar relationship. Can you list possible ways of treating her dental Class II? Specifically, can you discuss the advantages, and disadvantages, of various intra-arch and inter-arch Class II treatments for her?

A: *Intra-arch* Class II treatments include:

- Headgears: high-pull, straight-pull, or a cervical-pull headgear would distalize her maxillary molars through the maxillary alveolar process bone, restrict maxillary corpus forward growth, and allow the mandible to continue growing forward. All three effects will help correct Jasmin's Class II molar relationship. In addition, a high-pull headgear may reduce descent of her maxillary corpus and maxillary first molars, potentially further improving her anteroposterior correction by mandibular forward rotation [153–155]. A cervical-pull headgear would rotate her palatal plane down and back slightly and extrude (<1 mm) maxillary first molars compared to controls [154–156]. Neither of these cervical-pull headgear effects will help Jasmin. A straight-pull headgear (patient wears a combination of high-pull and cervical-pull headgears) will produce an effect somewhere between that of a high pull and a cervical pull. The advantage of using a headgear for Jasmin is that if she is compliant, we would readily correct her 2–3 mm Class II molar relationship. The disadvantage of using a headgear for Jasmin is that the skeletal effect resulting from differential anteroposterior jaw growth is unnecessary – her skeletal relationship is Class I.

- TADs: placed in the maxilla or infrazygomatic crest could act as anchors to permit retraction of the entire maxillary dentition into a Class I relationship. Or, TADs could be used to anchor palatal intra-arch Class II correctors (e.g. a pendulum appliance). The advantage of TADs is that patient compliance is minimized. The disadvantage of TADs is that placement is a minor surgical procedure.

- Extraction of maxillary first or second premolars: would provide space to retract Jasmin's maxillary canines into a Class I relationship with her mandibular canines. The advantage would be that our outcome is less dependent on patient compliance. Disadvantages include the loss of two maxillary

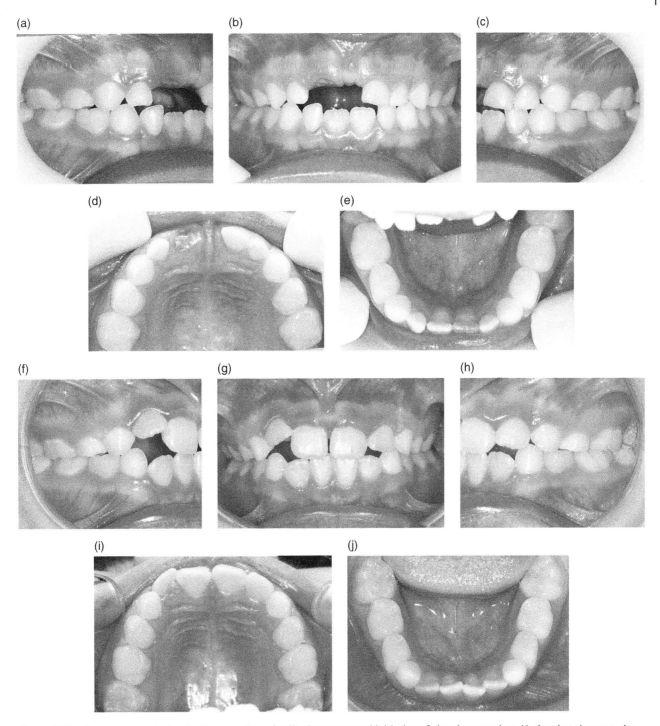

Figure 6.50 Progress records: (a–e) after cessation of split plate wear and initiation of chewing exercises. Notice that the posterior overjet has decreased as the overexpansion diminished; (f–j) following the eruption of permanent incisors.

premolars, and the need to execute maxillary arch mechanics that facilitate forward movement of maxillary posterior teeth to close the 7 mm premolar extraction space without simultaneously over-retracting the maxillary canines into a class III canine relationship.

Inter-arch Class II treatments include:

- Class II functional appliances: the effects of functional appliances include a tendency for restriction of maxillary forward growth, retraction of maxillary posterior teeth, uprighting of maxillary incisors, mesial movement of mandibular posterior teeth,

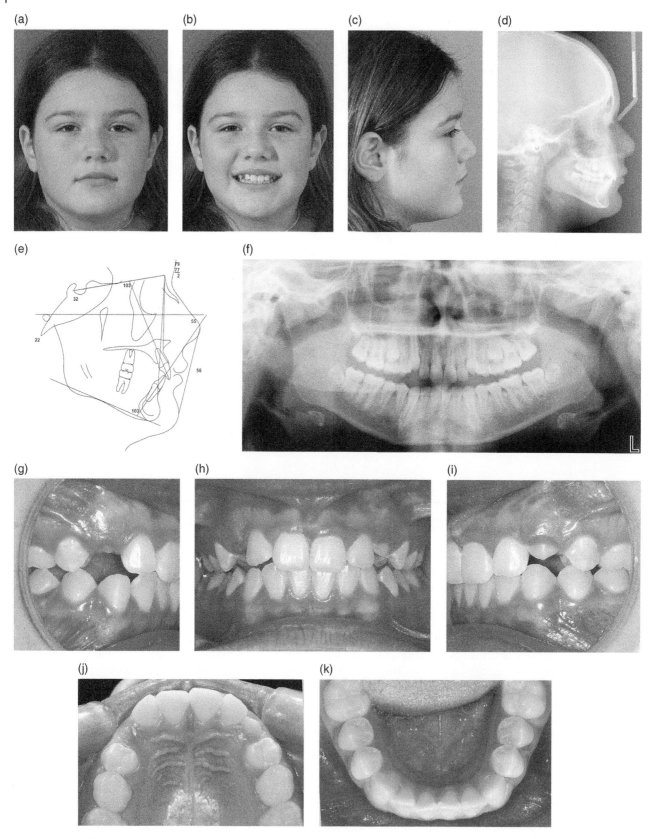

Figure 6.51 (a–k) Progress records of Jasmin at age ten years.

proclination of mandibular incisors, acceleration of condylar growth, and anterior displacement of the glenoid fossae [157, 158]. The tendency for retraction of maxillary posterior teeth, and mesial movement of mandibular posterior teeth, would be advantageous for Jasmin. However, proclination of already proclined mandibular incisors would be a disadvantage.

- Class II elastics: effects are mainly dentoalveolar – maxillary incisor eruption and lingual tipping, mandibular incisor labial tipping, and mandibular molar eruption/mesial movement [159]. The advantage of Class II elastics would be their ease of use and greater patient compliance. The disadvantage would be proclination of Jasmin's already proclined mandibular incisors.

Class II elastics have their place. Most orthodontists use them in Class II patients at some time. But be wary of using heavy Class II elastics in steep mandibular plane angle (MPA) patients for extended periods of time because the mandibular molars erupt – rotating the mandible down and back. *Principle of Class II treatment: avoid treatments that tend to rotate the mandible down and back (worsening the Class II relationship).*

- Class II compressed springs (e.g. Forsus™ appliance): effects include retraction of maxillary molars, mandibular molar mesial movement, mandibular incisor proclination, and mandibular incisor intrusion [160, 161]. Restriction of maxillary [160] growth has also been reported, but Forsus™ are not generally used for long enough periods of time for this effect to be significant. The advantage of Class II springs would be minimized patient compliance. The disadvantage would be mandibular incisor proclination.

Q: What treatment do you recommend?

A: Jasmin was placed on a high-pull headgear and was initially cooperative. Later, her cooperation waned. Once her maxillary canines and second premolars erupted, fixed orthodontic appliances were placed, arches were leveled/aligned, and the treatment finished.

Q: Deband records made at age twelve years are shown in Figure 6.52. Retention records (age twenty-two years) are shown in Figure 6.53. What changes do you note?

A: Changes include the following:
- Jasmin exhibits excessive gingival display in her deband posed smile (Figure 6.52b), but her smile

appears more exaggerated in her deband photo than in her earlier photo (Figure 6.51b).
- UDML and LDML are coincident and centered on the facial midline.
- A point – Nasion – B Point angle [ANB] angle has decreased to ANB = 1°.
- Maxillary incisors have proclined (U1 to SN = 110°).
- Mandibular incisors have uprighted (FMIA [Frankfort horizontal to mandibular incisor angle] = 58°).
- Skeletal lower anterior face height (LAFH) has increased by 1% (LAFH/TAFH [total anterior face height] × 100% = 57%).
- MPA has not changed (FMA [Franfort horizontal to mandibular plane angle] = 22°; SN-MP [Sella – Nasion to mandibular plane angle] = 32°).
- Roots appear parallel (Figure 6.52g).
- Right premolars and right canines were Class II by 1 mm at deband, but by age twenty-two years, her occlusion has settled into a Class I bilateral relationship (Figures 6.53d and 6.53f).
- Transverse correction has been stable.
- Overbite (OB) decreased from an initial 20% (Figure 6.51h) to a deband and long-term 10% (Figures 6.52i and 6.53e).
- Gingiva appears inflamed and hypertrophied at deband but improved at twenty-two years of age – except for the excessive fibrotic tissue remaining between the maxillary central incisors.

Q: I am confused. We noted that Jasmin was Class II by 1 mm on her right side at deband (twelve years of age) but Class I on her right side at twenty-two years of age. How can this be? Was this due to late asymmetric mandibular growth?

A: No, this change was not due to late (right) asymmetric mandibular growth. How do we know this? Jasmin's chin looks symmetric and her midlines remained coincident from age twelve to twenty-two years.

Q: Was this Class II to Class I improvement due to occlusal "settling" following deband? Can we expect occlusal settling like this post-deband? In other words, can we finish patients as Class II, or maybe Class III, and expect their anteroposterior relationship to improve with time?

A: No. *First principle of finishing: Complete treatment ideally, then maintain the patient in that position with lifelong retention.* Never expect post-deband occlusal improvements.

It is true that teeth will tend to erupt throughout life, tending to close vertical discrepancies (compare Figures 6.52h and 6.53d) and perhaps deepening the

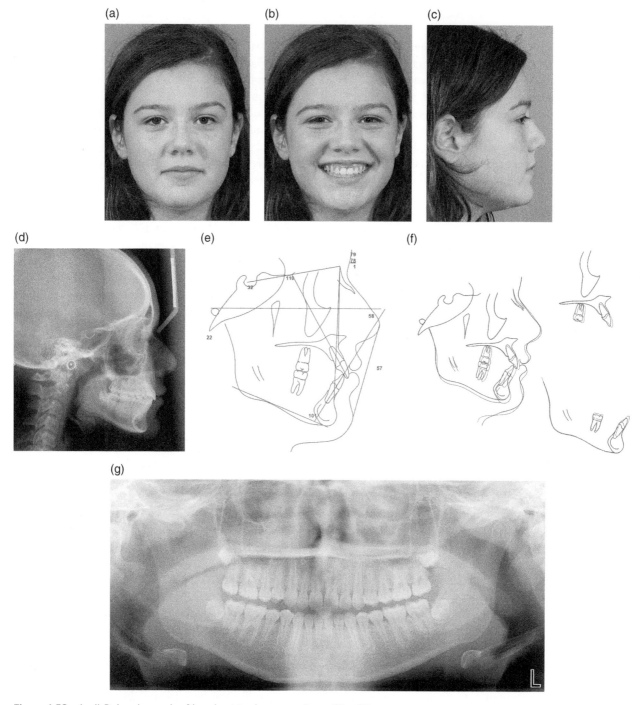

Figure 6.52 (a–l) Deband records of Jasmin at twelve years of age. CR = CO.

curve of Spee. And it is true that teeth will wear interproximally with function – and tend to shift anteroposteriorly. However, it would be speculation to state that the favorable change on Jasmin's right side was attributed to such factors. It may be true, but it is speculation. We cannot state with certainty how this improvement occurred. Jasmin should have been debanded with Class I canines, bilaterally.

Q: What retention protocol would you recommend for Jasmin?

A: Following deband, she was placed in removable Hawley retainers and asked to wear them at night for life. Lifelong retention is the only guarantee that the alignment of teeth can be assured. From the records made at age twenty-two years, it appears that Jasmin is being compliant during retention.

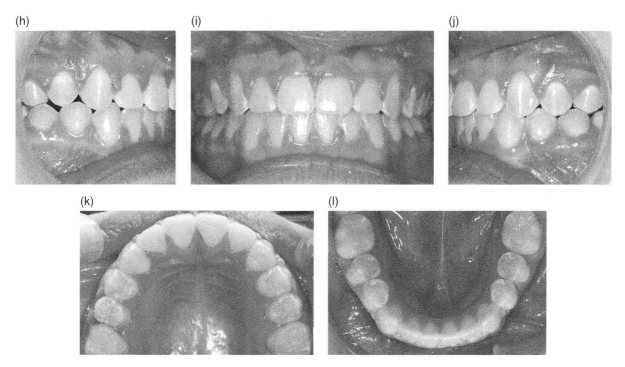

(h)   (i)   (j)

(k)   (l)

Figure 6.52 (Continued)

Q: Can you suggest "take-home pearls" regarding Jasmin's treatment?

A: "Pearls" include the following:

- Jasmin presented when she was five years old in the primary dentition with a right lateral CR-CO shift into a right lingual crossbite. When she was positioned in CR (Figure 6.48a), we observed that she exhibited inadequate bilateral posterior overjet, but was no longer in right crossbite. *If you learn only one thing from this textbook, it is this: check for a CR-CO shift on every patient at every appointment.* Why? *You cannot decide where to go with treatment if you do not know from where you are starting.*

- Her inadequate *bilateral* posterior overjet in CR was easier to treat than a unilateral crossbite. Why? Equal, but opposite, bilateral expansive forces were applied. Bilateral opposing forces (action/reaction) are generally easier to apply than unilateral forces. And, in CR, the magnitude of the right bilateral transverse problem was reduced by one half compared to when it was unilateral.

- Her right lateral CR-CO shift was eliminated using maxillary split plate expansion. Lateral shift elimination is important in preventing the development of a mandibular growth asymmetry.

- The split plate expansion was successful, but Jasmin's level of cooperation was very good. Such cooperation may not always be forthcoming. If treatment had been delayed until the permanent first molars erupted, then a cemented expansion appliance could have been used – minimizing the need for cooperation.

- Another option at age five years would be a fixed maxillary expander using the primary molars alone as anchorage. Midpalatal sutural separation could have been achieved if her facial skeletal resistance was low enough.

- If we could treat Jasmin again, then *we would not start treatment until the first permanent molars erupted.* Then, we would expand her maxilla with a *quad-helix or RME appliance.*

- If Jasmin's right posterior lingual crossbite had been caused by excessive asymmetric left mandibular growth, then the RME-corrected crossbite could have returned with continued excessive left mandibular growth unless unilateral Class III orthopedics were employed (e.g. TAD-supported left Class III elastic wear).

- Jasmin's primary dentition maxillary midline diastema disappeared with permanent tooth eruption. We had hoped for this closure because of the anticipated maxillary anterior space deficit following permanent incisor eruption.

- If you postpone placement of an LLHA, explain to the parent the need to return to your clinic in a timely fashion in order to have one fabricated/placed. This was not done.

- Jasmin's maxillary labial frenum appears to have migrated apically from the time we first saw her until she was twenty-two years old (compare Figures 6.47f

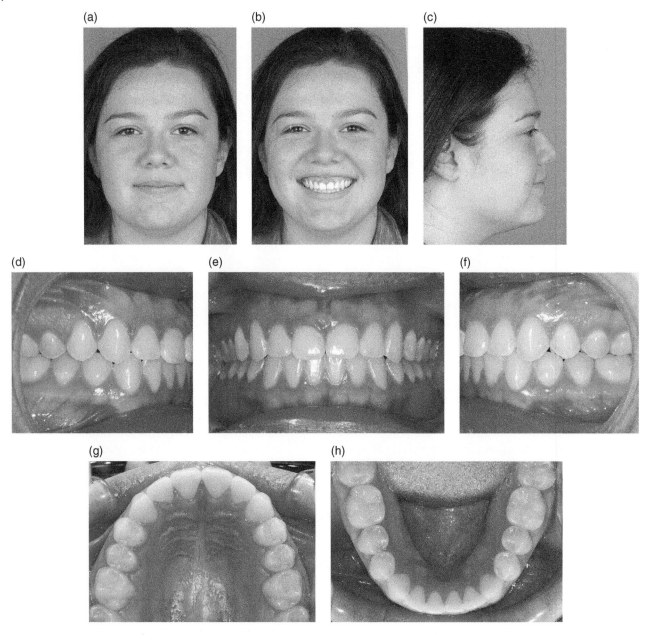

Figure 6.53 (a–h) Retention records of Jasmin made at age 22 years. CR = CO.

and 6.53e). This frenum migration obviates any need for a maxillary labial frenectomy. However, Jasmin will be referred to a periodontist for revision of her hypertrophic maxillary gingival tissue.

- *Principle of Class II treatment: Avoid treatments that tend to rotate the mandible down and back (worsening the Class II relationship).*
- *First principle of finishing: Complete treatment ideally, then maintain the patient in that position with life-long retention.*

Case Jenna

Q: Jenna is nine years and two months old (Figure 6.54). She presents to you with her parent's chief complaint, "Jenna's dentist says she has multiple problems and needs to see an orthodontist." Her PMH, PDH, periodontal evaluation, and TMJ evaluation are WRN. CR = CO. Compile your diagnostic findings and problem list for Jenna. Also, state your diagnosis.

A:

Table 6.6 Diagnostic findings and problem list for Jenna.

Full face and profile	**FRONTAL VIEW** Face is asymmetric with the right side longer than left (right-to-left lip cant disappears in the posed smile) Soft tissue LAFH WRN (soft tissue Glabella-Subnasale approximately equal to Subnasale – soft tissue Menton) 1–2 mm interlabial gap UDML ~1 mm left of the facial midline (Figure 6.54b) LDML ~2 mm right of the facial midline No gingival display in a posed smile **PROFILE VIEW** Straight profile (but tends toward convexity) Protrusive lips Upturned nose Acute NLA Chin projection WRN Obtuse lip-chin-throat angle Deep labiomental sulcus
Ceph analysis	**SKELETAL** Maxillary anteroposterior position WRN (A-Point lies on Nasion-perpendicular line) Mandibular anteroposterior position WRN (ANB angle = 3° with normal maxilla) Skeletal LAFH WRN (ANS-Menton/Nasion-Menton × 100% = 53%) Mandibular plane is flat (FMA = 18°; SNMP = 29°) with long posterior face height Effective bony pogonion (Pogonion lies on extended Nasion – B-Point line) **DENTAL** Proclined maxillary incisors (U1 to SN = 109°) Proclined mandibular incisors (FMIA = 52°)
Radiographs	Early mixed dentition Possible ectopic eruption of maxillary left permanent canine (crown appears to overlap maxillary left lateral incisor root)
Intraoral photos and models	Angle Class II division 1 in the early mixed dentition Iowa classification: II (3 mm) II (3 mm) II (2 mm) II (2 mm) OJ ~ 2–4 mm OB 20–30% 2.0 mm of maxillary incisor crowding is currently present 0.0 mm of maxillary arch crowding is anticipated following the eruption of all permanent teeth (if proper space maintenance is employed) 1.0 mm of mandibular incisor crowding is currently present 2.2 mm of mandibular arch spacing is anticipated following the eruption of all permanent teeth (if proper space maintenance is employed) Maxillary and mandibular arches are reasonably symmetric (Figures 6.54j–6.54k and 6.54p–6.54q) Maxillary right primary canine and right primary first molar in lingual crossbite Maxillary right permanent first molar is in lingual crossbite with distal of mandibular right primary second molar stainless steel crown (Figure 6.54o) Minimal posterior overjet of right permanent molars Maxillary posterior transverse compensations (first permanent molar buccal crown torque, Figure 6.54r) Mandibular posterior transverse compensations (first permanent molar lingual crown torque, Figure 6.54s) Labioversion of maxillary left central incisor Linguoversion and anterior crossbite of maxillary left lateral incisor (no damage noted)
Other	None
Diagnosis	Class II division 1 malocclusion with right posterior lingual crossbite and anterior crossbite

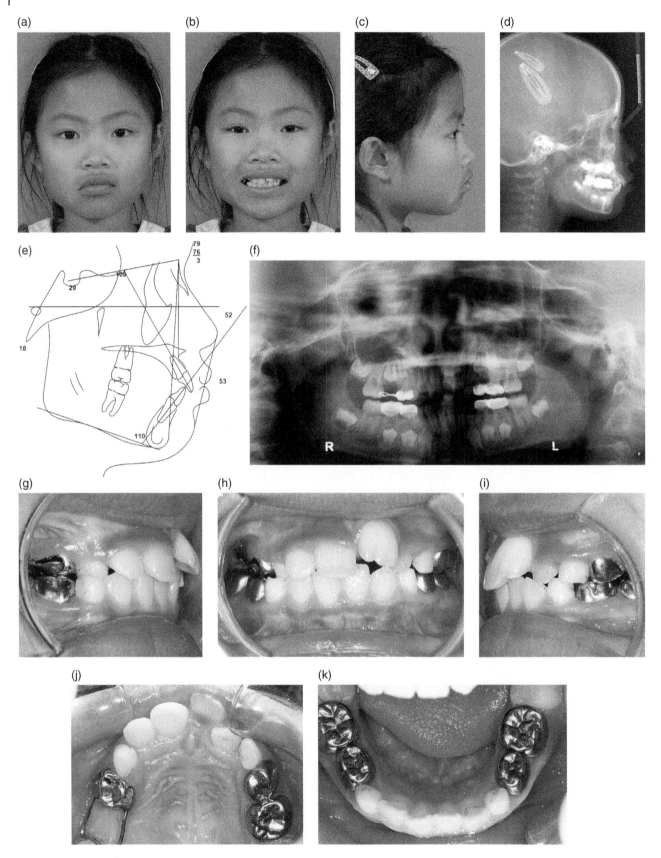

Figure 6.54 Initial records of Jenna: (a–c) facial photographs, (d–e) lateral cephalometric radiograph and tracing, (f) pantomograph, (g–k) intraoral photographs, (l–s) models.

(l)   (m)   (n)

(o)   (p)   (q)

(r)   (s)

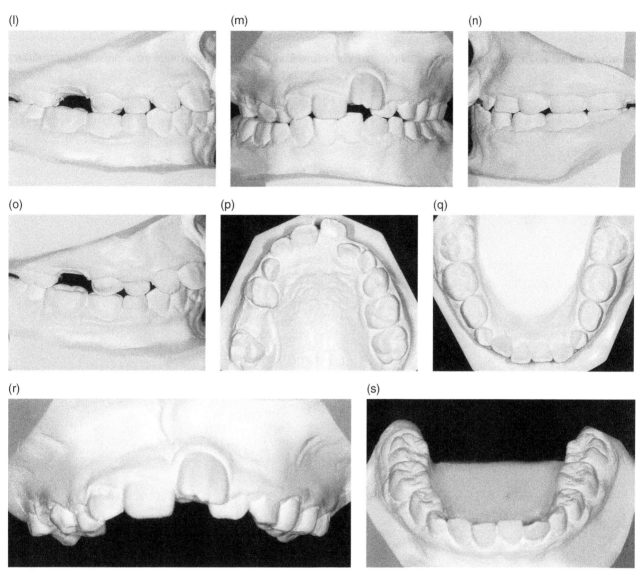

Figure 6.54   (Continued)

Q: Provide a detailed space analysis for Jenna's maxillary and mandibular arches. In other words, how were the anticipated 0.0 mm maxillary arch crowding and 2.2 mm mandibular arch spacing calculated (*if proper space maintenance is employed*)?

A:

Average mesiodistal widths of permanent teeth (mm): [152]

Maxillary central incisor	8.5	Mandibular central incisor	5.0
Maxillary lateral incisor	6.5	Mandibular lateral incisor	5.5
Maxillary canine	7.5	Mandibular canine	7.0
Maxillary first premolar	7.0	Mandibular first premolar	7.0
Maxillary second premolar	7.0	Mandibular second premolar	7.0
Maxillary first molar	10.0	Mandibular first molar	11.0
Maxillary second molar	9.0	Mandibular second molar	10.5

Average mesiodistal widths of *primary* teeth (mm): [152]

Maxillary central incisor	6.5	Mandibular central incisor	4.2
Maxillary lateral incisor	5.1	Mandibular lateral incisor	4.1
Maxillary canine	7.0	Mandibular canine	5.0
Maxillary first molar	7.3	Mandibular first molar	7.7
Maxillary second molar	8.2	Mandibular second molar	9.9

MAXILLARY ARCH (band and loop space maintainer has maintained second primary molar space)

-2.0 mm maxillary incisor crowding currently present

+2.0 mm of anticipated leeway space (1.0 mm/side)

Balance = -2.0 mm + 2.0 mm = 0.0 mm

MANDIBULAR ARCH

-1.0 mm incisor crowding currently present

+3.2 mm anticipated leeway space (1.6 mm/side)

Balance = -1.0 mm + 3.2 mm = +2.2 mm

That is, *0.0 mm of maxillary arch crowding and 2.2 mm of mandibular arch spacing is anticipated following the eruption of all permanent teeth (if proper space maintenance is employed).*

Q: In our previous patient (Jasmin), a right lateral CR-CO shift was present. Could an undetected right lateral CR-CO shift also explain Jenna's mandibular midline deviation? What should you check at your case presentation appointment?

A: A right lateral shift *could* explain Jenna's mandibular midline deviation to the right. For that reason, you need to check for a CR-CO shift again at the case presentation (and at every appointment). This was done, and we could not detect a CR-CO shift. Midline deviations can also result from dental arch asymmetries, crowding, etc.

Q: We noted the possible ectopic eruption of Jenna's maxillary left permanent canine. At this point, we cannot determine if the permanent canine is palatal or labial to the root of the permanent lateral incisor. However, as a general rule, when viewed on a panoramic radiograph, how is eruption success of a *palatally* displaced maxillary permanent canine related to the canine crown overlap of the permanent lateral incisor root?

A: The greater the permanent canine crown overlap, the less likely will be the chance that the canine will erupt successfully [162, 163].

Q: If, upon further investigation (manual palpation or 3-D radiography), we find Jenna's maxillary left permanent canine is palatally displaced, what can be done to improve the eruption of this tooth? Specifically, could extraction of Jenna's maxillary left primary canine guarantee successful eruption of her maxillary left permanent canine?

A: No, there is nothing you can do that would *guarantee* the eruption of any tooth. However, if Jenna's maxillary left permanent canine is palatally displaced, the literature suggests that extraction of the maxillary left primary canine, done in conjunction with space creation for the permanent canine (e.g. using headgear,

RME, extraction of the maxillary primary first molar, etc.), may increase the likelihood that her maxillary left permanent canine will erupt successfully [163–165].

However, extraction of the maxillary left primary first molar could *delay* the eruption of the maxillary left first premolar if the root of the first premolar is less than half developed. Delaying the first premolar eruption could delay permanent canine eruption.

Q: What are Jenna's *primary* problems in each dimension, plus other problems?

A:

Table 6.7 Primary problems list for Jenna.

AP	Angle Class II division 1
	Iowa classification: II (3 mm) II (3 mm) II (2 mm) II (2 mm)
Vertical	OB 20–30%
Transverse	Maxillary right primary canine and right primary first molar in lingual crossbite
	Maxillary and mandibular first permanent molars exhibit transverse compensations
Other	Maxillary anterior teeth malaligned
	Ectopically erupting maxillary left permanent canine
	Anterior crossbite

Q: Discuss Jenna in the context of three principles applied to every early treatment patient.

A:

1) The goal of early treatment is to correct developing problems – get the patient *back to normal for their stage of development* (including preventing complications such as resorption of adjacent tooth roots, reducing later treatment complexity, or reducing/eliminating unknowns). Preventing impaction of her maxillary left permanent canine (preventing root resorption of her maxillary left lateral incisor), correcting her Class II molar relationship, reducing her overbite, eliminating her right posterior crossbite, aligning her anterior teeth, and correcting her anterior crossbite would put Jenna back on track for her stage of development.

2) Early treatment should address *very specific problems with a clearly defined end point*, usually within six to nine months (except for some orthopedic treatments). Achieving eruption of her maxillary left permanent canine and correction of her Class II molar relationship are focused problems that may be much longer than six to nine months. Reducing her overbite, correcting her anterior crossbite, and aligning her incisors could be

accomplished with limited fixed orthodontic appliances in a few months. Her posterior crossbite could be readily corrected with RME.

3) Always ask: Is it necessary that I treat the patient now? *What harm will come if I choose to do nothing now?* If we are to prevent the impaction of Jenna's maxillary left permanent canine (and/or possible root resorption of her maxillary left lateral incisor), then we recommend addressing this problem now.

We anticipate no harm in delaying her right posterior crossbite treatment since she does not exhibit a lateral CR-CO shift. Nor do we anticipate harm in waiting a year to place an LLHA as the eruption of her mandibular canines and premolars is not imminent. Because no damage to her maxillary left lateral incisor exists, leaving it in crossbite and leaving her maxillary incisors malaligned should cause no harm.

Finally, Jenna is Class II by only 2–3 mm, and we have adequate time to correct her orthopedically to Class I if we place her on recall now and attend to this problem later during prepubertal or pubertal growth. Or, if we do not place an LLHA, then her molars may self-correct to Class I when the mandibular primary second molars exfoliate and the mandibular first permanent molars drift to the mesial.

Q: Jenna has a Class II molar relationship of 2–3 mm but normal maxillary and mandibular anteroposterior molar positions (i.e. flush terminal plane primary second molar relationships). Some orthodontists would recommend treating this relationship by *not* placing an LLHA and simply allowing mandibular first permanent molar mesial drift following exfoliation of mandibular primary second molars. The result could be a spontaneous molar improvement (correction) toward Class I. Other orthodontists would recommend orthopedics to achieve this molar correction (arguing that her profile tends toward convexity).

If Class II orthopedics is considered, can you state whether each of the following treatment effects would occur using a headgear or Class II functional appliance?
- Restriction of maxillary forward growth
- Distal movement of maxillary molars
- Acceleration of mandibular growth (not growth enhancement)
- Mesial movement of mandibular molars.

A: Treatment effects from appliances include:
- *Restriction of maxillary forward growth* – unequivocal short-term headgear skeletal effects include a small restriction in forward maxillary growth (SNA decreases 0.5–3 degrees) [166]. Inhibition of maxillary growth has also been reported with Herbst functional appliance treatment [167], and a tendency to restrict forward maxillary growth probably occurs with all Class II functional appliances.
- *Distal movement of maxillary molars* – a significant portion of headgear Class II correction is distal maxillary molar movement [166]. Distal movement of maxillary teeth has also been reported with Herbst functional appliance treatment [157], and a tendency to move maxillary teeth distally probably occurs with all Class II functional appliances.
- *Acceleration of mandibular growth (not growth enhancement)* – unequivocal short-term Class II functional appliance skeletal effects include a small forward positioning of B-point (1–2 degrees) [166]. However, functional appliances do *not* enhance mandibular horizontal growth beyond that found in control subjects [167]. Further, the acceleration in mandibular length gained by functional appliance treatment may not improve chin projection [168–171].
- *Mesial movement of mandibular molars* – Class II functional appliances demonstrate this effect [157].

Q: If Class II orthopedics is employed to correct her mild Class II molar relationship and increase chin projection, then would you begin orthopedics *now*?
A: First consider the *magnitude* of her skeletal discrepancy (apical base discrepancy) – which is mild. Since she is only nine years old, she is one year in advance of the average age for female onset of pubertal growth acceleration, and we should have an excellent chance of correcting her to Class I orthopedically – if she cooperates.

Now, let's talk about *when* to start. Generally, Class II orthopedic correction should be delayed until the patient is in the late mixed dentition, as opposed to the early mixed dentition [172–178]. Jenna is in the early mixed dentition stage of development – so it is a little early to begin with orthopedics.

However, even *if a patient is in the early mixed dentition, if the patient has good statural growth, then you should consider initiating Class II orthopedic treatment.* Jenna's parents state that she is not growing. Therefore, we do not recommend initiating Class II treatment.

Q: Is Jenna's right posterior lingual crossbite a dental, or a skeletal, crossbite?
A: It is a skeletal crossbite. Why? Ask what happens when we *upright her permanent molars transversely.* As we upright her buccally torqued maxillary permanent

molars (Figure 6.54r), their crowns will move lingually – worsening her transverse relationship and possibly placing her permanent first molars into lingual crossbite. As we upright her lingually torqued mandibular permanent molars (Figure 6.54s), their crowns will move buccally – worsening her transverse relationship and possibly placing her permanent first molars into lingual crossbite. Therefore, Jenna has a *skeletal* posterior crossbite. Her posterior skeletal bases do not relate well and removing compensations unmasks her true posterior transverse relationship.

Q: Should you start early treatment now or recall Jenna? If you start treatment, what treatment options would you consider?

A: Treatment options include the following:

- *Recall* (no treatment, monitor only) – *is not recommended due to the ectopically erupting maxillary left permanent canine.* If no treatment is rendered, then the ectopically erupting canine could become impacted and/or resorb the maxillary left lateral incisor root. No harm will come if we delay for one-year the correction of her maxillary left lateral incisor crossbite, maxillary incisor alignment, right posterior crossbite, or Class II molar relationship.

- *Limited fixed appliance treatment (maxillary 2x6 appliance) to align maxillary anterior teeth and correct maxillary left lateral incisor crossbite – is unnecessary.* Why? At this time, no damage is occurring to the lateral incisor, and maxillary incisor malalignment is not a concern to Jenna or her parents.

- *Extraction of maxillary primary canines and maxillary primary first molars – is not recommended.* Why? The roots of the maxillary first premolars appear to be *less than half developed* (Figure 6.54f). Extraction of maxillary primary first molars at this time could delay the first premolar eruption as scar tissue forms over them. Delayed first premolar eruption would delay providing room for eruption of the maxillary left permanent canine.

- *RME (Hyrax appliance) – is recommended* and would provide maxillary anterior *apical* space to aid eruption of the permanent canines. RME could also provide bilateral posterior overjet to eliminate the right posterior crossbite, upright maxillary and mandibular molars, and seat the posterior occlusion in a cusp-fossa relationship. The advantages of RME (Hyrax appliance) are that the appliance is cemented in place, thereby reducing the need for cooperation, and midpalatal sutural separation (skeletal expansion) is virtually guaranteed at nine years of age because facial skeletal resistance to expansion is small [41].

- *Maxillary expansion with quad-helix appliance* [40] – *offers no real advantage over expansion with a Hyrax appliance.* Midpalatal suture separation could occur with a quad-helix appliance, but facial resistance to skeletal expansion in a nine-year-old girl may be great enough to prevent midpalatal sutural separation with a quad-helix.

- *Maxillary expansion with a split plate – offers no advantage over expansion with a Hyrax appliance.* Facial skeletal resistance at nine years of age would likely prevent midpalatal suture separation/skeletal expansion with a split plate, and it is doubtful that enough lateral force could be generated to disarticulate the maxillary midpalatal suture.

- *LLHA to maintain uprighted mandibular first permanent molars.* For instance, if during RME, crossbite elastics are worn from the buccal of the Hyrax appliance to buttons on the lingual of the mandibular molars to upright the mandibular molars, then an LLHA could be fabricated later to hold the uprighted mandibular first molars in position. If a Schwarz expansion appliance is used to upright the mandibular molars, then it could be worn at night to maintain the uprighted molars. Or, an overexpanded LLHA could be used to both upright mandibular first molars and maintain them in an upright position.

- *LLHA to maintain space* – would provide 2.2 mm of arch spacing following the eruption of all permanent teeth. This spacing could provide room for slight mandibular incisor uprighting during comprehensive treatment. However, an LLHA would greatly reduce mandibular first permanent molar mesial drift during the transition to permanent dentition – drift which could improve Jenna's Class II molar relationship.

Q: What is your recommended treatment? How would you proceed?

A: The maxillary right band and loop appliance was sectioned – leaving the band on the primary first molar. A Hyrax appliance was fabricated with metal arms extending from the maxillary first permanent molar bands mesially, along the lingual surfaces of the primary teeth crowns, in the hope of adding additional expansion anchorage from these teeth. Maxillary expansion (0.25 mm per day) was initiated. The Hyrax appliance fractured and was replaced with another. As expansion proceeded, crossbite elastics were worn between the buccal of the Hyrax appliance and lingual buttons bonded to the mandibular first molars. Once the mandibular molars were uprighted, the crossbite elastics were worn at night to maintain the mandibular molars in the upright positions. Expansion continued until the maxillary permanent first molar lingual cusps opposed the mandibular permanent first molar buccal cusps.

Following expansion, we could palpate the developing crowns of the right and left maxillary permanent canines in the labial alveolar plate. We noted the developing crowns were in close proximity to the roots of the maxillary later incisors. In particular, the maxillary left permanent canine appeared to be more mesially positioned, overlapping the root of the left maxillary permanent lateral incisor along its anterior aspect. Therefore, we avoided bracketing maxillary lateral incisors so as not to move the lateral incisor roots into the developing maxillary canine crowns. Instead, maxillary central incisors were aligned using fixed orthodontic appliances. Brackets were removed (Figure 6.55), and a vacuum-formed clear retainer fabricated

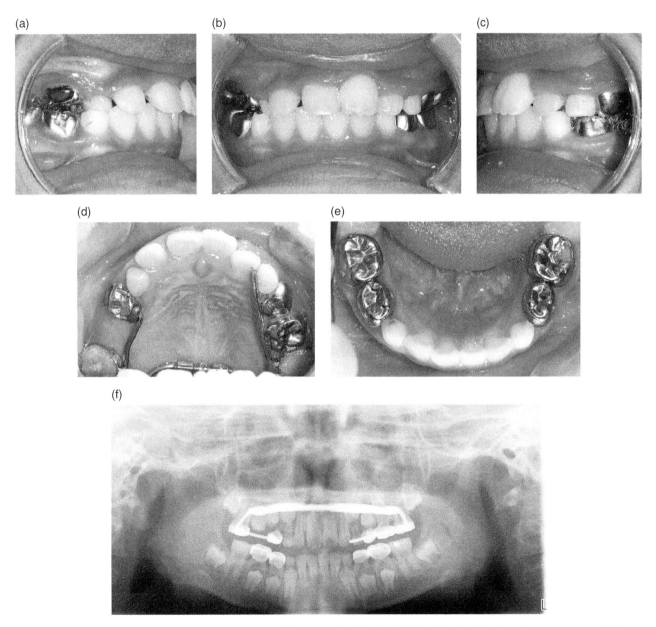

Figure 6.55 (a–f) Progress records at age ten years and three months following RME and limited fixed appliance treatment. RME proceeded until the maxillary permanent first molar lingual cusps opposed the *uprighted* mandibular permanent first molar buccal cusps. Note that the maxillary right primary canine and primary first molar remain in lingual crossbite and that the mandibular midline is still 3 mm to the right of the maxillary midline. Note that the maxillary left permanent canine overlaps the root of the maxillary left lateral incisor on the panoramic image, confirming our earlier diagnosis of labial canine displacement by palpation.

(extending mesially from the Hyrax appliance) to be worn at night to maintain maxillary central incisor alignment. Note that the maxillary right primary canine and primary first molar are still in lingual crossbite and that the mandibular midline is still 3 mm to the right of the maxillary midline.

Q: RME had proceeded until maxillary permanent first molar lingual cusps opposed uprighted mandibular permanent first molar buccal cusps. It would have been imprudent to expand further than this. However, Jenna's maxillary right primary canine and primary first molar remained in lingual crossbite, and our best chance for her maxillary right permanent canine and premolars to erupt into a normal transverse relationship would have resulted from moving the primary teeth buccally – out of crossbite. What could we have done to correct the maxillary primary canine and primary first molar crossbites?

A: The soldered RME appliance right metal arm, extending from the Hyrax appliance to the primary first molar, should have been extended further to contact the lingual of the maxillary right primary canine. Further, the maxillary right first primary molar should have been banded and included as part of the expansion appliance.

Q: Jenna's maxillary primary canines and primary first molars were never extracted. Was this a mistake?

A: No. We now know (by earlier palpation and Figure 6.55f) that the maxillary left permanent canine is in a much more favorable position than we thought initially (Figure 6.54f). Labial ectopic eruption of maxillary canines is, by and large, less problematic. Jenna's maxillary left permanent canine appears to be labially displaced but erupting. Its crown overlaps the left lateral incisor root less than before, and the primary canine and primary first molar roots are resorbing. It appears that the *anterior space created by RME* helped the labially displaced maxillary left permanent canine erupt without the need for primary tooth extractions.

Also, because the maxillary left first premolar roots were initially < half developed, extraction of the maxillary primary canine and primary first molar could have *delayed* eruption of the maxillary left first premolar. This delayed eruption could have had a negative impact on maxillary left permanent canine eruption.

Q: Jenna returned to our clinic at age eleven years (Figure 6.56). The Hyrax appliance was still cemented in place, but she had discontinued wearing her clear maxillary retainer. What changes do you note?

A: Changes include the following:
- Continued eruption of all permanent teeth including the maxillary left permanent canine.
- Adequate room appears for all erupting teeth.
- Maxillary right permanent canine and premolars appear to be erupting into lingual crossbite.
- Right permanent first molars are "end-on" (Class II by 1–2 mm).
- Left permanent first molars are now Class I.
- Discoloration of erupting maxillary premolars.
- Maxillary right second premolar is rotated.
- LDML is still 2–3 mm to the right of UDML.
- Excess overjet of maxillary left second primary molar and permanent first molar (Figure 6.56k).
- ~1 mm of mandibular anterior crowding is present.
- Mandibular first permanent molars spontaneously uprighted (compare Figures 6.54s and 6.56p).

Q: Why would Jenna's mandibular first permanent molars spontaneously *upright* transversely?

A: As RME expands the maxillary posterior dentition, it pushes the cheeks laterally and reduces cheek pressure against the buccal surfaces of the mandibular molars. Tongue pressure then uprights the mandibular molars as it pushes from them laterally.

Q: How would you now deal with the right Class II (1–2 mm) relationship?

A: We considered asking Jenna to wear a high-pull headgear which could correct her right molar relationship to Class I and overcorrect her left molar relationship to Class III. Space created by retracting her maxillary molars distally could then be used to upright her proclined maxillary incisors, and mandibular "E-space" could be used to upright her proclined mandibular incisors. Jenna had not achieved menarche. So, we anticipated adequate future growth.

Since Jenna was bimaxillary protrusive, we also considered different combinations of premolar extractions to provide space in order to upright her incisors and improve the right molar relationship. Extraction of her maxillary first premolars, mandibular left *first* premolar, and mandibular right *second* premolar would provide space to upright incisors in both arches and also move the mandibular right permanent molar more mesially than the left (improving the right molar relationship). We held discussions with Jenna and her parents, but they were adamantly opposed to premolar extractions and lip retraction.

Based upon the fact that her mandibular primary second molar crowns appeared large compared to the

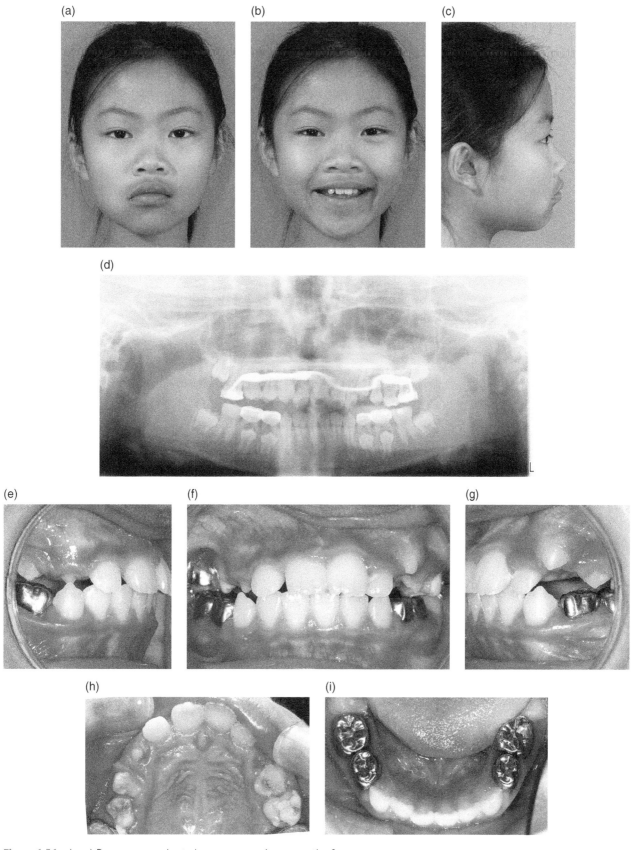

Figure 6.56 (a–p) Progress records at eleven years and one month of age.

(j)　(k)　(l)

(m)　(n)

(o)　(p)

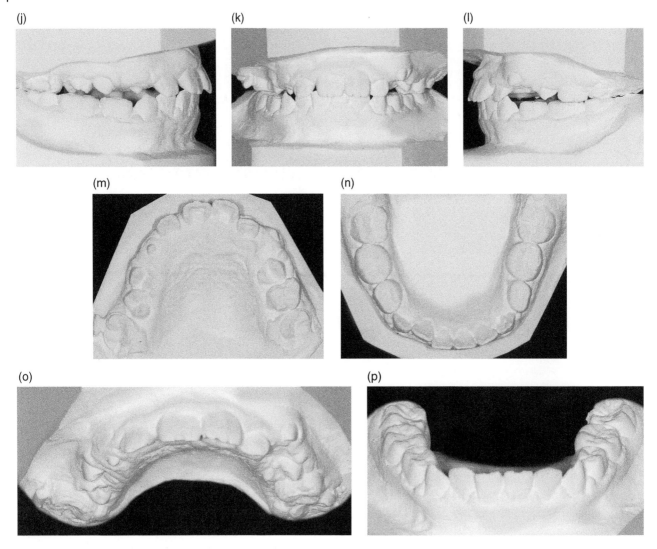

Figure 6.56 (Continued)

erupting mandibular second premolars (Figure 6.56d, large anticipated "E-spaces"), and based upon the fact that Jenna exhibited only mild mandibular anterior crowding, we decided to allow all her permanent teeth to erupt and to deal with the small (1–2 mm) right Class II relationship later.

Q: How would you proceed?

A: The Hyrax appliance was left in place, an LLHA was fabricated and delivered, and by the time Jenna was twelve years and six months old, all permanent teeth had erupted *(early treatment ended).*

Comprehensive non-extraction treatment began. Fixed orthodontic appliances were placed, and right crossbite elastics were worn to correct her right canine/premolar lingual crossbite. Orthodontic cement was placed on her maxillary first permanent molar occlusal

surfaces to open her bite enough to allow correction of her right lingual crossbite (Figures 6.57a–6.57e).

The right crossbite was corrected within two months, at which time the orthodontic cement and Hyrax appliance were removed, the maxillary first permanent molars were fitted with orthodontic bands, the arches leveled and aligned, and all spaces closed. Class II elastics were worn for a short period of time to achieve final cusp seating anteroposteriorly. Orthodontic finishing proceeded, Jenna was debanded, and a cosmetic dentist placed composite veneers on her maxillary lateral incisors to close small residual spaces and lengthen the lateral incisors.

Q: Final records of Jenna are shown in Figure 6.58. What changes do you note?

(a)   (b)   (c)

(d)   (e)

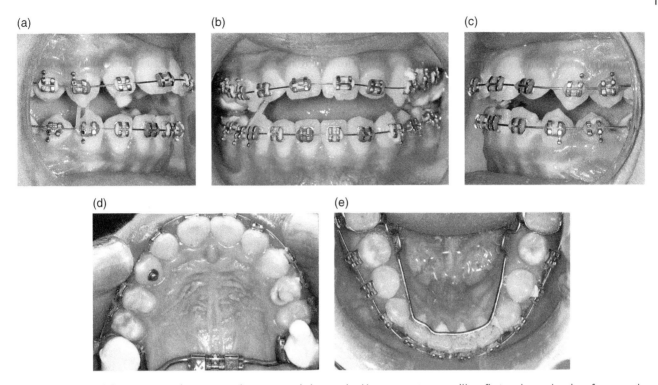

Figure 6.57 (a–e) Progress records at age twelve years and six months. Note cement on maxillary first molar occlusal surfaces used to prop open Jenna's bite so that her right canine/premolar crossbite could be treated with crossbite elastics. Also, note the residual "E-space" especially on the mandibular left side.

A: Changes include the following:
- Jenna now presents with a beautiful smile and a straight profile. She underwent significant downward and forward growth of her nose, lips, chin, maxilla, and mandible (Figure 6.58f). Her mandible grew forward more than her maxilla resulting in an ANB reduction from 3 to 2°. Molars and incisors erupted. Molars drifted to the mesial.
- Mandibular incisors uprighted (FMIA increased from 52 to 61°, IMPA [incisor mandibular plane angle] decreased from 110 to 101°).
- Facial cant (right side of face longer than left), including the right to left cant of lips, is still noted (Figure 6.58a).
- Slight occlusal cant noted relative to the interpupillary line (Figure 6.58b).
- UDML and LDML are now coincident but ~1 mm to the right of her facial midline (Figure 6.58b).
- OB has decreased from 20–30 to 10%.
- Discoloration of premolars is still noted.
- Gingival margin of the maxillary left central incisor is higher than the right central incisor (Figure 6.58i), but Jenna has a low smile line (Figure 6.58b) – so, this difference is masked.
- Roots of the maxillary right second premolar and left lateral incisor are not parallel (Figure 6.58g). Mandibular second premolar roots are not parallel.
- Root resorption (root apex "blunting") is observed in her mandibular second premolars and maxillary central incisors.
- Mild crowding has been eliminated.

Q: How was Jenna's right Class II molar relationship corrected?

A: Because her maxillary molars appear to have moved to the mesial more than her mandibular molars (Figure 6.58f), we conclude that her right Class II molar correction resulted primarily from greater forward mandibular growth than maxillary growth (differential jaw growth). However, the mesial drift of the mandibular right molar, and Class II elastic wear, also played a role.

Q: Is it unusual for a Class II molar relationship to self-correct?

A: As is true of so many orthodontic problems, the answer is a question of *magnitude*. Jenna had a mild right Class II molar relationship (1–2 mm Class II or approximately "end on" right molars).

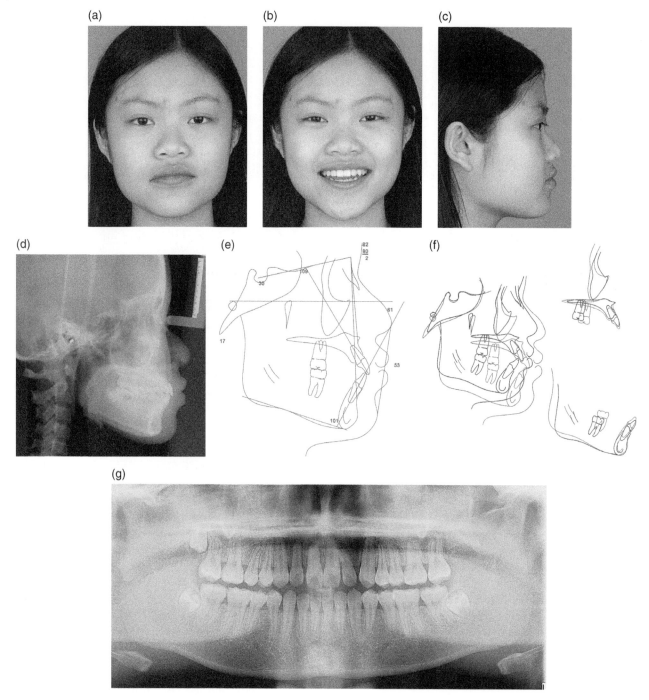

Figure 6.58 (a–l). Final records of Jenna.

If a patient in the primary dentition exhibits a *straight (flush) terminal plane*, then the permanent first molars will eventually erupt and drift into an ideal Class I relationship 56% of the time and in a Class II relationship 44% of the time. On the other hand, a *distal step* in the primary dentition (more severe Class II) always guides the erupting permanent first molars into a Class II relationship [179, 180].

Q: Jenna's final panoramic image (Figure 6.58g) revealed problems with root parallelism and root resorption. What did we fail to do during comprehensive treatment in fixed appliances? Could these problems have been avoided?

A: We *failed to make a progress panoramic image nine months into leveling/aligning arches with fixed appliances.* Such an image would allow us to identify errors of

(h)　　　　　　　　　(i)　　　　　　　　　(j)

(k)　　　　　　　　　(l)

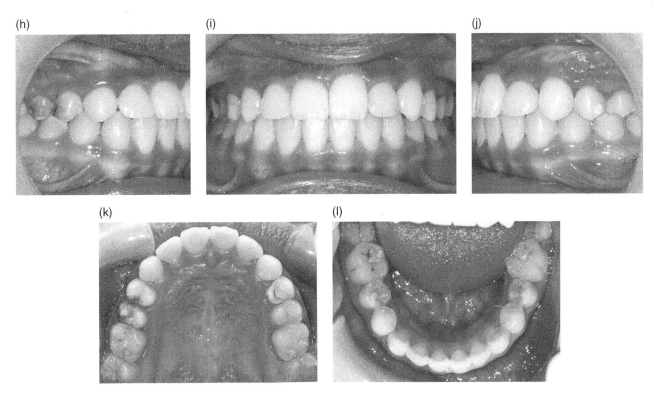

Figure 6.58　(Continued)

bracket positioning (root parallelism errors) and root resorption. The non-parallelism of roots could have been corrected using the progress panoramic image as a guide, but the root resorption may not have been avoided.

Q: Could Jenna's root resorption have been predicted?

A: No, at least not before treatment began, but *examining tooth roots radiographically six to nine months after the initiation of fixed appliance treatment appears to be a useful predictor of severe resorption at the end of treatment* [181]. A risk of severe root resorption post-treatment is seen in teeth with minor root resorption after six to nine months of treatment. On the other hand, severe root resorption is absent post-treatment in teeth without resorption after six to nine months. Again, we should have made a progress panoramic image of Jenna.

Q: Are there risk factors which could help predict apical root resorption?

A: Examples of factors that have been reported to be related to orthodontically induced root resorption include *total displacement of the root apex, treatment duration, and the presence of teeth with blunt or pipette-shaped roots* [181, 182]. Genetic factors account for at least 50% of the variation in root resorption, and future estimation of susceptibility to root resorption will likely require the analysis of a suite of genes, root morphology, skeleto-dental values, and the treatment method to be used – or essentially the amount of tooth movement planned for treatment [183].

Q: Jenna initially presented with non-coincident midlines, but she finished with coincident midlines. How was this correction made?

A: We suspect that she had an undetected right lateral CR-CO shift that was eliminated. We suspect this because the most dramatic improvement in her midline positions occurred as she wore right crossbite elastics (Figures 6.57a–6.57b). Further indication that the midline deviation was due to an undetected shift includes the fact that the midline improvement held after her right canine/premolar crossbite was corrected. In addition to CR-CO shift elimination, maxillary right space closure (Figure 6.57d) would have improved her midline relationship by shifting her maxillary midline slightly to the right, and mandibular left space closure (Figure 6.57e) would have improved her midline relationship by shifting her mandibular midline slightly to the left.

Q: Jenna finished treatment with a right to left occlusal cant relative to her interpupillary line (Figure 6.58b). How large must a right-to-left occlusal cant be in order to be noticed by lay persons?

A: At least 3 mm [184]

Q: What retention protocol would you recommend for Jenna?

A: She was placed in removable Hawley retainers and asked to wear them at night, for life. Only with lifelong retention can the alignment of teeth can be guaranteed. A mandibular fixed canine-to-canine retainer could also have been used, but we thought it best to place her in Hawley retainers to maintain her posterior transverse correction.

Q: Can you suggest "take-home pearls" regarding Jenna's treatment?

A: "Take-home pearls" include the following:

- Jenna initially presented when she was nine years old in the early mixed dentition with a Class II (2–3 mm) molar relationship, maxillary right primary canine and primary first molar lingual crossbite, ectopically erupting maxillary left permanent canine, and CR = CO.
- In spite of the fact that only two maxillary right primary teeth were in posterior crossbite, we concluded that Jenna had a *skeletal* (not dental) crossbite. Why?

During normal growth and development, mandibular first permanent molars erupt tipped to the lingual and upright with age. Maxillary first permanent molars erupt tipped to the buccal and upright with age [1]. Maxillary and mandibular molar uprighting are dependent upon maxillary width which increases during growth.

In normal transverse skeletal relationships, the maxillary and mandibular skeletal bases relate well. Orthodontic uprighting of posterior teeth moves them directly over their skeletal bases and positions maxillary posterior teeth directly over mandibular posterior teeth. In a transverse skeletal discrepancy, skeletal bases do not relate well, and uprighting posterior teeth tends to move them into crossbite. Therefore, to determine whether a transverse skeletal discrepancy exists between the jaws, you must visualize uprighting posterior teeth.

As we visualized uprighting Jenna's buccally torqued maxillary permanent molars, we saw that the molar crowns would move lingually – worsening her transverse relationship and possibly moving her permanent first molars into lingual crossbite. As we visualized uprighting her lingually torqued mandibular permanent molars, we saw that the molar crowns would move buccally – worsening her transverse relationship and possibly moving her permanent first molars into lingual crossbite. Therefore, Jenna had a *skeletal* posterior crossbite.

You cannot determine whether a posterior crossbite is of skeletal, or dental, origin simply by counting the number of teeth in crossbite. Even in the absence of a posterior crossbite, the transverse dental compensations may be so large that they mask an underlying skeletal discrepancy. Instead, you must visualize the effect of removing transverse compensations (uprighting posterior teeth).

- We did not initially detect a CR-CO shift in Jenna. But later, when she was placed on right crossbite elastics, her midline relationship improved dramatically leading us to believe that she had an undetected CR-CO shift.
- Jenna's mild Class II correction occurred primarily through differential jaw growth and without Class II orthopedic treatment (headgears or functional appliances). Mesial drift of the mandibular right molar, and Class II elastic wear, probably also played a role.
- Anterior space creation with RME appears to have helped Jenna's ectopically erupting maxillary left permanent canine change direction and begin to erupt normally (compare Figures 6.54f and 6.55f). If you detect maxillary permanent canine ectopic eruption (e.g. permanent canine crown overlapping maxillary permanent lateral incisor root on a panoramic image), consider additional measures to determine if the canine is displaced palatally or labially. If it is palatally displaced, creating a pathway and space for it to erupt by extracting the maxillary primary canine (and the maxillary primary first molar) may be prudent. Maxillary primary canine extraction alone may not resolve the problem – you must create adequate space for the permanent canine. Extracting maxillary primary first molars can accelerate first premolar eruption (moving them away from the permanent canine crowns/providing more space for the permanent canines to erupt) if the maxillary first premolar roots are ≥ half developed. You can also create space for the maxillary permanent canines with RME or headgear.
- Our best chance for Jenna's maxillary *right* permanent canine and premolars to have erupted into a normal transverse relationship would have been to have *moved the maxillary right primary canine and primary first molar laterally – out of crossbite during RME*. We failed to do this.

Case Jonathan

Q: Jonathan, a boy nine years and five months old (Figure 6.59), presents to you for a consultation with the parent's chief complaint, "Our family dentist says

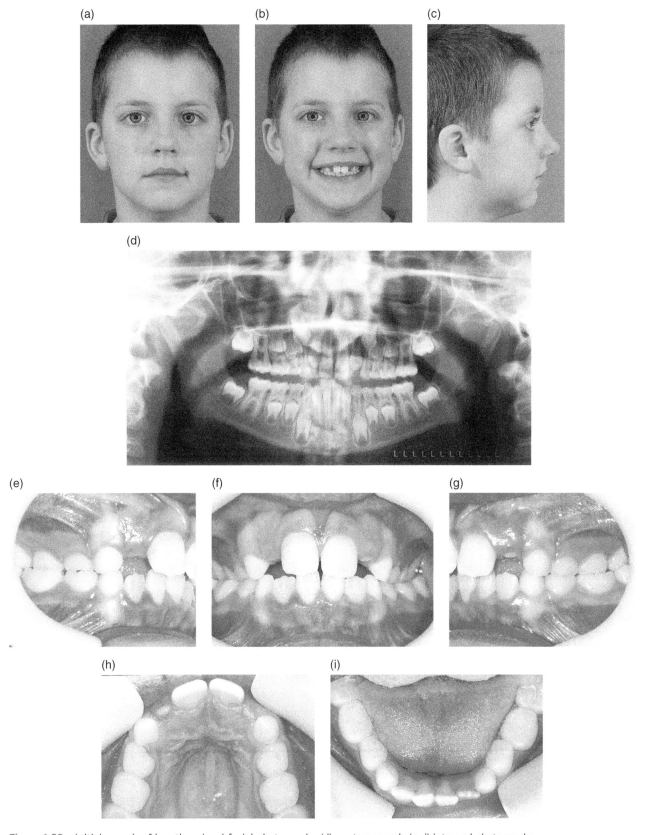

Figure 6.59 Initial records of Jonathan. (a–c) facial photographs, (d) pantomograph, (e–i) intraoral photographs.

Jonathan has a crossbite." PMH, periodontal, and TMJ evaluations are WRN. CR = CO. *Compile your diagnostic findings and problem list.* State your *diagnosis.*

A:

Table 6.8 Diagnostic findings and problem list for Jonathan.

Full face and profile	***FRONTAL VIEW*** Face is symmetric LAFH WRN (soft tissue Glabella-Subnasale = Subnasale – soft tissue Menton) Lip competence UDML 1–2 mm to right of the facial midline Incisal display during smile slightly inadequate (maxillary central incisor gingival margins slightly apical to maxillary lip) Moderately large buccal corridors ***PROFILE VIEW*** Convex profile Obtuse NLA Retrusive chin Obtuse lip-chin-throat angle Short chin-throat length
Radiographs	Early mixed dentition stage of development
Intraoral photos	Angle Class II molar relationship Iowa classification: II(4 mm) II(2 mm) II(2 mm) II(2 mm) Bilateral posterior lingual crossbite OJ 1–2 mm OB 10% LDML coincident with UDML Mandibular anterior attached keratinized gingival tissue WRN 2.4 mm maxillary anterior crowding is currently present (10.6 mm space but 13 mm needed for unerupted maxillary permanent lateral incisors) 0.4 mm of maxillary arch crowding is anticipated following the eruption of all permanent teeth (if appropriate space maintenance is employed) 2 mm mandibular anterior crowding currently present 1.2 mm of mandibular arch spacing is anticipated following the eruption of all permanent teeth (if appropriate space maintenance is employed) Maxillary arch symmetric (Figure 6.59h) Mandibular arch asymmetric with left posterior slightly ahead of right (Figure 6.59i)
Other	–
Diagnosis	Class II malocclusion with bilateral posterior lingual crossbite and mild mandibular anterior crowding

Q: Provide a detailed space analysis for Jonathan's maxillary and mandibular arches. How were the 0.4 mm of maxillary anterior crowding and 1.2 mm of mandibular anterior spacing calculated (if we employ space maintenance)?

A:

Average mesiodistal widths of permanent teeth (mm): [152]

Maxillary central incisor	8.5	Mandibular central incisor	5.0
Maxillary lateral incisor	6.5	Mandibular lateral incisor	5.5
Maxillary canine	7.5	Mandibular canine	7.0
Maxillary first premolar	7.0	Mandibular first premolar	7.0
Maxillary second premolar	7.0	Mandibular second premolar	7.0
Maxillary first molar	10.0	Mandibular first molar	11.0
Maxillary second molar	9.0	Mandibular second molar	10.5

Average mesiodistal widths of *primary* teeth (mm): [152]

Maxillary central incisor	6.5	Mandibular central incisor	4.2
Maxillary lateral incisor	5.1	Mandibular lateral incisor	4.1
Maxillary canine	7.0	Mandibular canine	5.0
Maxillary first molar	7.3	Mandibular first molar	7.7
Maxillary second molar	8.2	Mandibular second molar	9.9

MAXILLARY ARCH
+5.4 mm right lateral incisor space currently present (Figure 6.59h)
−6.5 mm anticipated space required for right permanent lateral incisor
+0.5 mm diastema space
+4.7 mm left lateral incisor space currently present
−6.5 mm anticipated space required for left permanent lateral incisor
+2 mm of anticipated leeway space (1 mm/side)
Balance = +5.4 mm −6.5 mm +0.5 mm + 4.7 mm −6.5 mm + 2 mm = −0.4 mm

MANDIBULAR ARCH
−2 mm of anterior crowding is currently present
+3.2 mm of anticipated leeway space (1.6 mm/side)
Balance = −2 mm + 3.2 mm = +1.2 mm

That is, *we anticipate 0.4 mm of maxillary arch crowding and 1.2 mm of mandibular arch spacing following the eruption of all permanent teeth (if we employ proper space maintenance).*

Q: What are Jonathan's *primary* problems that you must stay focused on?

A:

Table 6.9   Primary problems list for Jonathan.

AP	Angle Class II molar relationship Iowa classification: II(4 mm) II(2 mm) II(2 mm) II(2 mm)
Vertical	–
Transverse	Bilateral posterior lingual crossbite
Other	Mild maxillary and mandibular anterior crowding

Q: Is Jonathan's bilateral posterior lingual crossbite dental or skeletal crossbite?

A: It is a *skeletal* crossbite due to a narrow maxilla. Why do we conclude this? Jonathan's maxillary and mandibular molars appear upright (Figure 6.59f). Therefore, the narrow maxillary dental arch (relative to the broader mandibular dental arch) reflects a narrow maxillary skeletal base relative to a broader mandibular skeletal base. Also, his narrow maxilla and moderately large buccal corridors are seen when he smiles (Figure 6.59b). Jonathan has a skeletal crossbite.

Q: Discuss Jonathan in the context of three principles applied to every early treatment patient.

A:

1) The goal of early treatment is to correct developing problems – get the patients *back to normal for their stage of development* (including preventing complications such as resorption of adjacent tooth roots, reducing later treatment complexity, or reducing/eliminating unknowns). Correcting Jonathan's bilateral posterior crossbite and his Class II molar relationship would put him back on track.

2) Early treatment should address *very specific problems with a clearly defined end point*, usually within six to nine months (except for some orthopedic problems). Jonathan's posterior crossbite is a focused problem that could be corrected in a short time, but his Class II molar relationship (convex profile, deficient mandibular) could benefit from orthopedics which could take longer than nine months.

3) Always ask: Is it necessary that I treat the patient now? *What harm will come if I choose to do nothing now?* Jonathan is only nine-and-one-half years old, and it is improbable that he will reach puberty during the next year. Therefore, it is not necessary to perform RME now in order to maximize maxillary skeletal expansion. If we postpone RME (not creating additional arch space), then the maxillary lateral incisors may erupt malaligned. If Jonathan currently has good statural growth velocity, then we will potentially miss useful jaw growth for orthopedic correction if we recall.

Q: Jonathan lacks a CR-CO shift. If Jonathan had a *lateral CR-CO shift*, then how might this influence a decision to perform RME?

A: If he had a lateral CR-CO shift, then we would perform RME now in order to reduce the chances of his mandible growing asymmetrically.

Q: Regarding the timing of Jonathan's Class II orthopedic treatment, what should you consider?

A: You should estimate the time remaining until the average onset of pubertal growth acceleration in boys. For Jonathan, that estimate is ~three years [149]. You should ask Jonathan's parents if he is displaying statural growth (growing/getting taller).

If they say that he is growing now (i.e. he has good statural growth velocity), then you could initiate Class II orthopedic treatment now – even though he is in the early mixed dentition. If they say that he is not growing, or do not know if he is growing, then ask them to keep a monthly record of his height and inform you of what they find. Jonathan's parents state that Jonathan is *not* growing.

Q: Should you start treatment or recall Jonathan? If you start treatment, what treatment options would you consider?

A: Options include the following:
- *Recall (no treatment, monitor only) – is a viable option* because Jonathan:
  1) lacks a lateral CR-CO shift
  2) has years (probably) before entering puberty
  3) is in the early mixed dentition
  4) is not growing
- *RME (Hyrax appliance) – is a viable option* which would eliminate the bilateral posterior crossbite, reduce the size of Jonathan's buccal corridors, and provide additional room for eruption of his maxillary anterior teeth. The advantages of *Hyrax appliance* RME are that it is cemented in place (reducing the need for cooperation) and midpalatal sutural separation (skeletal expansion) is virtually guaranteed at nine years of age because facial skeletal resistance to expansion is small [41].

- *Maxillary expansion with a quad-helix appliance* [40] *or split plate – offers no advantage over expansion with a Hyrax appliance.* Facial skeletal resistance to expansion in a nine-year-old boy may be great enough to prevent midpalatal sutural separation with a quad-helix or split plate.
- *Class II orthopedics – is not recommended.* Class II orthopedics should be delayed until Jonathan reaches the late mixed dentition [166, 172–178, 185] or is reported to be growing. At that time, Class II orthopedics could include restriction of maxillary forward growth (headgear, Herbst functional appliance), distal movement of maxillary molars (headgear, Herbst functional appliance), acceleration of mandibular growth (Class II functional appliance), and mesial movement of mandibular molars (Class II functional appliance) [157, 166, 167, 169, 170, 185].
- *LLHA or Nance holding arch for space maintenance – is not recommended* because the eruption of Jonathan's permanent canines and premolars is not imminent. However, Jonathan and his parents should monitor the mobility of his remaining primary teeth and inform you of changes.
- *Extraction of primary teeth – is not recommended.* All of Jonathan's permanent teeth appear to be erupting normally, and primary tooth extraction would serve no definitive purpose.

Q: What if Jonathan's parents request mandibular incisor alignment? Would you extract his mandibular primary canines in order to achieve mandibular incisor alignment?

A: No – for three reasons. First, his mandibular incisor crowding is very mild (only 2 mm), and extractions to correct this crowding are unreasonable. Second, the eventual placement of an LLHA should result in spontaneous mandibular incisor alignment via leeway space – without the need for a minor surgical procedure (extractions). Third, be careful about allowing parents to dictate treatment. Although the evidence-based practice is based partially upon patient/parent desires, it is equally based upon the best science and upon your clinical experience. Parental input is important. But be careful about letting parents dictate treatment. If you decide to extract mandibular primary canines, then place an LLHA to prevent arch perimeter loss via mesial molar drift.

Q: At the conclusion of his consultation, Jonathan's parents ask for your recommendation. How do you respond? Do you have a "take-home pearl" for Jonathan?

A: We recommend:
- Recalling Jonathan in nine to twelve months.
- Asking his parents to record his height each month or to return to our clinic every two to three months so we can measure his height. If he begins to grow, we recommend initiating Class II orthopedic treatment and RME.
- Asking his parents to monitor the mobility of his mandibular primary teeth. If they become mobile, we recommend placing an LLHA.
- A "take-home pearl" is this – because Jonathan did not have a lateral CR-CO shift, there was no compelling reason to correct his crossbite immediately. We probably have years to correct the crossbite before puberty. If Jonathan had a lateral CR-CO shift, we would have corrected the shift with RME to prevent the possible development of a mandibular asymmetry.

Case Alaina

Q: Alaina is eight years and eight months old (Figure 6.60) who presents with her mother's chief complaint, "We would like a second opinion about our daughter's crossbite." PMH and TMJ evaluations are WRN. Periodontal and mucogingival tissues are WRN. She exhibits a minimal (~1 mm) left lateral shift from CR to CO. *Compile your diagnostic findings and problem list.* State your *diagnosis.*

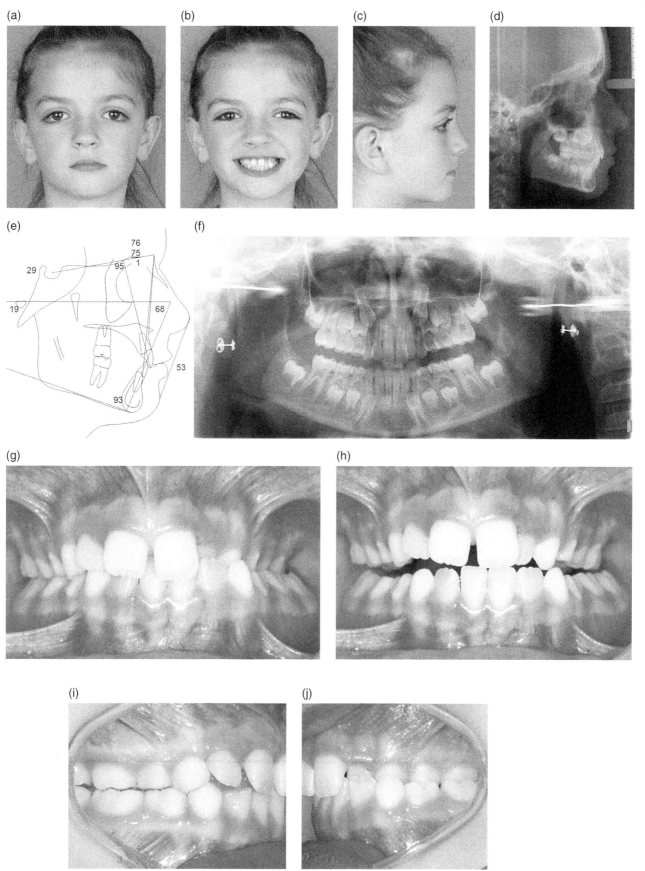

Figure 6.60 Initial records of Alaina. (a–c) facial photographs, (d–e) cephalometric radiograph and tracing, (f) pantomograph, (g) frontal intraoral photograph in CO, (h) frontal intraoral photograph slightly open in CR, (i–l) intraoral photographs in CO. Note: the photographs shown in G and H depict a minimal (~1 mm) left lateral shift from CR to CO.

(k)

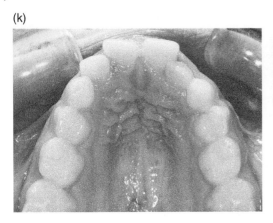

(l)

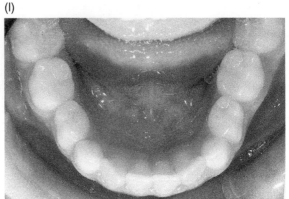

Figure 6.60 (Continued)

A:

Table 6.10 Diagnostic findings and problem list for Alaina.

Full face and profile	***FRONTAL VIEW***
	Chin deviation slightly to the left when occluding in CO
	LAFH WRN (soft tissue Glabella-Subnasale = Subnasale – soft tissue Menton)
	Lip competence
	UDML 1 mm to right of facial midline (Figure 6.60b)
	Incisal display during posed smile excessive (maxillary central incisor gingival margins lie below the maxillary lip)
	Moderately large left buccal corridor
	PROFILE VIEW
	Convex profile
	Obtuse NLA
	Lip-chin-throat angle WRN
	Chin-throat length WRN
Ceph analysis	***SKELETAL***
	Maxilla deficient anteroposteriorly (A-Point lies behind Nasion-perpendicular line)
	Mandible-deficient anteroposteriorly (deficient maxilla and a 5° angle exists between
	Nasion-perpendicular line and Nasion-B-Point line)
	LAFH WRN (LAFH/TAFH × 100% = 53%)
	Flat MPA (FMA = 19°, SN-MP = 29°)
	Effective bony pogonion (bony Pogonion ahead of the line extended from Nasion to B-point)

Table 6.10 (Continued)

	DENTAL
	Upright maxillary incisor inclination (U1 to SN = 95°)
	Mandibular incisor angulation WRN (FMIA = 68°)
Radiographs	Early mixed dentition stage of development
Intraoral photos and models	Angle Class II molar relationship in the early mixed dentition
	Iowa classification: II(1–2 mm) II(1–2 mm) II(1–2 mm) II(1–2 mm) in CR
	Unilateral left lingual crossbite from lateral incisors to permanent first molars
	OJ 1 mm
	OB 60%
	LDML to left of UDML by 3 mm in CO
	Thick mandibular anterior keratinized attached gingival tissue
	3.0 mm of maxillary anterior crowding is currently present
	1.0 mm of maxillary arch crowding is anticipated following the eruption of all permanent teeth (if appropriate space maintenance is employed)
	1.0 mm mandibular anterior crowding currently present
	2.2 mm mandibular arch spacing is anticipated following the eruption of all permanent teeth (if appropriate space maintenance is employed)
	Anteriorly tapered maxillary arch (Figure 6.60k)
	Maxillary and mandibular arches symmetric
Other	–
Diagnosis	Class II molar relationship with left anterior and posterior lingual crossbite and mild anterior crowding

Q: We noted that Alaina's mandible was deficient anteroposteriorly. However, her ANB angle = 1° which is a normal ANB angle. Can you explain?

A: As explained in the Appendix, we recommend using ANB angle to judge mandibular anteroposterior position only when the maxilla is normal anteroposteriorly. Because Alaina's maxilla is deficient, we recommend using the angle formed between *Nasion perpendicular* and the N-B line to judge the mandibular anteroposterior position. The reason is that A-Point would lie on this line if the maxilla was normal. Because the angle formed between Alaina's Nasion perpendicular and N-B line is 5° (normal angle is between 1 and 3°), we judge her mandible to be deficient (Figure 6.61). This judgment is corroborated by the fact that she has a convex profile.

Q: Why is the detection of a lateral CR-CO shift especially important in Alaina's case?

A: Because, with a left lateral CR-CO shift into a unilateral crossbite, her:

- Unilateral crossbite magnitude diminishes in CR into smaller *bilateral* inadequate posterior overjets.
- Transverse discrepancy can be corrected with balanced maxillary expansion.

- Left chin deviation will diminish/disappear with crossbite correction.
- Mandibular growth would be symmetric with crossbite correction.
- Chances of crossbite recurrence are unlikely after correction.

However, the absence of a left lateral CR-CO shift would leave Alaina with a true unilateral crossbite which is more difficult to treat and increases the chance that her mandible is growing asymmetrically. *If her left crossbite was due to asymmetric (relatively excessive right) mandibular growth, then we could end up chasing that left crossbite until she is finished growing* (Figure 6.62).

Q: In terms of possible asymmetric mandibular growth, what is an important observation to make from Alaina's lateral cephalometric radiograph (Figure 6.60d)?

A: *No asymmetry is noted* between the lower borders of her mandible or even between left and right molars. In other words, if asymmetric mandibular growth is present, then it is very small.

Q: Other than a mandibular growth asymmetry, can you think of any other reasons why Alaina could have such a large unilateral left crossbite without a CR-CO shift?

A: Two possible reasons might explain this finding: (i) Alaina's muscle memory for the functional shift cannot be "deprogrammed" during a clinical

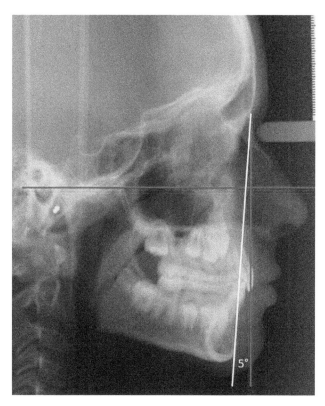

Figure 6.61 Because the angle formed between Alaina's Nasion perpendicular line (red vertical line) and N-B line (yellow line) is greater than 3°, we judge her mandible to be deficient.

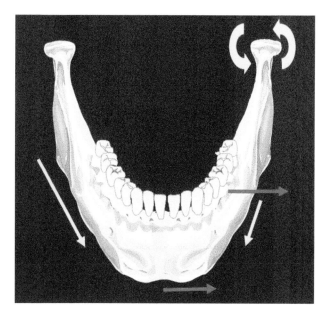

Figure 6.62 If Alaina did not have a left lateral CR-CO shift, then her left crossbite could be a result of asymmetric (relatively excessive right) mandibular growth (long right yellow arrow compared to left).

examination. Some patients require more aggressive methods that disclude the teeth for an extended period of time to reveal a functional mandibular shift. The use of a removable maxillary appliance with an anterior bite plane to disclude posterior teeth is an example of this approach. Without muscle memory deprogramming for these patients, the CR-CO shift remains undetected. (ii) Alaina may have had a larger functional shift into crossbite at an earlier age and has subsequently experienced adaptive growth of the condyles and glenoid fossae to the crossbite occlusion that reduced the mandibular shift.

Q: Provide a detailed space analysis for Alaina's maxillary and mandibular arches. How were the 1 mm of maxillary arch crowding and 2.2 mm of mandibular arch spacing calculated (if space maintenance is employed)?

A:

Average mesiodistal widths of permanent teeth (mm): [152]

Maxillary central incisor	8.5	Mandibular central incisor	5.0
Maxillary lateral incisor	6.5	Mandibular lateral incisor	5.5
Maxillary canine	7.5	Mandibular canine	7.0
Maxillary first premolar	7.0	Mandibular first premolar	7.0
Maxillary second premolar	7.0	Mandibular second premolar	7.0
Maxillary first molar	10.0	Mandibular first molar	11.0
Maxillary second molar	9.0	Mandibular second molar	10.5

Average mesiodistal widths of *primary* teeth (mm): [152]

Maxillary central incisor	6.5	Mandibular central incisor	4.2
Maxillary lateral incisor	5.1	Mandibular lateral incisor	4.1
Maxillary canine	7.0	Mandibular canine	5.0
Maxillary first molar	7.3	Mandibular first molar	7.7
Maxillary second molar	8.2	Mandibular second molar	9.9

MAXILLARY ARCH
    −4.0 mm maxillary lateral incisor crowding currently present (Figure 6.60k)
    +1.0 mm diastema space
    +2.0 mm of anticipated leeway space (1 mm/side)
    Balance = − 4.0 mm + 1.0 mm + 2.0 = −1.0 mm

MANDIBULAR ARCH
    − 1.0 mm of anterior crowding is currently present
    + 3.2 mm of anticipated leeway space (1.6 mm/side)
    Balance = − 1.0 mm + 3.2 mm = + 2.2 mm

That is, *1.0 mm of maxillary arch crowding and 2.2 mm of mandibular arch spacing is anticipated following the*

eruption of all permanent teeth (if proper space maintenance is employed).

Q: What are Alaina's *primary* problems that you must stay focused on?

A:

Table 6.11   Primary problems list for Alaina.

AP	Angle Class II molar relationship in the early mixed dentition
	Iowa classification: II(1–2 mm) II(1–2 mm) II(1–2 mm) II(1–2 mm) in CR
	Maxillary and mandibular anteroposterior deficiency
Vertical	OB 60%
Transverse	Unilateral left lingual crossbite from lateral incisors to permanent first molars
Other	~1 mm left lateral shift from CR to CO

Q: Is Alaina's left posterior lingual crossbite a dental, or skeletal, crossbite?

A: It is a skeletal crossbite. Looking at Alaina with her teeth slightly separated in CR (Figure 6.60h), her maxillary right permanent first molar exhibits slight buccal crown torque while her mandibular right permanent first molar exhibits lingual crown torque. If we upright these molars, then the maxillary right first permanent molar crown will move lingually and the mandibular right first permanent molar crown will move buccally. This will worsen her right transverse relationship. Her left posterior transverse skeletal discrepancy (maxillary deficiency) is obvious. Alaina has a *skeletal* crossbite, and her relatively narrow maxilla is reflected in her moderately large buccal corridors (Figure 6.60b).

Q: Discuss Alaina in the context of three principles applied to every early treatment patient.

A:

1) The goal of early treatment is to correct developing problems – get the patient *back to normal for their stage of development* (including preventing complications such as resorption of adjacent tooth roots, reducing later treatment complexity, or reducing/ eliminating unknowns). Correcting Alaina's left crossbite, CR-CO left lateral shift, left chin deviation, Class II molar relationship, and deep bite would put her back on track.

2) Early treatment should address *very specific problems with a clearly defined end point*, usually within

six to nine months (except for some orthopedic problems). Her left posterior crossbite, CR-CO shift, and chin deviation are focused problems that could be corrected with RME in a short time. The small (1–2 mm) Class II molar relationship is a focused problem but may take longer than six to nine months to correct depending upon growth (if orthopedics is employed). The deep bite could be readily corrected with fixed orthodontic appliances.

3) Always ask: Is it necessary that I treat the patient now? *What harm will come if I choose to do nothing now?* Delaying correction of the lateral shift could result in mandibular growth asymmetry. If orthopedics is employed to correct her Class II relationship, then we would recommend waiting to begin this treatment until she reaches the late mixed dentition (unless she exhibits good statural growth velocity now). The deep bite can be addressed during comprehensive treatment without harm.

Q: What unknowns do you face in treating Alaina?
A: Unknowns include an undetected left CR-CO shift, future jaw growth magnitude and direction, and treatment compliance.

Q: Should you start treatment now or recall Alaina? If you start treatment, what treatment options would you consider?
A: Treatment options include the following:

- *Recall* (no treatment, monitor only) – *is not recommended.* If Alaina's left lateral CR-CO shift into crossbite is not corrected, then her mandible could grow asymmetrically.
- *RME – is strongly recommended.* RME could eliminate the left posterior crossbite, provide overjet to upright the right permanent molars, eliminate the lateral CR-CO shift, and provide additional room for maxillary anterior teeth eruption. The advantages of a Hyrax appliance for RME are that the appliance is cemented in place (reducing the need for cooperation), and midpalatal sutural separation (skeletal expansion) is virtually guaranteed at eight years of age because facial skeletal resistance to expansion is small [41].

  Eliminating a left shift with RME could eliminate future asymmetric mandibular growth if such growth is caused by the shift. However, Alaina's parents should be informed that asymmetric mandibular growth may be the underlying cause of her left crossbite, such growth may continue, and such growth may have to be dealt with using orthopedics, masking (later), or surgery (later).

- *Maxillary expansion with a quad-helix appliance* [40] *or split plate – offers no advantage over expansion with a Hyrax appliance and is not recommended.* In an eight-year-old girl, facial skeletal resistance to maxillary expansion may prevent midpalatal sutural separation with a quad-helix appliance or split plate appliance.
- *Maxillary fixed orthodontic appliances (e.g. a 2x6 appliance) post-RME to correct her left anterior crossbite – is recommended* if the anterior crossbite does not self-correct during RME.
- *Class II orthopedics – is not recommended* at this time. There is no advantage in treating Class II relationships in the *early* mixed dentition (except for a possible decrease in incisal trauma as a result of excess overjet) [172–178] We subscribe to this guideline unless the patient shows good statural growth in which case we will begin Class II treatment in the early mixed dentition. Alaina's parents state that she is not growing, but they will begin monitoring her height and inform us of changes.
- *LLHA or Nance holding arch for space maintenance – is not recommended yet.* Why? Eruption of Alaina's permanent canines and premolars is not imminent, and the use of space maintainers should be reassessed after RME and the uprighting of mandibular first permanent molars.
- *Extraction of primary teeth – is not recommended* because Alaina's permanent teeth appear to be erupting normally, primary tooth extraction would serve no purpose, and RME will create additional maxillary space.

Q: Based upon the above options, what is your recommended treatment?
A: Treatment proceeded with RME followed by placement of a TPA (Figure 6.63).

Q: What do you note in Figure 6.63?
A: Several observations can be made:

- Alaina's LDML is now coincident with the mesial of her maxillary right central incisor. The left lateral CR-CO shift is corrected, and the shift may have been larger than we initially thought.
- The left posterior crossbite is overcorrected. To reduce this excess left first permanent molar overjet, a lingual button was bonded to her mandibular left permanent first molar and crossbite elastic worn between the lingual button and the buccal of her RME appliance.

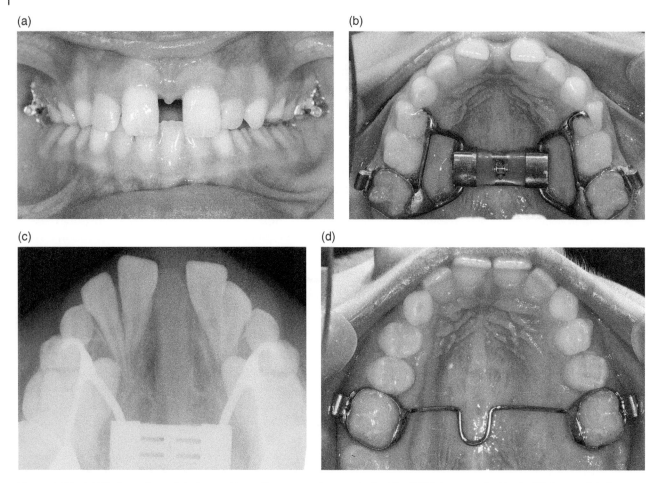

Figure 6.63 (a) Diastema formed during rapid maxillary expansion – note that the LDML is now coincident with the mesial of maxillary right central incisor; (b) RME appliance fully expanded; (c) occlusal radiograph illustrating midpalatal sutural separation; (d) TPA replacing RME appliance.

Permanent tooth eruption was monitored. A frontal progress photograph (Figure 6.64a) reveals that the diastema created by RME has closed, UDML and LDML are coincident, and the excess left posterior overjet has been reduced. At this time, a decision was made to extract Alaina's maxillary primary canines to help expedite the eruption of her maxillary permanent canines (Figure 6.64b). Alaina's Class II relationship was worsening.

She was placed on an high-pull head gear (HPHG) and corrected to Class I molars. All permanent teeth erupted except for the maxillary right canine (Figure 6.65). At this time, early treatment was complete and comprehensive treatment will begin.

Q: How do you recommend proceeding?

A: We will place fixed orthodontic appliances, level and align arches, trap a compressed open coil spring to create additional room for the maxillary right permanent canine, and monitor its eruption.

Q: Do you have any early treatment "take-home pearls" from Alaina?

A: "Pearls" include the following:

- Alaina was eight years old when she presented for correction of her unilateral left lingual crossbite which extended from her left lateral incisor to her left permanent first molars. The unilateral crossbite magnitude diminished in CR into smaller *bilateral* inadequate posterior overjets. Following visual uprighting of her molars, we concluded that her crossbite was a skeletal crossbite due to deficient maxillary transverse width – which was successfully corrected with RME. Her mild Class II relationship was corrected with HPHG.

- We cannot overstate the importance of carefully checking for a CR-CO shift. We initially detected a minimal (~1 mm) left lateral shift from CR to CO, but we suspect that a larger shift actually existed.

- We were grateful that Alaina had a left lateral shift because she ended up having a smaller

(a)

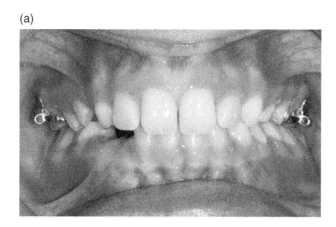

(b)

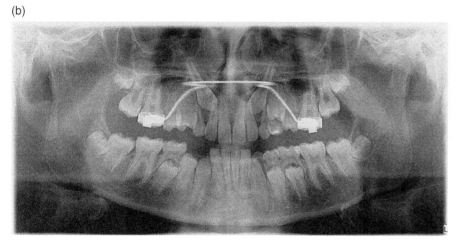

Figure 6.64   (a–b) Progress images of Alaina.

(a)   (b)   (c)

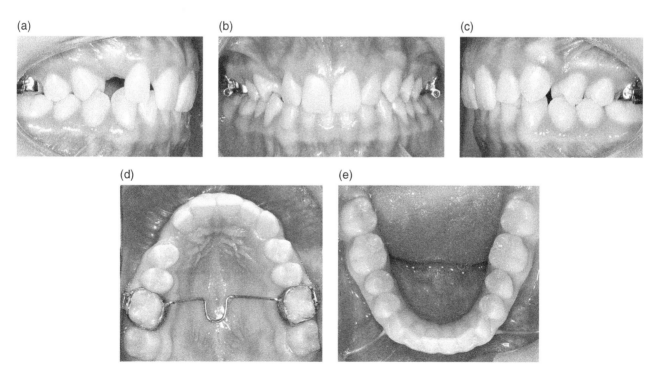

(d)   (e)

Figure 6.65   (a–f) Progress records of Alaina following Class II correction and eruption of all permanent teeth except for the maxillary right permanent canine.

(f)

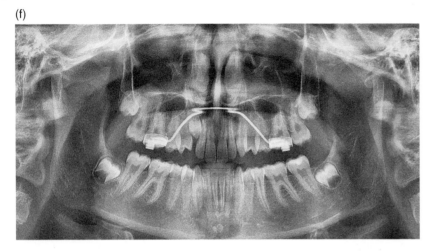

Figure 6.65 (Continued)

bilateral discrepancy that was readily treated with *bilateral* maxillary expansion. We were also grateful that her left posterior crossbite was not due to a mandibular growth asymmetry which could have required years of orthopedic treatment to correct and maintain.

Case Halee

Q: Halee is seven years and six months of age (Figure 6.66). She presents to you with her parents' chief complaint, "Our family dentist referred us to you." PMH and TMJ

(a) (b) (c) (d)

(e) (f)

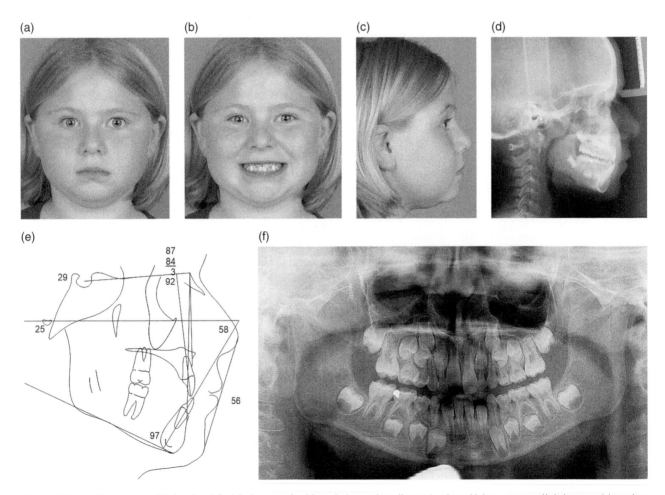

Figure 6.66 Initial records of Halee. (a–c) facial photographs, (d) cephalometric radiograph where Halee appears slightly open, (e) tracing, (f) pantomograph, (g) frontal photograph in CR, (h) frontal photograph in CO, (i–l) intraoral photographs, (m–s) model photographs.

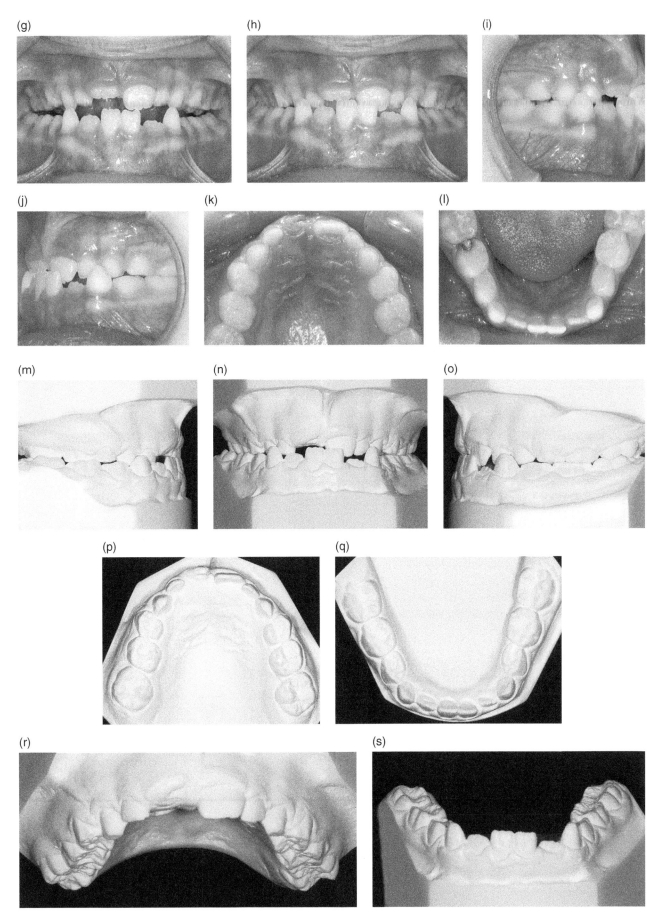

Figure 6.66 (Continued)

evaluations are WRN. Periodontal and mucogingival exams are WRN. A 1–2 mm anterior shift from CR to CO was detected (anterior shift only – *not lateral*).

Compile your diagnostic findings and problem list. State your diagnosis.

A:

Table 6.12 Diagnostic findings and problem list for Halee.

Full face and profile	***FRONTAL VIEW*** Face is symmetric LAFH WRN (soft tissue Glabella-Subnasale = Subnasale – soft tissue Menton) Lip competence UDML WRN Incisal display during posed smile inadequate (maxillary central incisor gingival margins apical to maxillary lip) Moderate buccal corridors ***PROFILE VIEW*** Straight profile Obtuse NLA Chin projection WRN (soft-tissue Pogonion projects forward of zero meridian line) Obtuse lip-chin-throat angle Chin-throat length WRN
Ceph Analysis	Maxillary anteroposterior position WRN (A-Point lies approximately on Nasion-perpendicular line) Mandibular anteroposterior position WRN (ANB angle = 3° with maxillary anteroposterior position WRN) Skeletal LAFH WRN (ANS-Menton/Nasion-Menton × 100% = 56%) Mandibular plane WRN (FMA = 25°; SNMP = 29°) Ineffective bony pogonion (Pogonion lies behind line extended from Nasion through B-Point) ***DENTAL*** Upright maxillary incisors (U1 to SN = 92°) Proclined mandibular incisors (FMIA = 58°)
Radiographs	Early mixed dentition stage of development
Intraoral photos	Angle Class I molar relationship Iowa classification: I I I I Unilateral right posterior lingual crossbite Anterior crossbite 50% overbite LDML approximately coincident with UDML Mandibular anterior attached keratinized gingival tissue WRN 4.0 mm of maxillary incisor crowding is currently present (7.3 mm space plus two primary lateral incisors of 5.1 mm width each, but 8.5 mm of space needed for right central incisor plus 6.5 mm of space needed for two permanent lateral incisors) 2.0 mm of maxillary arch crowding is anticipated following the eruption of all permanent teeth (if appropriate space maintenance is employed) 1.0 mm mandibular incisor spacing is currently present 4.2 mm of mandibular arch spacing is anticipated following the eruption of all permanent teeth (if appropriate space maintenance is employed) Right side of maxillary and mandibular dental arches appear slightly ahead of left sides (Figures 6.66k–6.66l and 6.66p - 6.66q) Attrition of mandibular left central incisor edge is noted (Figure 6.66g) Maxillary first permanent molars exhibit buccal crown torque (Figure 6.66r) Mandibular right permanent first molar is relatively upright (Figure 6.66s) Mandibular left permanent first molar exhibits lingual crown torque
Other	–
Diagnosis	Class I malocclusion with unilateral right posterior lingual crossbite and anterior crossbite

Q: Provide a detailed space analysis for Halee's maxillary and mandibular arches. How were the 2.0 mm of maxillary arch crowding and 4.2 mm of mandibular arch spacing calculated (if space maintenance is employed)?

A:

Average mesiodistal widths of permanent teeth (mm): [152]

Maxillary central incisor	8.5	Mandibular central incisor	5.0
Maxillary lateral incisor	6.5	Mandibular lateral incisor	5.5
Maxillary canine	7.5	Mandibular canine	7.0
Maxillary first premolar	7.0	Mandibular first premolar	7.0
Maxillary second premolar	7.0	Mandibular second premolar	7.0
Maxillary first molar	10.0	Mandibular first molar	11.0
Maxillary second molar	9.0	Mandibular second molar	10.5

Average mesiodistal widths of *primary* teeth (mm): [152]

Maxillary central incisor	6.5	Mandibular central incisor	4.2
Maxillary lateral incisor	5.1	Mandibular lateral incisor	4.1
Maxillary canine	7.0	Mandibular canine	5.0
Maxillary first molar	7.3	Mandibular first molar	7.7
Maxillary second molar	8.2	Mandibular second molar	9.9

MAXILLARY ARCH

+5.1 mm maxillary right primary lateral incisor width (Figure 6.60k)
−6.5 mm required for maxillary right permanent lateral incisor
+7.3 mm right central incisor space currently present
−8.5 mm required for maxillary right permanent central incisor
+5.1 mm maxillary left primary lateral incisor width
−6.5 mm required for maxillary left permanent lateral incisor
+2.0 mm of anticipated leeway space (1 mm/side)
Balance = +5.1 mm − 6.5 mm +7.3 mm −8.5 mm + 5.1 mm −6.5 mm + 2.0 mm = −2.0 mm

MANDIBULAR ARCH

+1.0 mm of incisor spacing is currently present
+3.2 mm of anticipated leeway space (1.6 mm/side)
Balance = + 1.0 mm + 3.2 mm = + 4.2 mm

That is, *2.0 mm of maxillary arch crowding and 4.2 mm of mandibular arch spacing is anticipated following the eruption of all permanent teeth (if proper space maintenance is employed).*

Q: What are Halee's *primary* problems that you must stay focused on?

A:

Table 6.13 Primary problems list for Halee.

AP	–
Vertical	50% OB
Transverse	Unilateral right lingual posterior crossbite
Other	Anterior crossbite

Q: Is Halee's unilateral right posterior crossbite a dental, or skeletal, crossbite?

A: It is a *skeletal* crossbite. Why? Halee's maxillary first permanent molars exhibit buccal crown torque (Figure 6.60r). Rotating them in the coronal plane (uprighting them) to normal buccolingual inclinations would tend to move their crowns *lingually* – worsening her transverse occlusal relationship. Her mandibular left permanent first molar exhibits lingual crown torque (Figure 6.60s). Uprighting it transversely would tend to move its crown *buccally* – worsening her transverse occlusal relationship.

Removing transverse dental compensations will therefore worsen her crossbite. This effect reflects an underlying transverse skeletal discrepancy between the jaws (a narrow maxilla relative to the mandible). Halee has a skeletal posterior crossbite.

Q: Halee's right mandibular first permanent molar (crossbite side) is relatively upright compared to her left permanent first molar (non-crossbite side). Is this typical? [29]

A: Yes, it is typical. Molar inclination on the *crossbite* side of a unilateral crossbite is generally more upright than molar inclination on the non-crossbite side. Why? The molar transverse inclinations on the crossbite side are not compensated buccolingually for the transverse skeletal disparity between the jaws, whereas the molar transverse inclinations on the non-crossbite side display buccolingual compensations (i.e. are less upright) in an attempt to maintain normal transverse molar occlusion.

Q: What unknowns do you face with Halee's orthodontic treatment?

A: An undetected lateral CR-CO shift, cooperation, and jaw growth (direction and magnitude). At age seven years, Halee should achieve midpalatal sutural separation if we perform RME.

Q: Discuss Halee in the context of three principles applied to every early treatment patient.

A:

1) The goal of early treatment is to correct developing problems – get the patient *back to normal for their stage of development* (including preventing complications, reducing later treatment complexity, or reducing unknowns). Correcting Halee's anterior crossbite, posterior crossbite, and deep OB would get her back to normal for her stage of development.

2) Early treatment should address *very specific problems with a clearly defined end point*, usually within six to nine months. Her anterior crossbite, posterior crossbite, and deep bite are specific problems which could be corrected readily with RME and fixed orthodontic appliances.

3) Always ask: Is it necessary that I treat the patient now? *What harm will come if I choose to do nothing now?* Mandibular left central incisor attrition has already occurred. If we do not correct Halee's anterior crossbite, then additional damage will most likely occur. Since there is not a lateral shift, it is not necessary to correct Halee's unilateral posterior crossbite yet. However, we will want to correct it before puberty. Once the anterior crossbite is corrected, there will be no harm in waiting to correct her deep bite.

Q: Should you start treatment now or recall Halee? If you start treatment, what treatment options would you consider?

A: Your treatment options include the following:

- Recall (no treatment, monitor only) – *is not recommended*. If we do not treat her anterior crossbite, then additional damage could occur to her incisors.
- *RME (Hyrax appliance) – is recommended*. RME could eliminate the right posterior lingual crossbite, deprogram Halee's masticatory muscle memory (allowing us to identify an undetected lateral shift), provide additional room for eruption of maxillary anterior teeth, and provide overjet to permit transverse molar uprighting. Considering the magnitude of the right posterior crossbite and the fact that Halee does not exhibit a lateral shift, we must anticipate bilateral expansion into a left posterior *buccal* crossbite before correction of the right posterior lingual crossbite occurs.
- *Maxillary expansion with a quad-helix appliance or split plate* [39–41] – *may provide adequate maxillary expansion*. Because Halee is only seven years old, her facial skeletal resistance to maxillary expansion (zygomatic buttress resistance) may be small enough

to permit midpalatal suture separation with a quad-helix or increased sutural growth (widening) with a split plate.

- *Enameloplasty of mandibular primary canine cusps – is reasonable* in order to permit unimpeded lateral movement of maxillary lateral incisors during maxillary expansion.
- *Anterior crossbite correction – is recommended*, but maxillary expansion should be performed first. Why? Anterior crossbites will sometimes self-correct during maxillary expansion (Figure 6.67). Further, RME will provide additional space for maxillary permanent canine crowns, reducing the likelihood that lateral incisor roots will impinge upon erupting permanent canine crowns during anterior crossbite correction.
- *LLHA or Nance holding arch for space maintenance – is not recommended at this time* because the eruption of Halee's permanent canines and premolars is not imminent.
- *Extraction of primary teeth – is not recommended* because her permanent teeth appear to be erupting normally. Further, if we proceed with RME, then additional space for permanent tooth eruption will be created in the maxilla.

Q: What is your recommended treatment?

A: We began with enameloplasty of the mandibular primary canine cusp tips. Compare the mandibular primary canine cusp tip lengths before enameloplasty (Figure 6.66g) to the lengths after enameloplasty (Figure 6.68a). RME followed (Figures 6.68b–6.68c).

Q: As anticipated, before RME could fully correct her right posterior lingual crossbite, Halee's maxillary left permanent first molar began to move into buccal crossbite. How would you manage this situation?

A: Recall that her mandibular left permanent first molar exhibited more lingual crown torque (more transverse compensation) than her mandibular right first molar (Figure 6.66s). By bonding a button on the lingual of her mandibular left permanent first molar and uprighting it with a crossbite elastic (Figure 6.69a), we reduced the left buccal overjet. This action prevented her from going into the left buccal crossbite (Figure 6.69b).

Following RME, the Hyrax appliance was removed and a TPA placed (Figure 6.69c) to maintain the expansion. Halee was also asked to wear a clear mandibular vacuum-formed retainer.

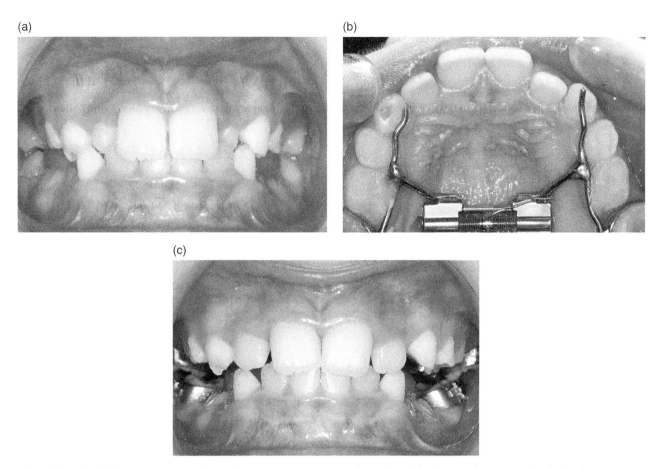

Figure 6.67 (a–c) A different patient who underwent spontaneous maxillary lateral incisor crossbite correction during RME.

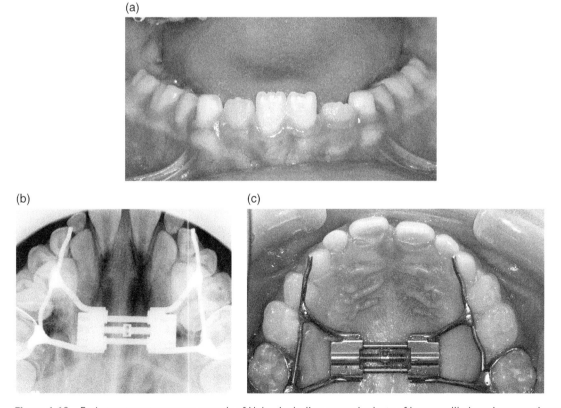

Figure 6.68 Early treatment progress records of Halee including enameloplasty of her mandibular primary canine cusp tips (a) and RME (b–c), which resulted in midpalatal suture separation. Note that the maxillary right metal arm has slipped over the maxillary right primary canine cusp. Both arms should have been bonded to the lingual of the maxillary primary molars.

(a)

(b)

(c)

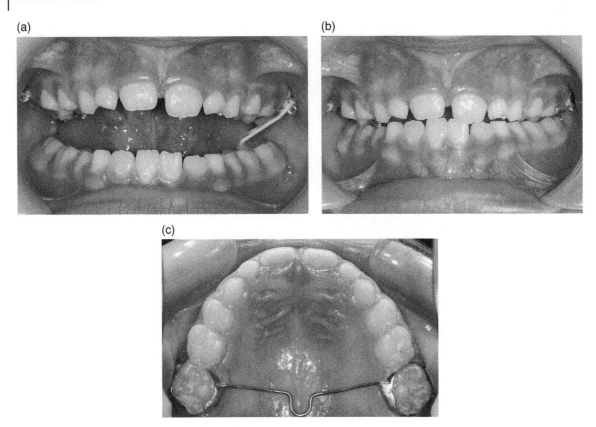

Figure 6.69 Progress records of Halee. (a) Crossbite elastic worn on the left during RME to upright the mandibular left permanent first molar and prevent the maxillary left permanent first molar from moving into buccal crossbite (b); following removal of the Hyrax appliance, a TPA was placed to maintain the maxillary expansion (c). Note that her maxillary primary lateral incisors are no longer in crossbite.

Q: How would you correct Halee's central incisor anterior crossbite?

A: Following RME, we asked Halee to bite on a soft suction tip as much as possible (Figure 6.70a). She was not compliant. We next fabricated a removable maxillary appliance with a finger spring to advance her maxillary left central incisor (Figure 6.70b). She was not compliant wearing it. Finally, we placed limited fixed maxillary appliances and advanced her left central incisor using open coil springs (Figures 6.70c–6.70e). Her anterior crossbite was successfully corrected and fixed appliances were removed (Figures 6.70f–6.70j).

We planned to place an LLHA when Halee's mandibular permanent canines and premolars are closer to eruption.

Q: Halee is now *back on track* for her stage of development, which was our early treatment goal. Initially presenting at seven years and six months of age, she was Class I with anterior and posterior crossbites. She was successfully treated with RME and limited fixed orthodontic appliances. Do you have any "take-home pearls" regarding Halee?

A: "Pearls" include the following:
- Mandibular permanent first molars on the crossbite side of unilateral posterior lingual crossbites are generally upright compared to molars on the non-crossbite side. That is, *molars on the non-crossbite side exhibit transverse dental compensations* that maintain normal transverse molar occlusion in the presence of transverse skeletal disparity between the jaws.
- If, during RME for a unilateral posterior lingual crossbite, you begin to overexpand into a buccal crossbite on the non-crossbite side, consider using a crossbite elastic (Figure 6.69a) to upright the mandibular molar on the non-crossbite side and reduce its posterior overjet.
- Always confirm that unilateral posterior crossbites are not the result of asymmetric mandibular growth. If asymmetric mandibular growth is the cause of the unilateral crossbite, then this growth must be addressed or the crossbite will likely return.
- Correction of anterior crossbites by asking the patient to bite on a soft stick, or to wear a removable appliance, requires more patient compliance than by using fixed orthodontic appliances. Talk to the

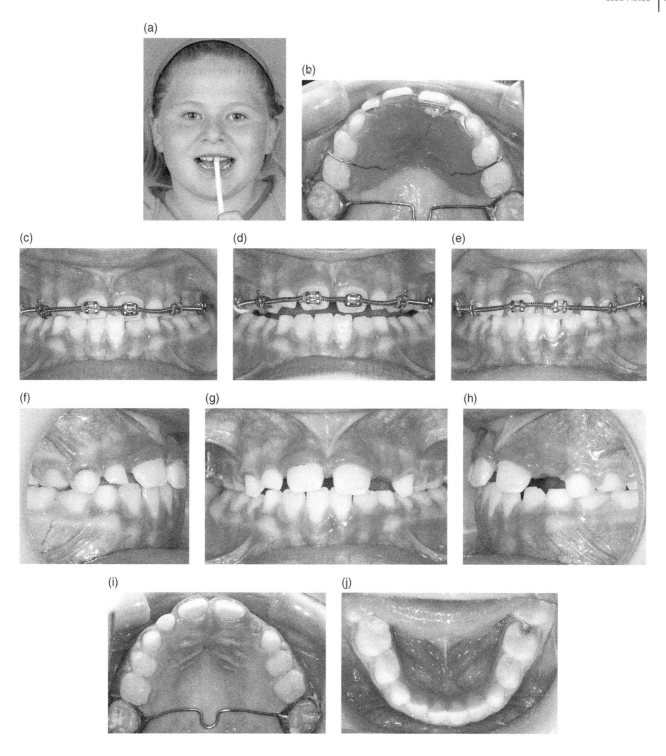

Figure 6.70 Correction of Halee's anterior crossbite following RME. (a–b) She was not cooperative when asked to bite on a soft suction tip nor when asked to wear a removable appliance with a finger spring; (c–e) anterior crossbite correction was finally achieved using fixed appliances, together with a temporary cement first molar biteplate (d), to open her bite and advance her maxillary left central incisor; (f–j) dentition following appliance removal.

patient before attempting the use of a bite stick. We talked to Halee first. She said she would use it, but she kept forgetting to use it.

Talk to the patient before your lab fabricates a removable appliance with fingerspring to correct a crossbite. We did, and Halee said she would wear it. But when we

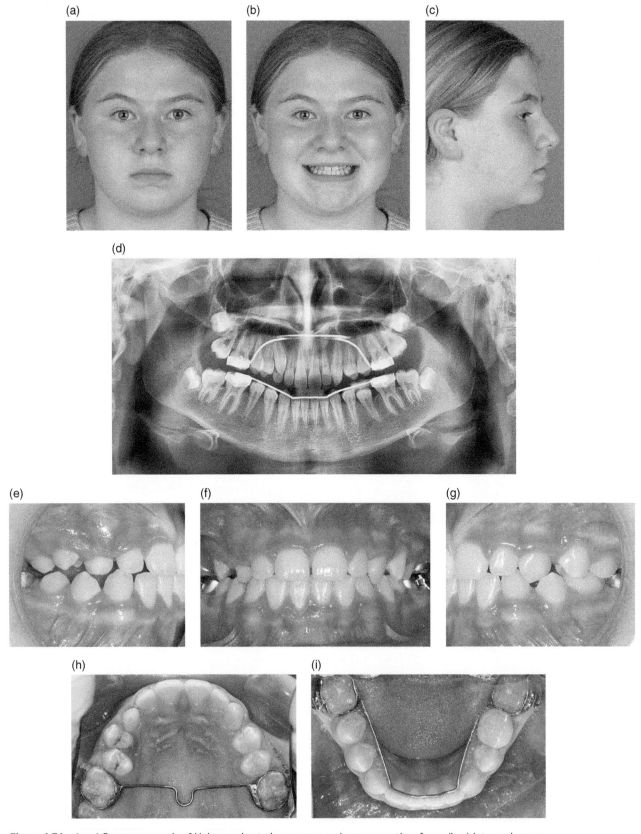

Figure 6.71 (a–p) Progress records of Halee made at eleven years and seven months of age. (j–p) Intraoral scans.

(j)

(k)

(l)

(m)

(n)

(o)

(p)

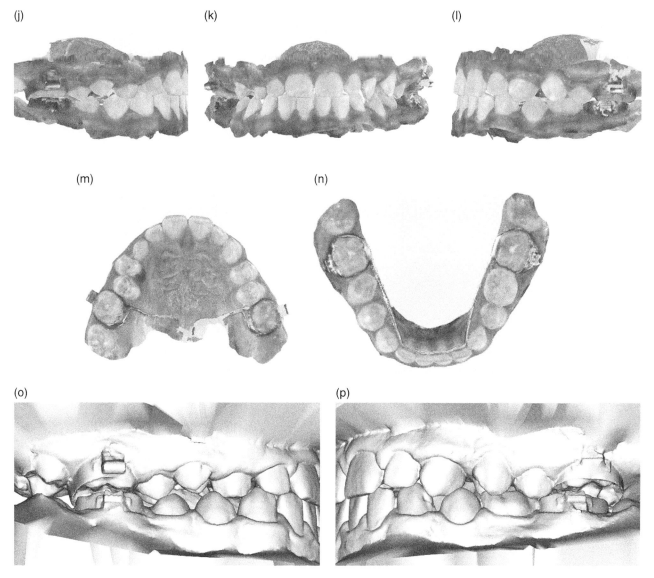

Figure 6.71 (Continued)

delivered it, she said that she could not wear it. We are very grateful to Dr. Edward Angle for inventing the fixed edgewise appliance to treat malocclusions, which required less compliance to correct Halee's crossbite.

Q: We placed an LLHA when Halee's mandibular primary canines became mobile. There was no additional early treatment. Records were made when she reached eleven years and seven months of age (Figure 6.71). What do you observe? How would you recommend proceeding?

A: Halee is close to exfoliating her remaining two primary teeth and entering her permanent dentition stage of dental development. She is Class I with approximately 10% OB. She has adequate OJ at her first permanent molars, but her maxillary right second premolar is in lingual crossbite. We will proceed with comprehensive orthodontic treatment using fixed appliances after her remaining permanent teeth erupt.

References

1 Marshall, S., Dawson, D., Southard, K.A. et al. (2003). Transverse molar movements during growth. *Am. J. Orthod. Dentofac. Orthop.* 124 (6): 615–624.

2 Tong, H., Kwon, D., Shi, J. et al. (2012). Mesiodistal angulation and faciolingual inclination of each whole tooth in 3-dimensional space in patients with near-

normal occlusion. *Am. J. Orthod. Dentofac. Orthop.* 141 (5): 604–617.

3   Thilander, B., Wahlund, S., and Lennartsson, B. (1984). The effect of early interceptive treatment in children with posterior crossbite. *Eur. J. Orthod.* 6 (1): 25–34.

4   Kutin, G. and Hawes, R. (1969). Posterior crossbites in the deciduous and mixed dentitions. *Am. J. Orthod.* 56 (5): 491–504.

5   Helm, S. (1968). Malocclusion in Danish children with adolescent dentition: an epidemiologic study. *Am. J. Orthod.* 54 (5): 352–366.

6   Hanson, M.L., Barnard, L.W., and Case, J.L. (1970). Tongue thrust in preschool children. II: dental occlusal patterns. *Am. J. Orthod.* 57 (1): 15–22.

7   Kurol, J. and Berglund, L. (1992). Longitudinal study and cost-benefit analysis of the effect of early treatment of posterior cross-bites in the primary dentition. *Eur. J. Orthod.* 14 (3): 173–179.

8   Lindner, A. (1989). Longitudinal study of the effect of early interceptive treatment in 4-year-old children with unilateral cross-bite. *Scand. J. Dent. Res.* 97 (5): 432–438.

9   O'Byrn, B.L., Sadowsky, C., Schneider, B., and BeGole, E.A. (1995). An evaluation of mandibular asymmetry in adults with unilateral posterior crossbite. *Am. J. Orthod. Dentofac. Orthop.* 107 (4): 394–400.

10 Pinto, A.S., Buschang, P.H., Throckmorton, G.S., and Chen, P. (2001). Morphological and positional asymmetries of young children with functional unilateral posterior crossbite. *Am. J. Orthod. Dentofac. Orthop.* 120 (5): 513–520.

11 Pirttiniemi, P., Kantomaa, T., and Lahtela, P. (1990). Relationship between craniofacial and condyle path asymmetry in unilateral cross-bite patients. *Eur. J. Orthod.* 12 (4): 408–413.

12 Myers, D.R., Barenie, J.T., Bell, R.A., and Williamson, E.H. (1980). Condylar position in children with functional posterior crossbites: before and after crossbite correction. *Pediatr. Dent.* 2 (3): 190–194.

13 Yoshikane, T.T., Pullinger, A.G., and Turley, P.K. (1987). Characteristics of functional posterior crossbites in the deciduous and mixed dentitions. Thesis. University of California, School of Dentistry, Los Angeles.

14 Hesse, K.L., Artun, J., Joondeph, D.R., and Kennedy, D.B. (1997). Changes in condylar position and occlusion associated with maxillary expansion for correction of functional unilateral posterior crossbite. *Am. J. Orthod. Dentofac. Orthop.* 111 (4): 410–418.

15 Nanda, R., Snodell, S.F., and Bollu, P. (2012). Transverse growth of maxilla and mandible. *Semin. Orthod.* 18 (2): 100–117.

16 Melink, S., Vagner, M.V., Hocevar-Boltezar, I., and Ovsenik, M. (2010). Posterior crossbite in the deciduous dentition period, its relation with sucking habits, irregular orofacial functions, and otolaryngological findings. *Am. J. Orthod. Dentofac. Orthop.* 138 (1): 32–40.

17 Marshall, S.D., Southard, K.A., and Southard, T.E. (2005). Early transverse treatment. *Semin. Orthod.* 11 (3): 130–139.

18 Betts, N.K., Vanarsdall, R.L., Barber, H.D. et al. (1995). Diagnosis and treatment of transverse maxillary deficiency. *Int. J. Adult Orthodon. Orthognath. Surg.* 10 (2): 75–96.

19 Moyers, R.E. (1973). *Handbook of Orthodontics*, 4e, 530–542. Chicago: Year Book Medical Publishers, Inc.

20 Higley, L.B. (1968). Crossbite mandibular malposition. *ASDC J. Dent. Child.* 35 (3): 221–223.

21 Clinch, L. (1966). Symposium on aspects of the dental development of the child. 1. The development of the deciduous and mixed dentition. *Dent. Pract. Dent. Rec.* 17 (4): 135–144.

22 Inui, M., Fushima, K., and Sato, S. (1999). Facial asymmetry in temporomandibular joint disorders. *J. Oral Rehabil.* 26 (5): 402–406.

23 Trpkova, B., Major, P., Nebbe, B., and Prasad, N. (2000). Craniofacial asymmetry and temporomandibular joint internal derangement in female adolescents: a posteroanterior cephalometric study. *Angle Orthod.* 70 (1): 81–88.

24 Kiki, A., Kılıç, N., and Oktay, H. (2007). Condylar asymmetry in bilateral posterior crossbite patients. *Angle Orthod.* 77 (1): 77–81.

25 De Clerck, H.J. and Proffit, W.R. (2015). Growth modification of the face: a current perspective with emphasis on Class III treatment. *Am. J. Orthod. Dentofac. Orthop.* 148 (1): 37–46.

26 Haas, A.J. (1961). Rapid palatal expansion of the maxillary dental arch and nasal cavity by opening midpalatal suture. *Angle Orthod.* 31 (2): 73–90.

27 Moore, T., Southard, K.A., Casko, J.S. et al. (2005). Buccal corridors and smile esthetics. *Am. J. Orthod. Dentofac. Orthop.* 127 (2): 208–213. quiz 261.

28 Jacobs, J.D., Bell, W.H., Williams, C.E., and Kennedy, J.W. III (1980). Control of the transverse dimension with surgery and orthodontics. *Am. J. Orthod.* 77 (3): 284–306.

29 Miner, R.M., Al Qabandi, S., Rigali, P.H., and Will, L.A. (2012). Cone-beam computed tomography transverse analysis. Part I: normative data. *Am. J. Orthod. Dentofac. Orthop.* 142 (3): 300–307.

30 Petrén, S., Bondemark, L., and Söderfeldt, B. (2003). A systemic review concerning early orthodontic treatment of unilateral posterior crossbite. *Angle Orthod.* 73 (5): 588–596.

31 Harrison, J.E. and Ashby, D. (2001). Orthodontic treatment for posterior crossbites. *Cochrane Database Syst. Rev.* 1: CD000979.

32 Schröder, U. and Schröder, L. (1984). Early treatment of unilateral posterior crossbite in children with bilaterally contracted maxillae. *Eur. J. Orthod.* 6 (1): 65–69.

33 Kantomaa, T. (1986). Correction of unilateral crossbite in the deciduous dentition. *Eur. J. Orthod.* 8 (2): 80–83.

34 Masucci, C., Cipriani, L., Defraia, E., and Franchi, L. (2017). Transverse relationship of permanent molars after crossbite correction in deciduous dentition. *Eur. J. Orthod.* 39 (5): 560–566.

35 Hicks, E.P. (1978). Slow maxillary expansion. A clinical study of the skeletal versus dental response to low-magnitude force. *Am. J. Orthod.* 73 (2): 121–141.

36 Murray, J.M. and Cleall, J.F. (1971). Early tissue response to rapid maxillary expansion in the midpalatal suture of the rhesus monkey. *J. Dent. Res.* 50 (6): 1654–1660.

37 Starnebach, J.K. and Cleall, J.F. (1964). Effects of splitting the midpalatal suture on the surrounding structures. *Am. J. Orthod.* 50: 923–924.

38 Storey, E. (1973). Tissue response to the movement of bones. *Am. J. Orthod.* 64 (3): 229–247.

39 Skieller, V. (1964). Expansion of the midpalatal suture by removable plates, analysed by the implant method. *Rep. Congr. Eur. Orthod. Soc.* 40: 143–158.

40 Bell, R.A. and LeCompte, E.J. (1981). The effects of maxillary expansion using a quad-helix appliance during the deciduous and mixed dentitions. *Am. J. Orthod.* 79 (2): 152–161.

41 Harberson, V.A. and Myers, D.R. (1978). Midpalatal suture opening during functional posterior cross-bite correction. *Am. J. Orthod.* 74 (3): 310–313.

42 Petrén, S., Bjerklin, P., Marké, L., and Bondemark, L. (2013). Early correction of posterior crossbite – a cost-minimization analysis. *Eur. J. Orthod.* 35 (1): 14–21.

43 Godoy, F., Godoy-Bezerra, J., and Rosenblatt, A. (2011). Treatment of posterior crossbite comparing 2 appliances: a community-based trial. *Am. J. Orthod. Dentofac. Orthop.* 139 (1): e45–e52.

44 Corbridge, J.K., Campbell, P.M., Taylor, R. et al. (2011). Transverse dentoalveolar changes after slow maxillary expansion. *Am. J. Orthod. Dentofac. Orthop.* 140 (3): 317–325.

45 Wertz, R.A. (1970). Skeletal and dental changes accompanying rapid and midpalatal suture opening. *Am. J. Orthod.* 58 (1): 41–66.

46 Garrett, B.J., Caruso, J.M., Rungcharassaeng, K. et al. (2008). Skeletal effects to the maxilla after rapid maxillary expansion assessed with cone-beam computed tomography. *Am. J. Orthod. Dentofac. Orthop.* 134 (1): 8–9.

47 Adkins, M.D., Nanda, R.S., and Currier, G.F. (1990). Arch perimeter changes on rapid palatal expansion. *Am. J. Orthod. Dentofac. Orthop.* 97 (3): 194–199.

48 Moss, J.P. (1968). Rapid expansion of the maxillary arch. I. *J. Pract. Orthod.* 2 (4): 156–171.

49 Moss, J.P. (1968). Rapid expansion of the maxillary arch. II. *J. Pract. Orthod.* 2 (5): 215–223.

50 Wertz, R. and Dreskin, M. (1977). Midpalatal suture opening: a normative study. *Am. J. Orthod.* 71 (4): 367–381.

51 Ghoneima, A., Abdel-Fattah, E., Hartsfield, J. et al. (2011). Effects of rapid maxillary expansion on the cranial and circummaxillary sutures. *Am. J. Orthod. Dentalfac. Orthop.* 140 (4): 215–223.

52 Isaacson, R.J. and Ingram, A.H. (1964). Forces produced by rapid maxillary expansion II. Forces present during treatment. *Angle Orthod.* 34 (4): 261–270.

53 Lines, P.A. (1975). Adult rapid maxillary expansion with corticotomy. *Am. J. Orthod.* 67 (1): 44–56.

54 Krebs, A. (1964). Midpalatal expansion studies by the implant method over a seven-year period. *Rep. Congr. Eur. Orthod. Soc.* 40: 131–142.

56 Krebs, A. (1959). Expansion of the midpalatal suture studied by means of metallic implants. *Acta Odontol. Scand.* 17 (4): 491–501.

56 Baccetti, T., Franchi, L., Cameron, C.G., and McNamara, J.A. Jr. (2001). Treatment timing for rapid maxillary expansion. *Angle Orthod.* 71 (5): 343–350.

57 Shetty, V., Cardid, J.M., Caputo, A.A., and Chaconas, S.J. (1994). Biomechanical rationale for surgical-orthodontic expansion of the adult maxilla. *J. Oral Maxillofac. Surg.* 52 (7): 742–749.

58 Tausche, E., Hansen, L., Schneider, M., and Harzer, W. (2008). Bone-supported rapid maxillary expansion with an implant-borne Hyrax screw: the Dresden Distractor. [article in French]. *Orthod. Fr.* 79 (2): 127–135.

59 Nienkemper, M., Wilmes, B., Pauls, A., and Drescher, D. (2013). Maxillary protraction using a hybrid hyrax-facemask combination. *Prog. Orthod.* 14 (1): 5.

60 MacGinnis, M., Chu, H., Youssef, G. et al. (2014). The effects of micro-implant assisted rapid palatal expansion (MARPE) on the nasomaxillary complex—a finite element method (FEM) analysis. *Prog. Orthod.* 15 (1): 52.

61 Goddard, C. (1893). Separation of the superior maxillae at the symphysis. *Dent. Cosmos* 35: 880–882.

62 Ferris, H.C. (1914, 56). Discussion of Dr. G.V.I. Brown's paper. *Dent. Cosmos* 218.

63 Brunetto, M., Andriani, J.S., Ribeiro, G.L. et al. (2013). Three-dimensional assessment of buccal alveolar bone after rapid and slow maxillary expansion: a clinical trial study. *Am. J. Orthod. Dentofac. Orthop.* 143 (5): 633–644.

64 Lagravère, M., Major, P.W., and Flores-Mir, C. (2005). Skeletal and dental changes with fixed slow maxillary expansion treatment: a systemic review. *J. Am. Dent. Assoc.* 136 (2): 194–199.

65 Haas, A.J. (1980). Long-term posttreatment evaluation of rapid palatal expansion. *Angle Orthod.* 50 (3): 189–217.

66 Chung, C.H. and Font, B. (2004). Skeletal and dental changes in the sagital, vertical, and transverse dimensions after rapid palatal expansion. *Am. J. Orthod. Dentofac. Orthop.* 126 (5): 569–575.

67 da Silva Filho, O.G., Boas, M.C., and Capelozza Filho, L. (1991). Rapid maxillary expansion in the primary and mixed dentitions: a cephalometric evaluation. *Am. J. Orthod. Dentofac. Orthop.* 100 (2): 171–179.

68 Sari, Z., Uysal, T., Usumez, S., and Basciftci, F.A. (2003). Rapid maxillary expansion. Is it better in the mixed or in the permanent dentition? *Angle Orthod.* 73 (6): 654–661.

69 Davis, W.M. and Kronman, J.H. (1969). Anatomical changes induced by splitting of the midpalatal suture. *Angle Orthod.* 39 (2): 126–132.

70 Chang, J.Y., McNamara, J.A. Jr., and Herberger, T.A. (1997). A longitudinal study of skeletal side effects induced by rapid maxillary expansion. *Am. J. Orthod. Dentofac. Orthop.* 112 (3): 330–337.

71 Lagravère, M.O., Major, P.W., and Flores-Mir, C. (2005). Long-term dental arch changes after rapid maxillary expansion treatment: a systematic review. *Angle Orthod.* 75 (2): 155–161.

72 Lineberger, M.W., McNamara, J.A., Baccetti, T. et al. (2012). Effects of rapid maxillary expansion in hyperdivergent patients. *Am. J. Orthod. Dentofac. Orthop.* 142 (1): 60–69.

73 Marshall, S.D., English, J.D., Huang, G.J. et al. (2008). Ask us. Long-term stability of maxillary expansion. *Am. J. Orthod. Dentofac. Orthop.* 133 (6): 780–781.

74 Zimring, J.F. and Isaacson, R.J. (1965). Forces produced by rapid maxillary expansion. 3. Forces present during retention. *Angle Orthod.* 35 (3): 178–186.

75 Schiffman, P.H. and Tuncay, O.C. (2001). Maxillary expansion: a meta analysis. *Clin. Orthod. Res.* 4 (2): 86–96.

76 Bell, R.A. (1982). A review of maxillary expansion in relation to rate of expansion and patient's age. *Am. J. Orthod.* 81 (1): 32–37.

77 Stockfisch, H. (1969). Rapid expansion of the maxilla – success and relapse. *Rep. Congr. Eur. Orthod. Soc.* 45: 469–481.

78 Davidovitch, M., Efstathiou, S., Sarne, O., and Vardimon, A.D. (2005). Skeletal and dental response to rapid maxillary expansion with 2- versus 4-band appliances. *Am. J. Orthod. Dentofac. Orthop.* 127 (4): 483–492.

79 Lamparski, D.G., Rinchuse, D.J., Close, J.M., and Sciote, J.J. (2003). Comparison of skeletal and dental changes between 2-point and 4-point rapid palatal expanders. *Am. J. Orthod. Dentofac. Orthop.* 123 (3): 321–328.

80 Cozzani, M., Guiducci, A., Mirenghi, S. et al. (2007). Arch width changes with a rapid maxillary expansion appliance anchored to the primary teeth. *Angle Orthod.* 77 (2): 296–302.

81 Greenbaum, K.R. and Zachrisson, B.U. (1982). The effect of palatal expansion therapy on the periodontal supporting tissues. *Am. J. Orthod.* 81 (1): 12–21.

82 Garib, D.G., Henriques, J.F., Janson, G. et al. (2006). Periodontal effects of rapid maxillary expansion with tooth-tissue-borne and tooth-borne expanders: a computed tomography evaluation. *Am. J. Orthod. Dentofac. Orthop.* 129 (6): 749–758.

83 Timms, D.J. and Moss, J.P. (1971). A histological investigation into the effects of rapid maxillary expansion on the teeth and their supporting structures. *Trans. Eur. Orthod. Soc.* 263–271.

84 Barber, A.F. and Sims, M.R. (1981). Rapid maxillary expansion and external root resorption in man: a scanning electron microscope study. *Am. J. Orthod.* 79 (6): 630–652.

85 Garib, D.G., Henriques, J.F.C., Janson, G. et al. (2005). Rapid maxillary expansion--tooth tissue-borne versus tooth-borne expanders. *Angle Orthod.* 75 (4): 548–557.

86 Weissheimer, A., Macedo de Menezes, L., Mezomo, M. et al. (2011). Immediate effects of rapid maxillary expansion with Haas-type and hyrax-type expanders: a randomized clinical trial. *Am. J. Orthod. Dentofac. Orthop.* 140 (3): 366–376.

87 Cohen, M. and Silverman, E. (1973). A new and simple palate splitting device. *J. Clin. Orthod.* 7 (6): 368–369.

88 Wendling, L.K., McNamara, J.A. Jr., Franchi, L., and Baccetti, T. (2005). A prospective study of the short-term treatment effects of the acrylic-splint rapid maxillary expander combined with the lower Schwartz appliance. *Angle Orthod.* 75 (1): 7–14.

89 Sarver, D.M. and Johnston, M.W. (1989). Skeletal changes in vertical and anterior displacement of the maxilla with bonded rapid palatal expansion appliances. *Am. J. Orthod. Dentofac. Orthop.* 95 (6): 462–466.

90 Asanza, S., Cisneros, G.J., and Nieberg, L.G. (1997). Comparison of Hyrax and bonded expansion appliances. *Angle Orthod.* 67 (1): 15–22.

91 Lagravère, M., Carey, J., Heo, G. et al. (2010). Transverse, vertical, and anteroposterior changes from bone-anchored maxillary expansion vs traditional rapid maxillary expansion: a randomized clinical trial. *Am. J. Orthod. Dentofac. Orthop.* 137 (3): 304–305.

92 Mosleh, M.O., Kaddah, M.A., ElSayed, F.A.A., and ElSayed, H.S. (2015). Comparison of transverse changes during maxillary expansion with 4-point bone-borne and tooth-borne maxillary expanders. *Am. J. Orthod. Dentofac. Orthop.* 148 (4): 599–607.

93 Little, R.M. (2002). Stability and relapse: early treatment of arch length deficiency. *Am. J. Orthod. Dentofac. Orthop.* 121 (6): 578–581.

94 Gianelly, A.A. (2003). Rapid palatal expansion in the absence of crossbites: added value? *Am. J. Orthod. Dentofac. Orthop.* 124 (4): 362–365.

95 Gryson, J.A. (1977). Changes in mandibular interdental distance concurrent with maxillary expansion. *Angle Orthod.* 47 (3): 186–192.

96 Frank, S.W. and Engle, G.A. (1982). The effects of maxillary quad-helix appliance expansion on cephalometric measurements in growing orthodontic patients. *Am. J. Orthod.* 81 (5): 378–389.

97 Sandstrom, R.A., Klapper, L., and Papaconstantinou, S. (1988). Expansion of lower arch concurrent with rapid maxillary expansion. *Am. J. Orthod. Dentofac. Orthop.* 94 (4): 296–230.

98 McNamara, J.A. Jr. (2002). Early intervention in the transverse dimension: is it worth the effort? *Am. J. Orthod. Dentofac. Orthop.* 121 (6): 572–574.

99 Bell, R.A. and LeCompte, E.J. (1981). The effects of maxillary expansion using a quad-helix appliance during the deciduous and mixed dentition. *Am. J. Orthod.* 79 (2): 152–161.

100 Handleman, C.S., Wang, L., BeGole, E.A., and Haas, A.J. (2000). Nonsurgical rapid palatal expansion in adults: report on 47 cases using the Haas expander. *Angle Orthod.* 70 (2): 129–144.

101 Lima, A.C., Lima, A.L., Filho, R.M., and Oyen, O.J. (2004). Spontaneous mandibular arch response after rapid palatal expansion: a long-term study on Class I malocclusion. *Am. J. Orthod. Dentofac. Orthop.* 126 (5): 576–582.

102 Blake, M. and Bibby, K. (1998). Retention and stability: a review of the literature. *Am. J. Orthod. Dentofac. Orthop.* 114 (3): 299–306.

103 Moussa, R., O'Reilly, M.T., and Close, J.M. (1995). Long-term stability of rapid palatal expander treatment and edgewise mechanotherapy. *Am. J. Orthod. Dentofac. Orthop.* 108 (5): 478–488.

104 Azizi, M., Shrout, M.K., Haas, A.J. et al. (1999). A retrospective study of Angle Class I malocclusions treated orthodontically without extractions using two palatal expansion methods. *Am. J. Orthod. Dentofac. Orthop.* 116 (1): 101–107.

105 Pollock, H.C. (1955). St. Louis and early orthodontics. *Am. J. Orthod.* 41 (11): 809–818.

106 Palaisa, J., Ngan, P., Martin, C., and Razmus, T. (2007). Use of conventional tomography to evaluate changes in the nasal cavity with rapid palatal expansion. *Am. J. Orthod. Dentofac. Orthop.* 132 (4): 458–466.

107 Wertz, R. (1970). Skeletal and dental changes accompanying rapid and midpalatal suture opening. *Am. J. Orthod.* 58: 41–65.

108 Haas, A.J. (1961). Rapid expansion of the maxillary dental arch and nasal cavity by opening the midpalatal suture. *Angle Orthod.* 31 (2): 73–90.

109 Wertz, R.A. (1968). Changes in nasal airflow incident to rapid maxillary expansion. *Angle Orthod.* 38 (1): 1–11.

110 Basciftci, F.A., Mutlu, N., Karaman, A.I. et al. (2002). Does the timing and method of rapid maxillary expansion have an effect on the changes in nasal dimensions? *Angle Orthod.* 72 (2): 118–123.

111 Bicakci, A., Agar, U., Sökücü, O. et al. (2005). Nasal airway changes due to rapid maxillary expansion timing. *Angle Orthod.* 75 (1): 1–6.

112 Buck, L.M., Dalci, O., Ali Darendeliler, M. et al. (2017). Volumetric upper airway changes after rapid maxillary expansion: a systematic review and meta-analysis. *Eur. J. Orthod.* 39 (5): 463–473.

113 Gordon, J.M., Rosenblatt, M., Witmans, M. et al. (2009). Rapid palatal expansion effects on nasal airway dimensions as measured by acoustic rhinometry. A systematic review. *Angle Orthod.* 79 (5): 1000–1007.

114 Behrents, R.G., Shelgikar, A.V., Conley, R.S. et al. (2019). Obstructive sleep apnea and orthodontics: an American Association of orthodontists white paper. *Am. J. Orthod. Dentofac. Orthop.* 156 (1): 13–28.

115 Timms, D.J. (1990). Rapid maxillary expansion in the treatment of nocturnal enuresis. *Angle Orthod.* 60 (3): 229–233.

116 Usumez, S., Işeri, H., Orhan, M., and Basciffci, F.A. (2003). Effect of rapid maxillary expansion on nocturnal enuresis. *Angle Orthod.* 73 (5): 532–538.

117 Doruk, C., Sokucu, O., Sezer, H., and Canbay, E. (2004). Evaluation of nasal airway resistance during rapid maxillary expansion using acoustic rhinometry. *Eur. J. Orthod.* 26 (4): 397–401.

118 Kurol, J., Modin, H., and Bjerkhoel, A. (1998). Orthodontic maxillary expansion and its effect on nocturnal enuresis. *Angle Orthod.* 68 (3): 225–232.

119 Brooks, L.J. and Topol, H.I. (2003). Enuresis in children with sleep apnea. *J. Pediatr.* 142 (5): 515–518.

120 Owens, J.A. and Witmans, M. (2004). Sleep problems. *Curr. Prob. Pediatr. Adolesc. Health Care.* 34 (4): 154–179.

121 dos Santos, B.M., Stuani, A.S., Stuani, A.S. et al. (2012). Soft tissue profile changes after rapid maxillary expansion with a bonded expander. *Eur. J. Orthod.* 34 (3): 367–373.

122 Stöckli, P.W. and Willert, H.G. (1971). Tissue reactions in the temporomandibular joint resulting from anterior displacement of the mandible in the monkey. *Am. J. Orthod.* 60 (2): 142–155.

123 McNamara, J.A. (1985). The role of functional appliances in contemporary orthodontics. In: *New Vistas in Orthodontics* (ed. L. Johnston). Philadelphia (PA): Lea & Febiger.

124 Woodside, D.G., Metaxas, A., and Aluna, G. (1987). The influence of functional appliance therapy on glenoid fossa remodeling. *Am. J. Orthod. Dentofac. Orthop.* 92 (3): 181–198.

125 Ruf, S. and Pancherz, H. (1998). Temporomandibular joint remodeling in adolescents and young adults during Herbst treatment: a prospective longitudinal magnetic resonance image and cephalometric radiographic investigation. *Am. J. Orthod. Dentofac. Orthop.* 115 (6): 607–618.

126 DeVincenzo, J.P. (1991). Changes in mandibular length before, during, and after successful orthopedic correction of Class II malocclusions, using a functional appliance. *Am. J. Orthod. Dentofac. Orthop.* 99 (3): 241–257.

127 Wieslander, L. (1993). Long-term effect of treatment with the headgear-Herbst appliance in the early mixed dentition. Stability or relapse? *Am. J. Orthod. Dentofac. Orthop.* 104 (4): 319–329.

128 Pancherz, H. (1997). The Herbst appliance: a powerful Class II corrector. In: *Biomechanics in Clinical Orthodontics*, 1e (ed. R. Nanda). Philadelphia (PA): WB Saunders.

129 Lande, M.J. (1952). Growth behavior of the human bony facial profile as revealed by serial cephalometric roentgenology. *Angle Orthod.* 22 (2): 78–90.

130 Subtelny, J.D. (1959). A longitudinal study of soft tissue facial structures and their profile characteristics, defined in relation to underlying skeletal structures. *Am. J. Orthod.* 45 (7): 481–507.

131 Sinclair, P.M. and Little, R.M. (1985). Dentofacial maturation of untreated normals. *Am. J. Orthod.* 88 (2): 146–156.

132 Feldmann, I., Lundström, F., and Peck, S. (1999). Occlusal changes from adolescence to adulthood in untreated patients with Class II Division 1 deepbite malocclusion. *Angle Orthod.* 69 (1): 33–38.

133 Carter, N.E. (1987). Dentofacial changes in untreated Class II Division 1 subjects. *Br. J. Orthod.* 14 (4): 225–235.

134 You, Z., Fishman, L., Rosenblum, R. et al. (2001). Dentoalveolar changes related to mandibular forward growth in untreated Class II persons. *Am. J. Orthod. Dentofac. Orthop.* 120 (6): 598–607. quiz 676.

135 Lager, H. (1967). The individual growth pattern and stage of maturation as a basis for treatment of distal occlusion with overjet. *Rep. Congr. Eur. Orthod. Soc.* 137–145.

136 Tai, K., Hotokezaka, H., Park, J.H. et al. (2010). Preliminary cone-beam computed tomography study evaluating dental and skeletal changes after treatment with a mandibular Schwarz appliance. *Am. J. Orthod. Dentofac. Orthop.* 138 (3): 262–263.

137 Bays, R.A. and Greco, J.M. (1992). Surgically assisted, rapid palatal expansion: an outpatient technique with long-term stability. *J. Oral Maxillofac. Surg.* 50 (2): 110–113. discussion 114-5.

138 Strömberg, C. and Holm, J. (1995). Surgically assisted, rapid maxillary expansion in adults: a retrospective long-term follow-up study. *J. Craniomaxillofac. Surg.* 23 (4): 222–227.

139 Lo, F.M. and Shapiro, P.A. (1998). Effect of presurgical incisor extrusion on stability of anterior open bite malocclusion treated with orthognathic surgery. *Int. J. Adult Orthodon. Orthognath. Surg.* 13 (1): 23–34.

140 Proffit, W.R., Turvey, T.A., and Phillips, C. (2007). The hierarchy of stability and predictability in orthognathic surgery with rigid fixation: an update and extension. *Head Face Med.* 3 (1): 21.

141 Sokucu, O., Kosger, H.H., Bıcakci, A.A., and Babacan, H. (2009). Stability in dental changes in RME and SARME: a 2-year follow-up. *Angle Orthod.* 79 (2): 207–213.

142 Joondeph, D.R. and Bloomquist, D. (2004). Mandibular midline osteotomy for constriction. *Am. J. Orthod. Dentofac. Orthop.* 126 (3): 268–270.

143 Alexander, C.D., Bloomquist, D.S., and Wallen, T.R. (1993). Stability of mandibular constriction with a symphyseal osteotomy. *Am. J. Orthod. Dentofac. Orthop.* 103 (1): 15–23.

144 Weil, T.S., Van Sickels, J.E., and Payne, C.J. (1997). Distraction osteogenesis for correction of transverse mandibular deficiency: a preliminary report. *J. Oral Maxillofac. Surg.* 55 (9): 953–960.

145 King, J.W., Wallace, J.C., and Scanlan, D. (2001). A new appliance for mandibular widening by distraction osteogenesis. *J. Clin. Orthod.* 35 (11): 666–672.

146 Mommaerts, M.Y. (2001). Bone anchored intraoral device for transmandibular distraction. *Br. J. Oral Maxillofac. Surg.* 39 (1): 8–12.

147 Malkoç, S., Işeri, H., Karaman, A.I. et al. (2006). Effects of mandibular symphyseal distraction osteogenesis on mandibular structures. *Am. J. Orthod. Dentofac. Orthop.* 130 (5): 603–611.

148 King, J.W., Wallace, J.C., Winter, D.L., and Niculescu, J.A. (2012). Long-term skeletal and dental stability of mandibular symphyseal distraction osteogenesis with a hybrid distractor. *Am. J. Orthod. Dentofac. Orthop.* 141 (1): 60–70.

149 Mellion, Z.J., Behrents, R.G., and Johnston, L.E. Jr. (2013). The pattern of facial skeletal growth and its relationship to various common indexes of maturation. *Am. J. Orthod. Dentofac. Orthop.* 143 (6): 845–854.

150 Bambha, J.K. and Van Natta, P. (1963). Longitudinal study of facial growth in relation to skeletal maturation during adolescence. *Am. J. Orthod.* 49 (6): 481–493.

151 Hunter, C.J. (1966). The correlation of facial growth with body height and skeletal maturation at adolescence. *Angle Orthod.* 36 (1): 44–54.

152 Wheeler, R.C. (1974). *Dental Anatomy, Physiology, and Occlusion*, 5e. Philadelphia: W.B. Saunders.

153 Firouz, M., Zernik, J., and Nanda, R. (1992). Dental and orthopedic effects of high-pull headgear in treatment of Class II, Division 1 malocclusion. *Am. J. Orthod. Dentofac. Orthop.* 102 (3): 197–205.

154 Baumrind, S., Korn, E.L., Isaacson, R.J. et al. (1983). Quantitative analysis of the orthodontic and orthopedic effects of maxillary traction. *Am. J. Orthod.* 84 (5): 384–398.

155 Elder, J.R. and Tuenge, R.H. (1974). Cephalometric and histologic changes produced by extraoral high-pull traction to the maxilla in Macaca mulatta. *Am. J. Orthod.* 66 (6): 599–617.

156 Kirjavainen, M., Kirjavainen, T., Hurmerinta, K., and Haavikko, K. (2000). Orthopedic cervical headgear with an expanded inner bow in Class II correction. *Angle Orthod.* 70 (4): 317–325.

157 Pancherz, H. (1997). The effects, limitations, and long-term dentofacial adaptations to treatment with the Herbst appliance. *Semin. Orthod.* 3 (4): 232–243.

158 Le Cornu, M., Cevidanes, L.H., Zhu, H. et al. (2013). Three-dimensional treatment outcomes in Class II patients treated with the Herbst appliance: a pilot study. *Am. J. Orthod. Dentofac. Orthop.* 144 (6): 818–830.

159 Janson, G., R, S., Fernandes, T.M. et al. (2013). Correction of Class II malocclusion with Class II elastics: a systematic review. *Am. J. Orthod. Dentofac. Orthop.* 143 (3): 383–392.

160 Franchi, L., Alvetro, L., Giuntini, V. et al. (2011). Effectiveness of comprehensive fixed appliance treatment used with the Forsus Fatigue Resistant Device in Class II patients. *Angle Orthod.* 81 (4): 678–683.

161 Heinig, N. and Göz, G. (2001). Clinical application and effects of the Forsus spring. A study of a new Herbst hybrid. *J. Orofac. Orthop.* 62 (6): 436–450.

162 Ericson, S. and Kurol, J. (1988). Early treatment of palatally erupting maxillary canines by extraction of the primary canines. *Eur. J. Orthod.* 10 (4): 283–295.

163 Power, S.M. and Short, M.B. (1993). An investigation into the response of palatally displaced canines to the removal of deciduous canines and an assessment of factors contributing to favourable eruption. *Br. J. Orthod.* 20 (3): 215–223.

164 Leonardi, M., Armi, P., Franchi, L., and Baccetti, T. (2004). Two interceptive approaches to palatally displaced canines: a prospective longitudinal study. *Angle Orthod.* 74 (5): 581–586.

165 Naoumova, J., Kurol, J., and Kjelberg, H. (2015). Extraction of the deciduous canine as an interceptive treatment in children with palatal displaced canines-part I: shall we extract the deciduous canine or not? *Eur. J. Orthod.* 37 (2): 209–218.

166 Southard, T.E., Marshall, S.D., Allareddy, V. et al. (2013). An evidence-based comparison of headgear and functional appliance therapy for the correction of class II malocclusions. *Semin. Orthod.* 19 (3): 174–195.

167 2005 AAO Council on Scientific Affairs (2005). Functional appliances and long-term effects on mandibular growth. *Am. J. Orthod. Dentofac. Orthop.* 128 (3): 271–272.

168 Pancherz, H., Ruf, S., and Kohlhas, P. (1998). "Effective condylar growth" and chin position changes in Herbst treatment: a cephalometric roentgenographic long-term study. *Am. J. Orthod. Dentofac. Orthop.* 114 (4): 437–446.

169 Araujo, A.M., Buschang, P.H., and Melo, A.C.M. (2004). Adaptive condylar growth and mandibular remodeling changes with bionator therapy – an implant study. *Eur. J. Orthod.* 26 (5): 515–522.

170 Ruf, S., Baltromejus, S., and Pancherz, H. (2001). Effective condylar growth and chin position changes in activator treatment: a cephalometric roentgenographic study. *Angle Orthod.* 71 (1): 4–11.

171 Rogers, K., Campbell, P.M., Tadlock, L. et al. (2018). Treatment changes of hypo- and hyperdivergent Class II Herbst patients. *Angle Orthod.* 88 (1): 3–9.

172 Proffit, W.R. and Tulloch, J.F. (2002). Preadolescent Class II problems: treat now or wait? *Am. J. Orthod. Dentofac. Orthop.* 121 (6): 560–562.

173 Tulloch, J.F., Proffit, W.R., and Phillips, C. (2004). Outcomes in a 2-phase randomized clinical trial of early Class II treatment. *Am. J. Orthod. Dentofac. Orthop.* 125 (6): 657–667.

174 Ghafari, J., Shofer, F.S., Jacobsson-Hunt, U. et al. (1998). Headgear versus functional regulator in the early treatment of Class II, division 1 malocclusion: a randomized clinical trial. *Am. J. Orthod. Dentofac. Orthop.* 113 (1): 51–61.

175 Keeling, S.D., Wheeler, T.T., King, G.J. et al. (1998). Anteroposterior skeletal and dental changes after early Class II treatment with bionators and headgear. *Am. J. Orthod. Dentofac. Orthop.* 113 (1): 40–50.

176 Dolce, C., McGorray, S.P., Brazeau, L. et al. (2007). Timing of Class II treatment: skeletal changes comparing 1-phase and 2-phase treatment. *Am. J. Orthod. Dentofac. Orthop.* 132 (4): 481–489.

177 O'Brien, K. (2006). Is early treatment for Class II malocclusions effective? Results of a randomized controlled trial. *Am. J. Orthod. Dentofac. Orthop.* 129 (4 Suppl): S64–S65.

178 O'Brien, K., Wright, J., Conboy, F. et al. (2009). Early treatment for Class II Division 1 malocclusion with the Twin-block appliance: a multi-center, randomized, controlled trial. *Am. J. Orthod. Dentofac. Orthop.* 135 (5): 573–579.

179 Bishara, S.E., Hoppens, B.J., Jakobsen, J.R., and Kohout, F.J. (1988). Changes in the molar relationship between the primary and permanent dentitions: a longitudinal study. *Am. J. Orthod. Dentofac. Orthop.* 93 (1): 19–28.

180 Barros, S.E., Chiqueto, K., Janson, G., and Ferreira, E. (2015). Factors influencing molar relationship behavior in the mixed dentition. *Am. J. Orthod. Dentofac. Orthop.* 148 (5): 782–792.

181 Levander, E. and Malmgren, O. (1988). Evaluation of the risk of root resorption during orthodontic treatment: a study of upper incisors. *Eur. J. Orthod.* 10 (1): 30–38.

182 Segal, G.R., Schiffman, P.H., and Tuncay, O.C. (2004). Meta analysis of the treatment-related factors of external apical root resorption. *Orthod. Craniofac. Res.* 7 (2): 71–78.

183 Hartsfield, J.L. Jr., Everett, E.T., and Al-Qawasmi, R.A. (2004). Genetic factors in external apical root resorption and orthodontic treatment. *Crit. Rev. Oral Biol. Med.* 15 (2): 115–122.

184 Kokich, V.O., Kiyak, H.A., and Shapiro, P.A. (1999). Comparing the perception of dentists and lay people to altered dental esthetics. *J. Esthet. Dent.* 11 (6): 311–324.

185 Hansen, K., Koutsonas, T.G., and Pancherz, H. (1997). Long-term effects of Herbst treatment on the mandibular incisor segment: a cephalometric and biometric investigation. *Am. J. Orthod. Dentofac. Orthop.* 112 (1): 92–103.

Appendix

Cephalometrics Primer

There are many cephalometric analyses. In this section, we present a straightforward analysis which has served us well.

Q: Lateral cephalometric radiographs provide valuable anteroposterior and vertical relationship information. What are the five most important relationships measured from lateral cephalometric radiographs?

A: As seen in Figure A.1, the five most important relationships are:

1) Maxillary anteroposterior (AP) skeletal position
2) Mandibular anteroposterior (AP) skeletal position
3) Vertical skeletal relationships
4) Maxillary incisor angulation
5) Mandibular incisor angulation

We wish to underscore one important concept: *Radiographic skeletal and dental relationships* (Figure A.2a) *should corroborate what you observe clinically* (Figure A.2b). For example, if a patient has a balanced maxillary and mandibular relationship, you should expect that he will have a relatively straight profile. If a patient has a deficient mandible, you should expect that he will have a convex (retrusive) profile, and so forth.

Q: How do you judge the *ideal* maxillary AP position on a cephalometric radiograph?

A: On the lateral cephalometric tracing, draw Frankfort Horizontal (FH) between *anatomic* Porion and Orbitale (Figures A.3a–A.3b). Next, draw a line downward from Nasion (N) passing perpendicular to FH (Figures A.3c–A.3d). An *ideal maxillary AP position is one in which A-Point lies on the Nasion perpendicular line* [1, 2]. Another means of explaining this is that a line drawn from Nasion to A-Point (N A line) makes a 90-degree angle with FH (i.e. angle FH-NA = 90°) when the maxilla is in an ideal AP position.

Q: If A-Point lies *nearly* on Nasion perpendicular, but not exactly on Nasion perpendicular, should the maxilla be

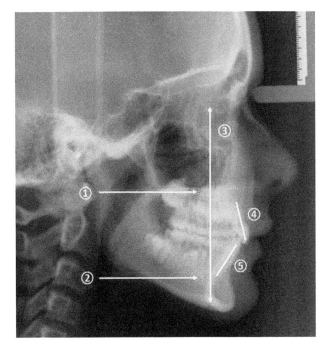

Figure A.1 Five important relationships determined from a cephalometric radiograph. Numbers 1–5 refer to definitions in the text.

classified as either AP deficient or AP excessive, but not normal?

Not necessarily. A *range of normal* exists in cephalometric analysis. If a patient presents with a cephalometric measurement that is close to normal, but not precisely normal, then that measurement may still be considered falling "within the range of normal" abbreviated WRN. In other words, if A-Point sits slightly behind or slightly ahead of Nasion perpendicular, then the maxillary AP position may still be considered WRN. Or, if the posterior-inferior angle formed by the N-A line and FH (NA-FH angle) is,

Practical Early Orthodontic Treatment: A Case-Based Review, First Edition. Thomas E. Southard, Steven D. Marshall, Laura L. Bonner, and Kyungsup Shin.
© 2023 John Wiley & Sons, Inc. Published 2023 by John Wiley & Sons, Inc.
Companion website: www.wiley.com/go/southard/practical

(a)　(b)

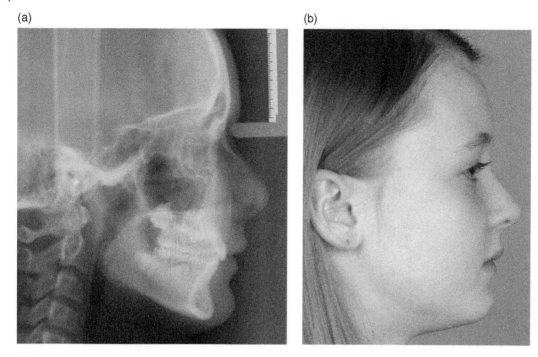

Figure A.2　(a) Cephalometric radiograph and (b) profile photograph of a twelve-year-old girl in the late mixed dentition stage of development.

say 89° or 91°, then the maxillary AP position may still be considered WRN.

Q: How would you describe the maxillary AP position in the cephalometric tracing shown in Figures A.4a and A.4b?

A: The maxillary AP position is very deficient (retrusive) in Figure A.4a. The maxillary AP position is very excessive (protrusive) in Figure A.4b.

Q: How would you describe the maxillary AP position in the cephalometric radiograph and tracing shown in Figure A.5?

A: In this patient, A-Point lies ahead of Nasion-perpendicular (NA-FH angle is 93°). This patient presents with maxillary AP excess (protrusion).

Q: How would you describe the maxillary AP position in the cephalometric radiograph and tracing shown in Figure A.6?

A: A-Point lies behind Nasion perpendicular (NA-FH angle is 85°). This patient presents with maxillary AP deficiency (retrusion).

Q: How do you judge the *ideal* mandibular AP position on a cephalometric radiograph if the maxillary AP position is WRN?

A: *If the maxillary AP position is WRN, then simply use the ANB angle.* As shown in Figure A.7a, when maxillary AP is WRN, the line N-A lies coincident with Nasion perpendicular. In this case, an ideal mandibular AP position will be found when a 1°, 2°, or 3° angle is formed between lines N-A and N-B (Figure A.7b and c), that is ANB = 1°, 2°, or 3°.

Q: How would you describe the mandibular AP position in the cephalometric tracing shown in Figures A.8a and A.8b and Figures A.8c and A.8d?

A: The mandibular AP position is deficient (retrusive) in Figures A.8a and A.8b. The mandibular AP position is excessive (protrusive) in Figures A.8c and A.8d.

Q: How do you judge the mandibular AP position when the maxillary AP position is *not* WRN? For example, how do you judge the mandibular AP position in Figures A.9a and A.9c?

A: Judge the mandibular AP position when the maxillary AP position is not WRN as follows:

- Just as you did when judging *maxillary* skeletal AP position, *relate the mandible to Nasion perpendicular.* Measure (estimate) the angle formed between Nasion perpendicular and the N-B line. What is the logic of doing this? This angle would match the ANB angle if the maxilla *was* WRN (if the N-A line was coincident with Nasion perpendicular).

- *If you measure the angle formed between Nasion perpendicular and the N-B line to be between 1° and 3°, then the mandibular AP position is WRN. Otherwise, it is deficient or excessive.* For instance, in Figure A.9a and b, the angle formed between Nasion perpendicular and the N-B line is 8°. Clearly, both the mandible and the maxilla are deficient. Most seasoned orthodontists would draw this same conclusion without measuring angles. Likewise, in Figure A.9c and d, the angle formed between Nasion perpendicular and the N-B line is −2°. The mandibular AP position is excessive (maxilla is deficient).

(a)

Porion

Orbitale

(b)

Frankfort horizontal (FH)

(c)

Nasion (N)

A-Point

(d)

Nasion (N)

FH

A-Point

Nasion
Perpendicular
(N⊥FH)

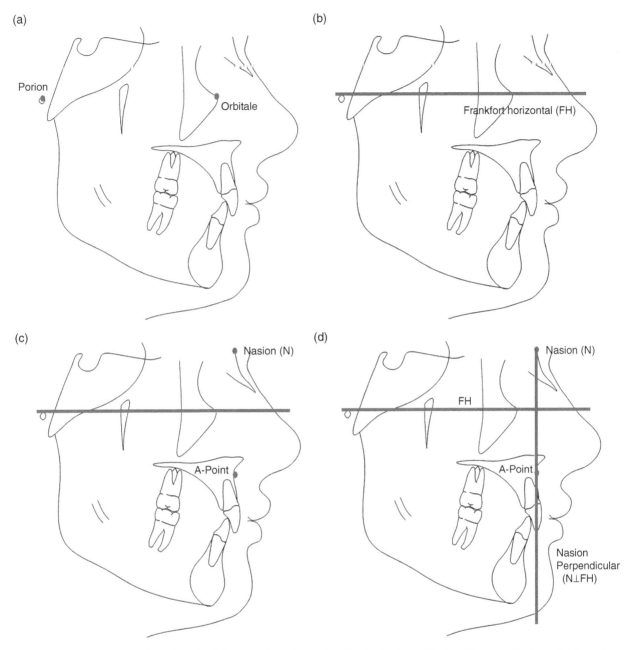

Figure A.3 (a–b) Construction of FH. (c–d) Construction of a vertical line beginning at Nasion (N) perpendicular to FH. For this subject, A-Point lies on Nasion perpendicular exemplifying an ideal maxillary AP position.

- As an alternative, you can often use logic to judge the mandibular AP position. For instance, if you measure an ANB angle to be 3°, but the maxilla is AP deficient, then logic would dictate that the mandible must also be deficient (ANB≥4°).

Q: How would you judge the mandibular AP position for the patient shown in Figure A.10?

A: Mandibular skeletal AP retrusion.

Q: How would you judge the mandibular AP position for the patient shown in Figure A.11?

A: Mandibular AP skeletal protrusion.

Q: How would you describe the maxillary and mandibular AP positions for the patient shown in Figure A.12?

A: Maxillary *and* mandibular AP skeletal retrusion (deficiency).

(a)

(b)

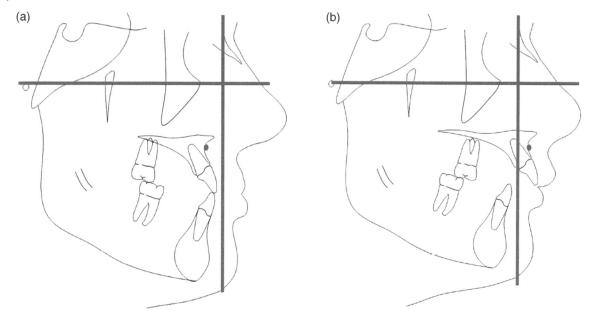

Figure A.4 (a) Cephalometric tracing where A-Point lies considerably behind Nasion perpendicular and the maxillary AP position is deficient/retrusive. (b) Cephalometric tracing where A-Point lies considerably ahead of Nasion perpendicular and the maxillary AP position is excessive/protrusive.

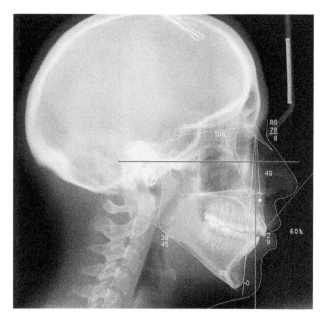

Figure A.5 Cephalometric radiograph and tracing where A-Point (yellow dot) lies ahead of Nasion perpendicular (NA-FH angle is 93°). This patient presents with maxillary AP excess (protrusion).

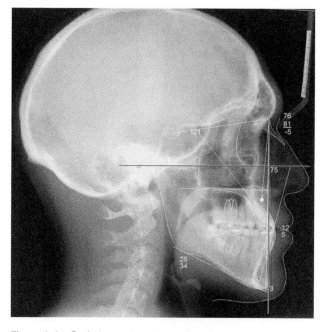

Figure A.6 Cephalometric radiograph and tracing where A-Point (yellow dot) lies behind Nasion perpendicular (NA-FH angle is 85°). This patient presents with maxillary AP deficiency (retrusion).

Q: How would you describe the maxillary and mandibular AP positions for the patient shown in Figure A.13?

A: Maxillary AP skeletal retrusion (deficiency) and mandibular AP skeletal WRN.

Q: Instead of using Nasion-perpendicular to judge maxillary and mandibular AP positions, why not use SNA and SNB angles?

A: *SNA and SNB angles are too dependent upon the vertical position of Sella* to be of value in judging maxillary and mandibular skeletal AP positions. For instance, normal values for SNA and SNB angles are 82° and 80°, respectively. But in Figure A.14a (a patient with normal maxilla and mandible but "high Sella"), SNA and SNB angles are 85° and 83°, respectively – incorrectly suggesting the

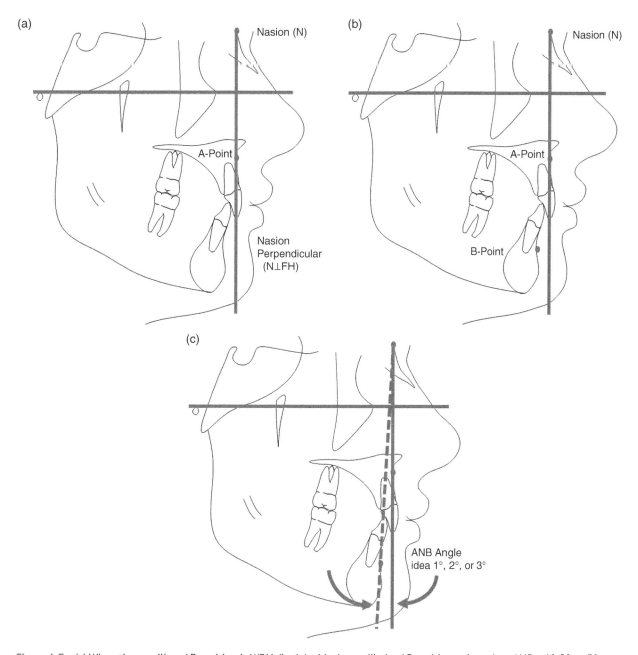

Figure A.7 (a) When the maxillary AP position is WRN. (b, c) An ideal mandibular AP position exists when ANB = 1°, 2°, or 3°.

maxillary and mandibular AP skeletal protrusion. Then, in Figure A.14b (the same patient, but low Sella), SNA and SNB angles are 77° and 74°, respectively – suggesting maxillary and mandibular skeletal retrusion. The use of SNA and SNB angles can be misleading.

Of course, you could argue that adjustments can be made to SNA and SNB to compensate for Sella being high or low. The normal angular difference between SN and FH is 7° (normal SN-MP = 32° and normal FMA = 25°, a difference of 7°). So, for the "high Sella" in Figure A.14a, where the angular difference between SN and FH is only 4° (SN-MP = 27° and FMA = 23°), you

could reduce SNA and SNB by 3°, making them 82° and 79°, respectively (indicating normal maxillary and mandibular AP positions). Conversely, for the "low Sella" in Figure A.14b, where the angular difference between SN and FH is 12° (SN-MP = 35° and FMA = 23°), you could increase SNA and SNB by 5°, again making them 82° and 79°, respectively.

Q: How do you judge *vertical* skeletal relationships from a cephalometric radiograph?

A: There are a number of measurements that can help make this assessment:

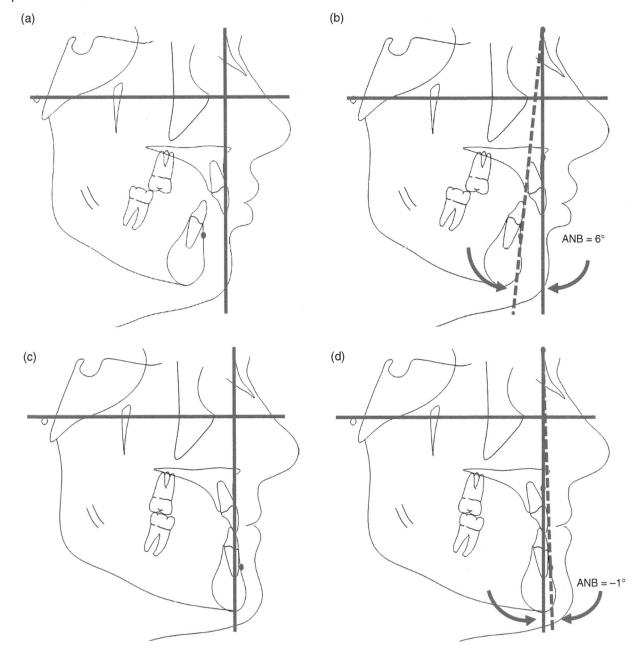

(a)

(b)

ANB = 6°

(c)

(d)

ANB = −1°

Figure A.8 Cephalometric tracings where the maxilla AP position is WRN: (a, b) mandibular AP deficiency (retrusion), (c, d) mandibular AP excess (protrusion).

- *The ratio of the lower anterior face height to total anterior face height*: measures the portion of the total height of the face contributed by the basal and alveolar portions of the jaws (Figure A.15). The average LAFH/TAFH × 100% ratio is 55%, with a 2% standard deviation [3].
- *The steepness or flatness of the mandibular plane*: measured as an angle between MP and either FH (FMA) or S-N line (SN-MP angle). These angular measurements are depicted in Figure A.16. Ideally,

FMA = 25° and SN-MP = 32°. Angle SN-MP values > 32° (FMA values > 25°) indicate increasing facial hyperdivergence, while angle SN-MP values below 32° (FMA values < 25°) indicate contracting facial hypodivergence.
- *The ratio of Posterior Face Height (PFH) to Anterior Face Height (AFH)*: the most common description of the PFH/AFH ratio is the quotient (Sella to Gonion distance)/(Nasion to Menton distance) as shown in Figure A.17 [4]. A ratio of 0.59 to 0.63 is

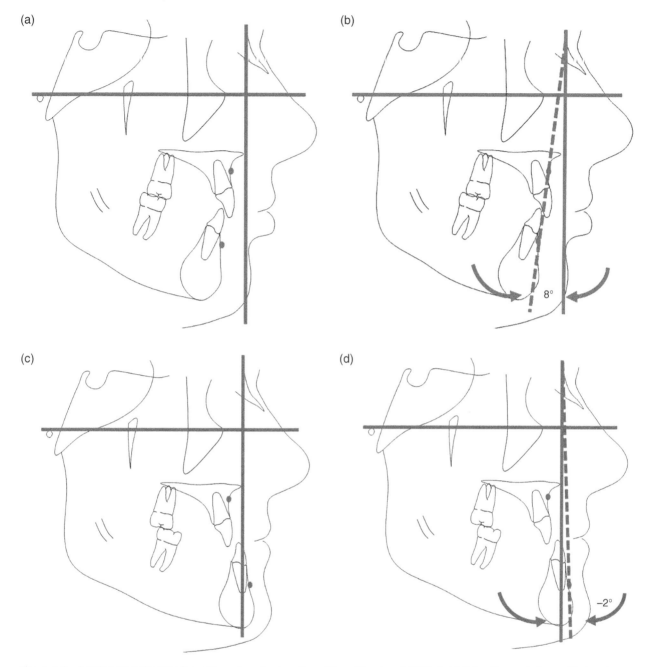

Figure A.9 Judging mandibular AP position when the maxillary AP position is not WRN: (a, b) Using the angle formed between Nasion perpendicular and the N-B line (8°), the mandible is judged to be deficient. (c, d) Using the same simple measurement, this mandible is judged to be excessive.

WRN. A ratio less than 0.59 indicates a hyperdivergent pattern tending toward skeletal open bite. A ratio greater than 0.63 indicates a hypodivergent pattern tending toward skeletal deep bite. Because the ratio is mathematically related to the angle SN-MP, we choose the SN-MP angle and FMA to describe the vertical relationship of the jaws instead of PFH/AFH.

Q: Evaluate the patient's vertical relationships in Figure A.18.
A: This patient's vertical relationship is normal and nearly ideal (LAFH/TAFH × 100% = 55%, FMA = 26°, SN-MP angle = 32°).

Q: Evaluate the patient's vertical relationship in Figure A.19.
A: She has a long skeletal lower anterior face height (LLAFH), LAFH/TAFH × 100% = 60% and a very steep MPA (FMA = 38°, SN-MP angle = 45°).

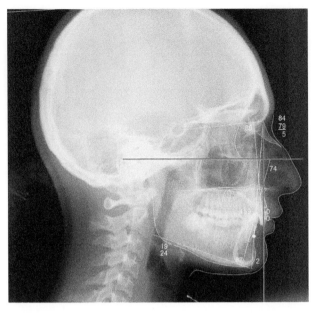

Figure A.10 Cephalometric radiograph and tracing where the maxilla is WRN (A-Point lies on Nasion-perpendicular), but the ANB angle is 5° (B-Point is indicated in yellow). The diagnosis is mandibular skeletal AP retrusion (deficiency).

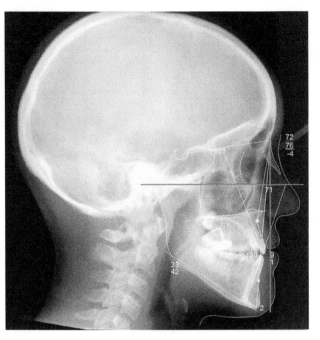

Figure A.12 Cephalometric radiograph and tracing showing an AP deficient maxilla (A-Point is quite distal to Nasion-perpendicular) and an AP deficient mandible (the angle formed by Nasion perpendicular and the N-B line exceeds 4°). A-Point and B-Point are indicated in yellow.

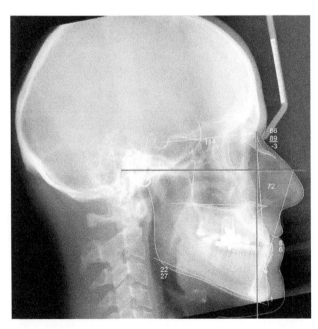

Figure A.11 Cephalometric radiograph and tracing where the maxilla is WRN (A-Point lies on Nasion-perpendicular), but ANB = −3° (B-Point is indicated in yellow). The diagnosis is mandibular AP skeletal protrusion (excess).

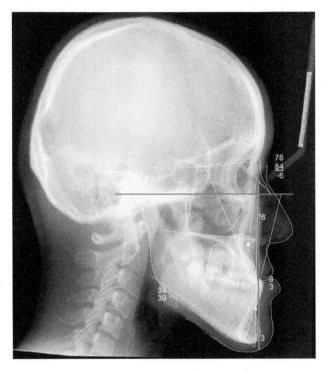

Figure A.13 Cephalometric radiograph and tracing showing an AP deficient maxilla (A-Point is quite distal to Nasion-perpendicular) and a mandible WRN (the angle formed by Nasion perpendicular and the N-B line is 2°). A-Point and B-Point are indicated in yellow.

(a)

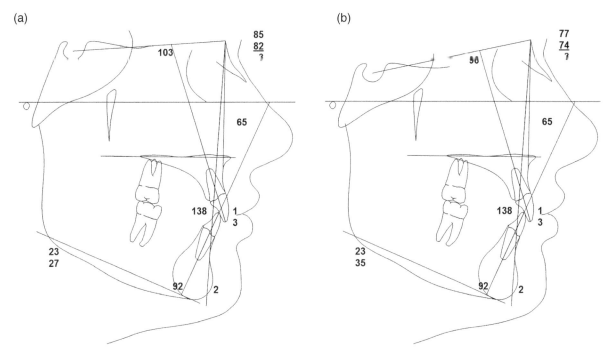

(b)

Figure A.14 Effect of Sella vertical position on 1̱-SN, SNA, and SNB. (a) A "high" Sella results in larger values of 1̱-SN, SNA, and SNB and (b) a "low" Sella results in smaller values. Note also that the ANB angle is independent of Sella vertical position.

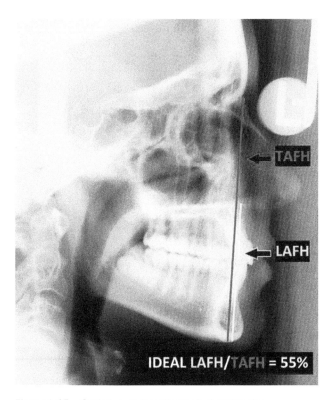

Figure A.15 Cephalometric radiograph showing the measurement of TAFH (distance from Nasion to Menton) and LAFH (distance along a parallel line from Menton to the projection of anterior nasal spine perpendicular to the Nasion-Menton line). The linear distances are combined into a percentage ratio LAFH/TAFH × 100%.

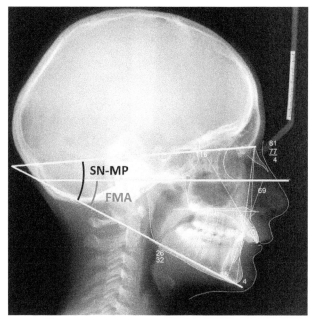

Figure A.16 Depiction of the angles formed by the Frankfort Horizontal and the mandibular plane (FMA) and by the Sella-Nasion line and the mandibular plane (SN-MP).

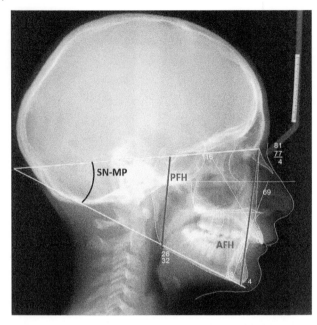

Figure A.17 Measurement of Posterior Face Height (PFH) and Anterior Face Height (AFH). For any individual, the ratio PFH/AFH is a mathematical relationship that defines the individual's SN-MP angle.

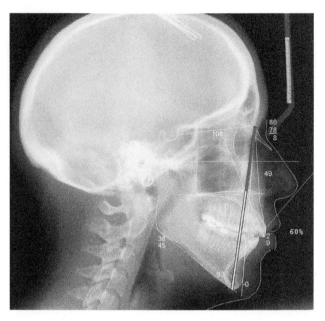

Figure A.19 Cephalometric radiograph and tracing illustrating an LAFH/TAFH (yellow/red) ratio × 100% = 60%, SN-MP angle = 45°, and FMA = 38°.

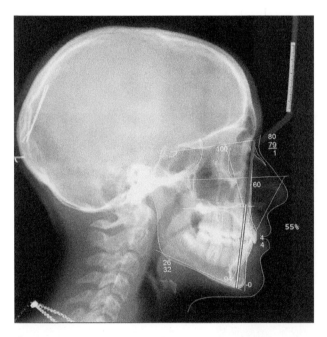

Figure A.18 Cephalometric radiograph and tracing illustrating an LAFH/TAFH (yellow/red) ratio × 100% = 55%, SN-MP angle = 32°, and FMA = 26°.

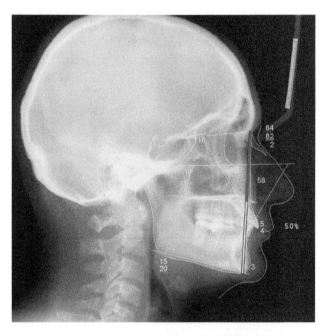

Figure A.20 Cephalometric radiograph and tracing illustrating an LAFH/TAFH (yellow/red) ratio × 100% = 50%, SN-MP = 20°, and FMA = 15°.

Q: Evaluate the patient's vertical relationship in Figure A.20.
A: She has a short skeletal LAFH (LAFH/TAFH × 100% = 50%) and a very flat MPA (FMA = 15°, SN-MP angle = 20°).

Q: How do you judge maxillary incisor angulation?
A: Maxillary incisor angulation is judged *using the angle formed by the axis of the maxillary central incisors and the Sella-Nasion line (U1-SN angle)*. This angle should lie within the range of 101–104°. U1-SN angles greater than 104° indicate proclined maxillary incisors. U1-SN angles

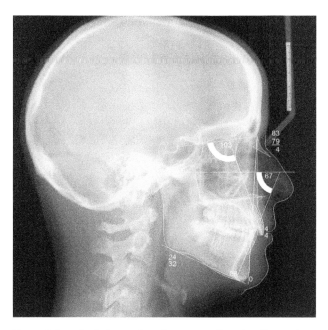

Figure A.21 Cephalometric radiograph and tracing illustrating normal maxillary and mandibular incisor relationships (U1 – SN = 103°, a line through the long axis of the maxillary central incisors projects through the distal of the orbits, and FMIA = 67°).

fewer than 101° indicate retroclined (upright) maxillary incisors. Also, *the long axis of the maxillary incisor should project close to, or through, the distal contour of the orbit* (Figure A.21). This position can not only vary with maxillary incisor inclination, but also with forward or backward maxillary skeletal AP position.

Q: How do you judge mandibular incisor angulation?

A: Mandibular incisor angulation is judged *using the angle formed by the axis of the mandibular central incisors and Frankfort Horizontal, termed the Frankfort Mandibular Incisor Angle (FMIA).* This angle should lie within the range of 65–68° (Figure A.21). FMIAs greater than 68° indicate retroclined (upright) mandibular incisors. FMIAs fewer than 65° indicate proclined mandibular incisors.

Q: We recommend using FMIA to judge lower incisor angulation. If instead, you use the angle formed by the intersection of the mandibular central incisor axis and the mandibular plane (incisor mandibular plane angle, IMPA) to judge lower incisor angulation, you must be careful. Why?

A: Imagine that the lower incisors are fixed in the mandible (lower incisors not moving relative to the mandible, IMPA fixed). Mandibular incisor proclination varies with the steepness of the MPA – which is reflected in changes in FMIA but *not* in IMPA. That is, as the mandibular plane is rotated upward and forward, the mandibular incisors are

increasingly uprighted with respect to the face. This will be reflected in increasing values of FMIA while IMPA remains fixed. Conversely, as the mandibular plane is rotated downward and backward, the mandibular incisors are increasingly proclined with respect to the face. This will be reflected in decreasing values of FMIA while IMPA remains fixed. We recommend using FMIA, not IMPA, to judge mandibular incisor proclination.

Q: Judge maxillary and mandibular incisor angulations in Figure A.5.

A: Proclined maxillary incisors, and proclined mandibular incisors.

Q: Judge maxillary and mandibular incisor angulations in Figure A.6.

A: Proclined maxillary and upright mandibular incisors.

Q: Judge maxillary and mandibular incisor angulations in Figure A.10.

A: Upright maxillary and mandibular incisors.

Q: Judge maxillary and mandibular incisor angulations in Figure A.12.

A: Normally inclined maxillary incisors, and upright mandibular incisors.

Q: Judge maxillary and mandibular incisor angulations in Figure A.13.

A: Proclined maxillary incisors, and upright mandibular incisors.

Q: This cephalometrics primer described an analysis using anatomic landmarks to define reference points and lines. However, there are other approaches to lateral cephalometric analysis. What is "natural head position" and what is the advantage of using natural head position in cephalometric analysis?

A: Natural head position is a standardized reproducible orientation of the head in space while focusing on a distant point at eye level [5]. This concept was introduced by Downs [6], Bjerin [7], Morrees, and Kean [8]. To obtain photographs or lateral cephalometric radiographs in natural head position, the subjects are typically seated in a relaxed state with the head unsupported and their eyes looking into their own image in a mirror [8]. An extracranial vertical line (true vertical) is used as a reference while interpreting lateral cephalometric radiographs and clinical photographs obtained in natural head position. The advantage of using natural head position is that it eliminates the biological variability inherent to anatomic reference points and lines. It is important to distinguish between natural head position and natural head posture. While the natural head position is fixed and standardized for all individuals, the natural head posture is a functional or postural position of the head for each individual [5].

Q: What is the estimated natural head position?

A: In scenarios when clinical photographs and lateral cephalometric radiographs are not obtained in the patient's natural head position, an "estimated natural head position" can be used. The photographs and lateral cephalometric can be "rotated" to the patient's natural head position [9, 10]. This is, however, subject to the judgment of the clinician.

Q: Can you offer any "take-home pearls" regarding cephalometric analysis?

A: "Take-home pearls" include the following:

- *Interpret cephalometric measurements in view of clinical impressions.* Your cephalometric skeletal analysis should always reflect what you observed clinically. For example, if you conclude (cephalometrically) that a patient has a mandibular AP skeletal deficiency, then this conclusion should be reflected in a retrusive (convex) photographic profile.

- *Never treat patients to satisfy cephalometric norms.* Deviation in cephalometric values away from average values can help compose your patient problem list, but these values alone should not dictate treatment. For example, if you determine cephalometrically that a patient has proclined mandibular incisors, then you may decide to leave the incisors proclined if the patient's profile is attractive and the mandibular incisors are reasonably aligned. You must take all factors into consideration when treatment planning, not just cephalometric values.

- All cephalometric analyses have their weaknesses. The weakness of the aforementioned analysis is that it relies on Nasion. If Nasion is shifted far backward or far forward for a particular patient, then the analysis we presented could result in misleading conclusions. After all is said and done, base your final judgments of maxillary AP, mandibular AP, and vertical skeletal relationships on clear thinking and clinical impressions.

Iowa AP Classification Primer

The permanent dentition occlusion depicted in Figure A.22 illustrates a nearly ideal AP dental relationship and interdigitation of posterior teeth. This is what Edward H. Angle would call Class I "normal" occlusion [11]. Even the distobuccal cusp of the upper first permanent molar occludes with the mesiobuccal cusp of the lower second molar, as suggested by Andrews [12]. When you state that this patient has a "Class I

occlusion," every orthodontist knows exactly what you mean and can visualize it.

The Angle classification scheme [13] describes malocclusion based largely on the variation of permanent first molar inter-arch anteroposterior relationships (variation from the maxillary first molar mesiobuccal cusp tip being aligned with the mandibular first molar buccal groove). Angle reasoned that the maxillary first molars were the most dependable reference from which to judge the position of other teeth:

> "So important is the influence of these teeth in the building of the dental apparatus that we believe Nature exercises the greatest care in locating them, especially the upper first molars – which we call the keys to occlusion – and so places them that the rest of the dental apparatus may be completed normally; the first permanent upper molar furnishes more nearly than any other tooth or point in the anatomy an exact scientific basis from which to reason on malocclusion." [13]

Expanding upon the three *bilateral* molar AP relationship categories (Class I, Class II, and Class III), Angle conceived of a seven-category classification system by adding subcategories for incisor inclination and unilateral inter-arch molar AP discrepancies:

- Class I
- Class II division 1
- Class II division 1 subdivision
- Class II division 2
- Class II division 2 subdivision
- Class III
- Class III subdivision

Although widely used today, Angle's classification scheme suffers from weaknesses:

- It constrains the diagnosis of inter-arch AP dental relationships to discrete categories. However, the variation of inter-arch AP dental relationships is *continuous*, not discrete.

- *It does not permit the orthodontist to clearly visualize the <u>magnitude</u> of the AP discrepancy.* In other words, a Class II malocclusion with a 4 mm discrepancy is classified the same as a Class II malocclusion with a 10 mm discrepancy.

- It does not classify inter-arch canine relationships. And yet canines are just as much keys of the dental arches as first molars are.

- It cannot classify malocclusions that are Class II molar on one side and Class III molar on the other.

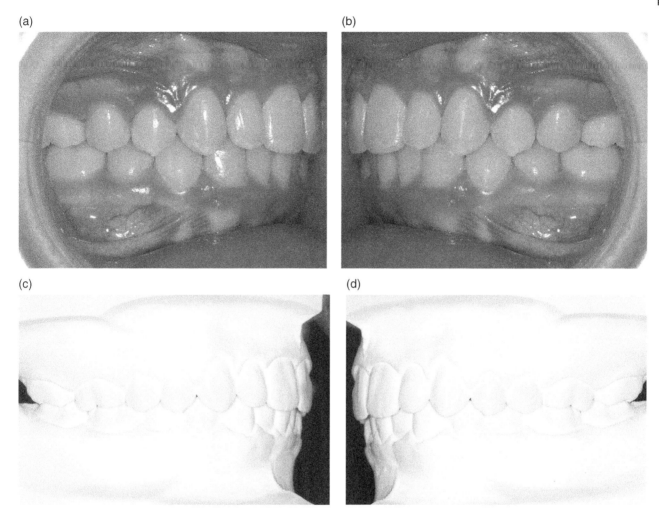

(a)
(b)
(c)
(d)

Figure A.22 (a–d) A patient with ideal Class I occlusion.

Consider the patient shown in Figure A.23. According to Angle's system, this patient would be classified as Class I malocclusion (with a 2 mm molar AP discrepancy, the mesiobuccal cusps of the maxillary first molars are not beyond one-half of the mesial cusp of the mandibular molars). This classification gives no indication of the severity of the AP inter-arch discrepancy, or even that there is a discrepancy. Simply put, with a diagnosis of Class I, you cannot infer whether the AP inter-arch discrepancy is nonexistent, mild (perhaps amenable to correction with inter-arch elastics), or severe (perhaps requiring orthognathic surgery for correction). Further, Angle's classification ignores canine relationships – which are at least as important as molar AP relationships in order to obtain maximum intercuspation.

To address these shortcomings, faculty at the University of Iowa (including ourselves and Dr. Robert Staley) developed a simple modification of the Angle classification system. This modification, which we call the Iowa Classification, is used throughout this text and consists of describing the patient's right molar, right canine, left canine, and left molar relationships in terms of millimeter deviation from Class I. The Iowa Classification system permits ready communication and visualization of the patient's AP relationship.

For example, the patient shown in 7.23 is reclassified in Figure A.24 according to the Iowa Classification as follows: Beginning with the right-side inter-arch first molar relationship, the AP discrepancy is measured to be Class II by 2 mm. The right-side inter-arch canine AP discrepancy is then measured to be Class II by 4 mm. The left-side inter-arch canine discrepancy is then measured to be Class II by 5 mm. And finally, the left-side inter-arch first molar AP discrepancy is measured to be 2 mm. The shorthand notation of the Iowa Classification for this patient is:

Right-side II (2 mm) II (4 mm) II (5 mm) II (2 mm) Left-side, or simply,

II(2) II(4) II(5) II(2); read as "Class II by 2, II by 4, II by 5, II by 2 mm"

Q: Classify the patient shown in Figure A.25.
A: III(3) III(3) III(3) III(3)

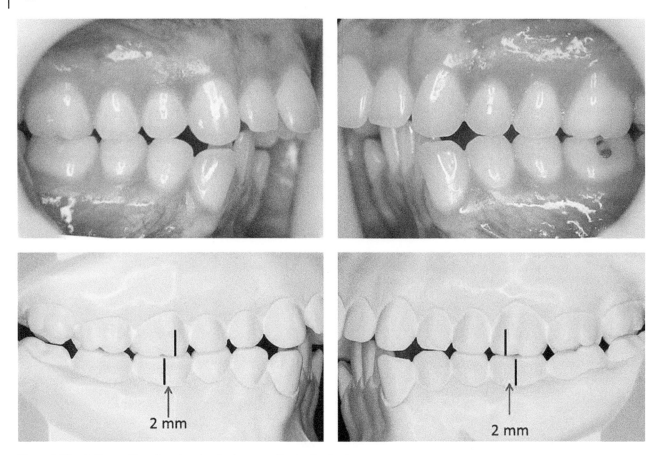

Figure A.23 Patient with a Class I malocclusion according to the Angle system.

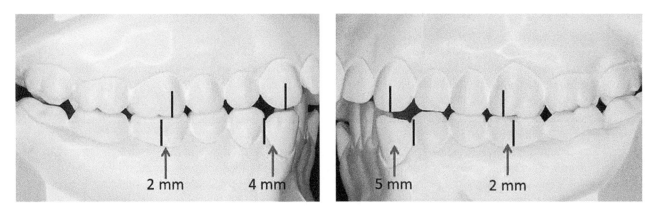

Figure A.24 The Iowa Classification measurements for the patient in Figure A.23. The shorthand notation for this classification is II(2) II(4) II(5) II(2).

Q: Classify the subdivision patient shown in Figure A.26.
A: II(3) II(3) I I

Q: Classify the late mixed dentition patient shown in Figure A.27.
A: Because the patient has exfoliated the maxillary primary canines, we will classify him as:
Iowa Classification: II(2–3 mm) X(canine missing) X(canine missing) II(2–3 mm)

Tables for Reference

The following Tables A.1 and A.2 are provided to you for use as a worksheet, or reference when treatment planning your own cases.

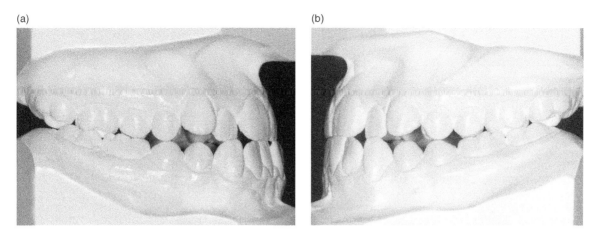

Figure A.25 (a–b) Patient who is Class III, bilaterally, by 3 mm at molars and canines.

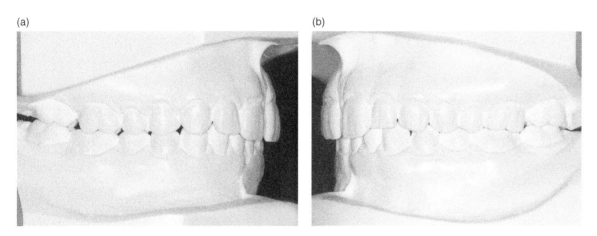

Figure A.26 (a–b) Subdivision patient.

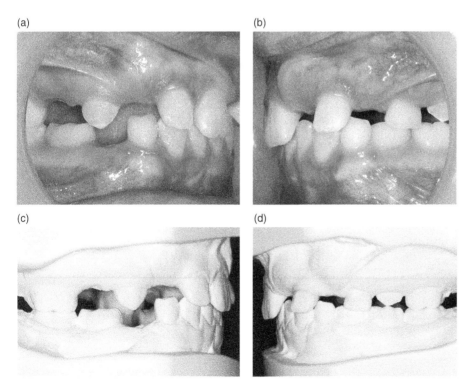

Figure A.27 (a–d) Late mixed dentition patient with missing (unerupted) maxillary permanent canines.

Table A.1 Template: diagnostic findings and problems list.

Full face and profile	FRONTAL VIEW
Ceph analysis	PROFILE VIEW
	SKELETAL
	DENTAL
Radiographs	
Intraoral photos and models	
Other	
Diagnosis	

Table A.2 Template: primary problem list.

AP
Vertical
Transverse
Other

Abbreviations

2X4	fixed orthodontic appliances (braces) placed on first permanent molars and incisors	LLHA	lower lingual holding arch
2X6	fixed orthodontic appliances placed on first permanent molars, canines, and incisors	LTSALD	lower tooth size arch length discrepancy
ADD	anteriorly displaced disk	Mn	mandibular
ANB	angle formed by A-Point – Nasion – B-Point	MPMO	multiple-piece maxillary osteotomy
ANS	anterior nasal spine	MP	mandibular plane
AP	anteroposterior	MPA	mandibular plane angle
BSSO	bilateral sagittal split osteotomy	Mx	maxillary
CC	chief complaint	NLA	nasolabial angle
CO	centric occlusion	OB	overbite
COS	curve of Spee	OJ	overjet
CPHG	cervical pull headgear	PDH	past dental history
CR	centric relation	PFE	primary failure of eruption
CW	clockwise	PMH	past medical history
CCW	counterclockwise	PNS	posterior nasal spine
FH	Frankfort horizontal	RME	rapid maxillary expansion
FMA	angle formed by Frankfort horizontal to mandibular plane	RPHG	reverse pull headgear
		SARME	surgically assisted rapid maxillary expansion
FMIA	angle formed by Frankfort horizontal to mandibular incisor	SN	Sella-Nasion
		SNA	angle formed by Sella-Nasion – A-Point
HPHG	high-pull headgear	SNB	angle formed by Sella-Nasion – B-Point
ILG	interlabial gap	SNMP	angle formed by Sella-Nasion to mandibular plane
IMPA	angle formed by lower incisor to mandibular plane		
IPR	interproximal reduction	TAD	temporary anchorage device
L1	lower central incisor	TAFH	total anterior face height (skeletal cephalometrically)
LLAFH	long lower anterior face height (soft tissue clinically or skeletal cephalometrically)		
		TMJ	temporomandibular joint
LAFH	lower anterior face height (soft tissue clinically or skeletal cephalometrically)	TPA	transpalatal arch
		U1	upper central incisor
		UDML	upper dental midline
LDML	lower dental midline	UTSALD	upper tooth size arch length discrepancy
		WRN	within the range of normal

References

1 Reidel, R.A. 1948. A cephalometric roentgenographic study of the relation of the maxilla and associated parts to the cranial base in normal and malocclusion of the teeth. Master's thesis, Northwestern University, 1948.

2 McNamara, J.A. Jr. (1984). A method of cephalometric evaluation. *Am. J. Orthod.* 86 (6): 449–469.

3 Wylie, W. and Johnson, E. (1952). Rapid evaluation of facial dysplasia in the vertical plane. *Angle Orthod.* 22 (3): 165–182.

4 Siriwat, P.P. and Jarabak, J.R. (1985). Malocclusion and facial morphology is there a relationship? An epidemiologic study. *Angle Orthod.* 55 (1): 127–138.

5 Moorees, C.F.A. (2006). Natural head position: the key to cephalometry. In: *Radiographic Cephalometry: From Basics to 3-D Imaging*, 2e (ed. A. Jacobson and R.L. Jacobson), 153–160. Chicago: Quintessence.

6 Downs, W.B. (1956). Analysis of the dentofacial profile. *Angle Orthod.* 26 (4): 191–212.

7 Bjerin, R. (1957). A comparison between the Frankfort Horizontal and the sella turcica-nasion as reference planes in cephalometric analysis. *Acta Odontol. Scand.* 1 5 (1): 1–12.

8 Moorees, C.F.A. and Kean, M.R. (1958). Natural head position, a basic consideration in the interpretation of cephalometric radiographs. *Am. J. Phys. Anthropol.* 16 (2): 213–234.

9 Jiang, J., Xu, T., and Lin, J. (2007). The relationship between estimated and registered natural head position. *Angle Orthod.* 77 (6): 1019–1024.

10 Moorees, C.F. (1994). Natural head position - a revival. *Am. J. Orthod. Dentofac. Orthop.* 105 (5): 512–513.

11 Angle, E.H. (1899). Classification of malocclusion. *Dent. Cosmos.* 41 (3): 248–264.

12 Andrews, L. (1972). The six keys to normal occlusion. *Am. J. Orthod. Dentofac. Orthop.* 62 (3): 296–309.

13 Angle, E.H. (1907). *Treatment of Malocclusion of the Teeth: Angle's System*. Philadelphia: SS White Dental Manufacturing Company.

Index

Practical Early Orthodontic Treatment: A Case-Based Review, First Edition. Thomas E. Southard, Steven D. Marshall,
Laura L. Bonner, and Kyungsup Shin.
© 2023 John Wiley & Sons, Inc. Published 2023 by John Wiley & Sons, Inc.
Companion website: www.wiley.com/go/southard/practical